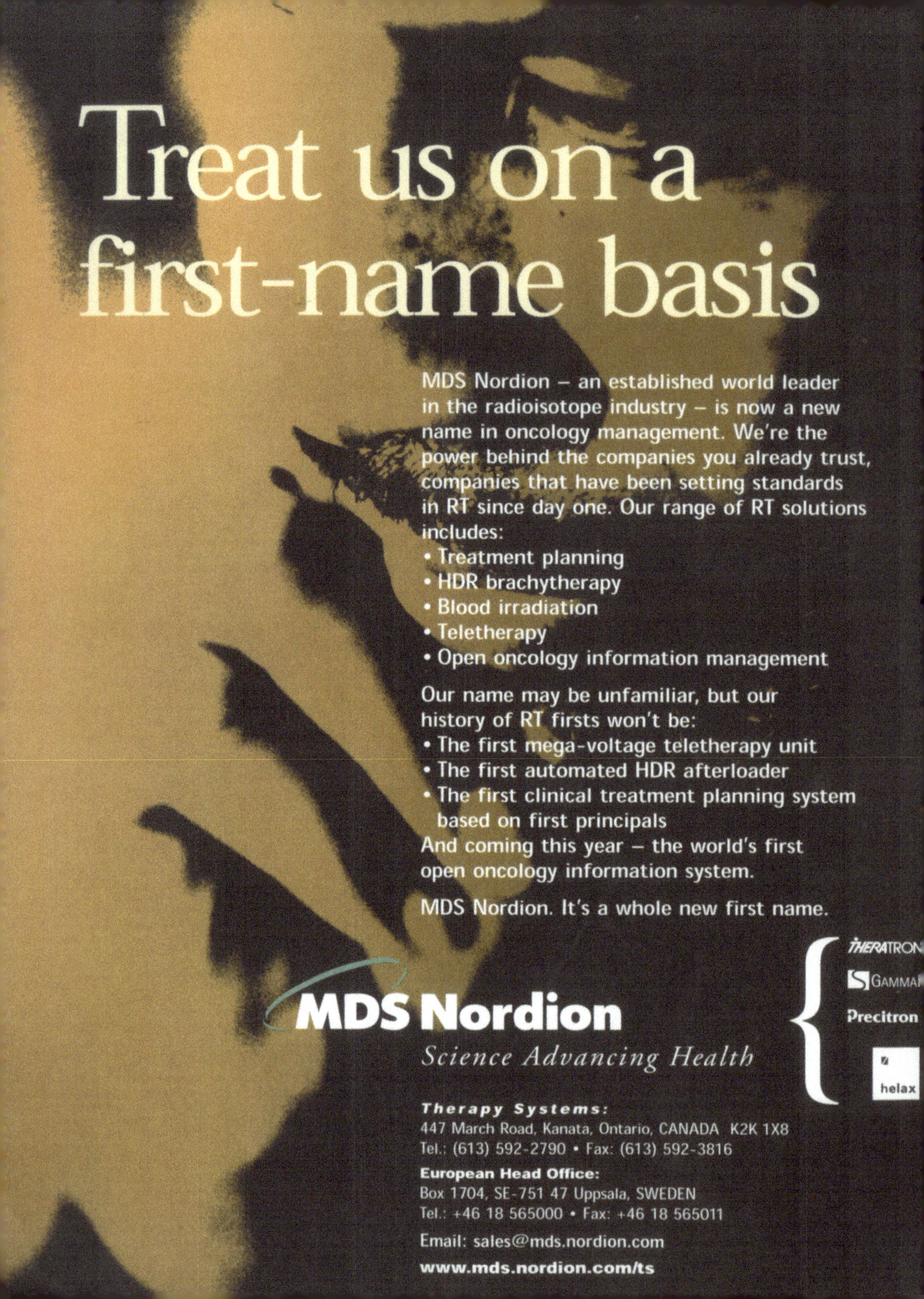
Treat us on a first-name basis
MDS Nordion – an established world leader in the radioisotope industry – is now a new name in oncology management. We're the power behind the companies you already trust, companies that have been setting standards in RT since day one. Our range of RT solutions includes:
• Treatment planning
• HDR brachytherapy
• Blood irradiation
• Teletherapy
• Open oncology information management
Our name may be unfamiliar, but our history of RT firsts won't be:
• The first mega-voltage teletherapy unit
• The first automated HDR afterloader
• The first clinical treatment planning system based on first principals
And coming this year – the world's first open oncology information system.
MDS Nordion. It's a whole new first name.
MDS Nordion
Science Advancing Health
THERATRON
GAMMA
Precitron
helax
Therapy Systems:
447 March Road, Kanata, Ontario, CANADA K2K 1X8
Tel.: (613) 592-2790 • Fax: (613) 592-3816
European Head Office:
Box 1704, SE-751 47 Uppsala, SWEDEN
Tel.: +46 18 565000 • Fax: +46 18 565011
Email: sales@mds.nordion.com
www.mds.nordion.com/ts

Schlegel, Bortfeld (Editors)
The Use of Computers in Radiation Therapy

XIIIth International Conference
Heidelberg, Germany
May 22–25, 2000

Springer

*Berlin*
*Heidelberg*
*New York*
*Barcelona*
*Hong Kong*
*London*
*Milan*
*Paris*
*Singapore*
*Tokyo*

Wolfgang Schlegel · Thomas Bortfeld
(Editors)

# The Use of Computers in Radiation Therapy

XIIIth International Conference
Heidelberg, Germany
May 22–25, 2000

Springer

Wolfgang Schlegel, Prof. Dr. rer. nat.
Thomas Bortfeld, PD, Dr. rer. nat.

Deutsches Krebsforschungszentrum (DKFZ)
Abteilung E0400
Im Neuenheimer Feld 280
D-69120 Heidelberg, Germany

Die Deutsche Bibliothek – CIP-Einheitsaufnahme
The Use of computers in radiation therapy: XIIIth international conference, Heidelberg, Germany, May 22–25, 2000/Wolfgang Schlegel and Thomas Bortfeld. – Berlin; Heidelberg; New York; Barcelona; Hong Kong; London; Milan; Paris; Singapore; Tokyo: Springer, 2000

ISBN 978-3-540-67176-3 ISBN 978-3-642-59758-9 (eBook)
DOI 10.1007/978-3-642-59758-9



Typesetting: Data conversion by Stürtz AG, Würzburg

SPIN: 10733443 21/3135 – 5 4 3 2 1 0
Printed on acid-free paper

# Scientific Council



# We thank the following referees for reviewing the abstracts

Dimos Baltas, Arthur Boyer, Anders Brahme, George Chen, Benedick Fraass, Michael Goitein, Marcel van Herk, Christian Karger, Mark Kessler, Peter Kneschaurek, Hanne Kooy, Anthony Lomax, Rockwell Mackie, Ben Mijnheer, Radhe Mohan, Fridtjof Nüsslin, Ulrich Quast, David Rogers, Ulf Rosenow, Lothar Schad, George Starkschall, Siegfried Stiehl, Randall Ten Haken, Steve Webb, John Wong, Peter Wust

The layout and technical realization of these proceedings were carried out by

*Oliver Jäkel*

*Gunilla Küster*

*Andreas Lüttgau*

*Andreas Mahr*

*Simeon Nill*

*Wilfried Schneider*

# Preface

*Wolfgang Schlegel and Thomas Bortfeld*

*Deutsches Krebsforschungszentrum (DKFZ), Department of Medical Physics, Heidelberg, Germany*

Radiation therapy was one of the first medical disciplines where computers started to play an important role: The first dose calculation systems were introduced more than 30 years ago. Today, computers are involved in practically all areas of radiation therapy: from tumour localisation with the help of tomographic imaging, 3D image segmentation, virtual therapy simulation, dose calculation, optimisation, treatment planning, to computer controlled delivery systems and verification. From the very beginning of computer application in radiotherapy, it has been a tradition that the International Conference on the Use of Computers in Radiation Therapy is held every three years. For us it has been a privilege and an honour to help organise the XIIIth ICCR in May 2000 in the beautiful southern German university town of Heidelberg.

The scientific program of the XIIIth ICCR is organised around plenary focus sessions, scientific sessions including a poster exhibition and poster session, as well as an exhibition and lunch sessions organised by industrial companies. This concept has evolved from the previous meetings and is largely based on the last meeting in Salt Lake City, which in our opinion was a great success. We also followed the ICCR tradition in providing the participants with the book of extended abstracts that is in your hands. We decided to limit each contribution to 3 printed pages, which we believe is an acceptable compromise between the amount of information that can be provided and the weight and size of this book. It also allowed us to include the abstracts of all posters. The resulting number of 596 pages is, however, the maximum that can be tolerated in terms of weight and cost of printing. It is our hope that this book will be a lasting reference for the participants as well as for other members of our community.

The number of abstract submissions (226) was again significantly higher than in the previous meetings. On the one hand, we are happy about this enormous interest in the ICCR. On the other hand, it had as a consequence that about 10% of the submissions had to be rejected, as we could not accept more than a total of about 200 papers and posters in order to avoid having more than two sessions in parallel. This was a hard decision. In spite of the careful peer review by expert referees, we are aware that abstract evaluation can never be perfectly objective, and one or the other rejection may be unjust. If this should have happened, we apologise.

One of our goals for the XIIIth ICCR was to strengthen the role of posters. We see posters as an equally important alternative to oral presentations. Some material is obviously better suited for poster presentation than for a talk. The referees have helped to make this decision. A good proportion of the 62 posters shows original scientific work of excellent quality. A special poster session is scheduled to view the posters in detail and to discuss their contents with the authors. As already mentioned, all poster abstracts are included at full length in this book. The best poster contribution will receive an award.

The topics of the submissions cover a wide range of applied physics and state of the art technology in radiotherapy. Some submissions are in fields such as hyperthermia and laser-neurosurgery. This is clearly far beyond the use of computers in radiotherapy. For future meetings, one may have to find a new name for the conference. Specifically, for the XIIIth ICCR we received a very large number of submissions in the field of intensity modulated radiotherapy (IMRT) and "inverse" planning, resulting in a total of 4 sessions with proffered papers and many posters. The big interest in IMRT is also reflected by the 4 invited focus sessions, which cover various aspects related to IMRT. Furthermore, we received an unexpectedly large number of submissions on Monte Carlo techniques. As a result there is a special Monte Carlo "Questions and Answers" session that was triggered by Dave Rogers and Radhe Mohan, as well as two session with proffered Monte Carlo papers plus numerous posters and presentations related to Monte Carlo in the other sessions. Besides these major topics, there are other sessions with highly interesting and original contributions. Among these we may find the answer to the question "What comes after IMRT?".

We hope that the XIIIth ICCR will give the opportunity to computer scientists, medical physicists, engineers and physicians involved in the field of radiation therapy from all over the world to exchange their experience and knowledge and to discuss the most recent advances in this exciting and steadily growing field of computer and high technology applications in medicine.

*Acknowledgement*

We wish to express our gratitude to the members of the scientific council for their advise in organising this meeting, for the organisation of focus sessions, and for evaluating the contributions to the young investigators and poster awards. We thank the referees for their careful and timely review of the abstracts. Financial support from the industrial companies is gratefully acknowledged. We are thankful to our colleagues who worked with us on preparing the conference and the proceedings, most of all the editorial team, who did an incredible job. Last not least we would like to thank the authors for submitting such a large number of original and significant contributions. We hope that they and all the other participants will be rewarded by stimulating discussions and lots of new ideas and visions for the second century of radiotherapy.

# The XIII$^{th}$ ICCR was sponsored by

*Direx Systems GmbH*
*Gammex-RMI GmbH*
*MDS Nordion Therapy Systems*
*Multidata Systems Deutschland GmbH*
*Physics in Medicine and Biology*
*Siemens Medizintechnik*
*Varian Medical Systems International AG*

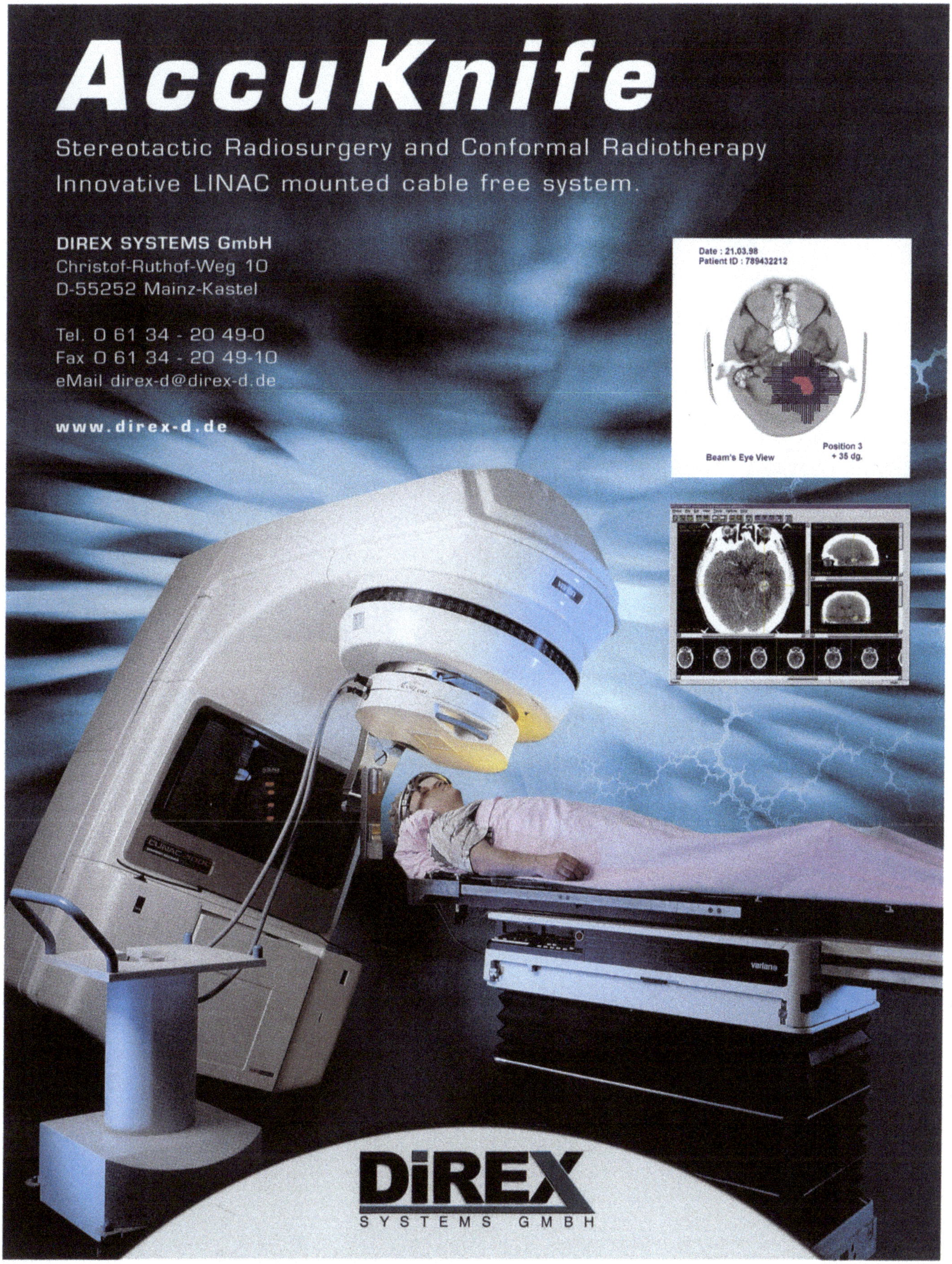
AccuKnife
Stereotactic Radiosurgery and Conformal Radiotherapy
Innovative LINAC mounted cable free system.
DIREX SYSTEMS GmbH
Christof-Ruthof-Weg 10
D-55252 Mainz-Kastel
Tel. 0 61 34 - 20 49-0
Fax 0 61 34 - 20 49-10
eMail direx-d@direx-d.de
www.direx-d.de
Date : 21.03.98
Patient ID : 789432212
Beam's Eye View
Position 3
+ 35 dg.
varian
DiREX
SYSTEMS GMBH

# Table of Contents

## Monday, 22 May 2000

### Focus Session: Inverse Planning (Steve Webb)



### Session: Optimization / Inverse Planning 1

## Session: Computer Science

## Focus Session: Monte Carlo-Based Routine Clinical Treatment Planning (David Rogers)



## Session: Computer Science / Imaging

## Tuesday, 23 May 2000

### Focus Session: IMRT Delivery: Theoretical Concepts and Clinical Reality (Arthur Boyer, Wilfried DeNeve)



### Session: IMRT Delivery Techniques

## Session: Dose Calculation & Biological Models

## Wednesday, 24 May 2000

### Focus Session: Quality Assurance in Treatment Verification of Conformal Radiation Therapy (Fridtjof Nüsslin)



### Session: IMRT Delivery & Verification

Wednesday, 24 May 2000

## Session: Other Treatment Modalities

## Session: Quality Assurance



## Session: Monte Carlo 1

## Thursday, 25 May 2000

### Focus Session: New Approaches in Patient Positioning - Strengthening a Weak Chain Link (Gig Mageras)



### Session: Optimization / Inverse Planning 2



### Session: EPID & Patient Positioning

# Inverse-planning for IMRT with a robotically-mounted linac: parameterisation of this ultimate (?) IMRT technique

**Steve Webb**

Joint Department of Physics, Institute of Cancer Research and Royal Marsden NHS Trust, Downs Road, Sutton, Surrey, SM2 5PT, UK.
email: STEVE@ICR.AC.UK

## 1. Introduction

Intensity-modulated external-beam radiotherapy (IMRT) is generally formulated in two distinct parts: (i) inverse planning to determine the intensity-modulated beam (IMB) profiles, followed by (ii) delivery (interpretation). Delivery can be by: (i) compensator, (ii) tomotherapy, (iii) multiple-static multileaf-collimator (MLC)-shaped fields (MSF), (iv) dynamic multileaf collimator (DMLC), (v) scanned photon beams, or (vi) scanned absorbers. At the time of writing, technique (ii) has treated more patients worldwide (excluding the historical [i]) but techniques (iii) and (iv) are gaining ground and have been heavily invested in by both industry and hospital physics departments. This is as it should be. The MSF and DMLC techniques in particular are practical and the problems are largely understood.

However, in performing inverse planning to "optimise" IMBs, many beam parameters are fixed ahead of numerical optimisation. Also the interpretation only generates an approximation to the IMBs from inverse planning because of equipment constraints. Ideally one would like to know what is the ultimate IMRT plan for a given case independent of delivery method and without too much pre-constraining. The aim of this work was to develop an inverse treatment-planning method which allowed a wide choice of beam orientation so that optimisation of beamweights essentially determined the most appropriate directions and for which the delivery technique exactly matched the planning assumptions. If one knew the "ultimate solution" for a problem then it would be possible to understand how close other, more common, IMRT techniques approach this ultimate solution. The study is presented as a contribution to the **Special Focus** debate "How good is optimal?"

## 2. Material and Methods: The robotically-mounted linac

The performance of a robotically-mounted in-line linac is simulated. The support (robotic arm) for the linac is specified by its direction ($\varphi,\vartheta$) in space and the "pointing" of the linac by the azimuth A and elevation E relative to this support (Figure 1). The linac has a circular collimator delivering a beam with a profile $1/(1+ (r/ r_B)^Q)$ at origin O which is 100 cm from source S. Q was set to 4. The beam profile was assumed to be zero beyond radius $r=d_C$ where $d_C \propto r_B$ (see Table 2). A central-axis TMR depth-dose with inverse-square law was used. Thus the pointing direction of the i-th linac-generated pencil beam is specified by the four parameters $(\varphi,\vartheta,A,E)_i$ and intensity modulation is created by the trajectory set of i-values each with weight $w_i(\varphi,\vartheta,A,E)_i$. These weights were determined by a conventional inverse-planning technique (iterative least squares minimisation of a r.m.s. importance-weighted dose-based quadratic cost function), the only complexity being provided by the unusual geometry. The sampled values of $A_i$ and $E_i$ were $180^0$ and $90^0$ ± a small range of A and E, respectively, so as to point at the spherical envelope of the planning target volume (PTV). The range was sampled with intervals $\Delta E=\Delta A$. These intervals depended on the beamwidth $r_B$. To study beam orientation and beamweight optimisation, $\varphi$ ranged over $360^0$ and $\vartheta$ ranged over $90^0 \pm \Delta\vartheta$ with equispaced sampling. In practice, because the links between dose-space and beam-space are too numerous to be stored and are also lengthy to calculate, the sampling of $\varphi$ and $\vartheta$ was discrete (see Table 1). The number of iterations was varied to maintain the "visitation frequency ($\approx 10$)" of potential trajectory components and hence the calculations for each plan took many days, some even weeks, on a DEC ALPHA computer. Further details and preliminary results with $r_B$=6.25 mm (fixed) were given by [1] for several planning problems. In this paper the work is developed to further study the effects of spatial sampling and of varying the beamsize. Delivery efficiency and other findings are presented.

## 3. Results and Conclusions

**(3.1) spatial sampling:** Allowing $\varphi$ and $\vartheta$ to vary continuously is computationally impossible. For the model problem shown in Figure 2, Table 1 shows the effect of changing the sampling of $\varphi$ and $\vartheta$ with $\varphi$ discretely distributed in 0-$360^0$ and $\vartheta$ in $90^0 \pm \Delta\vartheta$ and with $r_B = 6.25$ mm and $\Delta E = \Delta A = 0.5^0$. It is clear that conformality improves with increasing spatial sampling of potential beamspace. The 5th column shows the best computed conformality. The 3rd column *represents* the performance of a MIMiC-like tomotherapy delivery. The 1st column represents the delivery of 5 fixed fields via e.g. a compensator. More conformal IMRT stems from abandoning coplanarity.

**(3.2) effect of beamsize variation and under- and over-sampling beamspace:** Table 2 shows the effect of varying the beamsize of the elementary pencil. Columns 1,2,3 and 6 show that conformality improves as the beamsize decreases. For these inverse plans note that the sampling $\Delta E=\Delta A$ was carefully controlled so that elemental pencil beams have the potential to overlap and leave no "holes" in the dose distribution. As $r_B$ decreased so $\Delta E,\Delta A$ and $d_C$ were correspondingly reduced. Columns 4 and 5 show that over sampling A and E space is also acceptable but column 7 shows that under-sampling wrecks the conformality as one may expect. Figure 3 shows a central transaxial (x,z) slice corresponding to the data in column 6.

**(3.3) delivery efficiency:** Suppose there are N trajectory components each with beamweight $w_i$ delivered by $M_i$ monitor units. Suppose a dose of $D_{j,ref}$ is required at reference voxel labelled by "j" where the dose distribution $\Sigma_{i=1...N}\ {}_jf_i\ w_i = 1$ where ${}_jf_i$ is the dose contribution from the i-th beam component to the j-th dose voxel. Suppose the dose to a water phantom at depth $d_{max}$ from 100 MU's from a single robotic location is $D_{max,measured}$. Then the total number of monitor units required to deliver the complete irradiation is $M_{total} = \Sigma_{i=1...N} M_i = (100\ D_{j,ref} / D_{max,measured}) \times \Sigma_{i=1...N}\ w_i$. This will be an extremely inefficient delivery compared with other IMRT techniques. Unless a very-high output linac could be engineered it would not be a method of choice. The robotic linac is a *concept* to allow study of the limit to IMRT. Note the smaller the elemental beam the more inefficient is the delivery (see Table 2 values of $\Sigma_{i=1...N}\ w_i$ ; also $D_{max,measured}$ will decrease with decreasing beamsize).

**(3.4) practical robotic linac:** Several robotic photon linacs exist and two have been described [2,3]. However no robotic-linac IMRT has been performed yet and issues such as patient movement would need to be studied.

**(3.5) other findings:** The following have also been determined (space precludes illustration, proof and detail): (i) Conformal dose distributions to a convex PTV with adjacent OARs can be delivered as well with a robotic linac as with a conventional technique. (ii) It has been shown that the robotic linac efficiency relative to that of the NOMOS MIMiC has a lower bound $1/2N_E$ where $N_E$ is the number of transaxial irradiated slices. The corresponding lower bound relative to a compensator is $1/(N_E N_A)$ where $N_A$ is the number of required azimuthal locations. (iii) ($\varphi$,$\vartheta$,A,E) values could be converted to gantry angle G, couch twist T and couch shifts $\Delta x$,$\Delta y$,$\Delta z$ for the components to be delivered by a conventional accelerator fitted with a circular collimator. (iv) Inverse-planning with a limited spatially-sampled cost function is faster but results degrade slightly. In **conclusion:** (i) inverse-planning for robotic IMRT can (almost - limited by available CPU time) determine the ultimate external-beam IMRT, (ii) other, presently more practicable, IMRT techniques can be benchmarked against this. In the **Special Focus Session**, to the question "How good is optimal?" I shall answer with another question "How good do you want your IMRT to be? To the question "can one attain the ultimate IMRT conformality, i.e. the truly optimum solution?" I shall answer "no", because too many variables are still preset. However one can "almost" do so.

## References


[1] Webb S 1999 "Conformal intensity modulated radiotherapy (IMRT) delivered by robotic linac – testing IMRT to the limit?" *Physics in Medicine and Biology* **44**, 1639-1654

[2] Schweikard A, Tombropoulos R and Adler J R 1995 "Robotic radiosurgery with beams of adaptable shapes." *Computer Vision in Robotics and Medicine* ed A Ayache (LNCS 905), 138-149

[3] Fantini M, Benassi M, Arcangeli G, Begnozzi L, Bufacchi A, Soriani A, Orvieto A and Ciuffo P 1999 "Conformal irradiation by composition of narrow beams." *Physica Medica* **15** (3) , 213.


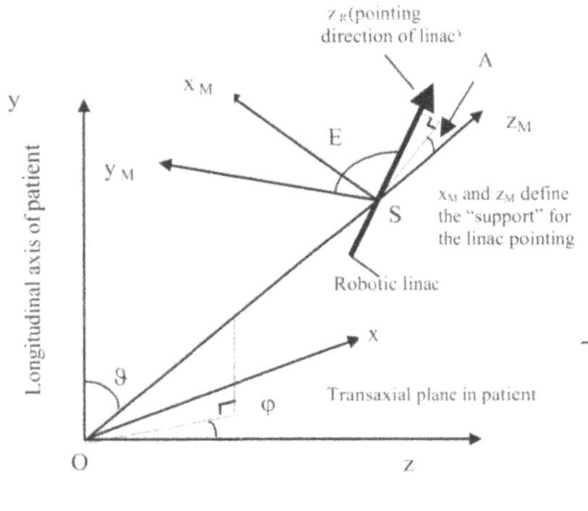


**Figure 1:** The robotic linac concept.

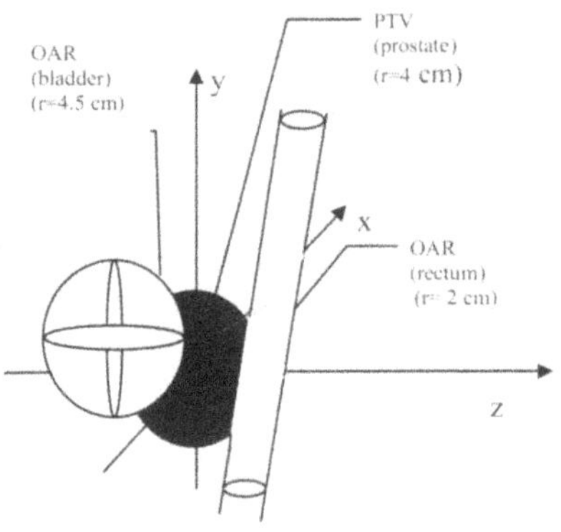


**Figure 2:** A model problem.

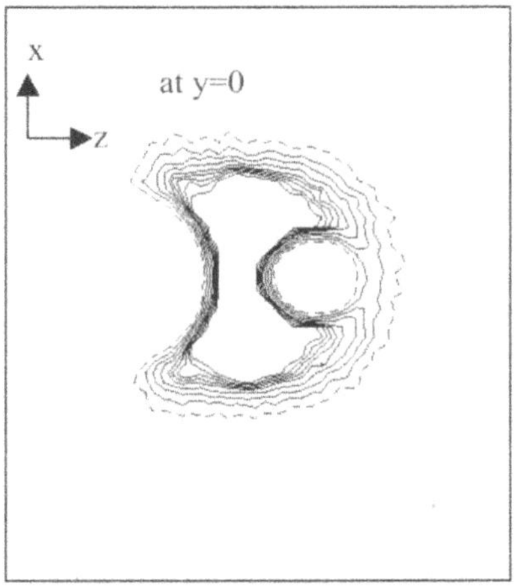


**Figure 3:** Transaxial dose distribution corresponding to data in Table 2 column 6.

| Number of φ values | 5 | 9 | 36 | 36 | 72 |
|---|---|---|---|---|---|
| Number of ϑ values | 1 | 1 | 1 | 9 | 17 |
| Number of iterations | 200k | 200k | 200k | 400k | 1600k |
| Δϑ range (degrees) | 0 | 0 | 0 | ± 40 | ± 40 |
| $PTV_{mean}$ (goal:unity) | 0.991 | 0.994 | 0.995 | 0.997 | 0.997 |
| $PTV_{max}$ | 1.084 | 1.086 | 1.084 | 1.046 | 1.052 |
| $PTV_{min}$ | 0.817 | 0.845 | 0.873 | 0.891 | 0.888 |
| $\sigma_{PTV}$ | 0.037 | 0.035 | 0.032 | 0.020 | 0.020 |
| $OAR_{mean}$ | 0.215 | 0.180 | 0.166 | 0.175 | 0.171 |
| $OAR_{max}$ | 1.026 | 0.988 | 1.003 | 0.942 | 0.945 |
| $OAR_{min}$ | 0 | 0 | 0 | 0 | 0 |
| r.m.s. $cost_{final}$ | 0.3164 | 0.2984 | 0.2909 | 0.2450 | 0.2436 |
| $\Sigma$ IMBs = $\Sigma_{i=1...N} w_i$ | 40.71 | 39.92 | 39.75 | 52.24 | 52.59 |
| $w_{i,max}$ | 0.28 | 0.23 | 0.11 | 0.10 | 0.07 |

Conformality increases as the sampled space increases →

**Table 1:** Simulated concave prostate + rectum + bladder problem (body outline: ellipse, semimajor axis 14 cm and semiminor axis 10 cm (larger than for corresponding table in [1])). Variation of conformality as a function of the number of equispaced φ and ϑ values allowed. The elemental robotic beams were sampled at $\Delta E=\Delta A=0.5^0$, $r_B$=6.25 mm, $d_C$=30 mm. (all units for dose and cost are in terms of planning for unit mean dose in the PTV)

| Radius of collimator $r_B$ mm | 12.5 | 9.375 | 6.25 | 6.25 | 6.25 | 3.125 | 6.25 |
|---|---|---|---|---|---|---|---|
| Sampling ΔE=ΔA | $1^0$ | $0.75^0$ | $0.5^0$ | $0.375^0$ | $0.25^0$ | $0.25^0$ | $1^0$ |
| Dose cutoff $d_C$ mm | 60 | 45 | 30 | 30 | 30 | 15 | 30 |
| Number of iterations | 100k | 180k | 400k | 800k | 800k | 1600k | 200k |
| $PTV_{mean}$ (goal:unity) | 0.994 | 0.995 | 0.997 | 0.997 | 0.997 | 0.999 | 0.987 |
| $PTV_{max}$ | 1.074 | 1.051 | 1.046 | 1.044 | 1.040 | 1.042 | 1.567 |
| $PTV_{min}$ | 0.851 | 0.871 | 0.891 | 0.880 | 0.891 | 0.952 | 0.551 |
| $\sigma_{PTV}$ | 0.032 | 0.026 | 0.020 | 0.020 | 0.020 | 0.011 | 0.094 |
| $OAR_{mean}$ | 0.231 | 0.205 | 0.175 | 0.173 | 0.173 | 0.143 | 0.202 |
| $OAR_{max}$ | 0.955 | 0.956 | 0.942 | 0.925 | 0.930 | 0.847 | 1.539 |
| $OAR_{min}$ | 0 | 0 | 0 | 0 | 0 | 0 | 0 |
| r.m.s. $cost_{final}$ | 0.2663 | 0.2536 | 0.2450 | 0.2414 | 0.2434 | 0.2343 | 0.3385 |
| $\Sigma$ IMBs= $\Sigma_{i=1...N} w_i$ | 13.5 | 25.31 | 52.24 | 54.38 | 53.29 | 189.95 | 41.85 |
| $w_{i,max}$ | 0.09 | 0.09 | 0.10 | 0.11 | 0.08 | 0.12 | 0.15 |

Conformality increases as elemental beam radius decreases →

Over-sampled in ΔE,ΔA

Deliberately under-sampled in ΔE,ΔA

**Table 2:** Simulated concave prostate + rectum + bladder problem (body outline as Table 1). Variation of conformality as a function of the radius $r_B$ of the elementary collimated beam (and linked dose cutoff value $d_c$) and of the sampling intervals ΔE=ΔA. For all cases there were 36 equispaced φ values and 9 equispaced ϑ values in $90^0 \pm 40^0$.

# Tomotherapy: Optimal coplanar radiotherapy

**T. Rockwell Mackie, Gustavo H. Olivera, Paul J. Reckwerdt and Harald Keller**

University of Wisconsin, Dept. of Medical Physics, Madison WI 53706 USA

Tomotherapy, literally "slice therapy", is intensity-modulated fan-beam rotational therapy. The NOMOS Peacock™ system is a serial (or sequential slice) tomotherapy system [1]. It is installed in more than 50 U.S. centers and has been used in the treatments of thousands of patients. Helical tomotherapy, like helical CT, has the fan beam continuously rotating around the patient as the couch is transporting the patient longitudinally through a ring gantry [2-7]. The Tomotherapy Research Group at the University of Wisconsin is assembling the first helical tomotherapy unit at the UW's Physical Sciences Laboratory at the Kegonsa Research Campus. Figure 1 is a photograph of the gantry for this unit while under construction.

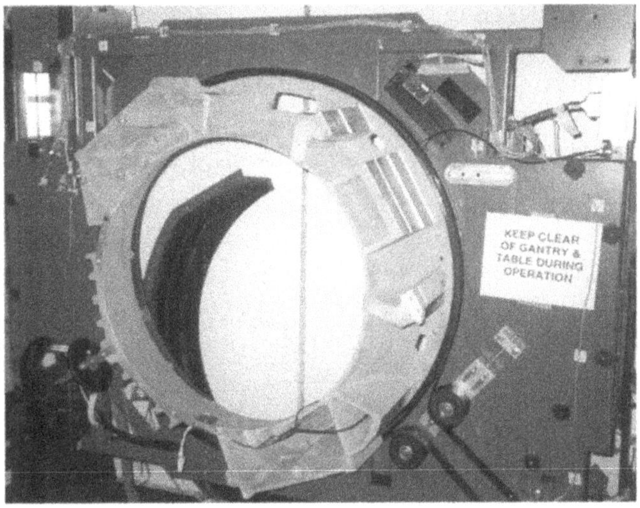


**Figure 1:** Photograph of the modified GE gantry for the first helical tomotherapy system.

## Material and methods

The NOMOS Peacock™ tomotherapy unit is designed to be an add-on unit to a conventional C-arm linear accelerator. Intensity modulated radiation therapy (IMRT) is provided by two multileaf collimator (MLC) banks, each with 20 small collimator leaves. Each bank of leaves can independently modulate two rotating fan beams of x-rays. The leaf movement is binary in that the leaf motion is provided by a pneumatic piston that quickly drives the leaves in or out of the field (closed or open) on a time scale of about 50 ms. The binary MLC system is light enough to be mounted by hand in the wedge tray of a C-arm gantry. There is a severe limitation in moving from the nominal couch position. This is to ensure that the treatment can be safely delivered without colliding with the couch. Very few Peacock™ treatments have been delivered with the couch moved away from the nominal position. The reason most often given is that the dose distributions that can be achieved using large-angle intensity-modulated coplanar arcs is so much better than conventional practices that there is felt to be little need to delivery the therapy in this way. We suspect as well that most users also prefer the convenience of not moving the couch and being able to more easily visualize the treatments being delivered in the same planes as acquired for CT or MRI.

The reluctance to use non-coplanar beams is not restricted to tomotherapy. In conventional non-IMRT practice very few patients receive radiation with the couch rotated from the nominal position. When it is done, it is usually done to provide better field border matching. This was standard procedure for breast treatments when more than a pair of tangential fields was delivered. With the use of independent jaws or half-beam blocks even this practice is less used. It was the hope of many developers of 3-D conformal radiation therapy treatment planning systems that the ability to visualize fully the delivery in 3-dimensions would lead to the use of more non-coplanar treatments. Except for the treatment of well-defined brain tumors this has largely not materialized. For treatments to the neck and body, non-coplanar delivery generally results in longer pathlengths through the patient that yields a corresponding increase in integral dose delivered. The goal, in part, of this paper is not to try to justify the use of coplanar beam directions but to accept it and present the design for a tomotherapy system that is deliberately constrained to delivering only coplanar treatments.

If one begins from the premises that 1) coplanar delivery is conventionally use for the vast majority of current treatments, 2) that IMRT provides excellent delivery of radiation therapy, and 3) more coplanar beam directions is never worse than fewer, a need presents itself for a dedicated treatment device that can optimize coplanar delivery.

Freedom from having to provide non-coplanar treatments presents opportunities to have tomographic verification images. Rather than using a C-arm gantry, coplanar treatments can best utilize the types of ring gantry used for CT or PET. In this geometry low-cost gantry bearings can provide more stable mechanical support for imaging systems. C-arm gantries are used in some single photon emission computed tomography (SPECT) imaging systems. Some vendors of SPECT systems choose to use C-arm gantries because they are perceived to be less claustrophobic than ring gantries. It is possible to get away with this in SPECT because of its intrinsically poorer resolution as compared to the other cross-sectional imaging systems.

It has been shown that it is possible to use a megavoltage (MV) beam to provide CT images that are acceptable for treatment verification. For the same dose delivered and using a detector system which is about 10% efficient, the low contrast resolution is not as good as conventional CT because there are fewer photons being detected resulting in noisier images. The limit of contrast detectable at a dose of about 5 to 10 cGy is about 1%. However, the high contrast resolution of MV CT is nearly as good as standard CT as long as the beam spot size and the detector resolution are comparable to those of standard CT.

## Results and discussion

### Mechanical Aspects

Helical tomotherapy can be viewed as a reengineering of radiotherapy equipment and processes to provide verifiable coplanar IMRT treatments. The clinical prototype is using a standard GE Highspeed™ CT gantry. For CT the gantry is capable of rotating at 60 rpm but for helical tomotherapy it has been slowed down to rotate at between 1 and 10 rpm. The gantry bore at 85 cm is somewhat larger than the 70 cm opening that is standard for diagnostic CT. The couch is from a standard GE CT with a treatment range of 1.2 m and a longitudinal precision of 0.25 mm. The table is capable of supporting a patient with a mass of 200 kg.

The pitch, as in helical CT (or as in the pitch of a thread), is defined to be the distance of translation per rotation divided by the slice width at the axis. A pitch of one corresponds to a translation equal to the slice width and a pitch of 0.5 is a translation equal to one half of a slice width so that each point would be irradiated throughout two rotations.

The gantry has slip rings to transmit power and communications to the rotating side of the ring. The slip rings on a GE Highspeed gantry can transmit 100 A of 500 VAC power on board. The communications uses a high-speed serial protocol and can transmit 100 Mbaud of data or commands.

Cooling for the magnetron, four-port circulator, radiofrequency load and linac is provided by chilled air moved by blowers on the stationary side blowing onto water-to-air radiators on the rotating side. The temperature of the air is provided at 14 °C and is flowing at a rate of 24 $m^3$/min.

The major challenge of the project was to repackage a linear accelerator onto a ring gantry. Our clinical tomotherapy unit uses a compact Siemens grided-gun 6 MeV linear accelerator. The linac is powered by a standard EEV (Model 5193) 2.9 MW peak-power magnetron. The length of the accelerator is 30 cm. The bremsstrahlung target has a unique design. It is a button of tungsten that is free to rotate in a stream of water. The photon beam is unflattened with a maximum dose rate of 8 Gy/min at the central axis. The length of the fan beam is 40 cm at the central axis and has a width that can vary between 0.5 cm and 5.0 cm.

The primary collimator and jaw pair, which defines the fan beam width, are immediately downstream of the target. In the forward direction, the total shielding thickness of the primary collimator and jaw is 22 cm of 94% purity tungsten. This allows the accelerator shielding to reduce the stray radiation for IMRT to levels comparable for conventional radiotherapy.

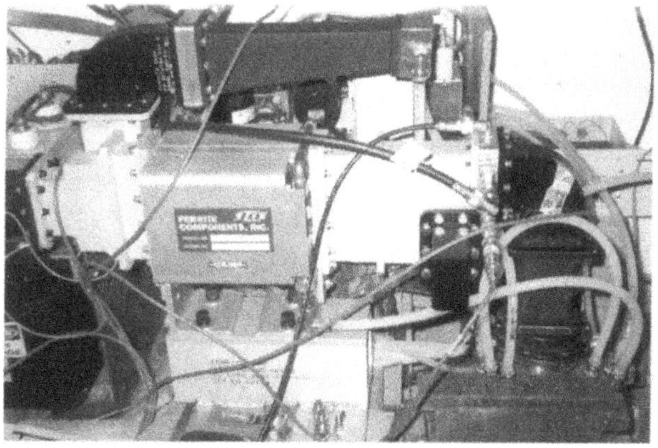

**Figure 2:** Photograph of the Siemens 6 MV linac used on the first helical tomotherapy unit.

There is a thin high-Z hardening foil just distal to the beam monitor to remove low-energy photons from the beam and to reduce the backscatter from the jaws to the beam monitor. The lack of a flattening filter and the presence of the hardening foil allows the head scatter to be minimized. Because it is unflattened, the dose rate is reduced at larger distances from the central axis such that it is about 60% of its maximum value at 20 cm from the central axis. This degree of non-uniformity is irrelevant for IMRT as long as this non-uniformity is taken into account in dose or monitor unit computations.

Like the NOMOS multileaf collimator, the leaves of the MLC are binary. Rather than the NOMOS's 40 leaves modulating two independent fan beams simultaneously, our MLC consists of 64 leaves modulating a single fan beam. The rapid stop of the leaves is cushioned by energy absorbing material. Consequently, the leaf movement noise is much reduced (it sounds like a typewriter). Additionally, the collimator system is inside the ring gantry cowling and so the sound is further reduced. The heights of the leaves are 10 cm of 94% tungsten alloy. They have a 0.15 mm tongue and a 0.3 mm grove in each of the leaves that enables the average leaf transmission to be less than 0.5%

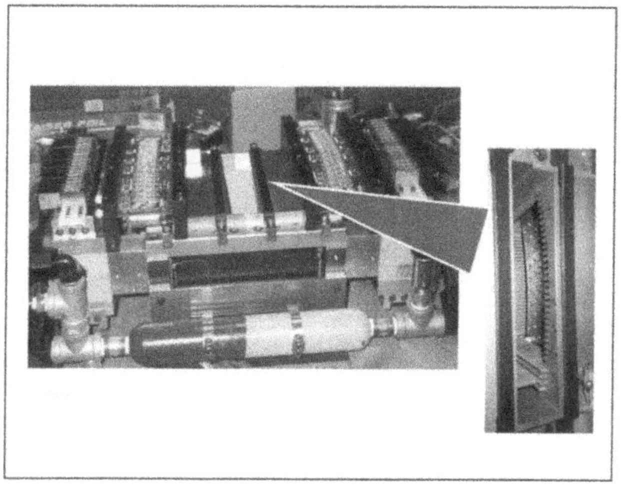

**Figure 3:** Photograph of our binary MLC system. The inset shows a detail of the guide fixture.

**Optimization**

The optimization techniques in helical tomotherapy use the convolution/superposition algorithm as the dose engine. This dose computation algorithm, even if slower than other available methods, provides accurate results in the presence of inhomogeneities, high gradient regions, and in electronic non-equilibrium situations.

Extensive discussion about optimization methodologies as applied to helical tomotherapy can be found in several publications [5,6,8,9]. Optimization for tomotherapy is currently based upon physical objective functions. Biological optimization is under development but is not being used in our implementation because of a lack of complete information on the necessary parameters and limited benchmarking of the biological models. We are using a group of optimization algorithms we refer to generically as iterative optimization techniques. These techniques take into account of the impact of individual pencil beams on the dose distribution. Different objective functions, constraints, and penalties based on dose-volume histogram (DVH) goals can be employed. The benefit of these methodologies is that they reduce the number of convolution operations necessary to perform the optimization and reduce considerably the memory demands [8].

The implementation of the dose computation and optimization algorithms is significantly easier for coplanar delivery. The partial ray sums for the ray tracing calculations to determine the radiological pathlength through the phantom can be precomputed, stored and is only a function of gantry angle. Additionally, the ray trace algorithm for image reconstruction is nearly the same as for the calculation of primary energy fluence. It is likely in the future that the same fast hardware can be used to perform both calculations resulting in faster dose computation.

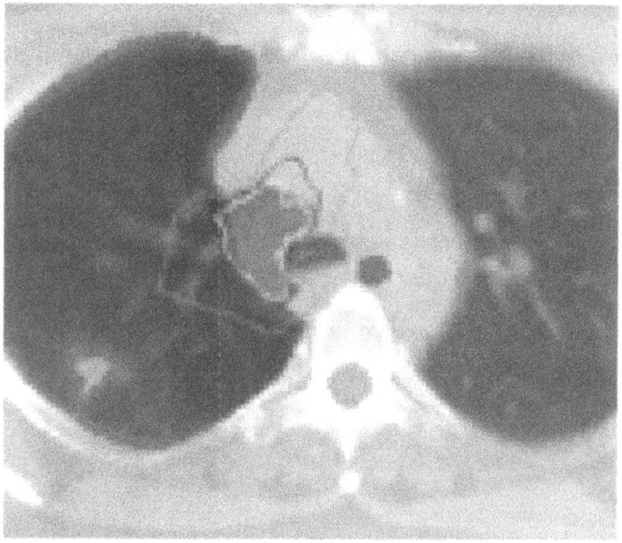

**Figure 4:** Tranverse view of a planned helical tomotherapy treatment for a lung tumor.

Figure 4 is a planned tomotherapy dose distribution for a lung tumor. The PTV is red. The superior vena cava is light blue. The esophagus is dark blue. The cord is green. The right lung and left lung are dark green and orange, respectively. The 95, 90, and 50% isodose lines are yellow, red and green, respectively. The objective for the plan was to avoid the sensitive structures and treat the tumor to a uniform dose. The superior vena cava had the highest avoidance weight.

## Conclusion

Helical tomotherapy, using only coplanar beam delivery can produce highly conformal dose distributions and avoid treating sensitive structures. Coplanar delivery on a ring gantry also provides an opportunity for tomographic-guided radiotherapy.

## Acknowledgements

We would like to thank the contribution of GE Medical System, Siemens Oncology Care Systems, TomoTherapy Inc. and NIH CA48902. TRM and PJR disclose financial interest in TomoTherapy Inc. that is commercializing helical tomotherapy.

## References

[1] Carol, M., H. Targovnik, et al. (1992). "3-D Planning and Delivery System For Optimzed Confomal Therapy." *Int. J. Radiat. Oncol. Biol. Phys.* **24**(Supp. 1): 159

[2] Mackie, T. R., T. Holmes, et al. (1993). "Tomotherapy: a new concept for the delivery of dynamic conformal radiotherapy." *Med. Phys.* **20**(6): 1709-19.

[3] Mackie, T. R. (1995). CT in Radiotherapy and Tomotherapy. Medical CT & Ultrasound: Current Technology and Applications. L. W. Goldman and J. B. Fowlkes. Madison, Wisconsin, Advanced Medical Publishing.

[4] Mackie, T. R. and e. al. (1997). Tomotherapy, Rethinking the Process of Radiotherapy. XII International Conference on the Use of Computers in Radiation Therapy, Salt Lake City, Utah, USA, Medical Physics Publishing.

[5] Mackie, T. R., J. Balog, et al. (1999). "Tomotherapy." *Sem. Radiat. Oncol.* **9**(1): 108-117.

[6] Olivera, G. H., D. M. Shepard, et al. (1999). Tomotherapy. Modern Technology of Radiation Oncology. J. Van Dyk. Madison, Medical Physics Publishing.

[7] Yang, J. N., T. R. Mackie, et al. (1997). "An investigation of tomotherapy beam delivery." *Med. Phys.* **24**(3): 425-36

[8] Olivera C.H., Shepard D.M., et al (1998) Maximum likelihood as a common computational framework in tomotherapy. *Phys. Med. Biol.* 43 3277-3294.

[9] Shepard D.M., Ferris M.C., et al. (1999) Optimizing the delivery of radiation therapy to cancer patients. *SIAM Review.* **41** 721-744.

# DMLC IMRT Is Sufficient for All Clinical Purposes

**Arthur Boyer, Lei Xing, Gary Luxton, Charlie Ma**

Stanford University School of Medicine, Stanford, California

## What is the DMLC IMRT Technique?

The development of Multileaf Collimators (MLCs) controlled by computer-driven motors has led to new technology for Radiation Oncology that allows the intensity of the x-ray fluence within the bounds of a treatment field to be modulated. Various forms of intensity modulation have been developed. One class of techniques can be called Dynamic Multi-Leaf Collimator (DMLC) Intensity-Modulated Radiation Therapy (IMRT). What is it?

Rotate/Translate Modulated Fan Beams. (Carol 1994) This IMRT technique (Figure 1) uses an accessory slot collimator containing a short-stroke MLC.

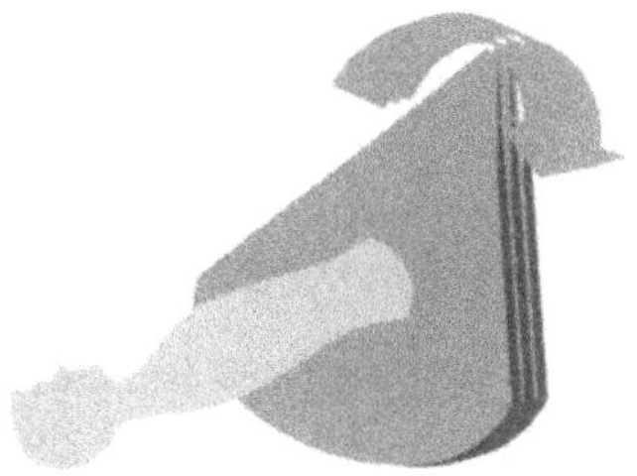

**Figure 1:** Multiple modulated fan beams seperated by longtitudinal translations of the patient (Peacock Tomotherapy).

The slot produces a fan beam. Inverse treatment planning seeks to determine the optimal dose distribution in each transverse slice of the patient and calculates and arc-angle dependent intensity pattern. This pattern is created by inserting short leaves across the slot. A leaf insertion sequence is delivered as a function of gantry angle for each axial slice through the target volume. The patient is translated longitudinally between each arc. This is not DMLC IMRT.

Modulated Spiral Fan Beam. (Mackie 1993) A low-energy linear accelerator waveguide is mounted along with a CT x-ray tube on a slip ring (Figure 2).

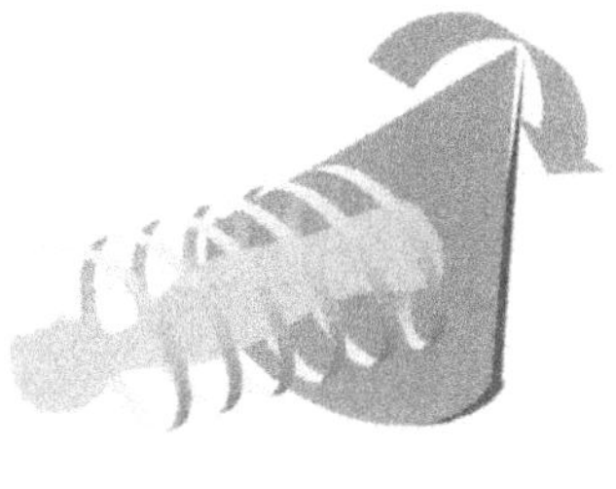

**Figure 2:** Spiraling modulated fan beam used in the tomotherapy concept (Tomotherapy Corporation).

The x-ray beam produced by the waveguide is collimated by a slot that is modulated by short-stroke MLC leaves. By integrating the CT scanner with the treatment delivery gantry, the CT scans of the patient can be acquired before each daily treatment to verify positioning. This is not DMLC IMRT.

Modulated Arc Beams. (Yu 1995) Cedric Yu proposed

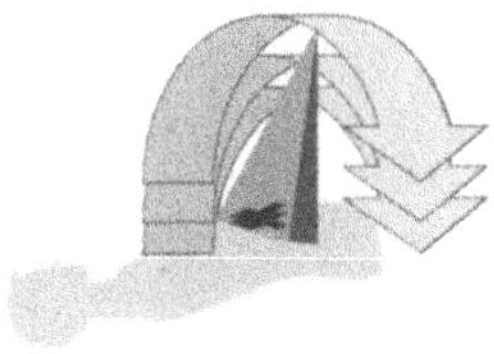

**Figure 3:** DMLC field sequences delivered as a series of arcs. This is the IMAT technique.

delivering a sequence of arced fields dynamically shaped by an MLC to produce the IMRT distributions (Figure 3).
Each arc would contain a window whose shape and size would change over the range of the arc. The shape and size would be determined by an inverse planning system. This is a form of DMLC IMRT.

Modulated Cone Beams. For a number of fixed-gantry field directions (Figure 4), a MLC window is swept between the boundaries of a field to modulate the intensity within those boundaries. The leaf sequence delivers the intensity modulation

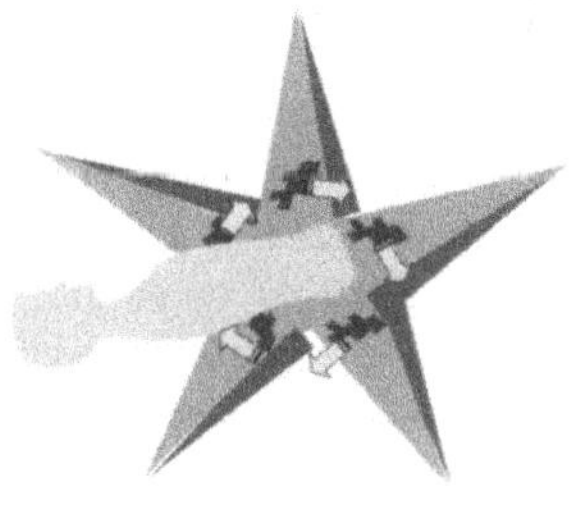

**Figure 4:** Fixed-gantry DMLC technique using dynam-ically swept windows or windows delivered by alter-nately setting the windows with the beam off and then delivering a dose increment with the leaves stationary.

computed by an inverse planning computation. This is another DMLC IMRT technique.
There are two features that seperate DMLC IMRT from tomotherapy. DMLC IMRT is a method used to deliver intensity-modulated beams using a multileaf collimator, with the leaves in motion during radiation delivery. The "sliding window" technique is a form of DMLC IMRT in which the gap, or window, formed by each opposing pair of leaves traverses across the tumor volume while the beam is on (Boyer 1999).

## Advantages of Clinical Application of DMLC

DMLC IMRT can produce three-dimensional dose distributions for complex-shaped target volumes that are superior to distributions that can be planned in equivalent times with conventional techniques (Figure 5). In this example, junction between lateral neck fields and AP/PA supraclavicular fields are entirely avoided (Carol 1996).
DMLC IMRT can be implemented immediately with available

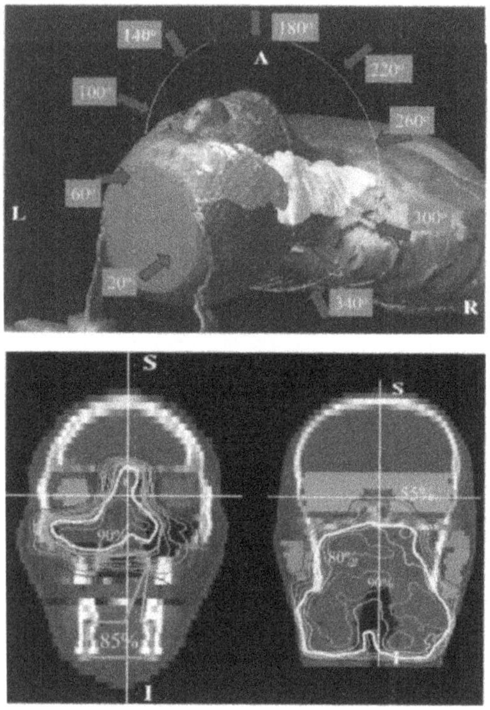


**Figure 5:** DMLC IMRT field configuration and resulting isodose distributions in coronal planes.

commercial products. The technology for treatment planning, treatment QA and documentation, and treatment delivery can be purchased from a number of competing vendors. Figure 6 shows a DMLC IMRT implementation at Stanford University based entirely on commercial products.

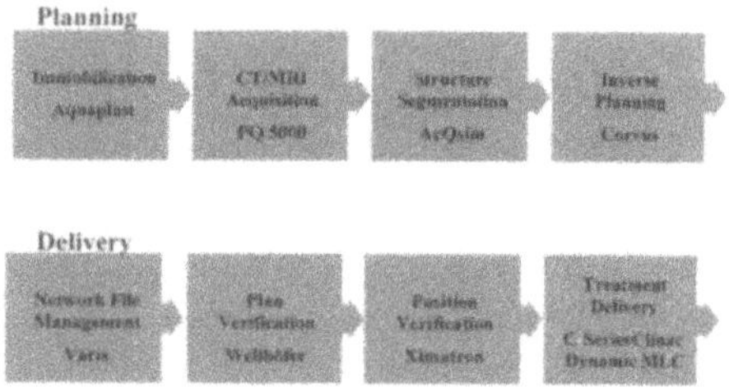


**Figure 6:** Flow diagram of treatment planning and treatment delivery for DMLC IMRT demonstrating the use of commercial products.

The functions of most of the products overlap with conventional and 3-Dimensional Conformal Radiotherapy. Therefore these systems can be used for both DMLC IMRT and for conventional treatments. Since not all treatment presentations require IMRT, the systems can be used in both cases.

Extensive hardware and software engineering are often required to develop a fully functional system for use in radiotherapy. Frequently problems with a system are not apparent to the designers, but become obvious only after extensive clinical application. Therefore, systems that have evolved out of a previously proven clinical system inherit much of the clinical robustness of the antecedent design. Since DMLC can be implemented with commercial products that have a long history of incremental development, it can be expected to be tolerant of the insults of clinical implementation and will be less likely to exhibit unanticipated behavior.

DMLC IMRT as implemented with these tools can be refined. There are a number of areas where improvements are apparent. It is more cost effective to pursue these refinements than to begin an entirely new engineering effort to develop competing technology that may or may not provide significant advantages over DMLC IMRT.

## Shortcomings and Remediations of DMLC

DMLC suffers from multileaf collimators whose transmission specifications were adequate for block replacement, but are suboptimal for IMRT. The MLCs in use are about 60mm thick. To provide shielding during leaf sequences, they need to be about 100mm thick. A change in the MLC design would remediate this deficiency. However, increasing the leaf thickness alone would reduce the clearance between the collimator and isocenter. The design would ideally be integrated with other refinements of collimator design.

The speed by which leaf sequences can be delivered is reduced by software, computer hardware, and mechanical hardware limitations. Conventional radiation therapy can be delivered at the rate of four patient treatments per hour. Systems designs should take advantage of cheaper and faster components as soon as is feasible so that DMLC IMRT for a large number of large fields can also be delivered in this time frame.

Most DMLC IMRT has been implemented using MLC leaves that are 1cm wide. One would expect that finer control of the intensity modulation patterns would provide a higher degree of conformality to target volumes and protection of organs as risk. Figure 7 presents the results of a computation study of smaller leaf widths and leaf step sizes that in most cases confims this expectation. Narrower leaves are being offered by some vendors.

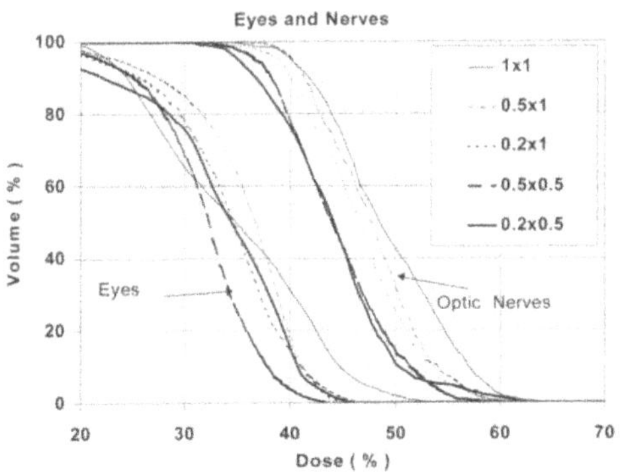


**Figure 7:** Comparison of DMLC IMRT plans using narrow leaves and small discrete steps.

## Future Potential of DMLC IMRT

The sweeping window DMLC technique can be adapted to proton and electron beams. The integration of Modulated Electron Radiation Therapy· (MERT) with photon DMLC IMRT opens new possibilities for improving radiation therapy delivery.

The accuracy of dose distribution calculations will improve with the integration of Monte Carlo simulations into the inverse treatment planning computation (Figure 8).

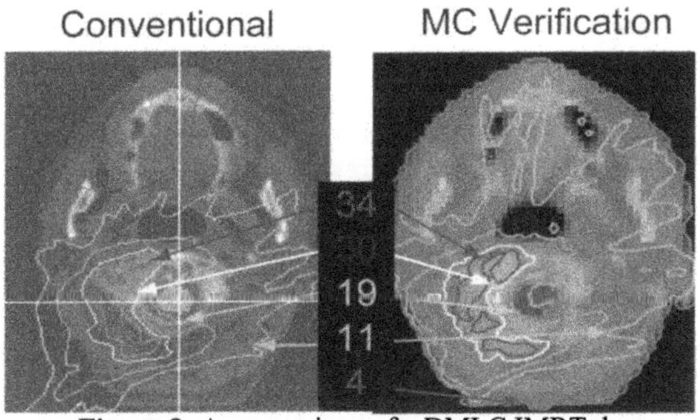


**Figure 8:** A comparison of a DMLC IMRT dose distribution computed using a superposition beam model and the same dose distribution computed using a Monte Carlo simulation. Differences are apparent.

DMLC IMRT will be fully integrated into the treatment planning and delivery systems of networked radiotherapy departments. The flow of large data sets between servers and client workstations will be more easily accomplished within the context of combined IMRT and conventional techniques.

## Summary

Perceived advantages of competing technologies over DMLC IMRT are largely an artifact of the ways technologies are compared. Given sufficient further refinement, DMLC IMRT can be implemented in the clinical environment along with other techniques to provide the most practical yet flexible advanced radiation oncology environment. DMLC IMRT fits within the development stream of widely disseminated technology. It can be implemented clinically since it is supported by collateral technology that is well developed commercially.

## References


Carol M P (1994). An automatic treatment planning system for linear accelerator based beam modulation radiotherapy. In: Hounsell AR, Wilkinson JM, Williams PC, ed. XIth Int. Conf. on the Use of Computers in Radiation Therapy. Manchester: ICCR: 172-173.

Mackie TR, Holmes T, Swerdloff S, Reckwerdt P, Deasy J O, Yang J, Paliwal B, et al.( 1993). Tomotherapy: A new concept for the delivery of dynamic conformal radiotherapy. *Med. Phys*. **20(6)**:1709-1719.

Yu CX (1995). Intensity modulated arc therapy with dynamic multileaf collimation : an alternative to tomotherapy. *Phys. Med. Biol.* **40**:1435-1449.

Boyer AL, Yu CX (1999). Intensity modulated radiation therapy with dynamic multileaf collimators. *Semin. Radiat. Oncol.* **9**:48-59.

Carol M, Grant III WH, Bleier AR, et al.(1996). The field-matching problem as it applies to the Peacock three-dimensional conformal system for intensity modulation. *Int. J. Radiat. Oncol. Biol. Phys.* **34**:183-187.

# Complex IMRT increases the potential for dose misadministration, and simple planning and delivery methods can achieve the same results with reduced risk of patient injury.

**James M. Galvin, D.Sc**

Thomas Jefferson University Hospital

Traditional radiation therapy planning uses rule-based application of treatment fields to obtain homogeneous dose distributions. Techniques for weighting fields and modulating their intensities with standard wedges are well understood. However, these methods have not been extended to address a number of problems that are now of great interest to Radiation Oncologists. For example, it is not obvious how they might be extended to plan targets with invaginations that surround critical normal tissues. Also, it is not easy to apply traditional planing methods to the situation where non-coplanar beams are used to spare healthy tissue. Instead of extending traditional planning techniques to handle these situations, a new planning paradigm was developed as an alternative. The new approach, called inverse planning, uses the desired dose distribution and critical structure constraints to calculate the beam intensity patterns needed to meet the prescription goals. These patterns are then approximated using intensity modulated dose delivery with a multileaf collimator. This talk makes the argument that there are distinct advantages to applying optimization algorithms to a modified version of the traditional forward planning approach. A major benefit of working in the forward direction is that intensity distributions are simplified relative to those produced by inverse planning. This is because the intensity maps, specified in the form of simple field segments within fields, are constructed based on rules that are a minor extension of the ones used for traditional planning. A relatively small number of segments are added to standard plans for the purpose of shaping the dose distribution to follow concavities in the target, and additional segments are added when missing tissue compensation is needed to improve dose homogeneity. Simplifying the intensity patterns is important for a number of reasons: First, since intensity patterns are specified as input to the optimization process, "interpreter" software is not required for dose delivery. This avoids approximations that are inherent in any translation process. Second, dosimetry is simplified because dynamic delivery is not needed and because the "small field" problem is reduced. Third, more fundamental quality control measures can be used to guarantee that the desired intensity map is actually achieved during patient treatment. Fourth, verification of the placement of the intensity pattern relative to the patient's anatomy can be accomplished using standard portal imaging techniques. Taken together, these advantages make the exporting of IMRT from major academic institutions to smaller clinics safe and reliable. For the work described here, the Cimmino algorithm is used to optimize field segment weightings to produce the desired dose distribution. The method has been implemented on both the CMS FOCUS and Precision Therapy Render-Plan planning systems by extracting dose matrices for each segment as well as contour descriptions, and using this information for the optimization of segment weights. The treatment plan is then recalculated to check the final result. Using this method shifts the problem to one of establishing the field segments on which the weight-optimization is performed. The simple rules used for this part of the process will be discussed.

# Using a dose-volume feasibility search algorithm for radiation treatment planning

**George Starkschall[1], Alan Pollack[2] and Craig W. Stevens[2]**

[1]Department of Radiation Physics, and [2]Department of Radiation Oncology, The University of Texas M.D. Anderson Cancer Center, 1515 Holcombe Blvd., Houston, TX 77030 USA

## Introduction

The widespread use of 3-D treatment planning has prompted the need for automated techniques to assist the treatment planner in selecting suitable plans. Approaches to treatment plan optimization are based on the presumption that a computer algorithm can rapidly search through the space of beam parameters to determine those parameters that yield the best treatment plan. Procedures for treatment plan optimization consist of two components. The first component is the definition of an objective function that quantifies the desirability of a treatment plan, while the second component consists of an algorithm that maximizes (or minimizes) the objective function. While the latter task is a relatively straightforward problem in mathematical optimization and is limited by execution time and computer memory, the more difficult task is that of defining the "best" treatment plan.

This paper proposes an approach to treatment planning that removes the necessity of defining a "best" treatment plan. The goal of the present work is to incorporate dose-volume constraints into a system for treatment planning that searches for any feasible plan that satisfies the dose-volume constraints. If no treatment plan can be found that meets the prescribed dose-volume constraints, the planner is advised of this, and is provided guidance as to how the constraints may be relaxed to achieve feasibility.

We apply a particular feasibility search algorithm, the cyclic subgradient projection (CSP) algorithm, to the problem of finding a treatment plan that satisfies dose-volume constraints. This method is applied to two representative treatment plans, a prostate plan and a lung plan. In the illustrated examples the initial set of dose-volume constraints yields no feasible solutions. The radiation oncologist must then modify these constraints in order to achieve feasibility.

## Material and methods

### Feasibility search algorithm

Define the cumulative dose-volume histogram function $DVH_j^D(\mathbf{W})$ as the fraction of anatomic structure $j$ receiving a dose greater than $D$. The dose-volume histogram is a function of the beam weights $\mathbf{W}$. Thus, a dose-volume constraint such as "No more than 30% of the left lung may be irradiated to a dose greater than 20 Gy" has the form $DVH_{lt\,lung}^{20Gy}(\mathbf{W}) < 0.30$, while a constraint such as "The dose to 99% of the PTV must be greater than 68 Gy" has the form $DVH_{PTV}^{68Gy}(\mathbf{W}) > 0.99$. The feasibility search problem is that of finding any beam-weight vector $\mathbf{W}$ so that all constraint equations are satisfied. A vector that satisfies all constraint inequalities is a feasible solution. Any feasible solution is considered acceptable.

The algorithm used to search for a feasible solution is the cyclic subgradient projection (CSP) algorithm [1]. The initial step is to select an arbitrary set of beam weights $\mathbf{W}^{(0)}$. The algorithm then iterates in the following manner:

$$\mathbf{W}^{(k+1)} = \mathbf{W}^{(k)} - \lambda^{(k)} \frac{g_i^+\left(\mathbf{W}^{(k)}\right)}{\left\|\mathbf{t}^{(k)}\right\|^2}\mathbf{t}^{(k)},$$

where

$$g_i^+ = \max\{0, g_i(\mathbf{W})\},$$
$$\mathbf{t}^{(k)} = \nabla g_i(\mathbf{W})\big|_{\mathbf{W}=\mathbf{W}^{(k)}},$$
$$0 < \lambda^{(k)} < 2.$$

The quantity $g_i(\mathbf{W})$ is identified with the dose-volume constraint. For example, for the dose-volume constraint $DVH_{lt\,lung}^{20Gy}(\mathbf{W}) < 0.30$, $g_i(\mathbf{W})$ would be equal to $DVH_{lt\,lung}^{20Gy}(\mathbf{W}) - 0.30$. The algorithm examines each constraint sequentially, updating the beam weights as needed with each constraint. One iteration cycle consists of an examination of each constraint. The iteration continues for a specified number of iteration cycles, or until a feasible solution is found.

Calculating the quantity $\mathbf{t}^{(k)} = \nabla g_i(\mathbf{W})\big|_{\mathbf{W}=\mathbf{W}^{(k)}}$ presents several problems. We first note that the gradient of the DVH as used in this context is not the derivative of the DVH with respect to the dose, but the derivative of the DVH evaluated at a specific dose with respect to each beam weight. The dependence of the DVH on beam weights is not explicit, consequently, the gradient of the DVH must be evaluated as a finite difference. A second problem occurs in calculating gradients of the DVH for a target volume. If the target volume is irradiated uniformly, the derivatives of the DVH at specified dose levels with respect to beam weights should be equal to zero almost everywhere. The quantity $\left\|\mathbf{t}^{(k)}\right\|^2$ that appears in the denominator of the iteration equation will then be equal to zero and the iteration will diverge. To prevent this from occurring, iterations where the dose-volume constraint refers to a target volume consist of either uniformly increasing or uniformly decreasing the beam weights until the dose-volume constraint is met.

**Patient selection and planning**

Two sample representative cases were selected to demonstrate the applicability of the feasibility search to clinical radiation treatment planning. The first case was a prostate case for which the PTV consisted of the prostate and seminal vesicles with a margin of 0.5 – 1.0 cm. The entire PTV was to be treated to 73.8 Gy with a maximum PTV dose of 79.0 Gy. Dose-volume constraints for the normal anatomic structures are indicated in Table 1. The patient was planned using six coplanar 18 MV beams at gantry angles of 50°, 90°, 130°, 230°, 270°, and 310°. Treatment portals were designed to encompass the PTV along with a margin of 0.5 cm to allow for beam penumbra. Five hundred randomly spaced point spanned the PTV while 250 points spanned all normal anatomic structures.

| Organ | Dose | % Volume |
|---|---|---|
| bladder | 60 Gy | 30% |
| bladder | 70 Gy | 20% |
| bladder | 85 Gy | 0% |
| rectum | 60 Gy | 35% |
| rectum | 70 Gy | 20% |
| rectum | 85 Gy | 0% |
| rt femoral head | 45 Gy | 15% |
| rt femoral head | 50 Gy | 5% |
| rt femoral head | 55 Gy | 0% |
| lt femoral head | 45 Gy | 15% |
| lt femoral head | 50 Gy | 5% |
| lt femoral head | 55 Gy | 0% |

**Table 1:** Dose-volume constraints for critical anatomic structures in prostate treatment planning. Each constraint gives the maximum volume that can exceed the specified dose.

The second case was a lung case. The CTV was outlined by the radiation oncologist and a PTV was defined to be the CTV plus a 1.0 cm margin. A prescription of 66 Gy to the entire PTV was specified, with a maximum PTV dose of 70.6 Gy, representing a 7% dose gradient across the PTV. Dose-volume constraints are indicated in Table 2. The patient was planned using six 18 MV beams with gantry angles and table angles summarized in Table 3. Treatment portals were designed to circumscribe the PTV with a 1.0 cm margin. Two hundred fifty points were used to span the PTV and each normal anatomic structure.

For each case, doses were calculated using an FFT-convolution algorithm [2,3] on a 0.5 cm dose grid. All calculations were done within the context of COPPERPlan, the 3-D treatment planning system developed at the M.D. Anderson Cancer Center [4].

The CSP algorithm was applied to each of the two cases to search for a set of beam weights that met the dose-volume constraints. Initial values of beam weights were determined by setting beam weights for all 6 beams equal and at a value so that the minimum dose constraint to the PTV was met.

| Organ | Dose | % Volume |
|---|---|---|
| rt lung | 20 Gy | 37% |
| lt lung | 20 Gy | 37% |
| esophagus | 65 Gy | 40% |
| esophagus | 70 Gy | 20% |
| esophagus | 75 Gy | 0% |
| spinal cord | 45 Gy | 0% |
| rt brachial plexus | 65 Gy | 50% |
| rt brachial plexus | 70 Gy | 20% |
| rt brachial plexus | 75 Gy | 0% |
| lt brachial plexus | 65 Gy | 50% |
| lt brachial plexus | 70 Gy | 20% |
| lt brachial plexus | 75 Gy | 0% |
| heart | 30 Gy | 50% |
| heart | 50 Gy | 20% |
| heart | 60 Gy | 0% |

**Table 2:** Dose-volume constraints for critical anatomic structures in lung treatment planning. Each constraint gives the maximum volume that can exceed the specified dose.

| Beam | Gantry Angle | Table Angle |
|---|---|---|
| PA | 180° | 0° |
| RAO | 320° | 20° |
| LPO | 140° | 20° |
| AP | 0° | 0° |
| RPO | 230° | -20° |
| LAO | 50° | -20° |

**Table 3:** Beam geometries for irradiation of the lung tumor.

## Results and discussion

**Prostate**

Feasibility was not achieved after the first set of 100 iterations. Table 4 illustrates the dose-volume relationships at the conclusion of the iterations. With the exception of the upper bound to the dose to the PTV, all constraints appeared either to have been met or violated by small amounts. The following modifications were made to the dose-volume constraints based on the clinical judgment of the radiation oncologist:

- Max dose to PTV raised to 81.2 Gy
- Max volume of rectum receiving 70 Gy raised to 25%
- Max volume of rectum receiving 60 Gy raised to 36%
- Max volume of femoral head receiving 50 Gy raised to 7.5%
- Max volume of femoral head receiving 55 Gy raised to 1%

Repeating the algorithm with these new dose-volume constraints achieved feasibility in 15 iterations with isocentric weights illustrated in Table 5.

| Constraint | Goal | Actual |
|---|---|---|
| 73.8 Gy to PTV | 100% | 100% |
| 79.0 Gy to PTV | 0% | 42.2% |
| 60 Gy to bladder | 30% | 10.4% |
| 70 Gy to bladder | 20% | 6.4% |
| 85 Gy to bladder | 0% | 0.0% |
| 60 Gy to rectum | 35% | 35.2% |
| 70 Gy to rectum | 20% | 24.4% |
| 85 Gy to rectum | 0% | 0.0% |
| 45 Gy to rt femoral head | 15% | 8.8% |
| 50 Gy to rt femoral head | 5% | 5.6% |
| 55 Gy to rt femoral head | 0% | 0.8% |
| 45 Gy to lt femoral head | 15% | 9.2% |
| 50 Gy to lt femoral head | 5% | 5.6% |
| 55 Gy to lt femoral head | 0% | 0.0% |

**Table 4:** Dose-volume relationships after 100 iterations of CSP algorithm to obtain feasible solution for prostate case

| Beam | Description | Isocentric Weight |
|---|---|---|
| 1 | RAO | 14.1 Gy |
| 2 | Rt Lateral | 14.0 Gy |
| 3 | RPO | 13.0 Gy |
| 4 | LPO | 12.8 Gy |
| 5 | Lt Lateral | 12.3 Gy |
| 6 | LAO | 13.4 Gy |

**Table 5:** Beam weights resulting from feasibility search in prostate plan

### Lung

Using the initial set of constraints, beam weights repeated themselves after 12 iterations without finding a feasible solution. This repetition of beam weights indicated that no feasible solution could be found. Two constraints were not met after these 12 iterations. These were that 36.4% of the PTV received more than 70.6 Gy and 40.4% of the left (ipsilateral) lung receibed more than 20 Gy. The maximum dose constraint on the PTV was then relaxed to allow 5% of the PTV to receive more than 72.6 Gy (10% more than the minimum PTV dose) and the constraint on the ipsilateral lung was relaxed to allow 46% of the lung to receive more than 20 Gy. After 7 iterations a feasible solution was found. Isocentric weights are illustrated in Table 6.

| Beam | Description | Isocentric Weight |
|---|---|---|
| 1 | PA | 12.2 Gy |
| 2 | RAO | 11.0 Gy |
| 3 | LPO | 12.7 Gy |
| 4 | AP | 12.9 Gy |
| 5 | RPO | 10.3 Gy |
| 6 | LAO | 11.6 Gy |

**Table 6:** Beam weights resulting from feasibility search in lung plan

## Conclusion

We have demonstrated a paradigm for radiation treatment planning that is based on finding a treatment plan that satisfies a set of dose-volume constraints. This paradigm is based on the clinical reality of dose prescription in which prescriptions are specified, either explicitly or implicitly, solely in terms of dose-volume constraints. We have presented a methodology that incorporates these constraints and searches through a space of beam parameters for any treatment plan that meets these constraints. If no plan meets these constraints, the program indicates which constraints cannot be met. The radiation oncologist has the option of accepting a solution for which the particular constraints are not met, or relaxing the constraints and reinitiating the search for a feasible solution. Unlike some constrained optimization schemes that allow for the relaxation of constraints, but assign a penalty to constraint violations, in this scheme, dose-volume constraints are viewed as "hard constraints" that can only be relaxed by respecifying the dose prescription. Applying this approach, the treatment planning task is closed-ended. The planner does not have to spend inordinate effort in searching for a solution that does not exist. Rather the onus is returned to the radiation oncologist, who must redefine the parameters of the problem, that is, the dose prescription, if a feasible solution is to be found. The present study indicates that application of a feasibility search algorithm provides a method for radiation treatment planning that enables the radiation oncologist to focus attention on the radiation dose rather than on the geometrical configuration of the radiation beams. Clinical implementation of this approach may effect a shift in the treatment planning paradigm.

## References

[1] Censor Y and Lent A 1982 Cyclic subgradient projections *Mathematical Programming* **24** 233-235

[2] Boyer A L and Mok E C 1985 A photon dose distribution model emplying convolution calculations *Medical Physics* **12** 169-177

[3] Boyer A L and Mok E C 1986 Calculation of photon dose distributions in an inhomogeneous medium using convolution *Medical Physics* **13** 503-509

[4] Starkschall G, Bujnowski S W, Wang L L, Shiu A S, Boyer A L, Desobry G E, Wells N H, Baker W L and Hogstrom K R 1991 A full three-dimensional radiotherapy treatment planning system *Medical Physics* **18** 647

# Dose-volume constrained radiotherapy optimization for a clinical treatment planning system

**Anders Gustafsson[1] and Mark Langer[2]**

[1]MDS Nordion Therapy Systems, Uppsala, Sweden, and [2]Indiana University Cancer Center, Radiation Oncology, Indianapolis, Indiana, U.S.A.

## Introduction

As MLC-based intensity modulated radiation therapy is becoming more clinically available, there is a simultaneous need for computer-assisted dose plan optimization.
Several treatment planning systems are currently providing the first generation of dose plan optimization tools. In general, the tools in the different TPS use similar objective functions, see e.g. [1]. The user is allowed to formulate a desired dose and acceptable dose variance in the target, a maximum dose or dose-volume requirements to the critical structures, and relative weighting factors for the different targets and critical structures to control the order in which the different requirements should be fulfilled.
Selection of relative weighting factors is however generally a trial-and-error process, and the user is often required to fine-tune one or several of the weighting factors to obtain a clinically acceptable dose plan. Normally, the optimal selection of weighting factors and dose limits is dependent on the treatment set-up, and if the beam directions, number of beams etc. are changed, the weighting factors and dose limits have to be adjusted to obtain clinically acceptable results for the new set-up. It is of course possible to have the computer determine sufficient parameters, and different approaches in this field have been developed, see e.g. [2], but these methods are more concerned with computational properties than with clinical considerations.
A more clinically relevant formulation of the optimization problem in radiotherapy is as follows:

*given a set of indispensable dose-volume constraints on the critical structures and a limit on target dose variance, maximize the minimum target dose.*

This alternate formulation, that could be denoted CCMTD (Critical structure Constrained Maximization of Target Dose), has already been applied by Langer and co-workers [3], where they have used mixed integer programming (MIP) algorithms to obtain optimized plans. One consideration that arises when using their approach, though, is that the algorithm applies to combinations of linear constraints and a linear objective function. However, the objective may not always be a linear function of dose. Furthermore, in some recently developed dose calculation models, dose is not a linear function of the compensating filter parameters [4], and hence so is not the objective function and constraints.
In this work, CCMTD has been applied to a more general dose calculation formalism. As will be shown, the novel approach provides plans with target doses equivalent to or higher than plans optimized using weighting factors, normalized to meet the constraints on the critical structures.

## Material and methods

### Method selection

There are at least four ways to generalize the CCMTD problem: (1) use a so-called MINLP (Mixed Integer Nonlinear Programming) algorithm, capable of handling both integer variables and nonlinear functions and constraints, (2) use MIP by making the objective function and constraints piecewise linear, with linear segments indexed by integer variables (3) use a multi-objective nonlinear programming (NLP) algorithm and solve the maximin problem (maximize the minimum of the dose distribution in target) or (4) reformulate the problem to fit a single-objective gradient based NLP algorithm, capable of handling continuously differentiable nonlinear objective functions and constraints, but not integer variables. In this work, the latter alternative has been selected due to the lack of sufficient MINLP and multi-objective NLP algorithms for large-scale problems such as intensity modulation optimization.

### Objective function and target constraints

Gradient based NLP algorithms generally require continuously differentiable objective functions and constraints, which are not available in the orginal formulation of the CCMTD problem.
On a discrete grid the target dose minimum function is only piecewise continuously differentiable. Therefore, the mean target dose is selected as the objective function instead. Provided dose is a continuously differentiable function of the intensity modulation, so is also the mean target dose function.
In general, it is desirable to control the target dose uniformity or variation. In the recent work of Langer and co-workers [3], target dose variation was taken as the quotient between maximum and minimum target dose, which is not a continuously differentiable function. In this work, the continuously differentiable dose variance (standard deviation squared) is applied instead.
The combination of target mean dose and variance does not offer the same control of the target dose as the original formulation where both minimum and maximum doses are explicitly accounted for. A cold spot might be produced. If a cold spot is seen, it might be possible to increase the optimization target volume to move the cold spot outside the clinical target volume.

To summarize, the objective function $F$ for one or more target volumes should be subject to *maximization* and is given by:

$$F = \sum_i \bar{D}_i = \sum_i \frac{1}{V_i} \sum_j v_{i,j} D_{i,j} \qquad (1)$$

where $V_i$ is the total volume of target with index $i$, and $v_{i,j}$ and $D_{i,j}$ are the partial volume and dose, respectively, of voxel $j$ in target $i$.
The dose variance constraint for target $i$ is given by:

$$\sigma_i = \frac{1}{V_i}\sum_j v_{i,j}(D_{i,j} - \bar{D}_i)^2 \le \sigma_i^{\max} \tag{2}$$

**Critical structure constraints**
For critical structures, one or more dose-volume constraints could be formulated, i.e. for the critical structure with index $i$ a maximum volume of $\hat{V}_{i,k}$ is allowed to absorb a dose higher than $\hat{D}_{i,k}$ ($k$ is the dose-volume constraint index). Mathematically speaking, this constraint can be formulated as:

$$V_{i,k} = \sum_j v_{i,j}\theta(D_{i,j} - \hat{D}_{i,k}) \le \hat{V}_{i,k} \tag{3}$$

where $\theta(x)$ is the Heaviside step function, equal to 0 when $x<0$ and equal to 1 when $x>0$. Unfortunately, inequality (3) is not suitable for gradient based NLP algorithms: the Heaviside function is discontinuous in $x=0$, and the gradient of inequality (3) is zero whenever $D_{i,j} \ne \hat{D}_{i,k}$. To overcome these difficulties, the Heaviside function $\theta(x)$ is approximated with the continuously differentiable function

$$\tilde{\theta}(x) = \begin{cases} 0, & x \le -1 \\ 1/2 + x + x^2/2, & -1 < x \le 0 \\ 1/2 + x - x^2/2, & 0 < x \le 1 \\ 1, & x > 1 \end{cases} \tag{4}$$

and the dose-volume constraint is expressed as:

$$\bar{D}_i \frac{V_{i,k} - \hat{V}_{i,k}}{V_i} \le 0 \tag{5}$$

where $\tilde{\theta}(x)$ is now used in the calculation of $V_{i,k}$. Apart from expressing the constraint in inequality (3), the lefthand side of inequality (5) also has the advantageous property to decrease with increasing mean dose in the critical structure.

## Results and discussion

To illustrate the performance of CCMTD a two-dimensional cervix geometry with critical structures rectum and bladder has been applied. The target is shaped to include potential microscopic tumor cell spread in the lymph nodes. Three intensity modulated beams are incident on the target from gantry angles 0°, 120° and 240°.
Optimization has been performed using the nonlinear programming code LSGRG2 [5], particularly suited for problems with many variables and nonlinear constraints.
For comparison with the new optimization approach, the intensity modulation has also been optimized with respect to a weighting factor objective function $F_w$. This function should be subject to *minimization* and is given by:

$$F_w = \sum_{i\in \text{tgt}} \frac{w_i}{V_i}\sum_j v_{i,j}(D_{i,j} - \hat{D}_i)^2 + \sum_{i\notin \text{tgt}} \frac{w_i}{V_i}\sum_j v_{i,j}\tilde{\theta}(D_{i,j} - \hat{D}_i)(D_{i,j} - \hat{D}_i)^2 \tag{6}$$

where $w_i$ is the relative weighting factor for target/critical structure with index $i$ and $\hat{D}_i$ is the desired and limit dose for target and critical structure, respectively.
Equation (6) is a simplified formulation of the objective function that is used in some clinical treatment planning systems. In its more general form, dose limits are replaced with dose-volume limits, but the principle is the same as in $F_w$; to a certain objective function cost, the dose-volume limits are allowed to be violated.

In this example, the dose limits for the critical structures have been selected the same for both optimization methods, as can be seen in Table 1.

| | $F_w$ | | CCMTD | | |
|---|---|---|---|---|---|
| | $\hat{D}_i$ / Gy | $w_i$ | $\hat{D}_{i,1}$ / Gy | $\hat{V}_{i,1}$ | $\sigma_i$ / Gy$^2$ |
| Target | 60 | 1.0 | - | - | 5 |
| Rectum | 40 | 0.1 | 40 | 0.2 | - |
| Bladder | 50 | 0.1 | 50 | 0.2 | - |

**Table 1:** Parameters in the $F_w$ and CCMTD optimizations.

The $F_w$ optimization has been executed a number of times with different target dose prescriptions and weighting factors, and target dose uniformity and critical structure avoidance in the different runs has been evaluated. The parameter set resulting in the most favourable optimized dose plan has been selected from these runs. For clinically relevant comparison of the two methods, the dose plan optimized using $F_w$ has been renormalized to exactly meet the specified dose-volume constraints (see Table 1) after completed optimization.
In the CCMTD optimization, the tolerance volumes for the critical structures and the target dose variance has been selected based on a clinical judgement.

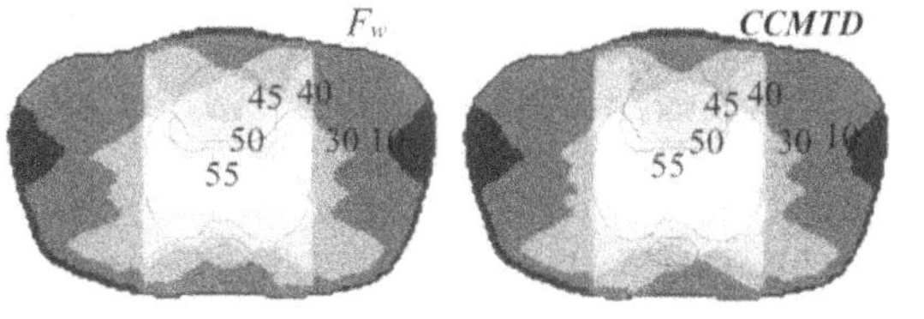


**Figure 1:** Dose distributions after $F_w$ and CCMTD optimization.

The results of the optimizations can be seen in Figures 1 (dose distribution), 2 (dose-volume histograms) and 3 (intensity modulation) for the two different optimization methods. From Figure 2 it can be clearly seen that despite the extensive search for sufficient weighting factors and target dose, the $F_w$ optimization has still lower target doses than the CCMTD optimization. In terms of minimum dose the difference is more or less negligible (47.5-Gy vs. 47.9-Gy) but in terms of maximum dose the difference is larger than a typical dose fraction (59.5-Gy vs. 61.8-Gy).

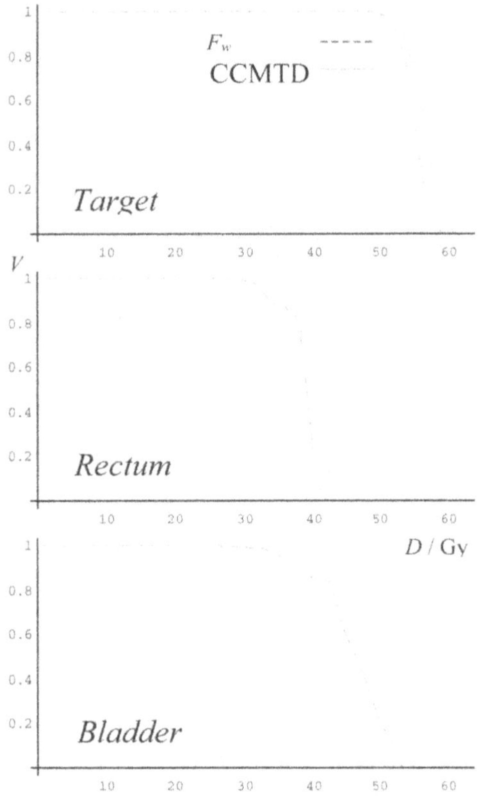


**Figure 2:** Dose-volume histograms for the two optimized dose plans.

From Figure 3 it can be seen that the level of complexity in the intensity modulation is about the same for both cases.

The treatment set-up was also changed to include five equidistantly distributed beams and the obtained optimized plans were normalized to meet the dose-volume constraints to the critical structures. For CCMTD optimization, the mean target dose was then increased to 67.3-Gy with minimum and maximum target doses 52.3-Gy and 75.1-Gy, respectively, whereas the target doses ranged from 48.8-Gy and 61.1-Gy for the $F_w$ optimization. The dose distributions to the critical structures were similar in both cases while the dose variance in the target was lower for the $F_w$ optimization, on the crucial expence of target dose level. The overall target dose levels can be increased for the $F_w$ optimization by adjusting the desired target dose parameter $\hat{D}_i$, but CCMTD has the advantage of maximizing the objective without repeating the optimization process with different parameters.

## Conclusion

The CCMTD formulation of the radiotherapy optimization problem presented in this work is well suited for clinically relevant optimization. The problem formulation is entirely concerned with clinical considerations in terms of tolerance doses and volumes, and involves no iterative search for computationally sufficient optimization conditions, such as selection of relative weighting factors and dose levels for different structures and volumes.

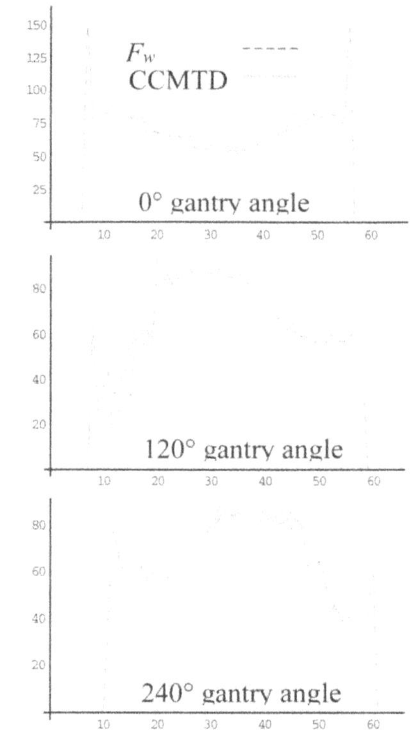


**Figure 3:** Intensity modulation for the two optimized dose plans, arbitrary length and modulation units.

The method is suitable for implementation in a clinical treatment planning system, since it does not rely on linearity in the dose calculation. From a clinical point of view, one drawback with the method is that it does not consider minimum target doses in particular, which is demonstrated in the examples above. The target volumes receiving these cold spots are however small, and the clinical effect might be reduced even further by sligthtly increasing the target size used in optimization, since the low doses generally appear on the target boundaries near critical structures.

## References

[1] Bortfeld T, Bürkelbach J, Boesecke R and Schlegel W 1990 Methods of image reconstruction from projections applied to conformation therapy *Physics in Medicine and Biology* **35** 1423-1434

[2] Xing L, Li J G, Donaldson S, Le Q T and Boyer A L 1999 Optimization of importance factors in inverse planning *Physics in Medicine and Biology* **44** 2525-2536

[3] Langer M, Morrill S, Brown R, Lee D and Lane R 1996 A comparison of mixed integer programming and fast simulated annealing for optimizing beam weights in radiation therapy *Medical Physics* **23** 957-964

[4] Ahnesjö A, Weber L, Nilsson P 1995 Modeling transmission and scatter for photon beam attenuators *Medical Physics* **22** 1711-1720

[5] Smith S and Lasdon L 1992 Solving large sparse nonlinear programs using GRG *ORSA Journal on Computing* **4** 1-15

# IMRT optimization based on the generalized Equivalent Uniform Dose (EUD)

**Qiuwen Wu[1], Radhe Mohan[1] and Andrzej Niemierko[2]**

[1]Dept. of Radiation Oncology, Medical College of Virginia Hospitals, Richmond, VA, USA, and [2]Dept. of Radiation Oncology, MGH and Harvard University, Boston, MA, USA

## Introduction

The purpose of this paper is to present the results of an investigation of an objective function based on "generalized Equivalent Uniform Dose (EUD)" for optimization of intensity-modulated radiotherapy (IMRT) plans. The concept of EUD for tumors was introduced by Niemierko,[1] and is defined as the biologically equivalent dose which, if given uniformly, leads to the same cell kill in the tumor volume as the actual non-uniform dose distribution. Niemierko generalized this concept to apply to normal tissues as well.[2]

In the early stages of IMRT optimization, many investigators utilized purely dose-based objective functions. Presently, most IMRT optimization systems employ dose- and/or dose-volume-based objective functions. The limitation dose- or dose-volume-based optimization criteria have led a number of investigators to propose models for predicting biological and dose-response indices, which could be used instead of or to supplement dose- and dose-volume-based criteria. There have been only a few rather limited studies in the use of dose-response-based objective functions for treatment plan optimization.

## Materials and methods

Previous attempts to define objective functions in terms of dose-response functions have generally used indices such as tumor control probability (TCP) and normal tissue complication probabilities (NTCP). In this paper we use the generalized version of EUD as the basis for defining the objective function for IMRT optimization. Recently, Niemierko suggested the generalized formalism

$$EUD = \left( \frac{1}{N} \sum_i D_i^a \right)^{\frac{1}{a}} \qquad (1)$$

for both tumors and normal tissues. In this expression, $D_i$ is the dose in the $i$'th voxel and $a$ is a parameter which is negative for tumors and positive for normal tissues. Values of parameter $a$ can be determined by comparing the calculated tumor and normal tissue responses based on this formalism either with observed responses or with those based on other models,[3,4] as has been done by Niemierko. In general, the value of EUD is between the mean and minimum dose for tumors and between mean and maximum dose for normal tissues. Figure 1(b) shows the EUD as a function of parameter $a$ for a sample DVH shown in Figure 1(a). In this work, we have made no attempt to determine the values of parameter $a$, but used it as a variable whose values for various tumors and organs were chosen and

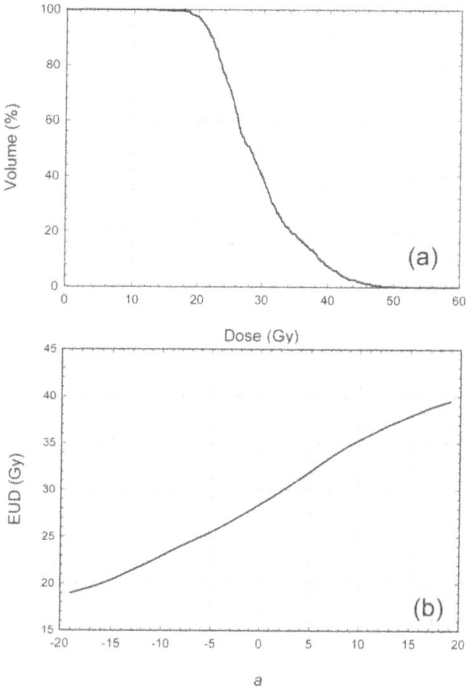


**Figure 1**: (a) Sample dose volume histogram. (b) EUD as a function of parameter *a*.

adjusted by trial and error. However, two important advantages of this formalism are that it has a biological bases and that it lends itself to an easy formation of an objective function suitable for optimization. In the work presented here, we used the objective function

$$F = \prod f_i \, , \qquad (2)$$

where the components $f_i$ may be either

$$f_T = \frac{1}{1 + \left( \frac{EUD_0}{EUD} \right)^n} \qquad (3)$$

for tumors, or

$$f_{OAR} = \frac{1}{1 + \left( \frac{EUD}{EUD_0} \right)^n} \qquad (4)$$

for normal tissues (organs at risk).

For target volumes, $EUD_0$ is the desired dose parameter, and for normal structures, it is the dose limit parameter. Parameter $n$ is like a weight/penalty function which indicates the importance of the structure. Contrary to the quadratic dose difference form typically employed in dose- and dose-volume-based criteria, where the goal of optimization is to minimize the objective function, in the work presented here, the goal is to maximize the objective function. A gradient method (steepest descent) is used for the optimization.

## Results and discussion

Figures 2(a) and (b) show objective function components for tumors and normal tissues respectively as a function of EUD for different penalty values. A value of 50 Gy for $EUD_0$ was

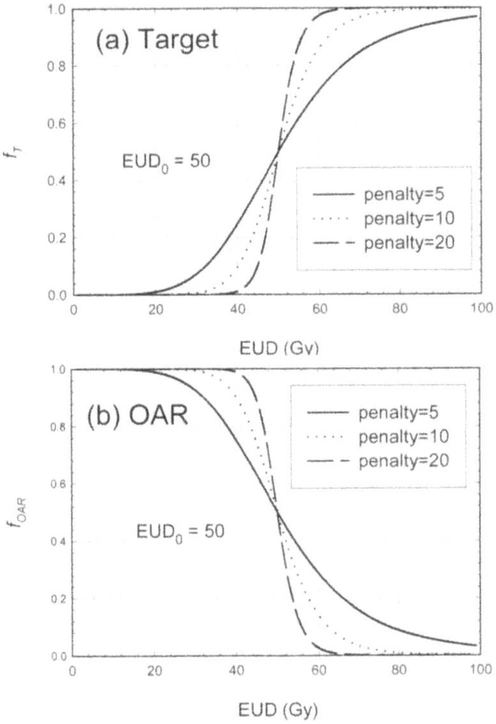


**Figure 2**: Objective function component for target (a) and organ at risk (b) with various penalties.

used. It is evident that for higher penalties, the rise (or drop) in the value of the objective function component is steeper.

Figures 3(a)-(c) compare dose distributions for IMRT plans optimized using dose-volume-based and EUD-based objective functions for a head and neck case with the same nine coplanar beams placed at equi-spaced gantry angles. The corresponding dose-volume histograms are shown in Figure 4. A significant reduction in normal tissue dose for a higher dose to the target and for about the same dose to the nodes results from the use of EUD-based objective function. Parameters used in the optimization are listed in Table 1.

| | Target | Target* | Brainstem | Cord | Parotid | Larynx |
|---|---|---|---|---|---|---|
| *a* | -8.0 | 4.6 | 4.6 | 7.4 | 5.0 | 7.4 |
| $EUD_0$ | 71 | 80 | 49 | 43 | 30 | 45 |
| *n* | 10 | 6 | 6 | 5 | 5 | 5 |

**Table 1:** EUD-based optimization parameters for target and selected critical structures. Target* denotes that it is treated as normal tissue. *a* and *n* are unitless and $EUD_0$ are in units of gray.

We should point out that the initial use of the EUD-based objective function with no constraint on high dose in the target volume resulted in a target dose distributions with a high degree of inhomogeneity. This is expected from the functional form of the EUD vs. dose inhomogeneity curve (i.e., vs. excess dose to a part of the target volume) which saturates rapidly. While the excess dose to the target may be considered beneficial to some clinical sites, it is generally not acceptable. There are several ways of overcoming target dose inhomogeneity. The method we used involved representing the target volume both as a target (with $EUD_0$ value of prescription dose) as well as a normal tissue (with a higher $EUD_0$ value as normal tissue constraint). This resulted in a significant reduction in target dose inhomogeneity, but at the expense of some increase in dose to normal structures (see Figure 3 (c)). Figure 5 compares DVHs for EUD-based plans with and without the assumption of the target. The EUD values[1] for the plans shown in Figure 3 were 70.5 Gy for the dose-volume-based plan, 72.6 Gy for the EUD-based plan with target dose inhomogeneity constraint, and 75.0 Gy for the EUD-based plan with no target dose inhomogeneity.

A possible reason that EUD-based optimization leads to greater normal tissue sparing may be the following: In dose- or dose-volume based optimization, it is typical to require the target

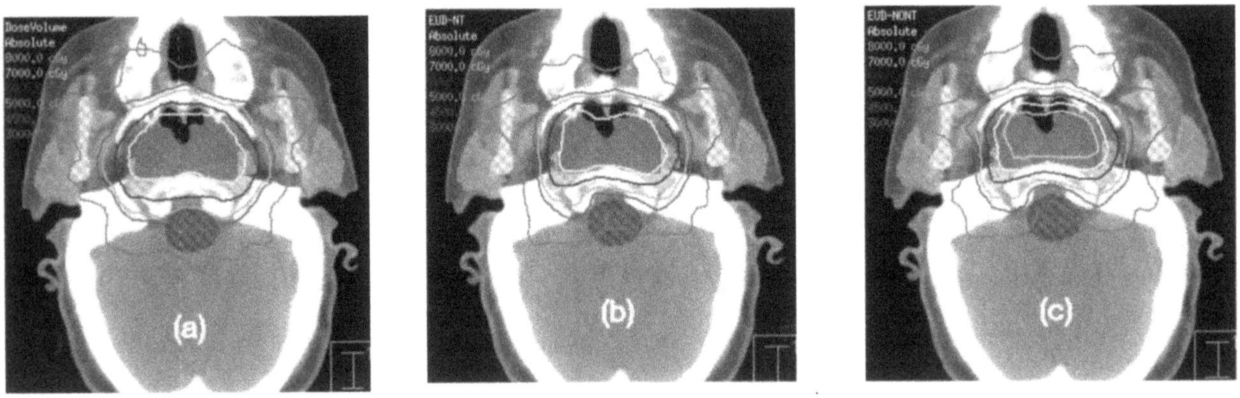


**Figure 3**: Dose distributions in an image section through the tumor for different optimization. (a) dose volume based objectives, (b) EUD-based objectives with dose homogeneity constraint, (c) EUD-based objectives without dose homogeneity constraint

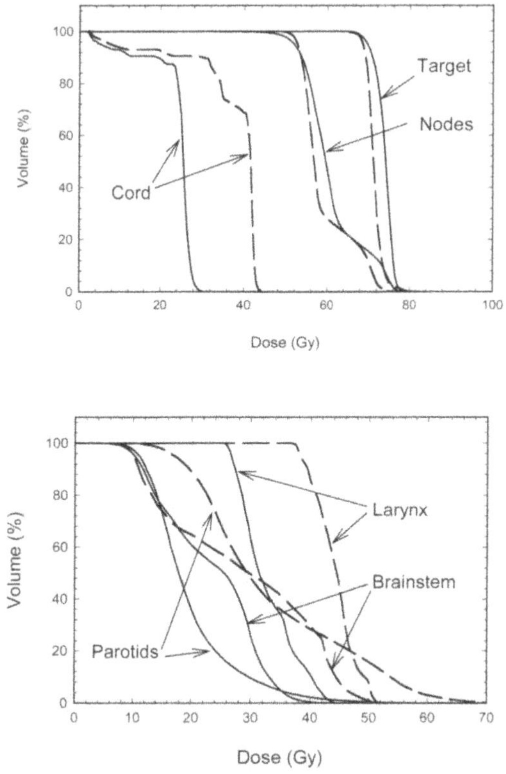


**Figure 4**: Dose volume histograms for target volume, electively treated nodes, and various critical structures. Solid lines are for EUD based optimization and dashed lines are for dose volume based optimizations

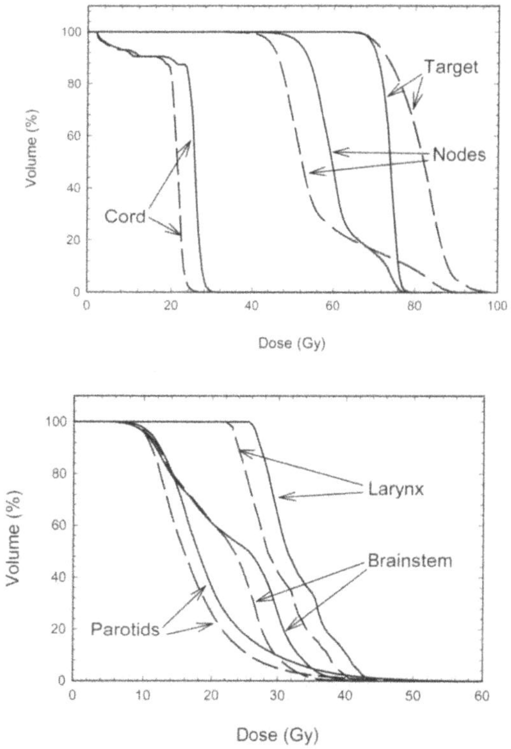


**Figure 5**: Dose volume histograms various structures. Solid and dashed lines are for EUD based optimization with and without target homogeneity constraints respectively

dose to be within a specified range of dose values. Points are penalized only when the dose value is outside this range. Similarly for an OAR, if the dose value is within the tolerance limit, no penalty is assessed. Therefore the optimization will not try to improve the plan once the specified criteria have been met. In contrast, EUD-based optimization will continue to improve the plan even beyond the required limits.

## Summary and conclusions

In addition to the head and neck case presented, we also applied the methods presented to a prostate case with similar results. In general, we found that EUD-based optimization provides improved sparing of normal tissues for the same or higher target dose, indicating that it is more robust, flexible, and clinically relevant. At this point, our results are too limited to draw any definitive conclusions regarding the value of EUD-based objective functions. However, results are consistent with previous studies using biology-based objective functions which indicated that such objective functions have the potential for improving treatment plans.

We should point out that there is considerable ongoing debate about the proper choice of objective functions. Some believe that specifying optimization criteria in terms of dose or dose-volume limits is adequate, while others stress that it is important to include dose-response criteria. Those who favor the former argue that the current dose-response data are sparse and unreliable, and that the models for computing dose-response indices and combining them into an objective function are simplistic and may not represent reality. Others have argued that the incorporation of even the limited information available, if used judiciously, is likely to lead to improved treatment plans. The controversy points to a clear need for further investigation.

By using a gradient technique, we have implicitly assumed that there are no multiple optima in the objective function. It is likely that they do exist in the type of objective function presented here. Our preliminary tests did not reveal any evidence of the optimization process getting trapped in a local optimum. This issue needs further examination.

## References

[1] A. Niemierko, "Reporting and analyzing dose distributions: A concept of equivalent uniform dose," Medical Physics **24** (1), 103-110 (1997).
[2] A. Niemierko, "A generalized concept of Equivalent Uniform Dose (EUD) (Abstract)," Medical Physics **26** (6), 1100 (1999).
[3] C. Burman *et al.*, "Fitting of Normal Tissue Tolerance Data to an Analytic Function," International Journal of Radiation Oncology, Biology and Physics **21** (123-135) (1991).
[4] B. Emami *et al.*, "Tolerance of Normal Tissue to Therapeutic Radiation," International Journal of Radiation Oncology, Biology and Physics **21**, 109-122 (1991).

# Investigation of ROC analysis for inverse treatment planning evaluation

**Catherine Dejean[1], Dimitri Lefkopoulos, Kalliopi Platoni, Pascal Grandjean, Laure Vieillevigne and Katia Kéraudy**

[1]Medical Physics Unit, Radiation Oncology Department, TENON Hospital, 4 rue de la Chine, 75 020 PARIS, France
email: catherine.dejean@tnn.ap-hop-paris.fr

## Introduction

We have experienced the inverse planning system in stereotactic irradiation using the singular value decomposition SVD [1, 2]. These last years, we have implemented this inverse planning module for IMRT, starting by an experimental environment [3] and then a clinical one.
Our objective function was the least square difference between the reconstructed and the prescribed dose distribution. Dose volume histograms were used for visual evaluation of the different reconstructed dose distribution.
We propose to examine a dose-volume histogram based evaluation methodology, the Receiver Operating Characteristics (ROC) analysis, already investigated by our group in stereotactic irradiations [4]. The ROC analysis treats very efficiently the conformity of dose distribution relatively to the target volume and can propose the most conformal prescription isodose.
We are going to use ROC analysis on inverse planning to evaluate quantitatively the proposed solution and to determine a prescription isodose (PI) that provides a good conformity, e.g. best matching of lesion surface with dose distribution.

## Material and methods

### Singular value decomposition and generalised matrix inverses

The inverse planning algorithm is based on the mathematical analysis of SVD. The SVD optimiser gives a number of solutions equal to the number of elementary beams and the goal was to determine the ideal solution that produces the best approximation to the prescribed dose distribution. In this study, we will consider physical solutions, i.e. negative values are forced to zero. More detailed information can be found in [3].

The intensity modulated profiles are given by:

$$W(r) = \left( \sum_{n=1}^{L} \frac{1}{\sigma_n^2} v_n v_n^T \right) M^T D,$$

where $\sigma$ is the singular value, v the singular vector, W weighting vector, M dose kernel matrix.
The singular value decomposition truncation (SVDT) is obtained by retaining only the r first singular components giving thus a solution W(r) of the order r. The reconstructed dose matrix is RDM(r)=MW(r).

### Choice of the best dose distribution

The objective function that serves as a measure of the goodness of the solution is calculated by summing the least square difference between the reconstructed dose matrix (RDM) of the order r and the prescribed dose matrix (PDM) [5]. The minimisation of the objective function gives the optimal RDM of the order r. It is calculated for each pixel of the dose matrix.

$$FCF(r) = \left\{ \frac{\sum_{i=1}^{NPIX} (RDM_i(r) - PDM_i)^2}{NPIX} \right\}^{1/2}$$

where NPIX is the number of pixel of the dose matrix.
The previous objective function FCF (full cost function) does not provide information about conformity of the dose distribution.

### Roc analysis

The ROC analysis defines the ROC space using the underdosed lesion factor (ULF) and the overdosed healthy tissues factor (OHTF) and thus creating a ROC curve. More details on the application of ROC analysis in conformal irradiations can be found in [4].
ULF is equal to

$$ULF = \frac{\text{volume of lesion receiving isodoses} < PI}{\text{lesion volume}}$$

OHTF to

$$OHTF = \frac{\text{volume of healthy tissues receiving isodoses} \geq PI}{\text{lesion volume}}$$

The geometric conformity factor (g) [2] is the sum of these two indices: g=ULF+OHTF.

The Youden index J is an important parameter of the ROC analysis describing the dose distribution conformity and is defined as J=1-(ULF+OHTF). Hence, the J index is the complement to one of the geometric conformity index g. The index g is the physical representation of the 3D matching of the lesion surface to an isosurface.

Another interesting point of ROC analysis is its ability to define the most conformal isodose for a given RDM(r). It appears that the PI could be situated at any point on the ROC curve. It is also obvious that some points on the ROC curve are preferable. Three techniques have been proposed for the radiosurgery [4], we consider the technique based on the maximisation of the Youden index. The prescription isodose proposed will provide a good geometric conformity. Actually, maximising Youden Index is equivalent to minimising the geometric conformity index g.

## Results

To assess the utility of ROC analysis for inverse planning in IMRT, we have used a simplified irradiation configuration (2D dose distribution and 1D beam profile). We have used parallel beam geometry and we take into account only primary dose.
The prescribed dose matrix (PDM) is defined in a single tomographic plane where the external contour of the patient is supposed to be elliptical (major axis: 40cm; minor one: 30 cm). Sixteen beams evenly spaced in $[0;2\pi]$ were used. Each beam size is 20 cm, divided into elementary beams of 1 cm (that is to say 320 elementary beams).
We used Brahme dose prescription [6] where the dose prescribed is 1 in the tumour (T), 0,15 in the organs at risk (OAR) and 0,3 in the healthy tissues (HT), as shown in figure 1.

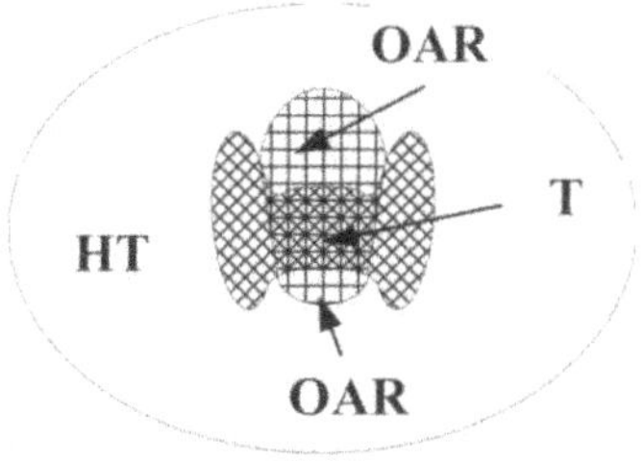


**Figure 1**: Brahme dose prescription

**The SVD dose distribution reconstruction**
The figure 2 shows the objective function as a function of the RDM order r. The optimal RDM order that minimises the objective function is equal to 180.

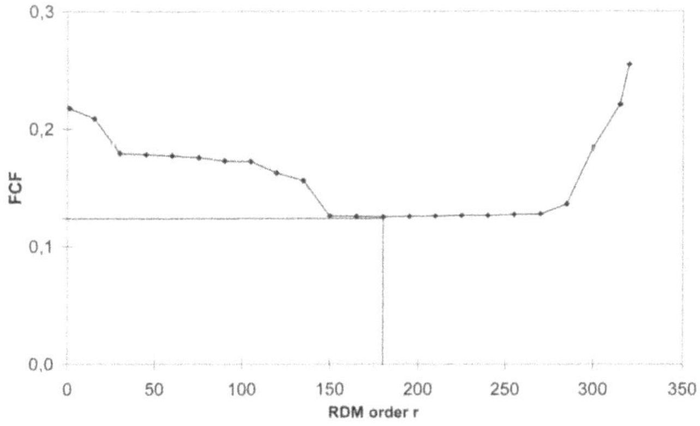


**Figure 2**: FCF for different RDM order r

The FCF curve can be divided into three parts:

- in the first part, we observe an improvement of the reconstruction precision expressed by the decrease of the FCF value until r=150,
- the second part represents a plateau where RDM of similar quality can be found,
- in the third part, the reconstruction precision is deteriorating because the FCF value increases : this is due to the very oscillatory singular components of this studied configuration.

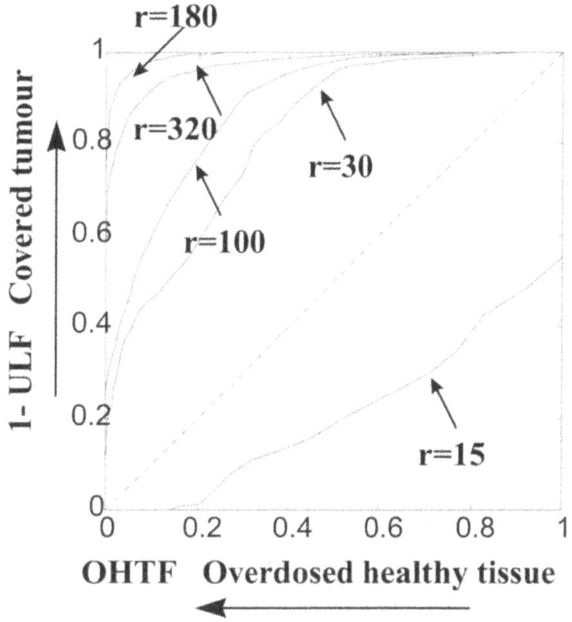


**Figure 3 :** Roc curves for different RDM order r

**The ROC analysis**
In the figure 3, we present the ROC curves into the ROC space for different RDM orders.

The shape of the ROC curve can describe the performance of the treatment plan quality. As the tumour coverage (1-ULF) and the healthy tissue protection (1-OHTF) improve, the ROC plot shifts upward and toward the left and thus the area under the plot increases. Therefore, the ROC curve can be considered as a tool to evaluate a treatment plan.
The different ROC curves presented in the above figure show that the optimal plan corresponds to the order r=180.

Applying now the prescription isodose research technique based on the Youden index maximisation, we present our results in figure 4. The interest of the J index curves as function of the prescription isodose is that we can simultaneously provide the most conformal RDM(r) and the corresponding PI. The J index curve corresponding to the five different order r clearly shows the optimal RDM order r=180 with the prescription isodose equal to 60%.
For the optimal order r=180, we have a good geometric conformity as J=0,91 but we have to evaluate the compromise between the underdosed lesion and the overdosed healthy tissue : ULF=0,04 and OHTF=0,05. It means that only 4% of the lesion volume is underdosed and 5% of the healthy tissue overdosed.
In figure 5, we present the maximum value of J index for different RDM orders and the corresponding prescription isodose. Although, numerically the optimum corresponds to the order r=180, we can notice that the maximum value is situated on a plateau and the corresponding prescription isodoses are very similar. We find that the optimal RDM range defined by the global FCF objective function is similar to the one defined by the conformity Youden index. This means that for the studied configuration a good global quality reconstruction (FCF) is accompanied by good isodoses conformity.

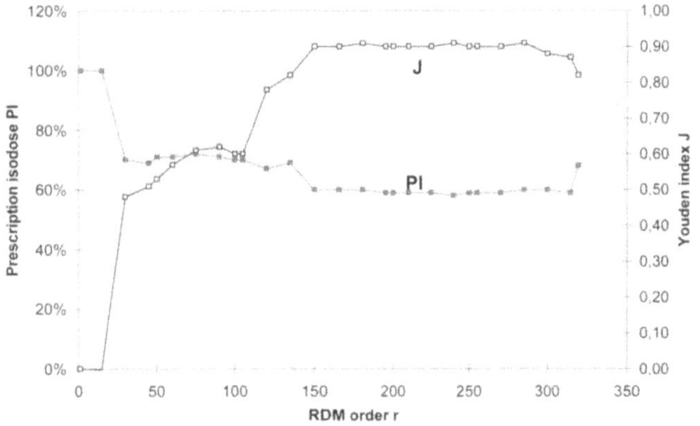


**Figure 5**: Maximum value of Youden index and corresponding prescription isodose for different RDM order r

## Discussion - conclusion

The study has shown an accordance between the least square difference between the reconstructed and the prescribed dose distribution and the geometrical conformity between the tumour surface and the isodose prescription surface. The ROC analysis can be complementarily used with a global FCF objective function to maximise the conformity of a plan and to define the corresponding prescription isodose.
The interest of the Youden index is that it can simultaneously attend these two previous goals. However, the acceptable RDM(r) proposed solution must correspond to a PI located in a clinically acceptable predefined range.
In the future, we can use SVD analysis to find an optimal mathematical solution and then ROC analysis to find the most conformal treatment plan taking into account clinical considerations and the compromise between underdosed lesion and overdosed healthy tissue.

Taking also into account clinical constraints, a compromise can be done between the maximum value of Youden index and the corresponding PI. A slight deterioration of the maximum J value (i.e. corresponding to the choice of a sub-optimal RDM order) could lead to a PI in the clinical range.
These preliminary results encourage us to continue these investigations into a clinical context (3D dose matrix, 2D beam profile), an improved dose model and different types of tumour.

## References


[1] Lefkopoulos D., Grandjean P., Laouar A., Schlienger M. 1995 Study of the ill-conditionning of a radiosurgical irradiation space using the singular value decomposition *Int J Imaging Sys Technol* **6** 104-13

[2] Grandjean P., Platoni K., Lefkopoulos D., Merienne L, Schlienger M. 1998 Use of a general inverse technique for the conformationnal stereotactic treatment of complex intracranial lesions *Int J Radiat Oncol Biol Phys* **41** 69-76

[3] Vieillevigne L., Lefkopoulos D., Grandjean P., Touboul E., Housset M. 1999 Intensity modulation optimisation by inverse planning into the SVD decomposition space: a preliminary study *Physica Medica* **XV** 11-19

[4] Platoni K., Lefkopoulos D., Grandjean P., Schlienger M. 1999 Study of the conformity degree of treatment plans using the Receiver Operating Characteristics Analysis *Journal of Radiosurgery* **2** 95-105

[5] Webb S. 1989 Optimisation of conformal Radiotherapy dose distribution by simulated annealing *P M B* **34** 1349-70

[6] Brahme A., Roose J., Lax I. 1982 Solution of an integral equation encountered in radiation therapy *Med Phys* **27** 1221-29


This work was partly supported by a grant of "Association de Recherche contre le Cancer".

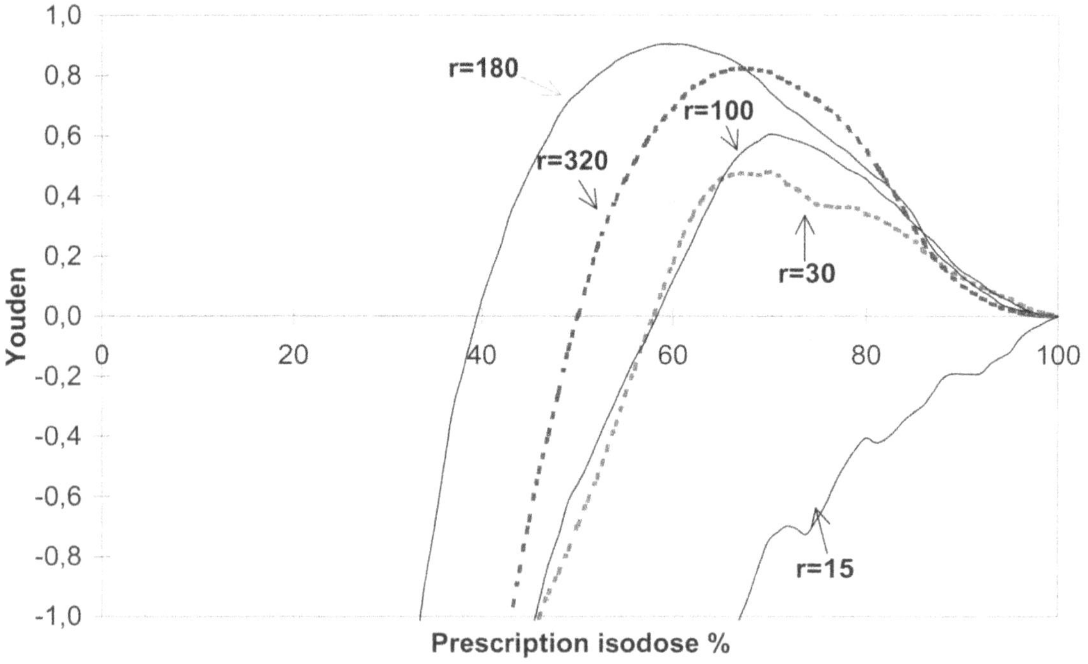


**Figure 4**: Youden index as function of prescription isodose for different RDM order r

# The use of the Maximum Likelihood Estimator and the Dynamically Penalized Likelihood methods in inverse radiation therapy planning

**Jorge Llacer[1], Timothy D. Solberg[2], Claus Promberger[3] and Alexander Kuzmany[3]**

[1]EC Engineering Consultants LLC, Los Gatos, CA, USA , [2]Dept. of Radiation Oncology, University of California, Los Angeles, CA, USA and [3]BrainLAB AG, Heimstetten, Germany

## Introduction

In November 1997, the first author of this paper published a description of the Dynamically Penalized Likelihood (DPL) method of inverse therapy planning[1]. It responded to the evident need at that time to treat voxels corresponding to Organs at Risk (OAR) in a manner different from those of the Planning Target Volume (PTV) by specifying for the former a desired maximum dose, for example, but otherwise allowing those voxels complete freedom to receive any dose lower than that maximum. Since that time, that need has been recognized by other workers, with perhaps the most used algorithm that incorporates that thinking being that of Spirou and Chui[2]. Since 1997 the DPL has evolved considerably and we feel that it is now nearly ready to be used in therapy in conjunction with a commercial therapy planning software package. This paper will describe the present form of the DPL, give a brief description of its theoretical foundation and describe its use together with the Maximum Likelihood Estimator (MLE) in order to achieve a useful degree of controllability. Two examples (a relatively "easy" and a "difficult" one) and the corresponding results will be given to facilitate the description of the algorithm.

## Algorithm foundation

### The DPL algorithm

The current DPL target iterative formula, excluding filtering terms, has the following form:

$$a_j^{(k+1)} = a_j^{(k)} \frac{1}{q_j} \left\{ \sum_{i \in D} F_{ij} \frac{d_i}{h_i^{(k)}} + \sum_{\substack{i \in S \\ (h_i^{(k)} - s_i) > 0}} F_{ij} \frac{s_i}{h_i^{(k)}} \right\} \qquad (1)$$

where

$$h_i^{(k)} = \sum_j F_{ij} a_j \qquad (2)$$

and

$$q_j = \sum_{i \in D} F_{ij} + \sum_{\substack{i \in S \\ (h_i - s_i) > 0}} F_{ij} \,. \qquad (3)$$

A beam weight $a_j$ at iteration $(k+1)$ is obtained from its value at iteration $(k)$ by multiplication by a normalized correction term, between the brackets of Eq.(1). This correction term consists of two summations, the first one over the voxels in the PTV's $(i \in D)$ and the second one over the voxels in the OAR's $(i \in S)$, but only for those voxels that receive a dose $h_i$ at iteration $(k)$ which is larger than the desired dose $s_i$. The desired dose in the PTV is given by $d_i$. The matrix elements $F_{ij}$ correspond to the dose delivered to voxel $i$ by beam $j$. One recognizes the form of Eqs. (1) through (3) as belonging to a MLE iterative step, but with the number of terms in the second summation changing dynamically as required to satisfy a desired dose distribution in the OAR's, within the limits of what the Physics of the problem can allow. The target function of the algorithm is, in effect, an adaptive function.

It was demonstrated in a paper by Llacer, Veklerov and Nunez[3] that a MLE solution is equivalent to a series of iterations in which the results of an iteration fulfill the role of prior information for the next iteration, in a statistical Bayesian sense. If we would take the results at iteration ($k$) and use Eqs. (1), (2) and (3) to calculate the optimization at iteration ($k$ + 1) and would then permanently fix the number of terms in the second summation of Eq. (1), the calculation of ($k$ + 2), ($k$ + 3), etc would proceed as a totally normal MLE estimation which leads to a single maximum[4]. Instead, we do not fix the number of terms in the second summation and we take the results of iteration ($k$ + 1) as prior information to calculate the results of iteration ($k$ + 2), etc with a variable number of terms.

The above discussion can be summarized by saying that the algorithm "thinks" that it is doing a bona fide MLE iteration at each one of the iterations, although the number of terms in the OAR summation can be different from iteration to iteration. The process has to lead to a stable single maximum and it appears to do so.

### The low rms surface

As will be discussed further in the first example below, optimizations with the DPL for an "easy" class of problems (those in which there is enough separation between the PTV and OAR voxels) lie in a rather flat surface in parameter space, the space of a dimension equal to the number of beam weights of a problem. That surface can be called a "low rms surface" because it has as its maximum the Maximum Likelihood point for an optimization of the PTV voxels only, i.e., using only the first summation of Eq. (1). In the context of the inverse therapy problem, Maximum Likelihood implies minimum square error between desired and delivered doses in the PTV.

When the problem is a "difficult" one (with OAR voxels adjacent or overlapping with the PTV), the DPL solutions may lie substantially below that low rms surface, depending on the values prescribed by the Therapist as desirable for the OAR's. As a result of those OAR doses, the resulting dose distributions in the PTV's may not be acceptable due, principally, to underdosing of PTV voxels. When that happens, a number of MLE iterations on the PTV only, starting from the DPL results, will bring the solution towards the low rms surface. The process can be stopped when the PTV dose distribution reaches acceptable characteristics.

What emerges is, then, a DPL method by which a therapist may define desired dose distributions for the OAR's, in the form of Dose Volume Histograms (DVH's), for example, inspect the resulting distributions in the PTV and backtrack, if necessary, to a satisfactory solution in the PTV. The MLE "knows" precisely which voxels in the OAR's have to be allowed to receive a higher dose than the original DPL results in order to achieve the satisfactory solution. Of course, the complete process can be done automatically, if desired.

## Results and discussion

### A relatively "easy" Problem 1

Figure 1 shows a pituitary adenoma, the PTV, close to but mostly not touching the brain stem, which is one of the OAR's. The two optical nerves were defined as two additional OAR's. Six ports were prescribed for the plan, with a total of 206 individual beams.

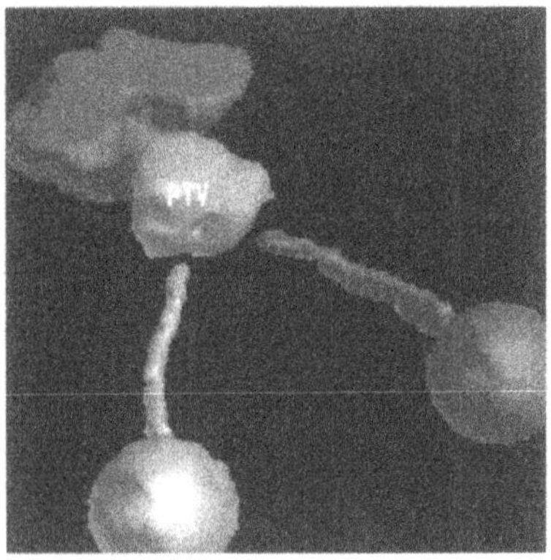


**Figure 1:** PTV and OAR's of Problem 1 (curtesy of Charité, Berlin).

Figure 2 shows the DVH's obtained by using the simple MLE iterative process on the PTV, with complete disregard to the OAR's. This sets an upper limit on the quality of the DVH that can be obtained for the PTV when a full optimization is carried out. It also gives an indication to the therapist about how low the desired OAR doses may be set. Based on the knowledge that there is little contact between the PTV and the OAR's, low dose DVH's for the OAR's were prescribed by indicating 4 points in the desired DVH curves, as described in Table 1.

| OAR | Max dose | Point 1 Dose | Point 1 Fraction | Point 2 Dose | Point 2 Fraction |
|---|---|---|---|---|---|
| Brain Stem | 30 | 15 | 0.1 | 10 | 0.2 |
| Optical Nerves | 20 | 15 | 0.2 | 10 | 0.3 |

**Table 1:** OAR DVH specifications for Problem 1. A fourth point at Dose = 0 and Fraction = 1.0 was automatically included.

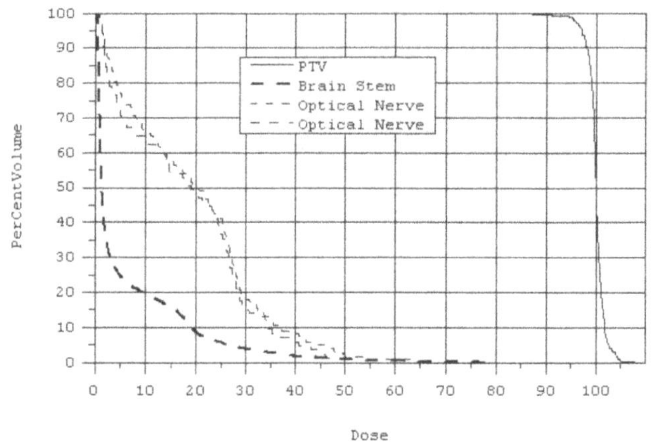


**Figure 2:** DVH's for Problem 1 after optimizing PTV only, i.e., disregarding the OAR's.

The resulting DVH's after the DPL steps are shown in Fig. 3. The procedure was stopped at a point where the average dose in the OAR's did not change by more than 1 part in $10^4$.

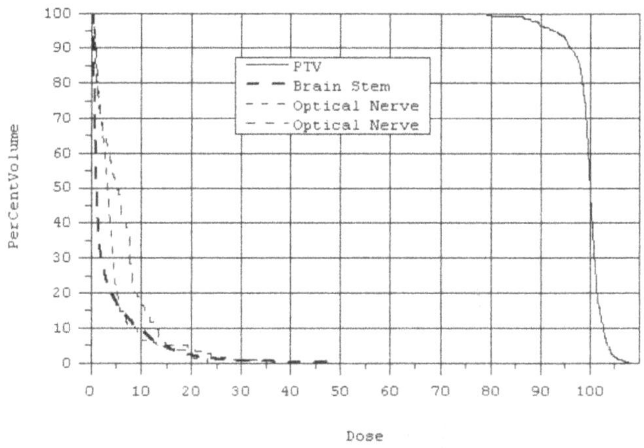


**Figure 3:** DVH's after DPL optimization.

We now illustrate the case in which the Therapist decides that the 7.4% of PTV voxels receiving less than a dose of 95 units shown by Fig. 3 is not acceptable, but a 5% volume would be. MLE iterations on the PTV only, starting from the DPL results and stopping as soon as the desired condition is satisfied yield the results of Fig. 4.

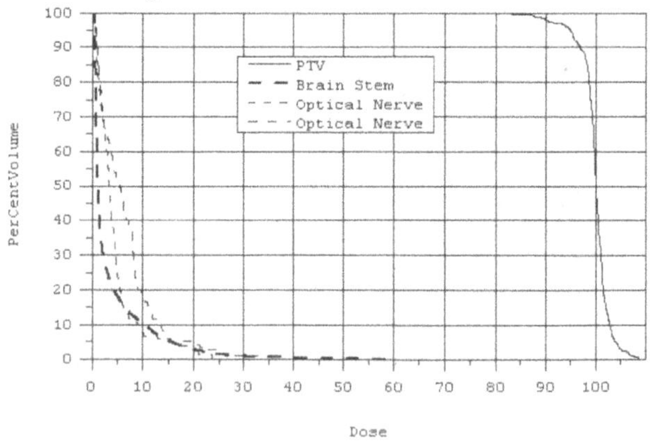


**Figure 4:** DVH's after further MLE processing.

There has been practically no change in most of the OAR characteristics, but a few voxels in the Brain Stem have increased their dose up to a maximum of approximately 58 units, from a value of approximately 47 before the final MLE steps. The results of Fig. 4 were obtained with 33 iterations of the MLE. Once this final iterative process reaches the low rms surface, which would have happened if the therapist would have specified an acceptable fraction of 3 to 4% at a dose of 95 units for the PTV, the backtracking process slows down considerably. To move from the results of Fig. 4 to those of Fig. 2, for example, may take thousands of iterations, indicating that the partial derivatives of the PTV portion of the target function with respect to the beam weights are very small, i.e., the surface in parameter space is very flat. It is then clear that, if the DPL solution lies already in the flat low rms surface, it may take a very large number of iterations to reach a particular desired PTV point. That would occur in very easy problems, in which the posterior MLE iterations would be unnecessary, anyway.

**A "difficult" Problem 2**

Problem 2 consists of a meningioma extending in two directions anteriorally and laterally from the spinal cord at the level of the cervical spine. Figure 5 shows a CT plane with the outlines of the two PTV's and the cord. Two isocenters, each with 5 beam ports, were used for the plan, for a total of 1207 individuals beams. The spinal cord was divided into two sections along the patient axis, for study purposes.

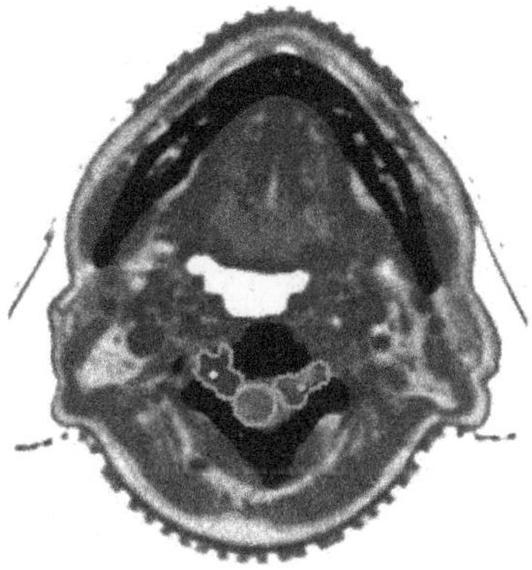

**Figure 5:** PTV's and OAR for Problem 2 (curtesy of Charité, Berlin)

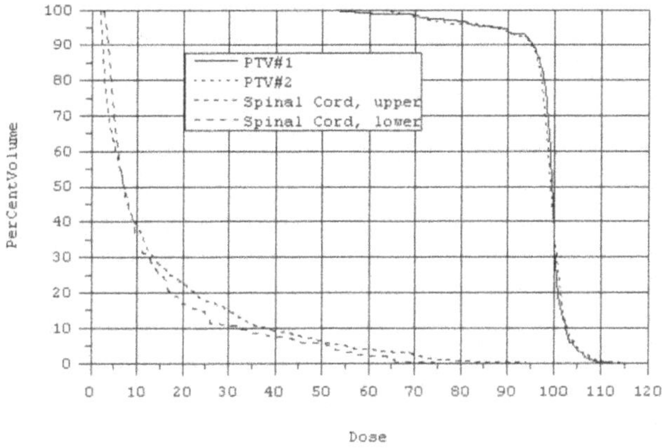


Figure 6: DVH's resulting after DPL optimization of Problem 2

Figure 6 shows the DVH's resulting after a DPL optimization with desired OAR doses that resulted in unacceptable PTV characteristics. Figure 7 shows the final DVH's when a condition that less than 1% of the PTV voxels were to receive less than 90 units of dose was placed on the final MLE iterations.

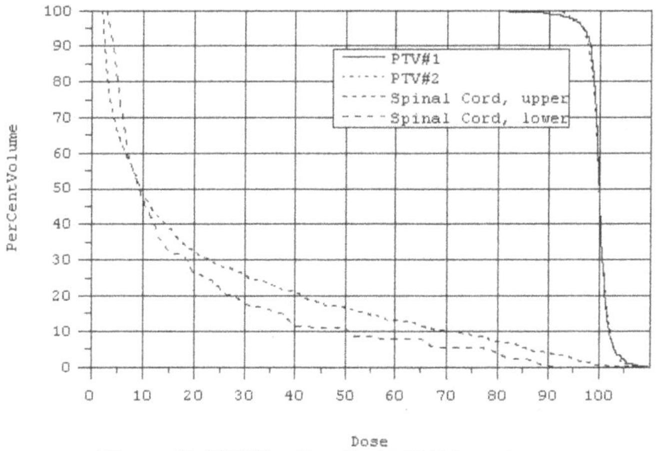


**Figure 7:** DVH's after final MLE iterations

As expected from the nature of the problem, it was not possible to retain a low maximum dose to the OAR's without damaging the distribution in the PTV. The final solution took 128 iterations of the MLE on the PTV only, with the speed of convergence slowing down substantially, indicating that the final solution is now close to the low rms surface.

## Conclusion and acknowledgments

This paper describes briefly a method of optimization based on the very stable Maximum Likelihood Estimator that has the power to deliver dose distributions whose characteristics can represent a tradeoff between the quality of the PTV and OAR dose distributions. The tradeoff is largely controllable by the Therapist, even in difficult optimization problems. At the time of this writing, the DPL-MLE package is being incorporated into the BrainScan software package of BrainLAB AG. We are showing in this paper the preliminary results of that effort. It can be expected that more sophisticated examples and more complete results will become available within the next few months.

The use of the MLE and DPL methods in inverse radiation therapy planning is covered by US Patent No. 5,602,892.

---

[1] Llacer J 1997 Inverse radiation treatment planning using the Dynamically Penalized Likelihood method, Med. Phys. **24,** (11), 1751-1764

[2] Spirou S V and Chui C S 1998 A gradient inverse planning algorithm with dose-volume constraints, Med. Phys. **25**, (3), 321-333

[3] Llacer J, Veklerov E and Nunez J 1989 Statistically based image reconstruction for emission tomography, Int. Journal of Imaging Syst. and Techology **1**, 132-148

[4] Shepp LA and Vardi Y 1982, Maximum likelihood reconstruction for emission tomography, IEEE Trans. Med. Imaging **MI-1** 113-121

# A multicriteria optimization approach for inverse radiotherapy planning

**Karl-Heinz Küfer[1], Horst W. Hamacher[1] and Thomas Bortfeld[2]**

[1]University of Kaiserslautern, Dept. of Mathematics, and ITWM, Dept. Optimization, Kaiserslautern, Germany; e-mail: hamacher, kuefer@mathematik.uni-kl.de; [2]DKFZ, Dept. of Medical Physics, Heidelberg, Germany; e-mail: t.bortfeld@dkfz-heidelberg.de

## Introduction

Today the inverse problem of radiotherapy planning is generally considered as an optimization problem, while some early approaches also looked at it as a feasibility search problem [1]. A variety of different objective functions $F$ have been defined for optimization of treatment plans. All of them evaluate the quality of a treatment plan and assign a quality index to it. This means that each treatment plan is characterized by a single number. Optimization procedures have been developed to minimize or maximize the cost or objective function, $F$.

This concept has led to some success in the past, especially when applied to intensity modulated radiotherapy (IMRT). Nevertheless, there are at least two major drawbacks of this approach:

1. It is often hard to balance overdoses in different critical structures against each other, let alone the sparing of critical structures against underdosing parts of the target volume.
2. There is little or no dynamics in the planning process. Instead of looking at two or more alternative plans one would like to see the tradeoff between over and underdosage.

One way to tackle the first point has been to break up the objective function into organ-specific functions $F_k$ and to define weight factors $w_k$ for each $F_k$,

(1) $$F = w_1F_1 + w_2F_2 + \ldots + w_KF_K,$$

where $F_1$ may stand for the objective in the target and $F_2$ to $F_K$ for the objectives in critical structures. Biological objective functions, in which $F$ is obtained as a product rather than the sum of the $F_k$, can be handled in a similar way.

Unfortunately, the determination of the weights $w_k$ is a time consuming trial and error process. Class solutions can be very useful here, but only for standard cases. The planning effort can be reduced by considering clinically relevant constraints such as dose-volume constraints [2,3,4,5]. Nevertheless, the principle problems remain: even with inverse planning one often has to compute several alternatives before an acceptable plan has been found, and that one gets only a more or less static answer to the planning problem (point 2).

To overcome these problems we propose to model the radiotherapy planning problem as a *multicriteria problem* with conflicting objectives. That is, we suggest to make the step from the conventional optimization approach (where each plan is characterized by a single real value defined by (1)) to a model where each plan is valued by a vector $(F_1, \ldots, F_K)$. We will show that it is possible and practical to find a *representative set* of so-called *efficient* (or *pareto) solutions* of the multicriteria problem. Once this set has been determined, the planner can search it interactively and find the most suitable treatment plan for the individual case. We will prove the general principle by applying the methods to a complex 2D example case using linear objectives $F_k$.

## Material and methods

Most of the approaches in inverse radiotherapy planning try to find a therapy plan whose dose distribution approximately meets some ideal physical dose bounds that guarantee a high probability of tumor control and a low probability of complications simultaneously: e.g. the dose in the target volume (indexed with 1) must be greater than some lower bound $L_1$ and the dose level for critical structure $k$ (critical structures are indexed with $2, \ldots, K$) must be smaller than some upper bound $U_k$.

For the sake of simplicity we assume in this paper that we are given a good irradiation geometry, i.e. a number of promising directions of irradiation. How to find such a geometry is the subject of current research, see [11]. Furthermore, we assume that the radiation beams are discretized in $N$ bixels in total and that the organs of interest consist of $M_k$ voxels ($k=1, \ldots, K$). Then, the dose distribution $D_k$ in organ $k$ for a given positive fluence vector $x$ can be described by matrix vector products $D_k = P_k x$, where the entries $p_{i,j}$ of the $M_k x N$- matrix $P_k$ reflect the contribution of bixel $j$ to the dose in bixel $i$ under unit intensity. (In this paper we assume that the matrices $P_k$ are given or can be easily calculated in a meaningful way.) Using this notation the ideal dose constraints can be written in the form

(2) $$P_1x \geq L_1 e, \quad P_kx \leq U_k e, \quad x \geq 0.$$

In general, the linear inequality system (1) will be inconsistent and we have to look for optimal approximations. In order to do this we extend system (1) by vectors $t_k$, $k=1, \ldots K$, measuring the deviations from the ideal dose bounds in (2)

(3) $$P_1x \geq L_1\,(e - t_1), \quad P_kx \leq U_k\,(e + t_k), \quad t_1, \ldots, t_K \geq 0,\ x \geq 0.$$

Here, $e$ is a vector with all entries equal to one. In contrast to (2), inequality system (3) is always feasible.

It is common to define organ-specific convex functions $F_k = F_k(t_k)$ that assign these deviations costs (positive real values) which are to be minimized. Typically, the functions $F_k$ are defined as $p$-norms of $t_k$ i.e. $F_k(t_k) = \|t_k\|_p$ ( [5] or [6] use, for instance, 2-norms and [2] uses maximum norms for all $k=1, \ldots, K$. Notice, that in our general approach nothing but convexity of the functions $F_k$ is required. This allows e.g. the use of different norms for different risks, such that organs of a parallel nature like lung or liver may have small $p$ values while more serial structured organs like esophagus or spinal chord

should have larger ones. For biologically meaningful values of $p$ we refer to [7,8].
In contrast to the well-known method that defines optimal approximations of (2) with the aid of weighted costs of type (1) we reflect the inherent multicriteria structure of inverse radiotherapy planning by a multicriteria optimization model:

(4) $F_1 \rightarrow Min,\ F_2 \rightarrow Min,\ F_K \rightarrow Min$
subject to (3).

A feasible solution $(x,t_1, \dots, t_K)$ of (3) is called an efficient or Pareto optimal solution of the multicriteria optimization problem (4) if there is no feasible solution $(x', t_1', \dots, t_k')$ of (3) that dominates $(x,t_1, \dots, t_K)$, i.e. $F_i(t_i') \leq F_i(t_i)$ for all $i=1, \dots, K$ where strict inequality holds for at least one index $j$ [9]. In other words, a feasible solution of (4) is efficient if it is not possible to improve some of the objectives $F_k$ without worsening some of the others.
The set of efficient solutions of (4) is in general a coherent (and infinite) subset of the topological boundary of the polyhedron of feasible solutions defined by (3) whose specific structure depends on the choice of the functions $F_k$.
For practical purposes it is not meaningful to characterize all efficient solutions but rather to find a good set of representative efficient solutions in which the decision makers, physician and dosimetrist, can search for an optimal treatment plan. Such a set of representative efficient solutions of (4) should have the following properties:

- Clinical relevance of each solution
- Appropriate neighborhood structure indicating pairwise interrelation
- Significant difference between interrelated solutions

One method (among many others) to generate such a set of representative solutions is given by the following two-step procedure:
*Initialization step:* For given positive ratios $r_2, \dots, r_K$ find a solution of the convex optimization problem:

(5) Find an efficient solution of problem (4) that fulfils:

$s \rightarrow Min$
subject to
$F_1(t_1) \leq s$
$F_k(t_k) \leq r_k s, \quad k=2, \dots, K,$

The ratios $r_k$ reflect different preferences of tolerating deviations from the ideal dose bounds (2) for different organs similar to the role of the weights $w_k$ in (1). In contrast to the weighted function (1) the outcome of (5) is however predictable: we will always find a solution that has the minimal relative costs (with regard to the choice of the $r_k$).
The solution of (5) serves as initial efficient solution of the set of representative solutions. Alternatively, if a good solution is known, e.g. from a clinical data base that contains a related case, this solution might be taken as initial solution.
*Recursion step:* Let $q \in (0,1)$ be a process parameter. For each representative solution $(x', t_1', \dots, t_K')$ already found and each index $j=1, \dots, K$ calculate a *j-neighbor* $(x, t_1, \dots, t_K)$ by solving the following convex optimization problem:

(6) Find an efficient solution of problem (4) that fulfils:

$F_j(t_j) \rightarrow Min$
subject to
$F_i(t_i) \leq F_i(t_i') + q/(K-1)\, F_j(t_j')\ ,\ i=1, \dots, K,\ i \neq j$
$F_j(t_j) \geq (1-q) F_j(t_j')$

By definition, $j$-neighbors of representative solutions have a significantly lower cost $F_j$ and have slightly higher costs regarding the other cost functions. The process parameter $q$ is chosen adaptively and will be dependent on actual representatives and $j$ in general. The recursion step is repeated until some stopping criterion (fixed number of iterations, cost or cost reduction lower than a given bound, etc.) is satisfied.
The set of representative solutions calculated by the procedure has the structure of a tree where the initial solution is the root node and the $j$-neighbors are the descendants of each node.
The representative set of efficient solutions of (4) is stored in an appropriate tree structured data base where each node carries the following information: the physical treatment parameters, visualizations of the dose distribution like isodose curves and dose volume histograms and the cost vector.
The final data base can be scanned by the physician and the dosimetrist in order to find a treatment plan that satisfies the individual planning requirements. It is not necessary that the physician evaluates and compares all efficient solutions in this data base. The search process starts with the initial solution i.e. the root of the tree. If the resulting radiation therapy plan is not acceptable, since the physician would like to see the dose constraints to be satisfied more tightly in some organ, say $j$, a corresponding treatment plan is found online in the data base as $j$-neighbor of the actual solution. If the new proposal is not satisfactory, the physician repeats this procedure until a satisfactory solution is found.

## Results and discussion

Observing the linear structure of the basic inequality systems (2) and (3) it is tempting to formulate the radiotherapy planning problem as a linear multicriteria programming problem in total. This is possible using a linear scale of cost functions

(7) $F_k(t_k) := \alpha ||x||_1 + (1-\alpha)\, ||x||_\infty,$

where $\alpha$ may be identical for all $k$ or different from organ to organ, depending on the specific organ's structure. Good values of $\alpha$ can be found by elementary curve fitting methods analogously to Niemierko's calculation of $p$-values in his scale of $p$ norms announced in [8].
It is the major advantage of a completely linear model that there is much known about the structure of the set of efficient solutions and about fast algorithms for calculating them [9].
We proved the potential of our multicriteria approach with a series of some critical clinical 2D examples and tested our algorithms with functions $F_k$ from (7) with $\alpha=1$, i.e. with pure maximum norm.
Here, we illustrate our method with a single 2D example from a cancer treatment department of a German hospital and show how the search in the set of representative solutions works. The example is taken from [10]. As initial solution we use the treatment plan that was used for the patient so far and which was calculated as a solution of an organ-weighted function of type (1). The screen shots show the dose distribution in the relevant organs. Notice, that the coloring of doses is done relatively to the maximal doses in the different organs. For the coloring of dose levels we use two scales shown at the top of the screen shot. The G-scale belongs to the organs at risk, the K-scale to the target. The numbers between the scales give the dose levels relative to the ideal dose. Under the screen shots we provide the $F$-vector of maximum relative deviations from

ideal doses and the $\Delta V$-vector that gives the overdosed (underdosed) relative volumina of the organs in %. The first entry corresponds to the target, the following entries correspond to the right eye and left eye.
*Example:* Nasal cavity tumor, eye balls and optic nerves as critical structures

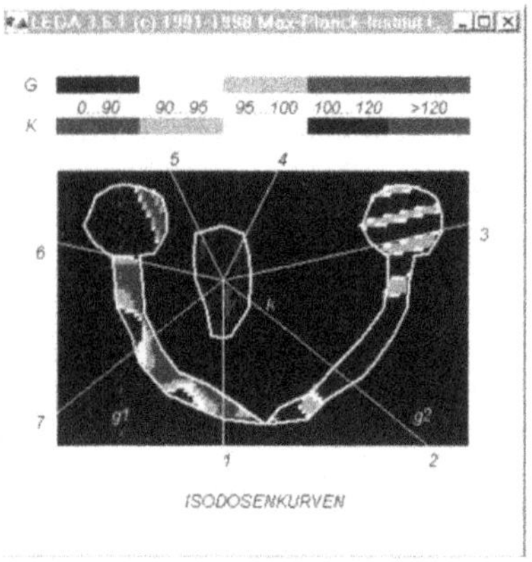


$F$-vector: ( 0 , 10 , 0 ) $\Delta V$-Vector: ( 0 , 46 , 0 )
**Figure 1**:Initial solution with weights: target 0.6, risks 0.2

We observe an initial solution that meets the ideal dose bounds in the target volume and the left eye while the right eye is overdosed by maximal 10% or 1 Gy in 46% of its volume.

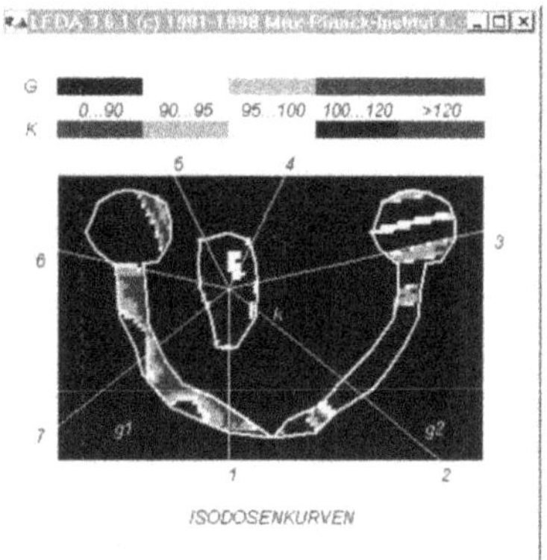


$F$-vector: ( 2, 7.2 , 2 ) $\Delta V$-Vector: ( 10 , 44 , 6 )
**Figure 2**: First search step: right eye neighbor solution, q=0,4

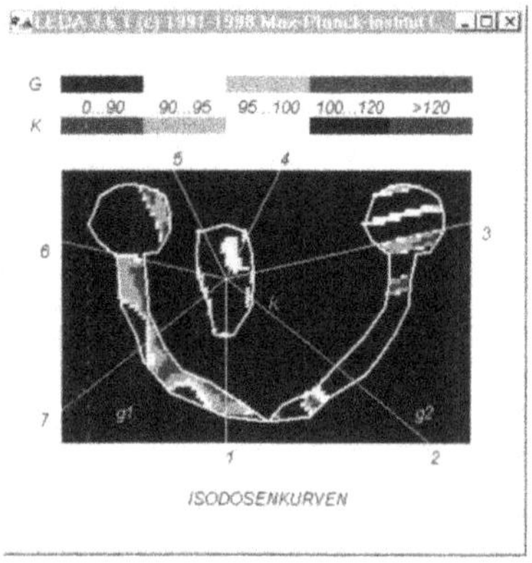


$F$-vector: ( 3.5, 5.3 , 3.5 ) $\Delta V$-Vector: ( 22.3 , 40 , 15 )
**Figure 3**: Second search step: right eye neighbor solution, q=0,4

In each steps the right-eye-neighbor solutions deliver successively better plans with regard to the right eye at the cost of a slight underdose of the target and a slight overdose of the left eye. A third improvement step in the direction of the right eye does not lead to a significant reduction of the maximum dose.

## Conclusion

The optimization problem in radiotherapy is inherently multicriteria. In this work a multicriteria optimization algorithm and search strategy has been developed that is adequate for this type of optimization problem. The merit of this approach as compared to conventional monocriterion optimization is threefold:

- It allows for interactive, computer based inverse planning once the representative set of efficient solutions has been found.
- It gives the planner a feel for the dynamics of the planning problem and its potential and limitations. It is also excellently suited for educational purposes.
- It does not require the introduction of trial-and-error based weight factors or penalties.

The numerical experience shows the potential of the proposed method: within reasonable computation time doctors and dosimetrists are provided a data base of relevant radiotherapy plans that allows a fast search and comparison of different clinically meaningful solutions.

## References

[1] Censor Y, Altschuler M D and Powlis W D 1988 A computational solution of the inverse problem in radiation therapy treatment planning *Appl. Math. Comput.,* **25** 57-87

[2] Langer M, Brown R, Urie M, Leong J, Stracher M and Shapiro J 1990 Large scale optimization of beam weights under dose-volume restrictions *Int. J. Radiat. Oncol. Biol. Phys.* **18** 887-893

[3] Langer M, Brown R, Kijewski P and Ha C 1993 The reliability of optimization under dose-volume limits. *Int. J. Radiat. Oncol. Biol. Phys.* **26** 529-538

[4] Bortfeld T, Stein J, Preiser K 1997 Clinically Relevant Intensity Modulation OptimizationUsing Physical Criteria *Proceedings of the XIIth ICCR, Salt Lake City 1997, D. D. Leavitt and G. Starkschall (eds.)* 1-4

[5] Spirou S V and Chui C S 1998 A gradient inverse planning algorithm with dose-volume constraints *Med. Phys.* **25** 321-333

[6] Bortfeld T, Bürkelbach J, Boesecke R and Schlegel W 1990 Methods of Image Reconstruction from Projections Applied to Conformation Radiotherapy *Phys. Med. Biol.* **35** 1423-1434

[7] Burman C, Kutcher G J, Emami B and Goitein M 1991 Fitting of normal tissue tolerance data to an analytic function. *Int. J. Radiat. Oncol. Biol. Phys.* **21** 123-135

[8] Niemierko A 1999 A Generalized Concept of Equivalent Uniform Dose *Med. Phys.* **26** 1100

[9] Steuer R 1985 Multicriteria Optimization: Theory, Computation and Applications. Wiley, NewYork.

[10] Hamacher, H W, Küfer, K-H 1998 Inverse radiation therapy planning – a multiple objective approach. Technical report 12, ITWM Kaiserslautern.

[11] Hamacher, H W, Küfer, K-H 1999 Finding irradiation directions using location theory models. Forthcoming

# Computer-Assisted Selection of Importance Factors in Inverse Planning

**Q.T. Le, J.G. Li, A. Pugachev, A. L. Boyer, and L. Xing**

Department of Radiation Oncology, Stanford University School of Medicine, Stanford, California 94305-5304, USA

## Introduction

Intensity modulated radiation therapy (IMRT) is being developed into an important radiation therapy modality. However, the clinical IMRT treatment planning process has been found to be labor intensive and time-consuming. This is due in part to the use of many free parameters, that constitute an additional muti-dimensional space coupled to the beam profiles. The formulation of the problem is deficient in that there is no effective feedback mechanism in the optimization process. The goal of this work is to establish a decision-making framework that allows us to adjust automatically the free parameters and to provide an efficient algorithm for the auto-selection of the importance factors in inverse planning.

## Material and methods

For simplicity, we will use a quadratic objective function defined by

$$F = \sum_{n} \gamma_\sigma (D - D_0)^2, \qquad (1)$$

where $\gamma_\sigma$ is the importance factor of a structure $\sigma$, $D_0$ and $D_n$ are prescribed and calculated doses, respectively. The clinical objectives are usually multifaceted and incommensurable. The importance factors are incorporated in the objective function to parameterize tradeoff strategies and to prioritize the dose conformality in different structures. Whereas the general formalism remains the same, different sets of importance factors characterize plans of obviously different flavor and thus critically determine the final plan. The determination of these parameters has been a "guessing" game because the influence of these parameters is not known until the plan optimization is completed. We now describe a two-step optimization which allows us to determine these parameters automatically.

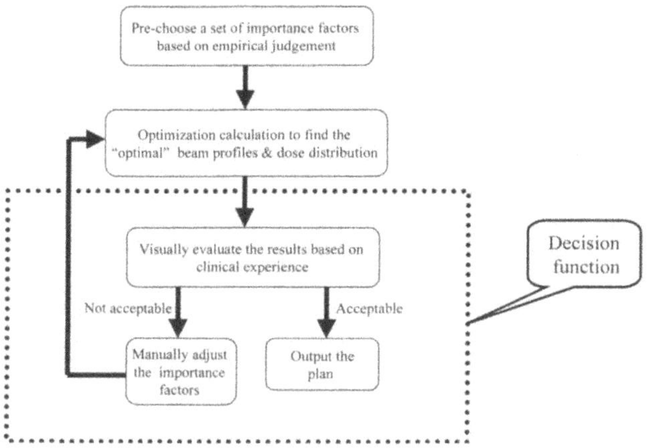


**Figure 1:** A flow chart of the two-step optimization process.

A conventional inverse planning process is sketched in Fig. 1. Given an objective function, it is common to start the inverse planning by assigning a set of initial importance factors $\{\gamma_\sigma\}$ empirically. The results corresponding to this set of importance factors are then evaluated by visual examination with the help of clinical experience. The "optimal" plan is either accepted or is further tuned by changing to a new set of importance factors until it is clinically acceptable. To use a computer algorithm to determine $\{\gamma_\sigma\}$, we introduce a decision function to score the "optimal" plans. The role of the function is to mimic the evaluation process of a planner in Fig. 1 (the elements in the dashed box). Since radiation effects can be measured by the volumetric information, we will define the score function $Q_\sigma(V)$ based on DVHs. The criterion used by the decision function is the "distance" between the calculated and the most-desired DVHs.

$$Q_\sigma(V) = \sum_{D,\sigma} \beta_\sigma [V_\sigma(D) - V_0(D)]^2, \qquad (2)$$

where $\beta_\sigma$ is the DVH trade-off parameter. It provides a measure of how far off a DVH is from the most-desired $V_0(D)$. $Q_\sigma(V)$ provides a quantitative measure of the "goodness" of an "optimal" plan corresponding to a given set of $\{\gamma_\sigma\}$.

We usually assume that the most desired target DVH corresponds to the DVH of the idealized case of a uniform target dose. The most-desired sensitive structure DVHs are chosen to be the ideal case in which the volume receiving non-zero dose is zero. To proceed, it is also needed to determine the DVH tradeoff parameters, $\{\beta_\sigma\}$, in the decision function. We wish to pre-determine a set of $\{\beta_\sigma\}$ that would at least yield a solution close to what would be considered as a "good" plan in an ordinary clinical situation. This "good" plan should possess the property that the DVH of a structure cannot be further improved without significantly sacrificing the others. In practice, such a set of $\{\beta_\sigma\}$ exists. By directly working in the DVH representation, we have the following advantages; (i) $\{\beta_\sigma\}$ provides a direct control in the tradeoff of different DVHs; and (ii) the correlation among $\{\beta_\sigma\}$ is weaker than that among $\{\gamma_\sigma\}$ because a DVH state is degenerate. Geometrically, the parameter $\beta_\sigma$ for a structure is related to the relative change in the area under its DVH curve when the DVH of another structure is varied. Although a trial-and-error may still be needed because of the subjective nature of the medical decision-making, the process of finding a clinical sensible plan becomes much more controllable. We usually set the parameter to unity for the target and 0.1 to a sensitive structure. We found that this choice mimics our clinical trade-off strategy very well.

Other types of decision functions can also be introduced to select the solution from the pool of the "optimal" plans corresponding to different sets of the importance factors. The important point here is that, in order to determine the importance factors in Eq. (1), it is required to use additional knowledge or an additional decision function. Generally, the parameters in the decision function are determined at a different representation which characterizes the plans using a set of higher level parameters. Hopefully, the higher level parameters are easier to determine either intuitively or empirically. The DVH decision function presented here is an example of this type of approach.

The remaining task is computational. Many algorithms can be used to optimize the system. For all their complexity, the algorithms to optimize a multidimensional function are routine mathematical procedures. Here an iterative algorithm (SIITP) reported in [1,2,3] was employed to optimize the beam profiles for a given set of $\{\gamma_\sigma\}$. In the following, we will focus on the description of the selection procedure of the parameters $\{\gamma_\sigma\}$.

The calculation begins with an initial set of $\{\gamma_\sigma\}$ and the corresponding "optimal" beam profiles. The "optimal" beam profiles are obtained using SIITP. The quality of the plan is then evaluated by the DVH decision function $Q_\sigma(V)$ given by Eq. (2). We then introduce a series of variations $\delta_\sigma$'s to one of the model parameters $\gamma_\sigma$ and move $\gamma_\sigma$ to the trial point, $\gamma_\sigma+\delta_\sigma$, which minimizes $Q_\sigma(V)$. The SIITP is invoked to re-optimize the beam profiles after the $\gamma_\sigma$ is updated to $\gamma_\sigma+\delta_\sigma$. The calculation proceeds to the next model parameter and the above procedure repeats. The first model parameter will be varied again after all model parameters are addressed. The iteration stops when the change of the DVH decision function is less than a pre-chosen precision (0.1% was used in our calculation). In general, we found that the calculation converges after four to five iterations and the DVH decision function saturates to its optimal value. Because the algorithm invokes the beam profile optimization for each variation in the model parameters, it is essential to use a fast algorithm for the beam profile calculation.

In the above calculation, the selection of the optimal plan could essentially be divided into two steps. The dose based preference function generates a pool of "optimal" solutions and the DVH decision function selects the final solution from the pool of the "optimal" solutions. In principle, it is possible to use the DVH decision function to select the solution directly from the pool of all physically realizable plans. The approach has two deficiencies. First, by directly optimizing the DVH decision function, we do not have any direct control over the dose distribution because of the degeneracy of a DVH state. Clinically, we sometime prefer one solution over others even though they all have the same DVHs. In other words, a formalism that allows us to incorporate prior knowledge is needed. The two-step optimization makes this possible. In this way, we can find a solution that does not simply optimize the decision function, but also consistent with the prior function. Secondly, it requires an calculation in the dose-volume space. Our previous experience has indicated the convergence of the iterative calculation for beam profile optimization was very slow; about several hundreds to a thousand of iterations in the dose-volume space were required to obtain the optimal solution[4]. Computationally, the approach proposed here is more feasible. The arguments here are perhaps even more true for other types of decision functions.

## Results and Discussion

The above algorithm was applied to study a six-field prostate case. The photon energy was 15 MV and the gantry angles of the incident beams were 180°, 225°, 270°, 315°, 45°, and 90°, respectively. Here the gantry angles were specified using Varian's convention (Varian Oncology System, Palo Alto, CA). The initial importance factors were chosen to be $\gamma_{target}=1$, $\gamma_{rectum}=0$, and $\gamma_{bladder}=0$, respectively. These choices of importance factors yield the best dose conformation to the target, but a penalty is paid in that there is no control on the dose delivered to the sensitive structures. The beam profiles corresponding to the initial $\{\gamma_\sigma\}$ were obtained using SIITP. The calculation proceeded with an iterative change of the importance factors, as described in the above section. In the upper row of Fig. 2 we show the gradual change of the DVHs with the iterative change of the importance factors. As can be expected, the best target DVH was achieved at the beginning of the importance-factor iteration (dashed curves), and the target dose inhomogeneity was increased slightly as the importance factors of the rectum and bladder deviated from zeros. But the rectum and bladder DVHs were improved significantly. The final solution compromised the requirements of the target and the sensitive structures (solid curves).

We found that it took only four to five iterations for the decision function to reach optimal, indicating that the correlation between the importance factors was not very strong. In addition, we noticed that the final solution became

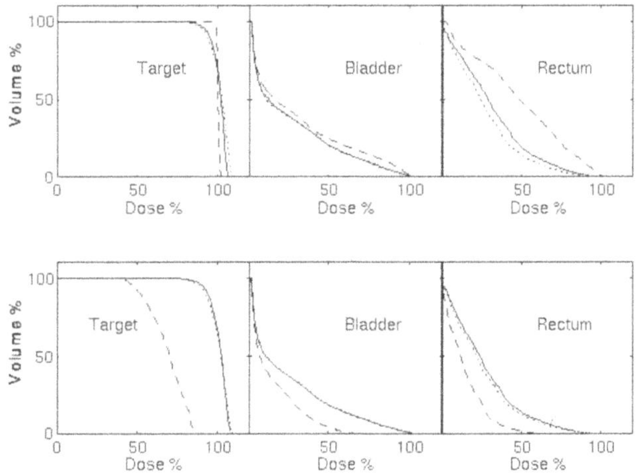


**Figure 2:** Systematic improvement of the DVHs with the iteration of the importance factors (IMs). The starting values of the IMs for the top three figures were $\gamma_{target}=1$, $\gamma_{bladder}=0$, and $\gamma_{rectum}=0$, respectively. The dashed curves represent the corresponding "optimal" DVHs. The algorithm auto-adjusted the importance factors and found the optimal DVHs (solid curves). The final IMs were found to be $\gamma_{target}=1.0$, $\gamma_{bladder}=0.06$, and $\gamma_{rectum}=0.04$, respectively. The dotted curves are the "optimal" DVHs in the third iteration. The bottom three figures showed the gradual improvement of the DVHs when the initial importance factors were set to be $\gamma_{target}=1$, $\gamma_{bladder}=0.2$, and $\gamma_{rectum}=0.2$ (dashed curves). The optimal DVHs (solid curves) converged to the same solution.

insensitive against a small change of the importance factors in the vicinity of the optimal solution. A small variation (1% to 3%) in one or more importance factors did not cause a noticeable change in the final dose distribution and DVHs. This observation suggested that the final solution was stable. The dotted curve in Fig. 2 represents the optimized DVHs of the system at the third iteration (the corresponding importance factors are $\gamma_{target}=1$, $\gamma_{rectum}=0.10$, and $\gamma_{bladder}=0.03$). Note that for every new set of $\{\gamma_\sigma\}$, the beam profiles have to be re-optimized using SIITP. The final values of the importance factors were $\gamma_{target}=1$, $\gamma_{rectum}=0.06$, and $\gamma_{bladder}=0.04$, respectively. The final plan was obtained after the beam profile optimization for this set of importance factors was done. The decision function saturated with further iteration of the importance factors. It is interesting to note that, as indicated by Fig. 2, the beam profile optimization converged fastest when $\gamma_{target}=1$ and the rest of importance factors were zero. The convergence became slower when the importance factors for the sensitive structures were increased because of the competition in the dose requirements of the target and the sensitive structures.

The initial and final isodose distributions of the system is shown in Fig. 3. Consistent with the evolution of the DVHs shown in the upper row of Fig. 2, the doses to the sensitive structures also showed significantly improvement with the iterative adjustment of the importance factors.

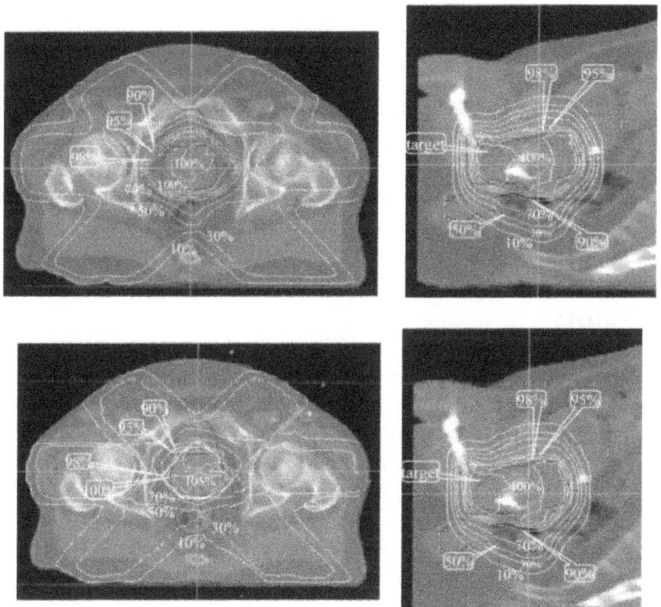

**Figure 3:** Dose distribution before and after the optimization with respect to the importance factors.

The behavior of the system when a different initial set of importance factors ($\gamma_{target}=1$, $\gamma_{rectum}=0.2$, and $\gamma_{bladder}=0.2$, respectively) was used is shown in the bottom row of Fig. 2. In this case, the target DVH was improved gradually as the importance factor iteration proceeded and the DVHs of the sensitive structures were compromised for the gain in the target dose conformation. The importance factors corresponding to the intermediate state (the dotted curves) were $\gamma_{target}=1$, $\gamma_{rectum}=0.04$, and $\gamma_{bladder}=0.08$, respectively. The system converged to the same DVHs and isodose distribution.

## Conclusion

Inverse treatment planning is a multi-objective decision making process in which there are conflicting clinical objectives. The tradeoffs between the objectives for various anatomical structures can be parameterized by a set of importance factors. How to determine the importance factors efficiently is an important problem in the plan selection. In the past, little attention has been paid to this issue. We have described an effective approach to determining the parameters. A decision rule or a score function is necessary in order to determine unambiguously the optimal importance factors. The response used to score the system can be based on experience, or simply a score function. A DVH based score function was introduced in our study to illustrate the methodology. Other types of score function based on, e.g., biological models, can also be introduced for this purpose. An iterative algorithm for automatically selecting the importance factors was demonstrated. In the two-step optimization the tradeoff strategy is specified in the DVH representation and the final solution, which assimilates the specified relative importance of different structures, is found in the scheme of the quadratic objective function. This approach allows us to incorporate prior knowledge into the optimization process and to take advantage of the useful features of each scheme. The algorithm was applied to a prostate case and the results indicated that the combined scheme of decision-making was effective and produced plan consistent with the planner's expectation. The approach has strong potential to automate the current trial-and-error IMRT treatment planning process and thus has widespread clinical implications.

The authors wish to thank R. J. Hamilton, D. Spelbring, C.A. Pelizzari, and G.T.Y. Chen for their efforts during the development of SIITP. This work was supported in part by grants from the Whitaker Foundation, Computerized Medical System (CMS), and the NCI (No. CA43840).

## References

[1] L Xing and G Chen. Iterative methods for inverse treatment planning. *Phys. Med. Biol.* **41**:2107--23, 1996.

[2] L Xing, R J Hamilton, D Spelbring, C A Pelizzari, and G Chen. Fast iterative algorithms for three-dimensional inverse treatment planning. *Med. Phys.* **25**, 1845-49, 1998.

[3] L Xing, J.G. Li, A. Pugachev, Q.T. Le, A. Boyer. Estimation theory and model parameter selection for therapeutic plan optimization, *Med. Phys.* **26**, 2348-58, 1999.

[4] D Togane, R J Hamilton, A L Boyer, and L Xing. Dose volume histogram based optimization for intensity modulated radiation therapy, *Med. Phys.* **25**:A118, 1998.

# Dose-Based Conformal Field Shaping using Automated Optimization

**Benedick Fraass, Daniel McShan and Marc Kessler**

Department of Radiation Oncology, The University of Michigan, Ann Arbor, Michigan, USA

## Introduction

Three-dimensional conformal radiation therapy (3DCRT) is typically performed using radiation fields which are shaped to create a high dose region which conforms to the shape of the target volume(s) in 3-D, while minimizing dose to normal tissues. Although this conformation should be performed using the dose distribution, often this dosimetric conformation is replaced with the use of simple geometric conformation of each field's aperture to the target projected in a Beam's Eye View (BEV) geometry, since simple automated aperture shaping algorithms[1-3] can be used to automate the process. This procedure, sometimes called "BEV targeting", results in a dose distribution which is generally shaped like the target, but does not optimize the conformality of the high dose volume to that of the target. True 3DCRT using forward planning (iterative plan optimization driven by the treatment planner) requires significant skill and effort by the planner to achieve the dosimetric conformation which is the aim of such 3DCRT. Up to this point, automated optimization of this process has not been possible.

Another method for the planning and delivery of 3DCRT involves the use of inverse planning and intensity modulated radiation therapy (IMRT). With this paradigm, dose- or dose-volume-based (or other) objective functions are used within the inverse planning system to arrive at an IMRT plan which achieves the desired plan objectives. Within the limits of the search engine and objective function which are used, these solutions are "optimal", i.e. the plan arrives at the best objective function score within the limits of constraints placed on the problem. Aside from the obvious difference that modulated intensities are used rather than flat conformally-shaped fields, inverse planned IMRT plans are qualitatively different from forward planned conformal plans in two additional ways: 1) automated searching through the parameter space is used, rather than iterative and interactive optimization by the dosimetrist, and 2) a quantitative scoring system is used to drive the plan optimization, rather than the qualitative and visual evaluation methods typically used by dosimetrists. It is reasonably clear, based on these various issues, that non-inverse planned flat conformal field treatment plans should not compare well to the inverse planned solutions, especially when compared using the quantitative measures which are often involved in the objective function used by the inverse planned method.

This work describes a method for the optimization of 3DCRT plans based on flat or segmental IMRT fields, using a combination of inverse planning driven by a sophisticated search engine (simulated annealing[4]) and a very general objectivie function method[5], combined with modification of the Edge/Octree dose calculation algoriithm[6] which has been used for photon dose calculations for many years. This new method, which we call Automated Dose-Based Conformal (ADBC) field shaping, results in the first possibility of truly optimizing routine conformal therapy. In addition, this technique makes possible the *quantitative* comparison of more sophisticated IMRT approaches and typical conformal flat fields used for normal 3DCRT. Finally, full utilization of this technique may also help fully automate field shape design for normal 3D conformal planning, one of the most time consuming and difficult parts of interactive 3-D treatment planning.

## Materials and Methods

The basic framework for the current work consists of the 3-D treatment planning system UMPlan[7-9] and the Edge/Octree photon dose calculation model[6,10], combined with several components of the in-house developed automated optimization (inverse planning) system UMOpt, including the simulated annealing search engine[4] and costlet-based objective function[5] components. The algorithm described here is fully integrated with all the 3-D treatment planning features contained in the planning system, including the 3-D anatomical description, beam parameters (including segmental and DMLC-delivered IMRT), and 3-D dose display, dose volume histogram (DVH) and NTCP/TCP evaluation capabilities. The algorithms used for this work have been implemented in FORTRAN and C, and are based on use of DEC/Compaq Alpha workstations using the OpenVMS operating system.

## Results

The photon Edge/Octree model[6,10], the standard photon calculation algorithm in UMPlan since 1986, was originally designed to provide very accurate and fast broad beam dose calculations, with particular emphasis on accuracy in calculations for conformal fields shaped with blocks or MLC. The clinical accuracy of this model has recently been demonstrated for multisegment IMRT[11]. The model has always included accurate handling of penumbra, scatter differences due to field shaping, varying transmissions for blocks, and 3-D patient and beam geometry. The main limitation of the Edge/Octree algorithm in the past has been its use of a modified equivalent path length density correction method, however, the newer version of this algorithm makes use of a correction method which can be described as a pseudo-3-D-ETAR type correction[12].

The Edge/Octree model is based on the differences of the experimental situation from a broad beam situation. All of the penumbra, scatter, and other aspects of the dose distribution of an individual field are modeled through the use of an "edge" function which is tied to changes in intensity (ie, edges) in the field. After modeling the dose inside the field with an intensity distribution (tied to the flattening filter) multiplied by the broad beam (very large field) depth dose, all other components of the dose distribution are handled by the integration of the edge function over all the edges, or intensity gradients. For calculational efficiency and speed, a non-uniform grid of points in a divergent beam geometry (represented by an Octree-like structure[10]) is used for all calculations.

The geometry and modeling used within this model make it particularly useful for the goal of this work: creation of a method of the automated optimization of dose distributions achieved with flat or segmental IMRT fields. As seen in Fig. 1, the model lends itself directly to the optimization of the position of leaves of a multileaf collimator (MLC) -shaped field. In order to recalculate the complete 3-D dose distribution of a new MLC shape D', the change caused by moving one MLC leaf can be directly and exactly calculated (within the accuracy of the model) using the equation below:

$$D' = D + K\,[\Delta P + \Sigma\, e_i + \Sigma\, (-e_j)\,] \qquad (1)$$

where D' is the new dose at point p, D is the original dose to point p, K is a function of depth and position, ΔP is the change in intensity (1 inside the field, 0 outside), and the sums are the integration of the edge function (e) over each of the changed edges (changed by the MLC leaf change). Therefore, recalculation of the full 3-D dose distribution for a change is reduced to a very fast summation of the differences between just a few terms of the original integration. This calculation is illustrated in Fig. 1 using the change in a single MLC leaf position.

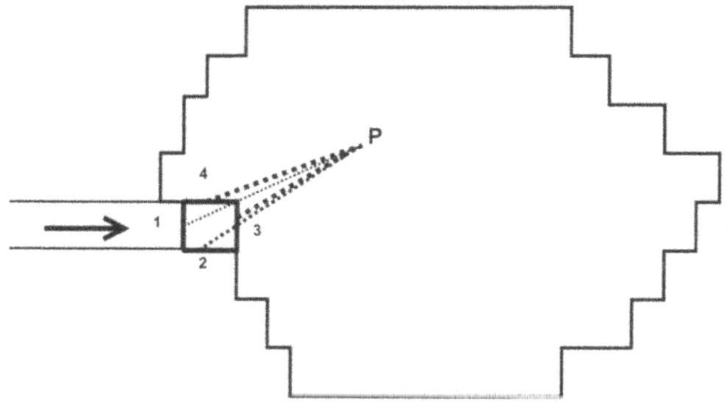


**Figure 1:** Change in dose to point p due to move of MLC leaf: edge functions for edges 1 and 2 are subtracted from edge functions for edges 3 and 4.

This approach is just a recasting of the implementation of the algorithm, which has been successfully been used for accurate and fast dose calculations for photon beams shaped with MLC and/or blocks for many years, and it retains all the accuracy of the older version. Various additional improvements to the basic algorithm have also been implemented, including a faster and more accurate integration around the edges which removes small artifacts due to sharp beam corners, an improved parameterization of the primary photon intensity due to the flattening filter to better model multicomponent and non-symmetric flattening filters, significantly improved modeling of the surface dose and buildup region dose contributions from contamination electrons[13-14], pseudo-3D-ETAR inhomogeneity corrections[12], use of a complete description of the collimator and head geometry which better takes into account MLC transmission, differences in penumbra due to tertiary collimators, and other issues. Finally, this algorithm is implemented for use with conformal fields, including segmental IMRT and IMRT delivered with dynamic MLC techniques.

Calculation speed is critical to the usefulness of any dose calculation algorithm in an automated optimization program. The current algorithm is approximately 1000 times faster than our convolution/superposition algorithm, while maintaining excellent accuracy for very complex field shapes. For use in the optimization algorithm, the speed is further improved: for 10,000 points (approximately 1000 points per structure used for optimization), each interation takes approximately 0.1 sec without any optimization of the code. This allows the optimization of a multi-beam plan (10 different segments spread over 5 beam directions) in less than 15 minutes, even with the non-optimized code. This calculation capability has also been implemented into the interactive planning system, and allows near instantaneous (about 0.5 sec) redisplay of isodose lines on multiple planes (e.g., axial, sagittal and coronal planes through the target) after interative movement of an MLC leaf (Fig. 2). Investigation of the usefulness of this capability for interactive planning will also be investigated, in addition to the studies planned for the automated optimization approach.

To illustrate the automated optimization of the dose distribution for a segmental IMRT plan, a comparison between three different IMRT plans will be described. The plan used as the basis for this comparison is a 5 field 10 segment non-coplanar treatment plan[15] clinically used to treat a grade 4 gliobastoma to 90 Gy on the UM brain dose escalation study[16]. This clinical plan, obtained with forward planning as described by Marsh[15] is also used as the basis for a beamlet IMRT plan consisting of the same 5 non-coplanar beam directions, planned with 1x1 cm beamlets using our optimization system[5,17]. The third plan involved in the comparison is the original 10 segment clinical plan, with the field shapes and segment weights optimized using the ADBC optimization method described here.

One of the critical parts of any quantitative plan comparison is the use of an appropriate and clinically relevant cost (or objective) function to drive the automated optimization. For this comparison, the clinically used plan ("segments") is the clinical plan, without automated optimization. The "beamlet IMRT" and "optimized segmental IMRT" plans have both been optimized using the same exact cost function, based on approximately 10 different costlets[5].

Dose volume histograms comparing the clinical segmental IMRT and beamlet IMRT (optimized) plans are shown in Fig. 2. DVHs for the central target volume (PTV1), and the two outer (and lower dose) target volumes (PTV2 and 3), as well as the normal brain (brain – PTV3) are shown. Both sets of DVHs satisfy the current clinical study protocol, but differences illustrate the kinds of differences which often arise between optimization performed interactively and optimization performed according to a specific cost function.

Fig. 3 shows the DVHs of the beamlet IMRT plan compared to the results of the initial optimization of the segmental IMRT plan. These DVHs show several important results. First, highest priority in the cost function, the dose inside PTV1, becomes nearly identical in the two optimized plans. The next priority, the PTV2 ring around PTV1, also

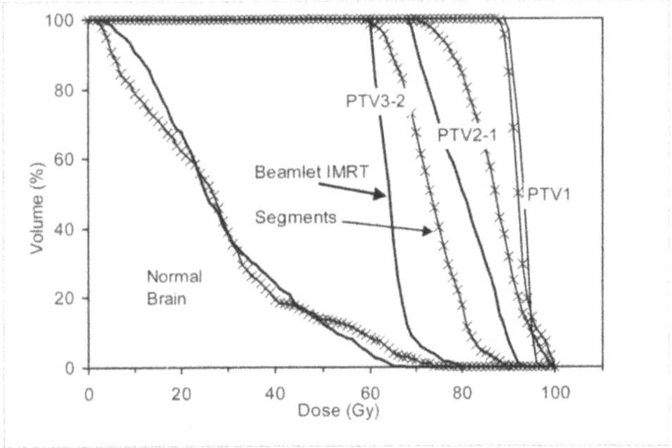


**Figure 2:** DVHs for beamlet IMRT and clinical segmental IMRT plan for brain treatment to 90 Gy.

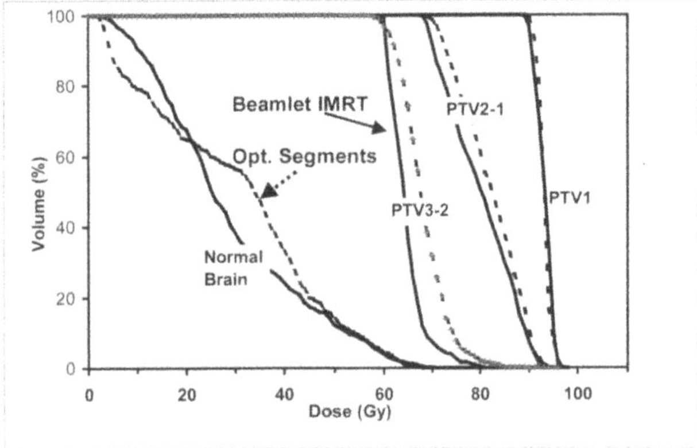


**Figure 3:** DVHs for beamlet IMRT plan and ADBC optimized segmental IMRT plan for brain treatment to 90 Gy.

achieves similar results, much closer than the original segmental plan. The higher dose part of the normal brain DVHs also agree quite well. Finally, the DVH for the PTV3 ring is also much closer to tbe beamlet IMRT as well.

Clearly, no conclusions can be drawn from a single plan comparison example. However, this example illustrates the potential power of the ADBC field shaping technique. Comparisons between flat conformal fields generated with forward 3-D planning and various IMRT delivery techniques can now be performed directly and quantitatively, using identical optimization capabilities and cost functions. The ability to formally optimize the flat conformal fields will allow the determination of the best results obtainable with specific beam arrangements, rather than being sensitive to the skill and/or persistence of the treatment planner. Finally, complete automation of the ADBC shaping technique should help make non-IMRT conformal planning much more efficient for routine clinical use. Studies investigating all these possibilities will be pursued in the near future.

## References

1. BA Fraass, DL McShan, KJ Weeks: Computerized beam shaping. In: Proceedings of the 1988 AAPM Summer School, Computers in Medical Physics, ed. Austin, TX, 1988, pp. 333-340.
2. DL McShan, BA Fraass, AS Lichter: Full integration of the Beam's Eye View concept into clinical treatment planning. Int J Rad Oncol Biol Phys, 18:1485-1494, 1990
3. L Brewster, G Mageras, R Mohan: Automatic generation of beam apertures. Med Phys 20: 1337-1342, 1993.
4. JJH Kim, N Dogan, DL McShan, ML Kessler: An AVS-based system for optimization of conformal radiotherapy treatment plans. 1995 Int. Advanced Visual Systems User + Developer Conf. Boston MA, 1995: 417-423
5. ML Kessler, JJH Kim, DL McShan, BA Fraass: A general framework for interactive and automated treatment plan optimization, Part I: evaluators, modifiers, and costlets. Med Phys 25: A178, 1998.[Abstract]
6. BA Fraass, DL McShan, RK TenHaken, KM Hutchins: 3-D treatment planning: V. A Fast 3-D photon calculation model. In: The Use of Computers in Radiation Therapy, ed. IAD Bruinvis, FH van_der_Giessen, HJ van_Kleffens, FW Wittkamper, North-Holland, Elsevier Science Publishers BV, 1987, pp. 521-525
7. BA Fraass, DL McShan: 3-D treatment planning: I. Overview of a clinical planning system. In: Use of Computers in Radiation Therapy, ed. IAD Bruinvis et al, North-Holland, Elsevier Science, 1987, pp. 273-276.
8. DL McShan, BA Fraass: "3-D treatment planning: II. Integration of gray scale images and solid surface graphics." The Use of Computers in Radiation Therapy, (ed) IAD Bruinvis et al. Elsevier Science Publishers BV, (North-Holland), 1987, pp. 41-44.
9. BA Fraass, DL McShan, KJ Weeks: 3-D treatment planning: III. Complete Beam's-Eye-View planning capabilities. In: The Use of Computers in Radiation Therapy, ed. IAD Bruinvis et al, North-Holland, Elsevier Science Publishers BV, 1987, pp. 193-196
10. DL McShan, BA Fraass: Use of an octree-like geometry for 3D dose calculations. Med Phys 20: 1219-27, 1993
11. MJP Brugmans, A van_der_Horst, JV Lebesque, BJ Mijnheer, DL McShan, ML Kessler, BA Fraass: Planning and dosimetric verification of a computer-optimized segmented irradiation technique for the prostate. Med Phys 25: A118, 1998.[Abstract]
12. MK Martel, BA Fraass, DL McShan: Study of limits of applicability of ETAR-like inhomogeneity correction methods. Med Phys, 1992.
13. BA Fraass, IAD Bruinvis: Calculation of accurate dose distributions in the buildup region of conformal fields using a simple model for electron contamination. Radiotherapy Oncology, 1996.
14. BA Fraass, IAD Bruinvis, JH Lanson, FW Wittkamper: Photon and electron contributions to the dose in the buildup regions for fields used in conformal therapy. European Society for Therapeutic Radiology and Oncology, 1994.
15. LH Marsh, RK Ten Haken, HM Sandler: A single plan approach for differentially dosing sequential target volumes. Medical Dosimetry 22: 275-81, 1997
16. RK Ten Haken, BA Fraass, AS Lichter, LH Marsh, EH Radany, HM Sandler: A brain tumor dose escalation protocol based on effective dose equivalence to prior experience. Int J Rad Oncol Biol Phys 42: 137-141, 1998.
17. DL McShan, BA Fraass, MK Kessler: Intensity modulation using beamlets. Med Phys 25: A149, 1998.[Abstract]

# Direct computation of the "step-and-shoot" IMRT plan

**Pekka Kolmonen[1], Jouko Tervo[2], Kai Jaatinen[1] and Tapani Lahtinen[3]**
[1]Department of Applied Physics, University of Kuopio, Kuopio, Finland, [2]Department of Computer Science and Applied Mathematics, University of Kuopio, Kuopio, Finland and [3]Department of Oncology, Kuopio University Hospital, Kuopio, Finland

## Introduction

A new approach for the IMRT using "step-and-shoot" MLC delivery method is presented. Leaf positions and the irradiation times of subfields are optimized directly without computation of intensity distributions over treatment fields. The output of the process is a simple and ready IMRT plan.

## Material and methods

The direct optimization of MLC parameters requires a model that combines a model for the MLC parameters (leaf positions and irradiation times) and the Fredholm integral equation of the first kind. The well-known integral equation is also called the pencil beam model in its discretized form.

To model the MLC leaf configuration and to include the head scatter of the leaves a modified Heaviside function was used. The model was fitted to data which was calculated using the Monte Carlo method [5].

The whole forward model for one leaf-pair is of the form $D(x) = \int_0^w h(x,u)H(u-a)H(b-u)du\delta t$, where $x$ is a point in patient space, $D(x)$ is the dose in point $x$, $w$ is the width of treatment field, $\delta t$ is the irradiation time, $h(x,u)$ is the dose deposition kernel and $H(u-a)$ and $H(b-u)$ are the modified Heaviside functions for left and right leaves respectively. Superposition of all leaf-pairs in all fields was used to compute the total dose.

In the model the dose deposition kernel $h(x,u)$ is needed. We have developed methods to determine a continuous approximation for the kernel using a discrete dose deposition matrix [6]. The discrete dose deposition matrix was computed using the commercial treatment planning system CADPLAN (Varian Medical Systems Finland, Espoo, Finland).

The technical limitations of the MLC can be taken into account in the course of optimization since all the parameters ($a$, $b$, $\delta t$) are included in the model. A notable point in the limitations is that subfields having too small $\delta t$ were neglected because they are difficult to deliver in practice.

A feasibility approach was used to include dose prescriptions for the Planning Target Volume (PTV) and Organs At Risk (OARs). This means that lower and upper dose limits were set for the PTV and upper limits were set to the OARs [2].

To determine a feasible solution two techniques were used. The first one was a home-made Projected Gradient Method (PGM) suitable for large systems of non-linear inequalities [3]. The second one was the limited memory algorithm L-BFGS-B [1]. L-BFGS-B was used as a reference method to verify the PGM.

When a solution was obtained intensity matrices were determined for each field to be used in CADPLAN for dose computations. Also an MLC file was written for the delivery of the feasible plan.

Both algorithm were written using F77 and were run on a HP J200/9000 machine with HP-UX 10.20.

A feasible plan was determined for a patient whose prostate was to be treated. The PTV dose was prescribed to be between 67 – 73 Gy. The dose inside the rectum volume was prescribed to be under 45 Gy. Figure 1 shows a transversal slice of the patient. Five equiangled coplanar fields were used. Each field had three subfields.

In the PTV there were 20205 voxels and in the rectum 513. The running time of the GPM was 774 seconds and of the L-BFGS-B 5003 seconds.

## Results and discussion

In figure 2 is the DVH of the feasible plan computed by the PGM. The maximum and minimum dose in the PTV volume were 79.2 Gy and 51.8 Gy respectively. Mean dose in the PTV volume was 70.0 Gy with standard deviation 5.6 %. The maximum dose in the rectum volume was 51.1 Gy. Both solution techniques gave similar dose distributions. The huge running time of the L-BFGS-B was due to the fact that the termination criteria were not the same as for PGM.

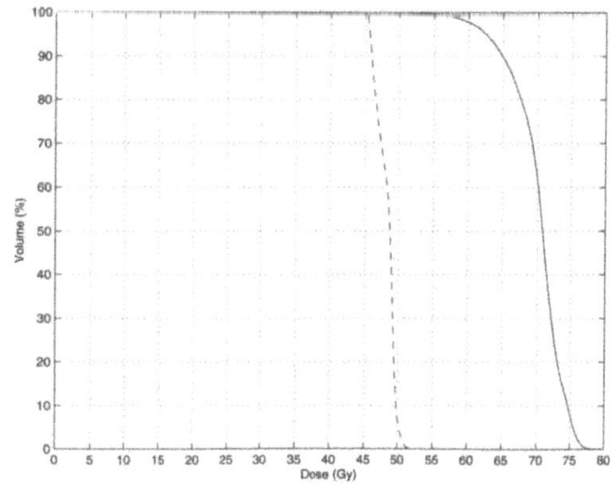


**Figure 2:** the DVHs of the feasible plan. The PTV is indicated by solid line and rectum by dashed one.

At the starting point the total amount of subfields was 15; when subfields having too small irradiation time $\delta t$ were left

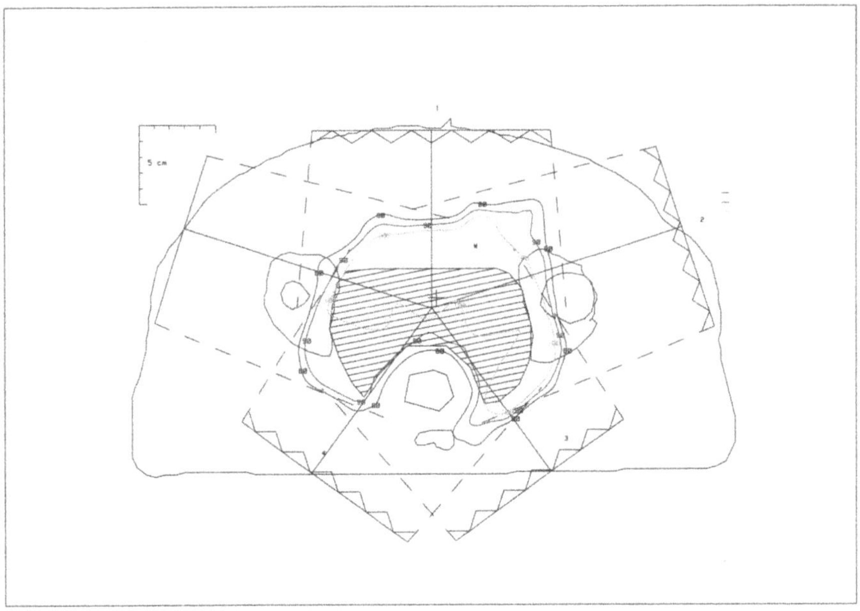


**Figure 1:** A transversal slice of the patient. Relative dose is indicated by 100, 90 and 80 % isodoses. 100 % equals to 70 Gy.

out there were 9 subfields. This partially explains the constraint violations in maximum and minimum dose. Fine detailed dose distribution requires large number of subfields.

## Conclusion

We have developed a complete system for producing 3D "step-and-shoot" MLC plans. The dose calculation and the MLC head scatter models are designed to meet the practical and technical demands set by clinical use and MLC mechanics/dosimetry. The output of the process is a ready treatment plan. The number of subfields is limited for easy verification of the plan.

Both methods that we have used to compute the plan were local optimizers. We are studying global optimization strategies to find the best plan that can be achieved. A global optimizer LGO is under test [4].

The dose volume constraints can be implemented in the system and are under test.

The model used can also be applied for dynamic MLC delivery. Then the velocity and acceleration of the leaves will place additional constraints to the solution. The output is, as with the "step-and-shoot", a ready IMRT plan.

## References

[1] Byrd R H, Lu P, Nocedal J and Zhu C 1995 A limited memory algorithm for bound constrained optimization *SIAM J. Scientific Computing* **16** 1190 – 1208

[2] Censor Y, Altschuler M D and Powlis W D 1988 On the use of Cimmino's simultaneous projections method for computing a solution of the inverse problem in radiotherapy treatment planning *Inverse Problems* **4** 607–23

[3] Censor Y and Zenios S A 1997 *Parallel Optimization: Theory, Algorithms and Applications* (New York: Oxford University Press)

[4] Pinter J D 1996 *Global Optimization in Action, Continuous and Lipschitz Optimization: Algorithms, Implementations and Applications* (Dordrecht – Boston – London: Kluwer Academic Publishers)

[5] Rogers D W O, Faddegon B A, Ding G X, Ma C-A and We J 1995 BEAM: A Monte Carlo code to simulate radiotherapy treatment units *Med. Phys.* **22** 505 – 24

[6] Tervo J and Kolmonen P 1998 Data fitting model for the kernel of integral operator from radiation therapy *Mathl. Comput. Modelling* **28** 59 – 77

# Beam orientations in IMRT: to optimize or not to optimize?

**Andrei Pugachev, Jonathan G. Li, Arthur L. Boyer and Lei Xing**

Department of Radiation Oncology, Stanford University School of Medicine, Stanford, California 94305-5304, USA

## Introduction

The goal of radiotherapy is to deliver a prescribed dose to the target while sparing the sensitive structures located in its vicinity. Intensity modulated radiation therapy (IMRT) allows one to achieve a better dose distribution by using intensity modulated beams. For conventional radiation therapy, the beam orientations can be determined with the help of a beam's-eye view (BEV). In IMRT, the situation is more complicated because the gantry angles are correlated with the intensity profiles. The X-ray beams sometimes have to go through sensitive structures in order to achieve an optimal compromise between the target and sensitive structure doses. In IMRT treatment planning, one usually selects a set of gantry angles empirically and then obtains the corresponding beam intensity profiles by inverse planning. Because the influence of a set of gantry angles on the final dose distribution is not known until the beam intensity profile optimization is done, several trial and error attempts are often needed in order to determine a set of adequate beam orientations.

Computer optimization of beam orientations allows one to select the best beam orientations automatically. However, the calculation is complicated by the highly non-convex dependence of the objective function on the gantry and couch angles. This requires a stochastic algorithm for the beam orientation optimization. The stochastic sampling and the greatly enlarged search space make the computational time prohibitively long and hamper its clinical application. In the past, some attempts have been made in developing techniques for the beam orientation optimization [1-3]. The results so far are controversial and non-conclusive. On one hand, it was argued that beam orientation optimization becomes non-significant when the number of beams is seven or more, since it only improves the dose distribution marginally. On the other hand, the reality is that the physicists are constantly frustrated by the lack of an effective tool for the beam orientation selection. In some complicated IMRT cases, considerable effort may be required to find a set of sensible beam orientations. The choice of the beam configuration for the treatment strongly depends on the planner's experience. Even under the best circumstances, there is no guarantee that the selected beam configuration is the best one.

In this work, we have developed a robust beam orientation optimization algorithm and systematically investigated the role of the beam orientations, including non-coplanar beams, in IMRT. We have applied the technique to the treatment of several types of clinical cases. In general, we have found that the importance of the beam orientation selection differs from site to site. In some cases, beam orientation optimization results in significant improvement in the dose distribution even when nine beams are used.

## Material and methods

Simulated annealing was used to search for the optimal set of beam orientations. To evaluate the quality of a trial set of beam orientations, beam intensity profiles have to be optimized in order to calculate the dose distribution and the corresponding objective function. Here, iterative inverse treatment planning technique was used for the beam intensity profile optimization for a given set of beam orientations. Dose calculation was done using the PLUNC treatment planning system. A quadratic dose-based objective function was used for this study [4,5].

The orientation of a beam was specified by the gantry and couch angles. The gantry and couch angle spaces were discretized in increments of 10°. Couch angles allowed for the beam positioning were limited from -40° to 40°. No limitations were imposed on the allowed gantry angles. To ensure good quality of the treatment plans, nine beams were used for all the cases. With more than nine beams, clinical delivery time becomes an issue. In addition, with increase in the number of beams the time required for the beam orientation optimization grows exponentially.

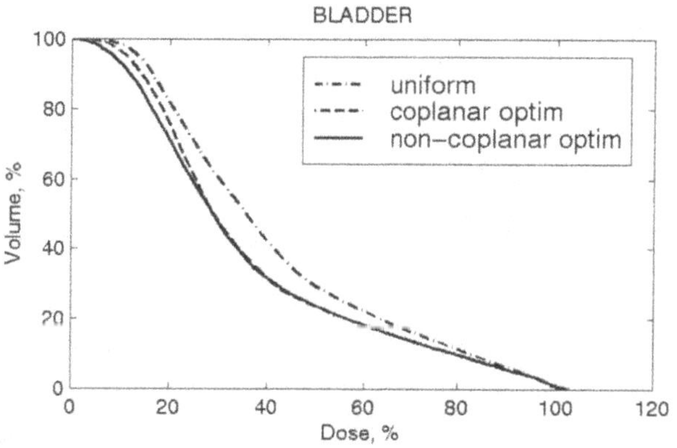


**Figure 1:** Comparison of the DVHs of the bladder for the treatment plans of a prostate case when using 9 equally-spaced coplanar beams (dash-dotted line), 9 coplanar beams with optimized beam orientations (dashed line), and 9 non-coplanar beams with optimized beam orientations.

Beam orientation optimization was performed for three typical clinical cases: a prostate cancer without regional lymph node involvement, a para-spine case, and a nasopharyngeal cancer. For each case, three types of optimization were done; (1) nine uniformly spaced coplanar beams. Beam intensity profiles were optimized. (2) Only coplanar beams were allowed. Beam orientations and beam profiles were optimized. (3) Similar to (2), but non-coplanar beams were allowed.

## Results and discussion

### Prostate

A prostate case without involvement of the regional lymph nodes was investigated first. Nine 15 MV photon beams were used. Figure 1 compares the DVHs of the bladder using the three methods described above. Beam orientation optimization resulted in only slight improvement of bladder DVH. Introduction of non-coplanar beam configurations to the search space did not improve the final dose distribution. DVHs for the target and the rectum were almost the same for the three cases. This finding is consistent with the previous study [3].

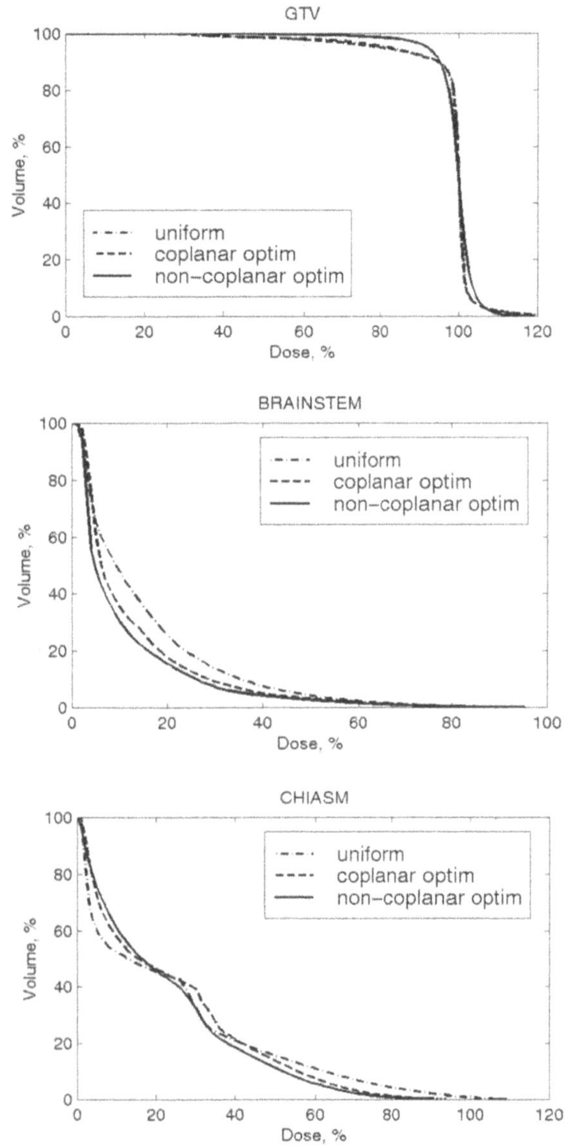


**Figure 2:** Comparison of the DVHs for the three treatment plans of a nasopharyngeal case.

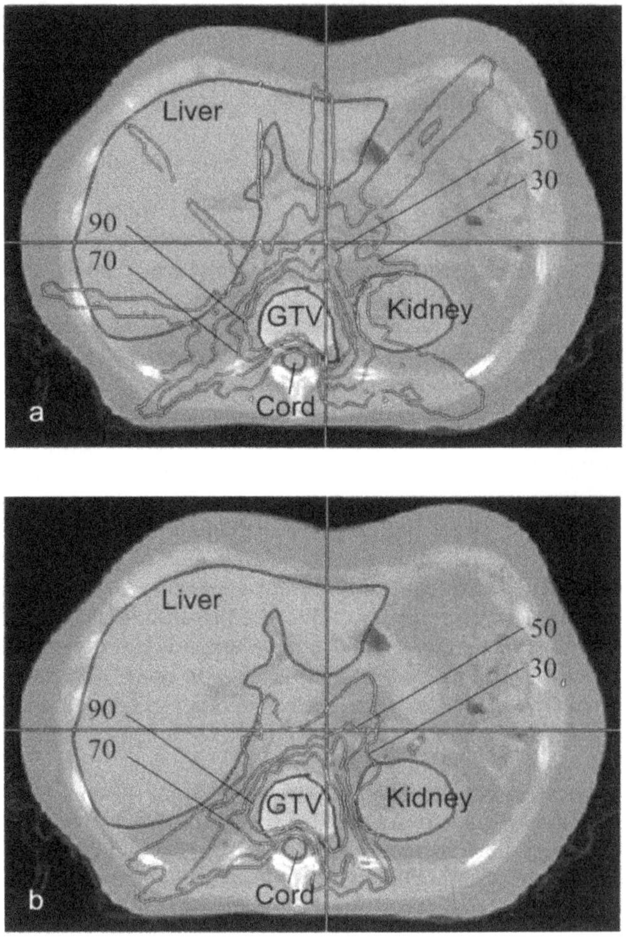


**Figure 3:** Calculated dose distributions for the para-spine tumor case. a) 9 uniformly-spaced coplanar beams were used. b) 9 non-coplanar beams with optimized beam orientations were used.

### Nasopharynx

Nine 6 MV photon beams were used in this case. The DVHs of the target and sensitive structures are shown in Fig. 2 for the three treatment plans. As can be seen from Fig. 2, beam orientation optimization resulted in more pronounced improvement of dose distribution. Maximum dose to the optic chiasm was reduced significantly. The use of non-coplanar optimized beams increased the minimum target dose and yielded noticeable improvement in the dose uniformity to the target as well.

### Para-spine treatment

Nine 15 MV photon beams were used in this case. In Fig. 3 dose distributions corresponding to a 9 uniformly spaced and optimized non-coplanar beam configurations are plotted. The DVHs of the GTV and the other sensitive structures are shown in Fig. 4 for the three different types of beam configurations. It can be seen that the optimization of beam orientations yielded some notable improvement in the final dose distribution. While improving the target dose, the reduction in the liver and kidney doses was significant.

## Conclusion

We have developed a robust beam orientation optimization algorithm and demonstrated that the sensitivity of treatment plans with respect to the selection of beam orientations varies from site to site, even when a large number of beams are used. For prostate case, the beam orientation optimization only resulted in a slight improvement of bladder dose and the use of non-coplanar beams did not give any noticeable advantage in comparison with coplanar beams. For other sites investigated here, such as the para-spine and nasopharynx, we found that the beam orientation optimization resulted in more significant improvement in the dose distribution, especially when non-coplanar beams were used.

## References

[1] Bortfeld T and Schlegel W 1993 Optimization of beam orientations in radiation therapy: Some theoretical considerations *Phys. Med. Biol.* **38** 291-304

[2] Söderström S and Brahme A 1995 Which is the most suitable number of photon beam portals in coplanar radiation therapy *Int. J. Radiat. Oncol. Biol. Phys.* **33** 151-159

[3] Stein J, Mohan R, Wang X, Bortfeld T, Wu Q, Preiser K, Ling C, and Schlegel W 1997 Number and orientations of beams in intensity-modulated radiation treatments *Med. Phys.* **24**(2) 149-160

[4] Webb S 1989 Optimization of conformal radiotherapy dose distributions by simulated annealing *Phys. Med. Biol.* **34** 1349-1370

[5] Xing L and Chen G 1996 Iterative methods for inverse treatment planning *Phys. Med. Biol.* **41** 2107-2123

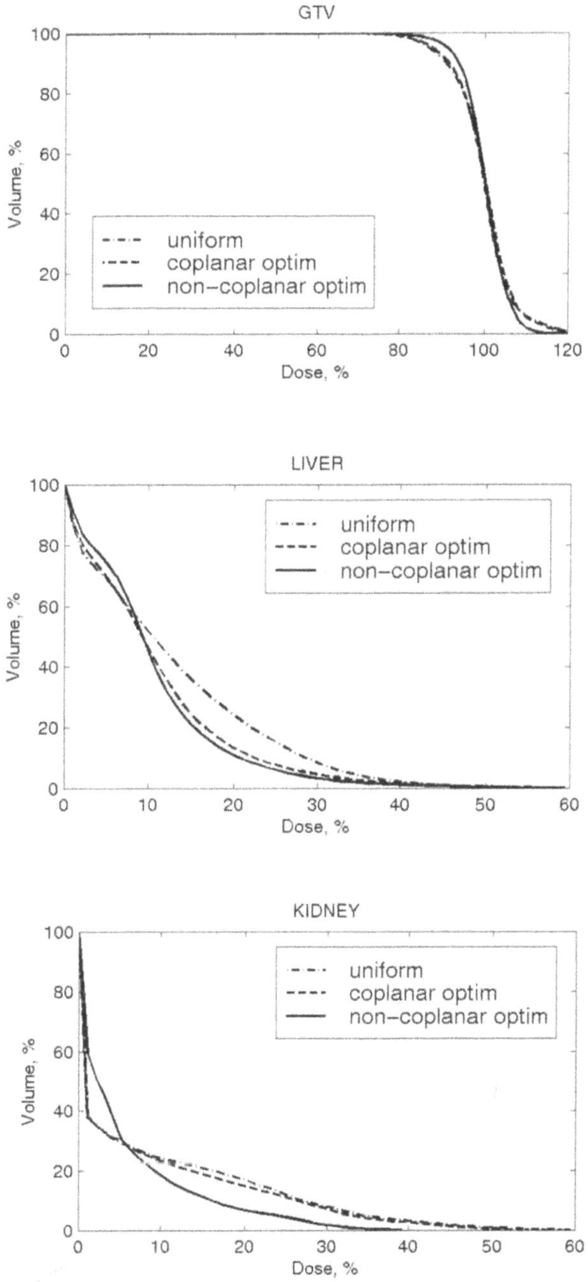


**Figure 4:** Comparison of the DVHs for the three treatment plans of a para-spine case.

# Inverse Treatment Planning for Gamma Knife Radiosurgery

**David Shepard[1], Michael Ferris[2], Lijun Ma[1], and Cedric Yu[1]**

[1]University of Maryland School of Medicine, Baltimore, MD, USA and
[2]University of Wisconsin, Madison, WI, USA

## Abstract

The goal of this project has been the development of an inverse treatment planning system for Gamma Knife radiosurgery. The techniques that have been investigated include nonlinear and mixed integer programming. These techniques have been applied to a variety of patient cases. The results indicate that an inverse planning approach has the potential to provide significant improvements in the quality of Gamma Knife treatment plans.

## Introduction

The Leksell Gamma Knife provides an advanced stereotactic approach to the treatment of tumors and vascular malformations within the head. Over 100 Gamma Knife units are installed worldwide, and more than 20,000 patients are treated each year[1].

Two hundred and one Co-60 sources are located in the shielded vault of the Gamma Knife treatment unit. The beams of radiation are focused so that they intersect at a single location in space. The result is a spherical region of high dose referred to as a shot of radiation. Four shot sizes are available with corresponding diameters of 4mm, 8mm, 14mm, or 18mm.

Each patient's treatment plan is developed by a neurosurgeon working in conjunction with a radiation oncologist and a physicist. Through an iterative process of trial and error, they determine the number of shots along with the size, the location, and the weight that is assigned to each.

When the treatment volume is small, the patient may only require one or two shots of radiation. For these patients, the treatment planning process is straightforward and can be accomplished in a few minutes. The planning process becomes much more complex when the tumor is large or irregularly shaped. For these patients, the development of a treatment plan can become very tedious, and the quality of the final dose distribution can vary from user to user. With this in mind, we have investigated a variety of inverse planning approaches that can be applied to the Gamma Knife.

## Material and methods

With inverse treatment planning, the user begins by outlining the tumor and any sensitive structures. Next, a series of treatment goals are defined. Based on these goals, an optimization algorithm determines the best possible treatment plan.

Each optimization incorporates both an objective function and a set of constraints. The objective function reduces an entire treatment plan into a single numerical value. The job of the optimizer is to either minimize or maximize the value of the objective function. The objective functions that we have tested include: (1) maximizing the conformality of the dose distribution, (2) minimizing the number of shots, and (3) minimizing the dose to a sensitive structure such as the brain stem or optic chiasm.

Each optimization also includes a series of constraints. A constraint is a condition that must be satisfied in order for a solution to be considered feasible. The constraints we have tested include: (1) placing a cap on the total number of shots, (2) specifying a minimum isodose line that must surround the entire tumor volume, and (3) setting a maximum dose for each sensitive structure.

The optimizations have been performed with the assistance of GAMS [2]. GAMS, the General Algebraic Modeling System, was chosen because of its strength as a tool for efficiently performing large-scale optimizations. GAMS is an optimization tool that allows the user to easily change between a wide variety of objective functions and constraints.

During our investigation, no single mathematical approach has proven to be clearly superior to all others. As a result, we have simultaneously pursued a variety of parallel paths. The goal is to find a technique that is fast, flexible, and robust.

The optimization process cannot begin until after the stereotactic head frame has been screwed into the patient's skull and MRI or CT images have been obtained. The optimization tool must be fast, because it is not practical to have the patient wait for hours during the planning process. Our goal is develop a system that optimizes in 20 minutes or less. Flexibility is also crucial, because the technique must be able to satisfy the personal preferences of each user. The system must also be robust. A robust technique is one that produces a high quality solution for treatment volumes of all sizes and shapes. A robust technique insures a high-quality result regardless of the quality of the initial guess.

The mathematical approaches that we have tested can be split into 2 main categories:

1. migrating shots of radiation
2. precomputed shots with fixed locations

**Migrating Shots**

With the migrating shot techniques, a limited number of shots are provided to the optimizer. Each of these shots has four corresponding variables: a x-coordinate, a y-coordinate, a z-coordinate, and a relative weight. The migrating shot

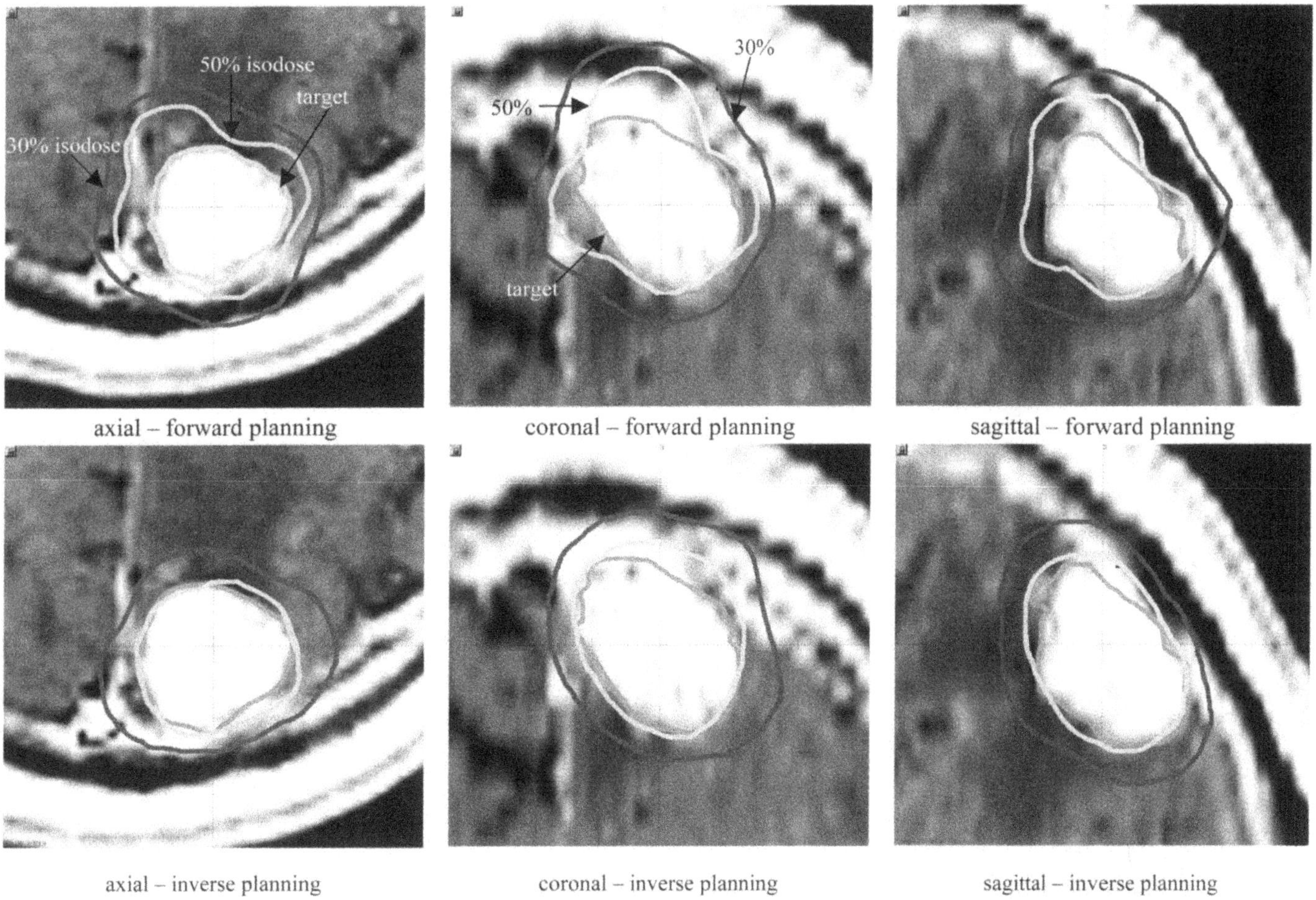


**Figure 1:** Top row: an axial, coronal, and sagittal slice from a patient's treatment plan developed using the conventional forward planning approach. Bottom row: the corresponding slices for the same patient optimized using a nonlinear programming approach . The innermost line shows the outline of the tumor. Both the 50% and 30% isodose lines surround it.

techniques have all been solved using a nonlinear programming approach.

We have tested a number of different implementations of the migrating shot approach. The simplest approach requires the user to specify both the number of shots and the size of each. This formulation provides a rapid path to an optimized solution. Unfortunately, it is difficult to predict a combination of shot sizes that will produce a conformal dose distribution. Consequently, the usefulness of this technique is limited to fine tuning an existing treatment plan.

A second migrating shot approach is to run a two-phase optimization. The first phase is used to determine an intelligent combination of shot sizes. In the second phase, an optimization is performed with the shot combination produced by the first phase. This approach can be realized by using continuous radii in the first phase of the optimization. After this optimization is complete, each radius is rounded to the closest available shot size. The second phase optimizes using the fixed shot sizes. An advantage of this approach is that the user does not need to assign the shot sizes. The disadvantage of this technique is that the rounding procedure could degrade the quality of the result particularly if the continuous radii fall midway between 2 available shot sizes.

A third migrating shot approach uses a number of shots of each shot size, but the optimization includes a constraint that limits the total number of shots. With this approach, the user does not need to specify the shot sizes. The disadvantage of this approach is that the time per iteration is increased as compared with the other migrating shot techniques. This is because the increased number of migrating shots leads to a longer dose computation time.

The primary disadvantage of the migrating shot approaches is that the dose calculation relies on the use of a nonlinear model. Consequently, there is a potential to get stuck in a local minimum. Our initial tests, however, indicate that a nonlinear programming approach can be formulated such that it produces a high quality dose distribution regardless of the initial guess.

**Precomputed Shots with Fixed Locations**

A second category of optimization techniques uses percomputed shots of radiation. With this approach, the dose

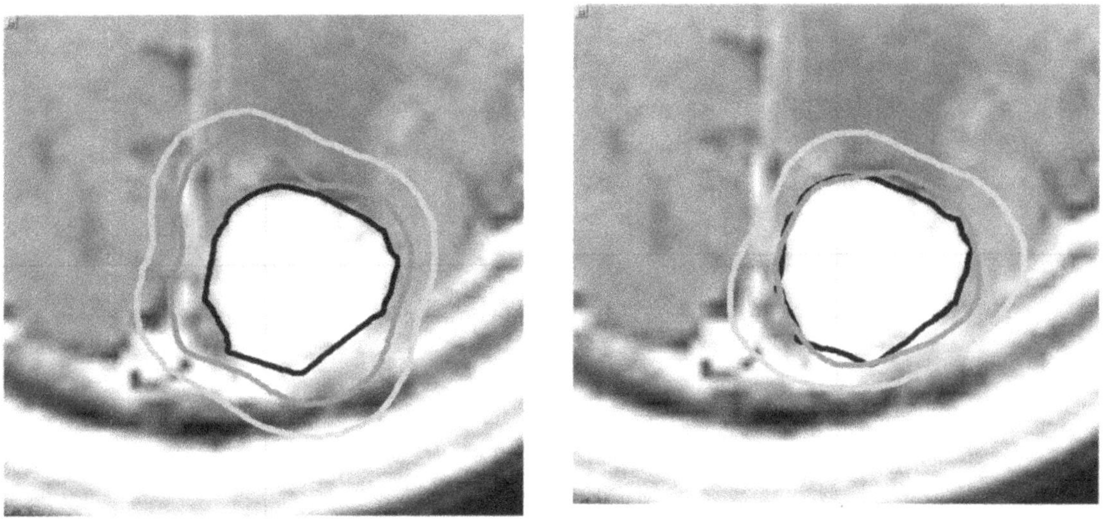

**Figure 2:** Left: an axial slice from a forward planned Gamma Knife Patient. Right: The same slice from an optimized plan produced using a nonlinear programming approach. The black line in each image is the tumor. The dark gray line is the 50% isodose line, and the light gray line is the 30% isodose line.

distributions for a very large number of shots are computed before the optimization. The location of each shot is fixed and does not move during the optimization.

With this approach, our primary focus has been on the use of a Mixed Integer Programming implementation. Mixed Integer Programming is a type of mathematical programming that permits the use of binary variables. In our case, each shot of radiation is assigned both a weight and a binary variable that indicates whether or not a shot is used. The binary variable is in essence a switch that turns a shot on or off. The sum over all of the binary variables is constrained to be less than the maximum number of allowable shots.

The primary advantage of this approach is that the dose calculation is linear in nature. This means that we can find the global minimum of the objective function. Consequently, the final result will not depend on the starting point of the optimization.

The disadvantage of this technique is that the total amount of data can become enormous. For example, imagine a treatment volume that is 4cm on each side. If we use a 1mm grid for the shot placement, the total number of precomputed shots will equal 256,000 (40x40x40x4). Consequently, there will be 256,000 dose distributions. The memory requirements for a problem of this size will exceed the capacity of most computers.

Although, the precomputed shot approach has proven successful for 2 dimensional problems, further work is necessary to make this approach practical as a clinical tool.

## Results and discussion

The top row of images in Figure 2 displays a sagittal, coronal, and transverse slice from a treatment plan developed using the conventional approach. Each image shows the tumor along with the 50% and 30% isodose line. The second row of images in Figure 2 shows the corresponding slice from a computer optimized treatment plan. The optimizer sought to maximize the conformality of the dose distribution subject to two constraints. The first constraint was that the 50% isodose line needed to surround the tumor volume, and the second constraint specified the maximum number of allowable shots. Note that a more conformal dose distribution has been obtained using an inverse planning approach.

In Figure 3, a comparison of axial slices is shown for a second patient. Again, the inverse planning system provides a more conformal result.

## Conclusion

An inverse treatment planning system has been developed for the Leksell Gamma Knife. Using a nonlinear programming approach, treatment plans have been produced for a series of patient cases. The results indicate that inverse planning can improve the consistency of care for Gamma Knife patients.

After further testing and refinement of the models, this tool should be able to produce optimized patient plans with the necessary robustness, speed, and flexibility.

## References

[1] http://www.elekta.com

[2] Brooke A, Kendrick D, and Meeraus A 1988 *GAMS: A User's Guide.* The Scientific Press, San Francisco, CA

# Heuristics for conventional planning

**Peter Dickof and Colin Ladyka**
Allan Blair Cancer Centre, 4101 Dewdney Avenue, Regina, Saskatchewan, Canada

## Introduction

Radiation therapy treatment planning is difficult in that the solution space of all treatment plans is very large, even for a relatively small number of beams. Despite this, therapy planning is a task routinely performed by humans who have been able to find reasonable, if perhaps sub-optimal, solutions. Humans have been successful because they have introduced tools which reduce both the dimensionality and range of the space of plans to be searched in such a way as to match the task to be performed with human capabilities. As examples:

- The exclusive use of coplanar beams reduces the search space and reduces many of the geometric tasks to two dimensions which humans understand better than three dimensional geometry.
- The use of parallel opposed pairs of beams (POPs) simplifies the task of obtaining dose uniformity in the target volume.
- The use of wedges allows the use of hinged pairs of beams and makes the production of dose uniformity easily understandable.
- Restricting the possible intensity distributions over the field to those produced by conceptually clear tools such as wedges, missing tissue compensators, and dose compensators.

Recent development of inverse planning has taken a much more general approach. The planning task is often specified using a solution space of very high dimensionality with a single objective function representing the goal. When this is done, the problem is so complex that even computerized search of the complete solution space is difficult.

We split this into three separate tasks with three separate solution spaces of lower dimensionality. The tasks are chosen so that humans can understand the problems to be solved and can use their visual scene recognition skills in their solution. Computerized tools are provided in areas where human skills are mismatched with the task.

## Material and methods

The three subtasks for a conventional plan require that we obtain: 1) high dose to the target region, 2) uniform dose to the target region, 3) low dose outside the target region in general and for specific organs at risk in particular.

### High dose to the target region

High dose to the target region can be obtained by ensuring that all beam hit the target - easily implemented by the choice of the target centroid as the isocentre.

### Uniform dose to the target region

Dose uniformity over some region is equivalent to stating that the dose gradient over that region is zero[9, 10, 11, 12, 7]. Sherouse showed that three parameters (wedge angle, collimator angle, and beam weight) for each of a given set of beams can be easily adjusted to minimize the dose gradient vector at a point[8] and reported that this problem is underdetermined; dose uniformity at a single point requires the solution of three simultaneous equations, but there are 3N parameters available for the N beams. This implies that there is an infinite number of essentially equivalent solutions to the problem of producing target uniformity for a given set of beams. Note also that the uniformity objective function is quasi-convex[4], since each beam's doses and dose gradient vectors at a point add linearly, thus

$$|\lambda\vec{g}_1 + (1-\lambda)\vec{g}_2| \leq \max(|\vec{g}_1|, |\vec{g}_2|). \quad (1)$$

This also implies that the region of the N-beam solution space for which the uniformity is zero is convex. It is thus not surprising that Sherouse found that "(t)he method ... induces very good dose homogeneity over the volume of crossfire of any 3D set of beams...". It is also clear that the use of a dose compensating filter can extend the region of low gradient over a relatively large volume.

We have implemented this algorithm with two minor modifications. We do not allow wedge angles other than the conventional set (0, 15, 30, 45, and 60 degrees). In addition, we allow the user to select which of the 3N parameters may vary and which are "locked". For a given iteration over all beams, the wedge and collimator angles may be modified once, then the residual gradient is used to calculate the required weight adjustment. When starting with no wedges this order ensures that the minimum wedge angle, (ie. the minimum gradient in the intensity for individual beams and thus uncertainty in the dose) tends to be used.

### Delineating the boundary

The boundary between the high dose and the low dose region is defined through the selection of appropriate beam orientations and outlines. Beam outlines are easily determined in each beam's eye view by expanding the bounds of the target volume by some adequate margin while shielding any organs at risk.

The role for beam orientation is now clear; an orientation is desirable when it allows shielding to be designed such that the boundary of the high dose and low dose region will lie between the target and any organs at risk (OARs), ie. the overlap between the target and OARs is minimized in the beam's eye view. Difficulty arises because even when the only OAR is just the non-target part of the patient, this objective function may have local minima[1]. The overlap can be assessed quickly by humans, but the beam orientation space is too large for an exhaustive search; even computerized calculation of the overlap at each point in the beam orientation space remains slow[6, 2, 5, 3]. We wish to find suitable beams without exploring the complete solution space by proposing orientations likely to be close to a local minimum.

Consider using infinite-SAD beams in the treatment of a spherical target inside a spherical patient with spherical OARs outside the target. For each OAR, draw the vector $\vec{O}_i$ from the centre of the target to the centre of the OAR. It is clear that the central axis of a beam which provides for maximum separation between the OAR and the target will lie on a plane through the centre of the target and perpendicular to $\vec{O}_i$. The direction of a non-coplanar POP of beams which maximally spares two OARs $i, j$ is then given by the cross product $\vec{B}_N = \vec{O}_i \times \pm\vec{O}_j$; an example is shown in Figure 1.

Similarly, for a cylindrical patient, beams perpendicular to a vector on the central axis of the cylinder $\vec{C}$ will spare the $i$th OAR when they are one of the coplanar POPs given by $\vec{B}_C = \vec{O}_i \times \pm\vec{C}$

Another group of potentially interesting beams are those given by $\vec{B}_A = \pm(\vec{O}_i - \vec{O}_j)$. In these cases, shielding can be given to the two aligned OARs simultaneously, at the expense of also shielding a portion of the target.

Convex shapes other than spheres are more complex because their boundaries may not lie perpendicular to the OAR vectors and concave shapes are more complex yet. Nonetheless the scheme outlined here identifies orientations likely to be close to a local minimum for a single beam.

We present the user with a list of all these beam orientations identified by their type (coplanar, non-coplanar, or aligned) and by which structures they spare. In the beam's eye view, the user can easily assess the degree of overlap of structures and also the direction of rotation required to minimize this overlap. For example, Figure 1 shows that OARs 1, 3 and 5 all overlap the target volume. It is clear that, if the current beam is rotated in the direction of the component of $\vec{O}_3$ perpendicular to the current beam, the overlap of OAR 3 will decrease. Similarly, if the rotation is defined by $-\vec{O}_1$ or $-\vec{O}_5$ components, the overlap of those OARs will decrease. We allow the user to define this tangent with the mouse; the planning system calculates the required couch and gantry angles.

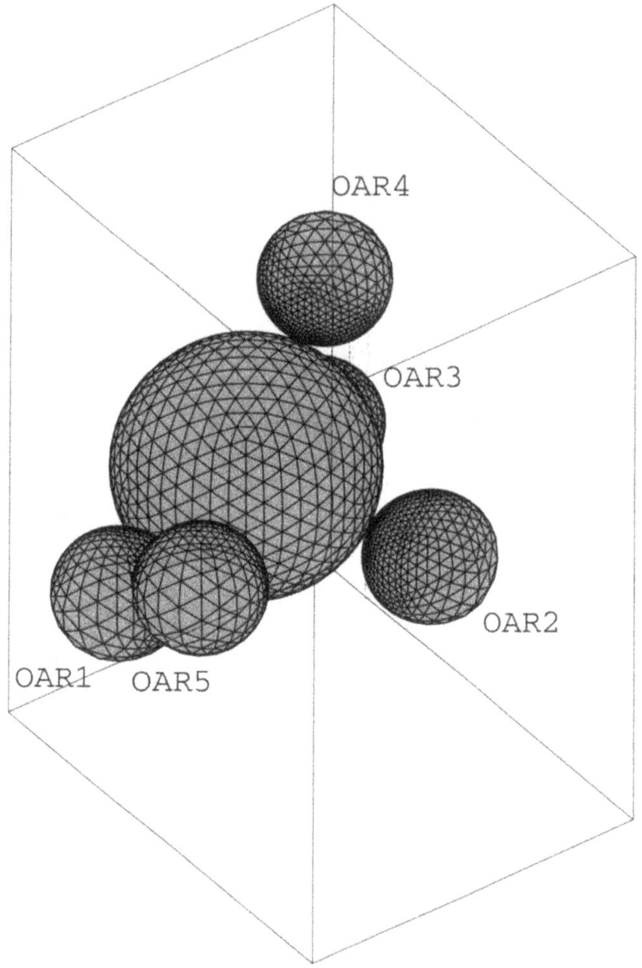


**Figure 1:** Spherical target and randomly placed touching OARs viewed from a beam's eye view where the beam's axis is perpendicular to the vectors from the target to OARs 2 & 4.

## Results and discussion

We have matched the treatment planning task to human capabilities in a number of ways:

- The three clinical goals of the conventional planning task are presented as three relatively independent operations selecting three relatively independent sets of beam parameters.
- We propose particular beam orientations to humans and identify the clinical goals (ie. which OARs would be spared) each orientation may be used to address and the strategy employed (eg. alignment of OARs to be shielded).
- Humans can quickly assess the degree of overlap of the target and OARs in the beam's-eye-view (the objective function), and also the direction of rotation required to modify these (the gradient of the objective function).

- Humans can not quickly calculate couch and gantry angles required for particular orientations; this calculation is easily performed by computer.

- Humans can not quickly perform the 3-D vector calculations required to obtain dose uniformity. The uniformity tool provides a solution within seconds. We have also observed that homogeneous solutions are easily found. We typically begin with equal beam weights and all collimator and wedge angles set to zero. After obtaining a solution providing uniformity, we set all collimator angles to the nearest of either 0 or 90 degrees (reversing wedge angles if necessary) to simplify treatment setup and search for another solution. We then outline the field boundaries and calculate the dose distribution. If we find the dose to some OAR to be too high, we identify the main contributing beams, reduce their intensity by the amount required and search for another solution. With four or five beams, solutions are quickly found at each stage.

## Conclusion

Conventional planning can, with the introduction of some extremely simple tools provide solutions which are easily found, easily understood, and easily delivered using beams with low dose gradients.

The solutions found with this scheme, even when not optimal, may well lie near optima and may provide suitable starting points for a more complete search. Orientations associated with other objective function components (eg. the principle moment of inertia for each OAR) could easily be added to the list of beams proposed.

## References

[1] Thomas Bortfeld and Wolfgang Schlegel. Optimization of beam orientations in radiation therapy: some theoretical considerations. *Physics in Medicine and Biology*, 38:291–304, 1993.

[2] George T.Y. Chen, Danny R. Spelbring, Charles A. Pelizzari, James M. Balter, Leon C. Myrianthopoulos, S. Vijayakumar, and Howard Halpern. The use of beam's eye view volumetrics in the selection of noncoplanar radiation portals. *International Journal of Radiation Oncology Biology and Physics*, 23(1):153–163, 1992.

[3] B.C.J. Cho, W.H. Roa, D. Robinson, and B. Murray. The development of target-eye-view maps for selection of coplanar or noncoplanar beams in conformal radiotherapy treatment planning. *Medical Physics*, 26(11):2367–2372, 1999.

[4] J.O. Deasy. Multiple local minima in radiotherapy optimization problems with dose-volume constraints. *Medical Physics*, 24(7):1157–1161, 1997.

[5] D.L. McShan, M.L. Kessler, and B.A. Fraass. Advanced interactive planning techniques for conformal therapy: high level beam descriptions and volumetric mapping techniques. *International Journal of Radiation Oncology Biology and Physics*, 33(5):1061–1072, 1995.

[6] L.C. Myrianthopoulos, G.T.Y. Chen, S. Vijayakumar, H.J. Halpern, D.R. Spelbring, and C.A. Pelizzari. Beam's eye view volumetrics: an aid to rapid treatment plan development and evaluation. *International Journal of Radiation Oncology, Biology, and Physics*, 23(2):367–275, 1992.

[7] George W. Sherouse. A mathematical basis for selection of wedge angle and orientation. *Medical Physics*, 20(4):1211–1218, 1993.

[8] George W. Sherouse. Dose homogenization using vector analysis of gradients. In A.R. Hounsell, J.M. Wilkinson, and P.C. Williams, editors, *Proceedings of the XIth International Conference on the Use of Computers in Radiation Therapy*, pages 248–249, 4513 Vernon Blvd, Madison, WI 53705 USA, 1994. ICCR, Medical Physics Publishing.

[9] A. Sonntag. Ein weg zur räumlichen Bestrahlungsplanung: I. Das Problem der Dosishomogenität innerhalb des Übershneidungsbereichs nichtkomplanar angeordneter Strahlenbündel, Basisuntersuchungen zu einen Optimierungsverfahren. *Strahlentherapie*, 150(5):507–520, 1975.

[10] A. Sonntag. Ein weg zur räumlichen Bestrahlungsplanung: II. Vektorielle Darstellung de räumlichen Dosisverteilung in einzelnen Strahlenbündel und erste Folgerungen für die Praxis. *Strahlentherapie*, 150(6):569–578, 1975.

[11] A. Sonntag. Ein weg zur räumlichen Bestrahlungsplanung: III. Näheres über das Verfahren zur Erzielung von Dosishomogenität bei nichtkomplanaren Strahlenbündelanordnungen und dessen experimentelle Überprüfung. *Strahlentherapie*, 151(1):10–25, 1976.

[12] A. Sonntag. Ein weg zur räumlichen Bestrahlungsplanung: IV. Beispiele aus der strahlentherapeutischen Praxis und Schlussfolgerungen". *Strahlentherapie*, 151(1):26–46, 1976.

# Hyperion - An integrated IMRT planning tool

**M. Alber, M. Birkner, W. Laub and F. Nüsslin**
Abteilung für Medizinische Physik, Universitätsklinikum Tübingen, D-72076 Tübingen

## Introduction

The IMRT planning process poses problems beyond conventional planning, and as yet not all confounding factors have been fully understood or countermeasures devised. It may thus be argued that the most prominent feature of IMRT software is its capacity for development.

We present a treatment planning system that is both modular and comprehensive in its design, which is centered around two features: evidence-based biological modelling and Monte Carlo dose computation. The aim of the biological objective modelling is to give both a high level of decision making support and control to the planner, at the same time safeguarding against hazardous dose levels to normal tissue. The Monte Carlo methods offers the flexibility to accomodate various types of beam modulation techniques to the same dose computation engine. This paper gives the details of the optimisation kernel and the beam modifier modules.

## Material and methods

The planning process is divided into two stages. The first stage permits user interference by the redefinition of the objectives and is designed for speed. The second stage translates fluence profiles into intensity modulation equipment parameters and is designed for precision, but does not allow user interference. Although both stages use the same optimisation algorithm, the set of optimisation parameters, constraints and the dose computation engine are different.

In the first stage, the necessary organs are defined. Each organ carries a set of complication measures which can be both predefined (from a data base) and user defined. These complication measures $g_i$ are tantamount to an iso-effective homogeneous dose (i.e equivalent damage) to a reference volume [1]. If so desired, physical constraints such as quadratic overdose penalties or DVH constraints may be used. For the quadratic penalties, the constraints are defined as the root mean square dose to that volume. Contrary to physical dose constraints, the biological constraints are specific to the volume effect of certain complications. In addition to the complications, organs contain information about inter- and intrafractional movement, margin generation and scatter cross-section data for Monte Carlo dose computation.

A special class of 'organ' are the target volumes which define the objective function. The objective function $f(\Phi)$ as a function of fluence $\Phi$ is the probability of clonogenic cell survival in the target volumes. Alternatively, quadratic underdosage penalties can be used. The optimisation follows the strategy to deliver the maximum feasible total dose under the constraints given. It is subject to three types of constraints:

- *biological constraints* are defined as organ and complication specific score functions. The user defines the maximum score for the given complication with the help of a data base.
- *hard physical constraints* are imposed by limitations of the treatment equipment, e.g. the minimum transmission or minimum inter-leaf distance. These constraints are peculiar to the chosen treatment modality and cannot be influenced by the user.
- *soft physical constraints* are intended to yield more practical fluence profiles, yet do not stipulate a certain condition if the cost in terms of target volume dose becomes too high. These constraints aim to minimise total beam-on times or shape the beams more expedient for verification. The user can specify the maximum cost they are willing to pay for these features.

These constraints are dealt with in different ways. Since they are taken into account by means of a restricted optimisation problem, there are no user-defined weights. If the user chooses to interfere with the optimisation, the biological maximum scores $c_i$ can be changed during the first stage of the optimisation.

The biological optimisation problem is transformed into an unrestricted problem by:

$$\max_{\lambda_i} \quad \min_\Phi \ \{f(\Phi) + \textstyle\sum_i \lambda_i \ (g_i(\Phi) - c_i)\}$$

$$\text{for} \quad \begin{cases} \lambda_i = 0 & : \quad g_i(\Phi) < c_i \\ \lambda_i > 0 & : \quad g_i(\Phi) \geq c_i \end{cases} .$$

The optimisation parameter $\Phi$ is the vector of all fluence elements, here defined on a regular grid for a given set of beam directions. The Lagrange parameters $\lambda_i$ are determined with a first-order update rule,

$$\lambda_i^{k+1} = \lambda_i^k \frac{(g_i^{-1})'(c_i)}{(g_i^{-1})'(g_i(\Phi^k))} \tag{1}$$

where $\Phi^k$ is the solution of the minimisation for the $k$-th vector of Lagrange parameters $\lambda^k$. The first iteration of the multiplier-update loop starts with $\lambda_i = 1$ for all $i$.

The physical constraints are defined in treatment equipment modules. These modules define constraints which assert that the fluence matrix is feasible with respect to some restrictions of the given equipment. This can be a relative minimum fluence constraint, i.e. the minimum fluence may not fall below a fixed fraction of the maximum fluence. For dynamic MLCs, it is an absolute minimum fluence constraint and constraints on the fluence gradient. Common to these constraints is, that they are all convex, i.e. do certainly not lead to local optimal solutions. They are taken into account by a penalty term whose weight factor goes to infinity with the number of iterations.

One soft physical constraint common to all modules acts as a 'noise filter'. This constraint aims to minimise the surface defined by the fluence distribution across the beam. This feature leads to shorter beam-on times for MLC techniques and less rugged compensators. A compensator/static MLC hybrid module allows to define the maximum thickness of the compensator as a soft constraint; modulations with greater amplitude are accomplished by delivering the field in subfields similar to the static MLC technique. This module allows to specify the maximum number of subfields as soft constraints. Common to all soft constraints is a treatment similar to the biological constraints with the difference, that the Lagrange multipliers $\kappa_j$ are adjusted with respect to the loss in total target dose incurred by these constraints, i.e. the optimisation starts with $\kappa_j = 0$ .

With these constraints, the first optimisation stage results in a fluence distribution which is feasible with respect to most practical limitations. The dose computation in stage one is a fast finite-size pencil beam algorithm with longitudinal density correction and lateral scatter. The optimisation is performed with a conjugate gradient algorithm and takes between 3 and 30 minutes on a 400MHz Pentium II PC with up to $10^4$ parameters on a $(3mm)^3$ dose grid.

The second stage of the optimisation is a refinement of the previously obtained fluence profiles with Monte Carlo dose computation. The compensator/static MLC hybrid module involves a translation of fluence profiles into field outlines and compensator thicknesses. Contrary to the first stage, the module now defines a projection operator in addition to the hard constraint. The translator acts as a projection operator in dose space rather than fluence space, i.e. the fluence is not projected onto a feasible fluence, but the dose distribution, which was found to solve the optimisation problem, is projected onto a Monte Carlo computed dose. The module can also alter the optimisation parameter space, i.e. deactivate, cluster or create new fluence elements. New fluence elements can be created which consist of clustered pencil beams to represent the static sub-fields. The biological constraints stay active and are handled the same way as during the first stage of the optimisation.

The second stage can be seen as computing small fluence updates on the basis of a feasible, Monte Carlo computed dose, such that a converging sequence of 'verification' dose distributions is constructed. The rationale for this separation of stages is the reduction of Monte Carlo computation time to the absolute minimum.

With a fast Monte Carlo code such as XVMC [3], computation times of around one hour on a PC can be achieved.

## Results and discussion

Independent of the use of biological or physical constraints, total user planning times can be substantially shortened due to the absence of user adjusted weights. Since all objectives are stated in units of dose (Gy) or per cent (damage or volume), they are intuitively accessible. If objectives have to be adjusted, the Lagrange multiplier value indicates the impact of the constraint onto the result, so that the effect of the change can be assessed a priori. The particular advantages of the biological objectives are demonstrated elsewhere [4].

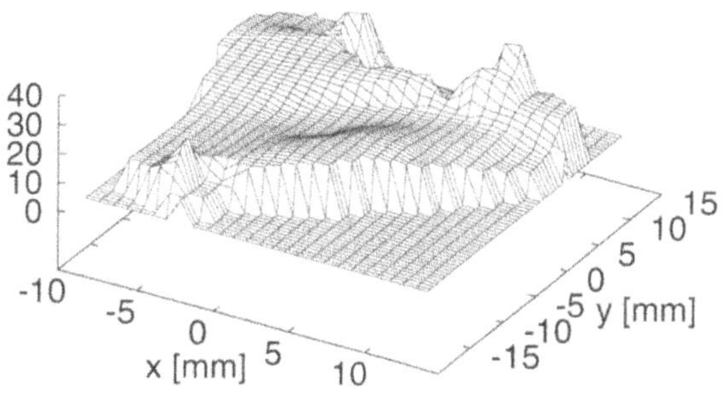


**Figure 1:** An intensity distribution optimised with Monte Carlo dose computation (here: EGS4) under certain constraints for the dMLC technique and a soft smoothing constraint. The peaks correspond to the positions of the sinuses, where dose loss due to the breakdown of secondary electron equilibrium is compensated for by primary fluence. The MLC was not included into the Monte Carlo computation

As compared to the a posteriori projection of fluence distributions onto equipment parameters the inclusion of the equipment constraints can sometimes lead to a reduction of beam-on times of 60 per cent. In many cases, the solution space allows sufficient freedom to find a feasible solution without relevant loss in target dose. (The iso-effective doses to the organs at risk would not change). One advantage of this technique is, that the dose to the organs at risk is under control at all times, so that the translation into equipment parameters cannot accidentially result in hot spots.

The two figures are taken from a stereotactic treatment case where the target volume is adjacent to the sinuses. One profile, shown in figure 1, was optimised with the dMLC constraints in place (yet without sequencing); the peaks in the profile correspond to the position of the sinuses and the nasal cavity and were not present in the Pencil Beam optimised plan. This is due to the incapability of the algorithm to compute lateral electron transport at low density surfaces and dose re-buildup effects. The Monte Carlo dose computation picked up these effects and compensated for the dose loss by an increased primary fluence form other directions.

Figure 2 shows the same field as a lead compensator which was restricted to 3 cm thickness.

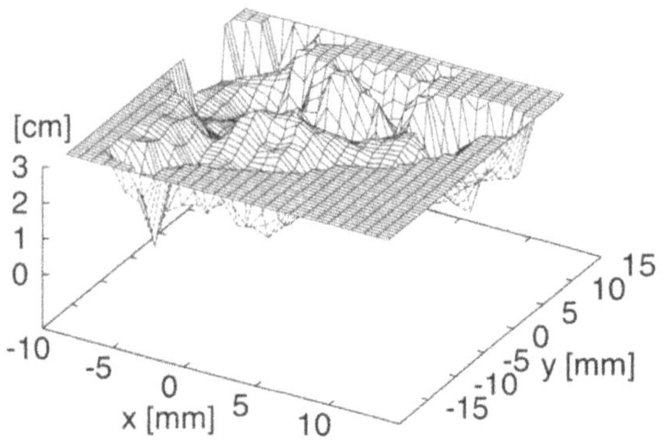


**Figure 2:** For the same field as in figure 1, a compensator is shown which was optimised to be at most 3 cm thick. Radiation transport through the compensator was modelled with a Monte Carlo algorithm during optimisation

## Conclusion

The great number of effects and constraints which have to be taken into account for IMRT optimisation makes it difficut to handle all at once. Furthermore, with a choice of treatment techniques which pose different problems in terms of practicality, the optimisation algorithm must have a high degree of flexibility. These considerations lead to the development of a modular architecture, which offers the possibility to link to a biological data base, compare different treatment techniques and use Monte Carlo dose computation for optimisation. To reduce total computation and user planning times, it is expedient to split the planning process into a fast stage which concentrates on the treatment objectives, and an unsupervised second stage, which centers around accurate dose computation and delivery. Although so far only one module, a compensator/static MLC hybrid technique, has been fully implemented, the design is flexible enough to accomodate the more intricate MLC techniques.

## References

[1] Alber M and Nüsslin F 1999 An objective function for radiation treatment optimization based on local biological measures *Phys. Med. Biol.* **44** 479–493

[2] Alber M and Nüsslin F Intensity modulated photon beams subject to a minimal surface smoothness constraint *submitted to Phys. Med. Biol.*

[3] Fippel M 1999 Fast Monte Carlo dose calculation for photon beams based on the VMC electron algorithm *Med. Phys.* **26** 1466–1475

[4] Birkner M , Alber M , Laub W and Nüsslin F Hyperion - An IMRT expert system *in this compilation*

# ORBIT: Optimization of Radiation therapy Beams by Iterative Techniques, a new optimization code

**Johan Löf, Bengt K Lind and Anders Brahme**

Medical Radiation Physics, Karolinska Institutet and Stockholm University, P.O. Box 260, S-171 76 Stockholm, Sweden

## Introduction

A new object oriented optimization code dedicated to radiotherapy optimization problems, has been developed. The philosophy of the program is to provide a framework for solving the very wide range of optimization problems encountered in treatment planning. The main design objectives has been to create a code that is possible maintain over a longer time span and that is easily extendible when new scientific problems need to be solved. Orbit is capable of handling complex optimization problems such as simultaneous optimization of intensity modulation and beam directions.

## Material and methods

Orbit consists of five main modules that are responsible for handling different aspects of the radiotherapeutic optimization process. The separation between these modules is strict and inter-communication take place via well defined interfaces. The module ***Machine*** is used to capture the physical characteristics and capabilities of the treatment unit. There may be several different machines involved in the treatment of a single patient. The ***Treatment technique*** module contains a description of the treatment in terms of specific settings of the available free parameters that control the treatment machine. Given a set of machine parameters, the *Treatment* module uses the associated *Machine* to produce the resulting irradiation of the patient. The quantity used to describe the irradiation depends on the type of treatment. For instance, in the case of an external beam this quantity is the energy fluence differential in energy and angle. A subset of the machine parameters may be registered for optimization and these are varied by the optimizer to obtain the best possible treatment. The ***Patient*** module provides a three-dimensional model of the patient, including it's anatomy and radiobiological characteristics of defined target volumes and organs at risk. For a given irradiation, the ***Dose*** component computes the resulting dose distribution in the patient. The optimization process itself is driven by the ***Optimization*** module which handles objective functions, constraints, decision variables and optimization algorithms. While utilizing the other components, the *Optimization* engine varies the decision variables, i.e. the free clinical parameters that have been defined in the *Treatment* component, iteratively in order to extremize the selected objective function while keeping the constraints that may be present in the problem formulation satisfied.

Several different objective functions have been implemented in Orbit. One set consists of the biological measures that describe the probability to achieve tumor control, the probability to cause normal tissue complications, and combinations of these such as the probability for complication free tumor control $(P_+)$[1] or the expectation value thereof $(\mathbf{E}P_+)$[2, 3, 4]. The purpose of considering the expectation value of the objective function is to be able to explicitly account for uncertainties that may be present due to organ motion, setup errors and variations in patient sensitivity. Another set constitutes the physical objective functions where one can directly define dose levels for the relevant structures and specify whether the desired dose should be less than, equal to, in between, or greater than these levels. It is also possible to specify explicit constraints, for example one might want to maximize $P_+$ while keeping the normal tissue complication probability below a certain level. Any of the implemented objective functions can also serve as a constraints and vice versa. Thanks to the object oriented design, new objective functions can easily be added.

## Results and discussion

In order to illustrate some of the capabilities of the present code, it is here first applied to a hypothetical two-dimensional cervix case to demonstrate the robustness of the beam direction optimization algorithm and then to a fully three-dimensional prostate case where the clinical importance of optimal beam direction selection is shown as well as the flexibility in specifying various objective functions and constraints.

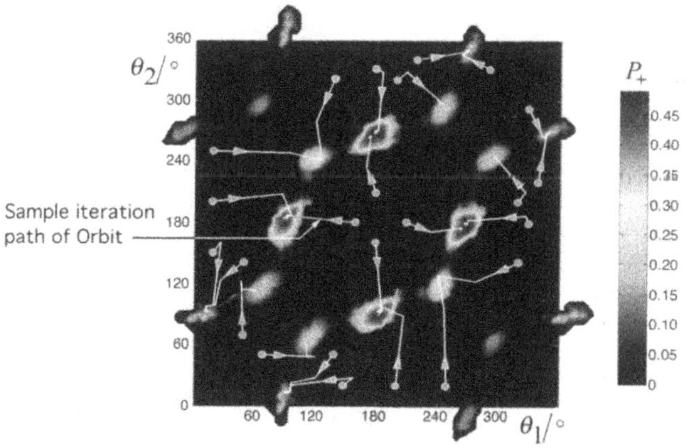


**Figure 1:** Map of optimal $P_+$ values for treatments using two intensity modulated beams with directions $\theta_1$ and $\theta_2$. Also shown are a few iteration paths for different starting points, that are denoted by a circle.

Figure 1 shows the variation of the optimal $P_+$ value with all coplanar 2-beam combinations for a cervix-like case that has a very complex concave target volume. Each point in this diagram corresponds to the maximum $P_+$ value that can be obtained with two fully intensity modulated beams whose angles of incidence are $\theta_1$ and $\theta_2$ respectively. It is seen that most beam configurations are of poor clinical value as there are large areas in the diagram that correspond to $P_+ = 0$. However, there are a few islands that correspond to higher values of $P_+$ and the problem is to find those beam directions without having to try every combination, as has been done to produce this diagram. Orbit is able to optimize beam directions simultaneously to any other beam variable that is subject to optimization, in this case the fluence profiles. In Figure 1 is also illustrated for a few different starting angles how this algorithm can locate a local optimum. Since there are only a few local optima, the global maximum is found by trying a number of starting angles. Automating the process of searching through the phasespace for the global optima is work in progress. It should be emphasized that the direction optimization algorithm is completely independent of the information produced by the exhaustive search (otherwise it would have been quite useless!), and this diagram has been made only to illustrate the workings of the algorithm. In Figure 2, four snap shots of the iterative process are shown. The initial gantry angles, $\theta_1 = 180°$ and $\theta_1 = 160°$ , are quite unfavorable since the beams enter through the sensitive critical structure rectum. Despite of this, the algorithm is able to separate the two beams and reach the global optimum at $P_+ = 51\%$.

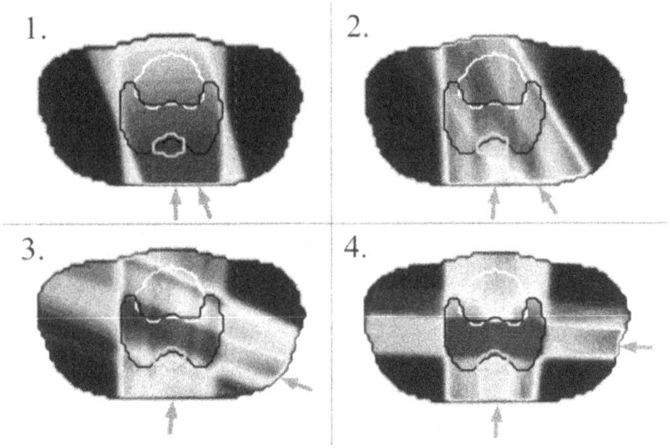


**Figure 2:** The dose distribution at four instances during simultaneous intensity modulation and beam direction optimization. These snapshots are taken along the iteration path that is indicated in Figure 1.

Next we apply the program to a clinical prostate case. Here the target volumes and critical structures have been defined in Pinnacle. After the initial beam setup has been made, Orbit is called from within Pinnacle and the optimization process can be followed in Pinnacle's ordinary visualization windows as the dose distribution and gantry angles etc. are updated after each iteration. Figure 3 shows a 7-field plan where both the beam directions and the intensity modulation has been optimized using $P_+$. As desired, the resulting dose distribution conforms very tightly to the internal target volume and spares the surrounding normal tissues well. The adjustments that the algorithm has made to the initial beam directions are shown as arrows in the figure. An important issue to address is how the treatment outcome varies with the number of intensity modulated beams[5,6]. The variation of $P_+$ with the number of beam portals is shown in Figure 4. In the lower curve the beams have been intensity modulated, but the gantry angles were manually preselected and kept fixed during the optimization. Quite expectedly there is an overall increase of $P_+$ with the number of beams. However, for badly chosen directions with parallel opposed beams, $P_+$ may even decrease locally (see for example the 6-field plan). The upper curve shows the results when the beam directions are subject to optimization in addition to the intensity modulation. This function is of course monotonically increasing and we see also that for lower number of beam portals the beam directions play a significant role. For nine beams, the equidistantly distributed beams give almost as good result as with optimized directions.

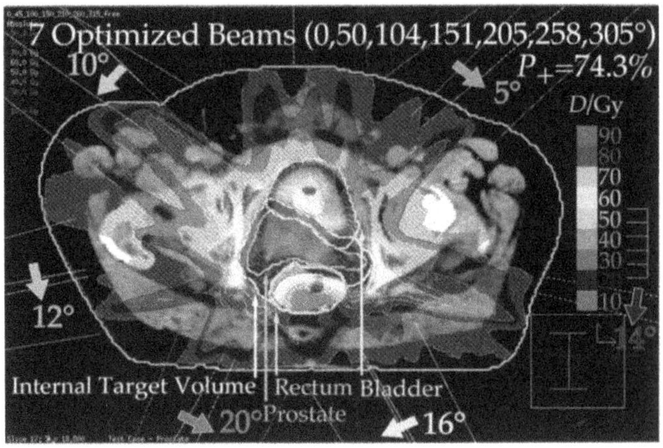


**Figure 3:** The dose distribution for a prostate case treated with seven beams for which the intensity modulation and coplanar orientations are simultanously optimized.

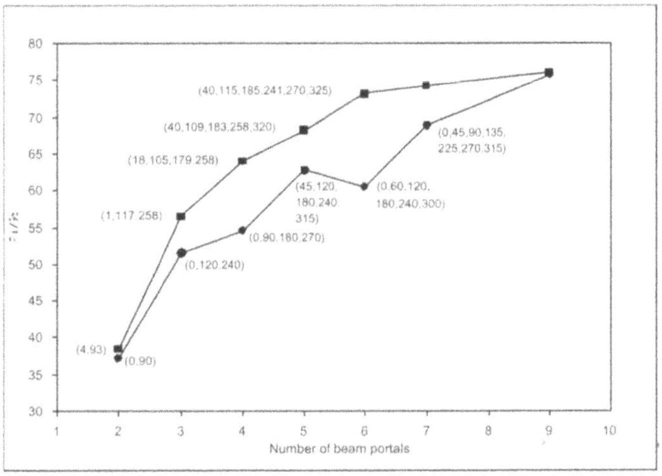


**Figure 4:** $P_+$ as a function of the number of intensity modulated beams. The solid circles show the results for fixed beam directions and the solid squares for optimized directions

Sometimes it is useful to be able to state explicitly upper limits on the acceptable risk of radiation induced injuries, for example when the clinical endpoints of tumor cure and the considered complications are incommensurable quantities. As an example, a 3-field plan for the prostate case results in a quite high risk of severe complications of the rectum (see Table 1). The case is rerun, but now with the constraint that the probability of complication in the rectum can't exceed 5%. This goal is achieved in the new plan but at the cost of higher complication risk in the small bowel and lower probability of tumor control.

| | Small bowel | Rectum | Bladder | ITV | Prostate |
|---|---|---|---|---|---|
| Unconstrained, $P_+ = 56{,}7\%$, gantry = (0, 117, 258°) | | | | | |
| $P_B, P_I$ / % | 13,3 | 10,4 | 0,6 | 85,8 | 96,1 |
| $P_I$(Rectum) ≤ 5%, $P_+ = 53{,}2\%$, gantry = (0, 115, 254°) | | | | | |
| $P_B, P_I$ / % | 14,1 | 5,0 | 0,6 | 80,2 | 95,2 |

**Table 1:** Response statistics for unconstrained and constrained optimization of a 3-field plan. Note that the beam angles are different for the two cases.

Finally we will illustrate how Orbit can be applied to physical optimization as well. In Figure 5 we see the dose distribution for a 5-field plan optimized with a least-squares objective function. The goal was to deliver 80 Gy to the ITV as uniformly as possible without causing excessive damage to the neighboring tissues. The relative standard deviation of the dose in the Prostate is 2.5% and 4% in the ITV. For comparison, the $P_+$-value was evaluated for this plan and the result was 39,8%. The corresponding value when $P_+$ *drives* the optimization process is 66,1%. The difference is due to the fact that the biological model allows for and utilizes inhomogeneous dose in the target.

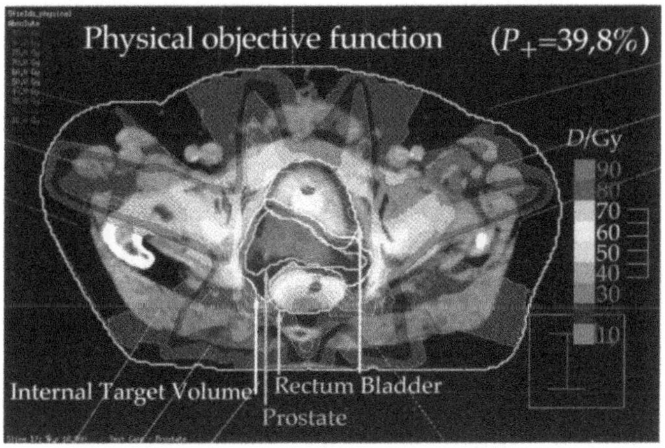


**Figure 5:** Prostate case treated with five equidistantly spaced intensity modulated beams. The objective function is least squares.

## Conclusions

It has been shown that Orbit can handle a number of difficult optimization problems in radiation therapy and its design makes it ideal to meet future challenges.

## References

[1] Källman P, Ågren A-K and Brahme A 1992 Tumor and normal tissue responses to fractionated nonuniform dose delivery *Int. J. Radiat. Biol.* **62** 249-62

[2] Löf J, Lind B K and Brahme A 1995 Optimal radiation beam profiles considering the stochastic process of patient positioning in fractionated radiation therapy *Inverse Problems* **11** 1189-209

[3] Löf J, Lind B K and Brahme A 1998 An adaptive control algorithm for optimization of intensity modulated radiotherapy considering uncertainties in beam profiles, patient set-up and internal organ motion *Phys. Med. Biol.* **43** 1605-28

[4] Kåver G, Lind B K, Löf J, Liander A and Brahme A 1999 Stochastic optimization of intensity modulated radiotherapy to account for uncertainties in patient sensitivity *Phys. Med. Biol.* **44** 2955-69

[5] Mohan R, Ling CC, Stein J, et al: 1996 The number of beams in intensity-modulated treatments (letter to the editor) *Int. J Radiat Oncol Biol Phys.* **34** 758-759

[6] Söderström S, Brahme A 1996 Small is beautiful-and often enough (letter to the editor) *Int. J Radiat Oncol Biol Phys.* **34** 757-758

# The Effect of PTV Size on PTV Dose Homogeneity

**Steven M. Morrill, J.E. Bayouth and Robin L. Kendall**

University of Texas Medical Branch, Dept. of Radiation Oncology, Galveston, TX

## Introduction

The Nomos CORVUS[1] System is a clinically-accepted method for IMRT treatment planning. Its dose calculation algorithm uses finite-area pencil beams with typical areas[2] of either 1 $cm^2$ (1 X 1), 2 $cm^2$ (1 X 2), or 0.5 $cm^2$ (0.5 X 1). In our particular system, a Siemen's PRIMART[3] linear accelerator using step and shoot static fields, we have selected a pencil beam area of 1 $cm^2$. For our optimization parameters, a pencil beam area of 1 $cm^2$ typically leads to 20 – 80 treatment segments. A smaller pencil beam area leads to better conformation with the given Planning Target Volume (PTV) and better PTV dose homogeneity, but also results in a larger number of beam segments generated by the inverse treatment plan optimization. The purpose of this investigation is to characterize the limitations of a 1 $cm^2$ pencil beam area by investigating the PTV dose homogeneity as a function of the size (diameter) of a given PTV.

## Material and methods

To investigate the dependence of PTV dose homogeneity as a function of PTV size, we generated a simplified geometry with a minimum number of confounding influences. An artificial PTV in the shape of a right circular cylinder was generated and placed near the center of a head and neck CT image set. PTV diameters were chosen to cover a range of PTV sizes that would involve additional pencil beams in the potential solution space. The set of PTV diameters included 7 diameters in the range of 2.0 – 6.0 cm (see Table1). The length of the PTV was fixed at 3.5 cm, which restricted the PTV to a portion of the skull having approximately a constant cross-sectional area. To minimize the confounding influences of conflicting optimization goals, the PTV was the only specific structure involved in the optimization. In this ideal scenario, the optimization parameters suggested by the manufacturer were used. They included the following constraints:

| | |
|---|---|
| PTV doses: | (minimum–47.5 Gy, maximum–55 Gy, 5% volume underdose allowed) |
| Tissue doses: | (minimum – 0 Gy, maximum – 50 Gy, no volume over dose), |

with an emphasis on meeting the PTV constraints. The treatment space was defined as 5 equally spaced fields at the vertices of an inverted pentagon. There were 5 intensity levels allowed for each pencil beam. Since there were no conflicting organ or structure constraints, this physical setup should give the best PTV dose homogeneity with some sacrifice in PTV dose conformity (i.e. the high dose region could extend slightly beyond the PTV borders).

## Results and discussion

The dose homogeneity data was extracted from the PTV dose-volume histogram (dvh) and is tabulated in Table 1. The PTV diameter, PTV dose range, and dose range for 5%-95% volumes of the PTV are shown. The 5%-95% volume was included because it corresponds directly to the PTV optimization constraints. It is obvious that there is a periodic nature to the solutions. Even in this idealized case, there is a difference of more than 4 Gy in the PTV dose homogeneity and a 1 Gy difference in the 5%-95% volume dose range as a function of the PTV diameter. Although a 2% difference (1 Gy) may seem minimal, this is a lower limit and realistic cases with conflicting constraints would be higher. With dose escalation using IMRT, a 2% effect could also become more significant. It should also be noted that the PTV dose range varies from 15% to 24%. Even in this idealized case, this is a large PTV dose inhomogeneity which would usually be considered unacceptable in conventional clinical cases.

The periodic nature of this data is illustrated in Figure 1 for the PTV 5%-95% volume dose range. Uncertainites are estimated from multiple optimization trials for a given PTV diameter. In this ideal situation, it appears as if the increase in the PTV 5%-95% volume dose range is linear with respect to the overlap with the outermost pencil beam.

| PTV Diameter (Gy) | PTV Dose Range (Gy) | 5-95%volume Dose Range (Gy) |
|---|---|---|
| 2.0 | 7.5 | 3.8 |
| 3.0 | 11.8 | 4.8 |
| 3.6 | 8.8 | 4.5 |
| 4.0 | 9.0 | 4.2 |
| 4.4 | 9.5 | 3.8 |
| 5.0 | 8.6 | 4.2 |
| 6.0 | 9.5 | 4.8 |

**Table 1:** Dose homogeneity parameters for the given PTV diameters

For this particular study, there is a correlation between the PTV size and the quality of the resulting solution. It also places a lower limit on the expected PTV dose range which can be achieved using this CORVUS system with 1 $cm^2$ pencil beams. This dose volume inhomogeneity can be reduced using smaller pencil beams, but only at the cost of approximately doubling the number of treatment segments.[4] This is clinically unacceptable for our static field technique.

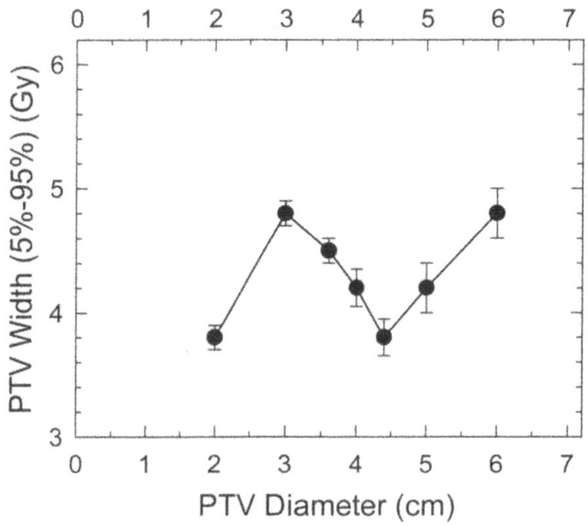


**Figure 1:** PTV dvh width as a function of PTV diameter.

## Conclusion

There is a correlation between the quality of the optimized solution and the PTV diameter using 1 $cm^2$ pencil beams. In our idealized case, a match between the PTV diameter and the 1 $cm^2$ pencil beams can reduce the width of the cumulative dose-volume histogram (dvh) by over 4 Gy (8%) and the width of the dvh 5%-95% range by 1 Gy (2%). These are lower limits since non-ideal cases will have confounding influences to degrade the solution.

## References

[1]CORVUS v3.0, Nomos Corporation, Sewickley, PA, USA.
[2]Larsen, S., Nomos Corporation, personal communication.
[3]Siemens Medical Systems, Inc., Concord, CA, USA.
[4]Larsen, S., Nomos Corporation, personal communication.

# Integration of the KonRad inverse planning tool into the iSis3D treatment planning system.

**Spiridon Papatheodorou[1], Luc Diot[1], Carsten Schulze[2], Geneviève Gaboriaud, Dominique Pontvert and Jean-Claude Rosenwald[1]**

[1]Institut Curie, Département de radiothérapie, Paris, France and [2]MRC Systems GmbH, Heidelberg, Germany

## Introduction

The purpose of this work was to integrate into a modern 3D treatment planning system the software tools that allow to implement radiotherapy with intensity-modulated beams (IMRT), based on the inverse method of treatment design and using a multileaf collimation system operating in the dynamic mode.

## Material and methods

In conventional forward planning, a given beam arrangement is used in order to produce a dose distribution that best meets the clinical goals. The treatment fields are set up manually and their parameters are modified by a trial and error procedure. Although such procedures may be adequate for simple planning problems, they are time-consuming and can be sub-optimal for difficult planning problems. Inverse planning, on the other hand, offers the possibility of automatically optimizing a number of parameters available for modification in conformal radiotherapy. KonRad[1] is an inverse planning tool for treatment planning with intensity modulated photon beams. This module considers a large number of pencil beams and seeks the best set of weights for these beams[1]. Thus, the output of the optimization is the intensity modulation pattern for each beam.

Converting the intensity modulation profiles to a leaf motion plan for practical delivery with dynamic collimators is a second software module. The software modules that perform this task are often called "leaf sequencing programs", "segmentation programs" or "interpreters"[1, 3, 5, 7, 8]. The purpose of such programs is to prepare the best MLC sequence so that the delivered fluence is as close as possible to the desired one. Other objectives, such as the minimization of the total beam-on time or the minimization of the overall treatment time are also considered. In our case we have used our home-made leaf sequencing program[5] that calculates the leaf trajectories, for practical delivery of the desired intensity, using the sliding window technique[7]. In this program, it is possible to correct for tongue-and-groove effects and, partially, for the transmission through leaves and the effect of rounded leaf tips.

Then, there is the need for a final "forward planning" step, which is the calculation of the dose distribution that will result when a particular arrangement of intensity modulated beams is applied to the patient. The purpose of the final dose calculation is to achieve good accuracy taking into account phenomena such as the leaf transmission and leaf penumbra, the variation of the output according to the collimator opening during the dynamic irradiation etc. In order to perform this task, the existing primary-scatter separation dose model had to be extended to account for intensity modulation generated by a dynamic multileaf collimator [4]. Therefore, a third software module, that calculates the expected (or generated) fluence corresponding to a given MLC sequence has been integrated.

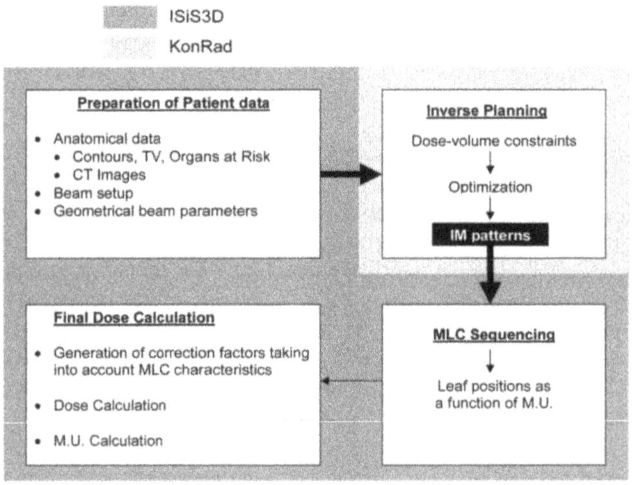


**Figure 1:** Integration of the KonRad add-on tool for IMRT Planning into the iSis3D treatment planning system.

## Results

All the above software modules and algorithm modifications have been integrated into the iSis3D[2] treatment planning system. The IMRT planning procedure was then applied for a study of a complex clinical brain tumor case, for which a 3D conformal radiotherapy plan already existed and has been used as a reference. Although the 3DCRT represents an improvement in comparison with previous "classic" non-conformal radiotherapy approaches, there are still some major difficulties with 3DCRT. In the example examined here, the shape of the PTV was concave and in proximity to the organs at risk. The normal tissue around the target volume presented limited tolerance. Such problems can be partially solved using a great number of beams and/or using non-coplanar beams. However in many cases (e.g. head) many beam entries are forbidden and the verification of non-coplanar beams by

[1] KonRad is developed at Deutches Krebsforschungszentrum (DKFZ), Heidelberg and commercialized by MRC Systems GmbH, Heidelberg, Germany.

[2] iSis3D is developed at Institut Curie, Paris and commercialized by Technologie Diffusion, Paris, France.

portals is not easy. Those constraints obliged an experienced physicist to perform a "manual" optimization of the available beam parameters. The limitations of 3DCRT justify the exploration of more complicated treatment methods. We made the hypothesis that for such tumors IMRT should allow to achieve a homogeneous dose distribution in PTV while sparing normal tissue around it.

**A study with a 5-field plan for brain tumor**

In the clinical example examined here, the target volume is a parasellar meningioma situated in the central-left part of the brain. The patient should receive post operative radiotherapy with a dose prescription of 54 Gy to the isocenter and a PTV dose ranging from 51Gy (Min PTV dose) to 57Gy (Max PTV dose).

Prior to starting the KonRad IMRT tool, the iSis3D treatment planning system is used to import patient images, contour normal anatomy and the target volume and position treatment fields. For the generation of the CT study, the patient was immobilized in the supine position using a thermoplastic mask. A total of 120 CT slices, 2.5mm thick (1mm close to the reference plane), have been used. The appreciation of the tumor extent has been facilitated by image fusion with MRI images and the injection of contrast material. The target delineation included the CTV (tumor volume/meningioma) and the PTV which is calculated by the application of a 3mm isotropic margin around the CTV. A number of organs at risk have also been outlined: brain stem, chiasm, cerebellum, temporal lobes, eyes, teeth, thyroid etc.

Then five equispaced coplanar beams have been set defining the beam entry angles and the beam energy. Information about the beam aperture shape does not need to be defined at this point since it is automatically optimized during the inverse planning phase. Then the control is handed over to KonRad where the planner can define clinical parameters such as the dose prescription to the target volume, the target volume dose heterogeneity constraints the maximum doses for the organs at risk and dose-volume constraints for the healthy structures (table I). A detailed description of the dose distribution optimization using KonRad is presented by Bortfeld et al and Preiser et al.[2, 6]

| Organ | Dose [Gy] | Volume [%] |
|---|---|---|
| Target Volume | 51 (min) | - |
| | 57 (max) | - |
| Brain Stem | 52 (max) | - |
| | 40 | 5 |
| | 30 | 10 |
| Right Temp. Lobe | 55 (max) | - |
| | 50 | 10 |
| | 40 | 20 |
| Chiasm | 55 (max) | - |
| | 50 | 5 |

**Table 1:** Maximum and minimum doses for the target volume and organs at risk as well as dose-volume constraints applied to the critical structures for the optimization of the dose distributions

Once KonRad has completed the generation of the intensity modulation matrices the user returns to iSis3D and generates the leaf motion plans for practical delivery of the desired intensity modulation with dynamic collimators[5]. At this point the computer files (DMLC files) that specify the leaf trajectories, i.e. the leaf positions as a function of the monitor units, are created and stored.

Then a 3D forward dose calculation is performed (figure 2). In our case, the final planning calculation is performed after the MLC sequence has been calculated and particularly using the information of the leaf motion plan in order to take into account the mechanical and dosimetric properties of the MLC. This information is taken directly from the computer files (DMLC files) that are used for controlling the MLC motion during the dynamic irradiation. The final planning dose calculation is based only on the DMLC files and can be performed independently of the origin of those files. Based on the information of the leaf motion, a 2-D matrix of correction factors in a plane perpendicular to the beam axis is precalculated for each beam. The dose calculation for the corresponding open field is then adjusted by these correction factors. The correction factors are used in order to weight both

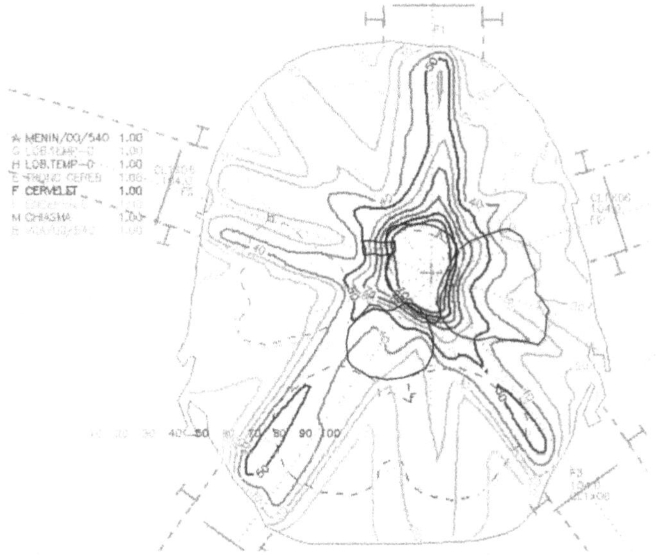


**Figure 2:** Screen capture of the iSis3D TPS illustrating a representative axial slice with the resulting optimized isodose lines conforming to the shape of the target volume. Note that the isodose lines indicate a higher dose gradient in regions where the PTV is in contact with an organ at risk.

the primary and the scatter component of the dose at a given point .

The generated "optimized" IMRT plan (figure 2) can then be compared with the "standard" 3DCRT plan in terms of dose distributions and dose-volume histograms (DVH).. Figure 3 illustrates such DVHs for the PTV and for the most constraining organs at risk in the plan, the chiasm and the brain stem. The results for the PTV are consistent with the clinical decisions concerning the minimum target volume dose. The maximum target volume dose has been slightly passed because

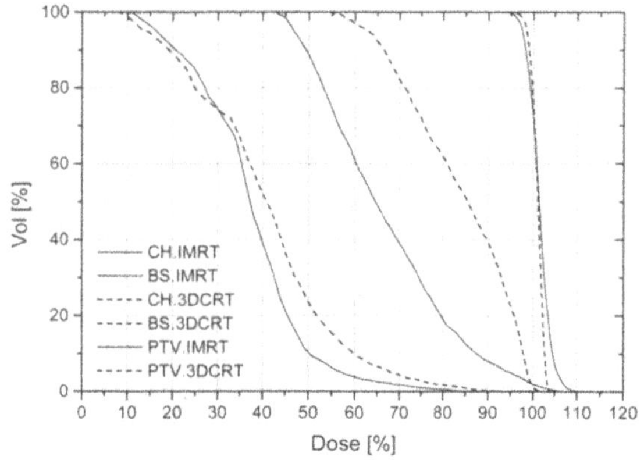


**Figure 3:** Comparison of cumulative Dose-Volume Histograms for the PTV, the chiasm and the brain stem. The DVHs corresponding to the IMRT plan are shown with solid lines, where those corresponding to the 3DCRT plan are shown with dashed lines.

the penalty value associated to this criterion was relatively small. On the other hand, IMRT helped us achieve improved normal tissue dose reduction for the chiasm and the brain stem. This is because the use of intensity modulated beams makes possible the creation of concave isodose surfaces and the creation of low dose areas surrounded by higher dose regions.

## Discussion and Conclusion

The results of the clinical case examined here, demonstrate the feasibility of using advanced IMRT planning techniques within the frame of a conventional 3D treatment planning system such as the iSis3D TPS. With the present implementation we were capable of planning optimized plans for brain tumors. Similar studies are also under way for other localizations such as prostate and head and neck tumors. The accuracy of dose calculations with intensity modulation has been also addressed with verification measurements[4] and the results are satisfactory for the cases tested so far.

The implementation of software modules for inverse planning, dynamic delivery and dose calculation of intensity modulated beams into an existing treatment planning system, is one more step for making intensity modulated radiotherapy more practical.

## References


[1] Bortfeld, T., Bürkelbach, J., Boesecke, R. ,Schlegel, W. 1990 Methods of image reconstruction from projections applied to conformal radiotherapy. *Physics in Medicine and Biology*. **35** 1423-34

[2] Bortfeld, T., Stein, J. and Preiser, K. 1997 Clinically relevant intensity modulation optimization using physical criteria. In: Proccedings of the XII ICCR. Salt Lake City, Utah, USA. 1-4

[3] Convery, D.J. and Rosenbloom, M.E. 1992 The generation of intensity-modulated fields for conformal radiotherapy by dynamic multileaf collimation. *Physics in Medicine and Biology*. **37** 1359-1374

[4] Papatheodorou, S., Rosenwald, J.C., Zefkili, S., Murillo, J., Drouard, J. ,Gaboriaud, G. 1999 Dose calculation and verification of intensity Modulation generated by dynamic multileaf collimators. *Medical Physics*. (submitted)

[5] Papatheodorou, S., Rosenwald, J.-C., Castellanos, M.E., Zefkili, S., Bonvalet, L. ,Gaboriaud, G. 1998 Utilisation d'un collimateur multilames pour la production de faisceaux modulés en intensité. *Cancer/Radiothérapie*. **2** 392-403

[6] Preiser, K., Bortfeld, T., Hartwig, K., Schlegel, W. ,Stein, J. 1997 A new program for inverse radiotherapy planning. In: Proccedings of the XII ICCR. Salt Lake City, Utah, USA. 425-428

[7] Spirou, S.V. and Chui, C.S. 1994 Generation of arbitrary intensity profiles by dynamic jaws or multileaf collimators. *Medical Physics*. **21** 1031-1041

[8] Stein, J., Bortfeld, T., Dörschel, B. ,Schlegel, W. 1994 Dynamic X-ray compensation for conformal radiotherapy by means of multi-leaf collimation. *Radiotherapy and Oncology*. **32** 163-173

# The influence of dose matrix and voxel dimensions for the dose calculation on inverse treatment planning for stereotactic radiosurgery

**Kalliopi Platoni[1], Dimitri Lefkopoulos, Pascal Grandjean and Katia Keraudy**

[1]Medical Physics Unit, Radiation Oncology Department, Tenon Hospital, 4 rue de la Chine, 75 020 PARIS

## Introduction

Brain tumours and arteriovenous malformations with simple elliptical or more complex shapes treated by stereotactic irradiation using converging beams of small dimensions (minibeams) could be regarded as candidates for precision conformal radiotherapy. In stereotactic radiosurgery, the development of new optimisation techniques are also crucial as in conventional radiotherapy. We propose as optimisation technique, the Singular Value Decomposition (SVD) [1-4]. The SVD analysis takes into account all the voxels of the 3D dose matrix for the calculation of the dose distribution and allows the measurement of the ill-conditioning of the stereotactic radiosurgery problem.

Planning radiation therapy using three dimensional patient data can be a time consuming process and that because of the 3D dose calculation in a volume of interest with a uniformly matrix of points. Some studies have been carried out comparing the efficiency of two commonly used sampling methods in the evaluation of treatments plans ; the regular grid point method (Cartesian method) and the pseudo-random number method [5-6].

The aim of this study is to examine how dose matrix and voxel dimensions (for regular Cartesian grids) influence the inverse treatment plan and the obtained dose distributions for stereotactic radiotherapy.

## Material and methods

### The irradiation and the dose space

The irradiation space (figure 1) is defined by two angular apertures: Anterior-Posterior = 180° and Right-Left = 180°.

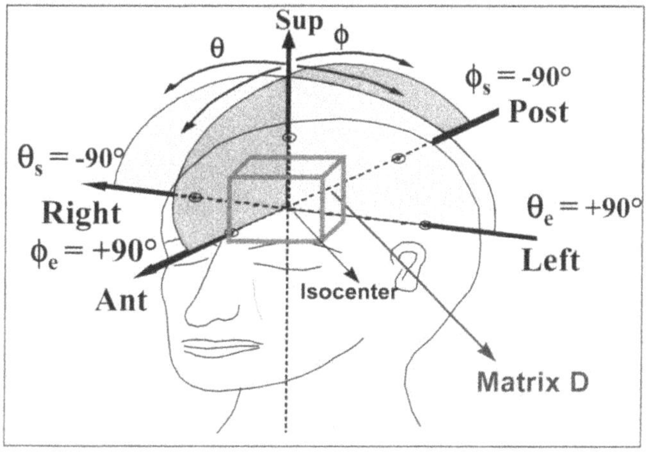


**Figure 1:** The irradiation space for a sitting patient position

The Anterior-Posterior aperture is sampled in arcs with an angular sampling of $\Delta\phi = 10°$. Each arc is sampled in elementary beams called minibeams with an angular sampling of $\Delta\theta = 10°$. Thus the irradiation is constituted of 361 minibeams.

The dose delivered by a set of minibeams is calculated in a dose matrix D (figure 1). In study A dose matrix dimensions varied from 16mm to 96mm, voxel dimension was constant to 2 mm (table 1). In the study of voxel dimension (study B), matrix dimension was constant to 80 mm while voxel dimensions varied from 1 mm to 8 mm (table 1).

| Study | *A* | *B* |
|---|---|---|
| Voxel size (mm) | 2 (constant) | 1, 2, 4, 8 |
| Matrix dimension (mm) | 16, 32, 48, 64, 80, 96 | 80 (constant) |

**Table 1**: the matrix and voxel dimensions of the studied values

### Modelling of convergent multi-arcs stereotactic irradiation

If the irradiation space is focused on to a volume, then the dose D delivered by NM converging minibeams at a same isocenter is described by the linear system of equations

$$D_\ell = \sum_{i=1}^{NM} M_{\ell,i} W_i \qquad \ell = 1,2,\ldots,NV \quad \text{and} \quad i = 1,2,\ldots NM$$

$\ell$: the index of the 3D dose matrix voxel

$D_\ell$: the calculated dose at this voxel

i: the index of the beams

$W_i$: the weight of beams

$M_{l,i}$: the kernel matrix M

$$\mathbf{D} = \mathbf{M} \cdot \mathbf{W} \longrightarrow \mathbf{W} = \mathbf{M}^{-1} \cdot \mathbf{D}$$

### Singular Value Decomposition and generalized matrix inversion

Any real NVxNM matrix M (NV>NM) may be expressed in the form : $M = USV^T$

$U^TU = V^TV = In$, and $S = diag(\sigma_1, \ldots \sigma_p)$, $\sigma_p > 0$, p=min NV, NF ,

$\sigma_p$: singular value, T : denotes matrix transpose.

### The condition number R of M

Inverse problems are usually ill-conditioned. The condition number R: ($R = \dfrac{\text{largest singular value}}{\text{smallest singular value}}$) measures the sensitivity of a solution of a linear system to different variations and gives an indication of the stability of the inverse problem (when the problem is ill conditioned, R is large).

**Regularization of the ill-posed problems**

The importance is to find the best rank L ($1 \le L \le NM$) matrix approximation to the matrix M which removes the noise :

$$W=(M^TM)^{-SVD} \cdot M^T \cdot D=\left(\sum_{n=1}^{L}\frac{1}{\sigma_n{}^2}V_nV_n{}^T\right)M^TD$$

**The methodology of a predefined weighting vector reconstruction**

Our approach to dose distribution optimisation is to recover estimates of beam weights from a well predefined dose matrix (PDM).

The procedure consists of:

i. choosing arbitrary anterior-posterior (AP) and right-left (RL) angular apertures to create a Predefined Irradiation Space (PIS) (ex. PIS : $(AA)_{AP}$ x $(AA)_{RL}$ = [-60° +60°] x [-50° +50°], figure 2.a),

ii. determining the weights for the beams which constitute the PIS. This beam weighting vector will be known as a Predefined Weighting Vector (PWV) (W = 1 for the beams ∈ ([-60° +60°] x [-50° +50°]) and W = 0 for the beams ∉ ([-60° +60°] x [-50° +50°]), figure 2.b)

iii. using the PWV we compute the corresponding PDM (figure 2.c) having as tool the ARTEMIS-3D TPS (the computation of PDM is a forward calculation),

iv. running the "SVD optimizer" software with the PDM as input data to find the Reconstructed Weighting Vector (RWV) closer to PWV (inverse calculation). The number of RWVs is equal to the number of the discretized minbeams. For each RWV the reconstruction error δ is computed

$$\delta_L=\sqrt{\sum_{\ell=1}^{NV}\frac{(PWV_\ell-RWV_\ell)^2}{NM}} \qquad L=1......NM$$

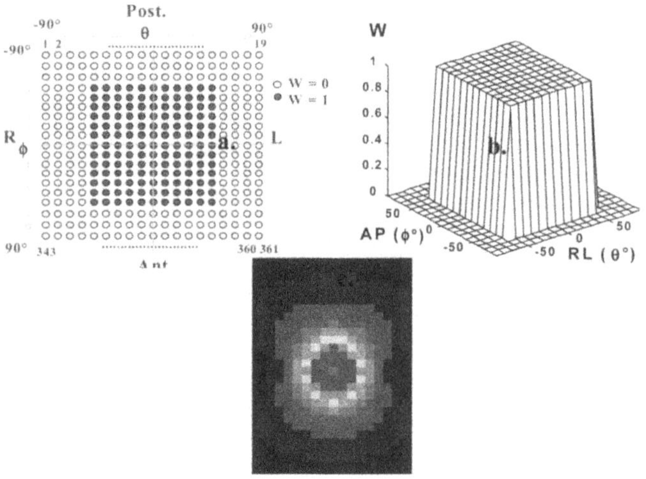


**Figure 2:** The definition of a) PIS, b)PWVand c) PDM (frontal plane)

# Results

**Singular Value Decomposition**

The superposition matrix $M^TM$

The shape of the superposition minibeams matrix $M^TM$ reflects the physical properties of each configuration. It is the shape and the complexity of each $M^TM$ that influence the ill-conditionning of the space. Figure 3 presents three $M^TM$ as function of the dose matrix dimensions. One observes that in the case of a 16 mm dose matrix (figure 3.a) the $M^TM$ is rather homogeneous as the dose is computed in a region very close the isocenter and thus the voxels deliver almost the same value. More the dose matrix dimensions are larger more the superposition matrix becomes inhomogeneous (figure 3.b, c) as the dose computation is realised in a larger 3D region which means that even the low interactions between the minibeams are computed.

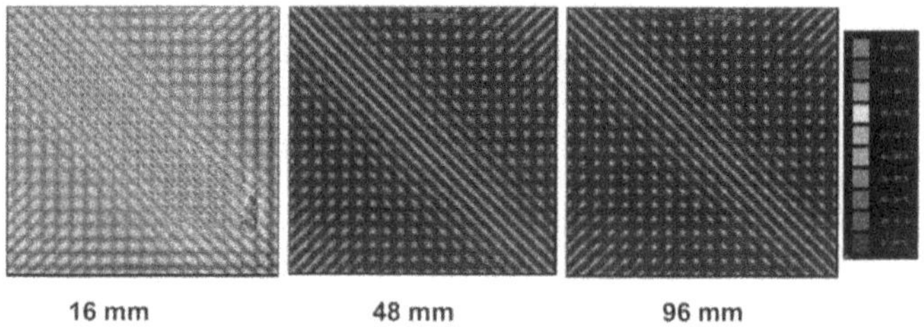


**Figure 3:** The minibeams superposition matrix for a ) 16mm, b) 48mm and c) 96mm dose matrix dimension.

In the study of voxel size the allure of the superposition matrix $M^TM$ was constant as the dose was computed always for the same region (dose matrix of 80mm).

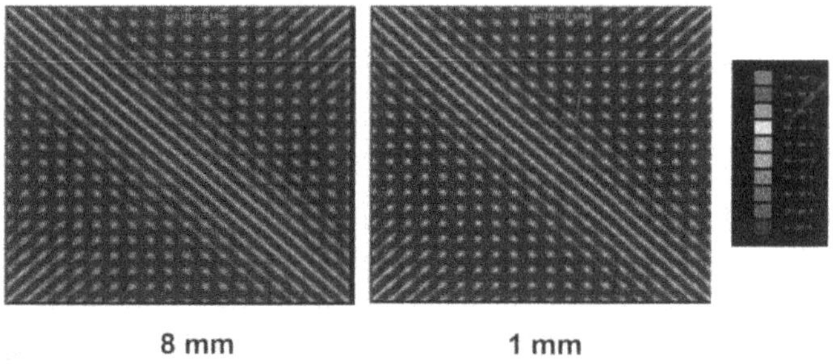


**Figure 4:** The minibeams superposition matrix for a ) 8mm and b) 1mm voxel size.

However, in the case of a small voxel size the superposition matrix is more detailed due to the larger number of coded information.

The singular values spectra and their condition numbers

The singular value spectrum of the matrix M for each configuration is presented in figure 4. The shape of the spectrum defines the condition number R (table 2 and 3).

The results showed that the conditioning is deteriorated by the decreasing of dose matrix dimensions and the increasing of voxel size.

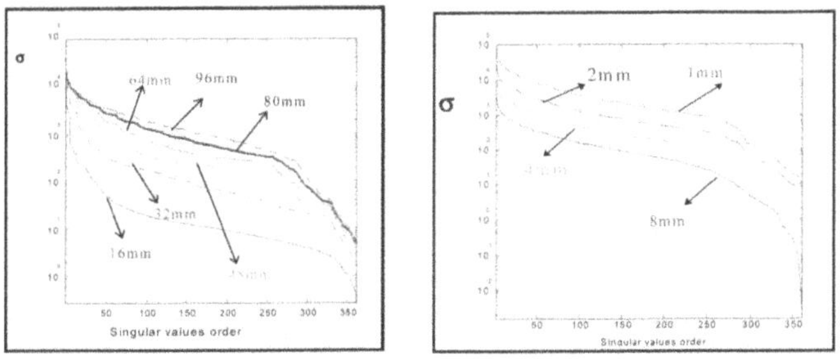


**Figure 4.** The singular values spectra as function of the a) dose matrix dimension and b) voxel size

| Dose matrix dimens. (mm) | 16 | 32 | 48 | 64 | 80 | 96 |
|---|---|---|---|---|---|---|
| max. singular value | 24,466 | 31,546 | 33,790 | 35,130 | 36,110 | 36,879 |
| min. singular value | 0.27 | 1.53 | 2.3 | 3.43 | 4.71 | 5.25 |
| condition number R | 89,622 | 20,589 | 15,127 | 10,241 | 7,657 | 7,011 |

**Table 2.** The condition number R as function of the dose matrix dimension

| voxel size (mm) | 1 | 2 | 4 | 8 |
|---|---|---|---|---|
| max. singular value | 102,071 | 36,110 | 12,785 | 4,293 |
| min. singular value | 10.28 | 4.71 | 1.24 | 0.0015 |
| condition number R | 9,928 | 7,657 | 10,307 | 2,768,589 |

**Table 3.** The condition number R as function of the voxel size

**Reconstruction**

To examine the influence of dose matrix dimension and voxel size on inverse treatment plan we studied the reconstruction of the PWV presented in figure 2.b.

For each configuration we computed and examined the reconstruction error curve δ as a function of the number of singular components. The study of the curves δ permits us to obtain the optimum value of the reconstruction error δ* for each configuration. Figure 5 presents the δ* for the different examined cases. The reconstruction of dose distributions revealed that an ill-conditioned problem (low value of dose matrix dimension and big voxel size) yields poor quality reconstruction.

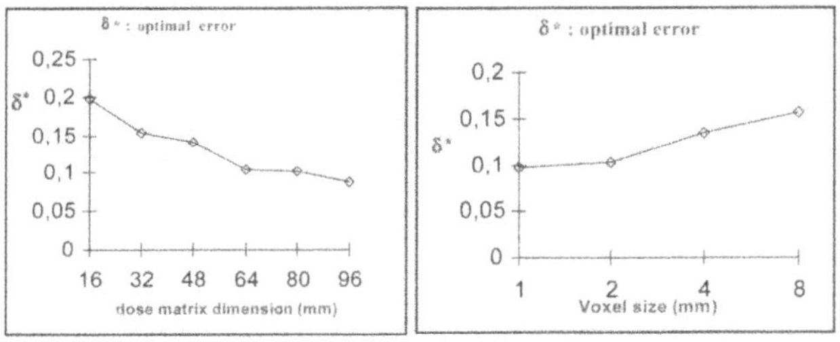


**Figure 5.** The optimum reconstruction error δ* as function of the a)dose matrix dimension and b) voxel size.

Figure 6 and 7 present the optimal reconstructed weighting vector (PWV) obtained by an inverse treatment planning in some configurations.

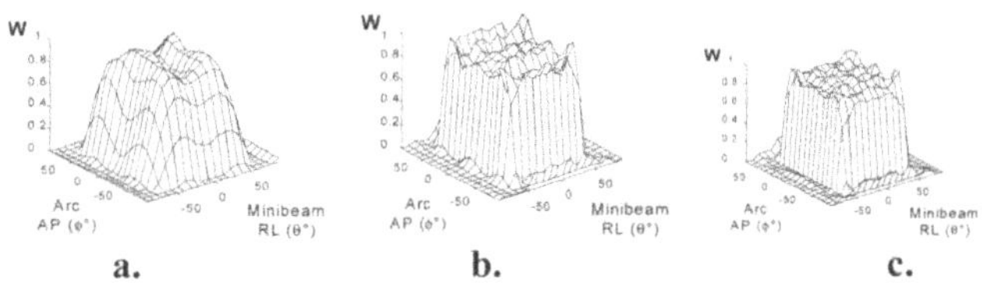


**Figure 6.** The RWV in the case of a) 16 mm, b)48 mm and c) 96 mm dose matrix dimension.

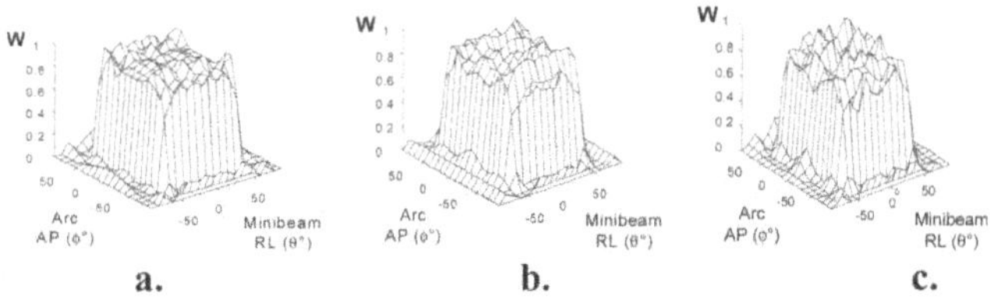


**Figure 7.** The RWV in the case of a) 1 mm, b)4 mm and c) 8 mm voxel size.

## Discussion - Conclusion

According to our results, the use of large dose matrix dimensions and a small voxel size do not improve the inverse optimization of dose distribution in stereotactic radiotherapy. A good compromise between quality of dose distribution, time calculation and hard disk memory is the use of a 64 $mm^3$ matrix dimension with a 2 $mm^3$ voxel size The validation of these results has to be made by the study of clinical cases.

## References

[1] Lefkopoulos D., Levier M., Bendada S., Touboul E. 1995 A general optimization procedure for stereotactic small beam multi-isocentric radiotherapy. *International Journal of Imaging Science and Technology* **6** 114-123.

[2] Lefkopoulos D., Grandjean P., Laouar A., Schlienger M. 1995 Study of the phase spece of pencil beam radiotherapy using singular value decomposition. *International Journal of Imaging Science and Technology*, **6** 104-113.

[3] Grandjean P., Platoni K., Lefkopoulos D., et al. 1998 Use of a general inverse technique for the conformational stereotactic treatment of complex intracranial lesions. *Int. J. Rad. Onc. Biol. Phys.* **41**(1) 69-76.

[4] Platoni K., Lefkopoulos D., Grandjean P., Schlienger M. 1999 Study of the ill-conditionning of Linac Stereotactic Irradiation Subspaces using Singular Values Decomposition Analysis. *Acta Oncologica* **38**(5) 581-590.

[5] Lu X-Q., Chin L.M. 1993 Sampling techniques for the evaluation of treatment plans. *Med. Phys.* **20**(1) 151-161.

[6] Niemierko A., Goitein M. 1989 The use of variable grid spacing to accelerate dose calculations. *Med. Phys.* **16**(3) 357-366.

# Cases Studies in Tomotherapy Optimization: Breast, Prostate, Mesothelioma and Nasopharyngeal treatments.

**P.J. Reckwerdt[2], G.H.Olivera[1,2], D.M. Shepard[1] and T.R. Mackie[1,2]**

[1]Department of Medical Physics, University of Wisconsin-Madison 1300 University Av. Madison WI 53706, USA, and [2]Tomotherapy Inc. 2228 Evergreen Road, Middleton WI, (53562-4241), USA.

## Introduction

Tomotherapy is a radiotherapy modality that includes planning, delivery and verification capabilities[1]. For the planning stage, it has an optimization code that uses an objective function to score the plan that includes set of penalties based on dose-volume consideration. The code produces a dose distribution that represents the physician's dosimetric requirements as close as possible.
As opposed to some other radiotherapy modalities, in tomotherapy is by necessary a large-scale optimization problem. Usually a tomotherapy treatment will have hundred of thousands of pencils beams for which intensity needs to be optimized. Moreover the number of voxels where the dose needs to be computed is on the order of 1,000,000.
The complexity and size of the optimization is a trade off paid in tomotherapy in order to obtain coplanar deliveries that are not limited by the number of directions and degree of modulation used during delivery. It is important to note, however, that because of the simplicity and capabilities of tomotherapy concept, a complex optimization plan will not lead to a complex delivery. The complexity on delivery is almost independent of the complexity on the optimization.
In the present manuscript several examples of large-scale tomotherapy optimization case will be presented. These include clinical cases of conformal and conformal avoidance treatment will be analyzed.

## Material and methods

At this stage of knowledge, optimization in tomotherapy is based on a physical objective function. Research on biological optimization is also being performed, however this will be not part of this discussion.
A key component in any planning optimization tool is the dose calculation engine. In tomotherapy, the convolution-superposition method is used. This allows inhomogeneities to be accounted for and also compute dose in non-electronic equilibrium conditions as presented in intensity modulated radiotherapy (IMRT). Specific implementations can be found elsewhere[2].
The results that will be presented are based on a quadratic objective function. A weighting scheme is used to establish the importance assigned to each region of interest (ROI). A set of penalties is used as soft constrain to control minimum, and maximum tumor dose and maximum dose in the regions at risk (RAR). Moreover, dose volume histogram penalties are also included as proposed by Bortfeld[3] and extended as proposed elsewhere[1].
The optimization can be performed with different delivery pitch. Axial optimizations are also possible. The results that will be presented were optimized with a pitch of 0.5. This pitch is adequate to minimize the junctioning problems in the inferior-superior direction that occur in other tomotherapy modalities[4, 5].
Another feature of the optimization is for cases where there are overlaps between tumor and RAR. The portion of the RAR that overlaps tumor is included as tumor in the objective function, but it plays a roll in determining the DVH penalty that should be applied to that RAR.
The optimizations were performed using the following geometry: 64 leaves, source to axis distance of 93 cm, leaf width of 0.625 cm. The jaw size used in this case was 1cm.
The photon beam was 4MV.

## Results and discussion

**Breast treatment**

DVH results for helical tomotherapy compared to 3D-planning for a breast case, are presented in figure 1. The conventional planning used a pair of 6 MV tangential fields, a supraclavicular 6MV field, and IMC fields using combined 12 MeV electrons and 6 MV photon beams.
The tomotherapy treatment was prescribed to at least 60 Gy for 90% of the breast volume. The nominal dose to the IMC node was 48 Gy to 90 % of the volume. The helical tomotherapy treatment was much more conformal and delivered less dose to the neighboring sensitive structures than the conventional treatment.

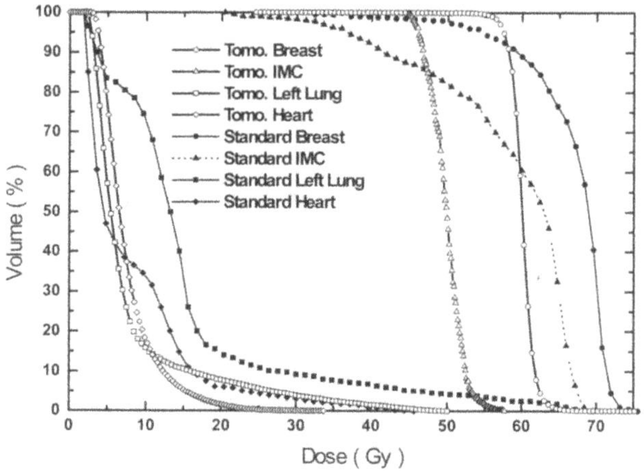


**Figure 1:** DVH comparison between standard and tomotherapy breast treatment.

Figure 2 a and b present sagittal and transversal slices respectively with isodose lines, and with the ROI indicated. As can be verified, the treatment is very conformal to the tumor, and the RARs are spared adequately. The IMC nodes were prescribed a lower dose. Moreover, they were included on the same treatment delivery. Therefore, junctioning problems will not appear in helical tomotherapy as they often do in standard radiotherapy.

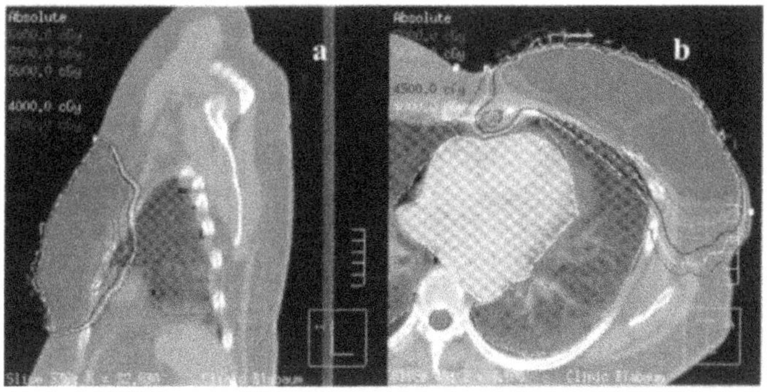


**Figure 2**: Sagittal and transverse dose distributions for the tomotherapy breast optimization.

**Prostate treatment**

In the prostate treatment, the prostate and seminal vesicles were both considered as tumor but outlined independently. The prescription was 75 Gy to 90 % of the volume in both case. The RARs were the rectum, bladder and the femur heads. Figure 3 shows the DVH for this optimization. The high dose regions in the bladder and rectum are because the DVH for these structures includes the part of rectum and bladder outlined as tumor. The dose to all the RARs are far below the allowed limits.

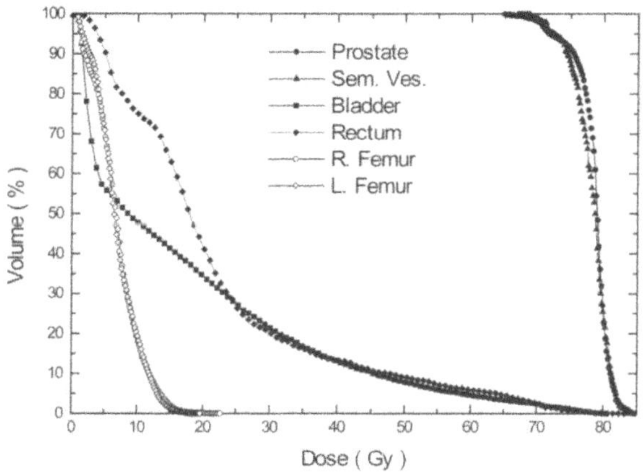


**Figure 3:** DVH plot for the tomotherapy prostate optimization.

Figure 4 a shows the isodose curves superimposed over the regions at risk. The isodoses are quite conformal to the tumor while sparing the RAR. Figure 4 b shows the isodoses plots over the CT. Even though 51 projections where used during this optimization, and all of them contribute, the radiation is largely incident from four angular sectors that resemble a four field oblique standard treatment.

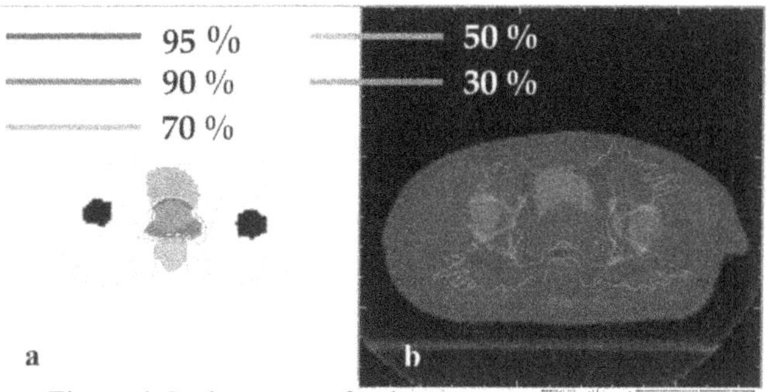


**Figure 4:** Isodose curves for the prostate optimization.

**Mesothelioma treatment**

This is a very complex treatment. This particular disease involved the pleural lining of the left lung. This region was prescribed a dose of 60 Gy to 90 % of the volume. Figure 5 a and b present the isodose distributions superimposed over the ROI's and CT, respectively. The right lung and the spinal cord were considered RARs. The internal part of the left lung was also considered as RAR. Therefore, it is necessary to have very high gradients to be able to obtain an adequate trade-off between tumor control and avoidance of the RAR. As can be inferred from the isodose lines there are extremely high gradients present in the left lung.

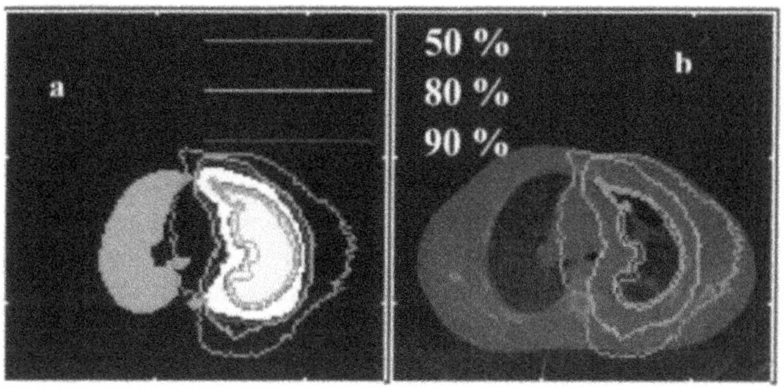


**Figure 5:** Isodose curves for the mesothelioma optimization.

Figure 6 is the DVH plot for this case. The uniformity of the dose in thetumor and the sparing of the RAR are both very good.

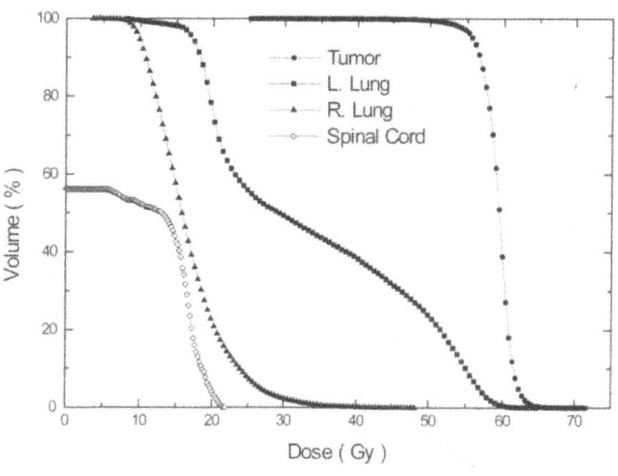


**Figure 6**: DVH plot for the mesothelioma optimization.

**Nasopharyngeal case**

Finally the DVH for a nasopharyngeal conformal avoidance treatment is presented in Figure 7.

The parotid glands can be easily distinguished, and in order to avoid xerostomia on the patient, the optimization for the regional fields was performed maintaining the levels of dose of the parotids glands within allowed limits. This treatment is a typical conformal avoidance case.

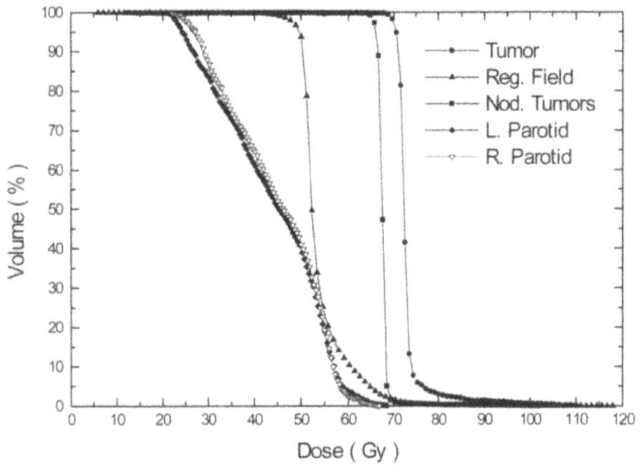


**Figure 7:** DVH plot for the nasopharyngeal optimization.

In this case there were several ROI's. There was a gross tumor prescribed to 75 Gy, a regional field covering the nodal region prescribed to 55 Gy, and several visible nodes in the MRI prescribed to 70 Gy. The RARs were the two parotid glands, the spinal cord, the lungs, the brain and the ear canals. Part of the parotid glands was included as tumor which can be seen as high dose levels in the parotid DVH. Therefore, part of the parotid will be in the tumor objective function while limiting the dose to the DVH of the parotids.

## Conclusion

Tomotherapy provides the opportunity to optimize very complex treatments that can be delivered without the difficulty of conventional multi-ports deliveries. Several optimization cases have been presented showing the types of delivery that can be achieved. The deliveries can be optimized as conformal or conformal avoidance treatments extending the flexibility of the optimizer.

**Acknowledgements**

The authors would like to thank Dr. Lynn Verhey, Dr. Mack Roach, and Pam Akazawa of the University of California, San Francisco for the images and contouring of the mesothelioma case and Dr. J. Stacy Aldridge for initial work on the breast and naso cases.

## References

[1] Olivera, G.H., D.M. Shepard, K. Ruchala, J.S. Aldridge, J.M. Kapatoes, E.E. Fitchard, P.J. Reckwerdt, G. Fang, J. Balog, J. Zachman and T.R. Mackie, *Tomotherapy*, in *Modern Technology of Radiation Oncology*, J. Van Dyk, Editor. 1999, Medical Physics Publishing: Madison. p. 521-587.

[2] Shepard, D.M., G.H. Olivera, P. Reckwerdt and T.R. Mackie, *Iterative approaches to dose optimization in tomotherapy.* Phys. Med. Biol., 2000. **45**: p. 69-90.

[3] Bortfeld, T., J. Stein and K. Preiser. *Clinically Relevant Intensity Modulation Optimization Using Physical Criteria.* in *XII International Conference on the Use of Computers in Radiation Therapy.* 1997. Salt Lake City, Utah, USA: Medical Physics Publishing.

[4] Balog, J.P., T.R. Mackie, P. Reckwerdt, M. Glass and L. Angelos, *Characterization of the output for helical delivery of intensity modulated slit beams.* Med. Phys., 1999. **26**(1): p. 55-64.

[5] Low, D.A., *Abutment region dosimetry for sequential arc IMRT delivery.* Phys in Med. and Biol., 1997. **42**: p. 1465-1470.

# Method of normalising and sensitivity to setup variations of IMRT treatment plans

**Anna Samuelsson[1], Karl-Axel Johansson[1] and Claes Mercke[2]**

[1]Department of Radiation Physics, Göteborg University, Sahlgrenska University Hospital, S-413 45 Göteborg, Sweden, and [2]Department of Oncology, Sahlgrenska University Hospital, S-413 45 Göteborg, Sweden

## Introduction

Inverse treatment planning for Intensity Modulated Radiation Therapy (IMRT) is an alternative approach to the traditional method of treatment planning. The inverse treatment planning procedure optimises the intensity distributions in the beams in the treatment plan. IMRT makes it possible to shape the high dose region so that it conforms closely to the prescribed target volume, even for target volumes with concave shapes, and hereby spare organs at risk in complex treatment geometries. This study is concentrated on head and neck tumours.
In conventional therapy the absorbed dose in the PTV is never uniform. With inverse dose planning the dose in the PTV and close to the normalising point is even more inhomogeneous and varies from one point to another. This implies that the result of the treatment plan is influenced by where the normalisation is done. The way of normalising and prescribing the dose is discussed for optimised dose distributions.
The optimised field fluences often have steep dose gradients inside the field. This gradient may have influence on the sensitivity to patient movements, organ motions and setup errors. The sensitivity for setup variations is investigated by simulation in the treatment planning system.

## Material and methods

The optimisation procedure used in this investigation is the dose-based conjugated gradient method developed at Memorial Sloan-Kettering Cancer Center[1]. It is based on delivering the optimised field fluence distributions with dynamic MLC using the sliding-window technique. The target volumes (CTV and PTV[2]) and organs at risk volumes (OAR and POAR[2]) have been delineated in multiple CT slices for some patients with head and neck tumours. The PTV was defined with a margin of about 0.35 cm added to the CTV and the POAR was defined with a margin of about 0.3 cm added to the OAR. The constraints for the PTV were always set to 95% and 105% of the prescribed dose. The treatment plans were evaluated with physical parameters such as dose volume histograms, the relative standard deviation in the target volumes and the volumes of the critical organs that receives more than the maximum dose constraint set for that particular organ.
Optimised treatment plans were compared with different normalisations such as normalisations to a point in the PTV, to the mean dose value in the PTV and to the modal dose in the PTV.
Interfraction setup variations were simulated by moving the isocenter, i.e. the beams, without changing the field fluence distributions. The dose distribution was recalculated with the same field fluence distributions and the new isocenter point. Setup variations of 0.5 cm were simulated in six directions; left, right, anterior, posterior, superior and inferior. Intrafraction geometric variations were also studied, moving one or a few beams. The setup variations were investigated for treatment plans with different numbers of beams i.e. different shapes of the field fluence distributions. The influence in the sensitivity for setup variations of sharp peaks and fast gradients in the field fluence distributions were investigated.

## Results and discussion

If the normalisation was set to a predefined point in the PTV, for example the isocenter point, it would be a quite random normalisation due to the dose variations close to the isocenter point. Figure 1 compares dose volume histograms (DVH) with different normalisations for one treatment plan optimised with different number of beams. In the DVH normalised to the mean dose in the PTV one can easily see the improvement of the

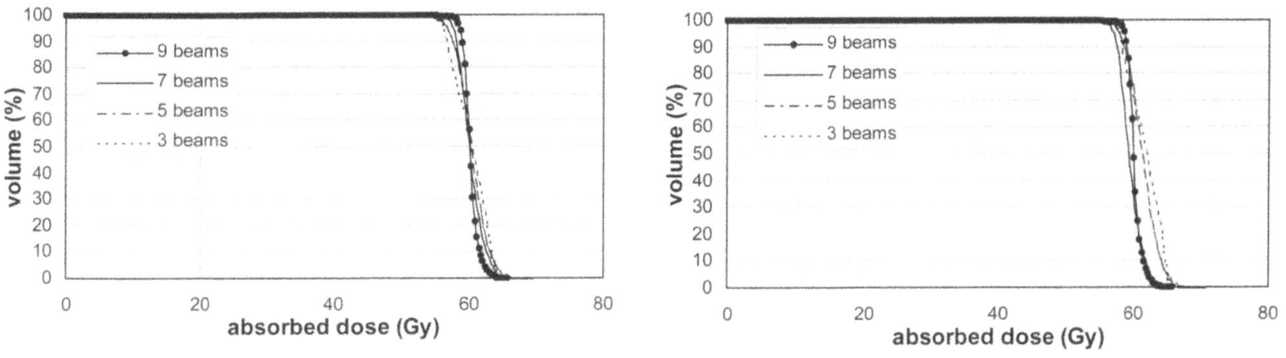


**(a)** **(b)**

**Figure 1:** Dose volume histograms for different number of beams normalised to (a) the mean dose in the PTV and (b) the isocenter point. The prescribed dose to the PTV was 60 Gy.

homogeneity in the PTV when the number of beams is increased. This is not obvious in the DVH normalised to the isocenter point. If the dose prescription was done to the isocenter point, the absorbed dose to the PTV would be random and somewhat arbitrary. Such a dose specification could not be reproduced in other treatment plans or in other institutions.
The result from interfraction setup variations of 0.5 cm in different directions simulated for one of the patients geometries studied is shown in table 1. The diagnosis for this patient was an advanced cancer in the base of tongue with the spinal cord set as the only organ at risk. The treatment plan was calculated with 7 beams. The sensitivity to setup variations in the dose distributions in CTV and OAR should be small since the dose distribution was optimised to PTV and POAR with an extra planning margin to take into account setup variations. The dose distribution for this patient geometry is only marginally affected of 0.5 cm setup variations when using field fluence distributions created with the optimisation algorithm used here. The peaks and gradients in the field fluence distributions are much larger for a treatment plan with fewer beams but this did not influence the sensitivity to setup variations of 0.5 cm for the target volume. However the sensitivity to setup variations for the critical organ is decreasing somewhat with increasing number of beams.

| Moved 0.5 cm in direction | Std dev in CTV (%) | Std dev in PTV (%) | Vol with dose > 42 Gy of OAR ($cm^3$) | Vol with dose > 42 Gy of POAR ($cm^3$) |
|---|---|---|---|---|
| not moved | 1.77 | 1.87 | 0 | 0.47 |
| left | 2.03 | 2.82 | 0.05 | 0.91 |
| right | 2.17 | 2.72 | 0.29 | 2.23 |
| ant | 1.93 | 2.8 | 0 | 0 |
| post | 1.79 | 2.17 | 2.67 | 6.36 |
| sup | 1.84 | 2.02 | 0 | 0.36 |
| inf | 1.91 | 2.20 | 0.02 | 0.56 |

**Table 1:** Setup variations for a treatment plan with 7 beams. The prescribed dose to the PTV was 60 Gy. The only critical organ in this geometry was the spinal cord and the dose constraint, the maximum dose accepted, was set to 42 Gy.

This investigation includes calculations with the inverse planning system. The project is now continuing with measurements of the MLC fields.

## Conclusion

The recommendations from ICRU[2] to normalise, prescribe and report doses to a reference point is not suitable for IMRT treatment plans since the dose variations are often several percent round the reference point. Normalisation and prescription to the mean absorbed dose value in the PTV is a stable and reliable way for a dose distribution with a reasonable (not too large) dose variation in the PTV.
The optimised dose distributions studied in this investigation are marginally affected by setup variations of 0.5 cm. The sensitivity to set up variations of the dose distributions is decreasing somewhat with increasing number of beams for the critical organ but the result for the target volume is not influenced. Even for beams with large dose gradients in the field fluence distributions the dose distributions in CTV and OAR are well within the acceptance tolerance for setup variations of 0.5 cm.

## References

[1] Spirou S V and Chui C-S 1998 A gradient inverse planning algorithm with dose-volume constraints *Med. Phys.* **25** (3) 321-333

[2] ICRU 1993 International Commission on Radiation Units and Measurements, Prescribing, recording and reporting photon beam therapy, ICRU Report 50 International Commission on Radiation Units and Measurements, Bethesda, Maryland

# Influence of the sampling of dose and beams spaces on the ill conditioning and on quality of inverse dose distribution for IMRT

**Laure Vieillevigne, Dimitri Lefkopoulos, Pascal Grandjean, Catherine Dejean and Frédéric Julia**

Medical Physics Unit, Radiation Oncology Department, Tenon Hospital, 4 rue de la Chine, 75 020 Paris

## Introduction

The main goal of intensity modulation radiotherapy (IMRT) is to conform the dose distribution to the shape of the tumour while sparing normal tissues. It improves accuracy of tumour coverage and protection of surrounding normal tissues. To plan IMRT, inverse optimised treatment planning is necessary. There are two components in an optimisation system [1]: (a) the optimisation model and (b) the optimisation algorithm.
Our group uses the singular value decomposition (SVD) optimisation technique, which is a powerful mathematical analysis that allows the measurement of the conditioning of the radiotherapy inverse problem and the examination of the influence of the irradiation parameters.
The aim of this work is to examine the influence of the discretisation parameters of the dose space (dose pixel size) and the beams space (bixel size) on the conditioning and the quality reconstruction of the dose distribution into a simplified irradiation context (2D dose matrix, 1D beams and primary dose calculation model).

## Material and methods

In the dose calculation model, the total number of beams is denoted by N and each of them is discretised into p elementary beams (bixels). A strip limited by two lines then constitutes the bixel. The dose matrix is quantized into a grid of $NPIX_x x NPIX_y$ pixels. The dose distribution is given by:

$$D_i = \sum_{j=1}^{NPIX} M_{ij} \cdot W_j$$

with i=1, NPIX ( $NPIX = NPIX_x x NPIX_y$ ),
where, NBIX = pxN, i is the index of the 2D dose matrix pixel, $D_i$ the value of the calculated dose at the pixel i, $W_j$ the weight of the bixel j and $M_{ij}$ is the kernel matrix whose row j contains the dose contribution of the bixel j in the 2D dose matrix.

More details on the SVD analysis are given in others papers [2, 3]. The reconstructed weighting vector W is given by

$$W(r) = \left(\sum_{k=1}^{r} \frac{1}{\sigma_k^2} v_k v_k^T\right) M^T D$$

where, $\sigma_k$ are the singular values, $v_k$ the singular vectors and r is the number of singular components used to obtain the $r^{th}$ solution. The number of W proposed by the SVD is equal to NBIX. The singular value decomposition truncation (SVDT) is obtained by retaining only the r first singular components giving thus a solution W of the order r. We define a truncation factor (TF)

$$TF = \frac{(NBIX - r)}{NBIX} x100$$

This factor represents the proportion of the singular components not useful in obtaining the $r^{th}$ solution.
The condition number that is the ratio between the larger to smaller singular values quantifies the conditioning of the inverse problem. To large condition numbers correspond ill conditioning situations.

The objective function FCF (" full cost function ") is calculated by summing the least square difference between the reconstructed dose matrix (RDM) of the order r and the prescribed dose matrix (PDM) [4]. The minimisation of the objective function gives the optimal $RDM^*$ of the order $r^*$.

$$FCF(r) = \left\{ \sum_{i=1}^{NPIX} (MDR_i(r) - MDP_i)^2 / NPIX \right\}^{\frac{1}{2}}$$

We calculate also a LCF (" limited cost function ") corresponding to a particular organ.

## Results

Sixteen equally spaced beams in 0-2π were used and each beam size was 20 cm. The X rays beam energy was 6 MV. The contour was elliptical with a major axis of 40 cm and a minor one of 30 cm. The studied configuration is the Brahme dose prescription [5] : the prescribed dose are 1 in the tumour (T), 0.15 in the organs at risk (OAR) and 0.3 in the healthy tissues (HT).

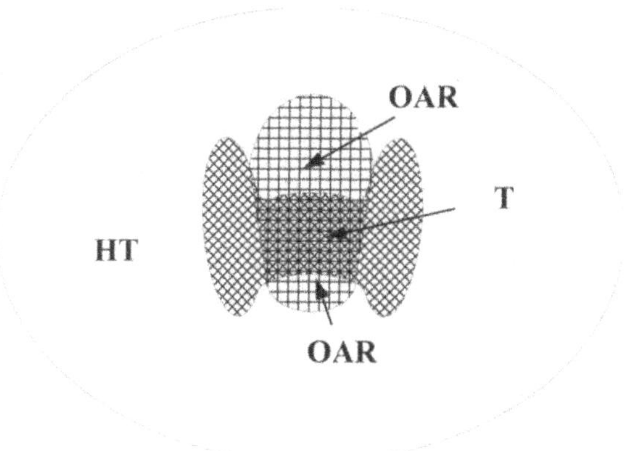


**Figure 1:** Prescripiton dose matrix (PDM) known as Brahme dose prescription

For the nine studied configurations (M1 to M9) the dose matrix size is of 40cmx40cm ; the dose pixel size (noted as pix) and the bixel size (noted as bix) take values of 0.2 cm, 0.5 cm and 1 cm (M1 : bix=0.2 cm/pix=0.2 cm ; M2 : bix=0.2 cm/pix=0.5 cm ; M3 : bix=0.2 cm/pix=1 cm ; M4 : bix=0.5 cm/pix=0.2 cm ; M5 : bix=0.5 cm/pix=0.5 cm ; M6 : bix=0.5 cm/pix=1 cm ; M7 : bix=1 cm/pix=0.2 cm ; M8 : bix=1 cm/pix=0.5 cm ;M9 : bix=1 cm/pix=1 cm )

**SVD analysis**

The condition numbers R for the nine configurations are given into the figure 2. The condition number variation shows that discretisation parameters influences the conditioning of the inverse problem.

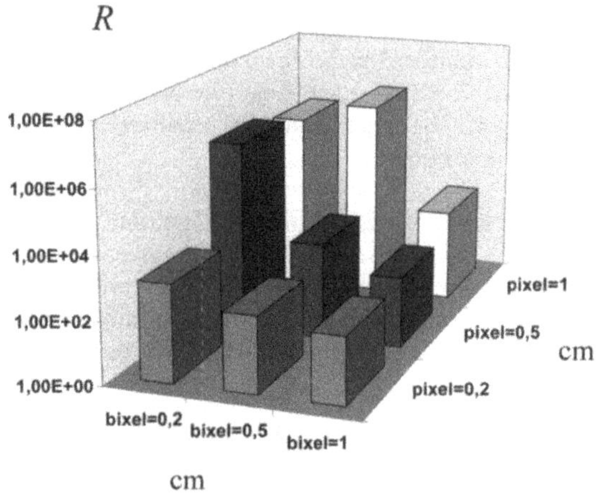


**Figure 2**: The condition numbers for the configurations M4 to M12

When the ratio between the numbers of pixels and bixels is not sufficiently large (> 4) the condition number are very large (order of $10^6$), because the sampling of the dose space is not sufficient. When the previous ratio is large the condition numbers are in order of $10^2$.

**SVD dose distribution reconstruction**

| pixel (cm²) / bixel (cm) | 0,2 × 0,2 | 0,5 × 0,5 | 1 × 1 |
|---|---|---|---|
| **0,2** | 43.75 *(0.1224)* *M1* | 77.90 *(0.1244)* *M2* | 86.03 *(0.1287)* *M3* |
| **0,5** | 45.31 *(0.1229)* *M4* | 53.12 *(0.1244)* *M5* | 67.69 *(0.1289)* *M6* |
| **1** | 37.50 *(0.1260)* *M7* | 43.75 *(0.1268)* *M8* | 53.12 *(0.1297)* *M9* |

**Table 1** : The truncation factors and in parentheses the FCF optimal values for the nine configurations.

The nine configurations M1 to M9 present a large range of discretisation parameters generating different levels of inverse problem conditioning (figure 2). The table 1 shows the power of regularisation of the SVD that can reconstruct optimal dose distribution with a similar precision independently of the level of ill conditioning. SVD optimizer imposes a larger truncation factor (TF) (table 1 and figure 3) when the ill conditioning is more important.

The modulated intensity profiles are very similar for the nine configurations. That means that independently of the dose space and beams space sampling the regularisation power of the SVD optimizer permits to obtain physically acceptable similar modulated intensity profiles. The figure 4 shows the reconstructed dose distribution for the M7 configuration.

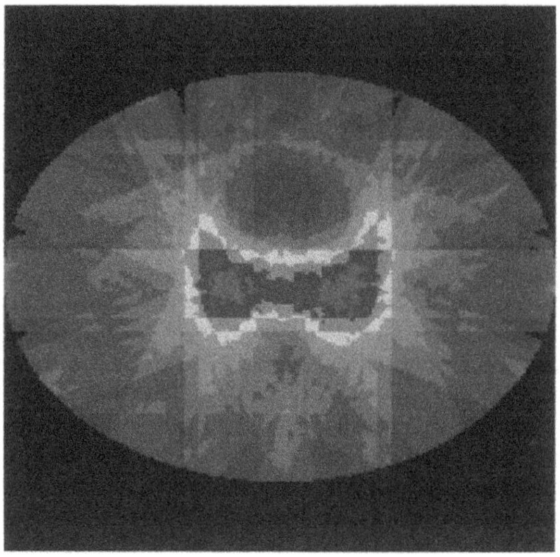

**Figure 4** : The reconstructed dose distribution for the M7 configuration.

The table 2 presents the similarity of the mean doses inside the tumour (T) and the OARs.

| | T | OARs |
|---|---|---|
| **M1** | 0,91±0,11 | 0,32±0,13 |
| **M2** | 0,90±0,11 | 0,32±0,14 |
| **M3** | 0,90±0,10 | 0,33±0,14 |
| **M4** | 0,90±0,12 | 0,32±0,14 |
| **M5** | 0,90±0,12 | 0,32±0,14 |
| **M6** | 0,90±0,11 | 0,33±0,14 |
| **M7** | 0,90±0,12 | 0,32±0,13 |
| **M8** | 0,89±0,12 | 0,33±0,15 |
| **M9** | 0,89±0,11 | 0,33±0,15 |

**Table 2:** The mean doses for the nine configurations.

## Discussion - Conclusion

This study corresponding to an experimental simplified environment has shown that the discretisation of the dose and beams spaces influences the ill conditioning of the IMRT inverse problem. Efficient regularisation is necessary to overcome this ill conditioning problem because simple inversion techniques, as Gauss inverse technique, cannot obtain optimal solutions. For other iterative techniques, as the gradient techniques, the knowledge of ill conditioning is a very useful information to prevent the difficulty to inverse a given irradiation configuration.
These previous studies must also be realised in clinical situations (3D dose matrix, 2D beams and clinical localisations). Our group has already started some clinical studies and their evaluation is at the moment in progress.

## References


[1] Bortfeld T. 1999 Optimized planning using physical objectives and constraints *Seminars in radiation Oncology* **19** 20-34

[2] Grandjean P., Platoni K., Lefkopoulos D., Merienne L, Schlienger M. 1998 Use of a general inverse technique for the conformationnal stereotactic treatment of complex intracranial lesions *Int J Radiat Oncol Biol Phys* **41** 69-76

[3] Vieillevigne L., Lefkopoulos D., Grandjean P., Touboul E., Housset M. 1999 Intensity modulation optimisation by inverse planning into the SVD decomposition space: a preliminary study *Physica Medica* **XV** 11-19

[4] Webb S. 1989 Optimisation of conformal Radiotherapy dose distribution by simulated annealing *P M B* **34** 1349-70

[5] Brahme A., Roose J., Lax I. 1982 Solution of an integral equation encountered in radiation therapy *Med Phys* **27** 1221-29


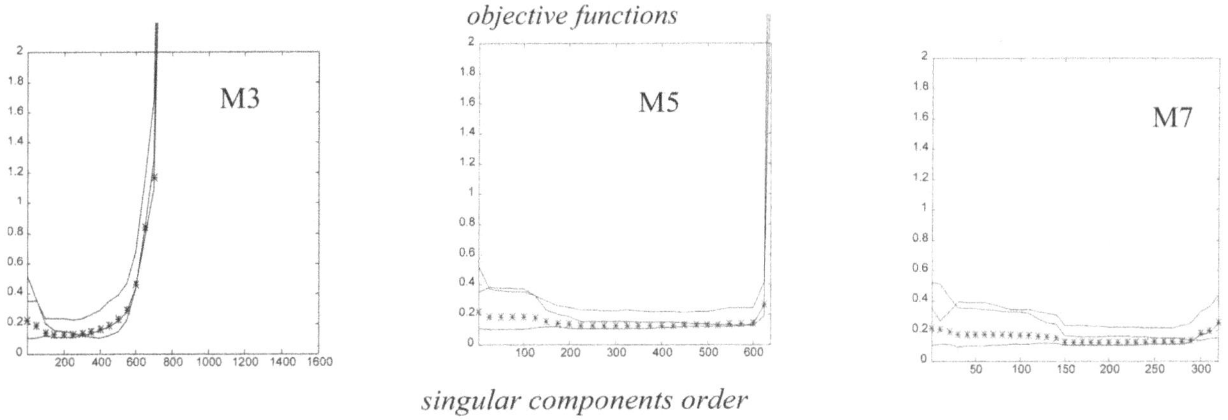


**Figure 3**: Variation of the FCF (stars) and the different LCF as function of the truncation factor for three configurations of different ill-conditionning degree M3, M5 and M7. (LCF(T): long dotted lines, LCF(OAR): short dotted lines, LCF(HT): continuous lines)

# Formal Safety Analysis of the Control Program for a Radiation Therapy Machine

**Jonathan Jacky**
Radiation Oncology, Box 356043, University of Washington, Seattle, Washington 98195-6043, USA

## Introduction

A central problem in software development is to assure that a complex program actually meets its requirements. This problem is most urgent in applications such as the control of radiation therapy machines, where execution of the program can have irreversible human consequences.

The problem is difficult for at least two reasons. First, there is the sheer mass of detail that must be handled correctly: the written requirements for our machine's control program comprise hundreds of pages of prose, and the printed program listing comprises hundreds of pages of programming language statements (code)[1]. The second difficulty arises because the two descriptions are so different. The requirements are expressed in English prose organized to be meaningful to the machine's users and maintainers, while the program is expressed in a machine-readable code organized to be efficiently executed by the computer. There is no obvious (simple, one-to-one) correspondence between the two. Yet we must somehow derive the code from the requirements. This is the *design* problem. Then we are obligated to show that the code satisfies the requirements — not approximately, but exactly, with no errors or omissions and no extra (undocumented) behavior. In the course of this effort we should discover and correct all errors that might have serious consequences. This is the *assurance* problem. How should we solve these two problems?

The usual approach to solving both problems is to create one or more intermediate descriptions between the requirements and the code. This description (or collection of descriptions) is usually called the *design*. It helps to solve both problems by replacing the huge leap from requirements to code with smaller steps, which should be easier to create (design) and justify (assure).

The choice of design method and notation is an active area of research and controversy. For this project we chose to use a *formal method* and express the design in a *formal notation*. This means that the design is a collection of mathematical formulas. In the literature this is usually called a *formal specification* (even though it often serves as the design).

We expected two benefits. First, we hoped to create a design document that was more concise and more clearly structured than we could achieve with prose or diagrams, so it would be more convenient to use as a guide for coding, test planning, and assurance activities (reviews). Second, we hoped to apply powerful assurance techniques that become possible when a formal specification is available. A formal specification is a kind of mathematical model, so it is sometimes possible to infer or calculate conclusive answers to questions about proposed system behaviors.

In particular, we hoped to demonstrate formally that the detailed design satisfies its safety requirements. The central safety requirement is that the beam can only turn on when the actual setup of the machine conforms to the prescription selected by the operator[2]. Checking this requirement might reveal errors that escape detection during testing and reviews. To make the safety analysis possible, the formal specification must explicitly describe the safe states. This information is not present in the program and cannot be inferred from the program.

Our innovation in this project, which we believe is a novel and significant scientific contribution, was to create a formal specification of a radiation therapy machine control program in sufficient detail that it could be implemented and also could be analyzed to determine whether it satisfies its safety requirements. We coded the program from the formal specification and it is now in use treating patients. We also experimented with formal assurance methods, but we relied primarily on traditional assurance methods: testing and code reviews.

## Material and methods

We developed a new control program for the isocentric treatment unit at the Clinical Neutron Therapy System (CNTS) at the University of Washington Medical Center in Seattle. Except for particle type, this machine is similar to a modern therapy linac with a leaf collimator. In July 1999 our new program replaced the manufacturer's original program which had been in use since the machine was installed in 1984 [1]. There was no re-use of design or code from the earlier program.

### Writing the requirements

The requirements express the properties that the system must have to be acceptable to its users, expressed in terms that they can understand and critique. The authors and reviewers include the physicist who defined the physical and clinical requirements for the original machine, engineers who installed and maintain the machine, and clinical users of the machine. Writing the requirements was a major

[1] Most project documents are available at `http://www.radonc.washington.edu/physics/cnts/`

[2] Other safety requirements are handled by hardware. Delegation of functions to hardware or software follows a hazard analysis not reported here.

portion of the whole project effort, not just a preliminary. It was an indispensable prerequisite to the formal specification.

### Writing the formal specification

The formal specification is a collection of mathematical formulas that express constraints on the values of a set of *state variables*.

The set of state variables must represent all pertinent features of the treatment machinery and the treatment session. Most obviously, there are state variables for all the inputs and outputs of the control hardware: the commanded and achieved values for all the leaves, etc. Other state variables represent the status of operations in progress (timers are one example). Still more state variables represent the prescribed settings (needed to check the safety requirement) and the patient and field identification used to select the prescribed settings from the prescription database. We identified 410 scalar state variables.

We wrote formulas to express the constraints that must hold among the values of the state variables at all times. These formulas are called *invariants*. All safety requirements can be expressed as invariants. The formulas are similar to the boolean expressions available in most programming languages: they evaluate to *true* in situations that satisfy the constraints and *false* otherwise. The English paraphrase of one invariant says: "If the beam is on, all leaves are within tolerance of their prescribed values". A condition that causes an invariant to evaluate to *false* violates a safety requirement. For example if any leaf is not within tolerance of its prescribed value when the beam is on, this invariant is violated[3].

The invariants express precisely what it means for the program to be in a safe state. Most of the value added to the project by the formal specification inheres in the invariants because they express information that is not present in the program and cannot be inferred from the program. The program code expresses a great many state transitions. With great effort, we might be able to analyze the code to determine the set of reachable states. But this cannot tell us if the reachable states are safe. The program might be able to reach an unsafe state, due to a designer's oversight or a programming error. In fact, the safety analysis is actually nothing more than checking that the set of reachable states is a subset of the set of safe states. For this we need an explicit description of the safe states which is independent of the program, and that is what the formal specification provides.

In addition to the invariants, we also wrote formulas to express the state transitions. Unlike the invariants, these formulas correspond closely to the program code. However they are written in the same mathematical notation as the invariants, and they are more concise than code because they only model its effects, not its details (for example there are no constructs corresponding to loops in the formal specification). Each operation is described by a formula called a *precondition* which describes the states where the operation can begin and another called a *postcondition* which describes the state after the operation completes (the postcondition can be a function of the precondition). We described 105 state transitions.

We wrote the formal specification in Z [2], a machine-readable notation for logic, set theory and arithmetic. Z defines many constructs that make it convenient to work with large numbers of state variables. We wrote 2103 lines of Z.

### Analysing the formal specification

A formal specification makes it possible to perform systematic analyses that can reveal design errors. Otherwise, these errors might not be detected until testing, and perhaps not even then. Some of these analyses can be performed automatically by a computer program.

We checked for syntax and type errors, using a tool similar to a programming language compiler. This reveals many of the clerical errors that can creep into large documents (such as different variables with the same name).

We also checked for *domain errors*, using an *automated theorem prover* [3]. This can reveal errors somewhat like array-out-of-bounds errors in programming languages, where a function is applied outside its domain.

We checked portions of the formal specification for *completeness* (there is a specified response to all possible inputs in all possible states) and *determinism* (there is just one response for each input in each state). It should be possible to automate much of this, but instead we inspected pertinent excerpts of the formal specification presented in a tabular format.

Our most important analysis was to check that the detailed design of the program code (the state transitions) satisfies its safety requirements (the invariants). To demonstrate safety we must show that every reachable state is safe. First, show that the initial states are safe. Then, for each state transition, show that if its starting state is safe, then its ending state is safe also. That's all. It is not necessary to consider the practically infinite collection of all possible program executions (we need not explicitly construct the entire (huge!) sets of safe states or reachable states). We need only consider the initial state (trivial) and then individually analyze each of our 105 state transitions (tedious but quite feasible). We check that each transition does not violate any invariants. It is not necessary to explicitly consider all possible values of the state variables because the transitions and the invariants are both represented symbolically (with variables instead of explicit values). We need only show that the formula that describes the transition implies the formula that expresses the invariants. This is usually a straightforward exercise in the simplification of

[3]The formula paraphrased *if p then q* is *false* when *p* is *true* and *q* is *false*, and is *true* in all other situations.

logical expressions. Again, it should be possible to automate much of this, but we used inspection (by eye) and a few pencil-and-paper calculations.

We also analyzed some of our design's tasking and timing properties with an exhaustive simulation technique called *model checking* [4]. We expressed portions of our design in a special programming language used by the checker. Then we expressed certain requirements in another formal notation called CTL that includes temporal operators such as *until* and *eventually* so it can check progress properties, not just invariance. The checker tool constructs the (very large but finite) set of states reachable by the (simplified) program, performing a simulation of all possible program executions. The tool checks that each simulated execution path satisfies the requirements expressed in CTL. If it does not, it prints the entire execution path that contains the error. This technique depends on constructing a much-simplified version of the program that nevertheless captures the requirements of interest.

### Writing and testing the program

The formal specification not only supported the safety analysis, it also served as the detailed design that guided coding and test planning. We used no other design notation.

Coding a program from a formal specification as detailed as ours is a straightforward exercise. State variables in the specification are implemented by program variables (of course there are many additional program variables: loop indices, etc.). State transitions are implemented by functions. Usually we can implement each Z construct in less than a page of C code so it is easy to confirm that the code correctly achieves the intent of its specification. We performed pencil-and-paper formal derivations of a few pages of code, but we derived most of the code by intuition and verified it by inspection, using methods recommended in a textbook [2]. The program is 15,786 lines of C code.

The formal analyses described in the preceding section were applied to the formal specification, not the code. It was intended to reveal design errors, and cannot reveal coding errors. Our development method should ensure that, at worst, the code only contains trivial logic errors. We used code inspections and testing to detect these errors.

Testing revealed 213 coding errors during development before the program was considered complete and 13 errors during testing of the completed program.

## Results and discussion

The new program began clinical operation in July 1999. In the first four months of use, six errors were revealed. All six involved incorrect warning messages or incorrect record-keeping by the program. At this writing (December 1999), no more errors have appeared. The program has never set up a field incorrectly or enabled the beam to turn on or remain on when the machine was not set up correctly.

## Conclusion

There is really only one way to show that a program possesses any invariance property (such as safety): show that the set of reachable program states is a subset of the set of acceptable (safe) program states. There are only two techniques that can show this conclusively: theorem proving and model checking. Both techniques require an explicit description of the acceptable states which is independent of the program.

Except for testing, all other effective assurance methods can be seen as more or less informal approximations to theorem proving or model checking. Our contribution in this project was to raise the level of formality, thereby (we believe) improving the effectiveness of the analysis. We have shown that it is feasible to create and use formal specifications for radiation therapy machine controls. However, our manual analysis effort was tedious and fallible. The obvious next step is to investigate the effectiveness of automated theorem provers and model checkers.

### Acknowledgements

Thanks to Rob Emery, Ira Kalet, Dave Reid, Ruedi Risler, and Peter Wootton for work on requirements, testing, installation and use, Michael Patrick and Jonathan Unger for work on the formal specification and code, Dave Reid also for work on code, and Mark Saaltink for help with Z/EVES.

## References

[1] Ira J. Kalet, Jonathan P. Jacky, Ruedi Risler, Solveig Rohlin, and Peter Wootton. Integration of radiotherapy planning systems and radiotherapy treatment equipment: 11 years experience. *International Journal of Radiation Oncology, Biology and Physics*, 38(1):213–221, 1997.

[2] Jonathan Jacky. *The Way of Z: Practical Programming with Formal Methods.* Cambridge University Press, 1997.

[3] Mark Saaltink. The Z/EVES system. In Jonathan P. Bowen, Michael G. Hinchey, and David Till, editors, *ZUM '97: The Z Formal Specification Notation*, pages 72 – 85. Tenth International Conference of Z Users, Springer-Verlag, 1997. Lecture Notes in Computer Science 1212.

[4] E. Clarke, O. Grumberg, and D. Long. Verification tools for finite-state concurrent systems. In J. W. De Bakker, W.-P. de Roever, and G. Rozenberg, editors, *A Decade of Concurrency*, pages 124–175, Noordwijkerhout, The Netherlands, 1993. REX School/Symposium, Springer-Verlag. Lecture Notes in Computer Science, vol. 803.

# Design Considerations for Intensity Modulated Proton Therapy Treatment Planning

**Hanne Kooy[1], Uwe Oelfke[2], Tony Lomax[3], Harald Paganetti[1], Wayne Newhauser[1], Thomas Bortfeld[2], Michael Goitein[1,4]**

[1]Dept of Radiation Oncology, Massachusetts General Hospital, Boston MA, USA, [2]Deutsches Krebsforschungszentrum, Heidelberg, Germany, [3]Paul Scherrer Institute, Switzerland, and University of Zurich, Zurich, Switzerland

## Introduction

Treatment planning for intensity modulated proton therapy, IMPT, or in general with heavy charged particles, poses significant computational problems in addition to those present in treatment planning for intensity modulated X-ray therapy, IMXT. IMPT has the additional degree-of-freedom of control in depth which permits control of intensity (fluence) at a point at the elemental dose delivery component [1]. IMPT and IMXT both control the intensity of the beam across a two-dimensional field aperture. IMPT, however, modulates this intensity at different energies within a single field. The IMPT computational problem is therefore an order of magnitude larger compared to IMXT, corresponding to the modulation at each energy level. In addition, dose deposition for heavy charged particles is, in general, a non-linear function of the spectral properties at that point. Thus, to be exact, conversion between RBE and energy deposition must be considered at the fundamental level. This results in a significant increase in information that must be maintained at a deposition point. These computational considerations require a thorough (re)evaluation of the data structures needed to support this additional complexity.

Proton therapy with intensity modulated beams, to be clinically effective, must rely on the integration of the knowledge base of the small group of practitioners of proton therapy. The design of IMPT treatment planning software must thus promote a modular and abstract design and support a network communication model to permit these practitioners to share algorithmic implementations and clinical data and results. In addition, such a modular system design of itself will directly support IMXT treatment planning.

## Material and methods

### System Design

The system design incorporates a comprehensive set of objects, encapsulating data and their operations, to model the IMPT process. These data structures emphasize computational completeness, i.e. inclusiveness of all the tasks necessary in the treatment plan optimization process, and efficiency to permit rapid evaluations of the score functions and progression to an optimal plan. The system design implements a client-server model. In this model, the "Task Manager" in the Figure 1 captures and manages the optimization process, while computational tasks (the "Clients"), which include dose computations and optimization algorithms, are defined as objects on the client-side that communicate through a Communication Manager (implemented with CORBA) with the server implementation of their computational methods. This design achieves a level of modularity where, given the object communication interface, one can develop and implement a new dose or optimization algorithm and include existing algorithms. The Task Manager and Clients request visualization and user interface services from the Visualization Manager.

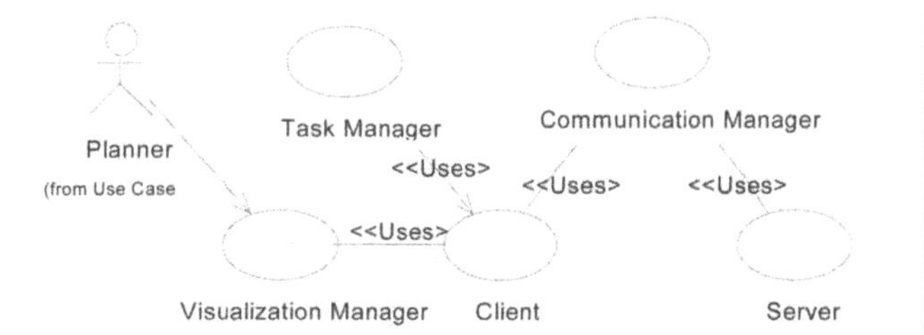


**Figure 1:** :Top level components of the IMPT system. The Task Manager manages functional Clients which execute their tasks in Server tasks through the Communication Manager. The Planner interacts through the Visualization Manager.

The system design extends its modular concepts by not including contouring or beam design capabilities. The system acquires such data from departmental databases which permit treatment plan and delivery data to be stored and retrieved.

### Data Objects

The object design emphasizes rapid computations through 1) the use of arbitrary point sets to reduce the need for full volumetric computations without loss of information [2], 2) pre-computations for elemental beams to decouple the dose computation from the optimization, 3) extensive indexing data structures to permit rapid access to computational data, 4) a fine-grained hierarchical definition of the object space, and 5) vector storage at each space point to permit calculation of RBE.

## Results

A particular example of the data object design, concerning data indexing considerations, is illustrated in Figure 2. The IMPT process operates on a fixed set of volumes and beams, i.e. we do not intend to optimize for the beam phase-space itself. (These are explicit design decisions.) The Planner manipulates the volume constraints and the optimization criteria to generate competing "optimal" plans. This problem decomposes into a set of arbitrary dose points, for which the elemental energy/dose distribution is computed, combined with a set of weights coupled to an optimization schema. Each optimization schema, or plan, has its own set of weights. The optimization task manipulates the schema weights to each dose deposition element to create a composite photon-equivalent dose in the "patient" and iterates until the optimization constratins are achieved. Clearly, a central problem in our design is thus the efficient indexing from an optimization schema with its set of weights to the individual dose points.

Our object hierarchy defines an optimization schema, OptScheme, which contains treatment Courses, which contain Beams, which contain DoseBusts (the dose and/or energy deposition elements). Sets of arbitrarily distributed points are stored in DoseStores. Each DoseStore maintains a vector at each member point to permit storage of energy/particle distributions and a scalar to store the photon-equivalent dose. Each Course maintains indices to the set of DoseStores that pertain to that Course. (The latter permits different Courses to consider different volumes in the optimization.) Each DoseBurst has a reference to each DoseStore point to which the DoseBurst makes a contribution. This contribution is pre-computed at the "unit" weight level and stored in the DoseBurst together with the reference to the point to which the contribution is made. The OptScheme links each of its weight to the corresponding DoseBurst. In the optimization iteration loop, the optimization schema directly manipulates the dose/energy contribution at the relevant points through a direct reference to the DoseBurst which has a direct reference to the points to which it contributes. Since the total number of points can be controlled by the user (through the choice of arbitrary distributions) the total number of references (and thus memory requirements) can be maintained at acceptable levels.

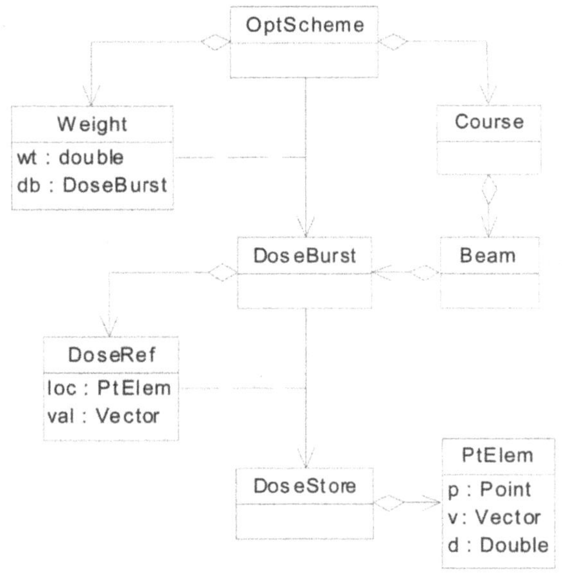


**Figure 2:** Class hierarchy of IMPT objects (see text). The optimization schema (OptScheme) has an association with the DoseBurst controlled by the Weight association class. The DoseBurst, in turn, references the computation points in a DoseStore through the DoseRef association class. Most objects are aggregate elements of the parent class as indicated by the diamond-arrow symbol..

## Discussion

The design of a software system is a non-trivial task. Firstly, one must consider existing components and evaluate their reusability. Often, within the context of radiation therapy, these comprise algorithmic components such as dose calculations, volume representations, and other legacy elements. Any new design should encapsulate these elements. Our approach is to incorporate these elements at the implementation level of data objects, which themselves are designed in a broader context and at a higher level of abstraction. The abstraction level is such that a data object can be manipulated at the client side, i.e. it physically resides with the Planner, while permitting ad-hoc implementation and runtime access of its services across the network as indicated in Figure 1.

It is clear that modern software technologies, such as network abstraction offered through CORBA, have great potential to provide a level of integration and sharing within our community that is not currently present or perhaps even conceptualized. Our particular application of IMPT especially benefits from such technology as we must be able to share data and results to properly evaluate the benefits of hadron therapy.

Software engineering has progressed from art to science. Good design principles certainly have always been available. What has changed is the availability of formal definitions and design tools that implement those principles. One such formal system, used by us, is the Unified Modeling Language [3] which is the basis of the Rose environment [4]. Such systems enforce a proper methodology, but still do not excuse the designer from not applying proper object designs.

Our effort is thus two-fold. Firstly, we must design a system that will operate over a world-wide network. This will require a top-level design as indicated in Figure 1 to promote a separation of the optimization process and the implementation of the computational elements. Secondly, we must design the computational objects which permit efficient algorithmic implementation of a severe computational problem and which permit the functional separation indicated in Figure 1.

## References

[1] Lomax A 1999 Intensity modulation methods for proton radiotherapy. Phys. Med. Biol. **44** 185-205

[2] Niemierko A and Goitein M 1990 Random sampling for evaluating treatment plans. Med. Phys. **17** 753-762

[3] The Unified Modeling Language Reference Manual Rumbaugh J, Jacobson I, Booch G, Addison Wesley 1998

[4] Rational Software Corporation, Cupertino, CA

# A delineation system for N modalities – software aspects

**Marcel van Herk, Katrien De Jaeger, Jan de Munck, Mischa Hoogeman, Jan Meinders, Lennert Ploeger and Lambert Zijp**

The Netherlands Cancer Institute / Antoni van Leeuwenhoek Huis, Amsterdam, The Netherlands. E-mail: portal@nki.nl

## Introduction

Target volume delineation is an important source of uncertainty in radiotherapy. The usefulness of image registration to improve the quality of target volume delineation for treatment planning is well established [e.g., 1, 2]. However, it is an unsolved problem how to best utilize multiple image modalities for target volume delineation. Mostly, users would switch back and forth between modalities, copying previously delineated contours, or target volumes are combined using Boolean operators. Some delineation systems can handle two scans simultaneously, using linked cursors [3]. When utilizing more than two image modalities for delineation, the image registration is difficult (how to build a consistent set of N matched images from arbitrary matched pairs), but also the user interface is complex (how to present several scans simultaneously). The aim of this study is to develop a software system that allows N different scans or image modalities to be used simultaneously for delineation (in short: the *system*). In this paper, the emphasis will be on the object oriented software constructs which were developed to implement such a complex system.

## Material and methods

The system is written in C++ (the image processing and image handling functions, and Borland Delphi (the user interface). It consists of the following components: data interface library, coordinate system manager, data flow manager, viewer component, and delineation and paintbrush controllers. Each of these components will be described in some detail. Finally, the integrated system will be presented.

### Data interface library

Image registration software is not included in the system. Instead, match results from our clinical image registration software [4, 5] are used as input. The system accepts scans from several sources, such as DICOM, AAPM RTOG and native files from a number of planning systems. All match results are stored in a text file (one per patient), of which an abbreviated example is shown in Fig. 1. Each match has a unique name and consists of two 'links' (similar to an internet address) to the registered scans, along with the transformation matrix which aligns one scan with the other. The links consist of a data type ('**dicom**' and '**pinnacle**' in this example), the physical location of the data, a patient identifier ('**patient_50**' and '**1**' in this example) and a scan identifier. The syntax of the links depends on the data format. For example, a link to a DICOM server contains an application entity name, an IP address, a port number, and unique DICOM identifiers that identify a scan (patient, study and series. When the user reads a match, both scans (pixel values and many other properties) indicated by the links are loaded into memory. However, the same scan is never loaded twice. The transformation matrix is passed to the coordinate system manager.

```
*******************************************************
Match: Example match 1

CT:     pinnacle:g:\patient_50:50.patient\iset1253.scan
MRI:    dicom:planning;127.0.0.1;104\1:1.patient\x.study\
        y.series\z.scan

transformation (mri to ct in scan coordinate system):
   0.9996     0.0130    -0.0252     0.0000
  -0.0129     0.9999     0.0029     0.0000
   0.0253    -0.0025     0.9997     0.0000
  -0.6816     0.7132    -4.3113     1.0000
*******************************************************
```

**Figure 1:** Abbreviated example of a match data file of our clinical image registration system. The data is stored in a simple text file with Internet address-like references to scans in different formats and stored on different physical location. The DICOM reference is abbreviated (unique identifiers are long!)

### Coordinate system manager

The system will accept match results of arbitrary image pairs in sequence and will build a consistent matched view of N scans, i.e., the system is able to compute transformation matrices between arbitrary scan pairs. When reading a match pair for which the transformation is already known, the system will report the inconsistency (change) in the match matrix.

To do this, an object-oriented software class was developed: the coordinate system manager. This manager works by maintaining a grid (with N rows and columns corresponding with matched coordinate systems in N scans) filled with all possible transformation matrices between the coordinate systems. Writing a particular transformation will update either a row or column with transformation matrices in the grid, depending on simple priority rules (which can be changed by the program). The changes are such that the whole set of transformation matrices is kept consistent. In particular this means that for any set of coordinate system (a, b, and c), the product of the transformation from a to b with the transformation from b to c will always be equal to the transformation from a to c.

In reality, the system maintains three coordinate systems for each scan, and two global coordinate systems are defined: a universal coordinate system (where, e.g., +x always points to the left side of the patient) and a view system which defines the patient orientation on the displays. Since, for practical reasons, the current limit on the number of scans is 10, a maximum of 32 coordinate systems (3 x 10 + 2) is defined in the system.

Suppose that N-1 scans are present in the system and a match pair is added between a new (Nth) scan and an already loaded scan. The following code then updates the grid of transformation matrices (this line is taken from the actual code that reads a match result between scans a and b):

```
W.Transform(Scan[b].Cmatch, Scan[a].Cmatch).assign(T),
```

where **W** is the coordinate manager software object, **Scan** is the array of scans in memory, **Cmatch** is the 'matched' coordinate system of a scan and **T** is the match matrix as read from the file such as shown in Figure 1. The **assign** method stores matrix **T** in the coordinate manager. This line of code results in a change of all transformation matrices that relate to matched **Scan[b]** (i.e., up to 32 matrices). One can imagine that keeping all program objects (e.g., display windows) that depend on these matrices consistent and up to date is a daunting task. A third important software construct, a data flow manager, has therefore been developed to automate this aspect.

**Data flow manager**

Almost all data objects used in the program (image data, transformation matrices, etc.) are derived from a base class that maintains a time stamp. To guarantee data consistency, the same mechanism is used as in the well known 'make' files for software projects: each object maintains a list of all other objects it is dependent upon. Each object has a make method, which performs the following actions:

- Invoke the make method of *all* objects on which this object depends
- If *any* object on which this object depends has a newer time stamp than the object itself:
  - ➢ Update the object (i.e., perform some computation)
  - ➢ Update the time stamp of the object

The result is that invoking the make method on a high level object (e.g., a viewer component) will cause a cascade of lower level computations, but only those that are required to make the end result up to date. In practice, all dependencies are pre-defined in the initialization part of the program, and a timer is used to regularly update the highest level components (all visible viewers). The result is that no client code is required to guarantee data consistency or update the displays. In the previous example, where 32 transformation matrices changed, only those display windows that depend on any of these matrices will update without writing a single line of code. Even though the timer triggers make events all the time (e.g., 100 times per second), computations will only be performed when needed, i.e., when any object has changed (when its time stamp was updated). Display windows which are invisible refrain from updating. In addition, the system automatically avoids unnecessary double computations which are often difficult to circumvent in event driven software.

**Viewer component**

The system contains a large number of display windows (see, e.g., Figure 2). Each of these windows is an instance of the same visual component: the viewer. This viewer is used in all our imaging applications and it is specialized for image fusion, i.e., it has multiple inputs that accept 3D data and a transformation matrix, and the slices are re-sampled and mixed as needed for display only. The viewer is capable of slicing orthogonal, slicing arbitrarily, adjusting level and window (using 8, 16 or 32 bit integer and floating point input data), zooming, fusing two volumes with color wash techniques, displaying overlays and contours, and cutting the display for side by side comparison of matched data. The viewer also contains a keyboard and a mouse interface for most common operations (e.g., zooming, slicing, adjusting level and window), and tools such as a ruler and a pixel value probe are built-in.

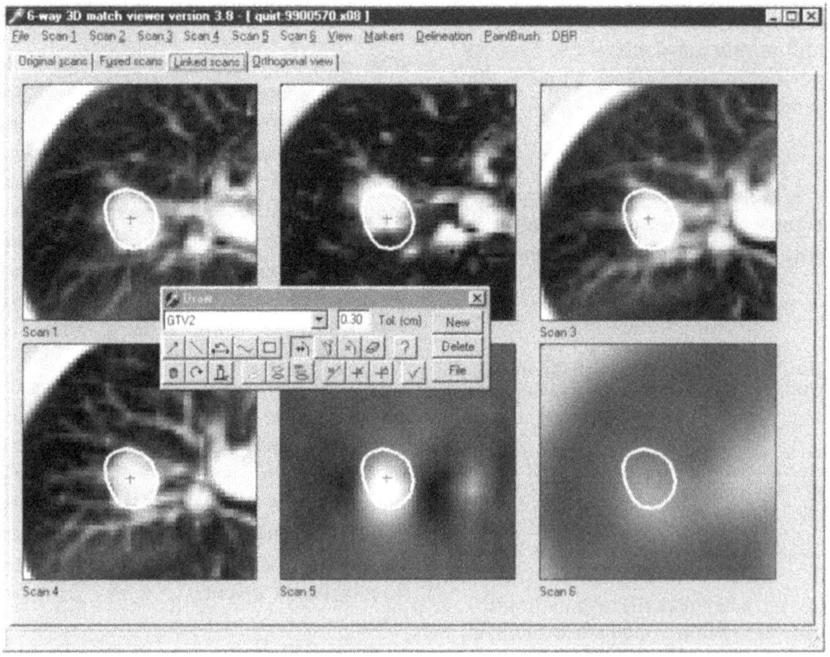


**Figure 2:** Example of the use of the delineation system for a lung case. Scans 1..4 are normal and helical CT scans in different phases of the breathing cycle (using voluntary breath hold). Scan 5 is a FDG PET scan, while scan 6 is the transmission PET which was used for matching. All scans were matched on bony anatomy and all displays are fully linked. Differences in tumor position are due to breathing.

**Delineation and paintbrush controller**

The delineation and paintbrush functionality is provided through tool windows that control all viewers simultaneously (the viewer component contains the software for delineation and painting, but no user interface). The delineation controller window (Figure 2) contains buttons for: getting information about a structure, drawing lines, capping structures, extruding structures, rotating structures, drawing rectangles, deleting details (lines and points), deleting details but keeping connections, sketching, interpolating structures between slices, scaling structures, moving structures, erasing, editing details, creating new structures, and deleting structures. The paintbrush controller window has buttons to set the paintbrush color, shape (circle, sphere, rectangle, cube), function (draw, erase, flood-fill) and size.

**The integrated system**

The complete system (Figure 2) contains, amongst others, up to 10 scan objects, one coordinate system manager, up to 10 viewer components displaying raw scans, up to 10 viewer components displaying linked scans, and one large display with fused data. Most code of the main program deals with reading and writing of views and handling menu items. The system provides concurrent processing and display of multiple (registered) image modalities. Actions performed on any display are reflected in real time in all other displays: such as slicing, zooming and panning. During delineation, every drawing action that is performed on, e.g., a CT display simultaneously occurs on, e.g., the MRI display and vice-versa. Note that this tool is similar to the "TOMAS" tool proposed by researchers of the DKFZ [3]. However, TOMAS only works with two scans, while our system accepts up to 10 scans.

## Practical application and discussion

The software system is currently in experimental use, and has already proven its use to answer a number of difficult clinical questions. We just started a study to accurately define treatment margins for lung cancer patients. Here, multiple CT scans are used from different phases of the breathing cycle, in combination with a PET scan to define narrow, patient specific, margins for breathing (Figure 2). Another use is recurrences. In case of a recurrence, it is imperative to know the location of the failure relative to the original dose distribution, in order to evaluate the source of failure and the possibility of re-irradiation. This system was used to provide the answer by matching the original planning CT, planning MRI, and dose distribution with a diagnostic follow-up CT. In this way, the recurrence visible in the follow-up CT is linked to the planned dose distribution. Similarly, we recently used the system to evaluate a case of rapid tumor growth, also for a brain case. It turned out that, during the first two weeks of irradiation, the tumor bulk and edema region had grown outside the high dose region. With this system, this situation could be identified quickly and the treatment fields were consequently adjusted.

The software constructs described in this paper significantly reduced the complexity of the system. Without the coordinate system manager and data flow manager, the software complexity would be $O(N^2)$, where N is the number of scans. Using the new software components the complexity is O(N), where each of the N scans is treated identically (i.e., in a loop). However, a disadvantage of automating the data flow is that it is sometimes difficult to understand the actions of the program and debugging becomes complicated. The use of a 'standard' data interface library and viewer component, makes that the client code has a modest size: about 3500 lines, where about half of this code deals with aspects not discussed in this paper.

## Conclusion

We have developed an advanced system for simultaneous delineation in up to 10 image modalities, which has already proven its usefulness for a few clinical cases. The complexity of this system was reduced by using pre-coded software objects, by automatically maintaining the relations between the numerous coordinate systems and by automatically maintaining data consistency using an algorithm based on time stamps and explicit dependencies.

## References

[1] Rasch C, Keus R, Pameijer FA, Koops W, de Ru V, Muller, S, Touw A, Bartelink H, van Herk M and Lebesque JV 1997 The potential impact of CT-MRI matching on tumor volume delineation in advanced head and neck cancer *Int J Radiat Oncol Biol Phys* **39** 841-848

[2] Rasch C, Barillot I, Remeijer P, Touw A, van Herk M and Lebesque JV 1999 Definition of the prostate in CT and MRI: a multi-observer study *Int J Radiat Oncol Biol Phys* **43** 57-66

[3] Pross J, Bendl R and Schlegel W 1994 TOMAS, A Tool for Manual Segmentation based on Multiple image data sets. *Proc. XIth International Conference on the use of computers in radiation therapy* 192-193

[4] van Herk M and Kooy H 1994 Automatic three-dimensional correlation of CT-CT, CT-MRI, and CT-SPECT using chamfer matching *Med Phys* **21** 1163-1178

[5] van Herk M, de Munck JC, Lebesque JV, Muller S, Rasch C, Touw A 1998 Automatic registration of pelvic computed tomography data and magnetic resonance scans including a full circle method for quantitative accuracy evaluation *Med Phys* **25** 2054-2067

# A new design for a DICOM-3 server

**Ira J. Kalet[1], Robert S. Giansiracusa[1] and Drora Avitan[2]**
[1]University of Washington, Seattle, Washington, USA, and [2]Soroka Medical Center, Be'er Sheva, ISRAEL

## Introduction

We describe a new design for programs using the DICOM-3 protocol [1], which we have implemented in a DICOM image storage server for our locally developed radiation treatment planning system, Prism [2]. This design is declarative, representing DICOM as a language for describing messages and sequencing of messages. The coding involved implementing an interpreter for this language. The resulting server program is small, simple, and extensible, because most of the details of the DICOM protocol are not hard coded but are in the rules and state table that the interpreter uses to perform all its functions.

Many DICOM implementations do nothing more than dump received data into files in the format specified by Part 10 of the DICOM standard. While this is simple from the implementor's point of view, it is useless to us. Prism has its own image storage and indexing system, and in order to use existing DICOM software, we would have to make major modifications either to Prism (to read DICOM files) or to the DICOM software (to write Prism files). We decided that the work involved in modifying software that was written in a totally different context would be at least as much as designing and implementing our own DICOM server from the beginning. We also saw an opportunity to experiment with an innovative design approach to this problem.

## Material and methods

The Prism DICOM Server (referred to here as "PDS") functions as a DICOM Application Entity. This section describes how PDS implements the DICOM protocol and selected DICOM services. In this and following sections, we assume the reader is familiar with the basic concepts of DICOM, as described in Bidgood [1]. We also assume familiarity with basic networking concepts, including the TCP/IP protocols, and the design of socket based clients and servers [3].

PDS is written in Common Lisp, as is the rest of the Prism system. It uses modules from the Prism system for reading and writing data in the Prism file system and for creating Prism image data objects. PDS follows the standard design of a connection-oriented, single-threaded TCP/IP server. PDS waits for an incoming connection, reads input from a TCP stream, decodes the information into DICOM messages, interprets those messages, performs operations on data, composes responses according to the protocol, and transmits those responses to the remote DICOM entity over the TCP stream. When a DICOM Image Object or set of Image Objects has been received, it is stored in the local file system as a Prism Image Set (or in the case of a single image, as part of an image set).

### The Prism DICOM state machine

The *DICOM Upper Layer Protocol* (DUL) specifies how *Application Entities* (DICOM clients and servers) use DICOM messages to communicate, to negotiate with each other, and to provide the complex services needed. The DICOM communication primitives that carry messages, commands, and data are called *Protocol Data Units* or *PDUs.* PDS uses a finite state machine to implement the DICOM Upper Layer Protocol, parsing incoming PDUs and generating outgoing PDUs using a production rule grammar.

We designed the state-machine and grammar rules to mirror closely the description published in the formal DICOM specification. These declarative representations and the underlying implementation are intended to be humanly understandable, self-documenting, and easily extensible. The rules document the PDU structures to the programmer wishing to extend our system to recognize additional data encodings (or commands, or message formats). PDS also uses a data dictionary, which describes the representation of data in DICOM objects. These entries are also human readable, extendable and machine interpretable.

Figure 1 shows a flowchart of the PDS design (above the TCP/IP layer). Packets are read until a complete PDU is received. The PDU is parsed using the parse rules, and the state table then determines the next action.

The standard defines the *control structure* or sequencing of actions via a *state table* which relates States, Events, and Actions. *States* name situations the system can be in (waiting for a certain PDU, sending data, etc), *events* name conditions triggering certain actions, and *actions* name the operation to be performed in the appropriate situation. A *state table* (or *state transition table*) is simply a table containing an entry for each legal state/event combination. Each entry indicates what action to perform under that condition and what state to enter for the next cycle.

Our representation of the DUL control structure is a direct translation of the standard's state table into a Lisp data structure consisting of a list of entries, each entry mapping a state/event combination to an action-function/next-state combination. Our state-table representation serves both to document the control structure of our system to the programmer and as machine-readable data to drive the sequencer directly.

The table entry shown in figure 2 indicates that `STATE-06` is the one for the purpose "Assoc. established, ready for data transfer" (a descriptive comment). In this state, the

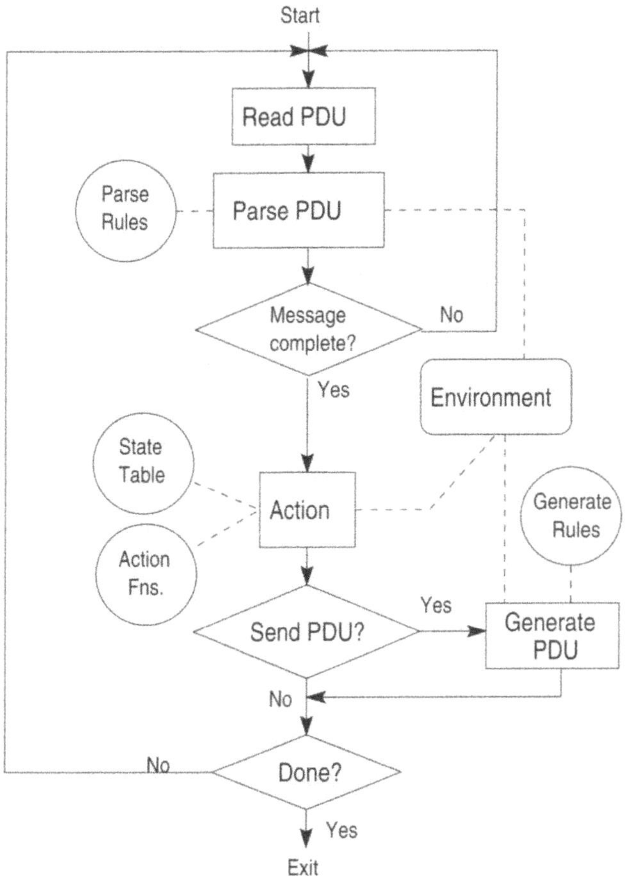


**Figure 1:** Prism DICOM server state machine design

```
(state-06
 "Assoc. established, ready for data transfer"
 ((event-09) dt-01 state-06)
 ((event-10) dt-02 state-06)
 ((event-20) dt-03 state-06)
 ((event-21) dt-04 state-06)
 ((event-11) ar-01 state-07)
 ((event-12A event-12B) ar-02 state-08)
 ((event-16) aa-03 nil)
 ((event-17) aa-04 nil)
 ((event-15) aa-01 state-13)
 ((event-03 event-04 event-06 event-13 event-19)
       aa-08 state-13))
```

**Figure 2:** State table entry for Data Transfer state

response to the signalling of **EVENT-09** is to invoke action function **DT-01** and to transfer next to **STATE-06**. Where several events are grouped in parentheses (for example, the row containing **EVENT-12A** and **EVENT-12B**), the meaning is that any of the listed events signals the invocation of the indicated action function and state transition.

The next state is listed last in each row. A next state of `nil` means that the server exits the DUL interpreter loop, closes the TCP connection to that client, and listens for another connection request.

## Parsing of PDUs via grammar rules

We implement parsing of incoming PDU data streams and generation of outgoing PDU data streams via rules which define the elements that must be matched in an incoming stream or placed in an outgoing stream. The rules contain variable references, allowing the substitution of data values for named variables during the parsing and generation process.

The rules define an *augmented context-free grammar*. It is *context-free* in that the legality of a structure depends only on its form and not on the context in which it appears, and *augmented* in that rules can contain embedded function calls to test decoded data values for appropriateness.

The elements of grammar rules are *tokens* (symbols naming constants or other rules) or *expressions* (an expression is a parenthesized list of tokens). Expressions can represent *variables* (data values that can be referred to by name in other rules), *function calls* (data values computed from simpler expressions), or *operators* (instructions to generate particular values, such as computing the length of the PDU currently being constructed).

As PDS parses incoming PDUs it extends an *environment* which stores these variables and their values. The environment is accessible to any operation that needs values of data fields in the decoded PDUs.

PDS uses rules in the same format to describe the generation and structure of outgoing messages. Generation rules can contain references to the same variables as do the parse rules, providing a simple mechanism to echo received values on transmission (or to output values computed from previously received data).

## Example of a Parse Rule

For parsing, a rule describes *conditions* for matching the incoming byte-stream and the *variable bindings* to be added to the environment as a result of such matches.

The rule shown in figure 3 (for parsing the *A-Associate-RQ* PDU) illustrates several element types, including tags, constants, ignored fields, variables, recursive rule invocations, and optional items.

The symbol **:A-Associate-RQ-PDU** is a *tag* and is returned as the result of decoding this PDU. It also serves to name the rule. This allows rules to be looked up by name in the list of rules.

The hexadecimal value **#x01** is a constant that must be matched by a single byte in the input stream.

The entries * for a single byte and (* 32) for a field of 32 bytes (and similar entries) indicate that the parser should account for byte field lengths but should otherwise ignore the content of those fields.

```
(:A-Associate-RQ-PDU
  #x01     ; Associate-RQ PDU Type tag
  *        ; Reserved field -- not used
  (* 4)    ; PDU Length [4 bytes]
  (>var Protocol-Version fixnum 2 :Big-Endian)
  (* 2)
  (>var Called-AE-Title string 16 :Space-Pad)
  (>var Calling-AE-Title string 16 :Space-Pad)
  (* 32)
  :Application-Context-Item-RQ/AC
  (:Repeat (1 *) :Presentation-Context-Item-RQ)
  :User-Information-Item-RQ/AC)
```

**Figure 3:** Parse rule for A-Associate Request PDU

`(>var Called-AE-Title string 16 :Space-Pad)` indicates that the data in the next 16 bytes should be interpreted as a character string, with space-padding stripped, and stored into a *variable* named `Called-AE-Title`.

`:Application-Context-Item-RQ/AC` means that a rule by that name should be used *recursively* to parse the next sequence of bytes (that is, rules can use other rules recursively to define their own components).

`(:Repeat (1 *) :Presentation-Context-Item-RQ)` indicates an item that may be present one or more times in the input data stream. *Which* item is indicated by its tag, and the minimum and maximum number of allowable repeats (including a minimum of zero for *optional* items) is indicated by the limits `(1 *)` (one to infinity in this case).

New kinds of messages can be supported by just adding rules and state table entries rather than adding to the code. Similarly, modifications to the DUL protocol can be accomodated by making the corresponding alterations in the rules and state table.

## Results and discussion

The entire server executable code consists of about 3000 lines of Common Lisp. The data dictionary, rules and state table account for another 3000 lines of Lisp expressions (in Lisp, code and data have the same form). Another 2000 lines of comments and blank space make the code and data easily human readable. The system has been thoroughly tested with four different types of image sources from different vendors. Because the data dictionary is complete, the parser should be able to handle just about any image source. The server is now operational and currently provides the C-ECHO (verification) and C-STORE operations.

Because the design puts details into rules and a state table, rather than hard coding them, it can easily be adapted to add other functions and support for additional objects such as radiotherapy plans. We plan to construct a DICOM-RT client for Prism and a DICOM-RT server for our Clinical Neutron Therapy System. These programs will reuse almost all of the code and data structures, requiring very little additional code. This also will enable us to send RT plan data to our computer controlled linear accelerators, when the accelerator manufacturer[1] provides DICOM-RT support. We believe the declarative language design is sufficiently general that it could be adapted to implement other network application protocols such as HL7 [4].

## Conclusion

The effort to produce our own server has resulted in a new design, which recasts DICOM as a declarative language for specifying messages and data, with the server essentially being an interpreter for this language. The design is easy to extend and adapt to other related applications. The entire code is available at the University of Washington Radiation Oncology Department web site[2].

It is a pleasure to thank Steven Moore of Washington University, St. Louis, for assistance in clarifying fine points of the DICOM protocol and for advice in using his CTN test programs. Thanks also go to Mark Phillips, Jon Jacky, and Homayoon Parsaei, University of Washington, Marv Kleven, David Haynor, and Steve Sutlief, Seattle VA Hospital, Pat Gavin and Hege Kippenes, Washington State University, and Yanai Krutman, Ludwig Avraham, and Gadi Gilon, Soroka Medical Center, for assistance in testing and debugging the server.

## References

[1] W. Dean Bidgood, Jr., Steven C. Horii, Fred W. Prior, and Donald E. Van Syckle. Understanding and using DICOM, the data interchange standard for biomedical imaging. *Journal of the American Medical Informatics Association*, 4(3):199–212, 1997.

[2] Ira J. Kalet, Jonathan P. Jacky, Mary M. Austin-Seymour, Sharon M. Hummel, Kevin J. Sullivan, and Jonathan M. Unger. Prism: A new approach to radiotherapy planning software. *International Journal of Radiation Oncology, Biology and Physics*, 36(2):451–461, 1996.

[3] Douglas E. Comer. *Computer Networks and Internets*. Prentice-Hall, Upper Saddle River, NJ, second edition, 1999.

[4] HL7 Working Group. Application protocol for electronic data exchange in healthcare environments, version 2.3.1, 1999. Available from the HL7 on-line bookstore, `https://www.hl7.org/library/bookstore.cfm`.

[1] Elekta Oncology Systems

[2] `http://www.radonc.washington.edu/`

# Implementing DICOM RT in a radiotherapy department

**Karsten Eilertsen, Lasse Sæten and Tor Olav Green**

The Norwegian Radium Hospital, Dept. of Medical Physics, Montebello, N-0310 Oslo, Norway

## Introduction

The computer network of the radiotherapy department should provide the technical infrastructure required for rapid transmission and exchange of data between the different modalities used for diagnosis, planning and treatment.

Until recently data export and import to and from the computer systems, have been managed by vendor proprietary solutions. In a multimodality radiotherapy department with equipment from different manufacturers, these solutions provide little flexibility and may jeopardise consistency as data must be reformatted to suit a given equipment specification. This creates a need for an additional maintenance level to assure data quality when for instance equipment is upgraded or replaced.

The DICOM v3.0 standard, including the radiotherapy extensions, supports fundamental network interactions, and the DICOM RT information objects provide a means for standardised transfer of most of the information that circulates in the radiotherapy department [1]. However, there are at present few manufacturers of radiotherapy equipment that fully support the DICOM RT standard.

We have therefore developed a DICOM RT engine that provides utilities for driving a DICOM based radiotherapy network in our department. The key features of this engine are a query/retrieve server and a DICOMDIR server that manages the storage of DICOM objects.

A graphical user interface (GUI) has been developed to run the engine. In addition, this interface allows a user to interactively browse the contents of the DICOMDIR storage.

The engine is currently used as the communication link between non-DICOM and DICOM applications. This is achieved by the use of custom made export and import applications that translate the vendor specific data into DICOM attributes or vice versa.

Thus, with the present system together with a commercially available DICOM RT conformant digital archive, the concept of a RT PACS system is near realisation.

## Material and methods

The DICOM RT engine applications (Figure 1) are mainly implemented in C. The MergeCom Toolkit (Merge Technologies Inc., Milwaukee, U.S.A.) has been used extensively for the core implementation of the low level network interaction. This enhances portability and ensures stability. The toolkit components have been subject to vigorous testing by several parties before they are put into use. At present the engine runs on a dedicated standard Pentium type computer, but it may run on any kind of platform that is supported by the MergeCom Toolkit.

The DICOM engine can act as Query/Retrieve Service Class User (Q/R SCU) and can connect to applications that can act as Query/Retrieve Service Class Providers (Q/R SCP), typically a digital archiving system. The query results received by the engine can subsequently be used to initiate a move of DICOM RT objects from the remote application to another destination e.g. the local storage of the engine itself (see next paragraph).

The DICOMDIR server consists of a Storage SCP that stores DICOM objects in a DICOMDIR folder/file hierarchy. This server also runs another process, a browser, to which user applications can connect in order to retrieve information about current contents of the DICOMDIR.

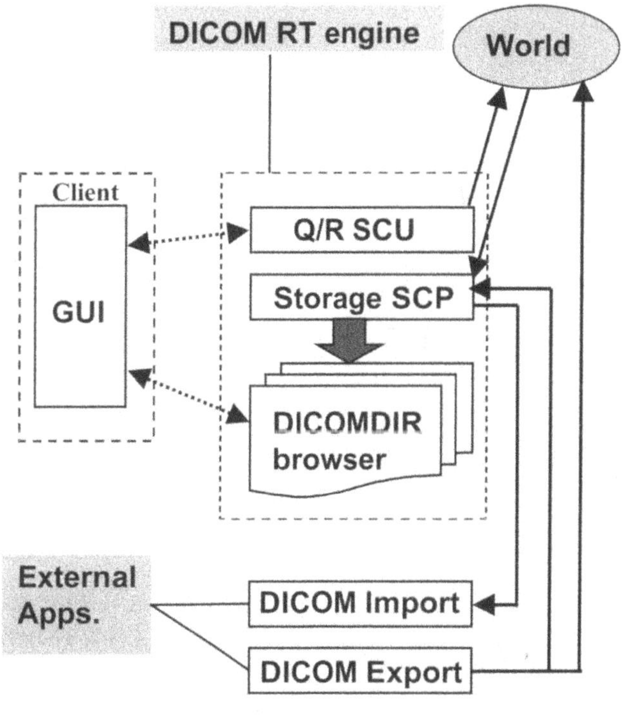


**Figure 1:** The DICOM RT engine.

The graphical user interface (Figure 2) has been developed in C++ using Microsoft Foundation Classes (MFC). This application may run as a client on PCs that are able to connect to the DICOM engine server via the hospital network. The client and the servers communicate by using Remote Procedure Calls (RPC), a communication mechanism supported by most operating systems.

The graphical user interface enables the user to select the archive to query as well as the move destination. The network and DICOM details required to establish the various connections are defined in a separate initialisation file. Furthermore, query model and query filters can be set from the

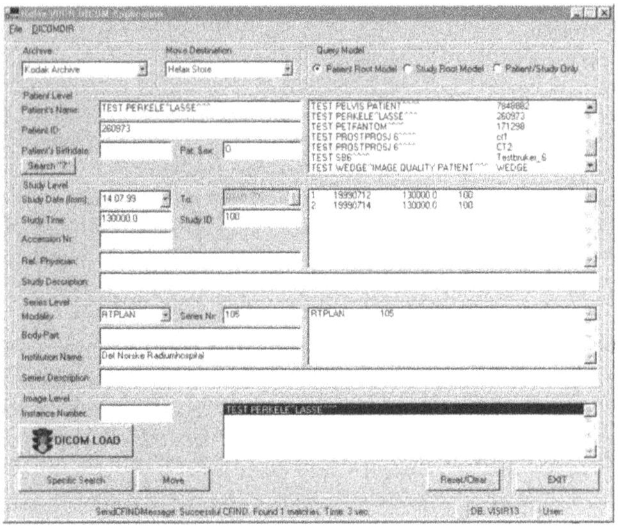


**Figure 2:** The Q/R graphical user interface

interface. The query results are displayed in separate lists that reflect the hierarchical DICOM data structure, i.e. patient – study – series – objects, according to the specified query model. One or more objects to move can be selected from any of the four levels, i.e. selecting a patient will cause the entire patient hierarchy to be moved, selecting a study will cause that study hierarchy to be moved and so forth.

The user interface is also designed to be started from within Windows NT based radiotherapy applications such as a verification and recording system or a treatment planning system in order to handle DICOM *export* and *import*. In either case demographics of the current patient can be transferred to the interface at start-up.

## Results and discussion

The described engine has been used to enable the exchange of DICOM objects between the different planning and treatment modalities in the department. These are the GE Advantage SIM v4.1 virtual simulator, the MDS Nordion family of products (the Helax IMCON v.1.1.1 digital simulator work station, the Helax TMS v.5.1 dose planning system, the Helax VISIR v1.3.a information and verification system), the Varian PortalVision v.5.23 electronic portal imaging system, the Varian Cadplan dose planning system, and finally the Kodak Archive Manager v3.5.1 picture archiving system.

From VISIR we were able to import RT Plans stored in the Kodak archive or the DICOMDIR. These plans were initially exported by the GE Adv. SIM, the TMS or Cadplan dose planning systems. We have also been able to export RT Plans to the Kodak archive, to the DICOM DIR Storage SCP, as well as to other remote applications.

Likewise, we have been able to import RT Plans and RT Images (referenced by the plans) to the IMCON system. The import of single RT Image objects requires the presence of an exposure sequence. Subsequently, when the image is displayed on the IMCON workstation, the collimator settings, beam shaping blocks and MLC settings appear as image overlays. We were also able to export RT Plans and an associated sequence of (referenced) RT Images to the Kodak archive and to the DICOMDIR Storage SCP. Each exported RT image was set to reference the associated RT Plan.

The import and export of data from the various radiotherapy systems involve the mapping of DICOM data attributes into the proprietary data format of each system and vice versa. For the MDS Nordion products, the mapping has been achieved by the use of a dedicated applications developed in close co-operation with the vendor.

The import/export of data to the VISIR and IMCON systems (as with any other non-DICOM compliant systems) represent a serious challenge. The DICOM object specifications do not contain every required data element and vice versa. One obvious solution to this problem is to extend the DICOM object definitions by introducing private attributes. However, this jeopardises the very idea of standardisation. So far we have been able to avoid using private attributes, but at the cost of sometimes having to ask the user to fill in required details.

One important side effect of the IMCON export facility is the linking of RT Plans and associated RT Images by utilising object referencing. This feature has been exploited by an in-house developed image registration software program. From this program, a plan and a reference image (e.g. simulator image or DRR) were retrieved from the Kodak archive. The image and the associated beam shape that was derived from the plan data, were subsequently compared to a portal image to verify the patient set-up. The portal image was exported as a secondary capture from PortalVision to the DICOMDIR Storage SCP and then picked up by the image registration program.

## Conclusion

The developed DICOM RT engine has proved to be a useful tool in the process of implementing DICOM RT in a radiotherapy environment. The engine has been used both to test the DICOM archive and to establish DICOM communication between different radiotherapy modalities. Although the mapping of radiotherapy data to and from DICOM has shown to be a very difficult and sometimes almost impossible task, we have been able to establish DICOM communication a long time before such solutions are commercially available.

However, DICOM does not provide any solutions of how to handle the logistics of the digital data flow in the department. Radiotherapy planning is an inherently complex process with several concurrent activities. It is therefore of vital importance that data consistency is maintained throughout. The next steps in our development of the DICOM programs will therefore be to improve the routines for data mapping and to implement locking mechanisms to handle concurrency problems.

## References

[1] Manens J P 1997 Exchange of medical imaging and data information in radiotherapy: needs, methods and current limits *Cancer-Radiother.* **1** 524-31

# The design and implementation of a multi-center volumetric and dosimetric database

**Mischa S. Hoogeman[1], Marcel van Herk[1], Lambert Zijp[1], Jan Meinders[1], Pietje Muller[1], Peter C. M. Koper[2], Liesbeth J. Boersma[1], and Joos V. Lebesque[1]**

[1]The Netherlands Cancer Institute/Antoni van Leeuwenhoek Huis, Plesmanlaan 121, 1066 CX Amsterdam, The Netherlands. E-mail: mischa@nki.nl. [2]University Hospital Rotterdam, Dr Daniel den Hoed Cancer Center, Groene Hilledijk 301, 3075 EA Rotterdam, The Netherlands.

## Introduction

In 1998, a Phase III study for prostate cancer has started applying three-dimensional conformal radiotherapy and randomizing between 68 Gy and 78 Gy. A total of 600 patients from various institutions in The Netherlands will be entered over a period of 4 years. The specific aim of the trial is to determine the relationships between the actual delivered 3D dose and local control and late complications, taking explicitly into account variations in clinical and physical parameters during the treatment period. The complexity of this study requires the development of a new type of database, which offers online access to all patient data and which can be used for sophisticated analyses without extensive user intervention.

We have designed and implemented such a database that offers direct access to CT images, dose distributions, delineated organs, Dose Volume Histograms (DVHs), treatment-variation and other data of eventually 600 patients. The data can be stored in different formats without increasing the complexity and the number of user interactions. Besides direct access to all data, the volumetric database offers elaborate analysis tools, which are absolutely necessary to perform the analyses of the dose-volume-effect relationships including treatment variations. In this paper, we will describe the structure of this new database type. Furthermore, we will illustrate the use of the database with some examples.

## Material and methods

### Structure of the volumetric database

Figure 1 shows a schematic diagram of the structure of the database. The central object of the database is the "Patient Tree". This patient tree visualizes how the data of each patient is stored in the memory. The data is formatted in a branching tree structure. This hierarchical patient description is very clear and flexible. As the structure of the tree is not fixed, the patient tree is easily extendible. All items in the patient tree can be accessed with the patient-tree user interface or in actual code using a uniformly formatted link.

A characteristic feature of the patient tree is that each item belongs to a certain modality. A modality is, for example, a scan, a contour, a 3D dose distribution or a DVH. Each modality type has some specific properties. The modality DVH, for instance, contains the following properties: the histogram itself, the maximum and minimum dose, Tumor Control Probability (TCP) and Normal Tissue Control Probability (NTCP) values according to different models, several dose-volume parameters, and many more. The properties will be used in the analysis of the data and can be exported to database tables. Properties can easily be added to a modality.

### Different data formats

All patient data is submitted to the volumetric database in

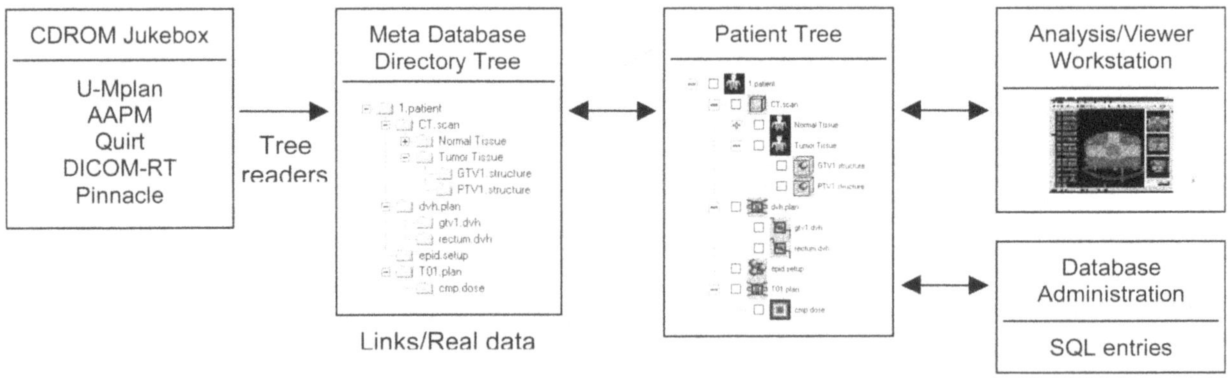


**Figure 1:** Schematic diagram of the volumetric database. The central part of the database is the "Patient Tree" which represents the structure, in which the data is formatted. The patient tree retrieves the data from the "Directory Tree". The directory tree contains real data and links to the data that is stored in the CDROM jukebox. Patient data, which is selected in the patient tree can be viewed and analyzed in the analysis workstation. The "Database Administration" is used to select patient groups and to export analysis results.

either a planning-system format or a standard data-exchange format. We have developed readers that interpret these formats. First, the readers construct the tree, which represents all available data of a patient. If an item in the tree is selected, the readers locate the requested data in the foreign format and load it into the computer memory. Readers have been developed for the U-Mplan and Pinnacle planning-system format, the DICOM-RT and AAPM-RTOG exchange format, and the local QUIRT image-database format.

Although the patient tree is easily extendible and can store new results, the planning-system and data-exchange formats are hardly extendible. Therefore, newly generated data, e.g. DVHs, TCP and NTCP values, are not stored in the original format, but in a so-called meta database. This meta database is a direct copy of the patient tree to a directory tree on a computer hard disk. The directory tree either contains real data (in our own format) or links to the data in the original format. If an item in the patient tree is selected, the tree will first look for real data in the directory tree and if that is not found, it will use the link to the data in the original format (stored, e.g., in a CDROM Jukebox). The meta database also allows a safe way of "fixing" the original data. If, for example, a contour is adjusted to improve the consistency of delineation, the adjusted contour will be stored in the meta database, while the link to the original contour is not removed. Thus the original contour can always be restored.

**Selecting patients and exporting results**

Extensive analyses of the patient data require searching and selecting of patients. Therefore, a Structured Query Language (SQL) database is used. This database makes it possible to select, for instance, patients randomized for the high-dose arm of the trial and treated at a particular institution. The analysis results (e.g., DVHs) are stored in the patient tree format. From these results, new database entries are prepared (e.g., TCP values), so that these entries can be used to select a new patient group. Furthermore, the use of a standard database makes it possible to export the results to almost any commercial database or analysis application.

**Analysis workstation**

The patient tree not only represents the patient data, but also contains a user interface. The interface is used in conjunction with an analysis workstation. We developed elaborate analysis tools for this workstation, such as delineation correction, automatic inner wall generation for the computation of Dose Wall Histograms [1], generation of DVHs, and incorporation of treatment variations (measurements and simulations). The workstation also incorporates the viewer of the Conquest EC project. The database entries are linked to the patient data, such that when a patient is selected (manually or automatically), the patient can be accessed immediately using the patient-tree interface.

**Treatment variations**

The specific aim of this project is to include treatment variations in the analyses of dose-volume-effect relationships for all 600 patients in a homogeneous way. The flexible format of the database allows the storage of measured and computed treatment variations. For this purpose, a treatment-variations object is assigned to each modality. This object contains all relevant variations, which can be obtained from direct measurements, simulations, or calculations. The treatment-variations object of a solid organ, for instance, contains for each fraction a translation and rotation. The set of translations and rotations describe the organ motion and is obtained from measured translation and rotation distributions (e.g., for the prostate [2]). The system uses the treatment-variations objects in the computation of the dose-volume-effect parameters, such as DVHs and TCP and NTCP values.

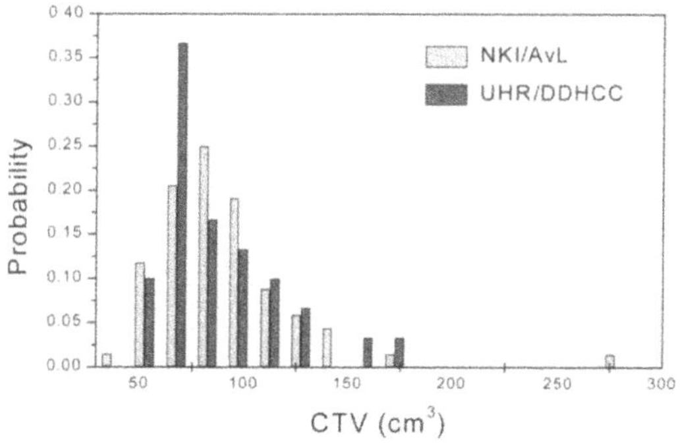


**Figure 2**: Volume distributions of the CTV (prostate + seminal vesicles) of 100 patients treated at the UHR/DDHCC and NKI/AvL.

## Results and discussion

At present, the database has been implemented at our institution and 200 patients have been added to the database. As an example of the use of the database, we present the analysis results of the first 100 patients. These first patients were planned at two different institutions and two different planning systems were used. Figure 2 shows the volume distributions of the Clinical Target Volume (CTV, prostate + seminal vesicles) of patients treated at the University Hospital Rotterdam/Dr Daniel den Hoed Cancer Center (UHR/DDHCC) and The Netherlands Cancer Institute/Antoni van Leeuwenhoek Huis (NKI/AvL), The Netherlands. To obtain these distributions, both patient groups were selected using a SQL query. Next, the property "Volume" of the contour "CTV" was exported to a database table. We observe no significant difference between the volume distribution of the CTVs delineated at the UHR/DDHCC and delineated at the NKI/AvL.

Figure 3 shows the distribution of the relative rectal wall volume, which received a dose equal or higher than 74 Gy (for 40 patients treated in the high-dose arm) compared to the relative rectum volume including filling. To obtain these distributions, the system automatically generated an inner wall for each patient using the model of Meijer *et al.* [1]. Next, the database calculated Dose Wall Histograms (DWHs) of the rectum wall and Dose Volume Histograms (DVHs) of the rectum including filling. The complete computation was performed automatically for the selected group of patients. No

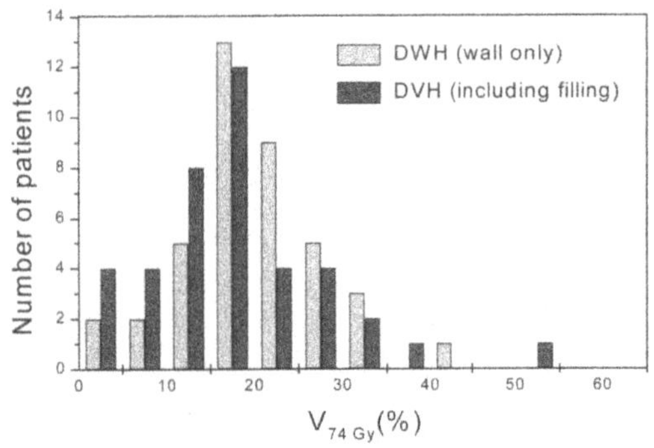


**Figure 3:** Distribution of the relative rectum wall volume and rectum volume including filling, which received a dose of 74 Gy or higher.

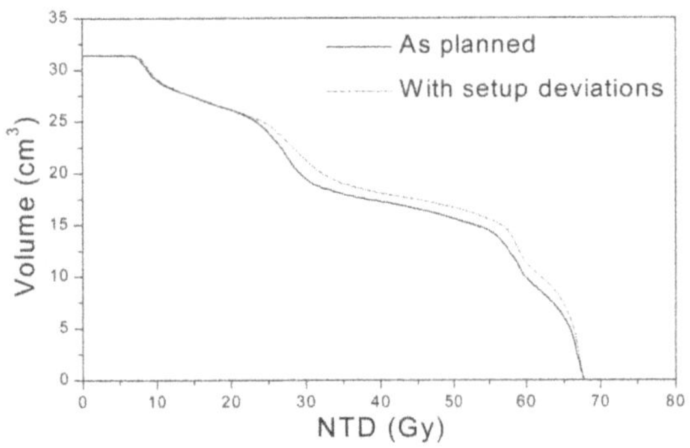


**Figure 4:** DWH of a rectum wall using the planned dose distribution and the dose distribution including setup deviations.

user intervention was needed for individual patients. The computation took 30 s per patient (on a 300 MHz Pentium II), which includes the automatic retrieval of the volumetric data from the CDROM jukebox. Thus the total analysis took 20 min.

From the stored DWHs and DVHs the requested parameter was exported to a database table and the two distributions are shown in Fig. 3. There is no significant difference between the distributions based on the DWHs and the DVHs. Only for one patient, the trial criterion that no more than 40 % of the rectum wall should receive a dose equal or higher than 74 Gy was exceeded. For this patient, the relative volume was 44 %. Note that these distributions do not show patient-specific differences between the DVHs and DWHs, but summarize the differences for the entire patient population. As soon as a sufficient number of patients have been added to the database, a more extensive quantitative comparison can be performed on these and other distributions.

The shown results are relatively simple examples of the use the volumetric database. The database has already been tested for more complex operations that include treatment variations. As an example, we present the DWH of a rectum wall, with and without taking the measured setup deviations into account. For each patient, about 10 setup measurements are available (from portal imaging). The setup deviations of the fractions without portal imaging were estimated by taking random samples based on the measured setup-deviation distribution. This distribution is estimated for each patient individually using the available portal images. Shifting the 3D dose distribution for each fraction and adding it to the total dose matrix, leads to an estimate of the 3D dose distribution including setup deviations. Figure 4 shows both DWHs, where the local dose per voxel was converted to a Normalized Total Dose (NTD) to take into account the differences in the dose per fraction ($\alpha/\beta$ = 3 Gy). The DWH of the actual delivered dose lies slightly above the DWH of the planned dose distribution.

## Conclusion

We have designed and implemented a multi-center volumetric and dosimetric database. The database facilitates complex analyses including the effects of various treatment variations, on a large group of patients, without extensive user intervention. All patient data (CT scans, 3D dose distributions, contours, treatment variations, etc.) is accessible online. The database maps the patient data to a tree structure, independent of the original format. Both the user and software engineer can access the patient data through uniform links, which hide the complexity of the different formats. The test results of the first 100 patients demonstrated the easiness and speed with which complex analyses can be performed on a large group of patients.

## References

[1] Meijer G J, van den Brink M, Hoogeman M S, Meinders J, Lebesque J V 1999 Dose wall histograms and normalized dose surface histograms for rectums *Int J Radiat Oncol Biol Phys* **45** 1073-1080.

[2] van Herk M, Bruce A, Kroes G, Shouman T, Touw A, Lebesque J V 1995 Quantification of organ motion during conformal radiotherapy of the prostate by three-dimensional image registration *Int J Radiat Oncol Biol Phys* **33** 1311-1320.

# Network-wide application sharing as part of an electronic patient referral system.

M Grossmann[1], A J Lomax[1], M Goitein[2,1].

[1]Division of Radiation Medicine, The Paul Scherrer Institute, 5232 Villigen-PSI, Switzerland.

## Introduction.

The current state-of-the-art in radiotherapy provides a rich variety of methods by which radiation can be applied to lesions. Patients can currently be treated with either fractionated photons and/or electrons (conventional or IMRT), protons (conventional or IMPT), or with stereotactically guided radiosurgery techniques. Within each of these groups, there are a wide spectrum of possible treatment methods. Taking stereotactic treatments as an example, there is currently the possibility of delivering conformal treatments with a LINAC, using either arc therapy or mini-multileaf collimated static fields, or alternatively with a dedicated radiosurgery system such as the GammaKnife. However, although each particular technique is often aimed at fulfilling a certain role in radiotherapy, it is also not necessarily the case that a particular treatment method will prove to be the most appropriate for *all* patients with a given indication.

Given the current diversity of treatments becoming available, it is extremely unlikely that any one institute can have access to all treatment possibilities. However, different treatment possibilities may well be available at other, possibly widely distributed treatment centres. If the potential of these specialised treatment centres are to be exploited, then it is necessary to put in place methods by which competing treatment methods can be assessed on a patient by patient basis across institutes.

Here we describe the use of network-wide application sharing software, in conjunction with radiotherapy data exchange standards, for the interactive assessment of treatment plans by two or more remotely situated treatment centres.

## Materials and methods.

At the Paul Scherrer Institute, we are currently treating patients with protons using the spot scanning technique. However, the institute itself is a physics research institute, and as such, we must rely on patients being referred from external radiotherapy clinics, within or outside of Switzerland. To facilitate the selection of patients, we have previously described an electronic patient referral system [1], by which 'core' radiotherapy data sets can be transferred between the proton planning system at PSI and a number of commercial planning systems that have installations in clinics within Switzerland. In this system, the results of evaluation plans performed at PSI, in the form of 3D dose distributions, can be electronically transferred back to the referring institute's planning system, where the proton plan can be carefully compared to the treatment possibilities at the local centre. However, there is inevitably still a need to discuss the competing plans and, if a patient is accepted for treatment, the details of the treatment itself, interactively with the referring clinic. For this purpose, we have started to use software for sharing applications over local and wide area networks. With this software, we can make available our proton therapy planning system to remote users, such that they can interact with it exactly in the same way as a user at our institute. That is, both the local and remote users can interact with the same program, thus facilitating meaningful discussions between the different parties.

Data conferencing standards have been defined by the International Telecommunication Union (ITU) in T.120 and H.323. [2] Software conforming to these standards has become available for a range of computer platforms. We are currently using Microsoft's NetMeeting on Win95/98/NT4.0. [3,4].

NetMeeting conforms to the above mentioned standards and allows application sharing and basic audio/video conferencing over TCP/IP. Data encryption for transfer over public networks is possible. NetMeeting can be downloaded from Microsoft's website along with a Resource Kit containing detailed technical documentation.

In a typical session we want to discuss patient data on PSI's therapy planning system with a remote referring institution [Fig. 1]. At both sites, a Windows PC with NetMeeting installed is connected to the Internet. The therapy planning system is typically running on a separate, VMS workstation. By running an X server on the PC and directing the workstation's display to it, we are able to take control over the planning system and, through NetMeeting, share it with the remote partner. Sharing in this context means not only that both sites may look at the same picture. Rather, that the remote site may completely take control over the planning application and, for example, modify VOIs.

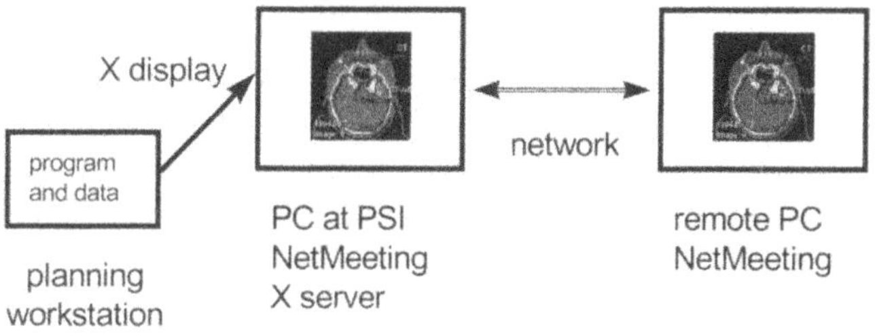


**Figure 1:** Sharing a therapy planning system over the network

At PSI we have set up one PC as a dedicated workstation for NetMeeting sessions [Fig. 2]. Along with the required software (Windows95, NetMeeting 3.01 and a X server) it has appropriate hardware (graphics card and a large monitor) to display medical images. A small camera (ViCAM from Vista Imaging, Inc.) transmits video images of the discussion partners. Close to the PC is a telephone with external microphone and loudspeakers. The PC is located in the room used for therapy planning where eventually required additional documents (MRI, CT) are readily available.

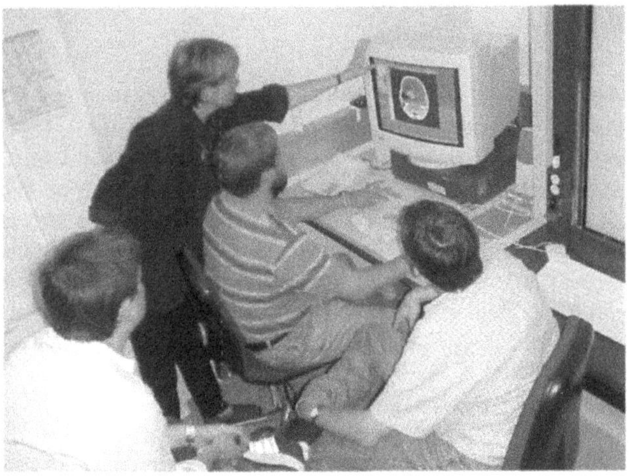

**Figure 2:** The NetMeeting workstation at PSI

## Discussion.

During 1999, NetMeeting in the configuration described above has been used frequently for the interactive discussion of patient data and therapy plans between PSI, referring clinics and other treatment centres. Inside Switzerland we could mostly rely on the Swiss academic network which offers bandwidths up to 155 Mbps. However, we also conducted interactive sessions over transatlantic links during busy hours or with dial-in links over analog telephone lines without problems.

Corporate TCP/IP networks often are not directly connected to Internet, but are protected by firewalls. This is not a big problem for application sharing. The NetMeeting documentation specifies which TCP and UDP ports have to be open to allow T.120 and H.323 traffic. At PSI, the NetMeeting station (PC in Fig. 1) is connected to the public internet, whereas the workstation holding the patient data is in the protected PSI subnet from which we allow outgoing X displays.

NetMeeting is capable of transferring audio data. However, we decided to use the normal telephone system for the audio connection. It proved helpful to have a parallel connection independent of the Internet link in case of problems.

## Conclusions.

As a treatment facility based outside the hospital environment, we rely totally on patients being referred from many different clinical centres. Being able to discuss potential cases before referral, as well as the planned treatment, both before and during delivery, is therefore an important part of our program. The ability of one or more remote partners to work interactively with our planning program has been found to make such discussion both more efficient and more meaningful. Subsequently, we believe such an approach could well benefit many centres where different treatment modalities are available, but only at difference locations.

## References.

[1] A. Lomax et al., submitted to Int. Jounal of Radiation Oncology Biology Physics
[2] http://www.itu.int/itudoc/itu-t/rec/t/t120.html and http://www.itu.int/itudoc/itu-t/rec/h/h323.html
[3] http://www.microsoft.com/netmeeting
[4] B. Sommers: Official Microsoft NetMeeting Book, The Microsoft Press, Redmond 1998. This book only covers version 2.1 of NetMeeting.

# Wide Area Networking for Radiotherapy Services

**Lindsay Tremethick, William Patterson**

Radiation Oncology Victoria
132 Grey Street, East Melbourne, Victoria, Australia
email: lindsay@tremethick.fam.aust.com, billpat@pipeline.com.au

## Introduction

In April 1999 Radiation Oncology Victoria (ROV) completed a nine month expansions to a 4 site practice, with centres located in metropolitan and country Victoria. The practice installed five new linear accelerators with MLC, changed the record and verify system (R&V) from Varian's RMS-2000 to VARiS and introduced new networking technologies.
This paper reports on our experiences.

The change in R&V software, at the time, not only addressed the Y2K problem, but also fully supported the introduction of MLC treatments. Unfortunately VARiS introduced a new problem. Without a patient import/export function like RMS-2000, the ability to move patients between sites, for events such as major breakdowns or service was severely limited.

The practice partners had developed a wish list that they felt would assist them in their day to day work. Ideally they wanted real time patient data access, the ability to review patient plans remotely, have access to internal and external email, have a video conferencing system for colleague support and finally internet access. It was felt that these additions would help resolve issues resulting from the increased movement of doctors between sites.

In addition to these desires there was still a need to support the existing local area network (LAN) applications such as the Picker AcQSim CT and Virtual Simulation system, ADAC's Pinnacle 3D treatment planning system and the important DBD Database Software (CAS) central patient information and billing system.

One solution which addressed all of the above requirements, was the establishment of a Wide Area Network (WAN) between centres. However the WAN had to remain financially viable whilst not degrading functionality.

## Method

Discussions were held with several networking consultants on various configurations of ROV's WAN, the major difficulty being that the frequency and quantity of data transfer had yet to be determined. Several different methods were investigated as a communication medium including Frame Relay, Wireless, ISDN, & ATM. Each method had strengths and weaknesses which played a major part in the choice of the final medium.
Although Picker, ADAC and DBD had previously established WAN's there was very little experience, even internationally, in building a WAN for VARiS, with only two sites in the US.

Unfortunately both sites offered very little guidence to the minimum bandwidth necessary for VARiS as both used T1 (~2Mbs) connections, which, in Australia, were economically unfeasible for the practice.

Although Frame Relay appeared to be the ideal medium, providing permanent connections with fixed costs that suited the bursty nature of network traffic, the very high costs of tails at two sites excluded it from consideration when compared to an ISDN solution. Wireless and ATM were eliminated due to geographical and/or high costs.

Having chosen ISDN, we had to test whether the WAN VARiS would function correctly given our limited bandwidth. With the assistance of our chosen networking consultants we conducted VARiS testing with a simulated bandwidth limited network. Our tests proved that the VARiS application would function satisfactorily at the minimum bandwidth available with ISDN. Further tests at higher bandwidths (256kbs) indicated that other network transfers such as CT data, file and screen update transfers could occur simultaneously provided the VARiS application had priority. Without traffic control VARiS was found to be unacceptably slow.

The WAN was established using Cisco routers (3600 & 2600) and the local telecommunication provider Telstra. Two BRI circuits (256kbs) were installed to each centre in a hub and spoke arrangement. To minimise communication costs between metropolitan centres one BRI to each centre was put on a calling plan that capped charges to a fixed cost each month. The WAN was designed as a two central file server arrangement. One server is dedicated to all of the metropolitan centres, yet has the ability to communicate with the second server at the country centre (Wodonga). This design was chosen, as a compromise between the practice needs for transferring patients between centres and the communication costs for the Wodonga connection. The Wodonga centre some 300kms north east of the city would act as a stand alone site with little or no movement of patients anticipated between it and the metropolitan centres.

A quartly review of the WAN operation, based on the response times of applications and the costs of connections, is used to identify whether further changes are necessary. The Cisco equipment chosen allows upgrading to Frame Relay should the reviews indicate it would be more cost effective.

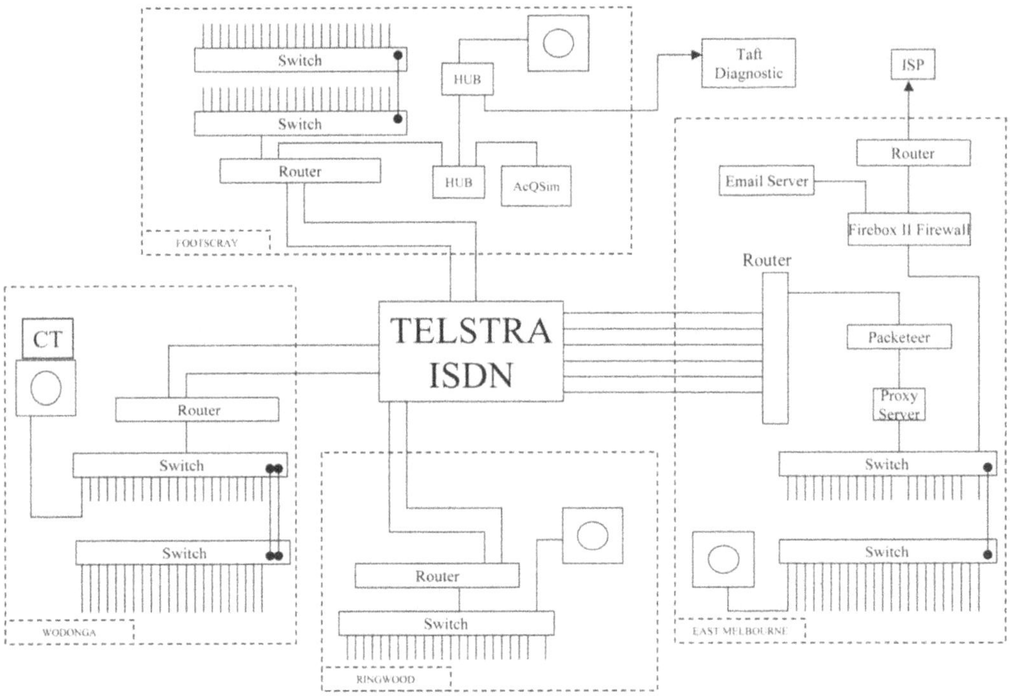


**Figure 1:** Block Diagram of Final ROV Wide Area Network.

Our prime concern was not to commit the practice to large recurrent communication costs before determining the actual data transfer requirements.

## Results and discussion

The topology of ROV's network is illustrated by figure 1 with the three sites (Footscray, Ringwood and Wodonga) connected to the main practice (East Melbourne) by 256kbs ISDN circuits. This final arrangement was the result of several adjustments to an initial network that displayed several problems.

Initially somewhat disappointing results were experienced whenever large data files were transferred. Although a queuing process had been implemented within the routers, to give priority to mission critical applications, there was insufficient refinement available on a dynamic basis to optimise bandwidth utilisation. The queuing process only worked adequately when the full bandwidth of the ISDN links where utilised. Several attempts at queuing optimisation were tried with little success. Additionally when all ISDN services were available the highest data transfer rate never approached the theorectical ~2MB per minute.
Not only were there WAN problems but also LAN problems now that all computer hardware had be connected through the new 100BaseT network. The Pinnacle planning workstations would loose communications with either printers and servers causing system lockups and unexpected error messages.

Although the LAN problems were easily rectified by returning all Pinnacle servers, workstations and printers to the network hub, this was a backward step failing to fully utilise the high speed network that had been installed. The actual cause of the problem was finally identified to correspond with the refresh time of the network switches address table.
As the switch dumped its address table, workstations would loose contact with each other and the printers causing crashes and lockups. By assigning secure addressing on the switch ports, each remains unique, and is not refreshed hence preventing the problem occuring.

Diagnosing and solving the WAN problems were somewhat more complicated.
Router queuing prioritises and distributes bandwidth to individual data flows, preventing low volume applications being swamped by large data transfers. However because the process is uni-directional it can only control how data moves from the LAN to the WAN. Data flowing into the router is only buffered, which results in packets being delayed and dropped.
Despite being able to identify all traffic using a network sniffer we had no way of controlling how each IP packet traversed the WAN from the router. We required an IP traffic manager that classified and controlled all IP traffic by address, port or application protocol.

The Packeteer, PacketShaper (IP Manager), not only allowed us to constantly monitor and identify network traffic, but also controlled all aspects of the TCP/IP traffic between sites allowing the network to be optimised. Each data connection is controlled at either end by the manager hence eliminating burstiness. Data may now be prioritised and bandwidth adjusted as per demand. It was also possible to implement time dependent protocols to utilise off-peak rates offered by the communication carrier for non urgent transfers.

Network traffic was now managed according to port number, application or IP but the performance was still disappointing. Data transfer rates were still inconsistent with the number of ISDN channels connected. Careful observation found that the router was not correctly aggregating the ISDN lines and hence was never able to transfer at the maximum rate. A new router reconfiguration has since appeared to solve this difficulty.

With the network finally functioning satisfactorily we were disappointed to find yet another problem. Up to this stage all IP traffic had passed either out-of or into the central site (East Melbourne) hence it passed through the traffic manager. Any traffic that is uncontrolled has the potential to swamp the mission critical applications of VARiS and CAS. We now found that data was being passed between other sites, such as between Footscray and Ringwood. Traffic that remained only in the WAN, was 'bounced' at the router and did not pass through the traffic manager.

When this data was bandwidth intensive, such as patient CT data files (up to 200MB) it swamped the traffic moving to and from the file servers at the central sight. It was therefore necessary to force all IP traffic through the packetshaper no matter what its final destination. The addition of the "proxy server", on the LAN side of the East Melbourne router, accepts all traffic from the WAN and forwards it either back to the WAN or into the LAN.

Although this arrangement appears to be an inefficient double handling of IP traffic, the network link between the PacketShaper and "proxy server" is 10Mbs which greatly exceeds the maximum throughput of the ISDN links. There is little or no appreciable delay in the IP data transmission.

Assessment of the current WAN configuration has shown that most of the initial design requirements have been achieved with only the Video Conferencing and email/internet access still to be implemented. It was necessary to delay these features until a stable platform for mission critical applications could be guaranteed under all circumstances.

Our approach for these remaining features is to use off the shelf, turn key solutions, to minimise the level of expertise required inhouse to maintain the services. The email server is the Cobalt Cube2 that will also act as the practices intranet and DNS server. The firewall between the practice and the ISP is a Firebox II with a software service contract that maintains the lastest defences against attack. The Firewall also provides Virtual Private Networking (VPN) access into the network from any site on the internet. We identified this as a better option than providing dial-in or dial-out access through multiple modem connections. Not only are the access points minimised but all data that passes through the firewall is tested against a set of rules that checks whether the transmission is permitted. The practice web server will be maintained by the ISP minimising the traffic on our link. It is expected that these will come online in the very near future.

The final choice of a video conferencing system has yet to be decided. However with the constant changes in the market, more capable systems are appearing each day, allowing the practice many more features for the same money when a system is finally purchased.

## Conclusion

Although this paper appears to report heavily on just the doom and gloom aspects of establishing the network it does illustrate what can be achieved with limited resources.

The WAN was primarily designed by one of the Physicists who had very little experience in network planning. When advice was sought from networking consultants they were unable to provide anything more than just a sketchy outlines, without having an idea of what sort, and how much data would be transferred between sites.

The WAN this paper describes, and illustrated by the block diagram, appears relatively simple. However when the individual components are considered the complexities of the WAN are revealed. There are:

6 WindowsNT servers, 2 SCO Unix servers
4 Sun Solaris Servers, 6 Unix terminals
4 Sun Work Stations, 45 WindowsNT desktop PC's
7 100BaseT switches, 6 routers
1 email server & 1 firewall

all of which are controlled by the Physics Department, who remain on a very steep learning curve.

Although the bandwidth of T1 connections would be extremely desirable, the configuration of our WAN proves that VARiS can coexist with other mission critical applications using bandwidth limited and low cost ISDN connections. It is envisaged that, should the practice choose to introduce Varian Vision products, an additional capped BRI circuit may be required to each site to support this product.

This paper has been written with the permission of the Board of Directors of Radiation Oncology Victoria.

# A Deformable Template Approach to Registration of Serial CT Studies for Dose Planning in Intracavitary Brachytherapy

J.Williamson[1], Peng Yin[2], G. Christensen[2], J. Dempsey[1], H. Bennet[1], C. Chao[1], P. Grigsby[1], K. Nguyen[1], and M. Vannier[3]

[1]Radiation Oncology Center ,Washington University, St. Louis, MO, [2]Dept. of Electrical and Computer Engineering, University of Iowa, Iowa City, IA, [3]Dept. of Radiology, University of Iowa, Iowa City, IA

## Introduction

CT and MR imaging have failed to replace the classical reference points and orthagonal film image as the basis for planning and evaluating intracavitary brachytherapy (ICT). - One serious obstacle is the substantial time-dependent displacement and deformation of pelvic soft tissue structures caused by multiple ICT insertions and removals, tumor regression, and normal tissue stenosis. This makes combination of dose distributions from different treatment components into a cumulative 3D dose distribution meaningfully correlated with the underlying anatomy all but impossible. We have adapted a deformable template model to map serial CT images, each representing one component of the treatment, to one another[1]. This provides a means to represent the cumulative dose distribution for a multiple-insertion course of ICT and external beam therapy registered to a single anatomical representation of the patient,. This approach, successfully applied to soft-tissue neuroimaging, uses continuum mechanics to model the non-rigid deformation of one CT study relative to another and to calculate a high-dimensional voxel-to-voxel transformation for bringing the two studies into registration[2].

## Material and methods

A clinical study, consisting of 20 patients with locally advanced cervix cancer receiving definitive RT, has been performed. CT compatible Fletcher-Suit applicators with afterloading tungsten shields[3] were used to obtain artifact-free images. Each patient undergoes five spiral CT studies, $I_i(\vec{x})$, before initiating treatment (i=1), just before (i=2) and after (i=3) the first ICT insertion and just before (i=4) and just after (i=5) placement of the second ICT. Each $I_i(\vec{x})$ denotes the Hounsfield intensity of the i-th serial examination at location $\vec{x} = (x_1, x_2, x_3)$ in the CT scanner frame of reference. Associated with each exam, i, is an ICT insertion or series of external beam fractions described by a 3D dose matrix, $D_i(\vec{x})$, in 1-to-1 correspondence with the image $I_i(\vec{x})$. To register each image $i \neq 3$, to the target image, $S(\vec{x}) = I_3(\vec{x})$ we need to compute a vector-valued transformation $h_i$: $\Re^3 \to \Re^3$ that maps each tissue voxel $\vec{x}$ in S to the corresponding voxel in $I_i(\vec{x})$, i.e., $I_3(\vec{x})$ and $I_i(h_i(\vec{x}))$ are image intensities of the same tissue voxel. Then the cumulative dose distribution, displayed in 1:1 correspondence with the subject image anatomy, $S=I_3$, is given by:

$$D_T(\vec{x}) = D_3(\vec{x}) + \sum_{i \neq 3}^{5} D_i(h_i(\vec{x})) \qquad (1)$$

Each 512-x512 image slice (resolution = 0.94 x 0.94 x 3.0 $mm^3$) was contoured manually to identify vagina, uterus, and cervix (as a single structure), rectum, colon, bladder and small bowel). The pelvic bones were segmented automatically by thresholding. To obtain a diffeomorphic (continuous, differentiable, and topology preserving) mapping $h(\vec{x})$ for a particular template and subject CT studies, **T** and **S**, the evolution of T into S as a time-dependent viscous fluid flow problem governed by a modified Navier-Stokes equation[1-2]:

$$\mu \nabla^2 \vec{v} + (\lambda + \mu) \vec{\nabla} (\vec{\nabla} \cdot \vec{v}) + \vec{b}(\vec{u}) = 0 \qquad (2)$$

where $\mu$ and $\lambda$ are viscosity constants, $\vec{u}(\vec{x}) = h(\vec{x}) - \vec{x}$ is the vector displacement field and $\vec{v}(\vec{x},t) = d\vec{u}(\vec{x},t)/dt$ is the velocity field. First, coarse registration was performed by rigidly matching the bony anatomy on the two studies. Then, each contoured studies **S** and **T** were represented as a multimodality image sets:

$$\mathbf{S}(\vec{x}) = \begin{bmatrix} S_1(\vec{x}) \\ S_2(\vec{x}) \\ S_3(\vec{x}) \\ S_4(\vec{x}) \\ S_5(\vec{x}) \end{bmatrix} \text{ and } \mathbf{T}(\vec{x}) = \begin{bmatrix} T_1(\vec{x}) \\ T_2(\vec{x}) \\ T_3(\vec{x}) \\ T_4(\vec{x}) \\ T_5(\vec{x}) \end{bmatrix}$$

$$\text{where } \begin{bmatrix} . \\ . \\ . \\ . \\ . \end{bmatrix} = \begin{bmatrix} \text{Gray scale CT image} \\ \text{Bladder binary mask} \\ \text{Vagina/uterus binary mask} \\ \text{Recto-sigmoid binary mask} \\ \text{Small bowel binary image} \end{bmatrix} \qquad (3)$$

where each binary mask image, $T_i(\vec{x}) = 1$ if $\vec{x}$ is in or on the contoured structure and is zero otherwise. The desired displacement field is that which minimizes the multi-modality image fusion cost function:

$$D(\vec{u}) = \sum_{i=1}^{4} \alpha_i \cdot \int_{\Omega} |T_i(\vec{x} - \vec{u}(\vec{x})) - S_i(\vec{x})|^2 d\vec{x} \qquad (4)$$

where the $\alpha_i$ are weighting constants. $D(\vec{u})$ will be minimized if only if the body force has the form $\vec{b}(\vec{x},\vec{u}(\vec{x},t)) = -\alpha \cdot (T(\vec{h}(\vec{x},t)) - S(\vec{x})) \cdot \vec{\nabla} T|_{h(\vec{x},t)}$ (i.e., is proportional to the mismatch between T and S at time t) and is reduced to zero by the deformation process In practice, the velocity field is assumed to be constant over the time interval, [t, t+$\Delta$t], and resulting linear PDE (2), given $\vec{v}(\vec{x},t)$, is solved for $\vec{v}(\vec{x},t+\Delta t)$ and $\vec{u}(\vec{x},t+\Delta t)$. This process of Euler integration in time continues until $\|\vec{b}(\vec{x},t)\|$ falls below a specified threshold, which takes 6-12 hours per pair of 3D CT studies on a UNIX single-processor workstation.

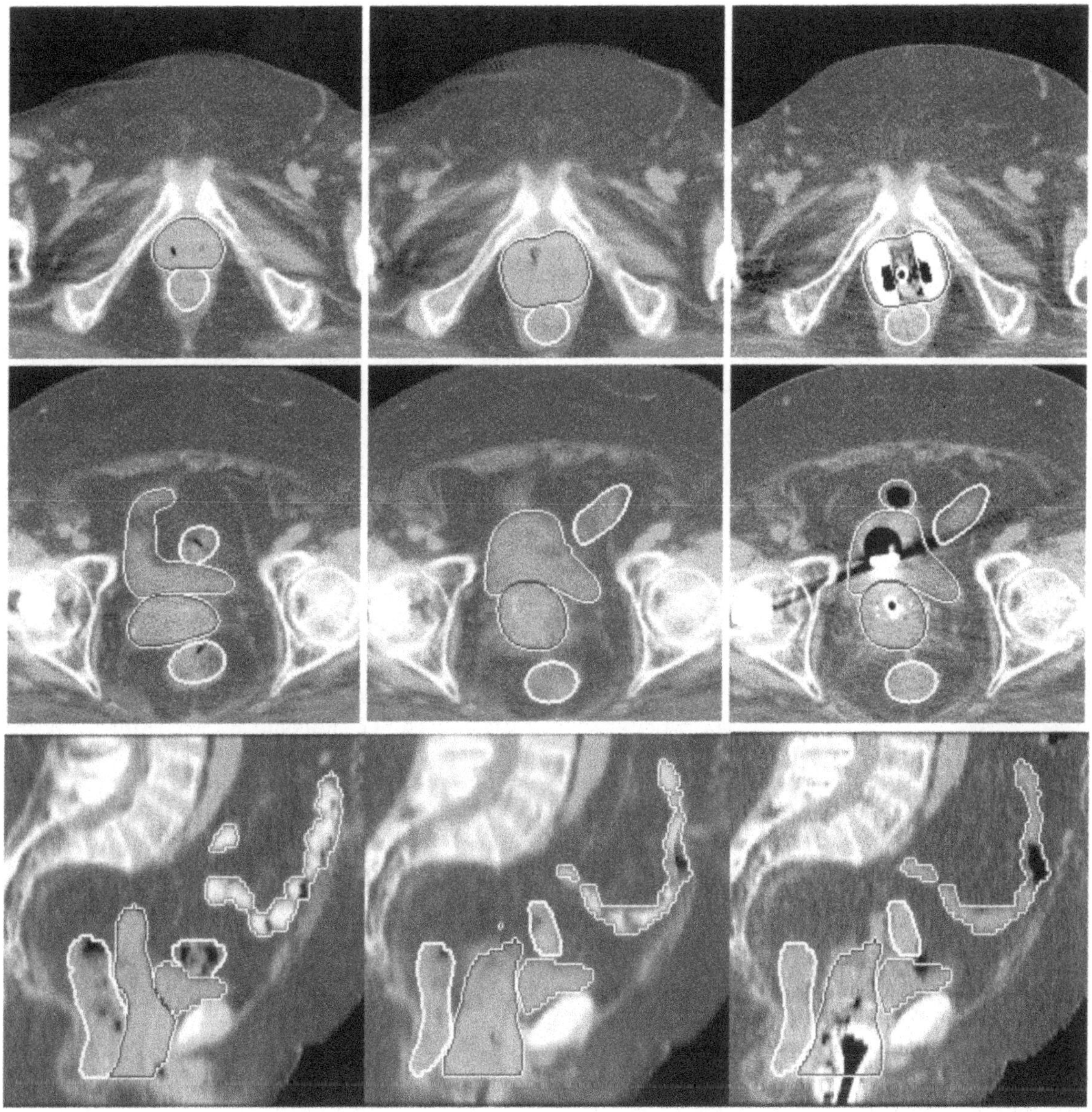

**Figure 1:** Use of viscous fluid model to register a pre-implant CT studies ($T = I_2$ = column 1) with study $S = I_3$ (column 3) obtained after the first ICT insertion. Column 2 shows the deformed template image, $I_2(h_2(\bar{x}))$, transformed so as to match the post-ICT images. The magenta, blue, yellow and red contours illustrate the small bowel, recto-sigmoid, vagina/uterus, and bladder respectively. Rows 1 and 2 show two transverse slices while row 3 illustrates the midline saggital plane.

We present the results from two patients. Several endpoints. Both pre-ICT to post-ICT and first-to-second ICT insertion registration problems were considered. The magnitude of the soft tissue deformation was quantified by calculating the linear displacement of each tissue voxel relative to the rigid alignment of bony structures. The effectiveness of the viscous fluid deformation was assessed by quantifying the conicidence index (CI) of each contoured organ, A, T after transformation to the S frame of reference, with the corresponding structure, B, on image S.

$$CI = \frac{Vol(h(A) \cap B)}{Vol(h(A) \cup B)} \qquad (4)$$

## Results and discussion

Figure 1 illustrates the voxel-to-voxel registration achieved by the visous fluid model for pre and post ICT insertion studies. The second column, showing the pre-insertion CT after transformation by the $10^7$ dimension mapping, h, accurately reproduces the changes in soft-tissue organ and shape due to insertion of the bulky Fletcher-Suit ICT system. Large changes in shape of the uterus, including AP expansion shortening, axial shortening, lower positioning in the pelvis and realignment relative to the large bowel, are all reproduced by the deformable template model. Despite significant change in bladder, rectal and uterine corpus shape, uncontoured soft-tissue details such as the ligaments supporting the uterus and the abdominal wall are properly duplicated on the transformed pre-implant CT study.

| Patient 1 | Pre-to-Post ICT 1 | | ICT 2 to ICT 1 | |
|---|---|---|---|---|
| Organ | Rigid | Viscous | Rigid | Viscous |
| Bladder | 0.733 | 0.995 | 0.538 | 0.991 |
| RectoSigmoid | 0.567 | 0.999 | 0.516 | 1.000 |
| Uterus/vagina | 0.734 | 0.997 | 0.666 | 0.996 |
| Sm. Bowel | 0.278 | 0.853 | 0.323 | 0.944 |
| Patient 2 | Pre-to-Post ICT 1 | | ICT 2 to ICT 1 | |
| Bladder | 0.503 | 0.999 | 0.368 | 0.995 |
| RectoSigmoid | 0.152 | 0.992 | 0.399 | 0.914 |
| Uterus/vagina | 0.330 | 0.985 | 0.567 | 0.974 |
| Sm. Bowel | 0.152 | 0.912 | 0.188 | 0.924 |

**Table 1:** Concidence Index, CI, for both rigid and locally deformable viscous fluid transformation.

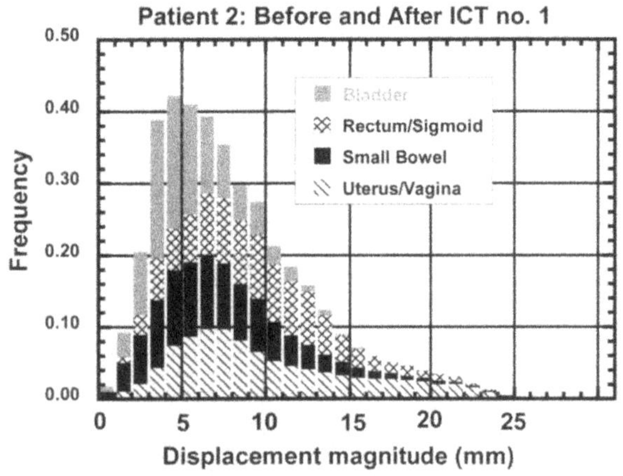


**Figure 2:** Histogram indicating the frequency of voxel displacement magnitures, relative to rigid alignment of the pelvic bones, due to application of the viscous fluid transformation.

Figure 2 shows that relative to global alignment of the pelvic bones, soft tissue deformation as modeled by the viscous fluid method, displaces tissue voxels on average by 4 mm to 10 mm and by as much as 15- 20 mm. Table 1 shows that rigid alignment, for both implant-to-implant and pre-to-post-insertion registration, results in very poor coincidence of the contoured anatomical structures. Bladder, rectum and uterus/vagina coincidence ranges from 0.3 to 0.7 while small bowel CI commonly ranges from 0.15-0.30. Application of the deformable template registration technique based upon the viscous fluid model usually improves coincidence to better than 0.99. The somewhat poorer registration results for small bowel are possibly due to difficulty in visualizing and contouring this structure on CT and inability to distinguish between individual bowel loops.

## Conclusion

Applicator insertion, tumor regression and vaginal stenosis---over the 7 week period needed to adminster definitive radiotherapy for locally advanced cervix cancer---produces significant deformation and displacemement of pelvic soft-tissue structures such as bladder, rectum, vagina and uterus. Relative to the rigid affine transformations currently used for image registration in radiotherapy, localized deformations result in tissue displacements averaging 5-10 mm and occasionally exceeding 20 mm. Deformable anatomic template registration, based upon continuum mechanics models of the deformation process, is a promising solution to this difficult problem. Future work will focus on using the high-dimensional voxel-to-voxel transformations to deform dose distributions into a single anatomically consistent frame of reference. This will permit rigorous registration of cummulative gynecologic brachytherapy dose distributions, summed over all treatment components, to the underlying anatomy.

## References

[1] Christensen, G, Rabbitt, R, and Miller, M, Deformable Templates using large deformation kinematics *IEEE Trans. Image. Processing.* **5** 1435-1447, 1996.

[2] Christensen, G, Rabbitt, R, and Miller, M 3D brain mapping using a deformable neuroanatomy *Phys. Med. Biol.* **39** 609-618, 1994.

[3] Weeks, KJ and Montana, GS, Three-dimensional applicator system for carcinoma of the uterine cervix *Int. J. Radiation Onocology Biol. Phys.* **37** 455-463, 1998

## Acknowledgment

This project is supported in part by grant RO1 CA 75371 awarded by the U.S. National Institutes of Health.

# Image Fusion in Radiotherapy

**Robert C. Krempien[1], Hartwig A. Grabowski[3], Wolfgang Harms[1], Sascha Daeubner[3], Frank W. Hensley[1], Arno Pernozzoli[2,3], Jakob Brief[2], Martina Treiber[1], Michael Wannenmacher[1]**

[1] Clinic for Radiology, Department of Clinical Radiology and [2] Clinic for Cranio-Maxillo-Surgery, University of Heidelberg, INF 400, 69120 Heidelberg, Germany and [3] Institute for Process Control and Robotics, Department of Computer Science, University of Karlsruhe, 76128 Karlsruhe, Germany

## Introduction

The emerging utilization of computer-assisted planning in pretherapeutic evaluation and therapeutic planning requires sophisticated imaging modalities [1,2,4,7,8,9,10,12]. Magnetic resonance imaging (MRI) has introduced several added imaging benefits that may confer an advantage over the use of CT such as improved soft tissue definition and unrestricted multiplanar and volumetric imaging however, MRI has not yet seriously challenged CT in radiotherapy planing [9]. The reasons for this include (1) the poor imaging of bone; (2) the lack of electron density information from MRI required for dosimetry calculations in radiotherapy; (3) the presence of intrinsic system-related and object-induced MR image distortions and (4) the paucity of widely available computer software to accurately and reliable integrate and manipulate MR images within existing therapy planning systems [9,14]. Frequently, information from multiple modalities or multiple scans of the same modality is important in planning a given case. In such instances, image registration may prove useful to allow synthesis of information from multiple sources into a single consistent coordinate frame [7,10,12]. Therefore a new system generating synthetic image modalities from matched and fused CT and MRI-data has been developed. The system presented consists of five modules serving for viewing, matching, segmentation, fusion and validation. With the presented new system manual or automatic image registration and fusion of CT and MR-images can be done, enabling the use of the imaging advantages of MRI and CT in pretherapeutic planing.

## Material and methods

For interaction with medical images a system is required which guides the user through several image processing tasks. For that reason a system consisting of six modules was developed. At each time during the image processing task the obtained results can be validated and, if necessary, the task can be repeated.

### System overview

***Viewing:*** At the beginning of a session, both volumetric data are loaded with the viewer module. This module is designed to exploit as much information as possible from the original slices. In two adjacent windows, the MR and CT images can be visualized in arbitrary planes, the slices can be interpolated, and a histogram-based gray value normalization can be performed. Other features like picking gray values or cutting regions are available.

***Registration:*** The presented registration algorithm uses a two step registration, first a voxel based method using a probabilistic approach for the detection of the initial transformation and second an approach based on voxel similarity measures using fast feature space calculations with a evaluation function based on mutual entropy [11]. Since this automatic registration approach was satisfactory only in the head area a manual transformation using manually set landmarks was used for coarse registration. This combination of manual and automated registration resulted in an average accuracy of the calculated transformation below 1 mm. The automatic registration takes about one to three minutes for two data sets of about 60 slices. The images can now be superimposed and visualized side by side within the same image slice (Fig. 1). This allows for the interaction of comprehensive anatomical mapping with functional distribution of the tissues within a single image set.

***Segmentation:*** In this module, the images can be segmented. Global thresholding and region-growing based seed-point segmentation is available. Up to 15 different structures can be segmented with an index-structure, so that one voxel can belong to two or more structures. Logical operations like (AND, OR, etc.) can be performed with the structures. All segmented structures can be visualized with different volume rendering techniques, like gradient shading, MIP (Maximum Intensity Projection) or SIP (Summarized Intensity Projection). The module consists of two modes, the *volume mode* and the *slice mode*. In the *volume mode* three dimensional region growing can be used to segment connected structures (Fig. 3). Since different structures are sometimes connected via thin regions, the size of the seed point can be chosen. In the *slice mode* fine segmentation can be performed slice by slice. For segmentation, polygon lines are used. The previously registered images are superimposed in one window, while it is possible to blend smoothly between the two images. In the superimposed image, interactive segmentation can be performed slice by slice (Fig. 3,4).

***Validation and Fusion:*** The gray values of the segmented structures can be copied and pasted from one volumetric image into the other (Fig. 3). In order to obtain high accuracy, the segmented regions are re-sampled before insertion. To avoid aliasing effects, the resampling can be performed with different rates. Additionally, the segmented regions can be copied and pasted without copying the gray values, thus enhancing the possibilities of the segmentation task. With the help of that technique, new imaging modalities can be created by a various fusion functions, like addition, subtraction, multiplication of gray values

The fusion function can be used for validation (Fig. 4). In the superimposition of the images under different fusion functions, the overall fitness of the obtained matching can be visualized transparently. Also technical validation like the average mean square distance between corresponding landmarks is possible.

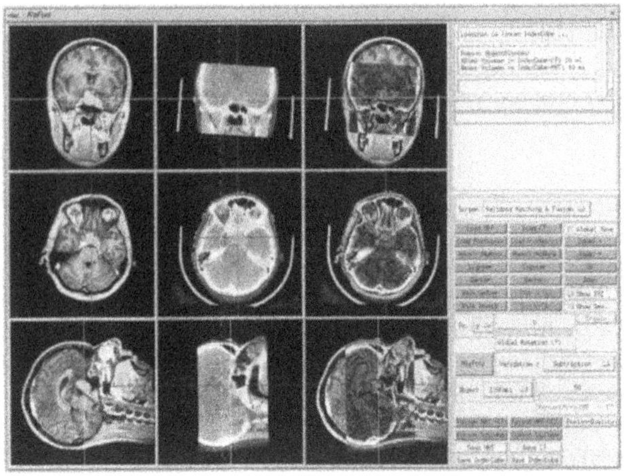

**Figure 1:**. In the registered images an interactive volume or slice by slice segmentation can be performed. The segmented structures can be visualized in both imaging modalities. The skull base tumor is segmented in the MRI (left images) and can be visalized in the correct anatomical position in the CT (middle, yellow structure). The result of the fusion obtained by addition, subtraction or multiplication of the gray values is used to validate the registration step. As seen in the right images the MR- and the CT images are fused by the fusion function *addition* (The gray values of both images are added after a certain kind of gray-value adaptation). Since bony structures are represented with high gray values in CT images, while these structures - giving no MRI-signal in T1w- and T2w-images - are represented with low gray values in MR images the result of the addition of both gray values can not exceed a certain threshold. Otherwise a high gray value in CT images corresponds to a high value in MR images which indicates an error in registration at the bony structures. As seen in the above image the bony structures and the skin contour fit well. Reconstruction of the fused images in different planes offer the possibility to validate the matching accuracy

## Results and discussion

The advent of cross-sectional image-based has introduced the possibility to individually adjust and optimize the dose description to anatomical structures. Studies with CT-based reconstruction showed a substantial benefit in the definition of the target volume and organs at risk and their respective dose prescription. Since CT is bound to axial scanning and offers limited soft tissue contrast, it is sometimes difficult to determine the exact tumor location and spread (Fig. 2) [9]. MRI has introduced several additional imaging benefits that may confer an advantage over the use of CT in radiotherapy planing however MRI has not yet seriously challenged CT in radiotherapy planing [9]. The reasons for this include (1) the poor imaging of bone; (2) the lack of electron density information from MRI required for dosimetry calculations in radiotherapy; (3) the presence of intrinsic system-related and object-induced MR image distortions and (4) the paucity of widely available computer software to accurately and reliable integrate and manipulate MR images within existing therapy planning systems and for brachytherapy (5) that MRI cannot visualize the dummy source positions required for detecting the source dwell positions needed for further planing [3]. One method of avoiding the problems associated with MRI is to integrate the superior tumor definition of MRI with the the electron density information and the geometric accuracy obtained from CT and in case of brachytherapy the accurate source localization. This allows for the integration of comprehensive anatomical mapping with functional distribution of the tissues within a single image set [10]. Manual methods of registering different image sets can be inefficient and error prone. In manual transposition of target information calculated mismatches of up to 8.5 mm between the volumes outlined by CT compared to MRI have been reported [2]. Automated approaches will reduce inter-operator variability and allow more accurate registration between multimodality systems [4]. Automated image registration requires the knowledge of a coordinate transformation between the two image studies which relates the patient position in each of them. It is necessary to be able to learn the orientation of the slices of each study with respect to some coordinate system fixed to the patient. The basis of this coordinate system can be intrinsic to the patient, meaning defined by some aspect of the patient anatomy, or it can be extrinsic, meaning added to the patient. Problematic for image registration are image distortions which may be present in MR-images [2,9,14]. The use of extrinsic registration methods requires either elimination of or correction for distortions since errors of several millimeters may be inherent in uncorrected MR-images especially in open low field MRI-systems and even when corrections are made, registration based on an external stereotactic frame in MRI may still be subject to errors on the order of millimeters [10,13]. One approach to addressing this problem is to use an intrinsic rather than extrinsic registration basis, that is to use the patient's anatomy as the basis of registration. Most methods identify anatomical homologies between the two image studies and attempt to find an interscan coordinate transformation which matches the homologous structures. Image registration and fusion additionally offers the possibility to use nonplaning diagnostic imaging in therapy planing. But distortion of anatomical structures due to patient movements or different positioning are problematic. The application of deformabel image models to use elastic registration procedures to wrap the images from nontreatment position to treatment position may here be a possible solution [5]. Initial results in computer assisted surgery planing procedures using finite element meshes seemed promising [6], but need further investigation in radiotherapy planing.

## Conclusion

The presented interactive system allows full automatic registration, based on voxel similarity measurements. After segmentation structures in the matched images can be copied from one image into the other. Structures of interest can be segmented in one imaging modality and then copied into the other thus enabling the use of the advantages of different imaging modalities or information of multiple scans i.e. pre- and postoperative, of the same modality therapeutic planning.

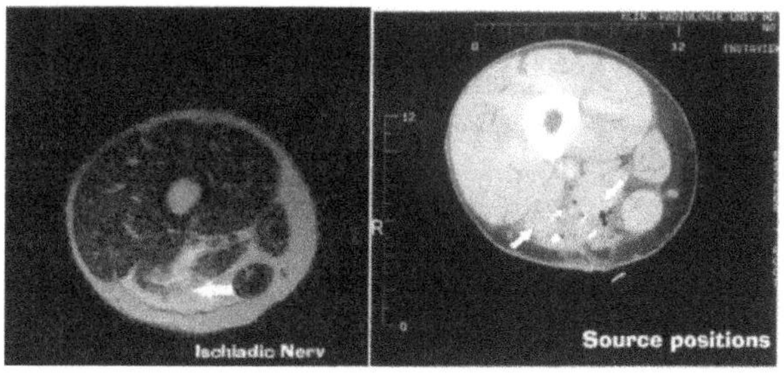


**Figure 2:** A patient with liposarcoma in the thigh showed a histological positive tumor margin to the ischiadic nerve. Intraoperativley the decision was made to implant brachytherapy guides for postoperative boost-radiation of the tumor-bed rather than resecting the nerve to preserve the function of the leg. CT (**right**) accurately localizes source positions (arrows) but due to the limited soft tissue contrast and the postoperative changes the nerve as the primary target structure was hardly detectable. The MRI (**left**) with its superior soft tissue contrast easily showed the nerve (arrow) but no source positions could be visualized.

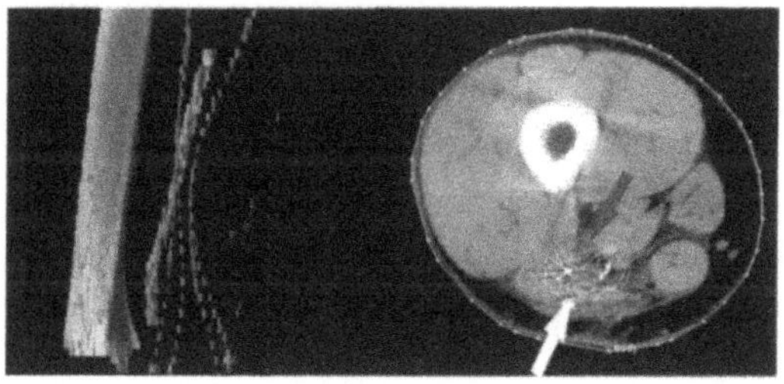

**Figure 3: Left:** The ischiadic nerve (yellow structure) is segmented in MRI and the segmented structure can be visualized and positioned in the CT image. The dummy source positions (red) and the femoral bone (blue) are segmented via seed point segmentation in CT. The Position of the nerve can now be visualized in comparison to the source dwell positions. **Right:** The fused synthetic images are added into the Plato brachytherapy planing system. The red circle (blue arrow) was the supposed nerve localization due to the planing CT, the turquoise circle (white arrow) due to the planing MRI. The 100 cGy isodose/pulse (yellow line) was the enclosing target volume isodose. The use of a CT alone for brachytherapy-planing would have resulted in a heavy overdose of the nerve with a high risk of radiation damage to the nerve in this slice position, in other places a actual miss of the target structure occurred which may have resulted in early tumor relapse.

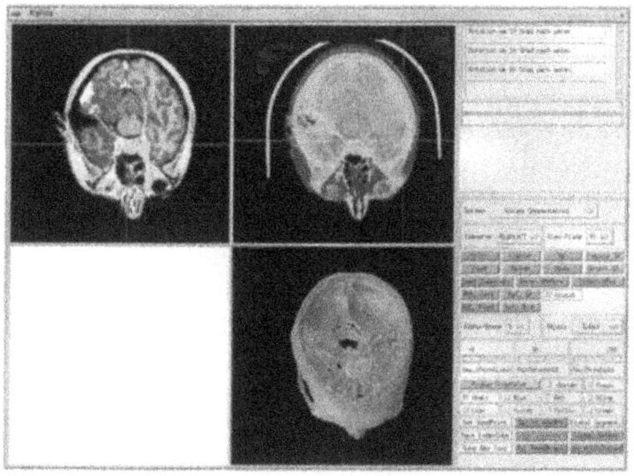

**Figure 4:** Segmentation: Combination of both segmentation modalities to obtain global alignment of tumor structure (yellow, manual segmentation slice by slice) and surrounding tissue (i.e. bony structures (red) by seed point segmentation). The gray values of the segmented tumor of the skull base are copied into the CT since further imaging processing is easier to handle using gray value images. If necessary artificial gray values can be assigned. These synthetic images can be used for further treatment planning.

# References

[1] Baltas D, Kolotas C, Geramani K et al. A conformal index (COIN) to evaluate implant quality and dose specification in brachytherapy. Int. J Radiat. Oncol. Biol. Phys. 1998; 40:515-524.

[2] De Salles AWT, Abe M, Kjellberg RN. Transposition of target information from magnetic resonance and computed tomography scan images to conventional stereotactic space. Appl. Neurophysiol. 1987; 50:23-32

[3] Dubois DF, Prestidge BR, Hotchkiss LA, Bice WS, Prete JJ. Source localisation following permanent transperineal prostate interstitial brachytherapy using magnetic resonance imaging. Int. J Radiat. Oncol. Biol. Phys. 1997; 39:1037-1041.

[4] van den Elsen PA; Pol EJ, Viergever MA. Medical image matching - a review with classification. IEEE Trans. Med. Biomed. Eng. 1993; 12:26-39

[5] Galvin JM, Han K, Noz ME et al. Warping CT scans from nontreatment to treatment position. Rad Oncol Invest 1997; 5:206-212

[6] Grabowski HA, Hassfeld S, Krempien R et al. Simulation of frontal orbital advancement. Virtual reality 1999; 3:1-6

[7] Hill DLG, Hawkes DJ, Crossman JE, et al. Registration of MR and CT images for skull base surgery using point-like anatomical features. Br J Radiology 64:1030-1035, 1991

[8] Kagawa K., Lee W.R., Schultheiss T.E., Hunt M.A., Shaer A.H., Hanks G.E. Initial clinical assessment of CT-MRI image fusion software in localization of the prostate for 3D conformal radiation therapy. Int. J. Radiation Oncology Biol. Phys. 38:319-325, 1997

[9] Khoo VS, Dearnaley DP, Finnigan DJ, Padhani A, Tanner ST, Leach MO. Magnetic resonance imaging (MRI): considerations and applications in radiotherapy treatment planing. Radiother. Oncol. 1997; 42:1-15.

[10] Pelizzari CA. Image processing in stereotactic planing: volume visualization and image registration. Medical Dosimety 1998; 23:137-145

[11] P. Pokrandt Fast Non-Supervised Matching: A Probabilistic Approach, Proceedings of the 10th International Symposium and Exhibition on Computer Assisted Radiology and Surgery (CAR'96), 1996

[12] Rosenman JG, Miller EP, Tracton G, Cullip T. Image registration: an essential part of radiation therapy treatment planing. Int. J. Radiation Oncology Biol. Phys. 1998; 40:197-205

[13] Sumanaweera TS, Adler JR, Napel S, Glover G. Characterization of spatial distortion in magnetic resonance imaging and its implications for stereotactic surgery. Neurosurgery 1994; 35:696-704

[14] Wesby G, Adamis MK, Edelmann RR. Artifacts in MRI: description, causes and solutions. In: Edelmann RR, Hesselink JK, Zlatkin MB Eds.: Clinical magnetic resonance imaging. Philadelphia, Pa: Saunders, 1996; 88-144

# Automated image registration using mutual information for both affine and thin-plate spline geometric transformations

**Marc L Kessler, PhD[1], Kelvin Li, MS[1], Charles Meyer, PhD[2]**

[1]Department of Radiation Oncology, and [2]Department of Radiology, The University of Michigan, Ann Arbor, MI 48109

## Introduction

In this presentation we describe the methodology and clinical implementation of a mutual information-based automated image registration system for conformal radiotherapy treatment planning. This system estimates the transformation that relates the coordinate systems of diagnostic MR or PET/SPECT image datasets with the treatment planning x-ray CT dataset. This transformation can then be applied to map volumes of interest, such as tumor volumes, defined on one dataset to the reference. Unlike many other studied registration systems, this system is not limited to affine transformations [1]. Instead, the option of a thin-plate spline warping transformation can also be applied to model possible distortions as a result of tissue deformations, as well as those that are imaging device related. This feature allows a wider range of imaging studies to be incorporated into the treatment planning process. Since the system uses the native image data rather than extracted surfaces or ridges, very little user interaction is required to perform the registrations.

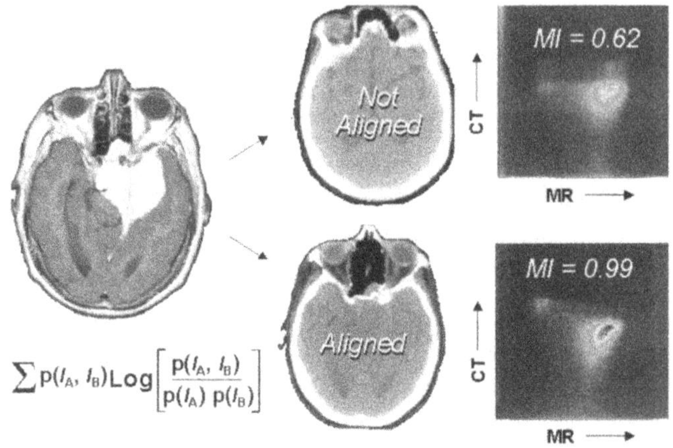


Figure 1: Two-dimensional grayscale histograms for aligned and misaligned MR and CT datasets. The MI is computed according to the equation shown.

## Material and methods

The registration process is implemented by using an optimizer, the Nelder-Mead simplex algorithm, to drive the positions of homologous control points in the homologous data set, i.e. the data volume to be mapped onto the reference volume, subject to maximizing the resultant mutual information (MI) between the reference volume and the transformed homologous volume [2].

The MI cost metric is computed from the bivariate histogram of gray values in the reference and reconstructed data set for geometrically corresponding voxels (**Figure 1**). Each optimization cycle is initiated by a random perturbation of the initial transformation vector. The trilinear interpolation process uses the original data set for each iteration instead of using previous interpolations to generate successive data. This approach prevents round-off and other undesired interpolation effects such as smoothing from accumulating across iterations.

For cases where the thin-plate spline bending energy [3] of a potential warping is small, nearly any evenly distributed, volumetric placement of control points (>4 and typically <10) in the reference volume is sufficient to compute a good registration. In typical use, only the first 3 homologous control points must be initially placed in the homologous volume corresponding to the approximate homologous loci of the first 3 reference points.

First, the six degrees of freedom (DOF) rigid body registration is computed by the optimizer's movement of the 3 control points in homologous space to maximize MI. Next, using the optimized rigid body model, the first 4 control points in the reference space are mapped into the homologous space, and then the 12 DOF, full affine registration is subsequently computed, again by optimizing MI through iterative movement of the 4 control points in homologous space. The optimized warping solution is initiated by using the previously optimized full affine solution to map all of the reference control points into the homologous volume. Finally, the algorithm optimizes the loci of all of the control points in the homologous space to compute the thin-plate spline registration that yields the maximum (global) MI between the reference and the geometrically transformed homologous data sets.

For cases where the warping is more severe, it may be necessary for the first transformation computed to be a low order warp in order to sufficiently approximate the geometric transformation necessary for the algorithm to capture the required deformation. Thus, the initial number of data point pairs to be placed in both reference and homologous data set is 5.

The entire registration system was implemented using the AVS, the Application Visualization System (Advanced Visual Systems, Wathham, MA) and the C programming language. All data management for treatment planning is handled by our 3D treatment planning system, U-MPlan.

## Results and discussion

We illustrate this system using an example of a registration of a diagnostic MR with a planning CT for a patient with a benign meningioma located near the base of the skull (**Figure 2**). As is often the case, the position of the patient's head in the two imaging studies is different (the patient is imaged wearing an immobilization mask during the CT procedure but not during the MR). The only user interaction required to initialize the registration system is the *approximate* placement of 3 or 4 homologous points chosen with a mouse. This usually takes 30-60 seconds. For brain cases, the centers of the orbits and top and back of the head are usually chosen.

Once the points are selected, the optimizer is started and no further user input is required. In this example, only 6 DOFs (3 rotations and 3 translations) were required to achieve an accurate registration. The entire registration process typically requires ~5 minutes of CPU time on a 550 Mhz Digital Alpha-based workstation running OpenVMS.

After the transformation is estimated, several tools are used to help assess the accuracy of the final transformation (**Figure 3**). One tool allows the user to compare images at equivalent anatomic levels from the reference and reformatted datasets by using the AVS supported module "IMAGE COMPARE." Another custom-written module allows the user to drag a rectangular window in which the complementary dataset is displayed. This type of display is coined the "MAGIC WINDOW" and was popularized by researchers at the University of North Carolina at Chapel Hill. Another approach provided is to allow the user to place any number of points within one dataset and display the corresponding (transformed) locations on the complementary dataset. Ultimately however, without knowledge of the ground-truth, the accuracy with which the transformation estimate can be used (for target volume transfer including margin specification) must be subjectively evaluated on a case-by-case basis.

For cases involving the brain, our experience to date has been that transformed data is accurate to within one or two pixels (< 2.0 *mm*). This degree of accuracy is representative of most anatomic feature-based registration systems in routine clinical use. These other approaches however usually require more user interaction and also a larger extent of the patient's anatomy to be imaged.

Finally, we demonstrate the results of applying the thin-plate spline option to register PET and CT datasets from the thorax (**Figure 5**). For this case, five initial points were placed in *approximately* similar regions on both the PET and the CT dataset (2 at lung apices, 1 in the lesion, 1 in the carina, and 1 on the chest, mid-sternum). After optimising the transformation using 5 points, 3 more points were *automatically* added and the registration optimised once more. Because of the larger number of degrees of freedom, significantly more iterations, and hence more time (~45 min.) were required for the overall registration computation. To demonstrate the extent of deformation computed, a rectilinear grid defined in the PET coordinate system is mapped to on display over the CT dataset.

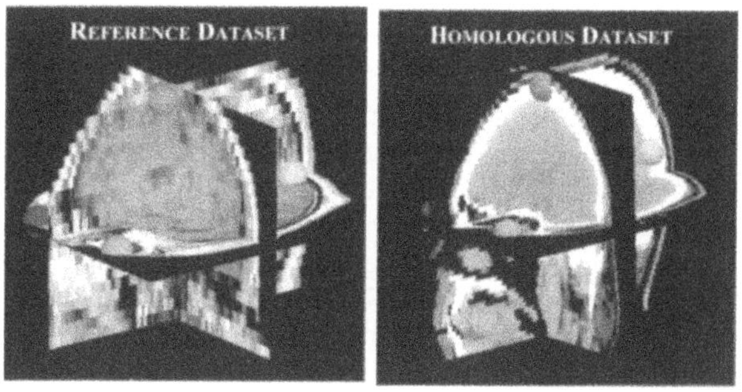


**Figure 2:** Initialization of registration of MR and Tx planning CT dataset using *approximately* placed homologous points.

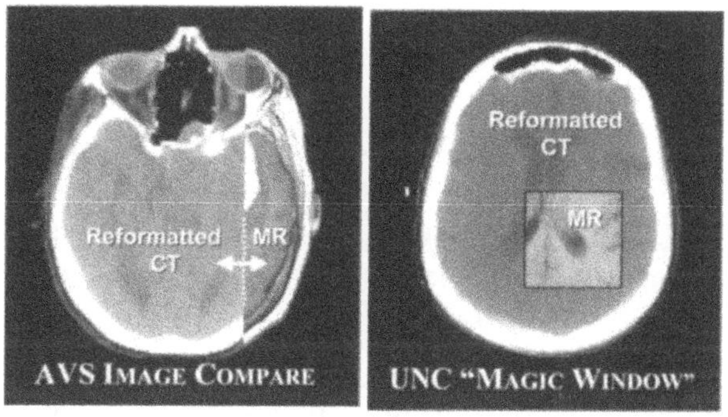


**Figure 3:** Visual validation of computed transformation results.

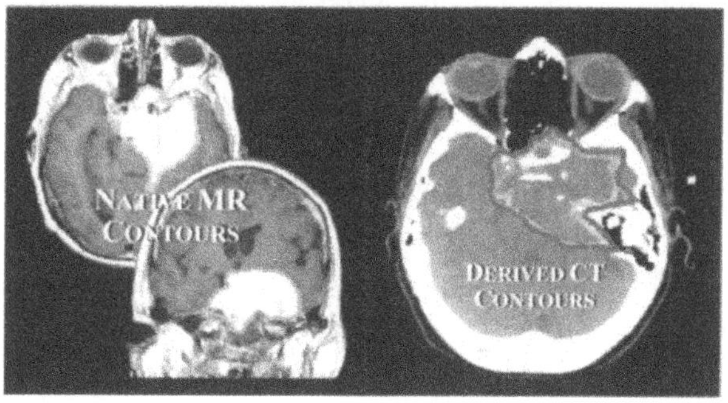


**Figure 4:** Left: contours drawn directly over the axial and coronal MR images. Right: contours derived by transforming, compositing, and intersecting the volumes created from the MR contours.

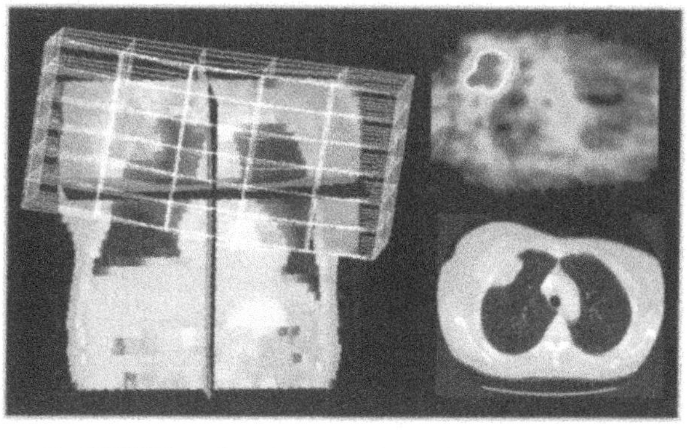

**Figure 5:** PET/CT registration applying thin-plate spline warping. Left: a rectilinear grid in the PET coordinate system is mapped to the CT dataset to demonstrate the affine and thin-plate spline components of the geometric transformation. Right: a native PET image at the center of the lesion and the corresponding reconstructed CT image.

## Summary

A mutual information-based automatic multimodality image registration system has developed and applied across a broad spectrum of volumetric data sets of various modalities and anatomies. One benefit with this system is the minimal user interaction and data pre-processing required. The major benefit, however, is the robustness of the MI algorithm to sparse or missing data and when registering anatomic data with functional data from PET/SPECT where precisely corresponding anatomic features are difficult to define. Finally, the option of using geometric warping in addition to affine transformations, to model certain tissue deformation and machine distortions greatly expands the range of imaging studies that can be incorporated into the treatment planning process.


## References


[1] Kessler M L, Pitluck S, Petti P L, Castro J R 1991 Integration of multimodality imaging data for radiotherapy treatment planning. *Int J Rad Oncol Bio Phys* **21**:1653-1667.

[2] Meyer C R, Boes JL,, Kim B, Bland B H, et al. 1997, Demonstration of accuracy and clinical versatility of mutual information for automatic multimodality image fusion using affine and thin plate spline warped geometric deformations. *Medical Image Analysis* **1**(3):195-206.

[3] Bookstein F L 1991. Morphometric tools for landmark data: geometry and biology. Cambridge Univ. Press: New York. 435 pp.

# Prostate Boundary Detection and Visualization in TRUS Images

**Steve T. Lam**[1], **Robert J. Marks II**[1] **and Paul S. Cho**[1,2]
[1] Department of Electrical Engineering, University of Washington, Seattle, WA 98195-2500, USA and [2] Department of Radiation Oncology, University of Washington, Seattle, WA 98195-6043, USA

## Introduction

Ultrasound imaging has been used extensively in various medical specialities. Transrectal ultrasound (TRUS) imaging is a valuable tool in analyzing the boundary of the prostate, the internal structure of the prostate and guiding the seed insertion during prostate brachytherapy surgery. Boundary determination of the prostate in the TRUS images is difficult due to noise inherent in ultrasound signals. Consequently, the prostate boundary is usually not well defined and often discontinuous. Even among the experts there likely exist variances in reading as to the exact location of the prostate borders. Currently, prostate boundary determination is very time consuming as it is performed manually.

A number of techniques has been applied to automate the process including neuronetworks [1], Laplacian edge operator [2], texture analysis [3], radial bas relief method [4], harmonics method [5], and snakes [6]. Of these the snakes technique appears to be most promising although it has not been fully automated. In this paper, we present the use of multiple snakes toward improved efficiency as well as a method of visualizing the prostate boundary with associated levels of confidence.

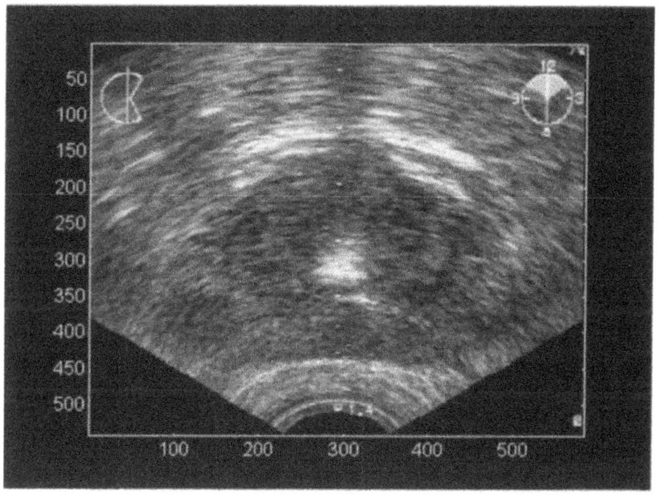


**Figure 1:** Original prostate ultrasound image.

## Materials and methods

Active Contour Model, first introduced by Kass, Witkin and Terzopoulos [7], is a model for representing image contours in a form that allows interaction with higher level processes. The initial snake points of the Active Contour Model provides general outline of object to be segmented and have been applied to numerous image analysis and computer vision problems including edge detection, shape modeling, segmentation [8], and motion tracking. Active Contour Model turns the problem of edge detection and linking into an energy minimization problem.

Let $V(s) = (x(s), y(s))$ represent the snake contour and the total energy of the snake by [7]

$$E(V) = \int_0^1 (E_{int}(V(s)) + E_{img}(V(s)) + E_{con})V(s)))ds \quad (1)$$

where $E_{int}$ is an internal enrgy of the snakes given by

$$E_{int}(V(s)) = \frac{1}{2}(\alpha(s)|V_s(s)|^2 + \beta(s)|V_{ss}(s)|^2) \quad (2)$$

where $V_s(s) = dV(s)/ds$ and $V_{ss}(s) = d^2V(s)/ds^2$.

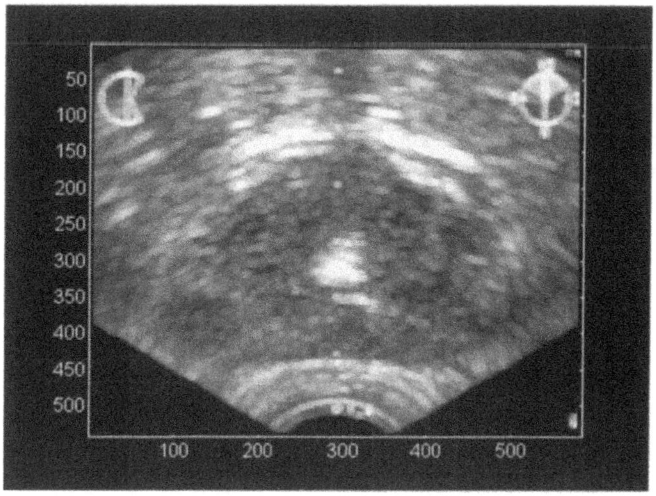


**Figure 2:** Sticks transform of the prostate image.

The first-order term controlled by $\alpha(s)$ makes the snake act like a membrane and the second-order term controlled by $\beta(s)$ makes it act like a thin plate that allows the snake to stretch, bend, or develop a corner. By adjusting these parameters, the snake can be controlled to deform according to prescribed mixture of membrane and thin-plate like behaviors.

$E_{img}$ is the image energy term that drives the contour to specific features in the image. $E_{con}$ is the energy component related to additional constraint applied to the contour.

Given an image with speckle noise, the Sticks transform has been shown to be effective in enhancing the structure edges [9]. The method superposes a line segment over the central pixel, $S_{ij}$, and sums all pixels along the segment, $\mu_s$. The maximum value of the sums among all orthogonal and diagonal orientations, $k$, is then used as the new value of the central pixel. Therefore,

$$\text{new}S_{ij} = \max_k \sum \mu_s. \tag{3}$$

Figure 2 shows the sticks transform of the prostate ultrasound image.

Snakes require initial starting point, the selection of which could be critical in the outcome of the final result. Carefully placed initial reference points would help achieve good results, but if time consuming, such an approach would defeat the purpose of computerized segmentation. In order to reduce the amount of manual intervention we have adopted a set of elliptical templates. The simple geometric templates can be quickly placed by the operator to approximately enclose the prostate as shown in Figure 3. By using multiple initial templates and launching snakes from each template plural solutions are obtained. However, the solutions are expected to converge in areas where the boundary is more distinctly defined.

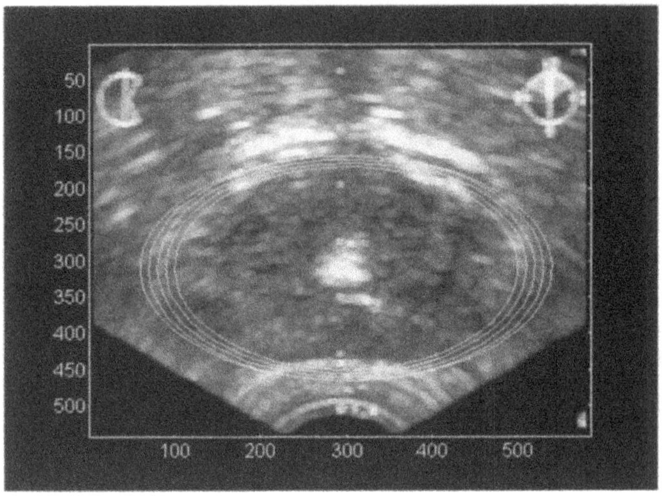


**Figure 3:** Initial elliptical reference contours.

## Results and discussion

Figure 4 shows the resultant snake contours overlayed on the original image. The results demonstrate strong-to-mild convergence of solutions for the top and the bottom portions of the prostate, whereas weaker convergence is observed for the side walls. The degree of congruence among the solutions can be interpreted as the level of confidence associated with the solution. For this reason, rather than forcing the decision as to which one of the solutions might be the "truth" we have opted to visualize the estimated prostate boundary in terms of a "range" of possible boundary positions. Such method of visualization may be useful in computer-assisted scheme by quickly providing the physician with an initial estimate.

In order to improve the level of confidence the signal to noise ratios of the image must be increased. To this end we are investigating the possibility of further contrast enhancement using recursive and variable length Sticks transforms. Another topic of investigation is the application of genetic algorithm in selection of the best final solution.

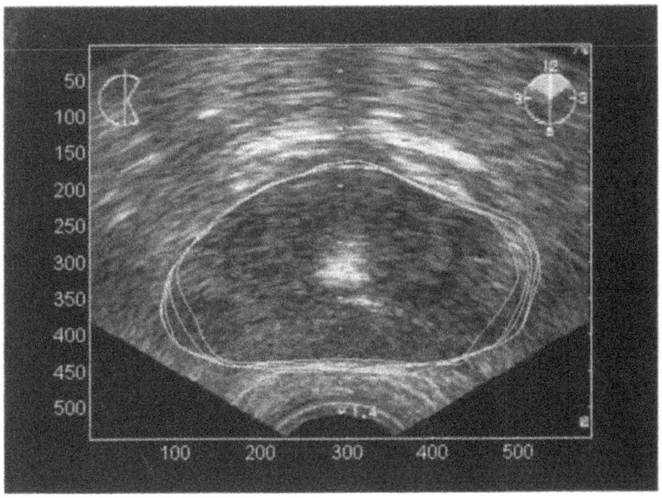


**Figure 4:** Results of boundary detection by multiple snakes. Good convergence of snakes (top and bottom portions) reflects high confidence in solution, while weak convergence as seen along the side walls represents a range of possible solutions.

## Conclusions

A method of computerized prostate boundary detection based on Active Contour Model was presented. The use of geometric templates helped minimize operator intervention in setting the initial conditions. Furthermore, satisfactory solutions were achieved by the multiple snakes method which demostrated varying degrees of convergence along the prostate boundary. Overall, our preliminary studies indicated that the technique can potentially provide the basis for determining the confidence level associated with the detected boundary.

## References

[1] Prater J S and Richard W D 1992 Segmenting ultrasound images of the prostate using neural networks *Ultrason. Imaging* **14** 159–185

[2] Richard W D, Grimmel C K, Bedigian K and Frank K J 1993 A method for three-dimensional prostate imaging using transrectal ultrasound *Comput. Med. Imaging Graph.* **17** 73–79

[3] Richard W D and Keen C G 1996 Automated texture-based segmentation of ultrasound images of the prostate *Comput. Med. Imaging Graph.* **20** 131–140

[4] Liu Y J, Ng W S, Teo M Y and Lim H C 1997 Computerised prostate boundary estimation of ultrasound images using radial bas-relief method *Med. Biol. Eng. Comput.* **35** 445–454

[5] Kwoh C K, Teo M Y, Ng W S, Tan S N and Jones L M 1998 Outlining the prostate boundary using the harmonics method *Med. Biol. Eng. Comput.* **36** 768–771

[6] Pathak S D, Aarnink R G, de la Rosette J J, Chalana V, Wijkstra H, Debruyne F M J and Kim Y 1998 Quantitative three-dimensional trans-rectal ultrasoud for prostate imaging *Proceedings SPIE Medical Imaging* 83–92

[7] Kass M, Witkin A, and Terzopoulos D 1988 Snakes: Active contour models *Int. J. Comput. Vision* 321–331

[8] Lam S T and Nguyen A G 1999 Object segmentation using active contour models and statistical methods of texture analysis *Proceedings DMS'99 Sixth International conference on Distributed Multimedia Systems* 182–188

[9] Czerwinski R N, Jones D L and O'Brien W D 1999 Detection of lines and boundaries in speckle images - application to Medical Ultrasound *IEEE Trans. Med. Imaging* **18** 126–136

# Multimodality image fusion and localisation environment for radiosurgery treatments of large AVMs.

**Yanic Bercier, Horacio Patrocinio, Phillipe Belanger, Dimitre Hristov**

Medical Physics Unit, Montreal General Hospital, McGill University, 1650 Cedar Avenue, Montreal, Quebec, H3G 1A4, CANADA

## Introduction

Radiosurgery is the preferred treatment for arteriovenous malformations (AVM) which are situated in deep brain locations such as close to the brain stem, or near critical areas such as the visual cortex[1]. The technique is commonly planned using multiple modalities, such as magnetic resonance (MR), computed tomography (CT) and digital subtraction angiography (DSA). T1 weighted MR images and CT images provide anatomical information but without additional contrast media, these techniques fail to provide adequate vascular information. For this reason, DSA images, which are obtained after contrast injection, are employed for target localisation. However, since these images are 2D projections of 3D structures, they may be inadequate for the 3D definition of large, complexly shaped AVMs[2]. Since the AVMs treated by radiosurgery are usually close to organs at risk, the dose must conform to the target and therefore accurate 3D target delineation may help achieve this goal.

Some of the non-invasive magnetic resonance angiography (MRA) techniques, such as the Time of Flight, provide volume data sets of the 3D vasculature. While such techniques may improve 3D AVM definition, they suppress stationary anatomical information and therefore, alone, are inadequate for radiosurgery planning. Therefore, fusing MRA to MR and/or CT (MR/CT) may be a solution to improve target delineation by combining the 3D MRA vasculature information and the 3D MR/CT anatomical information. By delineating the target on the MRA and the contours appearing on the MR/CT, a 3D target definition and anatomical verification can be obtained.

In this paper, a multimodality image fusion and localisation environment for radiosurgery treatment of large AVMs is presented. This environment consists of four major modules. Module 1 (Volume fusion) fuses the MRA and MR/CT volumes. Module 2 performs 3D target localisation and delineation within the fused volumes. Module 3 (DSA target localisation) determines the target position and the projection geometry. Module 4 (DSA/MRA correlation), in progress, correlates MRA and DSA data.

## Material and methods

The image fusion and localisation environment was implemented with the AVS 5.4 software (Advance Visual System Inc., Waltham, MA) running on a Pentium II processor (Intel Corporation, Santa Clara, CA) 400 MHz with 256 megs of RAM. The operational system employed is Red Hat Linux 6.0 (Red Hat Software Inc., North Carolina). The AVS software permits the programming of modules for specific tasks, which are then linked together in networks to complete application programs.

The environment supports both the Leksell and the OBT stereotactic coordinate system commonly used for radiosurgery. These stereotactic systems are established by fixing a rigid frame to the patient's head during all imaging procedures and the radiosurgery treatment. A series of fiducial marker plates, to be attached to the frame during imaging, exist for each modality in order to determine the frame position within the data sets.

The software comprises four main modules, as shown in Figure 1.

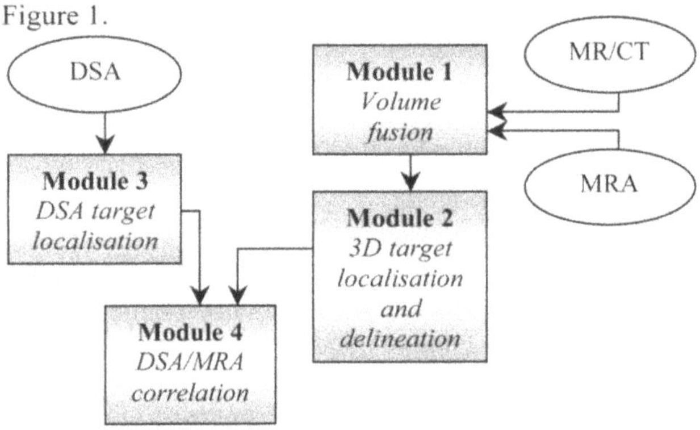


**Figure 1:** Four main modules of environment.

**Module 1: Volume fusion**

This module fuses the MRA and MR/CT volumes. The module consists of two sections, the first being the semi-automatic selection of fiducial markers and the second being the volume reformatting.

A) Fiducial marker selection

The CT and MR fiducial marker plates contain a series of N-shaped bars. The N-shaped bars, when imaged axially, give three collinear points. With three bars on each frame attachment, nine points are obtained on each slice as shown in Figure 2. These markers are selected semi-automatically. The user selects all fiducial markers on the first slice. The centre of mass (COM) of each marker is then determined, within the neighbourhood of the marker. Employing the neighbourhood of the points of the first slice, the COMs of the markers of slice 2 are determined, and so forth for the next slices of the volume. Additional rules are implemented to prevent confusion in the vicinity of the bar intersections. The user can then inspect the marker positions and perform corrections if any are needed.

The 3D space coordinates of the middle fiducial marker of each N-shaped bar cross-section are determined using ratios with respect to the extremity markers. The frame space coordinates of the middle fiducial markers $(x_1,y_1,z_1)$, $(x_2,y_2,z_2)$, $(x_3,y_3,z_3)$, along with their corresponding image coordinates $(u_1,v_1)$, $(u_2,v_2)$, $(u_3,v_3)$ are used to determine the frame transformation matrix (FTM). The FTM, which is specific to each slice, is obtained by the following expression:

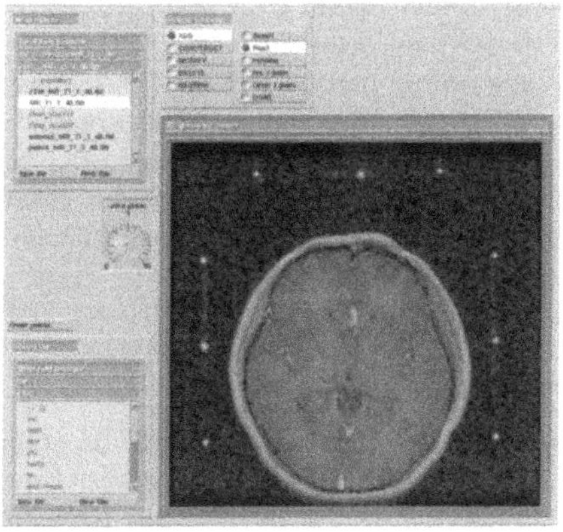

**Figure 2:** Panel for fiducial marker selection. The nine fiducial markers can be observed on the image slice.

$$\mathbf{FTM} = \begin{bmatrix} u_1 & v_1 & 1 \\ u_2 & v_2 & 1 \\ u_3 & v_3 & 1 \end{bmatrix}^{-1} \begin{bmatrix} x_1 & y_1 & z_1 \\ x_2 & y_2 & z_2 \\ x_3 & y_3 & z_3 \end{bmatrix}$$

The FTM allows the determination of the frame space coordinates (x,y,z) corresponding to the image space coordinates (u,v) and vice-versa, by the following transformations.

$$[x \quad y \quad z] = [u \quad v \quad 1] \cdot \mathbf{FTM}$$

$$[u \quad v \quad 1] = [x \quad y \quad z] \cdot (\mathbf{FTM})^{-1}$$

B) MR/CT and MRA volume reformatting

Using the FTMs, this module reformats and fuses the MRA and MR/CT volumes in frame space. This is necessary because subtle patient movements or scanning imperfections may lead to changes in the mutual orientation of image slices, as shown in Figure 3. Furthermore, reformatting is necessary to obtain the regular voxel array required for ray tracing in the DSA/MRA correlation module.

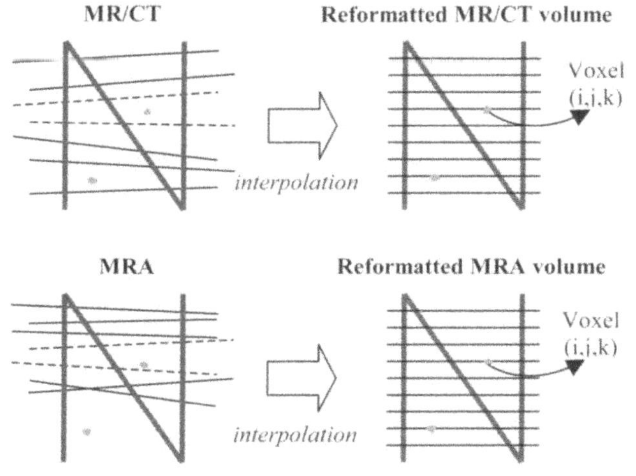


**Figure 3:** Slice orientation in frame space before and after reformatting (interpolation). The image slices may be arbitrarily oriented in frame space due to subtle patient movement or scanning imperfections. After reformatting, a regular voxel array is obtained. For the voxel (i,j,k), the nearest two slices which bracket the voxel are illustrated in dotted format.

The reformatting procedure is as follows. First, the frame space extents of MRA and MR/CT data sets are determined. These extents are then compared to determine a common *reformatting extent*, in order to proceed with the interpolation. For each data set, the extents along the x and y axis are determined by taking the intersection of the (x,y) extents of all image slices within the data set. The z extent is obtained by the minimum and maximum z values of the data set, as calculated from all the slices. The *reformatting extent* is determined by the union of the extents of the two data sets to be reformatted.

Given the *reformatting extent* and the voxel sizes ($v_x$,$v_y$,$v_z$) in millimetres as supplied by the user, a regular voxel array is built by interpolation. The intensity of each voxel (i,j,k) within the *reformatting extent* is interpolated employing the slices of each data set and their FTM. For each voxel (i,j,k) within the *reformatting extent*, which correspond to ($x_i$,$y_j$,$z_k$) in frame space coordinates, the nearest two slices which bracket the voxel are determined.. These slices are shown in dotted format in Figure 3. The intensity interpolation is then performed between the two slices. Points which are not between two slices or out of the corresponding data set extent, are padded with zeros. Since the *reformatting extents* are the same for both reformatted volumes, voxel (i,j,k) of the reformatted MRA volume data corresponds to voxel (i,j,k) of the reformatted MR/CT volume data. The fusion between the two volumes is therefore complete.

The frame space coordinates ($x_i$,$y_j$,$z_k$) corresponding to voxel (i,j,k) of the reformatted volume are determined by the use of the volume transformation matrix (VTM).

$$\begin{bmatrix} x \\ y \\ z \\ 1 \end{bmatrix} = \mathbf{VTM} \begin{bmatrix} i \\ j \\ k \\ 1 \end{bmatrix}$$

The VTM, a 4x4 matrix, accounts for translation, rotation and scaling between frame space and image space. Since the reformatted volume is aligned with the frame, the VTM is given by

$$\mathbf{VTM} = \begin{bmatrix} v_x & 0 & 0 & x_{\min} \\ 0 & v_y & 0 & y_{\min} \\ 0 & 0 & v_z & z_{\min} \\ 0 & 0 & 0 & 1 \end{bmatrix}$$

In the above expression, ($x_{min}$,$y_{min}$,$z_{min}$) represents the minimum of the (x,y,z) *reformatting extent* in frame space. The reformatting voxel sizes ($v_x$,$v_y$,$v_z$) determine the scaling between the two spaces.

**Module 2: 3D target localisation and delineation**

This module allows the user to localise and delineate the target in 3D after the reformatting. After the fusion of MRA and MR/CT data sets by the *Volume fusion* module, target contours, which are drawn on the reformatted MRA volume, can be simultaneously visualised on the reformatted MR/CT volume. Similarly, critical structures can be drawn on the reformatted MR/CT volume and simultaneously visualised on the reformatted MRA volume (Figure 4). The drawing of contours can be performed on transverse, sagittal or coronal slices of the reformatted volume. The frame localisation of the

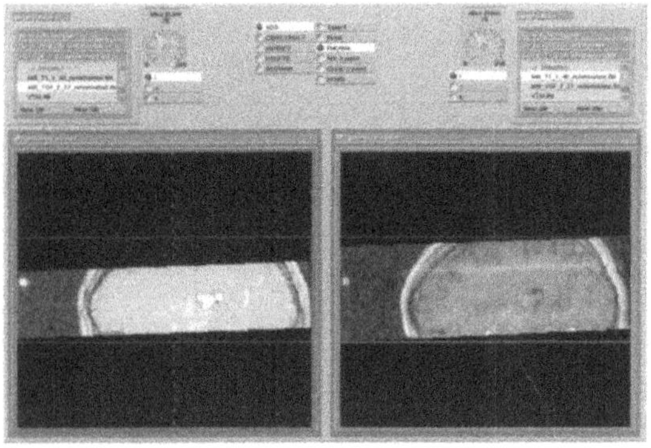

**Figure 4:** Panel for 3D target delineation. The user delineates the target on the MRA volume (left). The contours appear simultaneously in the MR volume (right).

drawn structures is performed by the use of the VTM, described earlier.

**Module 3: DSA target localisation**

This module allows localisation with a pair of DSA images. For this modality, the fiducial marker plates contain a series of lead beads on each side of the frame, which projected on the image plane, are selected by the user.

Two projections are taken. An anterior-posterior projection (AP) and a lateral projection (LAT) are taken. The subtraction of the non-contrast image from the contrast image provides the DSA images of vasculature. Using the contrast or non-contrast images, the user selects the fiducial markers on both projection images. This information allows the determination of the projection geometry of both views[7]. The user then traces the target on both DSA views to localise the target in frame space. The panel of this module is shown in Figure 5

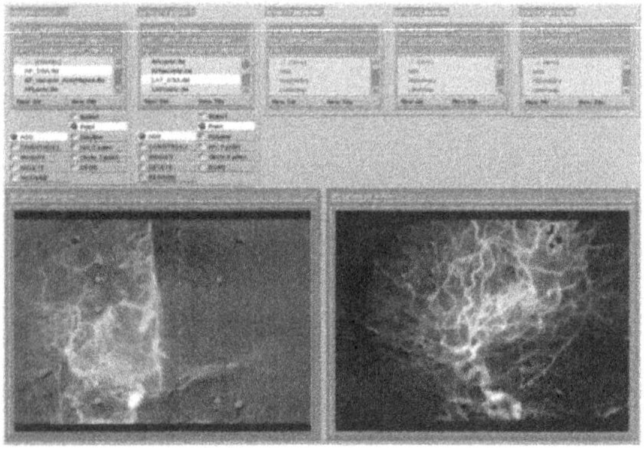

**Figure 5:** Panel for DSA target localisation. The user determines the target position on both views. The target position is then determined.

**Module 4: DSA/MRA correlation**

To help the user in the process of target delineation, this module correlates DSA and MRA data by the following two methods:

1. AP and LAT projection images of the reformatted MRA volume are obtained by ray-tracing, with the projection geometry used in the acquisition of the DSA images (determined in Module 3). These images are correlated with their DSA counterparts to examine possible inconsistencies between the DSA data sets and reformatted MRA volume which could arise from MR distortions or other sources of image artefacts.
2. MRA contours are projected onto the DSA images as they are drawn with the same projection geometry as above. This enables the correlation of the contoured 3D volume with the target extent observable on the DSA images. Thus, contours drawn on the MRA can then be modified accordingly.

## Summary

We have developed an environment for multimodality image fusion and localisation for radiosurgery treatment of large, complexly shaped AVMs. Within this environment, the fusion of MRA and MR/CT datasets combines vascular and anatomical information and therefore may help the physician in localising and delineating targets, especially when they are in close proximity to critical organs. The position of the target can also be determined with DSA images. To help the user in the process of target delineation, DSA and MRA are correlated. A study on patients that have previously undergone radiosurgery for AVM at our institution is underway to evaluate the clinical utility of this environment.

## References


[1] Pollock B E, April 1999, Stereotactic Radiosurgery for Arteriovenous Malformations, *Applications of Radiosurgery*, **10**(2) 281-290

[2] Levy R P, Schulte R W M, Frankel K A, Steinberg G K, Marks M P, Lane B, Heilbronn L H, Meinass H J, Galindo R A, Slater J D, Slater J M, 1996, Computed Tomography Slice-by-slice Target-volume Delineation for Stereotactic Proton Irradiation of Large Intracranial Arteriovenous Malformations: An Iterative Approach Using Angiography, Computed Tomography, and Magnetic Resonance Imaging, *Int. J. Radiation Oncology Biol. Phys.*, **35**(3) 555-564

[3] Guo W, March/April 1998, Application of MR in Stereotactic Radiosurgery, *Journal of Magnetic Resonance Imaging*, **8**(2) 415-420

[4] Ehricke H H, Schad L R, Gademann G, Wowra B, Engenhart R, Lorenz W J, 1992, Use of MR Angiography for Stereotactic Planning, *Journal of Computer Assisted Tomography*, **16**(1) 35-40

[5] Henri C J, Collins D L, Peters T M, Mar/Apr 1991, Multimodality Image Integration for Stereotactic Surgical Planning, *Medical Physics*, **18**(2) 167-177

[6] Peters T M, Henri C J, Munger P, Takahashi A M, Evans A C, Davey B, Olivier A, July/Aug 1994, Integration of Stereoscopic DSA and 3D MRI for Image-Guided Neurosurgery, *Computerized Medical Imaging and Graphics*, **18**(4) 289-299

[7] Siddon R L, Barth N H, Stereotaxic Localization of Intracranial Targets, *Int. J. Radiation Oncology Biol. Phys.*, **13** 1241-1246

[8] Tercier P, Coucke P, Frankhauser H, Mirimanoff R, Uske A, Valley J, 1997, Transfer of information between angiographic films and CT images: a Technique to Control the Drawing of Target Volumes, *Radiotherapy and Oncology*, **45** 263-269

# Computerized Segmentation of Clustered Seeds in Prostate Brachytherapy

**Paul S. Cho**
Department of Radiation Oncology, University of Washington, Seattle, WA 98195-6043, USA

## Introduction

Permanent interstitial implantation of radioactive seeds is widely recognized as a therapeutic option for early-stage prostate carcinoma [1]. One of presently active research areas associated with the procedure is intraoperative dose optimization designed to improve the delivered dose uniformity based on the anatomy under surgical condition [2]. The need for intraoperative optimization arises from the fact that the patient anatomy could change significantly under surgical condition due to positioning, anesthetically induced pelvic muscle relaxation, and swelling of the prostate due to the invasive nature of the procedure. Because of strict time constraint, intraoperative planning and dosimetry would require a computerized approach in image-guided components including prostate volume reconstruction as well as determination of implanted seed coordinates. This paper focuses on the latter aspect. Modality of seed image acquisition is projection x-ray captured with fluroscopy or film. There are three distinct steps in our approach, namely, (i) isolation of seeds from the background, (ii) grouping of segmented pixels into connected components, and (iii) determination of end coordinates of individual seeds. Steps (i) and (ii) have been previously presented [3]; here we will describe step (iii) in detail.

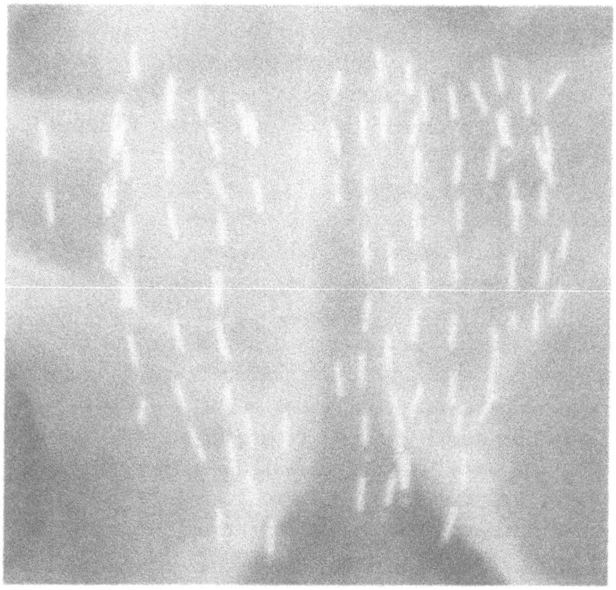

**Figure 1:** An example of implanted I-125 seeds: individually separated or clustered.

## Materials and methods

X-ray images of prostate brachytherapy often contain clusters of superposed seeds. This significantly complicates the task of image segmentation. An example of overlapping I-125 seeds is shown in Figure 1. Note that as many as four seeds are clustered together. Isolation of pixels representing the seeds from the background yields the binary image shown in Figure 2. The connected component analysis of the seed pixels provides geometric information such as area, maximum length, and perimeter. Using these parameters single seeds can readily be identified. Subsequently, the end coordinates of the seed can be estimated by finding the two pixels that are separated by the greatest distance.

When the geometric analysis has determined that connected pixels consist of multiple seeds, further processing is necessary to establish how the individual seeds are oriented. Exploration of overlapping regions based on grayscale value alone is generally not fruitful due to inherently low density resolution in these images. The grayscale information could, however, contribute to decision making process when ambiguity exists.

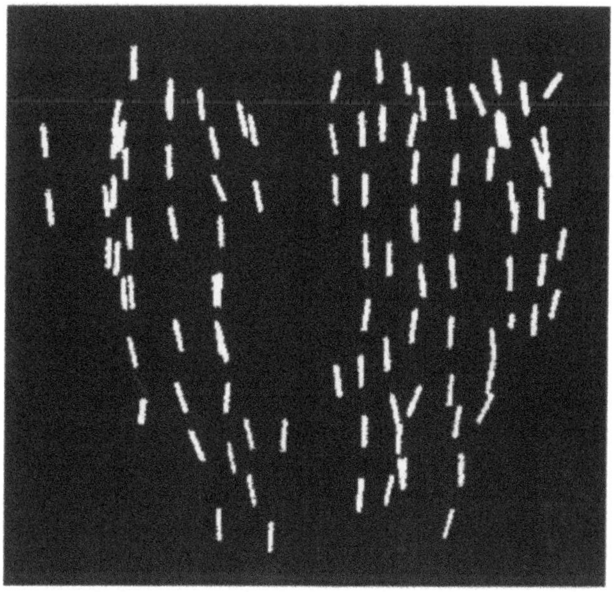

**Figure 2:** Isolation of seed pixels from the background.

Our method follows a morphological approach and seeks

to optimally pack the seed clusters with scalable templates. The templates are represented by a set of pixel coordinates $\{(x_i, y_i), (x_{i+1}, y_{i+1}), ...(x_{i+N}, y_{i+N})\}$ with each element transformable by

$$(x'_i, y'_i) = \left\{ \begin{array}{c} (x_i - x_o)cos\theta + (y_i - y_o)sin\theta, \\ -(x_i - x_o)sin\theta + (y_i - y_o)cos\theta \end{array} \right\} \quad (1)$$

where $i$ is the index corresponding to the standard seed dimensions. Template scaling is performed by incrementing the index at certain intervals. The angle $\theta$ represents the relative angular orientation of the template axis anchored at $(x_o, y_o)$.

By varying these parameters the seed template can be rotated, tranlated, and scaled. A score function representing the goodness of fit can be used to determine the optimal number of seeds and most likely orientation of each within the cluster. Stochastic optimization can be used to accomplish the search. Alternately, with the help of further image processing, the size of the solution space can be reduced so that exhaustive search becomes practical. We begin with an assumption that a cluster vertex corresponds to the long end of the seed. The vertices can then be used to anchor one end of the scalable template.

Identification of vertices is facilitated by morphlogical thinning of the binary image as shown in Figure 3. Subsequently, a connected component analysis is applied to the skeletonized cluster to identify the vertices. However, since the vertices of the medial axes do not necessarily coincide with those of the original due to erosion, the anchor coordinates need to be perturbed slightly. Once a cluster is filled with templates, the result must be examined for reasonableness of seed orientation and overlaps. Presently the notion of reasonableness is determined by simple metrics including the degree of congruence between overlapping seeds and grayscale information. Upon analysis, a template may be rescaled or eliminated. In the event that significant amount of void exists within the cluster, additional templates are spawned.

## Results and discussion

The seed segmentation algorithm was applied to the example I-125 seed image. The results are shown in Figure 4. The solutions are visualized graphically as crosses representing the end coordinates of the individual seeds. All the seeds were identified including those that are super- or juxtaposed. The end coordinates output by the program appears to be quite reasonable.

Input parameters needed to run the program are length and width of a single seed in pixel unit. These dimensions should be constant for given imaging system and geometry. In selecting these values, however, the magnification effects on the seeds located at varying distances from the image receptor must be considered.

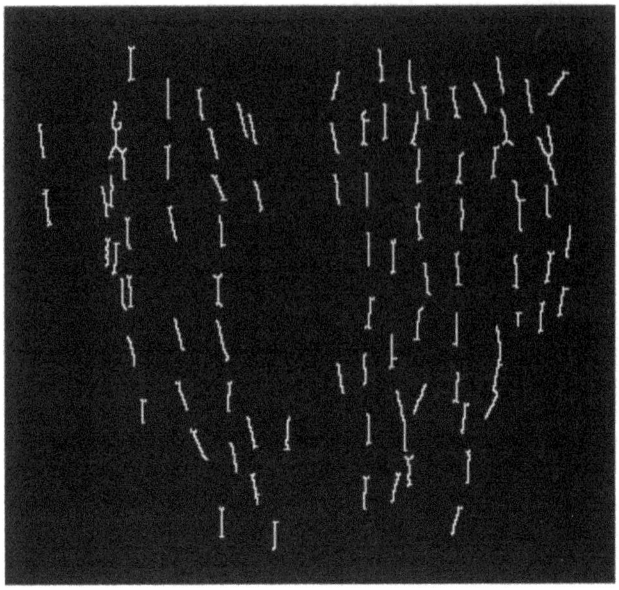

**Figure 3:** Processing by morphological thinning operation.

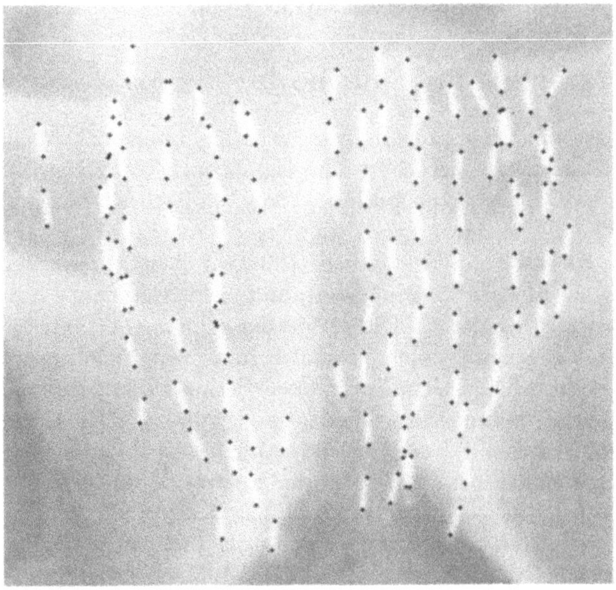

**Figure 4:** Results of seed segmentation. Crosses mark the seed end coordinates.

As an alternative method the idea of time-lapsed sequential imaging has been entertained. By performing the seed implantation in one coronal plane at a time and by imaging progressively, ambiguity due to seed overlaps should be resolved. In practice, however, fluidity of implanted seeds complicates the process, introducing the problem of image misregistration.

Our future work includes extensive testing and refinement of the algorithm using large number of synthetic data sets for which the seed configurations are exactly known. Efforts are also underway to extend the algorithm for Pd-103 seeds which exhibit much less pronounced aspect ratios than the I-125 sources. It is suspected that for highly ambiguous cases, it may be useful to adapt a probabilistic decision making mechanism.

## Conclusions

A computerized method of brachytherapy seed segmentation was presented. The technique utilizes geometric, morphological, and grayscale information as well as scalable template packing and connected component analysis to segment individual seeds. The algorithm's ability to segment both isolated and overlapping seeds was demonstrated using I-125 x-ray images. The proposed method will be useful in real-time intraoperative dosimetry and optimization.

## Acknowledgments

The author is grateful to Brian Adams for help in the early stage of connected component development and to Brett Heintz for providing the test images.

## References

[1] Blasko J C, Ragde H and Schumacher D 1987 Transperineal percutaneous iodine-125 implantation for prostatic carcinoma using transrectal ultrasound and template guidance *Endocurie. Hypertherm. Oncol.* **3** 131–139

[2] Messing E M, Zhang J B, Rubens D J, Brasacchio R A, Strang J G, Soni A, Okunieff P G and Yu Y 1999 Intraoperative optimized inverse planning for prostate brachytherapy: Early experience *Int. J. Radiat. Oncol. Biol. Phys.* **44** 801–808

[3] Cho P and Adams B 1999 Automated seed recognition for intraoperative prostate brachytherapy dosimetry *Med. Phys.* **26** 1146

# A quality control of a virtual simulation system including an inverse DRR software

**Hanna El-Balaa[1], Pascal Grandjean[1], Dimitri Lefkopoulos[1], Fredéric Julia[1], Jean-noël Foulquier[1], Emmanuel Touboul[1]**

[1]Tenon hospital, radiation-oncology department, 4 rue de la Chine, 75020 Paris.

## Introduction

The aim of this work was to define different quality control procedures so as to verify our virtual simulation system (1 Scanner PQ 5000, 2 virtual simulation system AcQSim/Picker). The Fox Chase center has already presented a phantom for the Picker simulation system in [1]. However, this phantom although interesting was considered by our team not sufficient to verify all the aspects of the system. More complete quality controls are presented in [2-4]. In this work, we present a complete procedure with new controls (see table 1) based on a cube phantom.

| Quality Control | Patterns |
|---|---|
| **QA1.** The data transfert between the scan and AcQSim. | Point landmarks. |
| **QA2.** The geometrical validation of the external and internal contours as well as the interpolation and the 2D and 3D margins. | 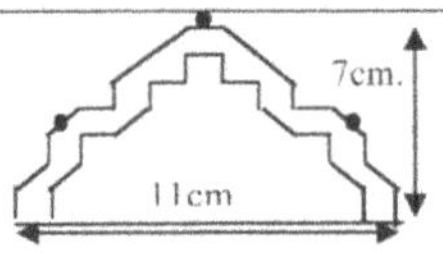 |
| **QA3.** The validation of the positioning of the "marked" and treatment isocenters as a function of the slice width. | Point landmarks. |
| **QA4.** The verification of the beam divergence for the 2 extreme SSD. | 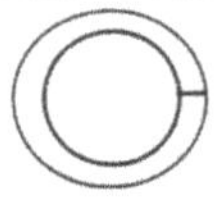 |
| **QA5.** The geometrical verification of the DRR : spatial linearity + field size. | 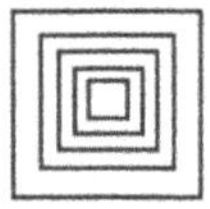 |
| **QA6.** The geometrical verification of the DRR : table + collimator rotations. | 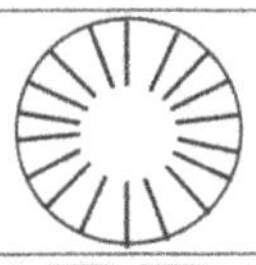 |
| **QA7.** The geometrical verification of the DRR : gantry rotation. | 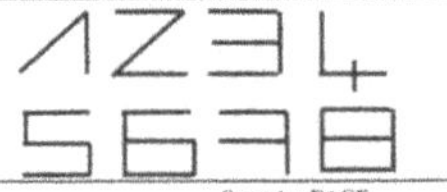 |
| **QA8.** The geometrical verification of the DRR : gantry + table rotations. | 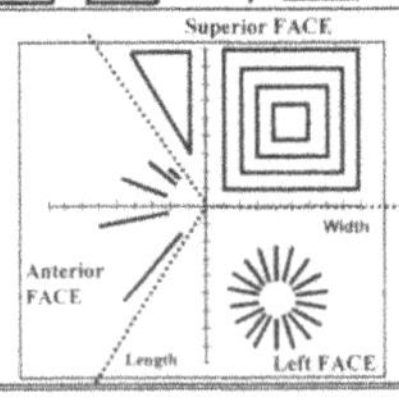 |

**Table 1:** The different patterns for the quality-control of the virtual simulation system.

## Material and methods

**The proposed phantom**

The phantom was a 20 cm plexiglas cube. The faces of the cube are removable and correspond each one of them to a control point. Their dimensions are 20 cm x 20 cm x 0.5 cm (anterior and posterior faces) 20 cm x 19 cm x 0.5 cm (right and left faces) ; 19 cm x 19 cm x 0.5 cm (superior and inferior faces).

The center of the cube is marked using three reference point landmarks positioned on the center of the faces.

Aluminium wires of 2 mm diameter were used to construct different patterns on the faces of the cube.

## Methods

**The data transfert between the scan and AcQSim (QA1)**

Firtsly; we compare the values of the longitudinal position, height of the table and the sagittal laser position corresponding to the three reference point landmarks on the scan and AcQSim. The position of each slice is also verified.

Secondly, we verify that the identification of the patient and the acquisition parameters are correct.

**The geometrical validation of the measuring and contouring tools of AcQSim (QA2)**

*External contours*

We carry out the external contour and verify using the measure tools the right-left and ant-post dimensions of the cube phantom.

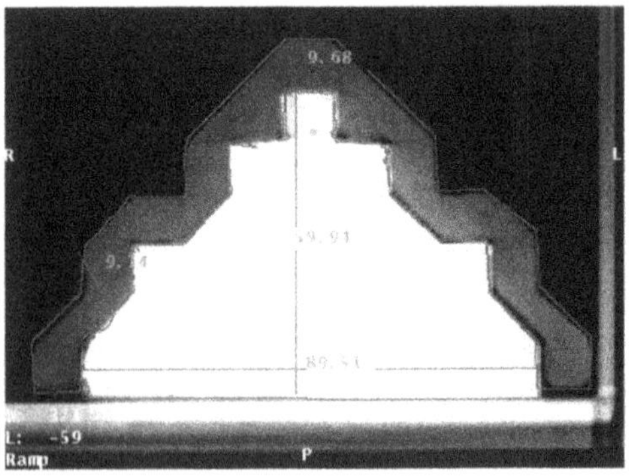

**Figure 1:** Internal contour composed of palavit M (pink) and margins composed of wax (red).

*Internal contours*
Two stairs shaped objects composed respectively of palavit and wax are precisely put inside the cube phantom (see figure 1). We compare the real distance of the these objects with the computed distance by AcQSim after contouring.

*2D, 3D margins*
The wax object represents the margin of 1 cm width in the right-left and sup-inf directions and varying from 1 cm to 7 cm in the ant-post direction.

**The validation of the positioning of the «marked« and treatment isocenters as a function of the slice width (QA3)**

The center of the cube phantom represents the «marked« isocenter and is marked using three coplanar reference point landmarks positioned on the center of the right, left and anterior faces.
The treatment isocenter is put on the center of the palavit volume representing the internal object. Three coplanar point landmarks are put on the wax objet to define this isocenter. Its position relative to the «marked« isocenter is : left = 4 cm, posterior = -6 cm and inferior = 6 cm).
On AcQSim, we marked the «marked« isocenter on the slice containing the three point landmarks. Then, we verify that this isocenter is on the center of the cube using measuring tools. After that, the treatment isocenter is positionned relative to the «marked« isocenter using the real relative deviations. We control that this isocenter is correct with the three treatment point landmarks.

**The verification of the beam divergence for the 2 extreme SSD (QA4)**
We put a circle of 6 cm on the anterior face and two circles of 6.6 and 8 cm on the posterior face of the cube phantom.
On AcQSim, we carry out the external contours so as to compute the SSD and print the DRR for the minimal SSD = 60 cm and the maximal SSD = 200 cm (figure 2).

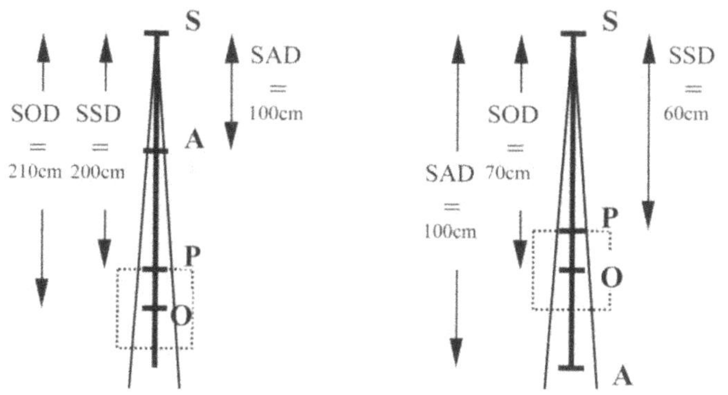


**Figure 2:** Schema of the beam divergence.

**The geometrical verification of the DRR**

*spatial linearity and field size (QA5)*
We construct a set of aluminium squares of different sizes (4, 6, 8, 10 and 14 cm) on the anterior and left faces centered on the center of the face.
On AcQSim, we set the treatment isocenter on the center of the cube.
To verify the spatial linearity, we control on the DRR the correct dimensions of the squares using measuring tools.
To verify the field size for the gantry angle of 0° and 90°, we use the different aluminium squares as a coordinate system. So, we may select in the AcQSim the field size for symmetric and assymmetric anterior and left fields.

*Collimator and table rotations (QA6)*
A star was constructed using wire lines with an angular spacing of 20°. Either we verify the collimator angle with the table angle equal to 0°, either we verify the table angle with the collimator angle to 0°. The beam axis must be superimposed with the correct aluminium line.

**The geometrical verification of the DRR using an original method of DRR phantom conception**
The aim is to choose patterns on the DRR plane easy to recognize, then via a back projection software (termed inverse DRR) to obtain the corresponding patterns on the phantom.

*Gantry rotation (QA7)*
We have designed on the DRR plane different numbers with dimensions 2 cm (right-left) by 4 cm (superior-inferior). Each number corresponded to a gantry angle : 1 to 10°, 2 to 20°, ..., 8 to 80°. Using the inverse DRR software, we have constructed the numbers 1 to 4 on the anterior face and 5 to 8 on the left face of the phantom. So, it was easy to control that the correct number is in the beam limits of 2 by 4 cm following the gantry angle (see figure 3).

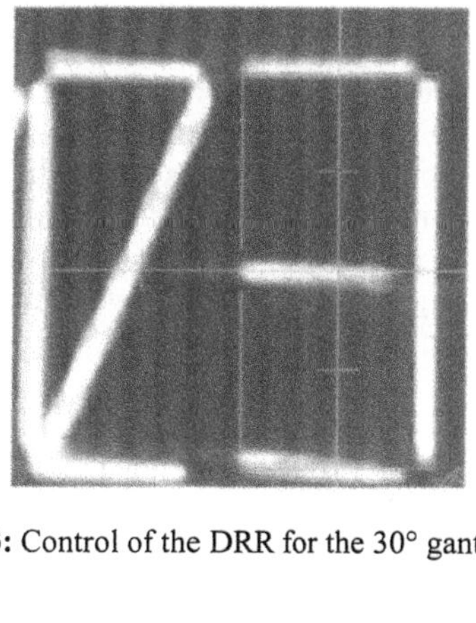

**Figure 3:** Control of the DRR for the 30° gantry angle.

*Non coplanar beams of 3D objects (QA8)*
We have chosen a non coplanar beam incidence of gantry=57.73° and table=45°. So, the beam axis passes from the anterior/left/superior corner through the center of the cube phantom to the posterior/right/inferior corner. The patterns designed on the DRR plane are presented in table 1. This plane is divided into 3 parts (dotted lines), each part corresponds to a face of the cube phantom : anterior, superior and left. In the inverse DRR software, the coordinates ($X_{DRR}$, $Y_{DRR}$) of each point of the patterns are entered and then these points are back

projected on the three faces of the cube. The resulting coordinates of the points are used to construct the aluminium lines on the faces of the cube phantom.
After scanning this cube, we compute the DRR with AcQSim and we compare this DRR with our initial patterns (see figure 4).

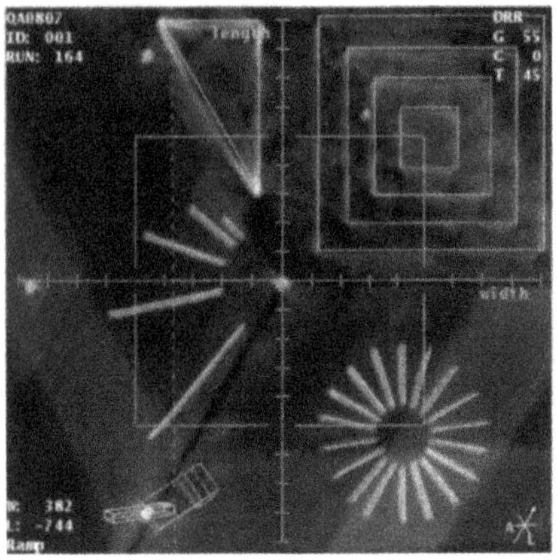

**Figure 4 :**Superpositon of the simple patterns on the DRR.

## Results &Discussion

In the control of the data transfert between the scan and AcQSim (QA1), no error is found.

Concerning the quality control of internal and external contours (QA2), the difference between the dimensions of the palavit M and wax objects are found inferior to 1 mm. The only problem which can be encountered in AcQSim concerns the posting of structures on the DRR when using copy and stretch tools of contours. Surprisingly, the problem doesn't appear in the 3D representation. In this case, it is required to modify the contours on CT slices to render contours more smooth and to eliminate if needed some additionnal contours which are visible only with a large zoom. In our case, we have found the posting of our structure two times larger on the coronal DRR than the real object.

Concerning the quality control of the marked and treatment isocenters (QA3), deviations are found along the head-feet direction. This deviation depends on the slice width, pitch factor and image index. In AcQSim, it is possible to choose either the real position of the isocenter or the position of the nearest slice. This is the second case which is selected due to our treatment planning system allowing only isocenters on CT slices. The deviation of the positionning of the isocenters is found inferior to the half of the slice width.

For the control of the beam divergence (QA4) The SSD of 60 and 200 cm are the limits fixed by AcQSim. We found a good superposition of the anterior and posterior circles for the two SSD.

For the validation of the field dimensions (QA5), the difference between AcQSim and aluminium lines is found inferior or equal to 1 mm. The difference may be explained by the fact that aluminium lines have on the DRR a diameter superior to the real diameter of 2 mm. The linearity is correctly controlled on the DRR images.

Concerning the rotation of the table and the collimator (QA6), the beam axis is correctly superimposed to the star pattern for every tested angles.

We have found a good geometrical reconstruction of the DRR (QA7 and QA8) in AcQSim compared to our back projection software. The minor differences are due to the manual construction and to the used material.

All these tests will be rapidly carried out for each new version of AcQSim.

## References


[1] Lawrence R. Coia, Timothy E. Schultheiss Gerald E. Hanks, 1995 A Pratical to CT Simulation *Madison Wisconsin.*

[2] H. El-Balaa 1998 Contrôle de la qualité d'une configuration intégrée de simulation virtuelle *Mémoire de diplôme d'études d'approfondies, Université de Toulouse III.*

[3] H. El-Balaa, Katia Keraudy, Frédéric Julia, Jean-Noël Foulquier and Dimitri Lefkopoulos 1999 Quality assurance protocol of an integrated virtual simulation system *5th Biennial ESTRO Meeting on physics for Clinical Radiotherapy ; Göttingen, Germany 6-11 April 1999 ; Radiotherapy Oncology* **51 suppl. 1** S12,.

[4] P. Grandjean, Dimitri Lefkopoulos, Hanna El-Balaa, Jean-Noël Foulquier, Katia Keraudy and Frédéric Julia 1999 Conception of an inverse digital reconstruted radiograph phantom *5th Biennial ESTRO Meeting on physics for Clinical Radiotherapy ; Göttingen, Germany 6-11 April 1999 ; Radiotherapy Oncology* **51 suppl. 1** S12 ,.

# Image fusion using mediated data displays

**A.N.T.J. Kotte and J.J.W. Lagendijk**
Dept. Radiotherapy UMC Utrecht, Heidelberglaan 100, 3584 CX Utrecht
kotte@radth.med.uu.nl

## Introduction

Treatment planning for radiotherapy is usually based on a single CT dataset. Diagnostic modalities such as MRI, CT, PET and SPECT, offer information, not found in the treatment planning CT data sets. Even different CT data sets (pre- and post-operative) complement each other. In the delineation process all the available information should be presented to the clinician in order to obtain optimal results.

The first step towards the combination of several image data sets is the registration. This procedure is often followed by the resampling of one or more data sets introducing resampling artifacts.

We have developed a flexible system which is capable of offering the use of data obtained from any number of imaging modalities without the resampling artifacts. Every data set is displayed using its own coordinate system in order to appreciate the special conditions used at acquisition time.

## Material and methods

Our system is build with two main modules: a data viewer and a mediator which acts as a communication channel between different viewers.

### Data viewer

Every data set is loaded in a single data viewer having its own coordinate system. Within this coordinate system every voxel centre has a unique position. The viewer presents three orthogonal slices through the volume, all having a single selected point in common. The user can change the selected point causing the three data slices to be updated. In Figure 2 the data display of two viewers is shown.

Within this viewer also a Volume Of Interest (VOI) can be displayed. The VOI is a geometrical three dimensional object, consisting of a collection of inter-connected three dimensional points. The simplest of such a geometry is a convex hull surrounding all the obtained points. All the points are defined in the global coordinate system of the viewer whereby the VOI is positioned relative to all the voxels constituting the displayed data set. The intersection of this VOI with the data slices is depicted in the three data slices and the addition of points to the VOI is allowed. Our software offers the possibility to import the patient data (anatomy and delineated regions) from the PLATO treatment planning system.

The delineation process in such a viewer is fundamentally different from the one presented by the PLATO environment. In our system arbitrary points can be added to the VOI while the PLATO system only supports the addition of points to a single contour, located in a single CT slice.

### Mediator

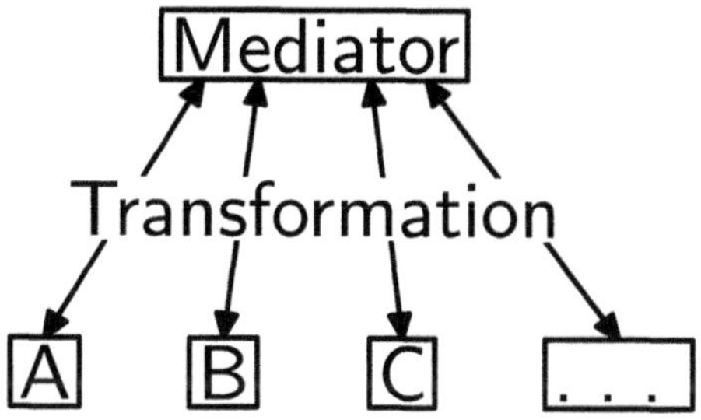


**Figure 1:** Component setup; each viewer has its own associated transformation

Single viewers can contact the mediator process. A state change in one of the connected viewers is forwarded to all the other connected viewers. Different state changes are supported:

- Generation of a new selected point
- Addition or removal of a new VOI
- Addition or removal of a new point to the selected VOI

Within each viewer, the user can select which state changes must be sent to or received from the mediator.

This setup allows any number of viewers to be synchronised, given the condition that the same coordinate system is used in all the viewers. Usually this single common coordinate system will not exist. To circumvent this problem a transformation can be applied by the viewer on the points communicated with the mediator process. The simplest transformation is given by a $3 \times 4$ matrix (the fourth column is needed to incorporate translations). Such a transformation can be defined interactively. More complex transformations could be obtained from a separate registration process and handled as a black box in our software.

## Results and discussion

We have build a system which can be used to delineate in a truly three dimensional fashion. In Figure 2 we can see the artifacts which can occur when the delineation process

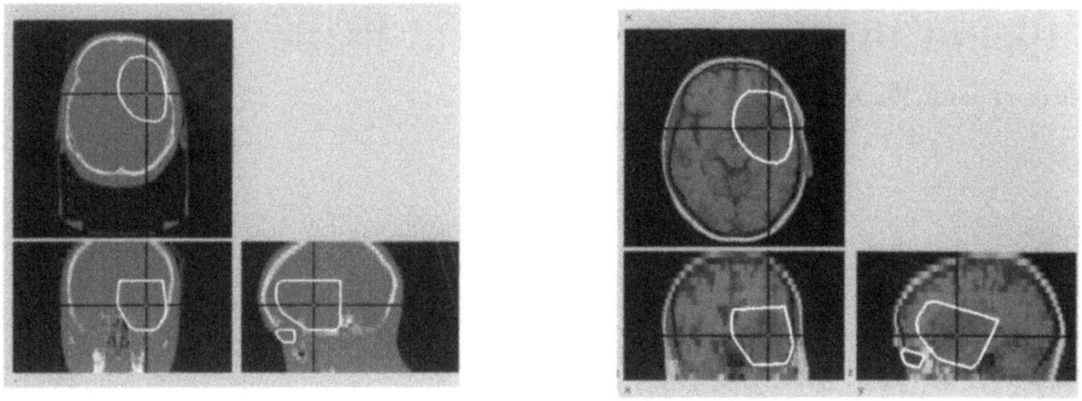

**Figure 2:** Example of the three slices presented to the user. Two VOI's are present. On the left a planning CT image is depicted while on the right an MR image of the same patient is shown

is done slice by slice only based on the planning CT: the eye contour looks very flat at the top as does the target volume. At the moment we only support convex hulls as the type of three dimensional point sets. We are working on the handling of concave hulls.

Convex hulls have the advantage of being defined solely by a set of points while a concave hull is dependent on the order of the points. When the user should be allowed to add and delete arbitrary points to and from the hull the unique reconstruction of the VOI from the point set is no longer trivial[1].

Data can be imported from the PLATO treatment planning environment: all VOI's, defined as contours in different slices, are transformed into our three dimensional format. Volumes of interest created using our system can be exported to the the PLATO environment by calculating the cross-section of the VOI representing hull with all the slices present in the planning CT.

## Conclusion

Without the support of concave hulls, the presented system is useful to correlate the patient anatomy, obtained from CT, to another data set of the same patient region, e.g. the calculated dose distribution.

Once the concave hulls are supported, the presented software system can be used to present all the available data to the clinician in order to aid the delineation process.

## References

[1] Veltkamp R.C. 1999 Closed object boundaries from scattered points *Ph.D. thesis, Erasmus University Rotterdam*

# A new approach for improved tumor volumetry

**Andreas Mahr[1], Malte Bahner[2], Sabine Levegrün[1] and Wolfgang Schlegel[1]**

[1]Department of Medical Physics, Deutsches Krebsforschungszentrum, INF 280, 69120 Heidelberg, Germany
[2]Department of Oncological Diagnostics and Therapy, Deutsches Krebsforschungszentrum, INF 280, 69120 Heidelberg, Germany

## Introduction

The tumor volume is an important parameter in the process of tumor diagnostics and therapy. In the ICRU 50 Report [1] the gross tumor volume (GTV) is defined as the visible or palpable volume of a tumor. In practice the GTV is calculated from the delineated tumor contours in CT or MRT image data sets. We showed in a previous study [2] that there are semiautomatic segmentation algorithms, which provide an acceptable accuracy for the determination of tumor volumes. The process of delineation incorporates several error sources, which prevent the exact calculation of the GTV. On the one hand, the result of a tumor volumetry is dependent on the user, who carries out the delineation of the tumor. On the other hand there are several quality factors of the image data (like image noise or tumor contrast), which influence the accuracy of the determination process. The neglect of this error can lead to misinterpretation and decisions based on wrong information. Since the error of the determination cannot be avoided, we developed a new approach to determine the accuracy of a tumor volumetry dependent on different influencing parameters.

## Material and methods

Our approach to describe the error of the volume determination process distinguishes two different variability factors by their origin:

- an user independent factor
- an user dependent factor

The user independent factor includes influencing factors of the object, the imaging modality, the image processing and the segmentation algorithm itself.
The user dependent factor reflects the variability of the segmentation results of a particular user. This variability is caused by different levels of proficiency as well as changes in the day-to-day performance of every user.

### Considered parameters

The first version of our system is designed to handle spiral CT data sets of the liver. This restriction allowed us for this first study to consider most of the imaging parameters as fixed values. As a conclusion of [1] we chose a region-growing algorithm as preferred method for tumor delineation.

The following parameters were considered to have substantial influence on the accuracy of the volume determination:

- tumor size
- contrast of the tumor in the CT data sets
- image noise
- intra-personal variability of the user

### User independent variability

To determine the influence of different object or imaging parameters, we developed a new CT phantom (see figure 1). The phantom consists of a hollow tube with 7 spheres installed into the tube. The size of the spheres ranged from 1 to 6 cm in diameter (volume: 0,52 ml to 113,1 ml). Varying contrast levels (10, 15 and 30 HU) were simulated by filling the tube with different dilutions of oral contrast medium. Varying noise levels were simulated by variation of the tube current (200 mA, 240 mA and 280 mA).

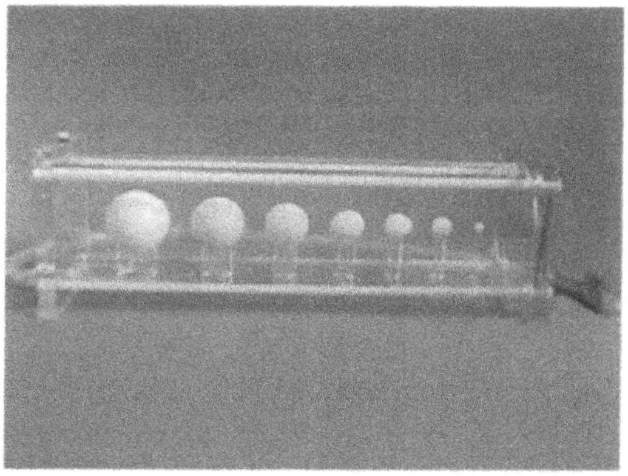

**Figure 1:** CT-Phantom

The acquired CT datasets (CT parameters: Siemens Somatom Plus 4, spiral mode, field-of-view 300x300 mm, pitch 1.5, filter AB50, tube voltage 120 kV, slice thickness 5 mm, interpolation SLIM2, z-axis increment 5 mm) were delineated using a region-growing algorithm. The different contrast and noise levels of the data sets are demonstrated in figures 2 and 3. To eliminate the user-influence on the segmentation results, the segmentation was repeated ten times and a mean value of the determined volume was calculated.

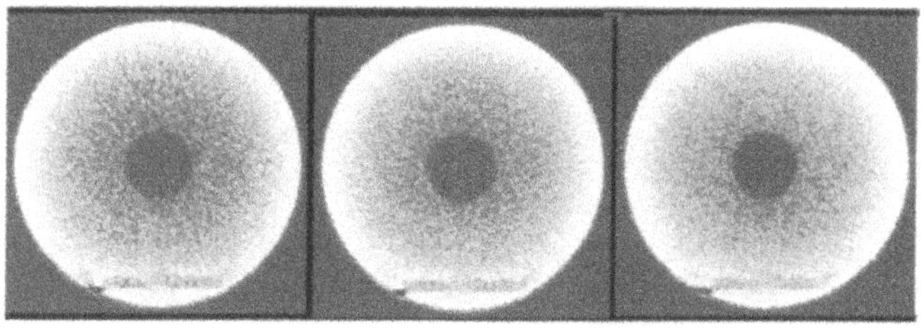

**Figure 2:** CT-images of the phantom with different noise-levels (from left to right: 200 mA, 240 mA, 280 mA tube current; pictures have been equalized for print)

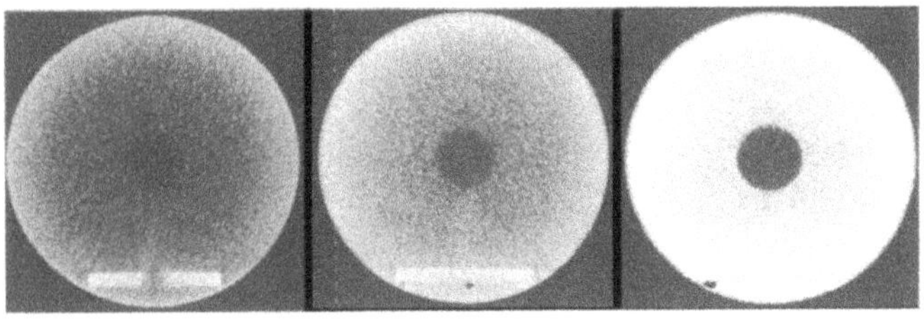

**Figure 3:** CT-images of the phantom with different contrast media (contrast from left to right: ~10 HU, ~15 HU, ~30 HU; pictures have been equalized for print)

Then the percental differences of the delineated volumes to the real volumes were calculated for each data set. Statistical tests (U-Test for different contrast and noise levels and Signed-Rank-Test for different volumes) were carried out to prove that there are significant differences in the accuracy of the volume determination.

We found significant results for different contrast levels and different sphere volumes. No significant result could be produced between the data sets with different noise levels. Therefore, the noise level was excluded as relevant parameter in the further considerations.

The model of user independent variability was then generated using a $\chi^2$–fit. Basic presumptions for the development of the model were the following dependencies:

- decrease in tumor size will lead to an increase of the error of the tumor volume determination
- decrease of the contrast level will lead to an increase of the error of the tumor volume determination.

With our data we found that the function

$$\sigma_i = \frac{2{,}9563}{contrast^2} + \frac{2{,}0704}{(delineated\ tumor\ volume)^2} + 0{,}0038 \quad (1)$$

best describes the dependence of the accuracy of the volume determination (see figure 4).

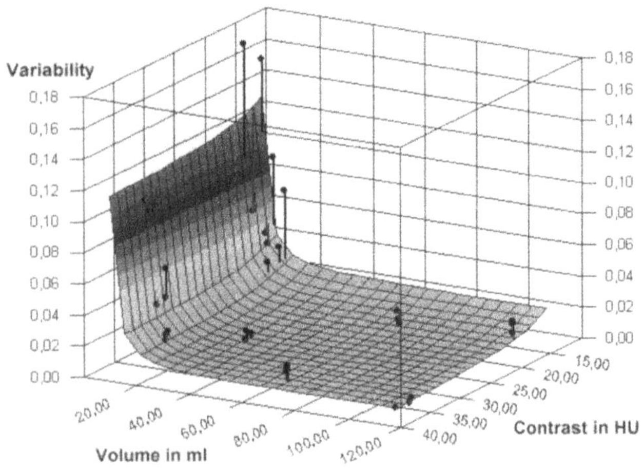


**Figure 4:** Fitted volumetry error function

### User dependent variability

For the determination of the user variability $\sigma_u$, we included a module for regular testing of the user performance. Every month each user has to delineate three typical clinical data sets (currently we are using two datasets with metastases with different sizes and one with a liver cyst). The results of these data sets are stored separately for every user. The user variability is calculated as standard variation of the previous segmentations. To consider a possible learning curve of the user over time, a maximum of twelve data sets is used to calculate the user variability.

## Results

### The new volumetry system: SaVT (*S*egmentation *a*nd *V*olumetry *T*ool)

The model of volume determination errors, which are dependent of the depicted parameters in this abstract, has led to the development of a new computer system for delineation and volume determination of tumors.

Using this new system, each user has to log in into a separate account. Then the user dependent variability factors are calculated using past result from the test data sets. After a successful delineation, the user independent error is estimated using the delineated volume and the contrast of the tumor as input factors for equation (1). The contrast of the tumor is determined as difference of the mean HU in the delineated tumor and the mean HU in a user defined reference region in the surrounding tissue. The estimation of the overall error is then displayed in the system as additional information to the determined tumor volume.

### Testing of the system

The delineations of our segmentation algorithm study [2] have been taken to check the plausibility of the error estimation function. In this study we delineated objects implanted into a bovine liver. Thus, the delineated volumes of our region-growing algorithm and the real volumes measured by water displacement were known. As shown in table 1, the error estimation in all cases enclosed the real volume of the objects, which means the system provided plausible results.

| object | con-trast | $\sigma_i$ | $\sigma_u$ | $\sigma_{overall}$ | $v_d \pm \sigma_{overall} * v_d$ | $v_{wd}$ |
|---|---|---|---|---|---|---|
| 1 | 43 | 0,0285 | 0,0213 | 0,0356 | 11,41±0,41 | 11,5 |
| 2 | 19 | 0,0285 | 0,0134 | 0,0315 | 37,74±1,19 | 38 |
| 3 | 10 | 0,0285 | 0,3091 | 0,3104 | 2,74±0,85 | 2,5 |
| 4 | 43 | 0,0285 | 0,0221 | 0,0361 | 11,12±0,40 | 11,5 |
| 5 | 19 | 0,0285 | 0,0135 | 0,0315 | 37,34±1,18 | 38 |

($\sigma_i$=user independent variability; $\sigma_u$=user variability; $\sigma_{overall}$=overall variability; $v_d$=delineated Volume; $v_{wd}$= volume measured by water displacement)

**Table 1:** Results of the plausibility test

We also tested the system with two clinicians and four medical data sets: one liver metastasis, one liver cyst and one metastasis before and after radiotherapy have been delineated with the new system.

The delineation of the metastasis (see table 2) shows results that differ significantly for the two users. Thus, the system could not compensate for the inter-personal variability. A correction of one of the delineations would be advised in this case.

| user | contrast in HU | $\sigma_i$ | $\sigma_u$ | $v_d \pm \sigma_{overall}$* $v_d$ |
|---|---|---|---|---|
| 1 | 67 | 0,0096 | 0,0209 | 20,09 ± 0,46 |
| 2 | 68 | 0,0102 | 0,0337 | 18,89 ± 0,67 |

($\sigma_i$=user independent variability; $\sigma_u$=user variability; $\sigma_{overall}$=overall variability; $v_d$=delineated Volume)

**Table 2:** volumetry of a liver metastasis

In the second case, the liver cyst, the results show a common range of possible volumes. The volume of the cyst is much smaller than the volume of the metastasis shown above. Therefore there is an increase in the variability of the result. The physicians can now decide, whether the result is accurate enough to use the volume information for further considerations.

| user | contrast in HU | $\sigma_I$ | $\sigma_u$ | $v_d \pm \sigma_{overall}$* $v_d$ |
|---|---|---|---|---|
| 1 | 72 | 0,0437 | 0,0209 | 7,25 ± 0,35 |
| 2 | 76 | 0,0405 | 0,0337 | 7,56 ± 0,40 |

($\sigma_i$=user independent variability; $\sigma_u$=user variability; $\sigma_{overall}$=overall variability; $v_d$=delineated Volume)

**Table 3:** volumetry of a liver cyst

In the last example, a very small metastasis has been picked to demonstrate that volume information cannot always be used to draw the right conclusions. Both physicians agree on the volume before therapy. After therapy, one physician determines a increase in volume by 16%. The other physician determines a tumor remission of almost 10%. Only with the additional information of the new volumetry system a more detailed statement can be made. The huge error estimation is mainly due to the small volume of the metastasis. Therefore a usage of the volume information for therapy monitoring is not advised in this case.

| user | contrast in HU | $\sigma_i$ | $\sigma_u$ | $v_d \pm \sigma_{overall}$* $v_d$ |
|---|---|---|---|---|
| 1, before therapy | 33 | 1,4958 | 0,0209 | 1,18 ± 1,77 |
| 1, after therapy | 57 | 1,1031 | 0,0209 | 1,37 ± 1,51 |
| 2, before therapy | 41 | 1,4925 | 0,0337 | 1,18 ± 1,76 |
| 2, after therapy | 66 | 1,8128 | 0,0337 | 1,07 ± 1,94 |

($\sigma_i$=user independent variability; $\sigma_u$=user variability; $\sigma_{overall}$=overall variability; $v_d$=delineated Volume)

**Table 4:** volumetry of a liver metastasis before and after radiotherapy (different contrast levels in identical data sets is caused by the user based determination of the contrast)

## Conclusion

Our new volumetry system can so far be used for liver tumor volumetry based on spiral CT data sets. The calculation of the error incorporated in a certain volume determination is a necessary improvement of current volumetry system, because:

- The assessment of the error of the calculated volume leads to a more conscious use of the given information.
- Decisions based on volume information can be made with a higher statistical certainty.
- Especially during therapy monitoring, the error information can be used to distinguish significant tumor remission from possible tumor stagnation.

## References


[1] International Commission on Radiation Units and Measurements, 1992, Prescribing, Recording, and Reporting Photon Beam Therapy, *ICRU Report* **50** 3-7

[2] Mahr A, Levegrün S, Bahner M L, Kress J, Zuna I and Schlegel W, 1999, Usability of Semiautomatic Algorithms for Tumor Volume Determination, *Investigative Radiology* **34** 143-150

[3] Elliot P.J. et al 1994 Covira Pilot System For Radiotherapy Planning, In: Covira: Computer Vision in Radiology, *The European Commission DG XIII, AIM Project A2003, Deliverable* **D5/2.5** 3-42

# Digital data exchange for multi-institutional clinical trials in 3D conformal radiation therapy and prostate brachytherapy

**John W. Matthews, William B. Harms, Sr., Walter R. Bosch, and James A. Purdy**

3D Quality Assurance Center, Mallinckrodt Institute of Radiology, Washington University School of Medicine, St. Louis, MO, 63110, USA

## Introduction

The 3D Quality Assurance (3DQA) Center was established at the Washington University School of Medicine in 1992 to provide quality control for multi-institutional 3D conformal radiation therapy (3DCRT) clinical trials being developed by the Radiation Therapy Oncology Group (RTOG). One of the challenges this presented was how to acquire the patient image, geometric, and dosimetric data 3DCRT protocols generated. At the previous ICCR meeting we presented a standard for the submission of digital data to the 3DQA Center for review [1]. We now present changes to the standard since the previous presentation and discuss the 3DQA Center's plan for migrating to the use of DICOM 3.0, which now includes RT objects, for digital data submission. More information can be obtained from our prior presentation [1] or from the 3DQA Center's web page [2]. Briefly, a data exchange submission consists of a set of files. The first file in the file set is a "directory file" describing all of the other "data files". The directory file consists of keyword and keyvalue pairs describing the data files contained in the submission.

## Material and methods

### Description of data submission

Figure 1 shows a block diagram of the process of preparing a submission of a protocol data set to the RTOG 3DQA Center. The first step is to obtain from the user (typically a dosimetrist or physicist) a specification of all the data to be included in the submission. We recognize that electronic data submission is laborious in the current implementation on most image-based planning systems. Continued work in the area of data exchange by the treatment planning system manufacturers is needed, and users are encouraged to contact the manufacturer of their treatment planning system and request improved system features that will simplify the data submission process. For example, a utility such as the graphical user interface (GUI) shown in Figure 2 that was designed and implemented by 3DQA Center staff could be provided that would allow the user to pre-select the data required for submission specific to the 3DCRT protocol. This utility would in turn create a button (or at most only a few buttons) on a GUI for submitting data.

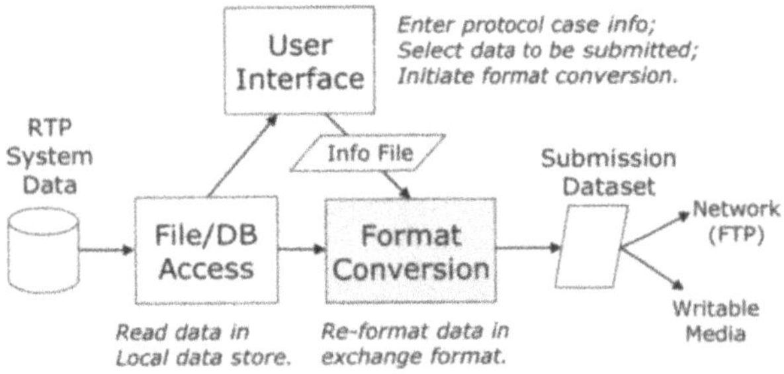


**Figure 1:** Block Diagram of Data Submission.

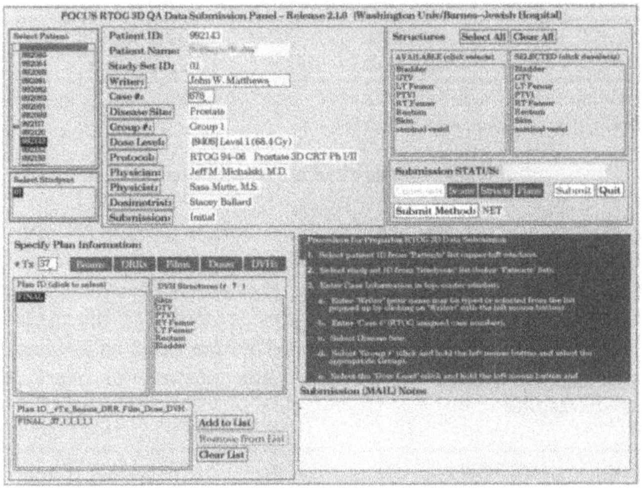

**Figure 2:** An example of the Graphical User Interface (GUI) used to aid correct and easy data submission.

When clicked on, the protocol data would automatically be selected and sent to the 3DQA Center. All of the additional edit features shown in our prototype GUI would be used only for exceptional submissions such as those correcting contour or planning problems in earlier submissions for the same patient in order to reduce the amount of data requiring resubmission. Currently, the GUI requires a dosimetrist to first select a patient ID and study-set. The interface then shows the data available for the selected patient study-set including CT scans, anatomical structures and treatment target volumes, and therapy plans. The individual submitting the data must input the RTOG case number, therapy protocol and stratification group number, treatment site, dose level, and physician, physicist, and dosimetrist involved with the protocol case. For therapy plans selected for submission, the GUI requires further selection of plan data to be submitted including beam or seed geometry, dose distributions, Digital Reconstructed Radiographs (DRRs), plan verification films, and DVHs. Clearly, new features are needed on treatment planning systems that make the submission process easier and also help in enforcing complete and correct protocol submission.

Under the current system, when the user is finished selecting data to be submitted, a button on the GUI initiates the submission process. The first step in this process is the generation of an "info" file . The info file is a short text file that specifies all the data that will be submitted; the info file is read by low level software that can access the treatment planning data of the treatment planning system and convert the appropriate data into the RTOG data exchange format files. Once converted the data are either written to a magnetic tape that is sent to the RTOG 3D QA Center, or more typically sent directly to the QA Center via the FTP protocol over the internet. The info file format has been augmented to include Brachytherapy Seed plan data objects as well as Ultrasound images. The format of the info file is shown in Figure 3.

### Data processing statistics

As of 10 December 1999, the 3DQA Center has processed 918 patient 3DCRT data sets. The processed data occupies 60 Gigabytes of storage. The network submission of data requires from a few minutes to about one hour depending on network performance for a given connection (depends both on peak bandwidth of the path and network traffic). Processing of a case at the 3DQA Center takes about two hours for a "clean case", i.e., all data are correctly submitted and the protocol is correctly followed. If there are errors, the case is scored but then corrections are made before the data are entered in the database [3]; this typically may take several days.

```
***************************************************************************
RTOG Case Number
Institution
Writer
Patient ID
Patient Name
Studyset ID
Site of Interest (Optional keyword for CT)
Number of Comment files
{Names of Comment files; one per line}
Number of CT files
{Names of CT files; one file name per line in descending order}
Number of MR files
{Names of MR files; one file name per line in descending order}
Number of US files
{Names of US files; one file name per line in descending order}
Number of anatomical/target structures
{Names of structures, one name per line}
Number of orphan films
{Name of orphan film file}
{Description of orphan film}
{repeat for each orphan film; two lines per film}
Number of Teletherapy plans
{Plan ID for 1st Teletherapy plan}
{Number of treatments for fraction group}
{Beam Geometry Flag}
{DRR Flag}
{Dose Flag}
{Number of beam "films"}
{File name of image}
{Beam number this image corresponds to}
{Beam description}
{repeat for each film; three lines per film}
{DVH File Name}
{repeat for each Teletherapy plan}
Number of Brachytherapy Seed plans
{Plan ID for 1st Brachytherapy Seed plan}
{Seed Geometry Flag}
{Dose Flag}
{DVH File Name}
{repeat for each Brachytherapy Seed plan}

{} indicates lines that appear only as necessary
```

**Figure 3:** Description of the "info" file which controls the generation of Data Exchange submission.

## Results and discussion

### Data processing for case submission

If the "Format Conversion" process in Figure 1 is structured properly, then the job of migrating to DICOM for data exchange can be more easily accomplished. The collection of data from the local RTP system is inherently vendor specific; while the reformatting of data into data exchange specified format is vendor independent. Segregating the code as much as possible gives two advantages: 1) writing RTOG data exchange format files is RTP system independent and can be reused by multiple vendors; 2) the output portion of the process could be rewritten to implement DICOM while preserving the data collection portions of the code. Example "C" code which indicates the requirements for RTP system data collection and implements output of the RTOG data exchange format is posted on the 3DQA Center web page [2].

### Data processing for permanent prostate implants

The RTOG 3DQA Center is currently adding the capability of supporting protocols for Transperineal Interstitial Permanent Prostate Brachytherapy (TIPPB). The additional data types needed to support these protocols are: ultrasound (US) images, MR images, and brachytherapy seed plans. US images and MR images data exchange issues are very similar to those posed by the already implemented CT image data exchange and thus will not be described here. The "Seed Plan" data type adds the following directory keywords: SEED MODEL, ISOTOPE, SEED STRENGTH, STRENGTH UNITS, DATE OF IMPLANT, and NUMBER OF SEEDS. The data file for "Seed Plan" consists of the spatial coordinates of the seeds. The RTOG 3DQA Center is now able to read TIPPB plans and we expect that multi-institutional protocol(s) will be developed shortly.

### Date exchange workshops

The 3DQA Center has held two workshops on the implementation of RTOG data exchange. The first workshop was held in March 1995 and was intended primarily for the original nine members of the RTOG 94-06 prostate dose escalation protocol. However the workshop was attended by the following RTP system vendors: ADAC, CMS, PTI, and Rahd. The second workshop was held in September 1999 and was attended by the following RTP system vendors: CMS, Elekta/PTI, Prowess/SSGI, and Varian/MMS. At the second workshop the RTOG data exchange specification including TIPPB objects (version 4.00) was finalized and the participants also discussed the future use of DICOM for data submission.

### DICOM for data submission

The 3DQA Center is committed to implementing the ability to receive DICOM data submissions within the next year. DICOM 3.0 now includes RT objects: RT image, RT dose, RT structure set, RT plan, RT beams treatment record, RT brachy treatment record, and RT treatment summary record. The usefulness of DICOM for submission of protocol data, however, depends on the extent to which RTP system manufacturers implement DICOM export mechanisms for all of the data objects needed for a complete protocol submission.

The first step for the 3DQA Center is to provide an Application Profile for DICOM data submission. A DICOM Application Profile defines a selection of choices at the various layers of the DICOM standard which are applicable to a specific need or context in which the standard is intended to be used. For the submission of data to the 3DQA Center, this profile indicates

- which DICOM information objects and associated service-object pair (SOP) classes will be used for protocol submissions and which are optional;
- the selection of a specific Media Format definition (from DICOM Part 12) including the selected Physical Medium, a specific associated Media Format and the mapping of this Media Format (or file system) services onto the DICOM File Service;
- the selection of appropriate Transfer Syntaxes; and
- other choices facilitating interoperability such as specific limits ( e.g., maximum file sizes, if necessary, support of options, if any).

One model for conversion to a DICOM based submission process makes use of DICOM Part 10 file-set specification. In a manner similar to the RTOG data exchange, DICOM information objects are encoded as files on physical media (disk or tape) with a DICOMDIR directory file describing the contents of the file-set. The recordable compact disc (CDR) is an attractive physical medium for protocol data submissions. A DICOM media storage model already exists for CDR using the ISO 9660 file system. This medium is inexpensive, small, and fairly rugged; its capacity (approximately 700 megabytes) is sufficient for the foreseeable future in terms of the data required for a single case. A CDR disk can be shipped to the 3DQA Center by mail or overnight delivery and the CDR itself serves as an archive of the submitted data (submitted data are currently archived to magneto-optic disks).

In addition to submission of DICOM Part 10 files using physical media, these file-sets can be transferred to the 3DQA Center over the Internet using FTP. While this method of exchange is not specified by the DICOM standard, binary-mode FTP transfers of properly encoded DICOM file-sets would work.

## Conclusion

The RTOG data exchange specification has been extended to include support for TIPPB protocols. However, the RTOG data exchange specification is clearly an interim standard. It is understood that it has a limited lifetime. This standard will ultimately be replaced by the RT information objects of DICOM 3.0 which themselves were motivated in part by this interim standard. However, this replacement must await the implementation of the RT information objects and their support by both commercial 3-D treatment planning companies and the 3DQA Center. The uncertainty of a time frame for broad acceptance and implementation of the DICOM RT objects (and because of the wider commercial implementation of the RTOG data exchange specification) suggests that it will continue to play an important role in support of 3DCRT multi-institutional trials for several more years.

## References

[1] Harms, W B, Bosch, W R, and Purdy J A 1997 An interim digital data exchange standard for multi-institutional 3D conformal radiation therapy trials *XII international conference on the use of computers in radiation therapy*, D D Leavitt and G Starkschall eds. 465-468

[2] http://rtog3dqa.wustl.edu

[3] Bosch W R, Lakanen T L, Kahn M G, Harms W B, and Purdy J A 1997 An image/clinical database for multi-institutional clinical trials in 3D conformal radiation therapy *XII international conference on the use of computers in radiation therapy*, D D Leavitt and G Starkschall eds. 455-457

## Acknowledgments

This work supported in part by NIH Grants 1 U22 CA81647 and CA60267 and DOD Medical Research Grant DAMD 17-98-1-8573

# The creation of a radiotherapy archive using Internet technology

**Oana Petrascu, Arjan Bel [*], Dirk Verellen and Guy Storme**

Department of Radiotherapy, AZ-VUB, Brussels, Belgium [*]currently at Nucletron, Veenendaal, The Netherlands

## Introduction

The electronic patient dataflow in a radiotherapy department is quite complicated. The main purpose of the computer network within the radiotherapy department is the sharing of computing resources and information (e.g. CT images, electronic portal images, isodose maps etc.). The Intranet is also used to facilitate working in groups (e.g. staff meetings). It uses TCP/IP, HTTP, and other Internet protocols and in general looks like a private version of the Internet.
The purpose of this study was to create an easily accessible radiotherapy archive using Internet technology.

## Material and methods

The computer network in our department consists of several UNIX workstations on which the GRATIS free-ware treatment planning system (TPS) is running. They are connected to several dedicated workstations with specific operating systems running commercial planning systems (Plato 14.0 for brachytherapy - IRIX, Peacock 1.12/ Corvus 3.0 for IMRT - Next/UNIX and Brainscan for radiosurgery - Windows NT), an Elekta SLS 25 simulator with CT option (sim-CT) and two electronic portal-imaging devices (EPID).
Our radiotherapy department has an electronic connection with the hospital information system used for receiving personal data about the patients to be treated. For the majority of patients the treatment is simulated first. During the simulation a pre-treatment planning is done in which the preliminary number of monitor units is calculated based on first principles. A final treatment plan is then made with the GRATIS-TPS, using either sim-CT or conventional CT-data. The CT images and the MR images (used for stereotactic or IMRT treatment planning) are received via a DICOM-3 connection from the radiology department.
Electronic links are connecting the UNIX workstations with the linear accelerators. This connection is used to export planning data such as the leaves' position of the multi-leaf collimator.
For most of the patients the EPID is used to check the treatment set-up before the dose delivery. Portal images can be made available in the network by exporting them via a DICOM connection.
At each step of the procedure information in different file formats is stored in a file-based database. Once a new patient is created in the treatment planning system the archive is updated automatically. The CT images are kept in the patient directory. Digital simulator images and the output of the pre-treatment planning made during the simulation are saved. General patient information such as name and identification is also stored on the hard disk together with treatment planning specific data. Isodose plots, dose volume histograms, output of the treatment plans (beam set-up and monitor units), digitally reconstructed radiographs etc. are directly accessible in electronic format due to the open architecture of the free-ware treatment planning system. The capacity of the disk space (32 GB) allows keeping patient information on-line for a long period of time (up to 2 years currently).

On the server workstation an Apache (Version1.3) server is running. Apache complies with the newest level of the Hypertext Transport Protocol, HTTP.
The users can access the database via conventional Web-browsers such as Netscape Navigator or Microsoft Explorer.
The common gateway interface (CGI) provides a consistent way to pass data back and forth between the Web server and the application program. When the user makes a request by clicking on a specific item (for example the isodose plots for a patient in the list), the server activates a CGI application to search in the database. The information is send back the to the server where another CGI application converts it to a Web page. The access to the information is restricted with a password so that security is maintained.

## Results and discussion

The archive is in use for three months. Initial results show an overall improvement of efficiency. The archive proves to be very useful in the daily staff meetings, as well as in the follow-up of the patients. It facilitates the quality assurance and quality control of different procedures encountered in daily practice of radiotherapy.
The archive is easy to use and easy to extend due to its modularity. Moreover, the access to the archive is platform independent therefore suitable to the diversity of operating systems existent in our department.
Future plans include the integration of the radiotherapy data into the hospital database.

## Conclusion

The digital archive provides multimedia reporting and increases the availability of the patient information specific for the radiotherapy department (simulation, planning and portal imaging data). The implementation was inexpensive since all software was in-house developed with free-ware tools.

# Questions for comparison of clinical Monte Carlo codes

**D.W.O. Rogers[1] and Radhe Mohan[2]**

[1]National Research Council of Canada, Ottawa K1A OR6 (dave@irs.phy.nrc.ca), and [2]Medical College of Virginia, Richmond VA 23298-0058 (rmohan@hsc.vcu.edu)

## Introduction

The use of Monte Carlo techniques for routine clinical treatment planning will soon be with us in the sense that various commercial producers of treatment planning systems are actively developing such systems. Since it has long been thought that Monte Carlo techniques represent the "ultimate" answer to the problem of accurate dose calculation, the commercialization of these techniques would appear to be highly desirable.

However we are now entering a particularly tricky stage in the development of routine clinical Monte Carlo techniques. The speed of the calculations is still an issue since if they take too long, Monte Carlo will never be used "routinely" in the clinic. A second issue concerns the accuracy of the calculations when actually implemented in a commercial system. Possible inaccuracies might come from two broad areas: (i) the calculation in the patient where compromises might be made to increase the speed or there might be bugs; and (ii) the specification or modelling of the clinical beam (including the patient specific shaping devices) which is essential for the overall calculation to be accurate.

We have arranged a session at the ICCR to which many of the major code developers have been invited and we have asked them some specific questions about their codes or algorithms. In the time permitted we have had to severely limit the topic and have chosen to emphasize the first two areas mentioned above, namely the speed issue and the accuracy issue. This does not imply that the beam modelling issue isn't important. On the contrary, it may prove to be the most difficult and important issue to resolve prior to useful clinical implementation. However, it is also the most difficult question to deal with in a short term comparative study.

In this paper we present the questions which the developers have been asked. These questions are by no means exhaustive and there are many other important questions to address but these could each be the focus of an entire session. For example: (i) How fast is fast enough? (ii) What level of accuracy and precision are clinically relevant and under what clinical circumstances? (iii) How do we prescribe dose for MC-based treatment planning? (iv) How do we evaluate MC treatment plans? (v) How do we calculate monitor units for MC-based treatments? (vi) How do we use MC for dose calculation for optimization of treatment plans? Time permitting we will discuss these and other questions in a panel discussion after the speakers.

## Question I: Speed of photon calculations

To define a meaningful comparison of dose calculations between codes it is important to specify a case which everyone will use. There are many, many possible variations but the case selected here is meant to represent a "typical" case which is both easy to implement and comparable to present day clinical practice using other algorithms. By presenting this case in some detail it can provide a specific benchmark against which others can also do a comparison.

The phantom is 30.5 cm×39.5 cm×30 cm deep and filled with 5 mm$^3$ voxels. The odd dimensions are to ensure a voxel on the central axis but otherwise represent a realistic size. The voxels are to be filled randomly with one of 4 materials (water, aluminium, lung (ICRU, $\rho$=0.26 g/cm$^3$) and graphite) although if a particular algorithm's speed does not make use of voxels being the same material, then using water everywhere is acceptable. The incident beam is to be a 6 MV spectrum from a point source at 100 cm SSD and collimated to 10×10 cm$^2$ at the phantom surface.

#### Statistical Uncertainties to be achieved

Any Monte Carlo timing comparison must specify what statistical precision has been achieved and the methods used to determine statistical uncertainties must be specified. If any smoothing procedure is applied it should be specified and its effects estimated but smoothing must not be used for the timing comparison.

Specification of precision is an evolving art. To avoid issues about the uncertainty on the uncertainty, a neutral way to specify precision is to sum in quadrature the estimated relative uncertainties in all voxels with a dose greater than some arbitrary lower dose limit, say $D_{max}/2$, and from this find the average relative uncertainty. For the timing comparison the precision sought is an average relative statistical uncertainty on these voxels of 0.02 or less.

#### I.a: How long?

The primary question is, how long does a code take to do the above calculation on an Intel P-III 500 MHz machine? To scale times from other machines the standard EGS4 timing benchmark can be used[1] as updated at http://www.npl.co.uk/npl/rad/egs/bench/bench.html. If additional scaling is needed one should just scale a given chip architecture by its clock speed. This approach is subject to uncertainties of the order of at least 20% due to variations in compilers, memory size, cache size etc which also play some role. Any special "tricks" used by a particular installation should be mentioned.

### I.b: Physics Approximations?

One way to increase calculation speed is to make some approximations in the physics. These should be listed and an estimate made of the effects of these approximations (i.e. will they lead to 1%, 3% or 5% errors and under what circumstances). The techniques used to verify this accuracy should be described. Obviously the ideal situation is to find better ways of doing things which lead to no decrease in accuracy, at least for the in-patient calculation for the energy range of interest in radiotherapy.

### I.c: Variance reduction used?

A strict definition of variance reduction techniques would be those techniques which are applied with no decrease in accuracy (e.g the use of forcing routines) but the term has been more generally used to include techniques which increase efficiency with negligible loss of accuracy (e.g. the use of range rejection to terminate a history when an electron cannot possibly escape from the current voxel). The variance reduction techniques used in a given code should be specified and the increase in efficiency ($= 1/(T_{cpu}\sigma^2)$) from each type of variance reduction should be estimated.

### I.d: Transport parameters used?

The transport parameters such as the energy cutoffs used in a Monte Carlo calculation play an important role in defining the speed and accuracy of the calculation. These cutoffs and other relevant transport parameters (eg ESTEPE step size limits or equivalent) should be specified and the methods used to determine that these parameters lead to accurate simulations should be specified.

### I.e Time scaling with voxel size, energy etc?

The case specified here is for a given voxel size and beam energy. If the variation of calculation time with voxel size and beam energy are known they should be specified.

## Question II: Speed of $e^-$ calculations

If the code system being developed is also capable of calculations for incident electron beams, the above questions should be answered for mono-energetic electron beams with energies of 6 MeV and 20 MeV. In this case beam energy is thought to be a more critical parameter and hence the use of the two extreme energies.

## Question III: Accuracy of calculations

The ultimate verification of code accuracy comes by comparison with experiment but this is very difficult to set up for comparison between codes because they require different inputs regarding beam characterization. As an initial step we propose that comparisons be against the EGS4/PRESTA code system. This provides a nominal way of demonstrating the accuracy of the in-phantom portion of the calculations and this well known code has been extensively benchmarked against experiment. The following cases have been set up to deliberately stress most codes without being too hard to implement. The results of the EGS4/PRESTA/DOSXYZ (ESTEPE=0.01(electrons) or default (photons), AE=0.521 MeV,ECUT=0.700 MeV) calculations are presented here graphically and are available in digital format on-line[4]. It is essential to show the absolute differences (or possibly ratios of results) between another calculation and the EGS4/PRESTA results because the expected differences are small.

Unlike the photon timing case where timing is not expected to be sensitive to the incident beam, here the incident beam is completely specified to avoid any differences due to different incident spectra.

To ensure fair comparisons, all parameters used for the timing comparisons in question I must be used for the accuracy comparisons in question III.

Both cases are for a $1.5\times1.5$ cm$^2$ beam from a uniform point source at 100 cm incident on the phantom and the dose is scored on the central axis in $5\times5$ mm voxels which are 2 mm thick in the beam direction.

### III.a: Photon case

The phantoms are the same outer dimensions as in question I but they are now slab phantoms. From 0 to 3 cm is water, 3 to 5 cm is aluminium, 5 to 12 cm is lung and 12 to 30 cm is water. The voxels are 5 mm$^2$ in the x-y directions but only 2 mm deep to increase the resolution. The photon beam is a uniform 18MV beam from a realistic clinical accelerator as calculated at NRC using the BEAM code[2] and is available on-line[4]. Fig 1 presents the results as calculated with EGS4/PRESTA and these are also available on-line. The statistical precision of this reference calculation is $\pm0.3\%$.

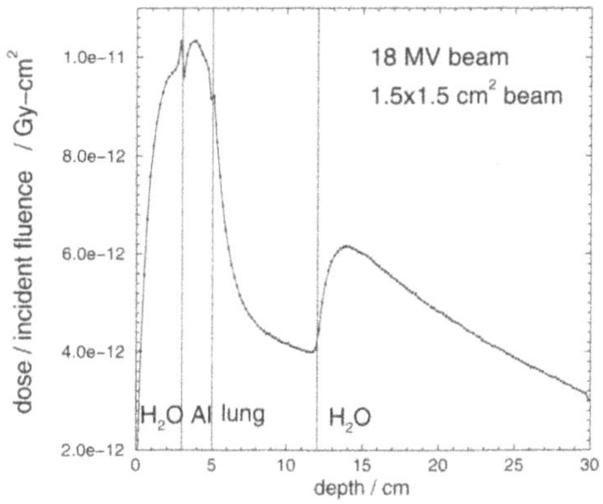


**Figure 1:** Depth-dose curves for the photon case as calculated by EGS4/PRESTA.

### III.b: Electron case

The phantoms are very similar to those for photon beams although compressed in depth because of the limited range of the incident 20 MeV mono-energetic electron beam. From 1 to 2 cm is water, 2 to 3 cm is aluminium, 3 to 6 cm is lung material and 6 to 30 cm is water. Fig 2 presents the results of the EGS4/PRESTA calculation in this case. Typical precision is 0.2% of dose maximum. This figure also shows a direct comparison to an EGSnrc calculation[3] (with no spin effects).

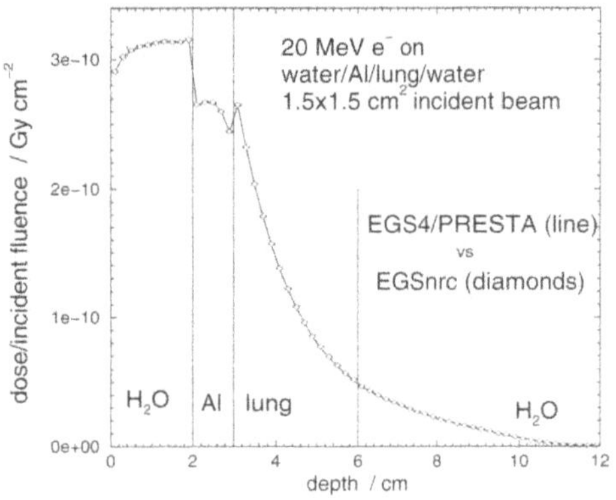


**Figure 2:** Comparison of depth-dose curves for the electron case as calculated by EGS4/PRESTA and EGSnrc (courtesy of Iwan Kawrakow).

The direct comparison in Fig 2 is not very informative since the differences are small compared to the scale whereas Fig 3 presents 2 other comparisons of the data. The absolute difference as a fraction of dose maximum shows that even for these two very slow codes there are some differences but they are limited to a few tenths %. Plotting the ratio of the two calculations vs depth shows that the codes diverge but this is for such small doses that it is not important. The presentation of the absolute difference in doses as a fraction of the total dose seems the most informative way to do the comparison.

## Question IV: Beam models

As discussed above, beam modelling may prove to be one of the most difficult problems to handle in implementing Monte Carlo techniques into routine clinical practice. Within the tight space limitations, the authors were asked to give a very brief overview of how they are handling this.

## Question V: CT conversion

Another important area, especially for electron beams, is the issue of converting CT numbers to materials and densities for the Monte Carlo calculations. The contributors were asked to briefly describe the techniques they use.

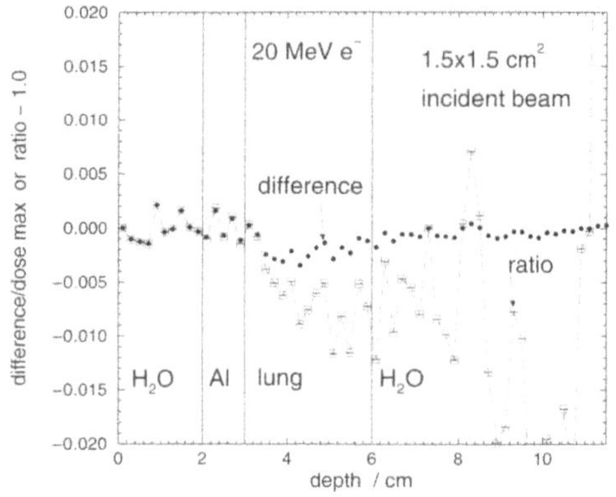


**Figure 3:** Difference in dose vs depth calculated by EGS4/PRESTA for the electron case less that calculated by EGSnrc as a fraction of the dose maximum (filled circles). Ratio of EGSnrc dose/EGS4-PRESTA dose -1.0 (open joined squares).

## Question VI: Commercial Links

At their discretion, the authors were asked to mention any links they have with commercial treatment planning companies.

## Summary/Acknowledgments

As the implementation of Monte Carlo techniques into routine clinical treatment planning proceeds, it will be necessary to develop standard tools for comparing various approaches and for assessing the speed of the calculations in a meaningful way. This is a first step in that direction and we thank the authors who have agreed to participate in this session at the ICCR. It must be emphasized that this is only a first step and there are many other important issues involved with the implementation of Monte Carlo into routine treatment planning in the clinic. We would like to thank Iwan Kawrakow for doing the EGSnrc calculations and for suggesting the criterion for statistical precision.

## References

[1] A. F. Bielajew and D. W. O. Rogers A standard timing benchmark for EGS4 Monte Carlo calculations. *Medical Physics*, 19:303 – 304, 1992.

[2] D. W. O. Rogers, B. A. Faddegon, G. X. Ding, C. M. Ma, J. Wei, and T. R. Mackie. BEAM: A Monte Carlo code to simulate radiotherapy treatment units. *Med. Phys.*, 22:503 – 524, 1995.

[3] I. Kawrakow. Accurate condensed history Monte Carlo simulation of electron transport. I. EGSnrc, the new EGS4 version. *submitted to Med. Phys.*, 1999.

[4] http://www.irs.inms.nrc.ca/inms/irs/papers/iccr00/iccr00.html

# MCDOSE – A Monte Carlo Dose Calculation Tool for Radiation Therapy Treatment Planning

**C.-M. Ma, J. S. Li, T. Pawlicki, S. B. Jiang and J. Deng**

Radiation Oncology Department, Stanford University School of Medicine, Stanford, CA 94305, USA

## Introduction

MCDOSE is an EGS4 [1] user code developed at Stanford University for radiation therapy treatment planning dose calculations. MCDOSE can be used to simulate the transport of photons and electrons in a patient geometry built from CT data. Realistic clinical accelerator beams can be used for any combinations of gantry angles, couch angles, collimator rotations, source skin distances (SSD) and beam modifiers. MCDOSE can be used to compute dose distributions for conventional treatment with photon and electron beams, beamlet distributions for inverse treatment planning, and the final dose distributions for intensity modulated radiotherapy (IMRT) using the multileaf collimator (MLC) leaf sequences generated by a treatment planning optimization system. The MCDOSE code has been implemented for clinical dose verification and treatment planning at Stanford since the end of 1998 [2].

In this talk, we describe the features of the MCDOSE code and present the results of the comparisons of the MCDOSE code with the DOSXYZ [3] code using the phantom geometry and beam setup recommended for the accuracy and timing study [4].

## Material and methods

### Simulation geometry

MCDOSE can simulate the transport of photons and electrons in a 3D rectilinear phantom geometry. The volume elements (voxels) in the phantom can have uniform or variable dimensions and the material in a voxel can be specified by the user or determined from the electron density data derived from the patient CT data. Tissue, bone and air are used to simulate the patient geometry based on the conversion of the electron density data on an existing treatment planning system. Other materials are used to simulate beam modifiers and metal inserts or dental fillings if present.

The beam modifiers are simulated by MCDOSE as a series of 3D objects stacked one above another; each modifier occupies a slab in space. Full particle transport is performed for the following modifiers: jaw, wedge, compensator, block and cutout. MCDOSE simulates the effect of a bolus by adding the bolus material to the patient geometry. Static MLC fields can be simulated by blocks and dynamic MLC and dynamic wedge are simulated by changing the particle weighting factors during a simulation. For IMRT dose verification, MLC leaf sequence files are used to reconstruct the photon intensity map for each treatment field and to account for the effect MLC leaf leakage. The accuracy of the beam modifier simulation with MCDOSE has been verified by comparisons with the EGS4/BEAM/DOSXYZ results [5].

### Source modeling and beam commissioning

MCDOSE uses a multiple source model for both photon and electron beams. For photon beams, our multiple source model [6] covers all the fixed components above the jaws in the accelerator head. For electron beams, the multiple source model [7] covers all the components down to the bottom scraper of the applicator. The source model parameters were derived from the measured data and verified using the phase space data simulated using the EGS4/BEAM system [8].

### Variance reduction techniques

Several variance reduction techniques have been implemented in MCDOSE including photon interaction forcing, Russian roulette, electron range/region rejection, and electron track repeating. The user can choose whether to apply these techniques in a patient dose calculation. No approximations are made in the patient phantom simulation. The effect of electron range/region rejection in the modifier simulation on bremsstrahlung production is estimated to be much less than 1% (ECUT = 2 MeV or smaller).

## Transport parameters

The EGS4 transport parameters used for the patient dose calculation are AE = ECUT = 700 keV (total energy) for electrons, AP = PCUT = 10 keV for photons and ESTEPE = 0.2 for electron transport. Default values are used for the PRESTA electron transport algorithm [9].

### Statistical analysis

The relative statistical uncertainty of the dose in a voxel is estimated by

$$\frac{\delta D}{D} = \sqrt{\frac{\sum e_i^2 - (\sum e_i)^2 / n}{(n-1)(\sum e_i)^2 / n}}$$

where $e_i$ is the energy deposited in the voxel in an energy deposition event and n is the total number of energy deposition events in the simulation.

A Mortran macro was implemented in DOSXYZ and MCDOSE to calculate the average relative statistical uncertainty [4] by summing in quadrature the estimated relative uncertainties in all voxels with a dose greater than $D_{max}/2$.

## Results

### The timing study

To compare the speed of the MCDOSE code and the DOSXYZ code, we have calculated doses in a 30.5 cm x 39.5 cm x 30 cm water phantom filled with 0.5 cm x 0.5 cm x 0.5 cm voxels. A point source of 6 MV photons has been used with a field of 10 cm x 10 cm defined at 100 cm SSD. This geometry is not the same as the one recommended by Rogers and Mohan [4], which consisted of a mixture of four materials. However, MCDOSE does not make use of voxels being the same material. To remove any inconsistencies in the simulation geometry and transport parameters, we have also performed dose calculations using DOSXYZ (from the BEAM98 distribution) under the same conditions. The MCDOSE results had an average relative statistical uncertainty of 0.019. More histories were needed by DOSXYZ to achieve the same precision. The dose distributions agreed very well (within the calculated statistical uncertainty). The CPU time required by MCDOSE was 10.5 min and by DOSXYZ was 284.3 min on a Pentium III 450 MHz PC (equivalent to 9.5 min and 257.2 min, respectively, on a Pentium III 500 MHz if scaled by the chip clock speed). The PC used in our timing study had 256 Mb RAM. The codes were compiled using the g77 compiler with an optimization level 2. In this case, the MCDOSE was estimated to be about 27 times faster than the DOSXYZ code. We also performed the same dose calculation with DOSXYZ using AE = 521 keV. The CPU time was 1198.1 min to achieve an average relative statistical uncertainty of 0.02. This means that we can speed up the calculation by a factor of 3 if we use 700 keV AE with respect to 521 keV AE. The difference in the dose distribution between the two AE values was found negligible for the cases investigated here.

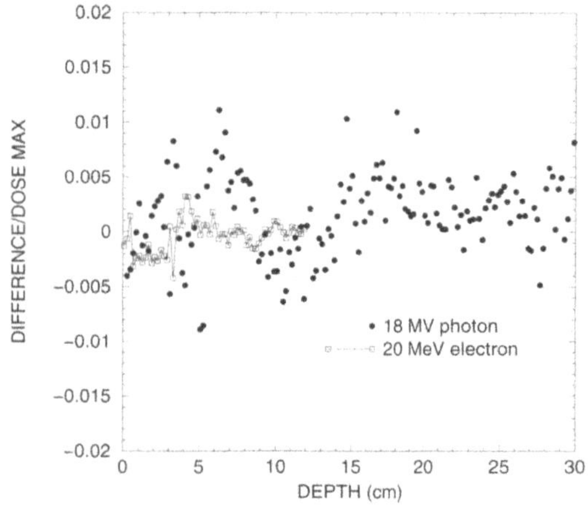


**Figure 1:** Difference in dose vs. depth calculated by EGS4/PRESTA/MCDOSE less that calculated by EGS4/PRESTA/DOSXYZ as a fraction of the dose maximum for a 18 MV photon beam (filled circles) and a 20 MeV electron beam (open squares).

### The accuracy study

For the accuracy comparison, phantoms of the same outer dimensions were used. A layered phantom was used for the 18 MV photon beam (1.5 cm x 1.5 cm field). From 0 to 3 cm is water, 3 to 5 cm is aluminum, 5 to 12 cm is lung and 12 to 30 cm is water. The voxels are 0.5 cm x 0.5 cm x 0.2 cm. For the electron beam comparison, a layered phantom was used. From 0 to 2 cm is water, 2 to 3 cm is aluminum, 3 to 6 cm is lung and 6 to 30 cm is water. A 20 MeV monoenergetic electron beam was used with a 1.5 cm x 1.5 cm field. Figure 1 shows the difference in dose vs. depth calculated by EGS4/PRESTA/MCDOSE [4] less that calculated by EGS4/PRESTA/DOSXYZ as a fraction of the dose maximum. The maximum difference in dose between the two codes is about 1% of the maximum dose for the two cases (the 1$\sigma$ statistical uncertainty on the MCDOSE results was about 0.3%).

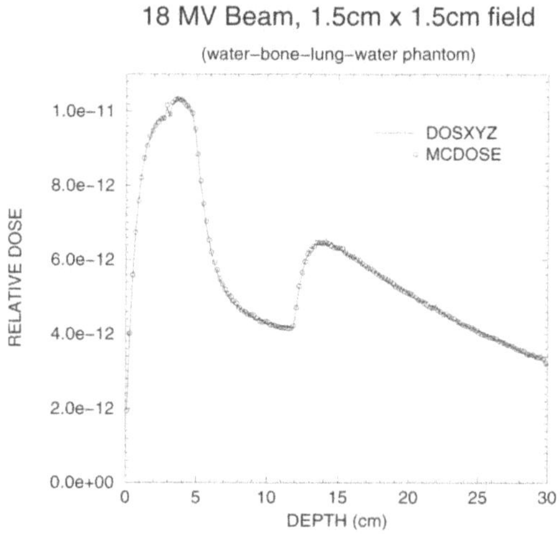


**Figure 2:** Central axis depth dose curves for a 18 MV photon beam as calculated by EGS4/PRESTA/DOSXYZ (line) and EGS4/PRESTA/MCDOSE (open circles) under the same conditions.

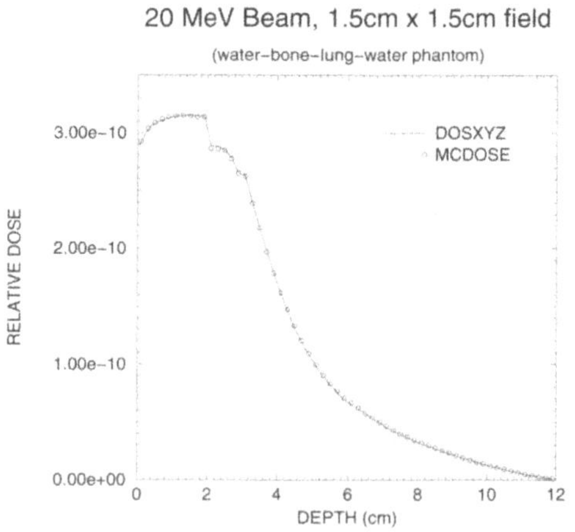


**Figure 3:** Depth dose curves for an 20 MeV electron beam as calculated by EGS4/PRESTA/DOSXYZ (line) and EGS4/PRESTA/MCDOSE (open circles) under the same conditions.

It is interesting to note that for the MCDOSE calculation, the EGS4 parameter AE was 700 keV while for the EGS4/PRESTA/DOSXYZ calculation AE was 521 keV [4]. To remove this inconsistency, we also performed dose calculations using both codes with AE = 700 keV. The same layered phantoms were used for a 18 MV photon beam and an 20 MeV electron beam except that the aluminum slab was replaced by a bone slab of the same thickness (because we usually use bone rather than aluminum in a patient geometry). Figure 2 shows the depth dose curves for the 18 MV photon beam and figure 3 shows the depth dose curves for the 20 MeV electron beam calculated by EGS4/PRESTA/DOSXYZ and EGS4/PRESTA/MCDOSE. The statistical uncertainty on the dose was about 0.5% of the maximum dose for both codes. Figure 4 shows the difference in dose vs. depth calculated, under the same conditions, by EGS4/PRESTA/MCDOSE less that calculated by EGS4/PRESTA/DOSXYZ as a fraction of the dose maximum. The results are consistent to within about 1% between the two codes.

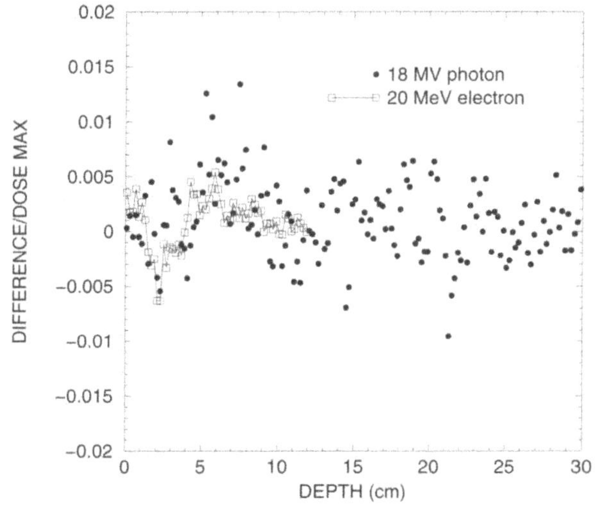


**Figure 4:** Difference in dose vs. depth calculated by EGS4/PRESTA/MCDOSE less that calculated by EGS4/PRESTA/DOSXYZ as a fraction of the dose maximum for a 18 MV photon beam (filled circles) and a 20 MeV electron beam (open squares).

## Conclusions

An EGS4/PRESTA user code, MCDOSE, has been developed for radiotherapy treatment planning dose calculations. The code has been implemented for clinical dose verification and treatment planning at Stanford Medical Center. Comparisons of the results calculated by EGS4/DOSXYZ and EGS4/MCDOSE have been made for various phantoms and beam setups. The MCDOSE results agreed in general with the DOSXYZ results to within 1% of the maximum dose for both photon and electron beams in heterogeneous phantoms consisting of tissue, bone, lung, air and aluminum. The MCDOSE code can run 10-30 times faster than the DOSXYZ code with the variance reduction techniques switched on depending on the beam energy and simulation geometry.

## Acknowledgments

This work is partially supported by NCI Grant No. CA 78331, DOD Grant No. BC971292, and a consortium agreement with NumeriX, LLC. We would like to thank other members of the Monte Carlo group at Stanford University, Arthur Boyer, Gary Luxton, Sam Brain, Ajay Kapur, Michael Lee and Grisel Mora for valuable discussions and comments on this work. We would also like to thank Todd Koumrian and Michael Luxton for computer hardware and software support.

## References

[1] Nelson R, Hirayama H and Rogers DWO (1985). The EGS4 code system, Stanford Linear Accelerator Center Report SLAC-265 (SLAC, Stanford, CA)

[2] Ma C-M, Pawlicki T, Li JS, Jiang SB, Deng J, Kapur A, Mok E, Luxton G, Boyer AL (1999). MCDOSE – A dose calculation tool for radiotherapy treatment planning, Med. Phys. 26: 1148 (Abstract)

[3] Ma C-M, Reckwerdt P, Holmes M, Rogers D W O, Geiser B, and Walters B, (1995) *DOSXYZ Users Manual*, NRCC Report No. PIRS-0509B

[4] Rogers DWO and Mohan R (2000). Questions for comparison of clinical Monte Carlo codes. These proceedings.

[5] Li JS, Pawlicki T, Deng J, Jiang SB, Ma C-M (2000). Simulation of beam modifiers for Monte Carlo treatment planning, These proceedings

[6] Deng J, Jiang S B, Kapur A, Li J S, Pawlicki T, Ma C-M (2000) Photon beam characterization and modeling for Monte Carlo treatment planning, Phys. Med. Biol. 45 in press

[7] Jiang S B, Kapur A and Ma C-M (2000) Electron beam modeling and commissioning for Monte Carlo treatment planning, Med. Phys. 27 (Jan) in press

[8] Rogers DWO, Faddegon BA, Ding GX, Ma C-M, Wei JS, Mackie TR (1995). BEAM: A Monte Carlo code to simulate radiotherapy treatment units. Med. Phys. 22: 503-25.

[9] Bielajew AF and Rogers DWO (1987), "PRESTA: The Parameter Reduced Electron-Step Transport Algorithm for Electron Monte Carlo Transport," Nuclear Instruments and Methods, B18: 165 – 181

# VMC$^{++}$, a fast MC algorithm for Radiation Treatment planning

**Iwan Kawrakow**[1] **and Matthias Fippel**[2]
[1] Institute for National Measurement Standards, National Research Council, Ottawa, Ontario K1A 0R6, Canada,
[2] Abteilung für Medizinische Physik, Radiologische Universitätsklinik, Hoppe-Seyler-Str. 3, 72076 Tübingen, Germany

This paper gives a short description of VMC$^{++}$, a recent C++ re-implementation of the VMC [1] and XVMC [2, 3] code systems that incorporates a variety of improvements, and answers the questions concerning speed and accuracy given in the paper by Rogers and Mohan [4].

## VMC$^{++}$, a short description

### Condensed history implementation

VMC$^{++}$uses a Class II condensed history (CH) scheme [5] for the simulation of charged particle transport (which is also employed in the popular EGS4 system [6]). That is to say, bremsstrahlung interactions that result in the creation of photons above an energy threshold $E_\gamma$, and inelastic scattering that sets in motion atomic electrons with an energy above $E_\delta$, are treated discretely by creation and transport. Sub-threshold inelastic processes are accounted for in a CSDA model. Angular deflections due to multiple elastic scattering are treated according to the theory of Ref. [7] with refinements presented in [8]. The electron-step algorithm (which relates the particle position at the end of a CH step to the step-length and the multiple scattering angle) employed in VMC$^{++}$will be discussed in details elsewhere [9]. Here we note that it has an $O(\xi^2)$ truncation error ($\xi$ is the 1st elastic scattering moment per step), exactly reproduces first order spatial moments and is therefore substantially more accurate than PRESTA [10] (for a detailed discussion of various CH electron-step algorithms and their truncation error see Ref. [11]). The main difference in the VMC$^{++}$' implementation of the CH technique compared to general purpose MC codes such as EGS4 is the boundary crossing algorithm employed. Steps are not terminated at interfaces as in EGS4 and EGS4/PRESTA as this procedure is now known to produce artifacts in certain situations [12, 13], but continue until the criterion that determined the step-length is satisfied, possibly passing several regions in a single CH step. This approach is also one of the main reasons for the speed improvement compared to EGS4.

CH step-lengths in VMC$^{++}$are determined from the maximum first elastic scattering moment per step $\xi_{max}$ (which controls the accuracy of path-length corrections and lateral correlations), the maximum energy loss per step $\Delta E_{max}$ (which determines the accuracy of local energy deposition along a CH step) and the delta particle production threshold energy $E_\delta$ (it does not make sense to take steps shorter than the range of cut-off electrons).

### Cross sections

Discrete charged particle inelastic scattering is modeled according to the Møller ($e^-$) or Bhabha ($e^+$) cross sections (CS). Bremsstrahlung production is based on the Bethe-Heitler [14] CS with an empirical correction factor chosen such as to reproduce ICRU recommended radiative stopping powers. Restricted stopping powers are calculated using the procedure adopted in ICRU report 37 [15]. Incoherent scattering is treated with the Klein-Nishina CS. Inclusion of bound effects and Doppler broadening is possible but not necessary for calculations in the external beam RTP energy range. Total pair/triplet production and photoelectric absorption CS are taken from the EPDL [16]. The differential pair production CS employed is the high-energy approximation by Bethe and Heitler [14]. Coherent scattering and atomic relaxations are ignored so far as they play no role in the external beam energy range of interest. Their inclusion will be necessary for calculations for low energy Brachy-therapy sources and is therefore scheduled for the next release of the system.

### Variance reduction techniques

The main speed improvement in VMC$^{++}$compared to EGS4 comes from the electron boundary crossing algorithm and the more accurate electron-step algorithm which permits longer CH steps. Depending on energy, voxel resolution, beam quality, cut-off energies and materials involved, these two aspects of the CH implementation give a factor of 5 to 30 compared to EGS4/PRESTA.

An additional factor of two results from the "history repetition" technique. In its original implementation in VMC this technique introduces a systematic uncertainty and limits the applicability of the algorithm to low $Z$ materials and the RTP energy range. The systematic error is estimated to be less than 1% in the energy range of interest in geometries that contain only human tissue. In VMC$^{++}$the "history repetition" technique is refined to remove any systematic uncertainties (and is therefore probably better referred to as STOPS – Simultaneous Transport Of Particle Sets). These refinements, discussed in detail elsewhere [9], make the application of the algorithm for arbitrary materials and energies possible with only a minor loss of calculation speed (20-30% in a phantom with 16 randomly distributed materials). This is demonstrated in Fig. 1 where the dose distribution in a lead phantom from a $10 \times 10$ cm$^2$ 20 MeV electron beam calculated with VMC$^{++}$is compared with EGSnrc [8] results.

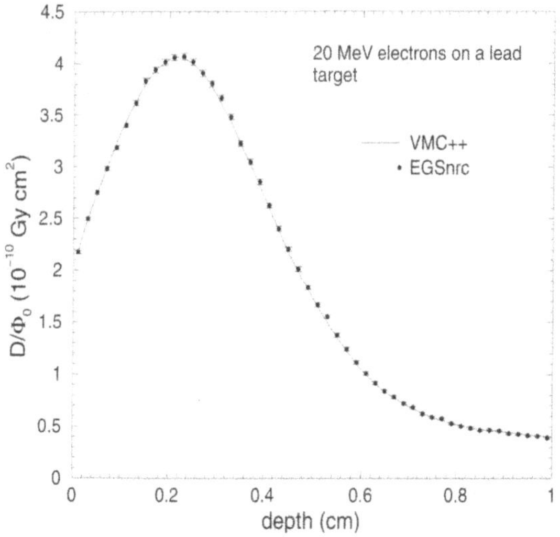


**Figure 1:** Dose distribution from a $10 \times 10$ cm$^2$ 20 MeV electron beam in a lead phantom.

The photon transport algorithm in VMC$^{++}$is taken from the most recent version of XVMC [3], see also the paper by Fippel *et al* in this volume. It employs a variety of variance reduction techniques (VRT) such as photon splitting, Russian Roulette, use of quasi-random numbers and KERMA approximation for scattered photons with energy below a user-defined threshold. The combined effect of these variance reduction techniques is a factor of 5 to 10 increase in calculation efficiency compared to a photon beam MC simulation without any VRT's employed.

## Statistical uncertainties and efficiency

Due to the use of a variety of variance reduction techniques, it is not possible to use a history-by-history statistical analysis in VMC$^{++}$. Statistical uncertainties are therefore estimated by subdividing the simulation into $N_b$ batches and calculating the dose variance at each point of the geometry. For the results presented in this paper 64 batches were used. To be consistent with the paper by Rogers and Mohan, the "overall" statistical uncertainty $\Delta\bar{D}$ of the simulation is defined as

$$\Delta\bar{D}^2 = \frac{1}{N}\sum\left(\frac{\Delta D_i}{D_i}\right)^2 \tag{1}$$

where $D_i$ is the dose in the $i$'th region, $\Delta D_i$ the associated statistical uncertainty (1 $\sigma$), the summation runs over all voxels with a dose greater than 50% of the maximum dose and $N$ is the number of such voxels. The efficiency $\varepsilon$ of the simulations reported in the subsequent sections is then

$$\varepsilon = \left(\Delta\bar{D}^2 T\right)^{-1} \tag{2}$$

where $T$ is the CPU time on a PC with a single 500 MHz PIII CPU. It is worth noticing that the efficiency as defined by Eq. (1-2) is independent of $N_b$ as long as $N_b >\sim 16$.

## Accuracy

A systematic approach for comparing dose distribution corrupted by statistical noise is presented in Ref. [3]. In this paper the accuracy if VMC$^{++}$will be demonstrated by presenting comparisons with results from EGSnrc calculations in the phantom-beam configurations described in [4]. We have chosen to compare VMC$^{++}$to EGSnrc instead of EGS4/PRESTA because of the observed parameter dependence of the EGS4/PRESTA calculated dose distribution and systematic differences to EGSnrc of 0.2-0.3% even for very small step-sizes (ESTEPE=1%) and low cut-off energies (AE=ECUT=521 keV, AP=PCUT=10 keV).

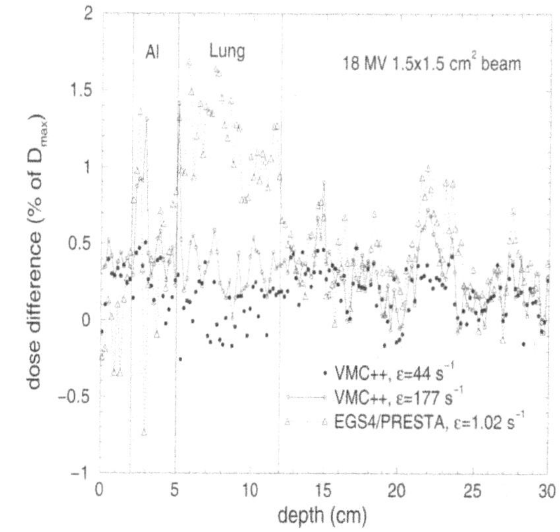


**Figure 2:** Dose differences (in % of the maximum dose) for VMC$^{++}$and EGS4/PRESTA compared to EGSnrc in a $1.5 \times 1.5$ cm$^2$ 18 MV beam incident on the water/aluminum/lung phantom described in [4]. Statistical uncertainties are of the order of 0.2% of $D_{max}$.

Fig. 2 shows the dose differences for VMC$^{++}$and EGS4/-PRESTA to EGSnrc along the central axis of a $1.5 \times 1.5$ cm$^2$ 18 MV photon beam incident on the water/aluminum/lung phantom described in [4]. The VMC$^{++}$calculation which agrees within 0.3% with EGSnrc ($E_\delta = 100$ keV, $\Delta E_{max} =$ 250 keV, $\xi_{max}$=0.1) has an efficiency of 44 s$^{-1}$, *i.e.* 40 times higher than EGS4/PRESTA with default step-sizes and AE=ECUT=700 keV. It is included in this figure in order to demonstrate that by selecting sufficiently conservative transport parameters it is possible to obtain a perfect agreement with EGSnrc. The VMC$^{++}$calculation with default parameters ($E_\delta = 500$ keV, $\Delta E_{max} = 750$ keV, $\xi_{max}$=0.25) is more than 150 times more efficient than EGS4/PRESTA for a comparable accuracy.

Fig. 3 shows a dose difference plot along the central axis of a $1.5 \times 1.5$ cm$^2$ 20 MeV electron beam incident on the water/aluminum/lung phantom described in [4] using default parameter for the VMC$^{++}$calculation which has an efficiency of 1400 s$^{-1}$.

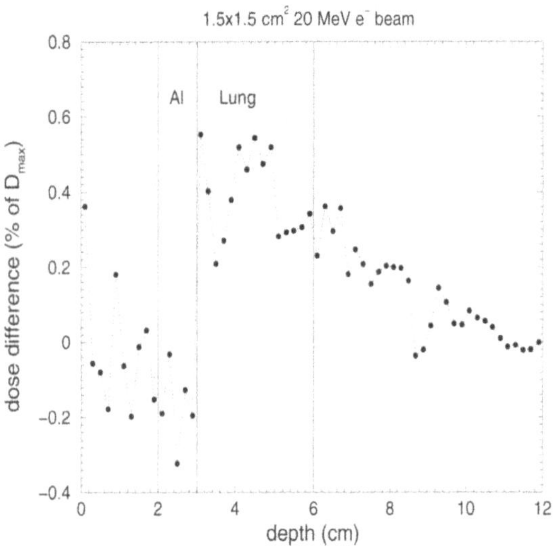


**Figure 3:** VMC$^{++}$to EGSnrc dose differences (in % of the maximum dose) along the central axis of a 1.5 × 1.5 cm$^2$ 20 MeV electron beam incident on the water/aluminum/lung phantom described in [4]. Statistical uncertainties are of the order of 0.2% of $D_{max}$.

## Speed

The VMC$^{++}$efficiency as defined in Eq. (1-2) for various $10 \times 10$ cm$^2$ beams incident on a $30.5 \times 39.5 \times 30$ cm$^3$ phantom made of $0.5 \times 0.5 \times 0.5$ cm$^3$ voxels and four randomly distributed materials (water, graphite, aluminum and lung) is summarized in Table 1 (*e*6 denotes a 6 MeV electron beam and $\gamma$18 a 18 MV photon beam). The efficiencies

| Q | e6 | e20 | $\gamma$6 | $\gamma$18 |
|---|---|---|---|---|
| $\varepsilon$ | 236 | 67 | 7.5 | 7.0 |
| $T$ | 10.6 | 37.3 | 333 | 357 |

**Table 1:** VMC$^{++}$efficiencies $\varepsilon$ (in $s^{-1}$) and CPU times $T$ for 2% relative statistical uncerty (in $s$) using a single 500 MHz PIII CPU) for various beam qualities. All beams are point sources collimated to 10 × 10 cm$^2$.

reported in this table result from the same transport parameter sets used in the accuracy comparisons. Note that if the cut-off energies were adapted to the larger voxel size the efficiencies increase by $\sim 20-30\%$. It is also worth noticing that if a 2-3% systematic accuracy is considered acceptable, an additional efficiency improvement by a factor of 2-3 is achievable by the appropriate selection of transport parameters.

## CT conversion

There are two possible approaches implemented in VMC$^{++}$ to convert Hounsfield numbers (HN) into scattering properties. The first approach, taken from VMC and XVMC (see Ref. [1] and [2] for details), uses fit formulae to calculate electron stopping and scattering powers and photon linear attenuation coefficients from the mass density or HN. The second approach uses a ramp of 16 materials which were selected from the 106 materials published in ICRU Report 46 [17] excluding non-body tissues such as urinary stones. The number of HN bins is determined from the requirement that the linear mass attenuation coefficient and the mass stopping power of all materials in the bin do not differ by more than 1%.

## References


[1] I. Kawrakow, M. Fippel, and K. Friedrich. *Med. Phys.*, 23:445 – 457, 1996.

[2] M. Fippel. *Med. Phys.*, 26:1466 – 1475, 1999.

[3] I.Kawrakow and M. Fippel. Investigation of variance reduction techniques for Monte Carlo photon dose calculation using XVMC . *submitted to Phys. Med. Biol.*, 1999.

[4] D.W.O. Rogers and R. Mohan. *this volume*, 2000.

[5] M. J. Berger. *Methods in Comput. Phys.*, volume 1, 135 – 215. Academic, New York, 1963.

[6] W. R. Nelson, H. Hirayama, and D. W. O. Rogers. The EGS4 Code System. Report SLAC–265, 1985.

[7] I. Kawrakow and A. F. Bielajew. *Nuclear Instruments and Methods*, 134B:325 – 336, 1998.

[8] I. Kawrakow. I. EGSnrc, the new EGS4 version. *submitted to Med. Phys.*, 1999.

[9] I.Kawrakow. *in preparation*, 2000.

[10] A. F. Bielajew and D. W. O. Rogers. *Nuclear Instruments and Methods*, B18:165 – 181, 1987.

[11] I. Kawrakow and A. F. Bielajew. *Nuclear Instruments and Methods*, 142B:253 – 280, 1998.

[12] B. J. Foote and V. G. Smyth. *Nucl. Inst. Meth.*, B100:22 – 30, 1995.

[13] I. Kawrakow. II. Application to ion chamber response simulations. *submitted to Med. Phys.*, 1999.

[14] W. Heitler. The Quantum Theory of Radiation. *(Clarendon Press, Oxford)*, 1954.

[15] ICRU. Stopping powers for electrons and positrons. ICRU Report 37, ICRU, Washington D.C., 1984.

[16] D. E. Cullen *et al. LLNL Report UCRL-50400, Volume 6, Revision 4 (Livermore, Calif)*, 1989.

[17] ICRU. Photon, Electron, Proton and Neutron Interaction Data for Body Tissues. ICRU Report 46, ICRU, Washington D.C., 1992.

# Performance benchmarks of the MCV Monte Carlo system

**Jeffrey V. Siebers, Paul J. Keall, Jong Oh Kim and Radhe Mohan**

Department of Radiation Oncology, MCV Hospitals, Virginia Commonwealth University, Richmond, VA, USA

## Introduction

The Monte Carlo group at the Medical College of Virginia has integrated Monte Carlo dose calculation directly into a commercial treatment planning system. The design basis for this system was to provide an integrated treatment-planning environment in which issues related to clinical implementation of Monte Carlo based treatment planning could be addressed. While this symposium addresses the speed and accuracy of MC dose calculation, our efforts have been directed toward the latter. Additionally, our efforts have addressed issues such as: What statistical accuracy is required for MC based treatment planning? What is the proper way to prescribe dose for MC based dose calculations? How do we compare MC dose distributions (that are dose to material) with other algorithms (that are dose to water)? What clinical advantages might be gained from use of MC in comparison with other dose algorithms?

These questions are the thrust of our research since we believe that, due to the increasing computer speed and more efficient algorithms (in a large part due to the efforts of the others included in this symposium), MC will have wide range clinical use within the next few years. When we have the ability to complete the task in a "fast-enough manner" on inexpensive computers, everyone will want the MC due to its superior accuracy.

## Brief Description of MCV

The Monte Carlo Vista (MCV) code, developed at the Medical College of Virginia, interfaces photon-electron Monte Carlo dose calculation algorithms directly to a commercial treatment planning system (Pinnacle[3*]). With MCV, Monte Carlo input files are auto-generated and auto-run on multiple unix-based computers. Following completion of the Monte Carlo simulation, results are automatically read back into the treatment planning system for display and analysis.

The radiation transport for MCV takes place in three stages. In the first stage, transport takes place through the patient independent portion of the beam line with phase space coordinates of exiting particles being saved to a phase-space file. This file is generated once for each energy of a given treatment machine. The second stage transports particles through the patient dependent portion of the treatment head. A slightly modified version of the EGS4[1]-based BEAM[2] user-code is used for this simulation. Different pre-generated executable files are required depending upon the configuration of beam modifiers located in the treatment head for the specific patient field. At the exit of the last beam modifier, particles are saved to a temporary phase space file that is used as input to the final patient/phantom calculation. The patient/phantom calculations are performed using either MCVRTP, a C++ Monte Carlo code provided by ADAC Laboratories[*] that uses many of the published algorithms of EGS4,[1] or it uses EGS4 directly with a slightly modified version of the user-code DOSXYZ[3] with the PRESTA[4] enhancements.

Since the MCV code can directly use the DOSXYZ code, agreement with the benchmark results provided should be expected.

## Benchmark Results

### Speed Benchmark

The speed timing benchmark was performed for a $30.5\times30.5\times30.0$ cm$^3$ homogeneous water phantom, with $0.5\times0.5\times0.5$ cm$^3$ voxels throughout the phantom. Source particles were sampled from a phase space input file for our Varian 2100c[5,6]. The break-down of the calculation time, scaled for a single 500 MHz Pentium III processor is listed in Table 1. Calculation times for the in-phantom portion of the calculation are given for both DOSXYZ and MCVRTP. Note that, although the total calculation time for a single PIII-500 is ~3 hours, using our current hardware configuration (32 computers of various speed), the calculation took ~10 minutes to complete (including the time to auto-generate the input files, convert the CT phantom, submit the MC jobs, sum all dose files, and load the dose file into the treatment planning system). Sampling particles from the source and transporting them through the blocks to the phantom surface uses <17% of the total calculation time. Using the simplified source proposed for the problem, this time is virtually eliminated, reducing the total calculation time to ~2.2 hours on a single PIII-500.

| | BEAM/DOSXYZ | BEAM/MCVRTP | Source/MCVRTP |
|---|---|---|---|
| Tx. Head | 0.47 | 0.47 | 0.02 |
| Phantom | 3.37 | 2.16 | 2.16 |
| Total | 3.84 | 2.63 | 2.18 |

**Table 1:** Time (in hours) for completion of the speed benchmark problem for a single Pentium III 500 MHz computer for various code configurations.

Our implementation uses few physics approximations. For both the beam-line and phantom calculations, the photon energy cut-offs (AP and PCUT) are set equal to 0.01 MeV while the electron total energy cut-offs (AE and ECUT) are set equal to 0.700 MeV. Range rejection is used to terminate electrons in jaws and wedges, with a kinetic energy cut-off of 3.0 MeV. Use of range rejection decreases the treatment head simulation time from 4.05 hours to 0.47 hours for the example case given here. No other variance reduction schemes are used in the beam-line simulation. The only variance reduction method used in the phantom calculation is the reuse of phase space particles. For a voxel with a volume of 0.2 cm$^3$, particles

[*] ADAC Laboratories, Milpitas, CA 95035.

are reused twenty times. For other voxel volumes, the number of times a particle is re-used is scaled inversely with the voxel volume. This method of reusing particles based on voxel volume allows us *a priori* knowledge of the statistical uncertainty of each beam. Re-using potentially correlated particles may have the effect of artificially reducing variance, however a study was performed which showed that no such correlation was observable for our implementation. The DOSXYZ code uses the standard PRESTA implementation, while MCVRTP does not use PRESTA. Differences between DOSXYZ and MCVRTP results are evaluated by comparing in-phantom dose distributions, with minimal differences observed between the two codes.

Statistical uncertainty for DOSXYZ is computed using the 'batch' statistical method. In MCVRTP, both the sum and the square of the sum of the energy deposited in each voxel of the dose grid by each source particle is used for the variance calculation. This, in effect, sets the number of 'batches' equal to the number of particles incident on the patient and minimizes the variance of the variance.

Figure 1 shows how computation time scales with voxel size for MCVRTP and DOSXYZ. Computations were run for equal statistical accuracy in the dose voxels. For MCVRTP, the computation time increases linearly with the inverse of the voxel volume. As voxel size decreases, the ratio between the DOSXYZ and MCVRTP calculation speed increases, presumably due to the use of the PRESTA algorithm in small voxels.

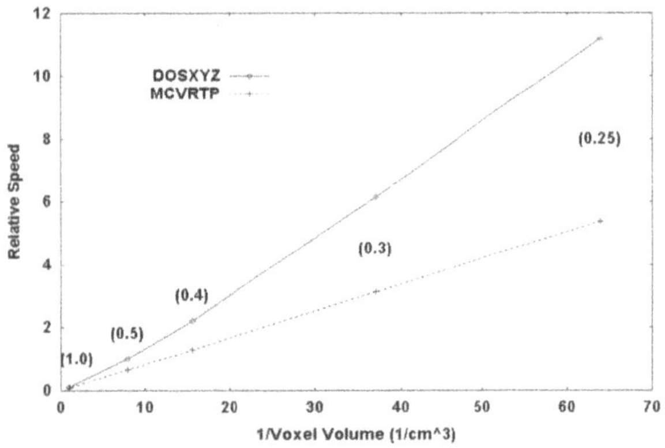


**Figure 1:** Scaling of calculation time with voxel volume for constant statistical precision with a 6 MV beam. Results are normalized to a value of 1.0 for a 0.5×0.5×0.5 $cm^3$ voxel with DOSXYZ. The length of a side of a cubic voxel is shown near the data points.

**Accuracy Benchmark**

The accuracy benchmark case was run using both the DOSXYZ and MCVRTP codes. To perform this benchmark, for our simulation, we replaced the phase space source usually used with the 18 MV NRC energy spectrum provided. The jaws were set to be much larger than the source size so as to not interact with particles. Due to the irregular materials included in this simulation, instead of using CTCREATE to create the phantom, we generated the phantom using a custom program. Figure 2 shows the depth dose profiles computed with DOSXYZ along with the "reference" dose profile provided. All calculations were done to ±0.3% statistical precision. The ratio of the dose values with respect to the reference standard is shown in Figure 3. The agreement of the DOSXYZ results is expected as our result essentially reproduces the reference calculation, except the electron energy cut-offs (AE and ECUT) are 700 keV instead of the 521 keV values used for the reference calculation, and a phantom file is used.

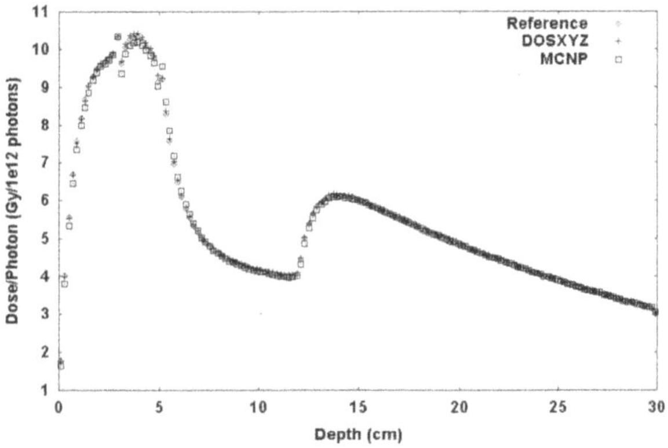


**Figure 2:** Photon beam depth dose curves for inhomogeneous phantom test case. Results are shown for DOSXYZ, and MCNP calculations, and the reference results provided..

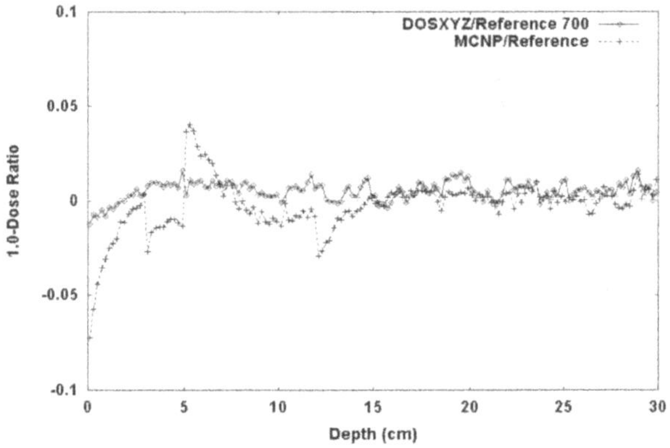


**Figure 3:** 1.0-Ratio of the dose results shown in Figure 1 with respect to the reference data provided.

To evaluate the accuracy of the "reference" calculation, we also performed this test with MCNP4b2.[7] Although MCNP is not part of our integrated treatment planning Monte Carlo system, this code is used to verify the accuracy of simulations for which we do not have measurements. MCNP is used for cross-checking since it, like EGS4, is a standard Monte Carlo code, however, its input data and methodology differs from EGS4. When EGS4 and MCNP agree, the confidence in a result increases, conversely, when they disagree, further investigation is merited. In this instance, the MCNP and DOSXYZ results show disagreements of up to 5% at the material interfaces. We are currently investigating the cause of these deviations.

**Beam models**

In our current implementation, the phase space of photons and electrons exiting the treatment head (incident upon the patient beam modifiers and then the patient) is derived directly from Monte Carlo simulations of the upper portion of the treatment head. That is, the phase space coordinates of particles exiting the treatment head are saved to a computer file, which is then used as input for simulations through patient beam modifiers and phantoms or patients. A typical phase space file is ~1.2 Gb and contains $\sim 7.5 \times 10^7$ histories. In order to match measured data for a given accelerator, the energy, energy spread, and radial distribution of electrons incident upon the bremsstrahlung target are adjusted (within realistic limits) to match depth dose and lateral beam profiles for several different field sizes. Direct phase space particles are used so as to avoid any inaccuracy introduced by beam models, and is practical in this era of inexpensive mass-storage devices.

**CT conversion**

To convert patient CT data into materials and densities for Monte Carlo calculations, we use the program CTCREATE.[3] The Hounsfield number to density conversion used is the same as that used by our treatment planning system. The materials assignments are similar to the CTCREATE defaults, with the addition of spongiosa (soft bone)[8] when the material density is between 1.1 and 1.4 g $cm^{-3}$. Soft bone was added because ICRP cortical bone[9] (density 1.85) has a much higher component of calcium than the sternum and other soft bones. Table 2 summarizes our CT conversion table. Though Monte Carlo has the advantage over commercial algorithms of being able to transport in patient representative materials rather than water, the density ranges of these materials are arbitrarily chosen, and the material composition will vary from patient to patient, and within a given patient. For this and other reasons, following completion of Monte Carlo dose calculations, the dose-to-material results are converted to dose-to-water.[10]

| PEGS4 Material name | Upper CT # | Min Density | Max Density ($g\ cm^{-3}$) |
|---|---|---|---|
| AIR700ICRU[8] | 98 | 0.0001 | 0.083 |
| LUNG700[8] | 544 | 0.083 | 0.50 |
| ICRUTISSUE700ICRU[11] | 1174 | 0.50 | 1.1 |
| SPNG (soft bone)[8] | 1620 | 1.1 | 1.4 |
| ICRPBONE700ICRU[9] | 3326 | 1.4 | 2.548 |

**Table 2:** Hounsfield number to material density and material conversion used for CT create.

**Commercial Ties**

Currently, MCV has no formal commercial ties regarding the development of Monte Carlo based treatment planning algorithms.

## Summary

The MCV integrated Monte Carlo code has been used to perform the photon beam test cases outlined. Monte Carlo dose distributions can be completed in 2-4 hours on a single 500 MHz PIII computer with a statistical precision of 2% for $0.5 \times 0.5 \times 0.5$ $cm^3$ voxels. Using multiple computers, this computation can be completed in ~10 minutes. As expected, our DOSXYZ calculations match that of the reference DOSXYZ calculations for the accuracy benchmark.

## Acknowledgements

The authors acknowledge the financial support of NIH Grant CA 74158-02. We thank ADAC for providing us with MCVRTP Monte Carlo code.

## References

[1]W. R. Nelson, H. Hirayama, and D. W. O. Rogers, "The EGS4 Code System," Report No. SLAC-265, Stanford Linear Accelerator Center, 1985.

[2]D. W. O. Rogers, B. A. Faddegon, G. X. Ding, C. M. Ma, J. We, and T. R. Mackie, "BEAM: a Monte Carlo code to simulate radiotherapy units," Med. Phys. **22** (5), 503-524 (1995).

[3]C.-M. Ma, P. Reckwerdt, M. Holmes, D. W. O. Rogers, B. Geiser, and B. Walters, "DOSXYZ users manual," Report No. PIRS-0509b, National Research Council of Canada, 1995.

[4]A. F. Bielajew and D. W. O. Rogers, "PRESTA-The Parameter Reduced Electron-Step Algorithm for electron Monte Carlo transport," Nucl. Instr. Meth. B **18**, 165-181 (1987).

[5]B. Libby, J. Siebers, and R. Mohan, "Validation of Monte Carlo generated phase space descriptions of medical linear accelerators," Med. Phys. **26** (8), 1476-1483 (1999).

[6]J. V. Siebers, P. J. Keall, B. Libby, and R. Mohan, "Comparison of EGS4 and MCNP4b Monte Carlo Codes for generation of photon phase space distributions for a Varian 2100C," Phys. Med. Bio. **44** (5) (1999).

[7]J. F. Briesmeister, "MCNP- A General Monte Carlo N-Particle Transport Code, Version 4B," Report No. LA-13181, Los Alamos National Laboratory, 1997.

[8]ICRU-44, "Tissue substitutes in radiation dosimetry and measurement," Report No. 44, International Commission on Radiation Units and Measurements, 1988.

[9]ICRP-23, "Reference Man: Anatomical, Physiological and Metabolic Characteristics," Report No. 23, International Commission of Radiation Protection, 1975.

[10]J. V. Siebers, P. J. Keall, A. E. Nahum, and R. Mohan, "Converting absorbed dose to medium to absorbed dose to water for Monte Carlo-based photon beam dose calculations," Phys. Med. Biol. Accepted for publication Dec 1999 (1999).

[11]ICRU-33, "Radiation Quantities and Units," Report No. 33, International Commission on Radiation Units and Measurements, 1980.

# Computer Automated Quantification of Respiratory Motion in a Fluoroscopic Movie

**Keatley EL, Mageras GS**

Memorial Sloan Kettering Cancer Center, New York, NY, USA

## Introduction

Organ motion uncertainty associated with respiration is a major factor affecting radiation therapy in the thorax and abdominal regions. A number of approaches have been developed to characterize and reduce this uncertainty [1]. These approaches share a common requirement: The need to measure internal anatomic motion in real time. Although quantitative measurements through fluoroscopic observation is often used in a research setting, the time and effort associated with such measurements precludes their clinical use on a routine basis. The development of a computer automated tool which would quantify fluoroscopic respiratory motion could greatly increase confidence in the these new treatment mechanisms.

Presented here is an automated fluoroscopic respiratory motion analysis tool based on the active contour algorithm. It reliably quantifies Superior/Inferior motion of both the diaphragm and upper chest wall with a calculation time of approximately one half a second per frame.

## Methods

### Theory

In general the term "active contour" refers to a deformable spline which varies it's position on an image under the influence of a score function. It is a member of the more general "deformable model" category of algorithms. Unlike many other members of this category, active contours do not require complex a priori shape constraints statistically derived from a set of training images. Shape information is often explicitly encoded into active contour models, and is usually simpler in form. Although less robust in general, this characteristic usually leads to faster execution times for applications in which such an approach is shown to be reliable. Active contours are especially appropriate for the segmentation of anatomy which are characterized by strong intensity gradients and lack structures of similar shape in the vicinity of the boundary of interest. Such is the case of the chest wall and diaphragm boundaries in fluoroscopic movies.

The behavior of active contours is determined by the form of its score energy function. The contour varies its position on the image until a local energy minimum is reached. The energy function is broken into two usually independent parts. The first is an external energy, such as an edge detection of the original image, which attracts the contour to features of interest. The second is an internal energy, which penalizes the contour's deviation from a preferred shape. The total energy of the contour can be expressed as the sum of the energies of it's vertices:

$$E_{total} = \sum_{i=1}^{n} \left[ E_{external}(v_i) + kE_{internal}(v_{i-1}, v_i, v_{i+1}) \right]$$

where $n$ is the number of vertices of the contour, and $k$ is a relative weighting factor. In this formulation, the external energy of a contour vertex depends only on it's own position, while the internal energy depends both on it's position and the relative position of it's neighbors, with special consideration for the end points of an open contour. In this active contour implementation, the energy image is generated by applying a 3x3 vertical edge detection operator to a median smoothed copy of the original. Median smoothing will preserve edges if the spatial extent of their curvature is large with respect to the kernel size, as is the case. The internal energy consists of two terms, one which acts to equispace the vertices of the contour, and one which penalizes deviation from a minimum energy angle each contour point forms with its neighbors. The penalty of both internal energy terms increases quadratically with the magnitude of the difference from the ideal.

The energy space is searched though the technique of dynamic programming [2]. The search for the local energy minima of the contour is done in iterations, and at every iteration the positional freedom of each vertex is restricted to a region of discrete locations about its current position. A multi-resolution technique is used to further increase execution speed.

### Steps of Execution

The program requires minimal user interaction. It begins by automatically determining the image scale and iso-center position from the cross hairs and graticule tray points, and extracts the extent of those artifacts so that they can be removed later, on a frame by frame basis. The fluoroscope aperture boundary is also found, and it determines the image field of view. Next the user roughly draws a contour near the anatomical boundary of interest, or simply marks the medial and lateral extent of that boundary. From this starting position a candidate contour converges and is displayed. If the user approves of the candidate contour, its shape is "memorized," and the program tracks the entire movie sequence without user interaction. Results are displayed graphically in real time (Figure 1) and saved to disk for later analysis.

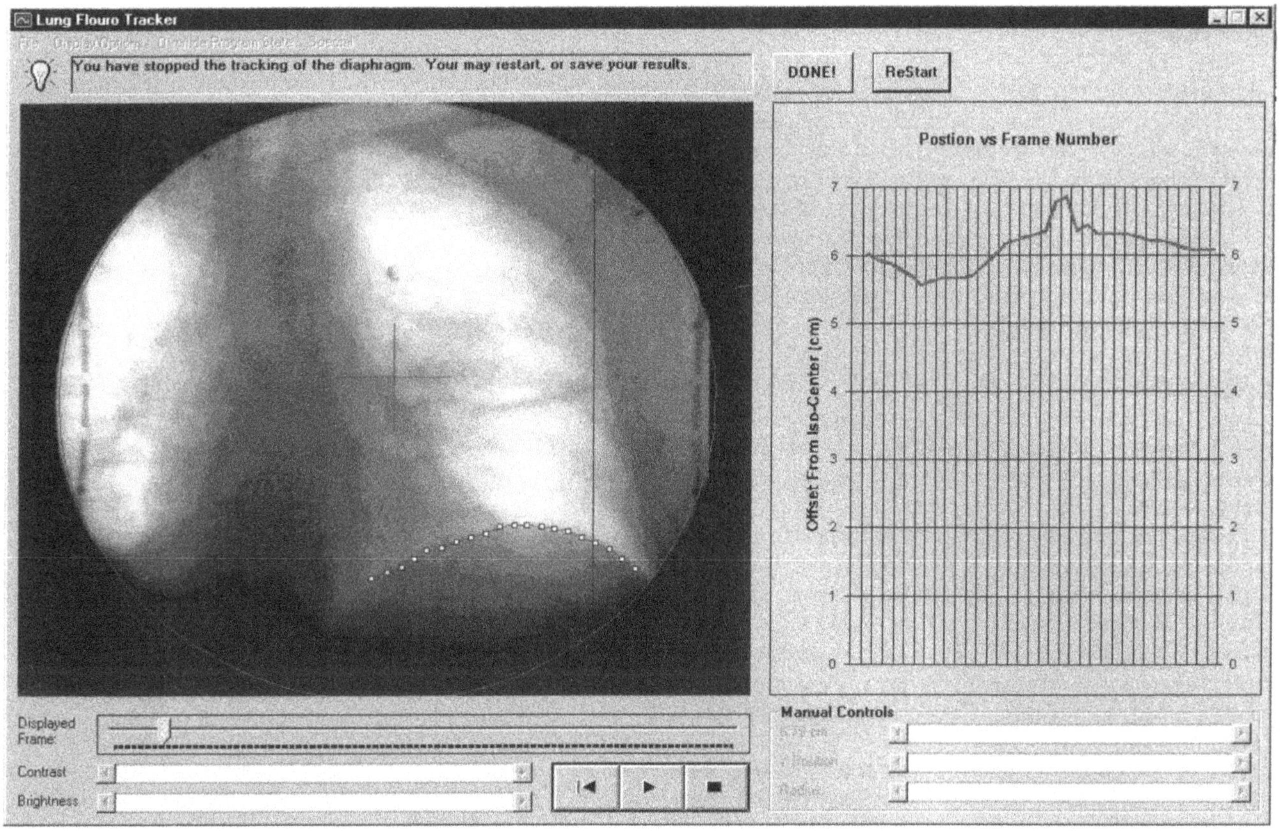


**Figure 1:** The program during diaphragm tracking.

## Results

Reproducibility was established by repeating analysis of the same movie five times, and examining positional variability of the tracked diaphragm apex. The average positional variation between each tracking at each point in time was 1 mm, or approximately 2 pixels.

The accuracy of automated tracking was directly compared (Figures 2, 3) to manually tracking using fluoroscopic studies of lung cancer patients under a deep inspiration breath hold maneuver [3]. Agreement is mostly within 1-2 mm with deviation being greatest (3 mm) at maximum inspirations. This difference at inspiration is likely the result of differences in the definition of the position of the diaphragm, since the manual tracking used an average of a number of positions along the diaphragm at each frame, while the automated tracking used only one.

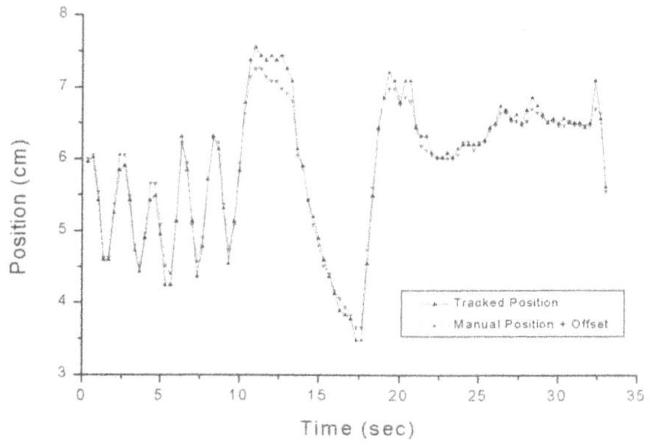


**Figure 2:** Comparison with manualy determined diaphragm position.

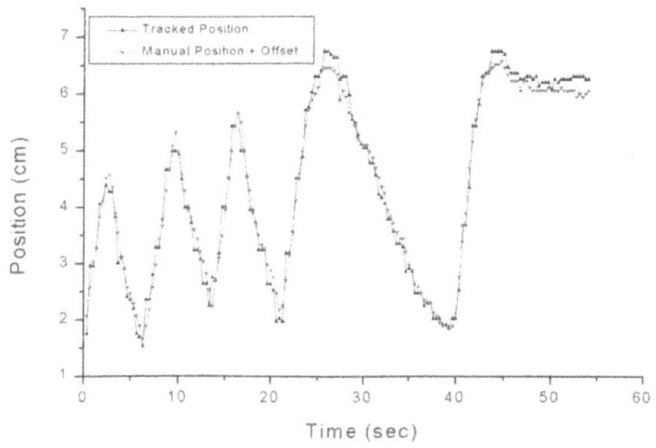


**Figure 3:** Comparison with manualy determined diaphragm position.

## Conclusion

The automated tool described here provides an accurate and robust means of quantifying respiratory organ motion in fluoroscopic studies. The program's speed and ease of use allow for fluoroscopic measurement of such motion in a clinical setting, in addition to providing a valuable research tool. Further computational optimization of the algorithm, combined with it's application to Anterior/Posterior motion, may lead to direct fluoroscopically gated treatment without the need for invasive procedures [4].

## References

[1] Gig Mageras. "Interventional Strategies for Reducing Respiratory-Induced Motion in External Beam Therapy," These Proceedings

[2]D. Geiger, A. Gupta, L. A. Costa, and J. Vlontzos. "Dynamic Programming for detecting, tracking, and matching deformable contours." PAMI, 17:294-302, 1995.

[3] Mah D, Hanley J, Rosenzweig KE, Yorke E, Ling CC Leibel SA, Fuks Z, Mageras GS "The Deep Inspiration Breath Hold Technique for the Treatment of Lung Cancer: The First 200 Treatments," Int. J Radit. Oncol. Biol Phys 45 Suppl 3: p206.

[4] Shirato H, Shimizu S, Shimizu T, Akita H, Kurauchi N, Shinohara N, Ogura S, Harabayashi T, Aoyama H, Miyasaka K. "Fluoroscopic Real-Time Tumor Tracking Radiotherapy," Int. J Radit. Oncol. Biol Phys 45 Suppl 3: p206.

# The use of artificial neural networks in mammographic screening

**Tomasz Kabarowski**

Department of Computer Science and Management, Technical University of Wroclaw, ul. Wybrzeze Wyspianskiego, Wroclaw, Poland
*mail address: ul. Sieradzka 7/104, 45-308, Opole, Poland*

## Introduction

Breast cancer is one of the most frequently observed cases of tumour among women. Recently, a number of Oncological Departments organises mammographic screenings for women from the regional institutions. Thousands of patients need to be separately examined for the individual diagnosis to be given. The aim of this project was to develop a specialised system, which could be used for the analysis and subdivision of the mammographic screenings into two following categories. One group would consist of images of healthy patients, while the other would gather all cases, which call for further investigation and individual diagnosis on the part of the specialist. At the same time, the second group would be automatically prediagnosed by the system.

## Assumptions

The possibility of cancer occurrence can be specified due to the observation of at least one of the typical pathologies, among which the commonest are approximately spherical or stellate shaped masses, microcalcifications, and asymmetry between breasts. The system was designed to examine the presence of the occurring pathologies so it should recognise them from the mammogram as the specialists do. The way to achieve this is to use artificial neural networks, which are most popular artificial intelligence mechanisms for pattern recognition. The data extracted as a result of the processesing of the mammographic image constructs an input layer of the neural network. After the neural processing the output of the network says if the case is suspicious of tumour existence or not.

## Preprocessing of digital mammogram

The data, which is presented to the system for diagnosis are two mamographic images (one for each breast, made in cranio-cadual projection) for each patient. The differentiated character of pathologies, which should be detected, made it necessary to create separate filters for each pathology. In every single method, an image or its fragment was initially filtered, with the use of median filter, in order diminish most of the artefacts. The following are short descriptions of pre-processing techniques used during detection of two pathologies being discussed here.

Spherical or stellate shaped mass: During the detection of this kind of pathology, only a part of a pictorial scene undergoes filtering. Such a fragment, after the most of redundant noises have been minimised, is high passed filtered, and by the time its histogram has been equalised, the number of the colours is reduced.

Histogram is a simple and very useful function, which makes it possible to depict an image globally. Formally, histogram is a function $h(i)$, where

$$h(i) = \sum_{m=0}^{M-1}\sum_{n=0}^{N-1} p\left(\frac{i}{(m,n)}\right), \qquad \text{where } i = 0,1,\ldots,2^B - 1,$$

$$\text{where } p\left(\frac{i}{(m,n)}\right) = \begin{cases} 1, & \textit{when} \quad L(m,n) = 1 \\ 0, & \textit{otherwise} \end{cases},$$

where $L$ is a gray level of pixel $(m.,n)$ on a 2D image.

If we assume that for the certain integers $m$ and $n$, which belong to the domain of the function $h(i)$, the conditions $h(m)>0$ and $h(n)>0$ and $h(i)=0$ for $m<i<n$ are fulfilled, then we should modify the points $m$ and $n$ in such a way to minimise the value $Q$, where $Q$ is:

$$Q = \left| \frac{\sum_{i=0}^{2^B-1} h(i)}{2^B - 1} - \frac{h(m)}{n-m} \right|.$$

Due to such filtering the potential suspicious object could be extracted and transformed into the input signals for the neural networks.

Process of graphical preprocessing of an example of image is presented on Image 1.

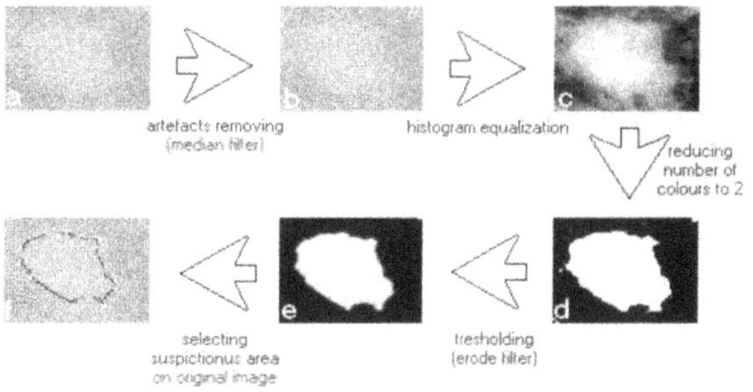


**Image 1** Detection of spherical shaped pathology – graphical preprocessing. Picture **a** – original "windowed" image fragment; picture **b** – image fragment after noise removing; picture **c** – after histogram equalisation; picture **d** – after reducing number of colours; picture **e** – after noise removing; picture **f** – image fragment with selected suspicious object.

After graphical preprocessing, if there are any suspicious object detected, system retrieves data about them from the image. Retrieved data is being scaled and presented as an input layer for the feed-forward neural network, which is to give an answer whether the selected object is a tumour or not. The object's data are:

- Feret's shape coefficient $R_F = \frac{L_h}{L_v}$, where $L_h$ is a maximum horizontal diameter and $L_v$ is a maximum vertical diameter
- Circular coefficients $R_c = 2\sqrt{\frac{S}{\pi}}$ and $R_D = \frac{L}{\pi}$, where $S$ is a field of the object, and $L$ is a circumference of the object
- Feret's diameters
- 4 Avg. edge gradients
- Region contrast
- Colour amplitude
- Average gray level
- Feret's width and height, each measured in 2 points placed proportionally to object size
- Object size
- Region contrast, color amplitude and average gray level extracted from symmetrically located fragment in the second mammogram of a patient

Those 20 features are served to an ANN as an input (after being scaled).

Microcalcification: The preprocessing process is very similar to the one used for detecting large objects. The main difference is the window size, which is much smaller. That's why, before a "windowed" fragment of an image is preprocessed, it is enlarged. It gives the possibility of using same scaling functions when counting network input values of extracted object. Number of network inputs is smaller this time, as it's not necessary to count additional values from symmetrically located fragment in the second mammogram.
As a microcalcification itself is not a pathology, if it is detected by a system, it does not necessarily mean that a patient is seek. The information about the found pathology is stored until the whole image has been processed. At that moment, the frequency of microcalcification occurence is being taken into account. If a number of microcalcifications on a certain area is too high, the system indicates that it might cause a pathology and classifies patient as "suspected of having cancer".
If there is just a few microcalcifications located on a large area, then it is classified as "normal" (and indeed it is normal).

## Characteristics of neural networks used

All three pathologies are ascribed to individual neural nets, which entails a new set of learning patterns. For instance, for the net that recognises the spherical or stellate shapes, the patterns appeared to be the fragments of numerous images, which did or did not include given pathology. The initial selection has showed, that the feed-forward neural network learned with a backpropagation method is the most appropriate for the system's demands. The input layer of the neural network was comprised of various inputs including Feret's shape coefficient of the examined object, Feret's diameter, Feret's dimensions measured in points which are placed proportionally to object's size, object's position, and similar data extracted from symmetrically located fragment of the second breast's mammogram, among the others. The network, which was learned by using backpropagation method consisted of two hidden layers. The output of the neural net pointed to the absence or presence of the pathology.

## Materials

322 films of 161 patients containing all kinds of pathologies, which have been digitised to 50 micron pixel edge by a Joyce-Liebl scanning microdensitometer, were provided by the Mammographic Image Analysis Society (MIAS). One projection (craniocaudal) was available for all patients.

## Results

The aim of this project was to develop a system, which would detect and classify most of the normal cases (those, which do not need specialist's further attention). This approach requires faultless analysis of those images that indicate traces of tumour. On the other hand, it may allow minor mistakes while analysing mammograms, which are normal cases. That is why the system must be consistent in detecting pathologies rather than categorising a particular image as a non-suspicious case. In the result of the tests, carried out on the mammograms of 160 patients from which 40% were suspected of having cancer, and allowing for the 0% negative-bad error, about 68% of examined cases was properly classified as normal ones. Such an outcome guaranties the shortening of physician's work time by much more than a half, and lowers the costs of all treatments as well.
The researches on this project are still being carried out, and it is believed to be successively expanded in the future. The results that have been reached so far are very promising.
The researches concerned with the usage of wavelet transform for the digital mammogram preprocessing are still carried out now. The initial results will be reached soon.

## References

1. E. Sorantin, F. Schmidt, H. Mayer, M. Becker, C. Szepesvari, E. Graif, E. Schuetz, P. Winkler *Automated breast cancer detection in digitized mammograms – An application of neural nets*, Univ. Hospital Graz, Austria, 1997
2. R. Zwiggelaar, J.E. Schumm, C.J. Tylor *The Detection of Abnormal Masses in Mammograms*, University of Manchester, UK, 1997
3. R. Gupta, P.E. Undrill *The use of texture analysis to identify suspicious masses in mammography*, University of Aberdeen, 1995
4. B.J.M. van Abel *Classification of Microcalcifications by Artificial Neural Networks*, master thesis: 424, Catholic University Nijmegen, 1997

5. T.C. Parr, R. Zwiggelaar, C.J. Taylor, S.M. Astley, C.R.M. Boggis *The detection of stellate lesions in digital mammography*, Univ. Of Menchester, UK, 1997
6. R. Tadeusiewicz, P. Korohoda *Komputerowa analiza i przetwarzanie obrazów*, WFPT Kraków, Poland, 1997

# Imaging *in situ* activated $^{15}O$ to study tumor hypoxia

**John Wong[1], Elwood Armour[1], Mark Oldham[1], Jeff Siewerdsen[1], Patrick Gavin[2], William Worstell[3], Valery Zavarzin[3], Steve Sutlief[4] and John Allen[5].**

[1]William Beaumont Hospital, Royal Oak, MI, USA; [2]Washington State University, Pullman, WA, USA; [3]Tomotronics Inc., Wayland, MA, USA; [4]VA Hospital at Puget Sound, Seattle, WA, USA; [5]Elekta Oncology Systems, Crawley, UK.

## Introduction

Advances in computer and imaging technologies in the last 5 years have made possible significant improvement in our ability to optimize and deliver a patient's treatment. The imaging information also enables us to have a better understanding of geometric treatment uncertainty and to develop effective strategies to ensure accurate treatment. Smaller planning target volumes and higher radiation doses can now be prescribed for improving local control. A comprehensive review of these advances has recently been published [1]. It is important to note that improvement in the geometric accuracy of treatment delivery does not necessarily result in an improvement in local control. Critical biological features of a tumor, such as the extent of micro-invasion, non-uniform cell doubling time and non-uniform radio-sensitivity are largely unknown and ignored in treatment planning. Consequently, important questions such as the merits of uniform or non-uniform dose distribution cannot be resolved. It is clear, as treatment becomes more accurate, efforts must now be directed to improving our understanding of the biological status of the tumor and its impact on treatment outcome.

One of the most important tumor characteristics is tumor hypoxia. To date, several experimental methods for identifying hypoxic regions in human tumors have been developed. These include the measurement of tumor oxygen tension with invasive electrodes [2,3], and the study of perfusion or the uptake of hypoxic cell affinic compounds using MRI [4] and PET [5] imaging techniques. Each has merits and limitations. However, none is practical enough to allow the necessary repeat analysis of the role of hypoxia, and re-oxygenation, in affecting the response of human tumors during a course of radiotherapy.

One promising method to study tumor hypoxia in conjunction with radiation therapy is by measuring the washout of accelerator activated $^{15}O$. The positron emitting radio-isotope $^{15}O$ is produced *in situ* from stable $^{16}O$ via the ($\gamma$,n) reaction using high energy photons (>20MeV). As oxygen exists mostly in the form of water in a tumor, the washout of $^{15}O$ is a surrogate marker of tumor perfusion, which in turn serves as a surrogate marker of tumor hypoxia. The method, originally proposed by Hughes et al in the late 1970's [6,7], was limited to simple volumetric coincidence counting due to the short 2 min half-life and the low activity produced at therapeutic dose levels (at ~ 0.1 μCi per cc per 200 cGy). Still, the earlier studies showed that there were mobile and non-mobile components to the $^{15}O$ washout, supporting the presence of poorly perfused or necrotic regions in the tumor. Unfortunately, the method was all but abandoned by the mid-80's, in part due to the method's inability to provide positional information, and in part due to the demise of most medical accelerators that were capable of producing the necessary high energy photon beam for $^{15}O$ activation.

In this article, we describe a new approach to study the washout of accelerator generated $^{15}O$ by imaging the variation of its spatial distribution with time.

## Material and methods

The operating characteristics of an Elekta SL-25 series accelerator were modified to allow the acceleration of electrons to an energy of ~ 29 MeV. The beam current was reduced. The RF power was increased. The current of the focussing magnet was adjusted to direct the electrons to strike the x-ray target. All filtration assembly within the collimation structure was removed from the beam-line to increase output.

In order to overcome the hurdle of low activity level and short half-life $^{15}O$, the new portable PET camera technology from Tomotronics, Inc. was employed [8]. The portable PET camera system consisted of a parallel-opposed pair of detector heads. Data were acquired with the camera heads stationary. The limited angle acquisition geometry was designed for single organ imaging, such as positron emission tomography. Three dimensional (3D) tomographic images were reconstructed by resolving the parallax information of the coincidence data.

A small portable PET system was provided by Tomotronics for imaging the spatial distribution of the in situ activated $^{15}O$. Each of the 2 camera heads consisted of 18 x 18 GSO crystals packed within a 6 cm by 6 cm housing. Each crystal had a cross-sectional area of 3 mm x 3 mm, and 8 mm long. Scintillation signal was acquired with an array of multi-channel PMTs. Utilities were implemented for energy and coincidence discrimination. The theoretical resolving power of the device was better than 3 mm FWHM for a single point source placed in the middle of a ~ 12 cm separation between the camera heads.

A pet dog with a spontaneous brain tumor was recruited for our feasibility study, with appropriate consent from the owner. The dog was anesthetized and immobilized in a body cast. The study volume was sandwiched between the 2 camera heads separated by 14 cm. The SSD was 62 cm. Activation was performed using a pencil beam and 2D slice beams. An activation dose of 300 cGy was employed, delivered in < 18 sec. Activities were produced in a plane parallel to the camera heads. The camera heads were left in treatment room during activation in order to facilitate data acquisition in < 5 sec after beam-off. Ten minutes of coincidence data were acquired. The simplified activation geometry greatly reduced background signal from out-of-plane activity and allowed reconstruction of a 2D image using simple back projection technique.

## Results and discussion

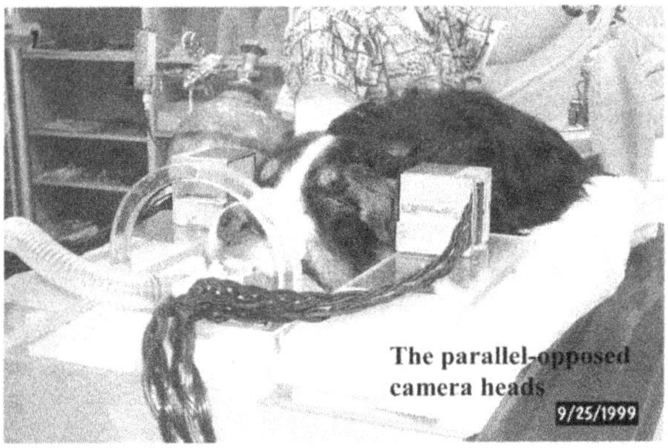


**Figure 1.** Study subject immobilized with dental cast and positioned between the PET camera heads.

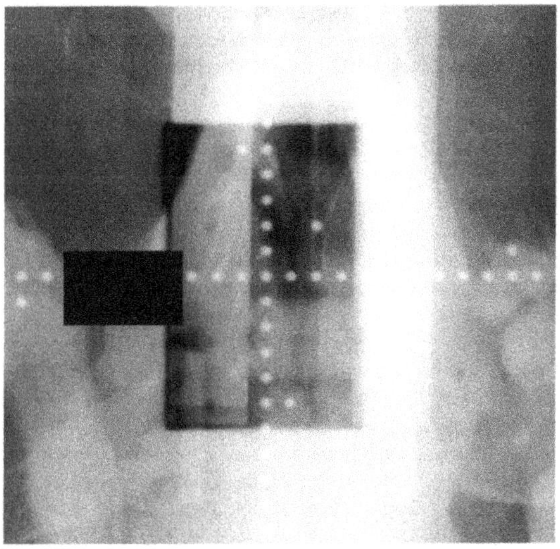

**Figure 2.** A double-exposed AP port film showing a pencil beam that was used for the activation study. The activation/ imaging session included other slice beams (not shown) and was performed in sequence.

Figure 1 shows the dog patient in the study position with the study volume sandwiched between the camera heads of the portable PET system. Figure 2 shows a double exposed AP port film depicting the position of a 1.2 cm x 1.2 cm activation beam. About 0.25 μCi of $^{15}O$ activity per cc was produced. A much smaller amount of $^{11}C$ activity was also produced, estimated to be less than 25 times that of the $^{15}O$ activity. The half-life of $^{11}C$ is ~ 20 min. Carbon atoms can be assumed to be entirely bounded in non-mobile biological molecules in tissue.

Figure 3 shows the 10 minutes of PET data presented in 5 time-binned images, with each image containing roughly the same number of counts. The portable PET system did not have the appropriate utility for the study of temporal information and the temporal division of the images after beam-off was estimated. Time-binned Image 1 spanned from 5 – 20 sec after beam-off; Image 2 spanned from 20 to 60 sec; Image 3 from 1 to 2 min; Image 4 from 2 to 4 min; and Image 5 from 4 to 10 min.

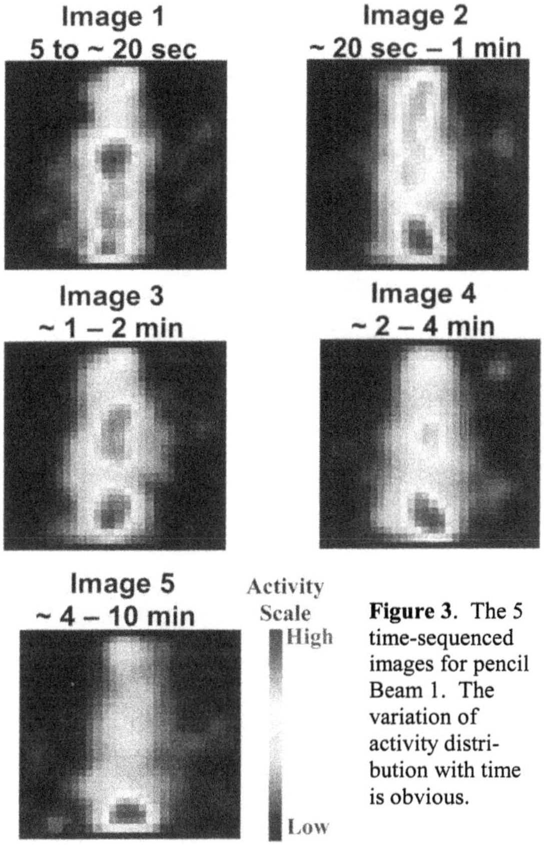


**Figure 3.** The 5 time-sequenced images for pencil Beam 1. The variation of activity distribution with time is obvious.

Quantitative analysis of washout parameters could not be made with the data from our feasibility studies. Qualitatively, Images 1 and 2 contain components of washout events that occurred relatively quick, as would be the case for normally perfused tissues. Images 3 and 4 depict washout events of moderate rates. Image 5 depicts the combined distributions of very slow washout events and non-mobile activities.

Figure 4 shows the activity distribution of time-binned Image 1 (top panel) and 5 (bottom panel) superimposed on the anatomic information of the MRI slice. The very slow washout events persisted in the region where the tumor resided.

## Conclusion

Our feasibility studies were very promising. Clearly, the accelerator-PET approach was capable of producing images of *in situ* activated $^{15}O$ in the dog brain and tumor. While our research emphasizes tumor perfusion, it was reassuring that the washout patterns corresponded with physiologically expected behavior. Results from other activated volumes using slice beams show that there are noticeable areas of fast washout, which are not surprising since the brain is a very well perfused organ. Slow washout regions seem to be associated with the presence of stable structure, such as those associated with nasal passages, bones and ventricles; but also most importantly, some regions of the tumor. However, any association of our washout results with tumor hypoxia will be premature and cannot be proven with the current data. It is clear that confirmatory experiments using $O_2$ electrode or immunohistochemical methods are needed to compare PET

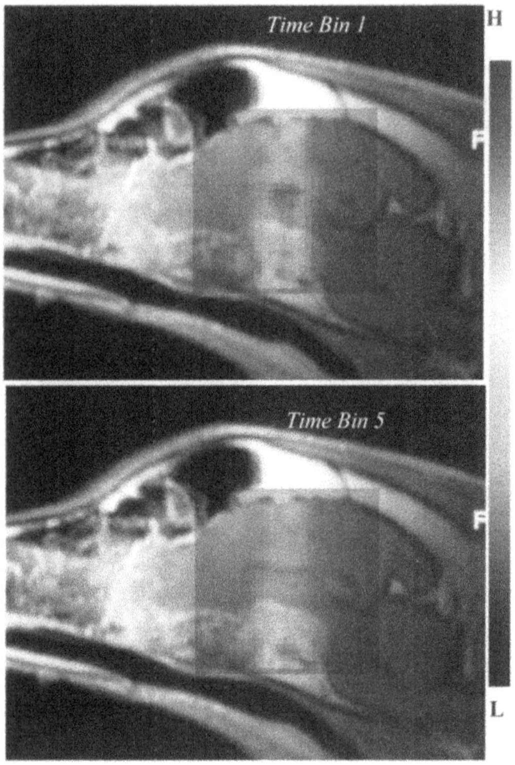


**Figure 4**. Activity distributions in time bin 1 (top) and 5 (bottom) overlaid on the irradiated MRI anatomy for the Pencil Beam study. H denotes high activity on the accompanying scale, and L denotes low activity.

images to the existence of hypoxia. These experiments are a critical part of our future study.

Our studies demonstrated the immense value of having spatial information in the form of an image rather than only having a single bulk value for $^{15}O$ washout. The information not only allows spatial characterization of the tumor, but also avoids the bias of results due to the regions of slow $H_2O$ movement in normal tissues that are also activated. Finally, because activation can be performed as part of the treatment, we are optimistic that our approach of imaging in-situ activated $^{15}O$ holds potential of becoming an important approach to study, or even to manage, tumor perfusion and hypoxia in the clinical setting.

## Acknowledgement

The authors wish to thank Dr. Steve Sapareto of the University of Arizona at Tucson for the valuable discussion on activation capability of the Elekta accelerator; and Mr. Kevin Brown for making available the technical resources of Elekta to support our study.

## References

[1]Radiation Therapy Treatment Optimization. 1999 T.R. Mackie, guest ed., J.E. Tepper, ed. *Semin Radiat Oncol* **9**.

[2]Hoekel M, Knoop C, Schlenger K, Vorndran Bm Baussmann E, Mitze M, Knapstein PG, and Vaupel P (1993) Intramtumoral pO2 predicts survival in advanced cancer of the uterine cervix. *Radiother Oncol* **26** 45-50.

[3]Kavanagh MC, Minkin S and Hill RP (1996) Comparing techniques of measuring tumor hypoxia in different murine tumors: Eppendorf pO2 histograph, [3H]misonidazole binding and paired survivial assay. *Radiat Res* **145** 491-500.

[4]Robinson SP, Howe FA, Rodrigues LM, Stubbs M and Griffiths JR (1998) Magnetic resonance imaging techniques for monitoring changes in tumor oxygenation and blood flow. *Semin Radiat Oncol* **8** 197-207

[5]Rasey JS, Koh WJ, Evans ML, Peterson LM, Lewellen TK, Graham MM and Krohn KA (1996) Quantifying regional hypoxia in human tumors with positron emission tomography of [18F]fluoro-misonidazole: a pretherapy study of 37 patients. *Int J Radiat Oncol Biol Phys* **36** 417-428.

[6]Hughes WL, Nussbaum GH, Connolly R, Emami B and Reilly (1979) Tissue perfusion rate determined from the decay of oxygen-15 activity after photon activation in situ. *Science* **204** 1215-1217.

[7]Ten Haken RK, Nussbaum GH, Emami B and Hughes WL (1981) Photon activation-$^{15}O$ decay studies of tumor blood flow. *Med Phys* **8** 324-336.

[8]Worstell W, Johnson O, Kudrolli H and Zavarzin V (1998) First results with high resolution PET detector modules using wavelength-shifting fibers. *Proc IEEE Trans Nucl Sci* **45** 2993-2999.

# Application to Lung Conformal Radiotherapy of a SPECT and Computerised Tomography (C.T.) Image Registration Method

**F. Courbon MD[1], O. Caselles PhD[2], Ph. Giraud MD[3], P. Francois[2], J.M. Bachaud MD[4], F. Arboucalot MD[5] A. Boneu MD[6]**

[1]Service de Médecine Nucléaire, [2]Unité de Radiophysique, [4]Service de Radiothérapie, [5]Service de Radiologie: Institut Claudius Regaud. 20-24 rue du Pont Saint Pierre 31052 Toulouse Cedex. [3]Service de Radiothérapie Hôpital de Tenon 4 rue de Chine 75020 Paris.

## Introduction

Owing to the proximity of the critical structures, conventional radiotherapy doesn't allow one to exceed the total dose of 65 Gy delivered to the target volume, which is notably insufficient (1). 3D conformal radiotherapy allows one to exceed this dose . Traditional simulation tends to be replaced by virtual 3 dimensional simulation. Dose Volume Histogram takes into account the quantity of pulmonary parenchyma included in the treated volume without keeping count of its functional characters (2). This has many consequences, because this treatment is frequently used in subjects with limited extension of tumour but inoperable .for the reason of insufficient respiratory condition. The purpose of this study is to validate a coupled exploration procedure, both scintigraphic (ventilation-perfusion tomo-scintigraphy) and tomodensitometric, applicable to radiotherapy of the lung (3.4.5) .

## Material and methods

Our work involves two stages: The first is a preclinical study has the purpose of validating the information links maintaining the transfer and the superimposition of images. The second stage is a study of clinical feasibility on a small group of patients with unresecable lung carcinoma. This second stage has the essential purpose of using an immobilisation system on a patient, allowing a strict and reproducible geometry for both the acquisition and the treatment.

### Preclinical study

- Phantom: elliptical Jaszczack's phantom (ECT Elliptical Phantom, DATA SPECTRUM Corporation, Hillsborough U.S.A.) This phantom contains full spheres or hollow spheres. The hollow ones can be filled with a solution of 3.3MBq/l of $^{99m}$Tc. The phantom is filled with an homogeneous solution of 3MBq/l of $^{99m}$Tc.
- Scintigraphy: HELIX® (ELSCINT, Haïfa, Israël) gamma camera, equipped with two large rectangular field detectors.
  °Tomographic mode over 360° with 60 projections of two minutes every 6°.
  °Matrix size : 128x128 pixels. The images are reconstructed by filtered back projection (METZ filter)
  °Image treatment computer Xpert-Pro ® (ELSCINT, Haïfa, Israël)
- Tomodensitometry : Philips SR7000 CT-scan (PHILIPS, Eindhoven, The Netherland) in spiral mode with a slice thickness of 10mm, a transfer speed from the test layer of 10mm/second and a pitch of 1.
- Image transfer : The CT images are converted to the DICOM 3.0 format and then transferred onto the Xpert-Pro® (ELSCINT Haïfa, Israël) workstation via the Ethernet network. The matrix size of the reconstructed slices is reduced to 128x128 pixels during the conversion into an Elscint proprietary format. The superimposition of the images is achieved using rigid fusion with the help of Xpert-match® software (ELSCINT, Haïfa, Israël).

### Study of clinical feasibility

- Patients : six patients suffering from respiratory failure with lung cancer are included.
- Immobilisation : Using radiotransparent support on which an expansive rubber polyurethane mould is mounted. The patient is placed in the mould in the treatment position during the acquisition of images (SPECT and CT), and for the duration of the irradiation.
- Tomoscintigraphic acquisitions : It is a SPECT double isotope acquisition (150MBq of intravenously injected $^{99m}$Tc radiolabelled microspheres CIS BIO INTERNATIONAL, $^{81m}$Kr gas MALLINCKRODT, Petten, Holland). $^{99m}$Tc radiolabelled markers are placed on the patients skin.. The position of these markers is indicated on the skin by felt tip pen.
- CT-scan acquisition. The acquisition is performed in spiral mode, with a delayed injection of contrast medium (1ml/kg, 1ml/minute flow) with the largest field of view (48mm). The thickness of the slices is 10mm, the transfer speed is 10mm/s, and the pitch of reconstruction is 1. Radio-opaque markers are placed according to the marked points on the skin.
- Treatment, transfer and image fusion. The translations, rotations, and scale changes allowing the matching of SPECT slices with CT images are therefore determined awing to the 3 visible landmarks on CT and perfusion SPECT images. The characteristic parameters are registered and applied to the ventilation SPECT data

### Results and discussion

Preclinical study: At the time of fusion, one doesn't observe any gap between the positioning of radioactive and radio-opaque markers. This procedure of superimposition of images, allows for an easy location of "cold volumes" corresponding zones of pulmonary hypoperfusion and hypoventilation, hereby validating the fusion process (Fig.1)

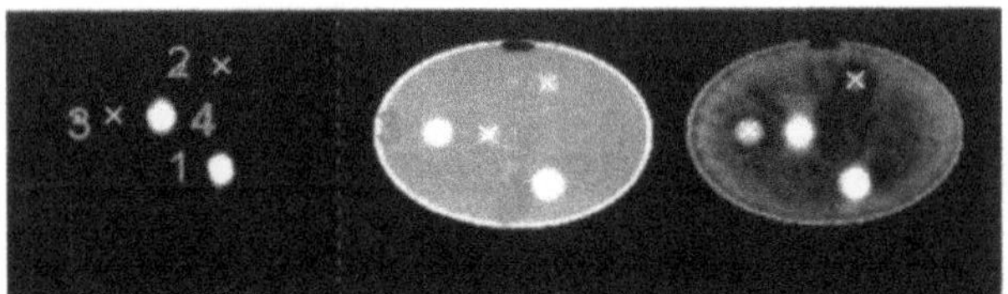


**Figure 1) ECT Phantom** (9.25MBq/l $^{99m}$Tc)
Radioactive spheres : n°1 (31.8mm) and n°4 (36mm)
Non radioactive spheres : n°2 (12.7mm) and n°3 (25.4mm)

**Clinical feasibility study.** The bulk of the immobilisation system and the reduced diameter of the gamma camera has led us to place patients prone. This position is well tolerated by all patients. For 5 out of 6 patients "hybrid" images are found to be satisfactory. One note the importance given to each of the test and the correct superimposition of the external markers (Fig. 2).

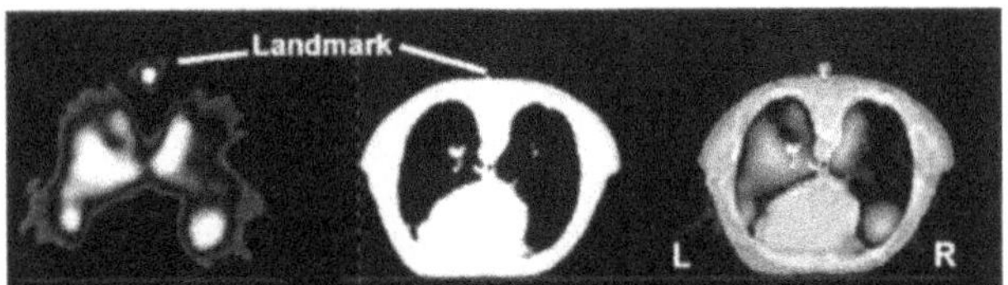


**Figure 2) Perfusion study + CT** $^{99m}$Tc tomoscintigraphy
Axial slices with external landmarks

Diaphragmatic domes and trachea (Krypton flow) are reliable landmarks (Fig3).

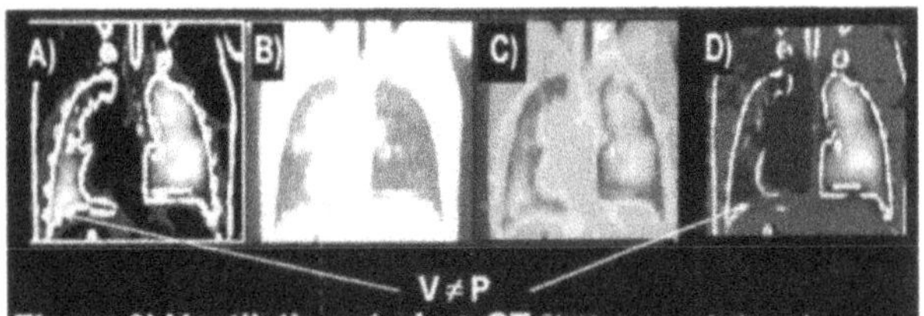


**Figure 3) Ventilation study + CT** $^{81m}$Kr tomoscintigraphy
Coronal slices A+B=C (D=Perfusion study coronal slice) ↙ $^{81m}$Kr flow

Scintigraphic information changed completely the ballistics (entry point and irradiation beam angle) of radiotherapy treatment in 5 out of 5 patients.
Scintigraphic ventilation data gave complementary information in 3 out of 5 patients. The total duration of the procedure is about 2 hours, which is compatible with routine clinical practice.

## Discussion

This procedure of images fusion seems operational and well tolerated. According to this preliminary study, it appears that scintigraphic information could be used to determine the beam geometry of the treatment of patients with respiratory insufficiency. The clinical relèvance of this procedure must be demonstrated by a prospective trial evaluating radiation tolerance

## Conclusion

We have highlighted a technique of superimposition of SPECT and CT images of the lung. This procedure should induce a better preservation of functional parenchyma This procedure is compatible with routine clinical practice. It seems useful for the choice of beam geometry for patient with respiratory insufficiency.
Integration of 3 dimensional scintigraphic images with dose volume histograms used for virtual simulation of conformational radiotherapy is still in progress. Depending from a prospective clinical trail using this procedure, ventilation-perfusion study could be of a clinical value for the conformal radiotherapy of the lung.

## References

[1] Arriagada R., Le Chevalier T., Quoix E. et al. Effect of chemotherapy on locally advanced non-small cell lung carcinoma: A randomized study of 353 patients. 1991. *Int J Radiat Oncol Biol Phys*; **20**:1183-1190.

[2] Rosenman J., Hazuka M.B., Martel M.K. Three-dimensional treatment planning in lung cancer radiotherapy. In Lung cancer: 1996 *Principles and Practice*, HI Pass, JB Mitchell, DH Johson, AT Turrisi eds. Lippincott-Raven, Philadelphia,:685-696,

[3] Damen E.M.F, Muller S.H., Boersman L.J., de Boer R. W. and Lebesque J. Quantifying local lung perfusion and ventillation using correlated SPECT and CT data. 1994 *Nucl Med*; **35**:784-792.

[4] Shinoara S., Arikawa K. Radioisotopic assessment on developpement of radiation pneumonitis and fibrosis. 1972 *Australia Radiol*,**16**:363-366

[5] Zwijnenburg A., Lebesque J., Roos C.M., Jansen H.M., Van der Schoot J.B., Marcuse H.R.. 1989 Early detection of irradiation induced lung damage using ventilation-perfusion single photon emission computed tomography. In : Zwijnenburg A ., ed. *Ventilation-perfusion studies using SPECT*. Amsterdam : Thesis;: 43-53

# FDG-PET Imaging for Radiation Therapy in Head and Neck Cancer

**Sunyoung Jang,[1] Peter Bloch,[1] Mijin Yun,[2] Timothy Zhu,[1] David Rosenthal,[1] Michael Needham,[1] Abass Alavi[2] and Bengt Bjarngard[1]**

Departments of [1]Radiation Oncology and [2]Radiology, University of Pennsylvania Medical Center, Philadelphia, PA 19104

## Introduction

Imaging of the accumulation of 18F-labeled fluoro deoxyglucose (FDG) using positron emission tomography (PET) is being used clinically for the evaluation of the physiological and pathological status of tissues *in situ*. FDG-PET imaging studies of patients with head and neck lesions have previously been shown to be useful for staging of the disease and for evaluating changes in tumor metabolism during a course of radiotherapy [1-3]. The purpose of this study is to evaluate the volume of elevated uptake of FDG in head and neck tumors and correlate these findings with the planning target volume (PTV) delineated on CT and MR images.

## Material and methods

FDG-PET imaging studies were preformed on 14 patients with 19 discrete head and neck tumors to determine the volume of elevated accumulation of FDG. The anatomical sites of these tumors are shown in Table 1. PET imaging studies were performed 1 hour following the injection of approximately 2.5 MBq/kg. The images were acquired using NaI(Tl) based PET scanners, UGM 240H or UGM CPET. The PET cameras are used clinically in the PET-Center at the Hospital of the University of Pennsylvania. A 3D-imaging data set consisted of images from the top of the skull to the shoulders at 4 mm slice interval. Acquisition time was 12 to 24 minutes. The spatial resolution of both PET cameras was approximately 6 mm [4]. The sensitivities of the UGM 240H and UGM CPET were 4.9 and 20.0 $cps.Bq^{-1}.cm^3$, respectively. The emission images were reconstructed using an ordered-subset expectation maximization algorithm (OSEM) [5]. The reconstructed 3D-imaging data consisted of cubic voxels with 4 mm on a side. The emission data was corrected for the radioactive decay and the variation in attenuation of the 511 keV annihilation radiation with depth. The attenuation correction was performed using Cs-137 gamma ray transmission images acquired with the PET scanner [6].

Standard uptake values (SUV) were measured in selected regions-of-interest (ROI). These ROIs were defined by a nuclear medicine physician as the volume containing the tumor $V_T$ and in a region within the same organ containing normal tissues $V_{NOR}$. The SUV was calculated using the following relationship:

$$SUV = \frac{\text{mean activity}(MBq/cm^3)\text{ in ROI}}{\text{injected activity}(MBq)/\text{body weight}(kg)} \quad (1)$$

| Tumor site | # Tumors | SUV | Tumor contrast | # PET Volumes elevated | # CT PVT | # MR PVT |
|---|---|---|---|---|---|---|
| Tongue | 6 | 2 | 4 | 1 | | 1 |
| Neck | 5 | 3 | 2 | 2 | 1 | 1 |
| Lymph node | 4 | 2 | 2 | | | |
| Mandible | 1 | | 1 | 1 | 1 | |
| Salivary gland | 1 | | 1 | | | |
| Naso-pharyngeal | 1 | | 1 | | | |
| Tonsil | 1 | | 1 | 1 | | 1 |

#: number of.

**Table 1:** Tumor sites and studies performed:

The conversion from counts to activity was previously determined for each PET scanner. The $SUV_T$ and $SUV_{NOR}$ were evaluated with eq. 1 for the ROIs including the tumor and normal areas in the same organ respectively. The SUVs were determined in 4 patients with 7 discrete tumor foci. The selected ROIs for a tumor in the neck and normal tissues are shown in Figure 1.

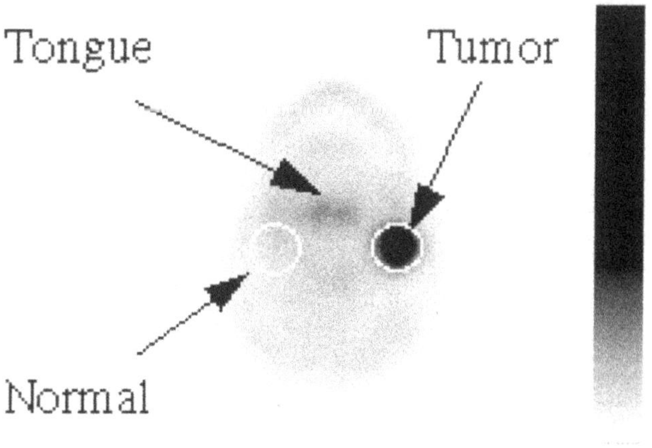


**Figure 1:** ROI measurements for SUV and tumor contrast.

A tumor contrast ratio ($C_T$) was evaluated for each study by

$$C_T = (N_T - N_{NOR}) / N_T \quad (2)$$

where $N_T$ and $N_{NOR}$ represent the number of counts in the ROI's corresponding to tumor and normal tissues, respectively.

The $C_T$ values were determined in 9 patients with 12 discrete tumor foci.

Radiation Oncology and Radiology physicians defined the PTV on CT or MR images. These imaging studies were acquired with pixel sizes of 0.5 and 1.0 mm with 5 mm slice thickness for the CT and MR images, respectively. A threshold method was used to evaluate the volume of tissue with elevated activity. The threshold SUV value was set at 0.4 times the maximum SUV found in the volume $V_T$. The number of voxels above this threshold was used to determine the tissue volume with elevated uptake of FDG. The PTV was compared with the volume of elevated SUVs.

## Results and discussion

The mean $SUV_T$ and $SUV_{NOR}$ in the tumor and normal tissue was 3.5 +/- 1.0 and 1.2 +/-0.7, respectively. These differences are statistically significant with a *p*-value less than 0.01.

The mean $C_T$ value measured for twelve head and neck tumors was $0.70 \pm 0.14$ with a range between 0.51 and 0.89. Tissues with $C_T$ greater than 0.5 are easily visualized on PET images.

In Table 2 the PTV defined on CT or MR images are compared with the volume of tissue having SUV above 40% of the maximum SUV in the tumor region. This preliminary data suggest that the volume of tissue with elevated SUVs are less than PTV. This may indicate that there are metabolically inactive regions within the PTV.

## Conclusion

The preliminary data demonstrated that in head and neck tumors there are regions with elevated metabolic activity as indicated by the accumulation of FDG. The uptake in the tumor regions is approximately 3 times greater than the normal regions. In general, the volumes of these regions with elevated FDG are less than the PTV defined on CT or MR images. This information may indicate active regions in the tumor may require additional radiation dose to control the disease. Escalating the dose to regions with elevated accumulation of FDG would require the use of conformal 3D dose delivery.

| Case | PET ($c\,m^3$) | CT ($c\,m^3$) | MR ($c\,m^3$) |
|---|---|---|---|
| Tumor 1 | 36.9 | 85.0 | — |
| Tumor 2 | 32.3 | — | 47.1 |
| Tumor 3 | 28.6 | 46.0 | — |
| Tumor 4 | 4.5 | — | 8.9 |
| Tumor 5 | 2.8 | — | 4.3 |

**Table 2**: PTV and volume of tissue with elevated FDG:

## References

[1] Rege S, Maass A, Chaiken L, Hoh C K, Choi Y, Lufkin R, Anzai Y, Juillard G, Maddahi J and Phelps M E 1994 Use of positron emission tomography with fluorodeoxyglucose in patients with extracranial head and neck cancers *Cancer* 73 3047-58

[2] Lapela M, Grenman R, Kurki T, Joensuu H, Leskinen S, Lindholm P, Haaparanta M, Ruotsalainen U and Minn H 1995 Head and neck cancer: detection of recurrence with PET and 2-[F-18]fluoro-2-deoxy-D-glucose *Radiology* 197 205-11

[3] Lindholm P, Minn H, Leskinen-Kallio S, Bergman J, Ruotsalainen U and Joensuu H 1993 Influence of the blood glucose concentration on FDG uptake in cancer -a PET study *Journal of Nuclear Medicine* 34 1-6

[4] Karp J S and Muehllehner G 1991 Standards for performance measurements of PET scanners: evaluation with the UGM PENN-PET 240H scanner *Medical Progress through Technology* 17 173-87

[5] Hudson H M and Larkin R S 1994 Accelerated image reconstruction using ordered subsets of projection data. *IEEE Transactions on Medical Imaging* 13 601-9

[6] Karp J S, Muehllehner G, Qu H and Yan X H 1995 Singles transmission in volume-imaging PET with a 137Cs source. *Physics in Medicine & Biology* 40 929-44

## Acknowledgement

The support of this study by Helax (Uppsala, Sweden) is gratefully acknowledged.

# Feedback and Interlock Triggering for Real-Time IMRT Verification

**Timothy Paul[1], Timothy Solberg[1], Min Leu[2], Peter Rosemark[2], Nzhde Agazarian[1], and James Smathers[1]**

[1]Dept. of Radiation Oncology, UCLA School of Medicine and Dept. of Radiation Oncology, Cedars-Sinai Cancer Center[2]

## Introduction

Intensity Modulated Radiotherapy or IMRT may lead to better clinical outcomes by highly conforming dose distributions to the tumor, while limiting doses to surrounding normal tissues. In dynamic IMRT, collimator leaf movement modulates the beam intensity while x-rays are being delivered. Dynamically delivered IMRT treatments are technologically complex with parameters changing during treatment. For example, the beam intensity at any position at a given point in time is a function of accelerator output, MLC leaf position, MLC leaf speed, collimator angle, gantry angle, beam number and beam weighting. The efficacy of highly conformal radiotherapy is dependent on accurate delivery. Thus, we must ensure accurate delivery of the dynamic IMRT treatment prior to and during the patient treatment.

Using the a-Si:H detector array as a transmission chamber provides an unobstructed view of the source. The analysis speed afforded by this simplified geometry and the high rate of image acquisition enables us to diagnose delivery errors before treatment has been completed. This is the key advantage to this method, but there is no point to a real-time verification system unless feedback can be provided to the operator. With that in mind, the aim of this research is to develop and evaluate feedback mechnisms for real-time verification.

## Material and methods

Beam imaging data is acquired with a 128 x 128 pixel amorphous silicon photodiode array with individual pixel size of 0.75 x 0.75 mm. The detector is provided by Wellhöfer Dosimetrie and has an active detector area of 9.6 x 9.6 cm. The minimum imaging capture time is 50 milliseconds. The Wellhöfer ADAS 128 system is held in a fixed into a reproducible position using a jig affixed to the accelerator's collimator bayonet fittings. Note that the detector array is placed between the source and the patient to monitor accelerator output and leaf position. The figure below shows the experimental set-up. The detector holder has slots for a number of detector positions, but it is positioned at 65 cm from the source. Beam attenuation measurements indicate uniform a uniform attenuation of five percent (5%). Thus, beam attenuation can be can accounted for in monitor unit calculations just like a blocking tray.

Leaf sequence files for dynamically delivered fields were created using a modified Bortfeld algorithm that accounts for leakage and transmission and minimizes tongue-and-groove effect [1,2]. IMRT fields were delivered dynamically on a Novalis accelerator. Verification of dosimetry and leaf position have been described previously[3].

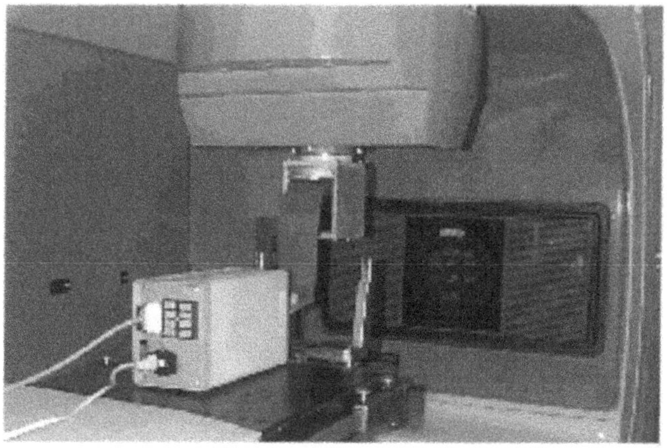

**Figure 1**. Experimental setup

UCLA's Novalis accelerator has been fitted with a gating interface by the manufacturer. The interface requires a switching device to open and control the switch. A computer controlled solid-state relay is used to control the switch. To enable the beam and dynamic IMRT delivery, the switch is closed. To disbable the beam and stop MLC leaf movement, the switch is opened. While designed as respiratory gating interface, this cicuit can be treated as a control/feedback system in the delivery verification of dynamically shaped IMRT. As described previously, images are acquired and analyzed during patient treatment. Errors exceeding preset tolerances trigger a software flag. This flag causes a DC signal to be generated by a digital-to-analog converter and outputed from the Intelligent Instruments' 20428 multifunction board to trigger to the solid-state relay to open the cicuit thereby disabling the beam and MLC leaf movement. A description of the radiation delay mechanism is provided by Ramsey et al [4].

Programmed delivery errors were intentionally introduced to dyamic IMRT leaf sequence file to trigger the feedback mechanism. The method was tested to determine sensitivity to error tolerance settings, time to stop the beam, radiation delivered and leaf movement during this time.

Leaf position for any given leaf i can be described by:

$$X_i(t) = a_i t^2 + v_{i,0} t + x_{i,0}$$

If we allow the beginning of the interval represent the beginning of a frame acquisition and start at t = 0, the change in position of leaf i in any small interval can be approximated by:

$$\Delta X_i(\Delta t) = X_i(\Delta t) - X_i(0) = a_i \Delta t^2 + v_i \Delta t$$

The total change in time over Δt is the summation of several parameters:

$$\Delta t_{Total} = \Delta t_{FrameAcquisition} + \Delta t_{Analysis} + \Delta t_{RelayTrigger} + \Delta t_{DisableBeam}$$

In a worst case scenario, $v_i = v_{max}$ or 2 cm per second for the Novalis accelerator. $\Delta t_{FrameAcquisistion}$ = 50 ms, $\Delta t_{analysis}$ = 38 ms, $\Delta t_{RelayTrigger}$ = 0.04 ms, $\Delta t_{DisableBeam}$ = unknown. Based on the known terms, we can estimate that during $\Delta t_{total}$, at maximum leaf velocity of 2 cm per second and a dose rate of 480 MU per min that the leaves may move 0.17 cm and 0.7 MU may be delivered.

## Results and discussion

Figure 2 shows surface plot of dose delivered in a 100 MU dynamically delivered IMRT treatment test field. The Field was defined by movement of the six central leaves of the mMLC.

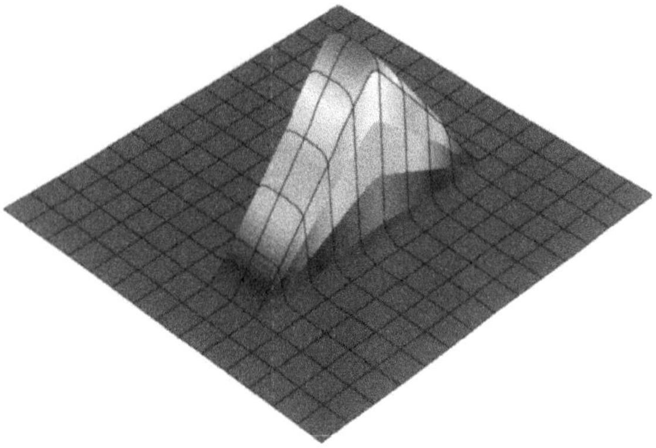

**Figure 2.** Surface plot of dynamically delivered IMRT treatment field delivered to 100 MU

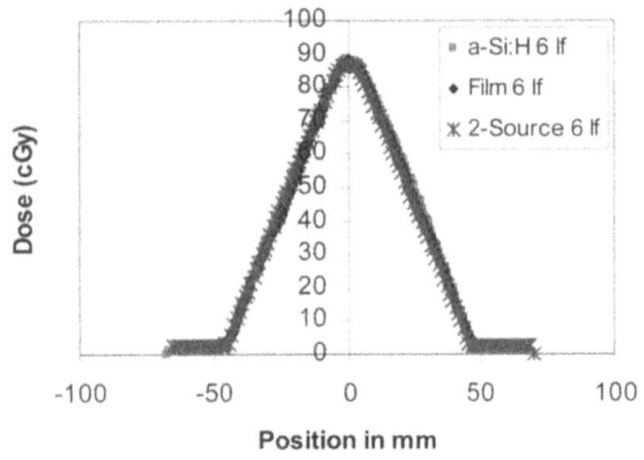


**Figure 3** Measured dose profile through central leaves of the dynamically delivered test pattern defined by six central leaves.

Figure 3 shows the measured dose profiles through central leaves of the deilvered field. Expect and measured dose profiles match within two percent and distance to agreement is within ± 1 mm in all regions of the field.
Figure 4 shows leaf position errors in the delivery of the above pattern. Generally, measured leaf position errors for this delivery are within ± 1 mm, with some measured errors exceeding this value significantly. These are a function of the initial leaf position; a hybrid method of leaf sequencing can minimize this effect. We start dynamic delivery with the leaves closed and for some fields, the leaves must race at maximum velocity to get to their next position. We use these points and others like them to generate out of tolerance flag positional errors.

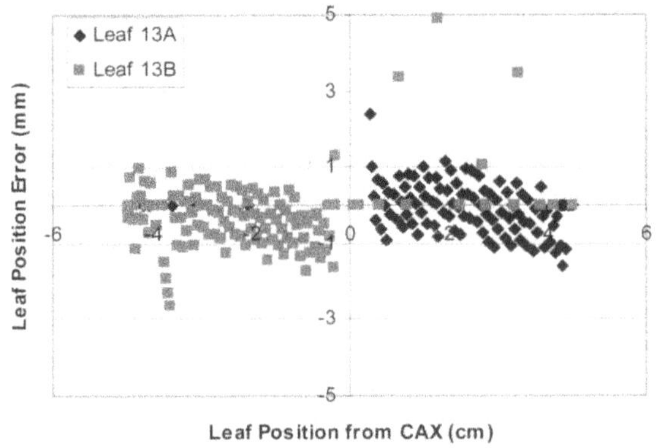


**Figure 4.** Measured leaf position error plotted against expected leaf position for pattern delivered in Figure 2.

## Conclusion

Results from the studies of the detector properties, dose map verification, leaf position verification and real-time feedback demonstrate that real-time verification is promising with this approach. Additionally, this approach has significant advantages over current methods, particularly in its ability to diagnose dynamic IMRT delivery errors and act upon them before the patient's treatment is completed. Feedback to the operator from a real-time verification system is an important stage in the process.

## References

[1] Bortfeld T R, Kahler D L, Waldron T J, Boyer A L. X-ray field compensation with multileaf collimators 1994 *International Journal of Radiation Oncology Biology Physics* **28** 723-730

[2] Agazaryan N, Solberg T D, Arellano A R, Paul T J. Leaf Sequencing for Fluence Modulated Radiation Therapy 1999 *Medical Physics* **26** 1139

[3] Paul T J, Solberg T D, Leu MY, Rosemark PJ, Smathers JB. Independent Real-Time Verification of Dynamically Shaped Intensity Modulated Radiotherapy (IMRT) using an Amorphous Silicon (a-Si:H) Detector Array 1999 *Medical Physics* **26** 1065

[4] Ramsey C R, Cordrel I L and Oliver A L 1999 A comparison of beam characteristics for gated and nongated clinical x-ray beams *Medical Physics* **26** 2086-2091

# Dynamic Opto-Electronic Body Surface Sensing & Computerised Surface Matching for Patient Positioning & Monitoring in Radiotherapy

**C.J. Moore[1,*], G. McVey[1], P.A. Graham[1,2], D. R. Burton[3], M. J. Lalor[3] and F Lilley[3]**

[1] North Western Medical Physics, Christie Hospital NHS Trust, Manchester, UK
[2] GCHQ, Cheltenham, Gloucestershire, UK
[3] Liverpool John Moores University, Coherent & Electro-Optics Research Group , Liverpool, U.K.

## Introduction

Radiotherapy treatments require the repeated delivery of doses of radiation to localised disease over sustained periods. During such fractionated treatment, the shape of a patient's body surface changes under the influence of internal and external forces. Conventional pre-treatment set-ups barely account for the three-dimensional shape of a patient and commonly rely on a few co-planar skin markers for beam alignment. Immobilisation devices fail to account for daily changes in the patient's shape and are in any case unsuitable when treating tumours executing quasi-periodic movement as in the lung.

Conformal radiotherapy techniques, using computer controlled multileaf collimators, MLC, have already proved to be extremely successful for cancer treatment [1,2]. However, clinicians and scientists are acutely aware that a lack of accurate patient positioning can compromise this approach [3,4]. No doubt dose conformation via MLC 'intensity modulation' will generally impact clinical practice in the near future. Thus a decade which has seen the evolution of smaller margins about a gross tumour volume will be complemented by the introduction of tight spatial tolerances around critical structures, adjacent to high dose volumes, in an effort to improve sparing of healthy tissues. Under these circumstances dose escalation will become an ever more attractive option in the quest to improve cure rates. Further progress in these techniques will require more detailed knowledge of the 3D patient body interface traversed by the various treatment beam configurations.

This paper reports progress in the development of an optical sensor demonstrator [5,6], to accurately measure the 3-D patient body surface, for use in computer assisted set-up and maintenance of patient body position in the treatment environment [7,8]. The 'live' treatment room body surface is compared to a refined patient body surface automatically defined from CT sections as part of pre-treatment planning. A two phase patient set-up and positioning technique is described, composed of manual approach and automated 'docking' using simulated annealing in 3D [9].

## Material and methods

Electro-optical sensing is based on a dual-fibre projection interferometer and camera image capture and analysis system. A helium-neon laser is used to launch an interference fringe pattern onto the body surface through pure silica optical fibres. This type of sensor is more resistant to radiation damage than systems which rely upon projection optics. A Fourier fringe analysis (FFA) method is used as the basic measurement technique. Several modifications have been made from standard FFA practice. Careful pre-processing of fringe data, frequency domain filtering and a novel technique for phase-to-height calibration are combined to create a robust measurement system that operates in near real-time. In addition, a practical calibration technique is employed that does not involve direct measurement of geometrical optical parameters.

Body surface detail acquired within the treatment room is compared to the body surface derived from CT cross sectional images taken for pre-treatment planning. An adaptive multi-point gradient boundary algorithm is used to generate continuous body contours from the CT planning sections. B-Spline skinning [10] of the contours then permits the computation of a high resolution three-dimensional surface which forms a planned *reference standard* against which the live sensor surface can be objectively measured. The changing optical sensor surfaces are rendered in 3D together with the CT *reference standard.* In parallel the mutual orientation of the two surfaces is objectively summarised within the region of any overlap by a simple colour-key accompanied by a histogram of colour frequencies. The dynamic, rendered 3D surfaces and colour coded surface overlays are used to guide manual approach to set-up. The residual movements required to complete an approximate set-up are determined using simulated annealing. This procedure iteratively applies affine transformations to the most recent optical sensor surface until a best fit to the CT *reference standard* is found.

## Results and Discussion

Though not state of the art in computer terms the prototype optical sensor-analysis system measures and displays in excess of 32,000 x,y,z triplets per second, with sub-millimetre accuracy. For images up to 128 x128 points this is near real time performance. The system has a configurable field of view very much greater than the typical 40cm x 40cm maximum irradiation beam size at a treatment machine isocentric distance of 1 metre. Figure-1a shows the laser fringes, on an anthropomorphic phantom during simulated set-up. Figure-1b shows the corresponding 3D surface data set extracted from the fringe pattern. Note the clear detection of the transverse boundaries between the slabs of the phantom, seen as lines running round the surface, and other sub-millimetre blemishes.

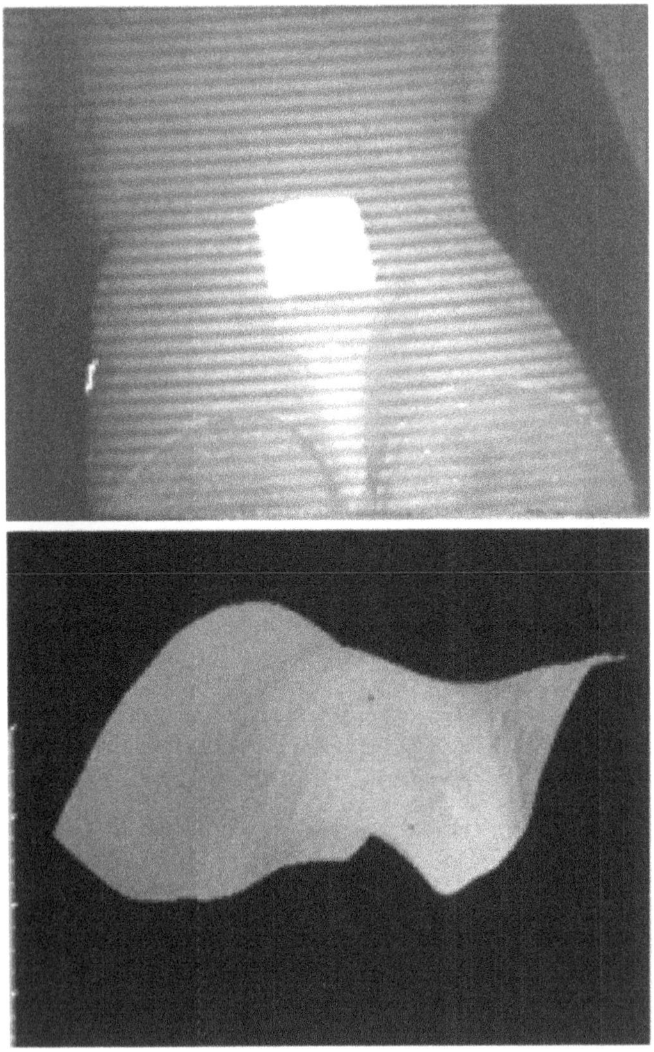

**Figure-1**

a. Upper Phantom showing laser fringe cover.
b. Lower 3D surface after fringe processing.

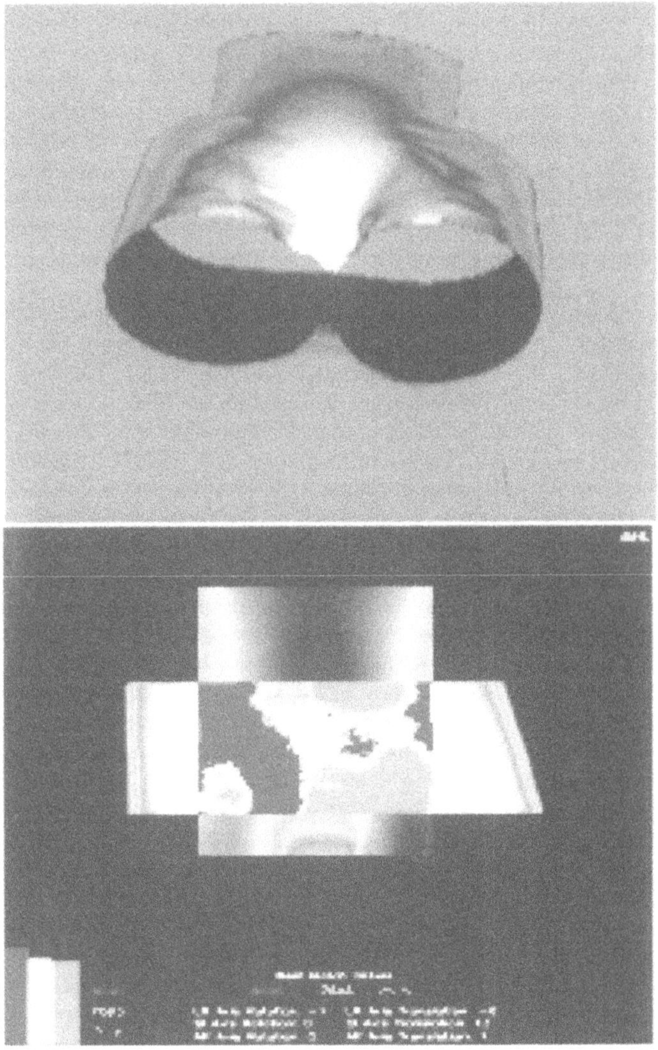

**Figure-2**

a. Upper 3D rendered CT-body & sensor surface.
b. Lower Objective information display during 'docking'.

Using some instantaneous views of a dynamic positioning process Figure 2 gives some idea of what an observer sees. Figure 2a shows one perspective view of the simultaneous 3D rendering of the dynamic, optically sensed surface as it is matched or docked with the 'wrap-around' CT planning reference surface. Figure 2b shows one still frame of the accompanying display providing objective information on where the sensed surface is above or below the ideal planning position. Note that in both the 3D rendered display and the objective information display the surface sensor provides a much larger inferior superior view than is available from the planning scan.

The matching facility has been tested using CT of real patients for whom data is available at weekly intervals. The initial week is the treatment planning scan, which when matched against itself produces the expected ideal fit. Simulated annealing consistently produces a better fit between surface sets than can be obtained using manual interaction. The sensing-matching strategy appears to be fast, practical and accurate. At the time of writing the sensor control software and surface matching code have been integrated in order to facilitate improved performance.

For in-treatment monitoring, the optical sensor software has been modified to include a data-logging mode with an option to save a video-stream to a Video For Windows (AVI) file. Off-line fringe processing of the male breathing pattern, of total duration 36 seconds, has been performed as part of early investigations into breathing motion reproducibility for an assessment of gating techniques in radiotherapy.

## Conclusion

A robust, fast and practical dynamic body sensor-matching system is described. The first steps to dynamic 3D automated patient set-up and monitoring have been taken. The authors are confident of the benefits to radiotherapy that will follow.

## Acknowledgements

This work has been funded by the EC Framework IV BIOMED2 programme. Project ARROW Contract: BMH4-CT98-03660.

## References

[1] Hounsell A R, Sharrock P, Moore C J, Shaw A, Wilkinson J M and Williams P, "Computer assisted Generation of Multi-leaf Collimator Settings for Conformal Therapy", *British Journal of Radiology*, 65, pp 321-326, 1992.

[2] Moore C J, "Computerised Conformal Radiation Therapy - A Critical Process", *IEE Computing and Control Engineering Journal*, Vol 6, No 5, pp205-210, 1995.

[3] Moore C J, Graham P A, MacKay R I and Sharrock P J, "Multi-modal Surface/Outline Projection and Simulation of Target/Critical tissue Movement", IEEE Computer Society, Proc Intl Conf on Information Visualisation, 10-17, London, England, August 1997.

[4] MacKay R I, Graham P A, Moore C J, Logue J P and Sharrock P J, "Concurrent Animation and Radiobiological Analysis of 3D Motion in Conformal Radiotherapy", (in press) Radiotherapy and Oncology.

[5] Burton D, et. al, "A Fibre Optic Interferometer for Fringe Projection Contouring", 2nd International Workshop on Automatic Processing of Fringe Patterns, pp242-248, Akademie Verlag, 1993.

[6] Lilley F, Lalor M J and Burton D R, "A Robust Fringe Analysis System for Body Shape Measurement." [in press] Jnl Optical Engineering.

[7] MacKay R I, Graham P A, Sharrock P J and Moore C J, "Patient Positioning using detailed 3D Surface Data for Conformal Therapy of the Prostate: A feasibility Study", (in press) ASTRO 1999.

[8] Moore C J and Graham P A, '3D Dynamic Body Surface Sensing & CT-Body Matching A Tool for Patient Set-up & Monitoring in Radiotherapy', (submitted) Jnl Computer Aided Surgery, Special Edition on Planning and Image-Guidance in Radiation Therapy, 2000.

[9] Press W H et al, *Numerical Recipes*, Cambridge U P, England, 1989.

[10] Jaillet F, Shariat B and VanDorpe D, "Periodic B-Spline Surface Skinning of Anatomic Shapes", *9th Canadian Conference on Computational Geometry*, Ontario, Canada, 1997.

# Monte-Carlo evaluation of a highly efficient photon detector for tomotherapy

**H. Keller[1], M. Glass[1], G. H. Olivera[1,2] and T. Rock Mackie[1,2]**
[1]University of Wisconsin, 1300 University Avenue, Madison, Wisconsin, USA 53706-1532,[2]TomoTherapy, Inc., 2228 Evergreen Rd., Middleton, Wisconsin, USA 53562

## Introduction

The aim of improving technology in radiotherapy is to close the loop of planning, delivery, and verification. Currently, the most common way to obtain information about the treatment is to image the patient's treatment volume on portal images. However, more accurate delivery techniques spur the need for improved patient imaging. In consequence, active research is going on in the optimization of current detector technologies combined with the modification of delivery systems. Dual-beam systems [1] and tomotherapy [2] are two approaches to achieve this goal.

Megavoltage images usually suffer from poor image quality. This is mainly due to two reasons [3]. First, the physical contrast between bone and tissue is low at MeV-energies, and secondly, portal images have a relatively high noise level, as only a small fraction of the incident x-rays interact with the detector geometry. The latter point implies that an improved megavoltage detector should exhibit a high intrinsic quantum efficiency.

The quantum efficiency (QE) defines an upper limit for the detective quantum efficiency (DQE) which also takes the noise properties of the system into account. The DQE of current detector technologies is on the order of only a few percent.

It has been shown that an arc-shaped xenon ionisation chamber is able to provide high quality image data (i.e. low noise, high resolution), even for high energy applications such as megavoltage imaging in tomotherapy. The reconstructed images delineate contrasts below 2% with resolutions of 2.0 mm with clinically reasonable doses ranging from 8 to 12 cGy [4]. At the same dose, high contrast objects as small as 1 mm can be resolved. Preliminary Monte Carlo calculations were employed to optimize the dimensions of the individual detector chambers for a future design of the detector.

## Material and methods

### The detector geometry

The detector in use at the UW Tomotherapy Benchtop is an arc-shaped CT xenon detector (General Electric), consisting of 738 ionisation chambers separated by tungsten septal plates. The distance between two plates is 0.32 mm, which is also the thickness of the plates. The plates are 5.4 cm long (in the beam direction), and the front and back plates are 0.5 cm and 0.1 cm thick (in the beam direction), respectively. The extension of the detector in lateral beam direction is also 5.4 cm. At every other plate a high-voltage (500 V) is applied. Therefore, the plates act as charge collecting electrodes for the ionisation chambers, which are filled with xenon gas under a pressure of 5 atm. The charge produced in two adjacent xenon cavities is collected together to yield a single pixel signal. The front face of the detector is placed 128.2 cm away from the photon source. As the radius of the detector arc measures only 103.6 cm, the detector is slightly off-focus with the source. The geometry is depicted in Fig. 1.

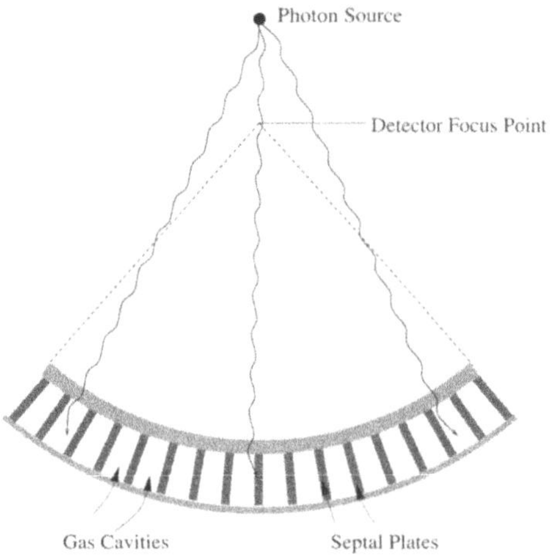


**Figure 1:** Simulation geometry.

### Monte Carlo calculations

The EGS4/BEAM Monte Carlo code [5] served as the computational tool for the particle transport through the detector geometry.

Different simulations were performed to investigate the particle transport within the detector geometry. First, the dose response of the ionisation chambers to a homogeneous 4 MV photon fan beam was calculated and compared to a measured response. Each single of the xenon cavities was assigned a dose scoring zone. The photon beam for the measured profile was produced by a 4 MV linear accelerator (Orion, Buc, France) and collimated to the size of the detector area.

Secondly, for the study of the quantum efficiency of the detector, simulations on one single tungsten plate were performed. To this purpose, EGS4/BEAM was modified to

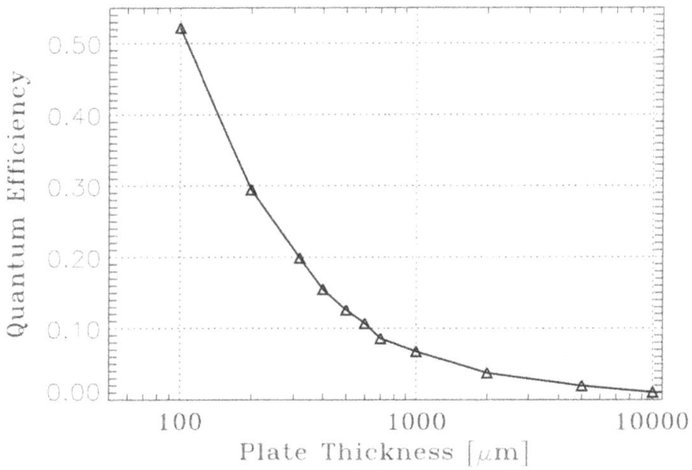


**Figure 2:** Quantum efficiency as a function of plate thickness.

study the particle transport through a rectangular parallelepiped of variable $X$, $Y$, and $Z$-dimensions. A rectangular photon beam of the same cross-section as the plate was directed perpendicular to one of its surfaces. In each simulation, a total number of $10^4$ photons were directed along the $Z$-axis towards the $X$-$Y$ surface, where the $X$-dimension of the plate varied between 0.1 mm and 2 cm. The thickness of the plate in $Z$-direction was always kept constant (5.4 cm). The particle cutoff parameters ECUT and PCUT were chosen as low as possible, i.e. 0.521 MeV and 0.01 MeV, respectively. The particle fluence exiting the plate in lateral direction was scored in a phase-space file.

The quantum efficiency QE can be defined as

$$QE = \frac{N_{el}^{out,0}}{N_\gamma} \tag{1}$$

where $N_{el}^{out,0}$ is the number of electrons leaving the septa plate (or "liberated") into a xenon cavity, and $N_\gamma$ is the number of photons incident on the tungsten plate. The "0" indicates, that only the first electron produced from each photon is counted.

Thirdly, in order to study the modulation transfer function (MTF) of the detector, a point spread function was generated from monoenergetic pencil beams of 1.37 MeV energy (corresponding to the mean energy of a 4 MV spectrum) directed on the center of the detector. The MTF was then obtained by simply taking the modulus of the Fourier transform.

## Results and discussion

Fig. 3 shows the result of the response calculation together with a measured detector scan. The lateral signal buildup was well reproduced. With increasing off-axis distance, the angle of incidence of the incoming photons is tilted more and more with respect to the septal plates, therefore increasing the geometrical cross-section and the relative signal. The field size of the measurement was slightly asymmetric with respect to the beam axis. This explains the difference between the measurements and the Monte Carlo calculations at the left beam edge in Fig. 3.

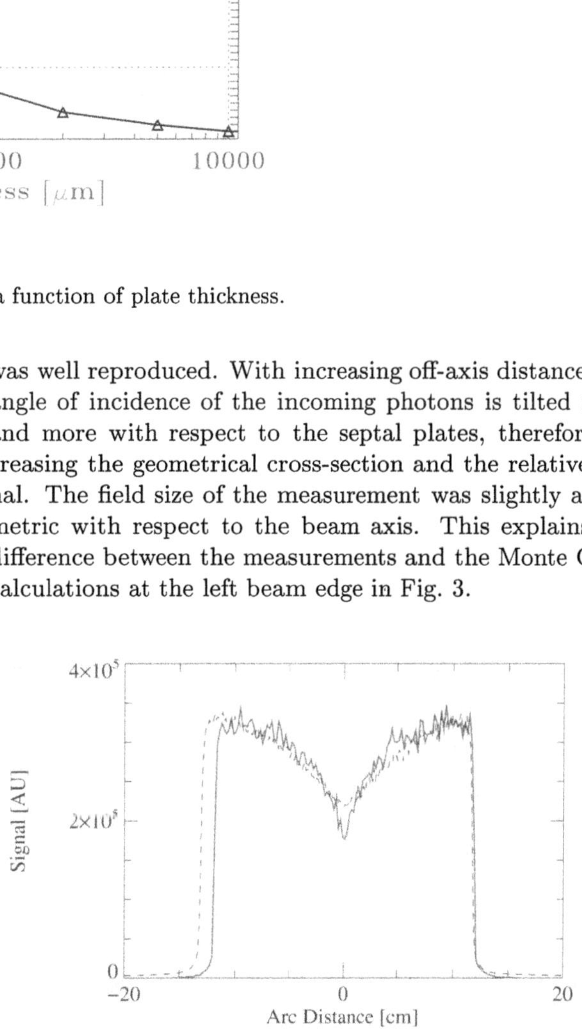


**Figure 3:** Calculated (solid) and measured (dotted) response of the detector to an incident fan beam of 4 MV photons.

In Fig. 2, the quantum efficiency according to Eq. (1) are plotted against the plate thickness. As over 99% of the incident photons interact in 5.4 cm tungsten, the resulting quantum efficiencies are very high. With decreasing plate thickness, the quantum efficiency is increasing dramatically. For the 0.32 mm thick plate the quantum efficiency is 0.19 and for the 0.1 mm thick plate the QE is 0.52. This is by

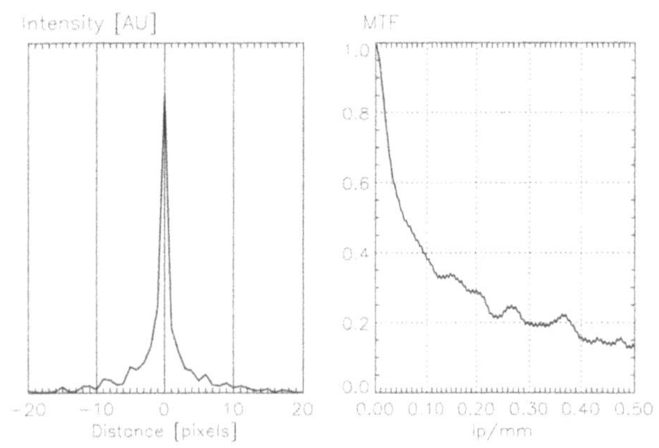


**Figure 4:** Calculated point spread function (left) and modulation transfer function (right).

far higher than in any other detector technology used for megavoltage imaging today. A separate calculation showed that these electrons contribute to over 95% of the absorbed dose in a xenon cavity. Therefore, for megavoltage radiation, the tungsten septal plates play the role of a very efficient signal amplifier.

The point spread function from $10^5$ monoenergetic 1.37 MeV photons is shown in Fig. 4. The width at an intensity level of 1% is about 20 pixels, which is fairly large. This is also expressed in the MTF, which decreases rapidly. The reason for this relatively poor response to an elementary beam is the fact, that all the photons of the pencil beam hit a tungsten plate and over 50% of the scattered photons in the tungsten leave the plate in lateral direction. Consequently, for MV radiation the septal plates only prevent cross-talk of the secondary electrons. This is in contrast to the situation in kV imaging, where the septal plates prevent inter-channel cross-talk of the photons. It may be hypothesized that the use of a lower-density metal instead of tungsten may decrease the number of side-scattered photons with respect to the number of liberated electrons. However, the MTF reflects the high quantum efficiency which should result in a high DQE [6]. Therefore, as the quality of the megavoltage imaging results in [4] indicates, the increased efficiency compensates effectively for the loss in spatial information.

## Conclusion

Monte Carlo calculations have the potential to effectively support design considerations for radiation detectors. Although this kind of detector has been used for tomotherapy applications, it could potentially be employed in imaging for radiotherapy in general.

## References


[1] Jaffray D A, Drake D G, Moreau M, Martinez A A, and Wong J W 1999 A radiographic and tomographic imaging system integrated into a medical linear accelerator for localization of bone and soft-tissue targets *Int. J. Radiat. Oncol. Biol. Phys.* **25** 773–789

[2] Olivera G H, Shepard D M, Ruchala K, Aldridge J S, Kapatoes J M, Fitchard E E, Reckwerdt P J, Fang G, Balog J, Zachman J, and Mackie T R 1999 Tomotherapy in Van Dyk J Ed. *Modern Technology of Radiation Oncology*, (Medical Physics Publishing, Madison, WI, 1999)

[3] Boyer A L, Antonuk L, Fenster A, Van Herk M, Meertens H, Munro P, Reinstein L E, and Wong J 1992 A review of electronic portal imaging devices (EPIDs) *Med. Phys.* **19** 1–16

[4] Ruchala K J, Olivera G H, Schloesser E A, and Mackie T R 1999 Megavoltage CT on a tomotherapy system *Phys. Med. Biol.* **44** 2597–2621

[5] Rogers D W O, Faddegon B A, Ding G X, Ma C-M, We J, and Mackie T R 1995 BEAM: A Monte Carlo code to simulate radiotherapy treatment units *Med. Phys.* **22** 503–524

[6] Kausch C, Schreiber B, Kreuder F, Schmidt R, and Dössel O 1999 Monte Carlo simulations of the imaging performance of metal/phosphor screens used in radiotherapy *Med. Phys.* **26** 2113–2124

# A 3D CT Software Platform for Radiotherapy

**Stefano Agostinelli**[1], **Franca Foppiano**[2]
[1]INFM and Physics Department of Genova - Via Dodecaneso 33 - 16146 Genova - Italy and [2]National Cancer Institute of Genova - Largo Rosanna Benzi 10 - 16132 Genova - Italy

## Introduction

Emerging radiotherapy treatment techniques such as conformal radiotherapy, intensity modulated radiotherapy and tomotherapy call for the introduction of a more accurate patient positioning and treatment verification paradigm [7]. While of primary importance in today clinical practice, the simple comparison of simulator Beam Eye Views (BEV), EPID supplied radiographs and computer generated Digitally Reconstructed Radiographs (DRR), is not able to fulfill the need of fully three dimensional (3D) verification as required by the treatment techniques outlined above.

To address this problem many authors are investigating comparison methodologies based on single-slice [1, 8, 9] and on multi-slice or 3D [5, 3] CT for radiotherapy devices. Basically the aim here would be to provide a reasonable tomographic reconstruction directly from the image output of radiotherapy simulators and linear accelerator portals instead of relying entirely on diagnostic scanners data. This approach would vastly improve the overall confidence on treatment correctness as well as offer to the physician a useful tool for evaluating the target morphology when it is really important to know it, i.e. during the simulation stage or just before the actual treatment, and to the physicist more appropriate attenuation data for on-line treatment planning and transit dosimetry.

We have been studying on-line three dimensional CT reconstruction in the radiotherapy field since early 1999. Initially our research involved cone-beam tomography from conventional radiotherapy simulators video output. The need for a user-friendly reconstruction system, easily upgradeable to support EPID radiographs, urged us to produce a software platform Strange Engine, capable to manage the entire reconstruction process: from the acquisition of data to visualization and exporting to Treatment Planning Systems (TPS). This paper describes Strange Engine capabilities pointing out its logical structure and user interaction by the way of its application to our research experience on radiotherapy simulators 3D CT.

## Material and methods

### The problem

Let's examine what kind of problem we are willing to solve. We have a X-ray source exposing the patient. The transmitted photons intensity is recorded on a two-dimensional detector (usually a fluoroscopic unit for simulators and an Electronic Portal Imaging Device for linear accelerators) in the form of projection images at different gantry angles. The 3D CT problem is then to reconstruct the $\mu(x, y, z)$, the attenuation coefficient volumetric distribution, from that set of projections. Once computed we can use this distribution to generate an on-line three-dimensional radiotherapy study and validate the treatment plan by using matching or correlation techniques on sinograms (see for example [2]).

### How to solve it

In the real world the problem outlined above is ill-posed and in general is not "exactly" solvable. This means that the solver, a reconstruction algorithm, has to introduce both some kind of approximation and regularization which depend typically on the trajectory followed by the source and the detector, on the signal to noise ratio of the projection images and on sampling and interpolation policies.

For this reason we often need to test the importance of these and other effects on a reconstruction algorithm; to this end it is very useful to be able to simulate X-ray exposition of analytical phantoms and apply the solver in case to the simulated set of projections. In conclusion we in practice need both a reconstruction algorithm, the so called backprojector, and a projecting algorithm, a.k.a. projector.

### Requirements

We can try to partition the 3D CT problem domain as in the simple scheme of figure 1 in which the backprojector and the projector play complementary rules by connecting projection space to volume space and vice versa.

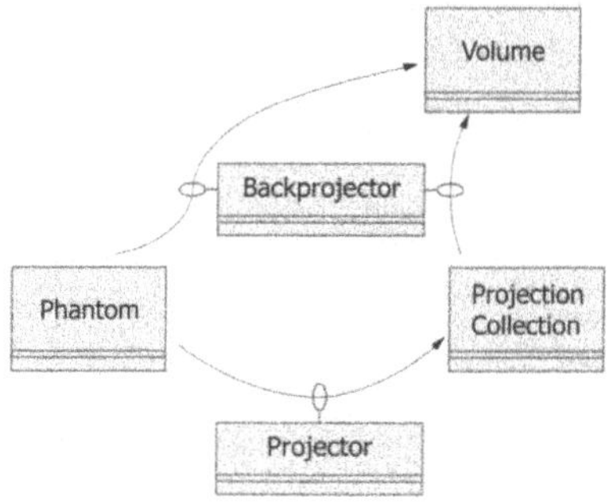


**Figure 1:** The minimal object abstraction for 3D CT.

Our software environment is required to represent the above object abstraction and to connect it to the real world: this should include the ability to load/save data from/to storage devices in industry standard formats, as required by EPIDs and TPSs, and to grab frames from video sources, as required by video based detectors.

### Strange Engine

Strange Engine (SE) provides an object oriented environment for 3D CT reconstruction. Basically SE implements the abstraction needed by reconstruction algorithms within a user-friendly visual Windows NT framework. The object paradigm pursued by SE is presented in figure 2.

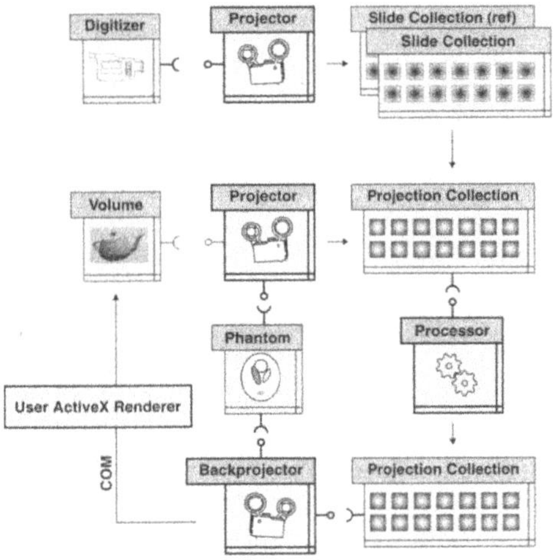


**Figure 2:** Strange Engine object framework.

One important thing to notice of our platform is that the user can plug into it his own reconstruction algorithm by encapsulation in a backprojector ActiveX component. In this way he can concentrate his efforts in writing an efficient reconstruction algorithm and let SE do the rest of the hard work, e.g. import/export of data, acquisition of video frames, visualization of projections and volume data, generation of simulated phantom projections, benchmarking of algorithm performance.

### Plug-ins and the COM interfaces

Backprojector plug-ins are written following the ActiveX control specification and must provide an implementation of the Strange Engine custom IBackProjectorRenderer COM interface. To this end plug-in writers can make use of the MFC framework or of the ATL COM/C++ wrapper. The IBackProjectorRenderer interface consists primarily of two abstract methods invoked by SE during the backprojecting rendering: the first one just asks for the rendering of a single projection while the second one passes directly the whole set of projections and should be implemented if the writer is willing to achieve a speed up in the rendering by exploiting groupal information contained in the projection set, e.g. geometrical symmetries.

Strange Engine can moreover show plug-in specific property pages which can be used to set configuration parameters of the encapsulated reconstruction algorithm. For example the *Agofdk* ActiveX control, included in the Strange Engine distribution, uses this feature to let the user configure the reconstruction filter and the interpolation policy.

### Import and export of data

While every object instance can be loaded/saved from/to disk in a proprietary binary file format (Lempel-Ziv compression is also used whenever it makes sense) interfacement to real world storage based data and medical devices is of course essential. To this end Strange Engine supplies import and export methods for matrix-based binary data and export methods to industry standard image formats including Windows Bitmap, Windows AVI Video, DICOM 3 and NCSA HDF. Moreover a digitizer object for Matrox Genesis frame grabber cards manages the acquisition of triggered video snapshots through on-the-fly hard-disk recording.

### User interface

The whole user input infrastructure is managed through the standard Windows Multi Document Interface. Object instances are represented either by Windows frames or by custom icons on the SE desktop. The desktop is designed to be quite similar to the Windows Explorer desktop and provides intuitive object interaction through drag and drop.

## Results and discussion

Let's now discuss the first application of our object oriented 3D CT environment we have been studying: a 3D CT extension for conventional radiotherapy simulators. The aim of our research was to investigate the real feasibility of multi-slice reconstruction from single-slice gantry rotation projection data. In fact while single-slice CT reconstruction is currently available from several manufacturers, it suffers a very evident problem: a useful (say at least 15 slices) multi-slice reconstruction is not achievable cause it would require too much time. Also most of the single-slice CT extensions available on market involve either a high radiation dose to the patient or cumbersome pre and post collimator setups. By using more efficiently the whole radiation beam 3D CT is probably able to solve these problems. Open questions are about reconstruction algorithm choice, backprojection time and overall CT quality as long as on-line radiotherapy treatment registration and verification are considered.

### The setup

The setup used by our prototype 3D CT extension consists of a conventional radiotherapy simulator, an acquisition personal computer and a reconstruction workstation. The radiotherapy simulator in argument is a Varian Ximatron C-Series equipped with the standard Ximatron fluoroscopic apparatus. This includes an input 12" phosphor plate, an image intensifier and a Newvicon CCIR video camera. The FWHM resolution of fluoroscopic radiographs is 1.3 lpmm: this means that in the usual radiotherapy geometry setup, SAD = 100 cm and plate-to-isocenter-distance of 50 cm, we are expecting a tomographic resolution of about 1 mm due to magnifying effect of the beam cone shape.

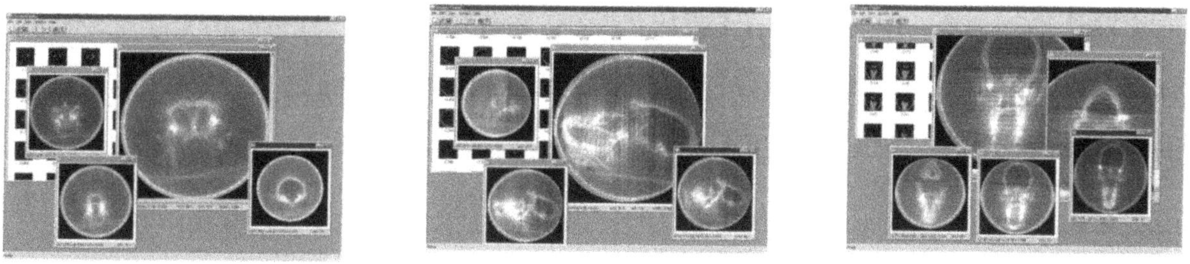

**Figure 3:** 3D CT provides in a single gantry scan not only trasversal but sagittal and coronal slices too.

The video signal is grabbed by the SE digitizer module as a 512 x 540, 8 bit image matrix on our acquisition PC. Currently we are able to grab and store in real time up to 300 frames per minute, in other words a frame is captured every 1.2° rotation of the gantry (a single-scan of the gantry requires one minute). This level of angular sampling should suffice to reconstruct on 256 x 256 slices [6].

### Pre-processing and reconstruction

The reconstruction is usually performed on a faster reconstruction PC connected to the acquisition PC by LAN. First of all grabbed images are converted to the Radon domain using the Lambert–Beer relation

$$I_\mu(x,y) = \ln I_0(x,y)/I(x,y)$$

where $I_0$ refers to in-air projections. Unfortunately, prior to reconstruction, it is necessary to correct projection distortions introduced by the imaging chain. In the case of our simulator fluoroscopic unit we have to correct some misalignment and a slight (about 3°) clock-wise rotation of the camera input window and image intensifier pincushion effects. While these distortions are probably of no relevance for 2D image analysis they can very severely affect 3D reconstruction quality so a pre-processing step is in fact almost essential. To this end SE introduces a processor module providing three basic image processing routines for rotation, shift and spherize corrections. At last we find the reconstruction step. With the actual simulator setup we produce a so called projection set on-a-circle: the X-ray source and the detector plane center move on circles. Currently we consider only full-width projections so in the typical clinical setup we can reconstruct only a 20 cm object positioned at the isocenter. The reconstruction algorithm chosen is based on the Feldkamp–Davis–Kress cone-beam formula [4]. While this formula provides only an approximated solution, in the case of small cone aperture angle vast amount of literature has proven that it provides satisfactory reconstructions comparable to more accurate algorithms. In our case the cone aperture angle is about 15°. Figure 3 shows a real-world reconstruction. This reconstruction was obtained as described in the preceding sections using ramp filtering without any make up. A high noise level is noticeable but we expect to reduce it substantially by introducing noise-depressing filtering, e.g. Shepp-Logan.

## Conclusions

We have presented Strange Engine, an object oriented software platform for 3D CT reconstruction. Strange Engine is particularly aimed at the radiotherapy field which nowadays is receiving a tremendous research impulse towards 3D CT on-line reconstruction for treatment verification and registration. To this regard we have showed its first application to multi-slice reconstruction from single-scan simulator projection data. Results are encouraging and we plan to continue its development to achieve better performance and integration within the radiotherapy clinical field.
Further information is available at:
http://www.geocities.com/SiliconValley/Campus/1694/.

## References

[1] D. Verellen et al. 1999 Characteristics and clinical application of a treatment simulator with a Ct-option *Rad. Oncol.* **50**

[2] E.E. Fitchard et al. 1999 Registration using tomographics projection files *Phys. Med. Biol.* **44**

[3] M.A. Shirazi et al. 1998 A cone-beam megavoltage CT scanner for treatment verification in conformal radio therapy *Rad. Oncol.* **48**

[4] L.A. Feldkamp et al. 1984 Practical cone-beam algorithm *J. Opt. Soc. Am.* **A1**

[5] B.M. Hesse and L. Spies and B.A. Groh 1998 Tomotherapeutic portal imaging for radiation treatment verification *Phys. Med. Biol.* **43(9)**

[6] A.C. Kak and M. Slaney 1989 Principles of Computerized Tomographic Imaging IEEE Press

[7] J.A. Purdy 1997 Advances in 3D Treatment Planning and Conformal Dose Delivery *Semin. Oncol.* **24(6)**

[8] P.H. van der Glessen et al. 1995 Commissioning & applications of a tomographic extension on a conventional simulator *Nucletron–Oldelft Activity Report* **7**

[9] S. Webb 1990 Non-standard CT scanners: their role in radiotherapy *Int. J. Radiat. Oncol., Biol., Phys.* **19**

# Magnetic resonance spectroscopy guided integrated boost irradiation for high grade gliomas using IMRT

**Andrea Pirzkall[1,3], Edward Graves[2], Tracy McKnight[2], David A. Larson[1], Penny K. Sneed, William M. Wara[1], Sarah J. Nelson[2] and Lynn J. Verhey[1]**

Departments of [1]Radiation Oncology and [2]Radiology, University of California San Francisco, San Francisco, CA / USA and [3]Clinic for Radiology, University of Heidelberg, Heidelberg, Germany

## Introduction

Although the prognosis for patients with high grade gliomas remains poor, early experience indicates that an increase in local dose to $\geq$ 90 Gy using accelerated mixed proton / photon irradiation may improve freedom from progression (FFP) and survival [1]. Such a high dose might cause serious complications unless limited only to clearly identified tumor; it is an absolute requirement when using such high dose that normal tissue be spared as much as possible. Intensity modulated radiotherapy (IMRT), a highly conformal delivery technique, not only provides a tool for sparing noninvolved tissue, thereby limiting side effects, but may also offer a means for delivering such high daily doses (2.5 - 3.0 Gy) to actively growing tumor while simultaneously treating the bulk of the tumor to a lesser dose (2.0 - 2.2 Gy).

Since the use of IMRT allows the creation of a steep dose gradient, it is critical that areas of active tumor (suitable for high dose) be identified separate from areas suspicious for tumor extension (suitable for a lower dose). Unfortunately, high grade gliomas are infiltrative tumors with margins that are difficult to delineate. The gadolinium enhancing lesion as seen on T1-weighted MRI is not always a reliable indicator of active tumor due to the existence of nonenhancing tumor tissue and to the presence of contrast-enhancing necrosis. Additionally, nonspecific effects such as edema or inflammation appear hyperintense in T2 weighted MR images, as does active tumor. Therefore, accurate assessment of the presence and the extent of viable tumor requires additional methods based on functional or metabolic aspects of the tumor. Techniques such as 3D multivoxel MR Spectroscopy (MRS) may provide information about tumor activity based upon the evaluation of cellular metabolite levels, which could then be used to identify areas that are appropriate for higher dose.

We therefore have developed a technique for incorporating 3D MR spectroscopy into the IMRT treatment planning process for accurate delineation of the gross tumor volume (GTV) in the treatment of brain tumors so as to assess the feasibility of delivering an MRS-guided integrated boost.

## Material and methods

Patients with previously diagnosed high grade glioma undergo contrast-enhanced CT scans after patient immobilization with an individualized, customized, thermoplastic mask. These CT images serve as the base images for both treatment planning and registration of the diagnostic MRI scans and MRS data. Magnetic resonance examinations are then performed on a 1.5 Tesla GE Signa Clinical Scanner (GE Medical Systems, Milwaukee, WI) without stereotactic fixation. At the conclusion of MR imaging, a 3D chemical shift imaging (CSI) MRS sequence is prescribed to encompass as much of the region of interest and surrounding tissue as possible while excluding areas of fat, bone, or other materials that might compromise the quality of the spectra. A point-resolved spectroscopy (PRESS) CSI sequence with a spatial resolution of 1 cc (1 cc voxels) is used for volume localization. The total MR examination time is approximately 1.5 hours, with the MRS sequence lasting approximately 17 min. The MRS data are then reconstructed using software developed previously at the UCSF Magnetic Resonance Science Center. The peak parameters for choline (Cho) and *N*-acetyl aspartate (NAA) are estimated and used in an automated statistical analysis to identify a control population of spectra. This population is used to identify and quantify the degree of abnormality on a voxel-by-voxel basis [2].

Computed tomography is acquired as the base image study for treatment planning due to its more accurate representation of tissue contour, the ability to use heterogeneity correction, and the lack of image distortion. In order to do coregister the CT and MR data, an automated alignment routine [3] that does not require manual extraction of features or identification of landmark points is used. When necessary, the alignment transformation returned by the algorithm is manually adjusted until correspondence between relevant features is judged to be clinically satisfactory. The identified transform is used to reconstruct the MRI and MRS data in the reference frame of the CT data. The registered MRS data are represented as a contour plot superimposed on the registered post-contrast T1-weighted MR images. Separate overlays show the degree of abnormality determined by the statistical technique.

These images are then transferred by ethernet directly to the radiation therapy planning workstation where they are once again coregistered with the planning CT using a null-set registration process (allowing the previously reformatted CSI data to remain unchanged). Using the CT, MR and 3D MR Spectroscopic data, an optimal segmentation of target (GTV, CTV), organs-at-risk, and tissue contour is performed; GTV is defined as the spectroscopic voxels suggestive of tumor spectrum, CTV is designated to include the contrast enhancing regions on CT and MR as well as any suspected area including microscopic disease, organs at risk are identified first on MR and then validated against the CT, and tissue contours are segmented based on the CT using an autocontour tool.

The IMRT treatment plans for delivery with a MIMiC or a MLC are then created with a goal of delivering concurrently 90 Gy to the actively growing tumor, 66 Gy to the region suspicious for tumor while appropriately dose limiting organs-at-risk. The energy and intensity modulating device, as well as coplanar or noncoplanar fields, are chosen based upon the size of the CTV, the location of the target volumes, and the proximity of organs-at-risk.

## Results and Discussion

The technique and a series of examples will be presented. The integration of coregistered MRS information into the inverse treatment planning process appears to allow a more effective integrated boost irradiation to metabolically active areas within high grade gliomas. However, this approach is not without limitations. First, because the IMRT treatment plans are by definition highly conformal to both the GTV and the CTV, it is critical that these volumes be localized precisely. This means that the use of immobilization systems with an accuracy of better than 2 mm is required. Second, signal-to-noise constraints necessitate a spatial resolution of 1.0 cc for MRS; this must be considered when outlining target volumes. Third, given the inherent difficulties in MRS visualization of targets adjacent to bone or fatty compartments, this technique should be limited for the present time to supratentorial tumors. Finally, even the use of IMRT and precisely identified target volumes does not remove the inherent limitation imposed by the delivery devices; the achievable dose gradient may limit the ability to deliver the desired dose to the target if complications from over dosing organs-at-risk are to be avoided.

## Conclusion

The radiobiological concept of such a dose escalation of primarily radioresistent tumors like glioblastoma multiforme using IMRT may yield superior treatment outcomes compared to conventional irradiation techniques. A randomized trial for the conformal treatment of high grade gliomas using this technique should be considered.

## References

[1] Fitzek MM, Thornton AF, Rabinov JD, et al. Accelerated fractionated proton/photon irradiation to 90 Gy cobalt gray equivalent for glioblastoma multiforme: results of a phase II prospective trial. *J Neurosurg* 1999; **91**:251-260.

[2] McKnight TR, Noworolski SM, Dillon WP, et al. Statistical classification of metabolites in low grade gliomas with H1 MRSI. *Proc ISMRM* 1999; 1398.

[3] Nelson SJ, Nalbandian AB, Proctor E, et al. Registration of images from sequential MR studies of the brain. *J Magn Resonan Imag* 1994;**4**:877-883.

# A full 3-D verification technique for static field IMRT

**Fang-Fang Yin, Huaiqun Guan and Jae Ho Kim**

Department of Radiation Oncology, Henry Ford Health System, Detroit, MI 48202

## Introduction

Intensity-modulated radiation therapy (IMRT) has emerged as a critical tool for dose escalation in three-dimensional (3-D) conformal therapy. Although several IMRT techniques have been tested for clinical application, the mechanism for 3-D verifying conformal radiation delivery relative to specific patient anatomy has not been fully established. Only limited quality assurance procedures and verification methods have been proposed and tested for IMRT (Refs.1-5). Current investigation on the verification methods using portal CT is very encouraging (Refs.6-9). However, some critical issues remain to be resolved. For example, it requires too many conventional projections for reconstruction, which, in turn, involves excess radiation to patient and long imaging time. There is no dosimetry information related to the reconstructed anatomy. As a result, they are not feasible for clinical application of IMRT with static fields.

We have been developing a novel portal CT reconstruction technique that leads to a full 3-D verification technique for IMRT with static fields. In this new approach, the treatment beams are used for image reconstruction so that radiation treatment can be truly verified.

## Material and methods

Our solution to the problem of static-field IMRT verification is to use treatment beam projections in combination of a limited number of conventional CT projections to reconstruct both portal CT anatomy images and portal CT dose images. Use of treatment beams for portal CT reconstruction reduces the number of conventional CT projections (equivalent to dose reduction to patient) and correlates the treatment beams to the treated anatomy. Also, the relative dose distribution can be reconstructed using treatment beam projections so that it can be overlaid onto the portal CT anatomy images.

In order to reduce the number of projections for portal CT reconstruction, and improve the efficiency of 3-D portal verification, an adaptive portal CT reconstruction technique is developed to reconstruct portal CT images. The conventional CT beams will be set at different orientations from treatment beams for minimum geometrical correlation and maximum complementary information. A pilot simulation study was conducted to test adaptive portal CT reconstruction concept. A total of 24 fan projections were acquired from a Shepp-Logan phantom as shown in Fig.1a. The x-ray source to isocenter distance was set to 100 cm and isocenter to detector distance was 60 cm. The matrix size of the phantom is 256x256 pixels with a pixel size of 1 mm. For simplicity, we assume 12 projections were acquired using conventional CT beams and the other 12 projections were acquired using treatment beams. The second 12 projections were truncated to cover only a portion of the whole phantom (similar to real treatment beam) and redo the reconstruction using both 12 full projections and 12 truncated projections.

Portal verification requires not only the anatomical information but also the relative dose distribution with respect to the treated anatomy. We developed a dose reconstruction technique using treatment beam projections to estimate the relative dose distribution inside the reconstructed portal CT image. In this method, radiation delivered by each IMRT beam is recorded using a portal detector. Two portal images, one with treatment object and the other without treatment object, are acquired for each IMRT beam. The detected exit beam intensities are then back-projected to reconstruct dose distribution. The reconstructed dose is then normalized to a reference point to yield relative dose distribution.

## Results and discussion

Figures 1b and 1c show the reconstruction images from 12 projections and 24 projections, respectively. An example of reconstructed image is shown in Fig.1d for truncated data covering only 2/5 of the original projection around the isocenter. It is obvious that the image quality in Fig.1c is much better than that in Fig.1b because of the doubled projection number. Figure 1d shows that the image quality within the central region is similar to that in Fig.1c. However, the peripheral area of the phantom shows poor quality as seen in Fig.1b because of truncation. Quantitatively evaluations using root mean square difference, correlation coefficient, and gray-level histogram between the reconstructed and standard images indicate that the adaptive CT image is very comparable to reconstructed image with full projections.

A computer simulation study is conducted to test whether treatment beam projections can be used to generate 3-D relative dose distribution inside the treatment object with the technique described above. The phantom image and the reconstructed relative dose distribution are illustrated in Fig.2a (phantom image) and 2b (reconstructed relative dose distribution), respectively. For comparison, the planned relative dose distribution is shown in Fig.2c. The preliminary results indicated that the method is capable of generating 3-D relative dose distribution that is consistent with the planned distribution inside the treatment object.

## Conclusion

An adaptive portal CT reconstruction technique has been developed to perform full 3-D treatment verification of IMRT with static fields. This technique has three advantages. (1) The projection data from the treatment beams will locally improve the CT image quality around and inside the tumor without additional dose to patient. (2) The location of the treatment beams inside the patient geometry can be obtained. (3) The relative dose distribution can be reconstructed from treatment beam projections and can be overlaid onto the anatomical portal CT image such that one can correlate dose to anatomy.

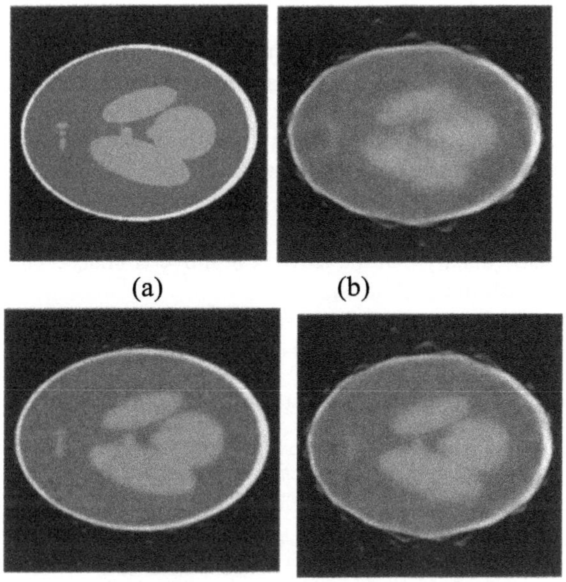

(a) (b) (c) (d)

**Figure 1:** (a) A Shepp-Logan phantom. Reconstructed images using (b) 12 full projections, (c) 24 full projections, and (d) 12 full projections plus 12 truncated projections.

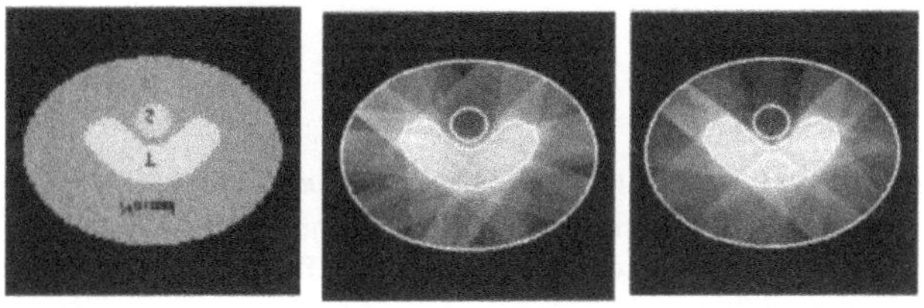

(a) (b) (c)

**Figure 2:** (a) A phantom image. Relative dose distribution images generated using inverse planning method (b) and reconstructed from projections (c).

## References


[1] L. Xing, B. Curran, R. Hill, T. Holmes, L. Ma, K. Forster, A. Boyer, Dosimetric verification of a commercial inverse treatment planning system, Phys. Med. Biol. 44, 463-478 (1999).

[2] R. Mohan, Q. Wu, M. Arnfield, R. Schmidt-Ullrich, Intensity-modulated radiotherapy, ASTRO Refresh Course (1998).

[3] X. Wang, S. Spirou, T. LoSasso, J. Stein, C. Chui, R. Mohan, Dosimetric verification of intensity modulated fields, Med. Phys., 23, 317-327 (1999).

[4] D. A. Low, R. L.Gerber, S. Mutic, and J. A. Purdy, Phantoms for IMRT dose distribution measurement and treatment verification, Int. J. Radiat. Oncol. Biol. Phys. 40, 1231-5 (1998).

[5] M. Oldham, I. Bauster, C. Lord, T. A. D. Smith, M. Mcjury, A. P. Warrington, M. O. Leach, S. Webb, An investigation into the dosimetry of a nine-field tomotherapy irradiation using BANG-gel dosimetry, Phys. Med. Biol. 43,1113-1132 (1998).

[6] H. Guan and Y. Zhu, Megavoltage computed tomography (CT) using a multilevel scheme algebraic reconstruction technique (MLS-ART) and an electronic portal imaging device (EPID), Phys. Med. Biol. 43, 2925-2937 (1998).

[7] M. A. Mosleh-Shirazi, P. M. Evans, W. Swindell, S. Webb, and M. Partridge, A cone-beam megavoltage CT scanner for treatment verification in conformal radiotherapy, Radiother. Oncol. 48, 319-28 (1998).

[8] K. Ruchala, G. Olivera, T. Mackie, Can MLC leakage and transmission be used to obtain CT images during treatment, Med. Phys. 26, 1086 (1999).

[9] J. Kapatoes, G. Olivera, H. Keller, P. Reckwerdt, E. Fitchard, K. Ruchala, T. Mahcies, Dose reconstruction in tomotherapy, Med Phys 26, 1104 (1999).

# IMRT by Dynamic MLC

**Arthur Boyer, Lei Xing, Gary Luxton, Yan Chen, Charlie Ma**
Stanford University School of Medicine, Stanford, California

## Summary of IMRT Delivery Options

The development of Multileaf Collimators (MLCs) controlled by computer-driven motors has made feasible new technology for Radiation Oncology that allows the intensity of the x-ray fluence to be modulated within the bounds of a treatment field (Kallman, 1988). Limitations on applications possible with each MLC depend upon the technical construction and control of the MLC.

Different control mechanisms are used to position the leaves during an MLC treatment sequence. In general, a description of the positions of the leaves as a function of time or monitor units is drawn from a computer file and loaded into a control computer. The control computer directs the leaves to move to the specified positions and verifies that the leaves move to the correct locations during the treatment sequence.

Delivery methods which have been proposed include the use of specially manufactured high-Z compensators for each field, "tomotherapy" which is dynamic arcing IMRT with either contiguous fan beams (Carol 1994,1995) (Peacock MIMiC[c] ) or continuous spiral arcs (Mackie 1993), "stop and shoot" static IMRT using multiple MLC fields (Bortfeld 1994, Boyer 1997, Xia 1998, Pickett 1999), dynamic IMRT with velocity modulated MLCs from fixed beam directions (Convery 1992, Chui 1994, Ling 1996), and intensity modulated arc therapy using a full-field MLC (Yu 1995) (IMAT).

## A dynamic leaf-setting algorithm

In order for the leaves of a MLC to modulate the intensity of a x-ray beam, the leaf control mechanism must be engineered to position the leaves accurately at precise increments of the dose-delivery sequence. Let $\Phi(x)$ be the fluence along the trajectory x of the leaf pair. An example profile is given in Fig. 1.

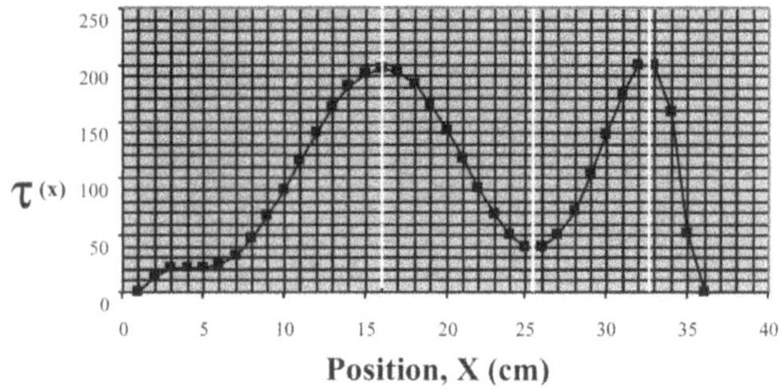


**Figure 1**

One may deliver a beam with such an arbitrary profile section by sweeping two MLC leaves across a track aligned with the profile (Convery 1992, Spirou 1994). In order to deliver the fluence one must determine the arrival times tA(x) for Leaf A at x, and tB(x) for Leaf B at x. The units of the arrival times can be seconds or they can be expressed as Monitor Units. Indicate the irradiation time interval at x between the opening of the ray by Leaf B and the shielding of the ray by Leaf A as

$$\tau(x) = t_A(x) - t_B(x) = \Phi(x)/\Phi_0 \qquad (1)$$

The maximum velocity that the leaves can move is $\upsilon max$ . The velocity modulation equation is,

$$\upsilon(x) = \upsilon max /[1 \pm \upsilon max \cdot (d\Phi/dx)/ \Phi 0] \qquad (2)$$

The resulting leaf-setting sequence is given in Fig. 2.

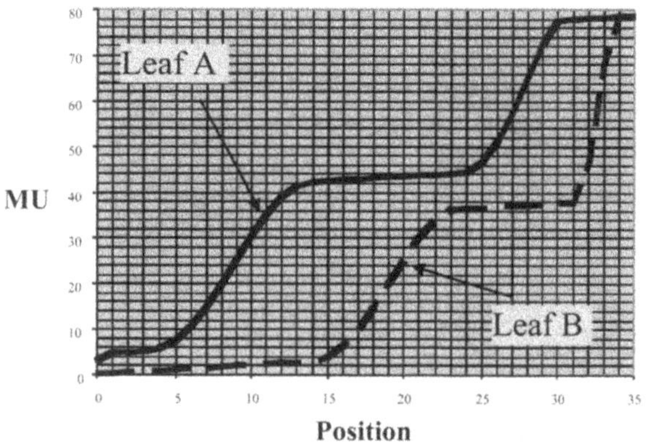


**Figure 2**

The leaves start the sequence closed at the left side of the field and end the sequence closed together at the right side of the field. In a region in which the original fluence gradient is positive, the leading leaf, Leaf B, moves with a constant slope determined by the maximum velocity and the trailing leaf A moves along the trajectory given in Eq. (2). In those regions in which the fluence gradient is negative, the trailing leaf, Leaf A, moves with the maximum velocity while the leading leaf moves along the trajectory given in Eq. (2). This can be used to generate the velocity modulation required to deliver the fluence profile starting with the leaves closed together at one side of the profile and ending with the leaves closed together again at the other. The results are ideal and exact. In order to deliver a predictable dose distribution, a number of other refinements are needed in an accurate dynamic MLC sequence to account for effects such as field flatness, relative output factor of the MLC leaves, penumbra, phantom scatter effects, leaf leakage, rounded leaf ends (Spirou 1994) and back-scatter into the transmission ion chamber.

Another type of leaf-sequencing algorithm may be described as a step-and-shoot method applied to individual leaf tracks (Bortfeld 1994). For a modulated field to be delivered at some gantry angle, each component profile along the center of the leaf pair must be rendered into a leaf trajectory. Fig. 3 depicts a simple example of an intensity pattern. The intensity in a 6-cm x 4-cm field is expressed using five discrete intensity levels.

[c] Peacock MIMiC is a trademark of NOMOS Corporation, Sewickley, PA

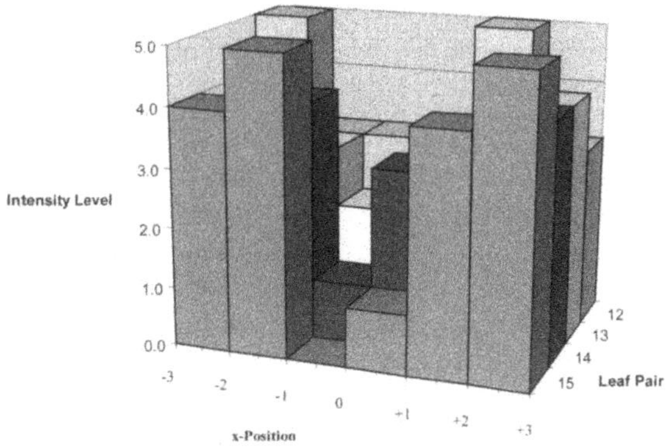


Figure 3

Four 1-cm wide leaves (numbered 12, 13, 14 and 15) are to be used to generate the intensity pattern. The profiles that each leaf pair must generate are shown in the individual graphs in Fig. 4.

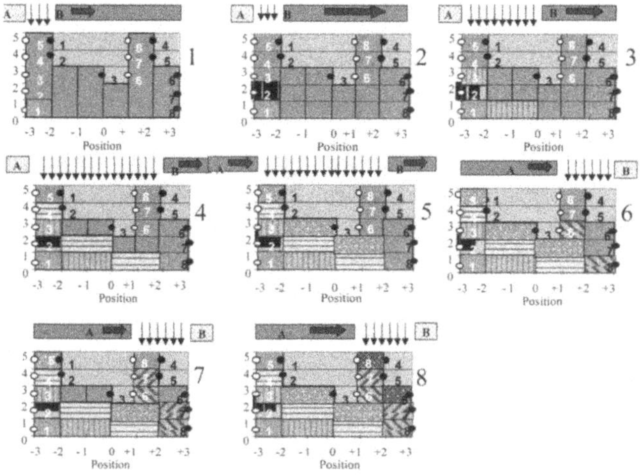

Figure 4

The profile required of leaf pair 12 is used to illustrate how a leaf-sequence can be computed. One assumes that one will modulate the intensity along the profile by sweeping the leading leaf, 12B and the following leaf, 12A, from left to right along the X-axis.

The first step in this procedure is to divide the total beam intensity into a number of equal intervals of width $\Delta\Phi$ as indicated in Fig. 4-1. The number of intervals selected to span the range of the intensity is NL=5 in this example. The second step in the procedure is to find the intersection of the centers of these profile increment bins with the profile. Circles in Fig. 4. indicate these points. The algorithm requires that an even number of such points be found. The third step is to divide the coordinates of these points into two groups. One group consists of those points lying on an ascending slope of the profile where there is a positive gradient (open circles in Fig. 4), and the other group consists of those points lying on a descending slope of the profile where there is a negative gradient (filled circles in Fig. 4). The fourth step is to rank order the points in each group as indicated in Fig. 4. The numbers indicated are the i-index for the sequence for the 12$^{th}$ pair of leaves. Pairing together the coordinates of equal rank order and assigning the coordinates to each pair of leaves produces the desired leaf sequence for the kth gantry angle position, $\{xA_{i,j,k}, xB_{i,j,k}\}$ where the index i ranges from 1 to $NI_j=8$ in this example. The number of steps required to create the trajectories will not be the same for all profiles that make up a field. Steps must be added to the shorter sequences with the leaves abutting beneath a jaw at one end of the profile so that all sequences for a field will have the same number of steps (Fig. 5).

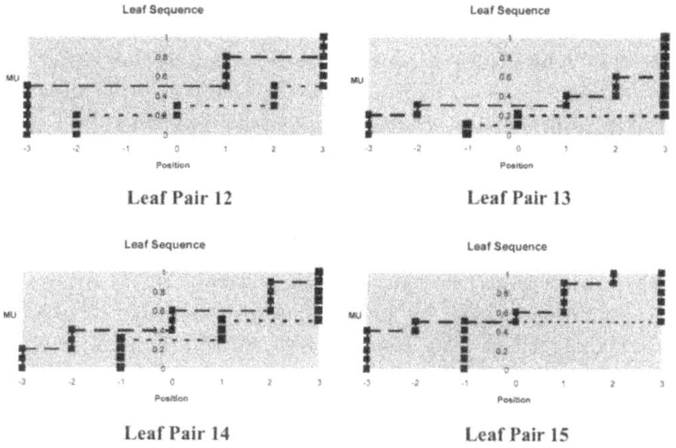


Figure 5

Another leaf-sequencing approach used to produce IMRT can be explained with the aid of the pattern of integers as shown in the Fig. 6.

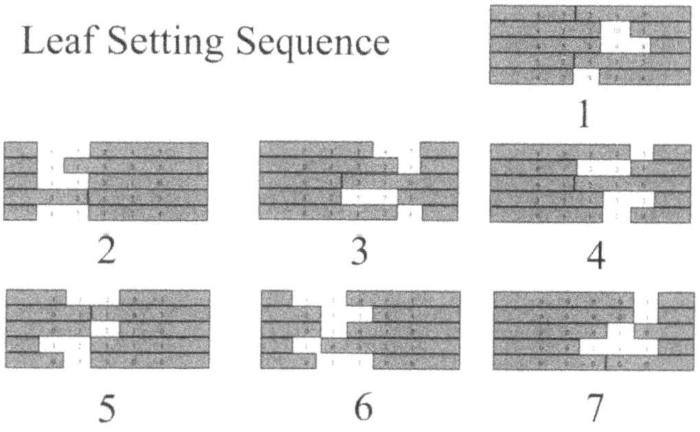


Figure 6

This pattern represents an intensity pattern to be delivered by this leaf-setting sequence. The 5-cm x 5-cm field is to be delivered with a maximum beamlet intensity of 10 and minimum beamlet intensity within the field of 1. The underlying principle of the algorithm for determining the sequence is that the most efficient way to subdivide a sequence is by halves (Xia 1998). The sequence is to be delivered by increments that are powers of 2. In this case, the increments are 8, 4, 2, and 1. The first step is to set the leaves in a pattern that can deliver an exposure of 8. There are four beamlets with intensities of 8 or more. They are not contiguous, but leaves can be set to form two windows around the two regions that each delivers an intensity of 8. This is step 1 in Fig. 6. After this exposure,a leaf pattern can be found that exposes beamlets that require a residual exposure of 4 or more. However, two such regions exist that require two separate sets of leaf-settings. These are steps 2 and 3 in Fig. 6. The residual intensity then contains values up to 3 that can be reduced by exposures of 2. Again, in order to expose all the beamlets, two leaf patterns are required, each delivering exposures of 2. These are steps 4 and 5 in Fig. 6. Then all the beamlet positions have either received their full exposure are have a residual of 1. Two more leaf patterns are required to reach all the 1 positions and reduce the residual intensity to zero. In all seven steps are required to deliver the intensity pattern. The single profile step-and-shoot leaf-setting algorithm requires 13 steps to deliver this pattern.

## Implementation Considerations for IMRT

Leaf Transmission. The delivery sequencing algorithms must take the leaf transmission into consideration in order to select a sequence that will accurately deliver a desired intensity pattern. The transmission through the leaves limits the dose minima that can be created by dynamic MLC delivery sequences. Determination of the transmission by direct and indirect measurements is an important feature of the DMLC commissioning process. The leakage dose delivered along the profile can be computed once a first approximation of the sequence has been computed. This leak-age is a dose profile of relatively low intensity. The leakage dose profile can be sub-tracted from the desired profile and the leaf-setting sequence recomputed using the corrected profile.

Leaf Position Calibration. The system that positions the leaves must be accurately calibrated in order for accurate intensity-modulation to be achieved. The design of the system determines the calibration process. Curved leaf ends create a displacement between the light field and the nominal edge of the radiation field (Figure 7).

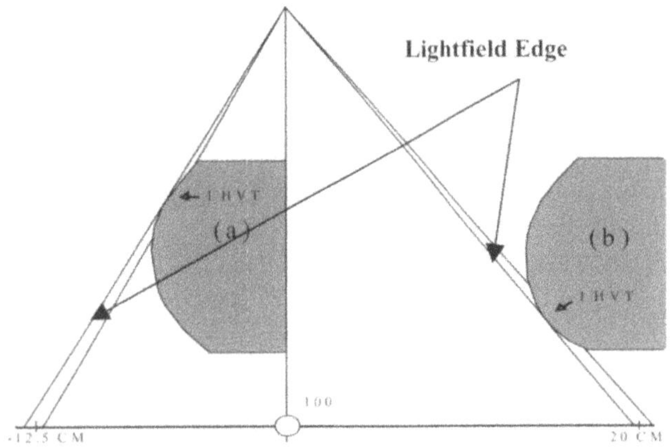


Figure 7

Understanding corrections for this displacement implemented by the vendors is necessary in order to set the calibration parameters.

Leaf Position Offset. For dynamic and step-and-shoot algorithms, an offset may be necessary between the leaf position specified for conventional MLC settings and the position specified for DMLC IMRT to avoid gaps or overlaps between superposed beamlets, or an incorrect positioning of leaves dynamically that can lead to significant dose delivery errors. Profiles obtained with a series of different offsets between ajoining subfields are shown in Figure 8.

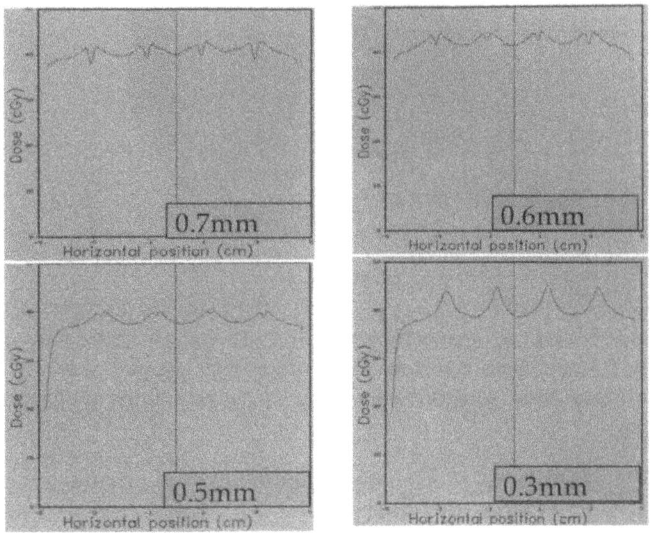


Figure 8

The physicist should understand the origin of this offset and have a means to determine the optimal offset when comissioning DMLC systems.

Tongue and Groove Corrections. Other modifications of the leaf-setting sequence must be made to correct for specific effects that come about as consequences of the physical construction of the MLC leaves such as the tongue-and-groove effect (Van Santvoort 1996, Webb 1997). Small, narrow strips of underdose can be caused by the tongue and groove construction of the leaf sides. The effect is understood and corrections can be made in the leaf sequence to remove the strips (see Figure 9).However, the corrections lengthen the leaf sequences.

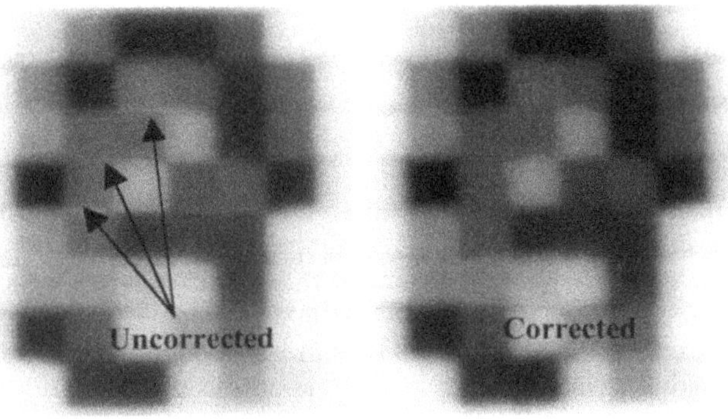


Figure 9

Transmission Monitor System End Effects. Since the IMRT sequences require the dosimetry system to continuously turn the beam on and off for very short intervals, the potential for cumulative end effect errors must be investigated and corrected.

Dose Rate Effects. The dose modulation systems provided with different linear accelerator systems can exhibit significant dose rate effects. Means to detect these effects and to determine operating conditions that avoid them are important to the IMRT comissioning procedure. An example of a test of this effect by delivering strips that should have equal weights is given in Figure 10.

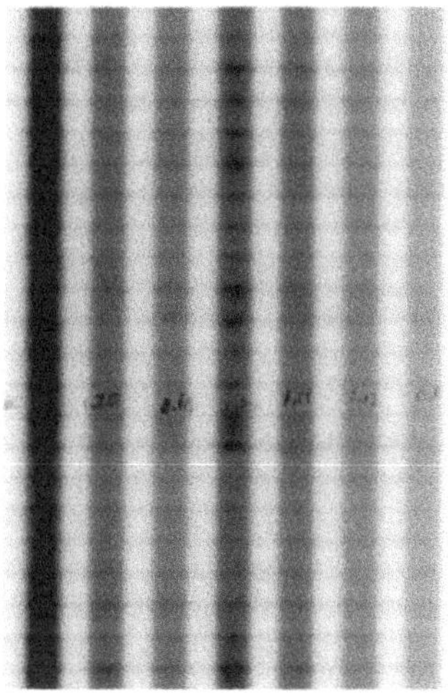

**Figure 10**

## Summary

Medical physicists around the world are developing techniques made possible by the computerization of MLC leaves and the integration of the leaf motion into the delivery sequence. The technology offers a rich area for research and holds the promise for significant improvements in the management of malignant disease by radiation therapy. Understanding of the technology is essential for its successful application.

## References


Bortfeld T, Kahler DL, Waldron TJ, Boyer AL(1994). X-ray field compensation with multileaf collimators. *Int. J. Radiat. Oncol. Biol. Phys.* **28** 723-730.

Boyer A, Geis P, Grant W, Carol M (1997). Modulated beam conformal therapy for head and neck tumors. *Int. J. Radiat. Oncol. Biol. Phys.* **39(1)** 227-236.

Carol M. P. An automatic treatment planning system for linear accelerator based beam modulation radiotherapy. In: Hounsell AR, Wilkinson JM, Williams PC, ed. XIth Int. Conf. on the Use of Computers in Radiation Therapy. Manchester: ICCR, 1994: 172-173.

Carol MP. Integrated 3D conformal planning/multivane intensity modulating delivery system for radiotherapy. In: Purdy JA, Emami B, eds. 3D Radiation Treatment Planning and Conformal Therapy. Madison, Wisconsin: *Medical Physics Publishing*; 1995:435-445.

Chui C S, LoSasso T, Spirou S (1994). Dose calculation for photon beams with intensity modulation generated by dynamic jaw or multileaf collimations. *Med. Phys.* **21(8)** 1237-1244.

Convery D J, Rosenbloom ME (1992). The generation of intensity-modulated fields for conformal radiotherapy by dynamic collimation. *Phys. Med. Biol.* **37** 1359-1374.

Kallman P, Lind B, Eklof A, Brahme A (1988). Shaping of arbitrary dose distributions by dynamic multileaf collimation. *Phys, Med. Biol.* **33(11)** 1291-300.

Ling C, Burman C, Chui C, Kutcher G, Leibel S, LoSasso T, Mohan R, et al. (1996). Conformal radiation treatment of prostate cancer using inversely-planned intensity-modulated photon beams produced with dynamic multileaf collimation. *Int. J. Radiat. Oncol. Biol. Phys.* **35(4)**721-730.

Mackie TR, Holmes T, Swerdloff S, Reckwerdt P, Deasy J O, Yang J, Paliwal B, et al.( 1993). Tomotherapy: A new concept for the delivery of dynamic conformal radiotherapy. *Med. Phys.* **20(6)** 1709-1719.

Pickett B, Vigneault E, Kurhanewicz J, Verhey L, Roach III M (1999). Static field intensity modulation to treat a dominant intra-prostatic lesion to 90 Gy compared to seven field 3-dimensional radiotherapy. *Int. J. Radiat. Oncol. Biol. Phys.* **43(4)** 921-929.

Spirou SV, Chui CS (1994;). Generation of arbitrary intensity profiles by dynamic jaws or multileaf collimators. *Med. Phys.* **21** 1031-1041.

Van Santvoort JPC, Heijmen BJM (1996). Dynamic multileaf collimation without 'tongue-and-groove' underdosage effects. *Phys. Med. Biol.* **41** 2091-2105.

Webb S (1991). Optimization by simulated annealing of three-dimensional conformal treatment planning for radiation fields defined by a multileaf collimator. *Phys. Med. Biol.* **36(9)** 1201-26.

Webb S (1992). Optimization by simulated annealing of three-dimensional, conformal treatment planning for radiation fields defined by a multileaf collimator: II. Inclusion of two-dimensional modulation of the x-ray intensity. *Phys. Med. Biol.* **37(8)** 1689-704.

Webb S, Bortfeld T, Stein J, Convery D (1997). The effect of stair-step leaf transmission on the 'tongue-and-groove problem' in dynamic radiotherapy with a multileaf collimator. *Phys. Med. Biol.* **42**:595-602.

Xia P, Verhey L (1998). MLC leaf sequencing algorithm for intensity modulated beams with multiple static segments. *Med Phys.* **25(8)** 1424-1434.

Yu CX (1995). Intensity-modulated arc therapy with dynamic multileaf collimation: an alternative to tomotherapy. *Phys. Med. Biol.* **40** 1435-1449.

# INTENSITY-MODULATED ARC THERAPY: Clinical Implementation and Experience

**Cedric Yu, Dong-Jun Chen, Allen Li, Lijun Ma, David Shapard, and Mehrdad Sarfaraz**

University of Maryland School of Medicine

## I. INTRODUCTION

Intensity-modulated arc therapy, or IMAT, is one of the methods for delivering intensity-modulated radiation treatments to achieve high dose conformity. Instead of delivering intensity-modulated beams with fixed gantry angles [1], IMAT delivers optimized dose distributions by rotating the radiation beam around the patient. During delivery, the field shape, which is formed by a multileaf collimator (MLC), changes constantly as determined by the required intensity distributions at different beam angles. Intensity distributions at all angles around the patient are achieved with multiple overlapping arcs of different field apertures and gantry speed. Therefore, IMAT is also different from tomotherapy[2,3], which use intensity modulated fan beams rotating around the patient to delivery the treatment slice-by-slice. As with tomotherapy, IMAT combines intensity modulation and rotational delivery. Detailed description of the technique was reported by Yu in a previous article [4].

We have implemented the IMAT technique in our clinical practice for treating patients with cancers of the head/neck. The purpose of this paper is to describe the issues in the implementation and in clinical usage of this technique. Clinical examples of IMAT treatments will be presented to illustrate the dosimetric advantages of rotational delivery.

## II. METHODS AND MATERIALS

As with conventional treatment techniques, IMAT involves treatment planning and delivery. It has been demonstrated that treatment plans developed for tomotherapy treatment delivery can be converted into multiple arcs and delivered with IMAT [4]. However, since the treatment plans were developed for fan beam delivery with little constrains on the smoothness of the beam intensities, the beam intensity distributions are overly modulated. As a result, a plan with 2-3 intensity levels would require 3-8 arcs to deliver.

To overcome such inefficiency, we implemented IMAT into clinical use with a combination of forward and inverse planning. From simulation CT images, the target and surrounding normal structures are delineated on a commercial 3D treatment planning system (RenderPlan, Precision Therapy, Inc.). Arcs are approximated as multiple shaped fields spaced every 10 degrees around the patient. The ranges of the arcs are chosen manually to give the desired dose distributions. Multiple coplanar or non-coplanar arcs are allowed. Wedges can also be used. The initial plan is then read by an external software that optimizes the beam weights. The optimized weights are written back to the 3D planning system and the dose distributions are re-evaluated. The final treatment plan is put into a leaf-sequencer, which simply copies the MUs for each of the beams and shapes the fields with MLC leaves. Such MLC prescriptions are sent to the MLC controller for dynamic leaf motion. During beam delivery, the linear accelerator is programmed to deliver arc treatments and the MLC is programmed to dynamically step through a sequence of field shapes.

To verify the clinical value of such a simplified process, we have compared the treatment plans using 1 to 3 forward planned arcs with the plans generated by conventional techniques and by a commercial inverse planning system (CORVUS by NOMOS Corporation, Inc.) for multiple head and neck treatments. Both the conventional plans and the IMAT plans are presented to the physician. For most cases, the IMAT plans provide greater sparing of normal brain and critical structures. In comparison to the plans generated with inverse planning, we found that, in general, the forward planned arcs provide smoother dose distributions in the target while the inverse planned arcs can give sharper gradient at the critical structure boundaries.

Dosimetric accuracy of the entire process was verified with phantoms before IMAT is used clinically. Angular spacing of the shaped fields used for approximating an arc was investigated with drastically changing field shapes on a cubical phantom. It was found that spacing of the fields from 5 degrees to 20 degrees does not change the central axis dose for the same total MU. The accuracy of the 3D treatment planning system for IMAT planning was also verified with a humanoid phantom, which was modified to allow an ion chamber to be placed at different lateral positions of different sites at the isocenter depth. Central axis dose as well as the dose distributions were measured.

For all IMAT treatments, a dry run is conducted to assess the geometric and dosimetric accuracy and to eliminate possibilities of technical problems such as setup difficulties and MLC movement constraints. The dry run is conducted by copying the patient plan parameters including field shapes and MUs to the same site of the modified humanoid phantom. Both the central axis dose and the dose distribution on a plane are measured and compared to that generated by the planning system. As the gantry is rotating around the patient and the radiation beam is on, it is important that the field shapes of adjacent beam angles do not require the MLC leaves to travel very long distances. For most clinical cases, the field shapes vary slowly between angles. Treatments can be delivered with the highest machine dose rate determined by the linear accelerator based on the maximum speed of gantry rotation, resulting in very short beam time. Occasionally, constraints on MLC leaf speed may require a reduced machine dose rate to avoid radiation pauses during delivery. Determining the proper machine dose rate is also part of the dry run QA procedure.

So far, only patients with head and neck cancers are treated with IMAT. Most patients are treated with one to three arcs.

We are in the process of comparing treatment plans and evaluate potential advantages of using IMAT for other sites.

## III. RESULTS

The time needed for creating a satisfactory treatment plan is found to be comparable to conventional 3D conformal plans for complex cases. This is largely due to the use of convenient features in the planning system such as the application of template plans, and auto-field shaping. However, due to the need for creating phantom plans for the dry run, and to recalculate dose after beam weight optimization, the overall planning time doubles. The dry run QA procedure also take additional 1-2 hours per course of treatment. We hope that after a large number of patients have been treated, the dry runs can be replaced with alternative QA procedures.

The IMAT delivery was implemented using an Elekta's linear accelerator equipped with a MLC, which replaces the upper collimator jaw. Pre-clinical dose verification revealed that the measured doses at the isocenter is always of 2-3% lower than the calculated values. This systematic error was found to be due to the over estimation of head scatter factor by the treatment planning system. As MLC is used for shaping the fields, the head scatter should be determined by the irregular MLC-shaped fields. However, the treatment planning system uses the rectangles circumscribing the irregular field to estimate the head scatter factor. Since the field sizes used for head and neck treatments are relatively small, an over estimation of the equivalent field size by 2 cm can cause more than 2-3% error. After the corrections were made for all the field shapes, all absolute dose measurements were found to be within 2% from the calculated values (most within 1%).

Isodose distributions on transverse planes were also measured with films. Figures 1 and 2 show a clinical example of the planned and measured isodose distributions. Figure 1 is the dose distribution predicted by the planning system in the patient. By spreading lower doses to a greater volume, the 95% isodose covers the tumor uniformly and the dose drop off from 95% to 50% is very sharp. The plan is applied to the modified humanoid phantom for the dry run. Figure 2 is the isodose distribution measured with a film exposed by sandwiching it between two transverse slices of the phantom and delivering the treatment to the phantom. We set an acceptance criterion that the predicted and measured 95% isodoses in the phantom must match with 2mm and the 50% isodose lines must agree within 5mm.

Besides the superior dose distribution as compared with conventional techniques, the delivery time using IMAT is generally shorter than conventional treatments. This is due to the reduced number of beams when each arc is counted as one beam. Most treatments use less than three arcs. The same cases would require 4-7 fields with complex wedge arrangements to achieve an acceptable dose distribution. Although the beam time of each arc is longer than that for a fixed field, the number of patient setups is reduced.

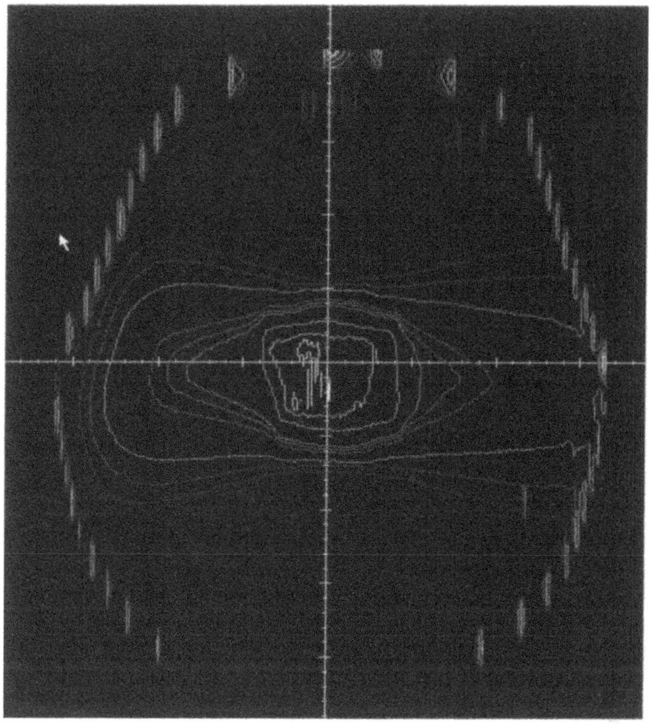

**Figure 1**

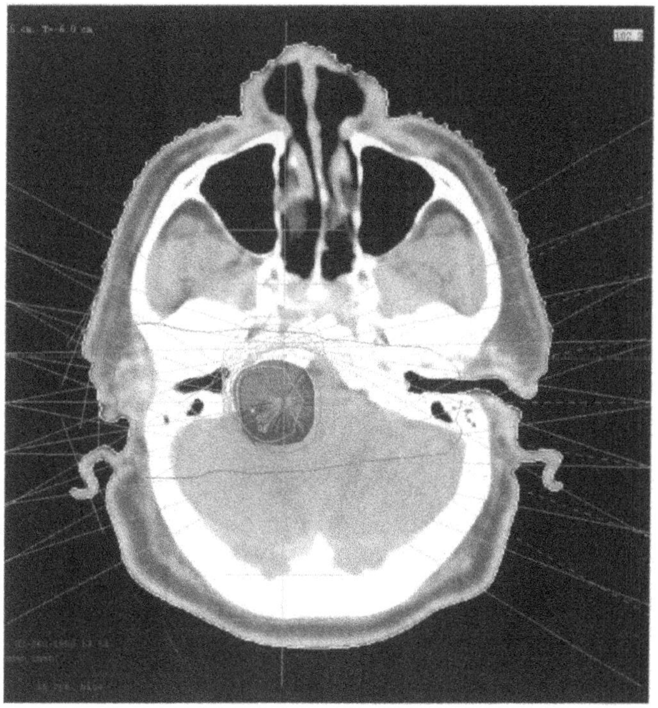

**Figure 2**

## IV. DISCUSSION

We have demonstrated the clinical feasibility by delivering IMAT treatments to patients with head and neck cancers. The number of arc needed to achieve conformal dose distribution is relatively low. The combination of forward planning and beam weight optimization is a practical solution to the existing drawbacks of the inverse planning system. If treatment plans can be optimized for IMAT cone beam delivery, we expect IMAT technique to achieve dose distributions that rivals both slice based techniques [Carol et al 1993, Mackie et al 1993] and the use of non-rotational intensity-modulated beams. In comparison with the sliced delivery schemes, IMAT has many advantages. It is implemented on existing linear accelerators equipped with an MLC. Since it does not collimate the beam into a slit, most of the target will be in the beam during the delivery, maintaining a high efficiency in utilizing the photons generated in the x-ray target. No additional patient transport mechanisms are required to move the patient from slice to slice. Eliminating the slicing also eliminates the problem of beam abutment between slices, and the cold and hot spot associated with the abutments. Finally, since the intensity modulation in tomotherapy relies on a set of leaves to open or close the slit beam, the resolution of the beam intensities is the slit width by the leaf width. For IMAT treatments, both the leaves and the jaws travel continuously, resulting in tighter conformity at the target boundaries.

## V. CONCLUSION

A new treatment technique, intensity modulated arc therapy (IMAT), has been implemented in our clinical practice. Initial clinical results demonstrated the feasibility and accuracy of such treatment. The complexity of the IMAT is not significantly greater than existing arc therapy from the operator point of view. A typical IMAT treatment can be delivered in less time as compared with conventional treatments.

## References

[1] Bortfeld T R, Kahler D L, Waldron T J, and Boyer A L 1994 X-ray field compensation with multileaf collimators *Int. J. Rad. Oncol. Biol. Phys.* **28(3)**, 723-730

[2] Carol M P 1994 An automatic 3D conformal treatment planning system for linear accelerator based beam modulation radiotherapy *Proceedings of the XIth International Conference on the Use of Computers in Radiation Therapy* Ed: Hounsell A R, Wilkinson J M, and Williams P C, 172-3

[3] Mackie T R, Holmes T, Swerdloff S, Reckwerdt P, Deasy JO, Yang J, Paliwal B, Kinsella T 1993 Tomotherapy: a new concept for the delivery of dynamic conformal radiotherapy *Med. Phys.* **20(6)**, 1709-19

[4] Yu, C X 1995 Intensity-modulated arc therapy with dynamic multileaf collimation: an alternative to tomotherapy. Phys. Med. Biol., **40** 1435-49

# Clinical Implementation of IMRT by MLC Technology

**W. De Neve, M.D., Ph.D., F. Claus, M.D., W. De Gersem, Ir., G. De Meerleer, M.D. and C. De Wagter, Ir., Ph.D.**

Division of Radiotherapy, University Hospital, Gent (R-UZG), Belgium

The case in favour of IMRT is made as IMRT allows to shape the dose distribution in such a way that at least three challenges in clinical radiotherapy can be addressed. These are i) conforming dose to concave PTV shapes (i.e. head and neck (H&N), paraspinal, cervix, some prostate tumours); ii) reducing the volume of surrounding tissues irradiated to intermediate dose levels by using beam combinations with restricted hinge angles (lung, mediastinal tumours) and iii) generating controlled 3D-inhomogeneous dose distributions (i.e. prostate, paranasal sinus tumours). The two largest groups of patients that we treat with IMRT are H&N and prostate cancer patients.

From September 1996 till September 1999, 31 patients received IMRT as primary treatment or as a re-irradiation of H&N cancer. According to site, the patient group was composed of 7 (6/7) hypopharynx; 8 (3/8) nasopharynx; 1 (1/1) oropharynx; 8 (0/8) paranasal sinus; 1 (1/1) salivary gland; 2 (0/2) thyroid and 4 (0/4) cancers from other sites (in brackets: re-irradiated). The aim of IMRT was to spare nervous system structures (brainstem, spinal cord, optic structures) in all cases, to spare bony structures and parotid gland in selected cases and to avoid underdosage of difficult to reach regions like the area between the optic nerves, the retropharyngeal space, the lateral pharyngeal and deep jugulary chain nodes.

From July 1998 till December 1999, 31 patients received IMRT for prostate cancer to a prescription median dose of 76 Gy in 36 fractions. The main goal of IMRT was to keep the maximal rectal dose at 72 Gy. No acute toxicity above grade 2 was observed. The IMRT planning strategy with forward (class solution)2 and inverse (desired dose distribution decomposition; intensity optimization (W. De Neve, Presidential Course, ASTRO 1999)) elements3,1,2 lead to IM-beams consisting of superposed unmodulated segments. At the final stage of planning, segments were linked for fast sequencial delivery by an SL-18-MLCi or SL-25-MLCi (Elekta), with a dynamic multileaf collimator forced in step and shoot mode2. For head and neck tumours, a treatment session involved the delivery of 20-50 segments and took 12-22 minutes, including the time required for patient setup and portal imaging. QA-QC was described previously2. Prostate IMRT (13-20 segments) was delivered in less than 6-12 minutes depending on the ease of patient setup and on portal imaging. More follow-up is needed to evaluate long-term side effects and efficacy.

## Discussion

Our IMRT planning method creates less segments than the more common bixel-based (inverse) planning methods, which is important to minimize treatment delivery time. It maximizes segment size and is inherently suitable to create sharp dose gradients in anatomically predefined regions. IMRT planning is largely automated by a class solution approach. Actually, about 10% of our patients receive IMRT. The projected total number of IMRT treatments for the year 2000 will be about 100; albeit a small number but sufficient to consume most part of our human and material research resources. Like the vast majority of other centers that use IMRT (with large MLCs i.e. not NOMOS MiMiC) clinically, we have solved the IMRT planning problem in-house. This means that development, maintenance, quality assurance and clinical use of IMRT planning tools is a do-it-ourselves business, which is expensive. We expect that this situation will persist until a commercial IMRT planning system matches our clinical and interfaces with our delivery equipment.

## References

[1] De Gersem W., Derycke S., Colle C., De Wagter C. and De Neve W.; Inhomogeneous target-dose distributions: a dimension more for optimization? *Int. J. Radiat. Oncol. Biol. Phys.* **44**, 461-468 (1999).

[2] De Neve W., De Gersem W., Derycke S., De Meerleer G., Bate M.-Th., Van Duyse B., Vakaet L., De Deene Y., Mersseman B. and De Wagter C.; Clinical delivery of intensity modulated conformal radiotherapy for relapsed or second-primary head and neck cancer using a multileaf collimator with dynamic control. *Radiother. Oncol. 50*, 301-314 (1999).

[3] De Wagter C., Colle C.O., Fortan L.G., Van Duyse B.B., Van den Berge D.L. and De Neve W.J.; 3D-conformal intensity modulated radiotherapy planning: interactive optimization by constrained matrix inversion. *Radiother. Oncol. 47*, 69-76 (1998).

# Quality Assurance of IMRT

**Chen-Shou Chui and Thomas LoSasso**

Memorial Sloan-Kettering Cancer Center, New York, NY 10021, USA.

## Introduction

Intensity-Modulated Radiation Therapy (IMRT) differs from conventional therapy in that the intensity distribution of each field is non-uniform. This intensity distribution is typically determined by an optimization algorithm so that, whcn combined with other fields, an optimum dose distribution can be obtained. The delivery of an intensity-modulated field can be accomplished with a physical compensator, a special multileaf collmator (MLC) such as MIMIC, or a conventional MLC. To ensure accurate and safe delivery of IMRT in the clinic, it is prudent to implment additional quality assurance procedures to those that are already used for conventional therapy. In this wrok, we describe the procedures used in our hospital that are specific to the delivery of IMRT with a conventional MLC.

## Material and methods

There are two types of QA tests involved in IMRT, those concern the machine performance and those verify the accuracy of patient dosimetry. These tests and their frequency are described below.

### Machine Performance

*Film Test* This test[1] was designed to provide a quick and easy check on the accuracy of leaf positions. A special leaf motion file was designed which contains a sequence of all leaf positions that form a pattern so that, when exposed on a film, any error in leaf position in the order of 0.5 mm can be easily detected by eye. This test is performed weekly.

*Gap Test* This test checks the accuracy of the leaf speed and the gap between opposing leaves. A small gap, say 5 mm, is formed by the opposing leaves and the gap is scanned over a flat phantom at a pre-selected constant speed. A chamber is used to measure the dose delivered by such a scanning gap. A nominal dose can be calculated for a given gap width and a scanning speed. An error of 0.1 mm can be easily detected by the chamber reading. This test is performed monthly and can be done at different gantry and collimator angles to evaluate the effects of gravity.

*Log File Analysis* A log file containing the detailed information of all leaf positions, beam-on-time and beam status during beam delivery is produced by the MLC computer. A program was written to analyze these data and compare with those specified in the leaf motion file to ensure that leaf motions are accurately carried out. This test is done periodically or when there is a new software release or IMRT is applied to a new treatment site.

### Patient Dosimetry

*Independent MU Check* For conventional therapy, independent beam-on-time (MU) can be calculated by hand. For the delivery of IMRT with an MLC, hand check is not practical due to its complexity. An independent program was written to verify the MU. The program takes the leaf motion file and the total MU and calculated the delivered intensity distribution. This calculation includes the effects of the rounded leaf end, extended source, and transmission through the leaves. Based on this intensity distribution, doses are then calculated in phantom. These can be checked against the results produced by the treatment planning system. This test is performed for each beam for each patient.

*Portal Image* For conventional therapy, a field is either defined by the jaws or by the aperture of a block. For IMRT delivered with an MLC, we use the most extended position of each leaf as a representation of the field, that is, the left-most positions of all left leaves and the right-most positions of all right leaves. This test is performed weekly for each beam for each patient.

*Record-and-Verify* In addition to checking all other beam parameters such as gantry angle, couch position, etc., the record-and-verify system also checks the initial and final positions of all leaves against those stored as a reference. The initial positions are checked to ensure that the correct leaf motion file is used and the final positions are checked to ensure normal completion of the delivery. This check is performed for each beam delivery.

*Chamber and Film Measurement* Dose delivered from an intensity-modulated field to a point or to a plane in phantom is measured with a chamber or a film. This measurement verifies the accuracy of the calculated dose. This test is performed periodically, or for a new software release, a new treatment site, or when there is a significant discrepency between the independent MU check and treatment planning system.

## Results and discussion

*Film Test* Figure 1 shows an example of the film test. In this example, all leaf pairs are positioned to form 1-mm bands at 1 cm intervals. Figure 1(a) shows that under normal conditions, when all leaf positions are accurate, solid dark lines are seen on the film. In Figure 1(b), positioning errors of 0.5 mm were intentionally introduced to some leaf pairs, the anomalies in the dark lines can be easily seen.

*Gap Test* Figure 2 shows the results of the gap test over a period of more than 18 months. The arrow on the right of the figure indicates a variation in the gap width of 0.2 mm.

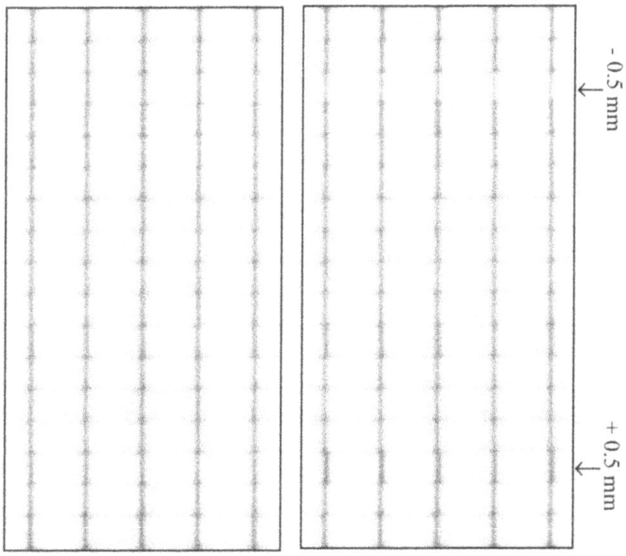


**Figure 1(a):** normal conditions **(b):** errors introduced

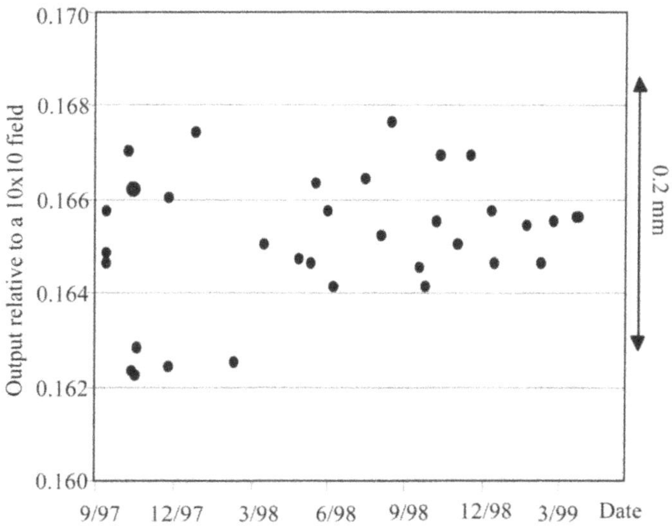


**Figure 2:** Gap test, variation of measured output vs. time

*Independent MU Check* Figure 3 shows the comparison of measured (in solid lines) and calculated (in dotted lines) isodose distribution for one of the fields used in a nasopharynx case. Measurement was made with film and the calculation was done with the independent MU check program based on the leaf motion file and the beam-on-time. In general, the agreement is within 2% in dose or 2 mm in distance. Note that the doses are absolute doses in Gy.

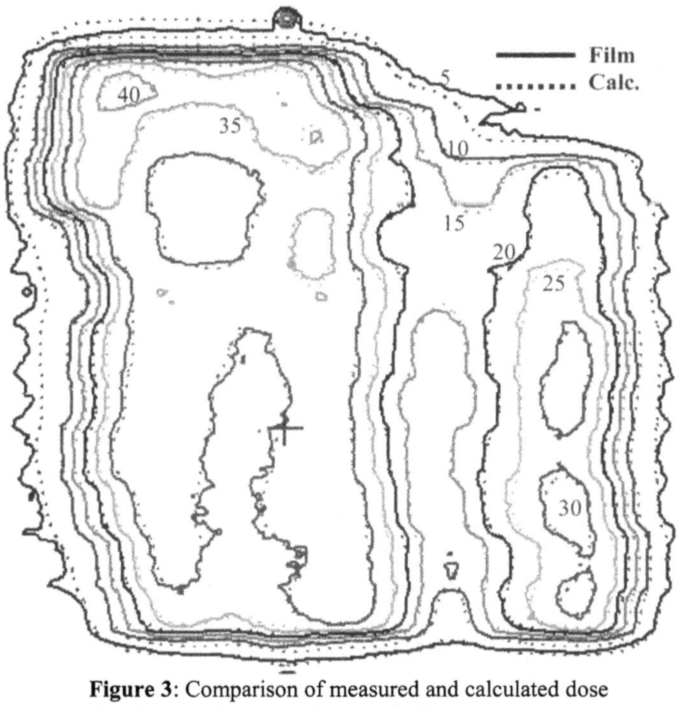


**Figure 3**: Comparison of measured and calculated dose distributions for a nasopharynx field

*Chamber Measurement* Figure 4 shows the results of chamber measurement for almost 400 prostate patients. Each dot represents the raio of measured dose to the calculated dose for all 5 fields for a patient. The agreement is within ±2% for most patients. The mean value of the ratio was 0.993 with a standard deviation of 0.8%.

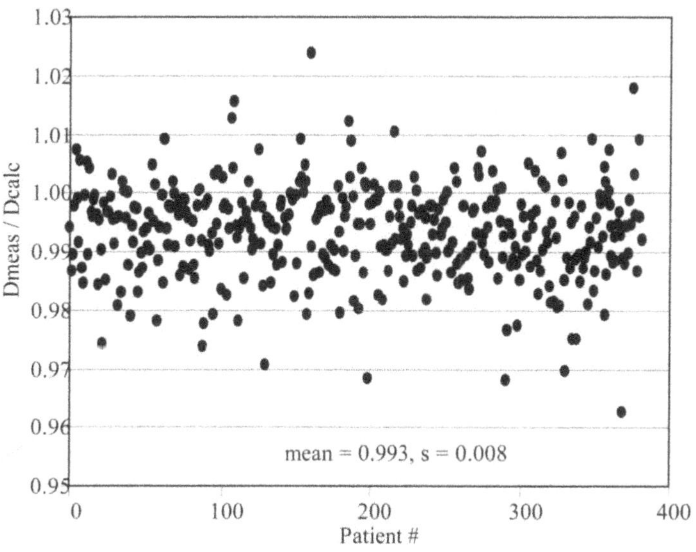


**Figure 4**: Dose of 5 IMRT fields for prostate treatment

## Conclusion

To ensure accurate and safe delivery of IMRT with a conventional MLC, comprehensive QA procedure both for machine performance and for patient dosimetry should be implemented. In general, agreement between calculated and measured doses within 2% or 2 mm can be achieved.

## References

[1] Chui C S, Spirou S V and LoSasso T 1996 Testing of Dynamic Multileaf Collimation *Med. Phys.* 23 635-641

# Monte Carlo studies of energy modulated radiotherapy

**Bruce Faddegon, Judith Balogh, Bob Mackenzie, Yee Ung, and Mark Ruschin**

Toronto-Sunnbrook Regional Cancer Center, 2075 Bayview Avenue, Toronto, Ontario, Canada, M4N 3M5

## Introduction

Our overall goal is to improve the management of head, neck, and breast cancer. Achieving local control is important as a considerable proportion of patients who die, do so with uncontrolled local disease [1]. Moreover, failure to eradicate local disease may serve as a nidus for distant dissemination [2], with local control linked to a reduction in the incidence of distant metastases for a variety of cancers [3-6]. Energy modulated radiotherapy (EMRT) will provide us with the ability to vary energy and intensity over the target and this may lead to improved target coverage with less normal tissue irradiated.

Our best opportunity to evaluate the clinical impact of EMRT is to develop technology that can be put in place at reasonable cost and effort at radiotherapy clinics, since large patient numbers are required for clinical assessment. We intend to make use of standard equipment widely available to radiation oncologists and adapt this equipment to conformal therapy. We have restricted ourselves to the use of linear accelerators (linacs) equipped with scattering foils and commercially available treatment planning systems. To insure that the clinical impact of EMRT is fully and rigorously assessed, treatment planning and dose delivery techniques must be accurate and provide a high level of conformation to the target volume. This will be achieved through research in conformal dose delivery techniques and Monte Carlo inverse planning.

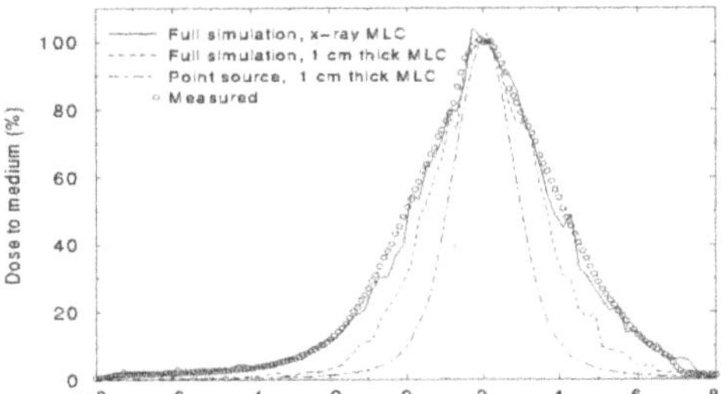


**Figure 1:** BEAM simulations of Philips SL20 15 MeV electron 1.5 cm x 8 cm strip field. Field defined by MLC 70 cm upstream of isocenter. Comparing x-ray MLC with dual scattering foils to thin MLC with either both foils or single foil (point source).

Research in improving the conformation of electron dose distributions to the target volume has included consideration of a motor-driven MLC [7,8], either with conventional linacs [9], or the Scanditronix MM50 racetrack microtron [10-13].

The published work on dose calculation in EMRT [14-17] has been restricted to algorithms known to be in error by more than ±10%/5mm, for standard fields in clinical sites that involve heterogeneities such as air cavities and bone (see Samuelson et al, 1998, [18] and references therein). The accuracy is likely worse in planning the irregular, narrow, segmented fields of conformal therapy. Monte Carlo is the most accurate practical method of dose calculation available, capable of calculating absorbed dose to 4%/4mm in a selection of arbitrary geometries [19-23]. We have developed and commissioned our own electron treatment planning based on the EGS4 Monte Carlo system [24-25]. We have integrated our system with commercial planning systems (Picker ACQSIM and Theratronics Theraplan Plus to take advantage of the interactive, 3-D planning capabilities that these systems offer. Similar systems are under development elsewhere [26-32].

Our current research in EMRT is directed to extending our Monte Carlo RTP system to automated, inverse treatment planning, to establishing energy modulated dose delivery techniques on conventional linacs equipped with scattering foils, and to assessing the clinical impact of EMRT. We present our preliminary results.

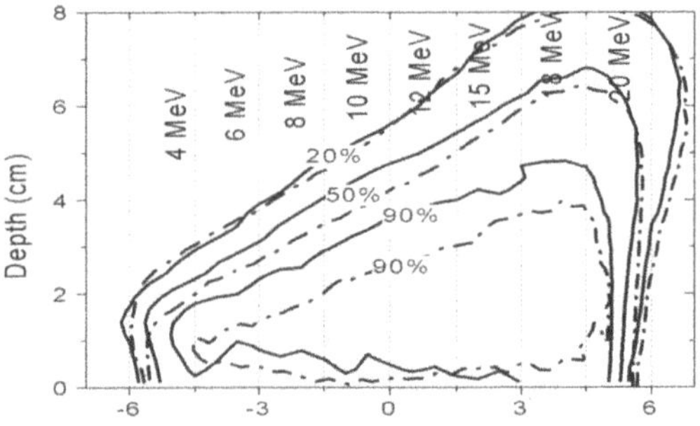


**Figure 2:** BEAM/MCRTP simulations of Philips SL20 wedge field comprised of 8 strip fields of 4-20 MeV. Comparison of dose distributions with two different MLC positions: 5 cm upstream of water surface (solid lines) and 50 cm upstream (dot-dashed lines).

## Material and methods

To investigate the use of conventional accelerators for EMRT, we have considered MLC thickness and placement above the patient, the use of a single scattering foil, and helium in place of air in the treatment head. We have relied on Monte Carlo treatment head simulation with BEAM [21] and dose calculation with MCRTP [24], both EGS4 user codes. We have assessed the accuracy of this approach by comparing measured and calculated dose distributions of 1.5 cm wide, asymmetric strip fields of 4-20 MeV delivered with a Philips SL20 linac and shaped with either the x-ray MLC, 70 cm upstream of the patient, or shields placed on the applicator 5 cm upstream. The accuracy of the calculation was 3%/3mm.

To demonstrate the feasibility of inverse planning EMRT treatments with Monte Carlo, a dose distribution was defined by 8 abutting, 1.5 cm wide field segments, with energies varying from 4-20 MeV across the field. Beam weights were iteratively adjusted to achieve a uniform dose distribution in a wedge shape.

Finally, we have used Monte Carlo inverse planning to study the clinical value of EMRT for a variety of sites. The patient shown here required treatment of the upper third of the esophagus.

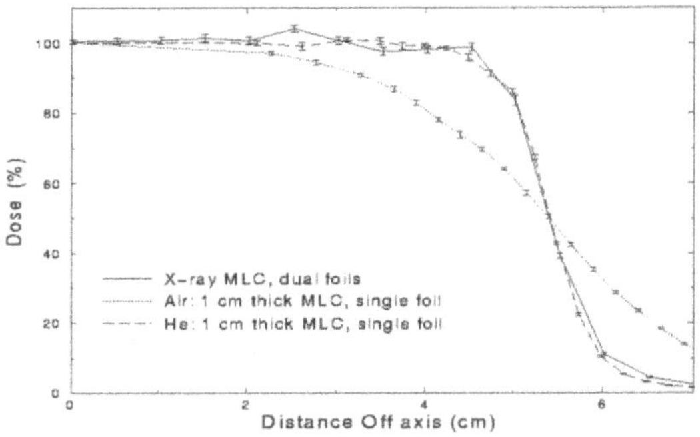


**Figure 3:** BEAM/MCRTP simulation of SL20 15 MeV beam comparing 2 cm depth profile from conventional MLC and scattering foils with profiles from thin MLC and single scattering foil with either air or helium atmosphere in the treatment head.

## Results and discussion

Electron fields shaped with the x-ray MLC of the SL20 have broad profiles, limiting the spatial resolution for field shaping to 4.3 cm for the 15 MeV beam (Figure 1), much larger at lower beam energy. A thinner MLC, with reduced scattering off of the shield edge, improves this somewhat. A single scattering foil further sharpens the field edge dramatically, providing 2.0 cm resolution in field shaping, with the MLC at the level of the x-ray MLC.

The wedge-shaped EMRT field delivered with two different MLC placements of 5 cm and 50 cm above the patient, given a point source 100 cm above the patient, are compared in Figure 2. A single shield placed near the patient is required to sharpen the field at the outermost edge of the combined EMRT field segments. Moving the MLC downstream increases the slope of the dose profile at the edge of the field segment, providing for increased resolution in field shaping, while making beam junctioning more difficult. Effective EMRT field segment shaping is possible with an MLC 50 cm above the patient, with air in the treatment head. This simplifies EMRT design, since the MLC leaves and control mechanism (motors) can be placed well upstream of the patient.

An atmosphere of helium in the treatment head sharpens the penumbra, allowing the use of the jaw-level MLC without the fixed applicator (Figure 3). Mixed modality treatment would be easier to deliver without the electron applicator, eliminating the need for room entry between fields. The x-ray MLC may provide an effective means of field shaping, eliminating the need for a separate electron MLC.

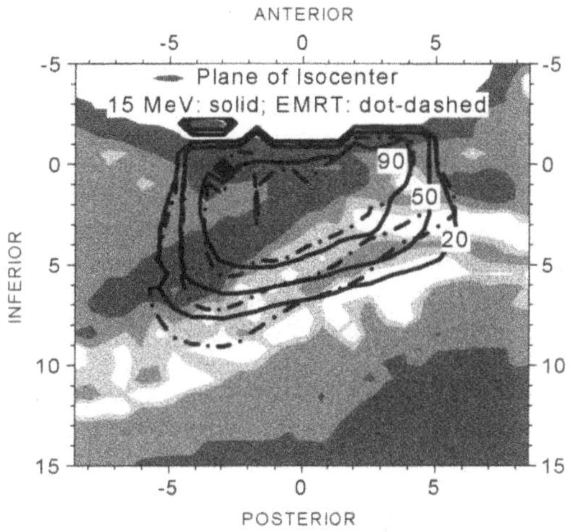


**Figure 4:** Electron therapy of upper third of esophagus. Comparing dose distribution calculated using BEAM/MCRTP in sagittal plane through isocenter for single 15 MeV beam and EMRT field consisting of 3 adjacent strip field segments of 10, 15, and 20 MeV (superior to inferior).

The EMRT treatment of the upper third of the esophagus, shown in Figure 4, is a considerable improvement over a single energy beam. The latter treatment overdoses the spinal cord in the superior portion of the field while underdosing the treatment volume in the inferior portion. In this case we limited the beam energy to 20 MeV, the maximum energy available on our SL20. A higher energy delivered to the inferior portion of the field would further improve conformation of the dose distribution to the treatment volume.

## Conclusion

This study provides further evidence of the feasability of EMRT with a conventional scattering-foil based linac and demonstrates the feasibility of Monte Carlo inverse planning for this application. EMRT provides for much improved conformation to the treatment volume, for example, in the treatment of superior regions of the esophagus.

## References

[1] Brady LW, Markos AM, Mically B, Fischer SA, Lann F, 1990, Innovative Techniques in Radiation Oncology, Cancer 65:610-624

[2] Leibel SA, Ling CC, Kutcher GJ, Mohan R, Cordon-Cordo C, Fuks Z, 1991 {The biological basis for conformal three dimensional radiation therapy, Int J Radiat Oncol Biol Phys 21:805-811

[3] Fuks Z, Leibel SA, Wallner KE, Begg CB, Fair WR, Anderson LL, Hilaris BS, Witmore WF, 1991, The effect of local control on metastatic dissemination in carcinoma of the prostate - long term results in patients treated with I-125 implantation, Int J Radiat Oncol Biol Phys 21:537-547

[4] Leibel SA, Scott CB, Mohinddin M, Marcial VA, Coia LR, Davis LW, Fuks Z, 1991, The effect of local-regional control on distant metastatic dissemination in carcinoma of the head and neck - results of an analysis from the RTOG database, Int J Radiat Oncol Biol Phys 21:549-556

[5] Arriagada R, Rutquist LE, Mattsson A, Kramar A, Rotstein S, 1995, Adequate locoregional treatment for early breast cancer may prevent secondary dissemination, Journal Clinical Oncology 13:2869-2878

[6] Anderson P, Dische S, 1980, Local control and the subsequent incidence of distant metastases, Int J Radiat Oncol Biol Phys 7:1645-1648

[7] JL Humm, A Larsson, EP Lief, 1996, Dosimetric properties of a scanned beam microtron at low monitor unit settings: Importance for conformal therapy, Med Phys 23(3):329-335

[8] EE Klein, Z Li, DA Low, 1996, Feasibility study of multileaf collimated electrons with a scattering foil based accelerator, Radioth and Onc 41(2):189-196

[9] M G Karlsson, M Karlsson, C-M Ma, 1999, Treatment head design for multifleaf collimated high-energy electrons, Med Phys 26(10):2162-2167

[10] A Brahme, 1987, Design principles and clinical possibilities with a new generation of radiation therapy equipment Acta Oncologica 26:403

[11] M Karlsson, H Svensson, H Nystrom, and J Stenberg, 1988, The 50 MeV race-track accelerator -- a new approach to beam shaping and modulation, Proc of Dosim in Radioth 2:307-320

[12] M Karlsson, H Nystrom and H Svensson, 1992, Electron beam characteristics of the 50 MeV racetrack microtron, Med Phys 19(2):307-315

[13] JL Humm, A Larsson, EP Lief, 1996, Dosimetric properties of a scanned beam microtron at low monitor unit settings: Importance for conformal therapy, Med Phys 23(3):329-335

[14] S Hyodynmaa, A Gustafsson, and A Brahme, 1996, Optimization of conformal electron beam using energy and fluence modulation, Med Phys 23(5):659

[15] M Asell, S Hyodynmaa, A Gustafsson, and A Brahme, 1997, Optimization of 3D conformal electron beam therapy in inhomogeneous media by concomitant fluence and energy modulation, Phys Med Biol 42(11):2083

[16] MA Ebert and PW Hoban, 1997, Possibilities for tailoring dose distributions through the manipulation of electron beam characteristics, Phys Med Biol 42(11):2065-2081

[17] M G Karlsson, M Karlsson, and B Zackrisson, 1998, Intensity modulation with electrons: calculations, measurements and clinical applications, Phys Med Biol 43:1159-1169

[18] A Samuelson, S Hyodynmaa, and KA Johansson, 1998, Dose accuracy check of the 3D electron beam algorithm in a treatment planning system, Phys Med Biol 43:129-1544

[19] KR Shortt, CK Ross, AF Bielajew, DWO Rogers, 1986, Electron beam dose distributions near standard inhomogeneities, Phys Med Biol 1, 235

[20] H Neuenschwander and EJ Born, 1992, A macro Monte Carlo method for electron beam dose calculation, Phys Med Biol 37, 107

[21] DWO Rogers, BA Faddegon, GX Ding, CM Ma, J We, TR Mackie, 1995, BEAM: A Monte Carlo code to simulate radiotherapy treatment units, Med Phys 22, 503

[22] BB Sorcini, S Hyodynmaa, and A Brahme, 1995, The role of phantom and treatment head generated bremsstrahlung in high-energy electron beam dosimetry, Phys Med Biol 40, 1135

[23] M Fippel, I Kawrakow, and K Friedrich, 1997, Electron beam dose calculations with the VMC algorithm and the verification data of the NCI working group, Phys Med Biol 42, 501

[24] BA Faddegon, 1998, MCRTP: A new EGS4 user code for Monte Carlo electron treatment planning, Med Phys 25(6):1073 (abstract)

[25] BA Faddegon, J Balogh, R Mackenzie, and D Scora, 1998, Clinical considerations of Monte Carlo for electron radiotherapy treatment planning, Rad Phys and Chem 53, 217

[26] SP Teng, DW Anderson, and DG Lindstrom, 1986, Monte Carlo electron-transport calculations for clinical beams using energy grouping, Appl Radiat Isot 37(12):1189-1194

[27] AA Al Beteri, DE Raeside, 1992, Optimal electron beam treatment planning for retinoblastoma using a new three-dimensional Monte Carlo-based treatment planning system, Med Phys 19: 125

[28] H Neuenschwander, TR Mackie, PJ Reckwerdt, 1995, MMC – a high-performance Monte Carlo code for electron beam treatment planning, Phys Med Biol 40: 543

[29] PJ Keall and PW Hoban, 1996, Super-Monte Carlo: A 3-D electron beam dose calculation algorithm, Med Phys 23: 2023

[30] I Kawrakow, M Fippel, K Friedrich, 1997, Improved modeling of multiple scattering in the VMC model, Med Phys 24: 505

[31] CL Hartmann Siantar et al, 1997, Validation and clinical implementation of the Peregrine Monte Carlo dose calculation system for photon beam therapy, Medical and Biological Engineering and Comput 35, supplement part 2: 1102 (abstract)

[32] JJ DeMarco, TD Solberg, and JB Smathers, 1998, A CT-based Monte Carlo simulation tool for dosimetry planning and analysis, Med Phys 25(1), 1

# Modulated Electron Beams for Treatment of Breast Cancer

C.-M. Ma[1], T. Pawlicki[1], M.C. Lee[1], S.B. Jiang[1], J.S. LI[1], J. Deng[1], B. Yi[2], E. Mok[1] and A.L. Boyer[1]

[1]Radiation Oncology Department, Stanford University School of Medicine, Stanford, CA 94305, USA,
[2]Asan Medical Center, University of Ulsan, College of Medicine, Seoul, Korea

## Introduction

Photon beams have been an effective modality for breast cancer treatment in radiation therapy while electron beams are occasionally used for a boost dose when the photon beams are intentionally placed to miss part of the target in order to reduce the dose to the lung and heart. Although such conventional treatment with tangential photon fields has been successful, the following problems (or potential areas of improvement) remain: (1) the inclusion of the lung and other normal tissues, and sometimes of a small volume of the heart in the high-dose volume due to tumor location, patient size or in the case of chest-wall treatments; (2) lower dose near the skin surface due to lack of electron build-up in a photon beam; and (3) high exit or scatter dose to normal structures such as the lung and heart, and more importantly the contralateral breast, which may be a major cause for the occurrence of secondary cancer in the contralateral breast for women under the age of 45.

Advances in the state of the art of computer-controlled medical linear accelerators have recently become available so that, along with newly-developed treatment planning techniques, significant improvementscan be made in the delivery and control of external beam radiation through beam-intensity modulation. Using the modulated electron radiotherapy (MERT) technique [1-3], problem (1) above may be significantly improved and problems (2) and (3) maybe almost eliminated due to the nature of the electron beams. In this work, we investigate the feasibility of optimizing energy- and intensity-modulated electron beams for breast cancer treatment.

## Material and methods

### A prototype electron MLC

We have developed a prototype electron MLC for MERT beam delivery (Fig. 1). The electron MLC consists of 30 steel leaf pairs. Each leaf is 0.476 cm wide, 20 cm long and 2.54 cm thick with straight edges and ends. The leaves were mounted on a steel frame attached to the bottom scraper of a 25 cm x 25 cm electron applicator on a Varian Clinac 2100C (Varian Oncology Systems, Palo Alto, CA). The leaves can slide in the steel frame and the leaf positions can be easily set using a pre-cut cardboard for a beam segment. The field shape is maintained by tightening the screws from the side. The largest light field available using the electron MLC was 15.7 cm x 15.7 cm projected at 100 cm source-surface distance (SSD).

### Monte Carlo simulations

We have used the EGS4[4] user code BEAM[5] for the accelerator head simulation. A detailed description of the clinical implementation of the Monte Carlo method at the Stanford Medical Center was given in a previous publication[6]. For this work, we have used the previously simulated Monte Carlo beam data[6] for 6, 12 and 20 MeV electron beams from a Varian Clinac 2100C linear accelerator and for 6 MV photon beams from a 2300CD accelerator (Varian Oncology Systems, Palo Alto, California). The phase-space data were scored at a plane directly above the lowest scraper. Field shaping by the electron MLC was further simulated using the BEAM component module MLC. In the simulations of the electron beams collimated by an electron MLC, the leaves were placed on the bottom scrapper of a 25 cm x 25 cm applicator with a 7 cm air gap between the bottom surface of the MLC and the isocenter.

An EGS4 user code, MCDOSE, was used in this work for the dose calculations. MCDOSE was designed for dose calculations in a 3D rectilinear voxel geometry. Voxel dimensions were completely variable in all three directions. Every voxel (volume element) could be assigned to a different material. The mass density of the material in an MCDOSE calculation was varied based on the patient's CT data. Several variance reduction techniques have been implemented in the MCDOSE code to improve the calculation efficiency. These include photon interaction forcing, particle splitting, Russian roulette, electron range rejection and region rejection, particle track displacement and rotation, and correlated sampling. For patient dose calculations, the simulation phantom had up to 128 x 128 x 128 voxels (uniform in any dimensions). The side of a voxel varied from 0.2 to 0.4 cm. To simulate the dose distribution of a finite size beamlet used by the inverse planning process, particles were transported to the MLC plane and only those within the beamlet area were allowed to go through. After optimization, a leaf sequence was generated using a "step and shoot" algorithm. The final MERT dose distribution was computed based on the leaf sequence and the bremsstrahlung leaf leakage effect was included in the final dose calculation using pre-calculated leaf leakage data for 1.5 cm thick tungsten leaves. The EGS4 transport parameters were ECUT = AE = 700 keV, PCUT = AP = 10 keV and ESTEPE = 0.04. The number of particle histories simulated ranged from 2

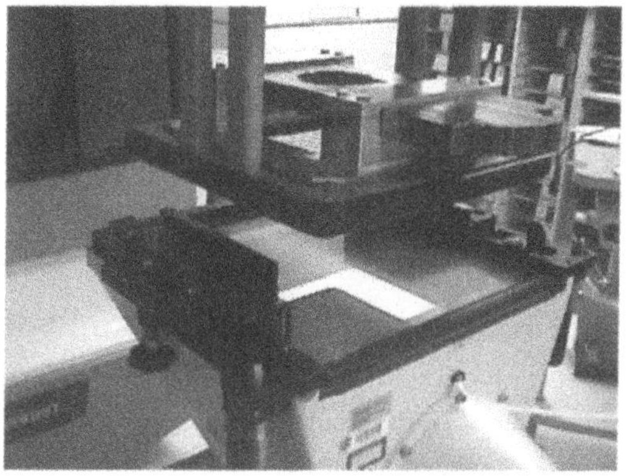

**Figure 1:** A prototype electron MLC and the Beam Imaging System.

million to 30 million for a MERT treatment. The 1-σ statistical uncertainty in the dose was generally 2% or smaller of the maximum dose. The CPU time required for a MERT simulation was about 1 - 3 hours on a Pentium III 450 MHz PC with the variance reduction option switched on.

### The optimization process

The treatment planning optimization system used in this work is developed in-house. First, the dose deposition coefficients, defined as the dose contribution from a beamlet to a point, are calculated using the MCDOSE code. Second, using the calculated dose deposition coefficients as input, the optimal intensity profile for each beam is achieved by using the center-of-mass method(guided by the Zangwill's penalty function) to minimize the augmented objective function. An improved conjugate vector method has been investigated. For the target area, a quadratic form of objective function is specified. In addition, two target dose-uniformity constraints are used to ensure a uniform target dose distribution and to distinguish the clinical importance of cold and hot spots. For the critical structures, maximum-dose constraint and several levels of dose-volume constraints are assigned to each structure. For each objective function and constraint, an importance weight relative to the target objective function is assigned. All the constraints are mathematically transformed to the penalty functions of quadratic forms. The augmented objective function, which should be minimized, is a combination of the original objective functions and all penalty functions. The results of the optimization process are the intensity profiles for the individual fields. Each beamlet within a given field can vary in intensity and incident energy.

## Results and discussion

### Characteristics of MLC collimated electron beams

Figure 2 shows the electron fields collimated by the prototype electron MLC for 6, 12 and 20 MeV electron beams on a Varian Clinac 2100C machine. For convenience, a photo showing the MLC leaf positions for the field shape is also included. The MLC-to detector distance was 10 cm. It is found that for a 20 MeV electron beams, 0.5 cm leaf shapes are still distinguishable on the surface but become much blurred at the

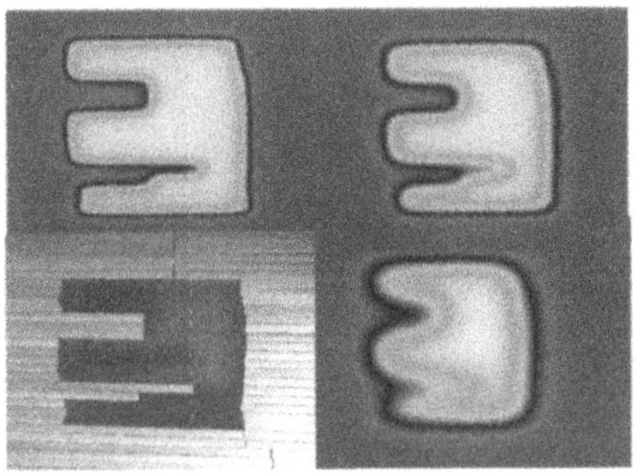


**Figure 2:** Electron fields collimated by an electron MLC measured using a Beam Imaging System.

2 cm depth. For a 6 MeV electron beam, however, the effect of electron scattering becomes so severe that a leaf width smaller than 1.0 cm will not result in any improvement in the spatial resolution. However, a small leaf width may have the advantage of defining the field more precisely in the direction perpendicular to the leaves.

We further performed Monte Carlo simulations of electron fields collimated by 1 cm wide leaves to study the effect of material type and leaf thickness. Although the beam penumbral widths did not change significantly for leaf thicknesses smaller than 2 cm the beam intensity outside the field was affected by the leaf thickness and the atomic number of the leaf material. For 1.5 cm copper, 1.5 cm of lead and 2 cm of steel, the electron fluence was about 2.5% of the central axis value for a 20 MeV beam. The electron fluence was reduced to about 1.5% if the leaves were made of 1.5 cm tungsten. If we increased the tungsten leaf thickness to 2 cm the electron fluence would be reduced to less than 1% of the central axis value and the photon leakage would be reduced to about 50% of the central axis value.

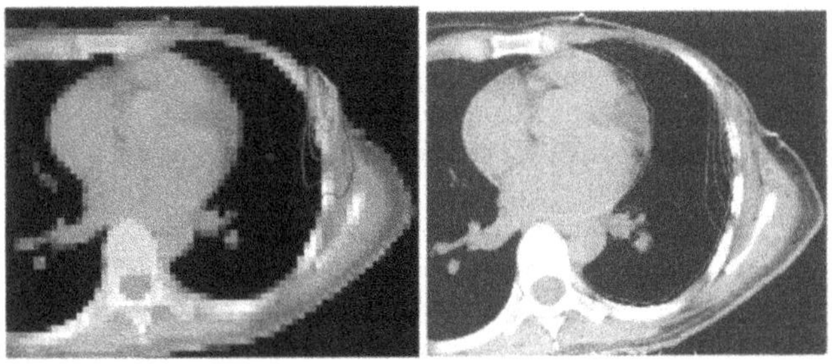

**Figure 3:** Electron beamlet distributions calculated by Monte Carlo (left) and the FOCUS 3D pencil beam algorithm (right).

### Comparison of beamlet distributions

The accuracy of the beamlet distribution calculation may play an important role in the treatment planning optimization process. We have computed the beamlet dose distributions using the 3D pencil beam as implemented in the FOCUS treatment planning system (Computerized Medical Systems, St. Louis, MO) and compared with the Monte Carlo calculated beamlets. For beamlets with normal incidence, the difference in the dose distributions in the heart was evident: the Monte Carlo calculated isodose lines varied with the heart contour while the pencil beam isodose lines remained symmetrical despite the change in material densities. The beamlet distributions differed significantly in the lung for oblique incidence (Fig. 3). The axis of the beamlet was intentionally placed to go through soft tissues and bones. The pencil beam isodose lines seemed to stretch according to the beam axis pathlength and showed no signs of electron build down near the low density material.

### Comparison of a breast plan

To demonstrate the possibility of improving the dose homogeneity in the target and the reduction of the dose to the lung and other normal tissues, we compare the dose distributions of a typical breast treatment plan using tangential photon beams and MERT (Fig. 4). The MERT plan was achieved with normally incident 6, 12 and 20 MeV electron beams. The beamlet size was 1 cm x 1 cm. The dose

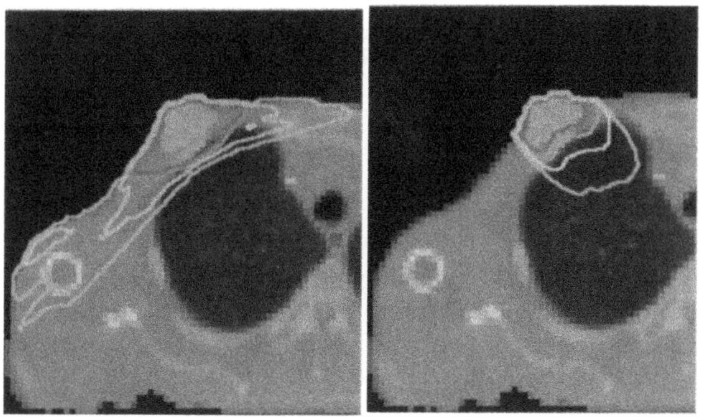

**Figure 4:** Breast treatment plans using tangential photon beams (left) or MERT (right).

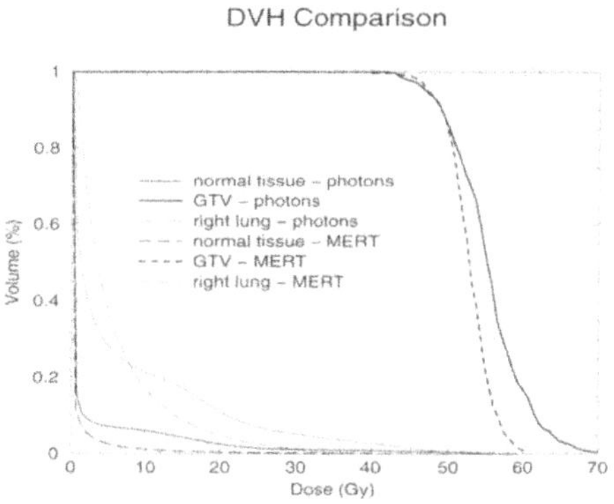


**Figure 5:** Electron fields collimated by an electron MLC measured using a Beam Imaging System.

distributions for both plans were calculated using the Monte Carlo method. The isodose lines (90, 70, 50 and 30%) were normalized in such a way that the 90% isodose surface would receive the prescribed target dose of 50 Gy. For the photon plan, the 90% dose line also included a 1 cm margin between the target and the lung to account for the effect of patient breathing. This was not needed for the electron plan as electron beams were incident from the front and the dose distributions were not expected to vary significantly with breathing. Figure 5 shows the dose volume histograms (DVH) for the breast treatment plans shown in Fig. 4.

It is clear that MERT provided much better dose homogeneity in the target region than tangential photon beams. Tangential photon beams produced hot spots in the target and cold spots near the skin (Fig. 5), MERT also significantly reduced the dose to the lung than tangential photon beams; the maximum dose to the lung was reduced from 50 Gy for a tangential treatment to 35 Gy for MERT. However, MERT increased the volume of the lung that received lower dose (10% more volume received 5 Gy and 20% more volume received 2 Gy) compared to tangential photon beams. The clinical significance of the increased lung volume that received such low dose needs to be investigated. Another clear benefit with MERT is the exclusion of the normal tissue from the high dose volume. Over 1000 $cm^3$ of normal tissue received 10 - 30 Gy less dose in a MERT plan compared to a tangential photon plan. This can significantly reduce normal tissue complications in a breast treatment.

## Conclusion

We have investigated the feasibility of optimizing energy- and intensity-modulated electron beams for breast cancer treatment. A multileaf collimator (MLC) specially designed for MERT was investigated both experimentally and by Monte Carlo simulations. An inverse-planning system based on Monte Carlo dose calculations was developed to optimize electron beam energy and intensity to achieve dose conformity for target volumes near the surface. The results showed that an MLC with 5-mm leaf widths could produce complex field shapes for MERT. Focused leaf ends reduced the electron scattering contributions to the dose compared to straight leaf ends. There were significant differences in the beamlet distributions calculated by an analytic 3-D pencil beam algorithm and the Monte Carlo method. A breast treatment was compared using tangential photon beams and MERT to demonstrate that MERT had the potential to improve the target dose coverage and reduce the dose to the surrounding healthy tissues for treatment of breast and other tumors near the skin.

This work was supported in part by a grant from the Department of Defense US Army Breast Cancer Research Program BC971292 and NIH grant CA78331 and a consortium agreement with the NumeriX, LLC.

## References

[1] Hyodynmaa S, Gastafsson A and Brahme A (1996) Optimization of conformal electron beam therapy using energy- & fluence-modulated beams, Med. Phys., 23: 659-666

[2] Åsell M, Hyödynmaa S, Gustafsson A and Brhma A 1997 Optimization of 3D conformal electron beam therapy in inhomogeneous media by concomitant fluence and energy modulation Phys. Med. Biol. 42: 2083-100

[3] Karlsson MG, Karlsson MK and Ma C-M (1999), Treatment head design for multileaf collimated high-energy electrons, Med. Phys. 26: 2125-32

[4] Nelson R, Hirayama H and Rogers DWO (1985). The EGS4 code system, Stanford Linear Accelerator Center Report SLAC-265 (SLAC, Stanford, CA)

[5] Rogers DWO, Faddegon BA, Ding GX, Ma C-M, Wei JS, Mackie TR (1995). BEAM: A Monte Carlo code to simulate radiotherapy treatment units. Med. Phys. 22: 503-25.

[6] Ma C-M, Mok E, Kapur A, Pawlicki T A, Findley D, Brain S, Forster K and Boyer AL (1999) Clinical implementation of a Monte Carlo treatment planning system for radiotherapy, Med. Phys. 26: 2133-43

# Monte Carlo Simulations of Multileaf Collimated Electrons

**Michael C. Lee[1], Steve B. Jiang[1], Byong-Yong Yi[2], and Chang-Ming Ma[1]**

[1]Department of Radiation Oncology, Stanford University School of Medicine, Stanford, CA 94305, USA, and [2]Asan Medical Center, University of Ulsan, College of Medicine, Seoul, Korea

## Introduction

There has been growing interest in the use of intensity modulated electron beams in conjuction with intensity modulated photon beams to obtain optimal dose distributions for radiation therapy. A number of methods have been proposed, including the use of scanned beam systems[1] as well as utilizing the existing photon multileaf collimators for electron therapy. Studies by Jansson *et al.* have used matched photon and electron beams from the intrinsic MLC of a microtron (MM22, Scanditronix Medical AB, Uppsala, Sweden) to improve dose distributions for breast cancer treatment.[2] Experimental work by Klein *et al.* has shown that in a standard Varian 2100C, an SSD of no greater that 70 cm is required for a clinically acceptable field[3]. Recently, Karlsson *et al.* utilized Monte Carlo simulations to conclude that for a 9 MeV beam, an acceptable dose penumbra could be acheived by replacing the beam axis atmosphere with helium to reduce in-air scatter, or by lowering the photon MLC by at least 11cm[4]. This study uses a combination of Monte Carlo simulations and film measurements to extend these studies to a greater energy range (6, 12, and 20 MeV) and presents data that suggets that for low energies, an electron specific multileaf collimator is necessary for intensity modulated electron beam therapy.

## Material and methods

### Monte Carlo Simulations

Electron beam simulations of a Varian Clinac 2100C (Varian Oncology Systems, Palo Alto, CA) were performed using the EGS4/BEAM Monte Carlo code[5]. Vendor supplied geometries were used in the component-wise simulation, leading to a previously demonstrated agreement with measured data of better than 2% in transverse profiles and depth dose curves[6]. Two different phase space files were obtained below the photon jaws (set for a 25x25 applicator) for each energy: one in which the ambient atmosphere of the treatment head and air gap was standard air ($1.205\times10^{-3}$ g·cm$^{-3}$), and one in which it was replaced with helium ($1.663\times10^{-4}$ g·cm$^{-3}$). These files were used as sources for MLC simulations. This and all simulations utilized electron and photon cutoffs of 0.700 MeV and 10 keV total energy respectively. The number of initial electron histories ranged from $150\times10^{6}$ for 6 MeV to $50\times10^{6}$ for 20 MeV.

The photon MLC in this study was an idealized MLC with tungsten leaves of the same thickness as the Varian 52 leaf MLC, but with ends and sides always singly focused to the photon source, regardless of leaf position. This was set for an exact 10x10 cm$^2$ field or a specific leaf sequence.

To select an optimal electron MLC design, simulations were performed with the MLCs completely replacing the last scraper of a 25x25 cm$^2$ applicator. Different materials and thicknesses were simulated, and phase space files obtained immediately at the back surface of the MLC. Three construction materials were considered in this investigation: steel (8.06 g·cm$^{-3}$), copper (8.933 g·cm$^{-3}$), and tungsten (19.30 g·cm$^{-3}$). The copper and tungsten MLCs were limited to 1.5cm in thickness, and the steel MLC was 2.0cm in thickness. Simulations were also performed for single leaves in a 20x20 cm$^2$ field to determined optimal leaf widths.

In all cases, dose was calculated using the EGS4/DOSXYZ user code[7] with homogeneous water phantoms. The voxel geometry for penumbra calculations were 3mm x 15mm x 2mm, for isodose curves 3mm x 3mm x 2mm, and for leaf width simulations 1mm x 40mm x 2mm.

### Prototype electron MLC

Based on the results of the theoretical study, a prototype of an electron MLC was designed and built. The MLC comprised two sets of 30 leaves, each leaf 2.54 cm in thickness and 0.48 cm (0.53 cm projected at 100cm SSD) in width. Both ends and sides were constructed parallel with the beam axis, ie. unfocused. Leaf positions could be set manually and allowed a maximum opening of 15.7x17.6 cm$^2$ at 100cm SSD with complete leaf overrun allowed. The MLC was designed to fit into the cutout mounting frame in the last scraper of a 25x25 applicator used by a Varian Clinac 2100C linear accelerator such that the bottom face of the leaves are supported at 3.03cm above the applicator scraper.

The geometry of this prototype was simulated using BEAM and phase space files were obtained for a representative set of leaf positions and dose calculations conducted with DOSXYZ.

The MLC was then installed onto the treatment head and film (Kodak X-omat V, Eastman Kodak Company, Rochester, NY) measurements were taken at the surface, located at 100 cm SSD) and at the surface and solid water depths of 1.5cm, 3cm, and 3cm for 6, 12, and 20 MeV respectively. The film was scanned using a Vidar scanning system (VIDAR Systems Corporation, Herndon, VA) and the RIT315 software package (Radiological Imaging Technology, Colorado Springs, CO) was then used to generate isodose distributions.

## Results and discussion

### Electron beams collimated with the photon MLC

The 90-10 dose penumbras of photon MLC collimated electron beams were computed at depths of 0.75, 2.0, and 3.0 cm for 6,

12, and 20 MeV respectively, and the results displayed in Table 1. At all energies, a substantial difference was observed in the penumbra width between the standard setup and systems in which a helium atmosphere was present. At 6 MeV, the difference was 52% while at 20 MeV it was a smaller, though still significant, 26%.

Furthermore, the data suggests that within the SSDs of interest, in particular those that are clinically acheivable, there is a linear relationship between SSD and penumbra size. This is clearly seen in Figure 1, where a least squares linear fit has been overlaid on the data. This will be employed in a later section to illustrate the advantage of a specialized electron MLC.

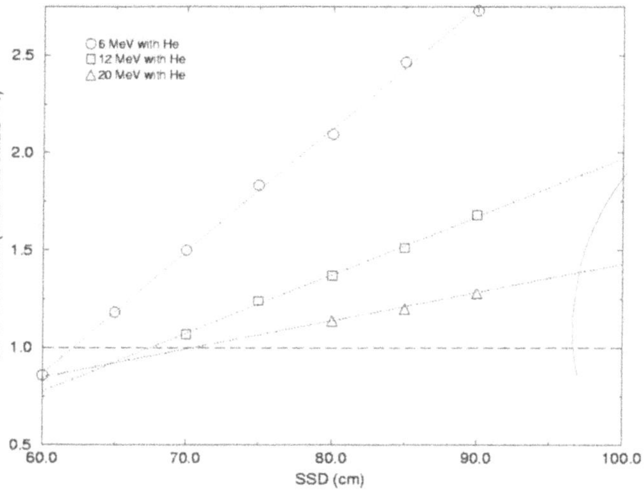


**Figure 1:** Dose penumbras for a 10x10 $cm^2$ electron beams, normalized to the 90-10 penumbra of the electron MLC.

| | 80 cm (air) | 80 cm (He) | eMLC |
|---|---|---|---|
| **6 MeV** | 46.7 | 27.6 (40.9) | 13.2 (52.2) |
| **12 MeV** | 26.0 | 18.6 (40.0) | 13.6 (26.9) |
| **20 MeV** | 22.3 | 16.5 (26.0) | 14.5 (12.1) |

**Table 1:** 90-10 penumbras, expressed in mm, for a photon MLC with SSD = 80 cm with and without helium, and the ideal electron MLC model. The numbers in the parentheses are the percent improvement for helium over air, and the eMLC over helium.

### Design considerations for an electron MLC

In Monte Carlo simulations of the proposed designs, the tungsten leaves exhibited a background electron leakage of 1.5% of the central axis fluence (scored immediately at the back of the eMLC), while both the steel and copper models exhibited greater than 2.0% leakage. Additionally, the tungsten leaves resulted in a steeper drop at the field edge, corresponding to a reduction in the passage of high angle electrons through the leaf ends.

The production of bremstrahlung photons by the interaction of high energy electrons in the leaves was also considered. As expected on the basis of the material bremstrahlung production cross-sections, tungsten again exhibits the best fluence profile, presenting less than half the photon leakage of the copper or steel MLCs. Use of the BEAM code's "latch bit" settings to track particle interaction histories demonstrated that this photon leakage was primarily bremstrahlung production. Indeed, 1.5 cm tungsten was sufficient to stop all but 15% of the total direct leakage. As expected, the bremstrahlung photons from the tungsten leaves were of a slightly higher energy (5.3 MeV for tungsten and 4.3 MeV average for steel and copper), but the overall photon energy fluence from the tungsten leaves remains significantly below that of the other materials. Based on this information, the tungsten leaf design was chosen as the model of what is hereafter referred to as the "ideal" electron MLC.

Further Monte Carlo studies were performed to analyze the leaf width that provides the highest degree of resolution while minimizing the number of leaves so as to reduce interleaf leakage, mechanical complexity, and cost. Of particular interest were the maximum dose reduction acheived at $d_{max}$ and the width of the dose "valley" produced by this single leaf. The results are plotted in Figure 2 with a cubic least squares interpolation. At an energy of 6 MeV, it was found that a leaf width of 8.82 mm projected at 100 SSD, or 8.58 mm at the level of the MLC, would produce a dose reduction of 50%. Not unexpectedly, the critical leaf width for the 20 MeV beam was much smaller, and the same dose reduction of 50% could be acheived by a leaf width of 4.90 mm projected, or 4.77 mm at the MLC. It was observed that the 75% dose width scaled linearly with the leaf width. We thus conclude that a leaf width of less than 1cm at 100cm SSD are not useful for defining the shape of a low energy field, though a leaf width of 5mm will provide maximal resolution definition of high energy fields and will also be useful in defining the lateral position of the field.

Additional simulations were performed to compare the ideal eMLC with the prototype eMLC. At all energies, lowering the MLC resulted in a reduction 20-21% reduction of the 90-10 penumbra. Therefore, we conclude that any production eMLC should follow the design recommendations described above, in particular with respect distance from the surface and construction material.

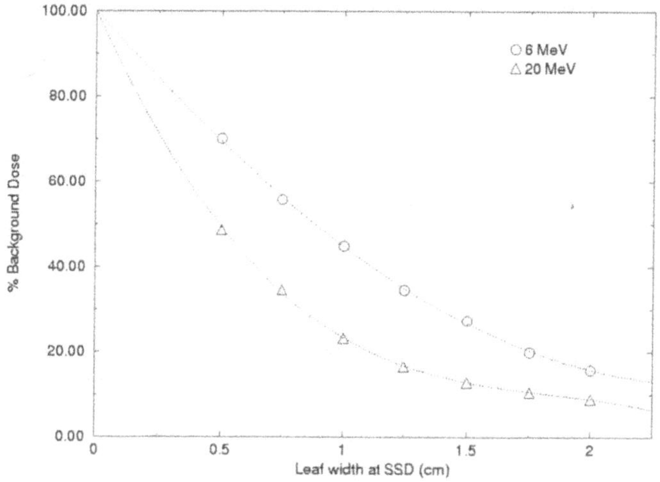


**Figure 2:** Dose reduction as a function of leaf width. A single leaf was inserted into a 20x20 $cm^2$ field collimated by an electron MLC.

**Measurements and Monte Carlo Simulations**

Studies were conducted to examine the ability of Monte Carlo calculations to accurately simulate an electron MLC. A comparison was made between the isodose curves generated from simulations and film scans. The agreement between the two is excellent at all energies, with a maximum deviation of less than 2mm at 3cm depth for 12 and 20 MeV and 1.5cm depth for 6 MeV. It is therefore concluded that the Monte Carlo method is capable of simulating dose distributions from an electron MLC in homogeneous media.

**Comparison of electron and photon MLC shaped fields**

Calculations were performed to compare the dose penumbras from the eMLC to those from the photon MLC. As shown in Table 1 and Figure 1, even in the presence of helium, using the electron MLC reduces the 10x10 $cm^2$ 90-10 penumbra from 12.1% (20 MeV) to as much as 44.6% (6 MeV). However, the absolute change from 20 MeV was only 2 mm. Extrapolating from the existing data points, one can calculate the SSD required for the penumbra from the photon MLC to match the electron MLC. It was determined that, the required SSDs for 6, 12, and 20 MeV are, respectively, 65.5, 68.0, 69.8 cm. In a standard air atmosphere, the required SSDs are all less than 65cm, which is clearly unacheivable in any practical system.

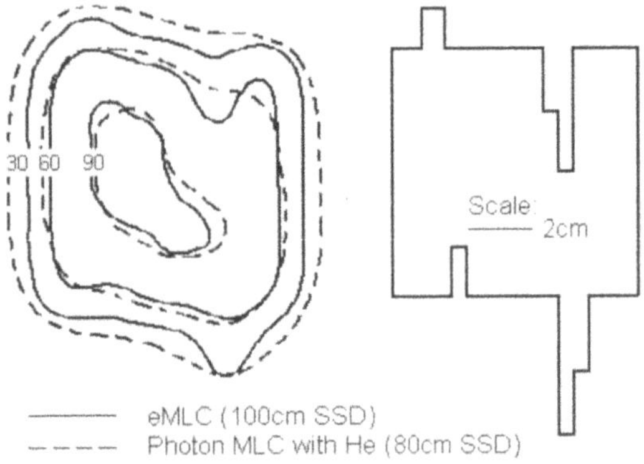


**Figure 3:** (left) Isodose curves at 1.5cm depth from a 6 MeV beam (right) The projected leaf sequence at phantom surface

In Figure 3, the Monte Carlo simulated isodose curves for a 6 MeV field collimated by the prototype electron MLC and an equivalent photon MLC with He are shown. It is seen that at this energies, the eMLC is more faithful to the original leaf pattern than the photon MLC. At 12 and 20 MeV, the shapes of both fields are comparable, with the 90% isodose lines agreeing to within 3mm. However, penumbras differ along the trend shown in Figure 1.

## Conclusion

It has been demonstrated that the in-air scattering of the electron beam makes the photon MLC a poor choice for generating complex shapes needed for intensity modulated electron therapy. This is partially ameliorated by filling the treatment head with helium (a non-trivial task of engineering) and placing a helium filled bag between the patient and the treatment head. Indeed, for such a system, at 12 and 20 MeV at an SSD of 80cm, the isodose curves are within 3 mm of the equivalent electron MLC field. However, at 6 MeV the isodose curves are no longer comparable, and adding helium to the beam axis atmosphere does not improve the situation. We therefore conclude that an electron specific MLC constructed of tungsten leaves of 15mm thickness and 5 mm width, would be minimally sufficient for use in intensity modulated electron beam therapy. This MLC would optimally be part of a specially designed electron applicator, although experiments have indicated that an MLC designed as an applicator accessory also provides significant improvement in dose distribution over the photon MLC. Additionally, it has been demonstrated that Monte Carlo simulations provide an accurate means of calculating dose distributions from such a collimation system.

This work was supported in part by a grant from the Department of Defense US Army Breast Cancer Research Program BC971292 and NIH grant CA78331. MCL was supported in part by the NIH Training Grant 2T32GM08294-11.

## References

[1] Brahme A 1987 Design principles and clinical possibilities with a new generation of radiation therapy equipment *Acta Oncologica* **26** 403-412

[2] Jansson T, Lindman H, Nygärd K, Dahlgren C V, Montelius A, Öberg-Kreuger S, Asplud S and Berg J 1997 Radiotherapy of breast cancer after breast-conserving surgery: an improved technique using mixed electron-photon beams with a multileaf collimator *Radiotherapy and Oncology* **46** 83-89

[3] Klein E E, Li Z and Low D A 1996 Feasibility study of multileaf collimated electrons with a scattering foil based accelerator *Radiotherapy and Oncology* **41** 189-196

[4] Karlsson M G, Karlsson M and Ma C-M 1999 Treatment head design for multileaf collimated high-energy electrons *Med Phys* **26** 2161-2167

[5] Rogers D W O, Faddegon B A, Ding G X, Ma C-M, We J and Mackie T R 1995 BEAM: A Monte Carlo code to simulate radiotherapy treatment units *Med Phys* **22** 503-524

[6] Kapur A, Ma C-M, Mok E C, Findley D O, Boyer A L 1998 Monte Carlo calculations of electron beam output factors for a medical linear acclerator *Phys Med Biol* **43** 3479-3494

[7] Ma C-M, Reckwerdt P, Holmes M, Rogers D W O, Geiser B, Walters B 1995 DOSXYZ users manual *National Research Council of Canada Report PIRS-0509b* (Ottowa: NRC)

# Applicability of a multi-hole collimator for scanned photon beams: A Monte Carlo study

**Gunilla Küster and Thomas Bortfeld**
DKFZ, Dept. of Medical Physics, Im Neuenheimer Feld 280, D-69120 Heidelberg

## Introduction

One possibility to deliver intensity modulated fields is to use a scanned photon beam, i.e. to build the intensity profile from narrow photon beam spots. The photon beam is moved across the radiation field by scanning the incident electron beam above the bremsstrahlung target. The target has to be designed such that a narrow photon intensity distribution is produced. This technique has been investigated for 50 MeV electrons by Svensson et al. [1, 2, 3], where photon beams with a width of about 3 cm at 100 cm source to axis distance (SAD) were generated with an optimized target. In order to achieve steeper dose gradients, the scanning of the narrow bremsstrahlung beam was also combined with static multileaf collimator settings. In a recent study the feasibility of the scanned photon beam technique has been investigated at lower electron energies of around 20 MeV [4]. As expected, the photon beam width behind the bremsstrahlung target is significantly higher than for 50 MeV electrons. With a thin beryllium target beam widths of around 4 cm can be realized. Since this resolution is not sufficient for many IMRT applications, the applicability of a multi-hole collimator has been investigated in the present work (patent pending). The use of this collimator eliminates the rather large penumbras that are observed if the narrow bremsstrahlung lobes are superimposed without collimation.

## Material and methods

The Monte Carlo system GEANT 3.21 developed at CERN [5] was used for the calculations. The physical processes were chosen such that for photons Compton scattering, photoelectric effect, Rayleigh effect and pair production were considered. For the secondary electrons bremsstrahlung, annihilation, multiple scattering and continuous energy loss with generation of $\delta$-rays were included. The cutoff energy was set to 10 keV both for photons and electrons. The stepsizes and the permitted fractional energy loss were calculated automatically by GEANT.

The width of the photon distribution behind the bremsstrahlung targets was calculated theoretically as given by Nordell and Brahme [6] and also simulated with Monte Carlo. The intensity distribution behind the collimator was calculated with GEANT only. For these simulations an effective photon source was used that yields a Gaussian intensity distribution.

To produce the desired intensity pattern at isocenter, the photon beam is scanned such that it sequently transmits all holes that contribute to the field. Depending on the type of collimation that is employed, the scanning has to fulfill different criteria (cf. below).

The collimator was simulated as a tungsten plate of thickness $H$ with square holes. A section and top view are shown in figure 1. If the ratio of the hole size $R$ to the hole distance $D$ is chosen suitably for the given source to collimator distance, adjacent positions of the spots at isocenter can be achieved while at the same time transmission through the neighbouring holes is kept low.

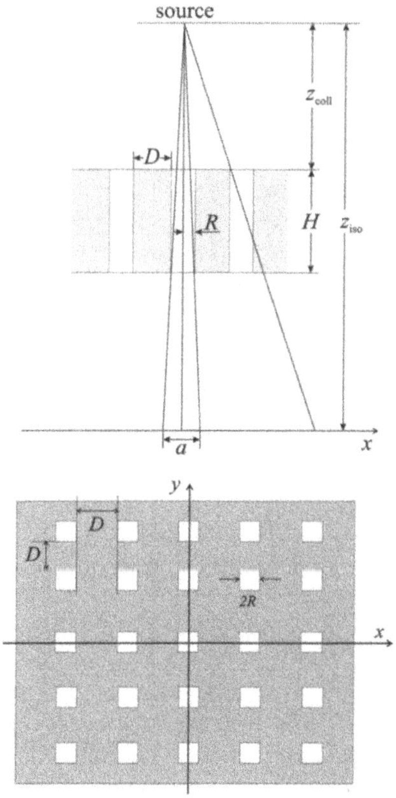


**Figure 1:** Section and top view of the collimator plate with square holes. Source denotes the position of the bremsstrahlung target. In this study the distances were $z_{coll} = 15$ cm, $z_{iso} = 100$ cm and $H = 10$ cm.

In order to allow transmission of the pronounced forward photon intensity through the collimator, the electrons have to leave the scanning magnet parallel to the central axis. This requires a more advanced scanning technique – either by using additional dipoles or by employing a scanning magnet similar to figure 2.

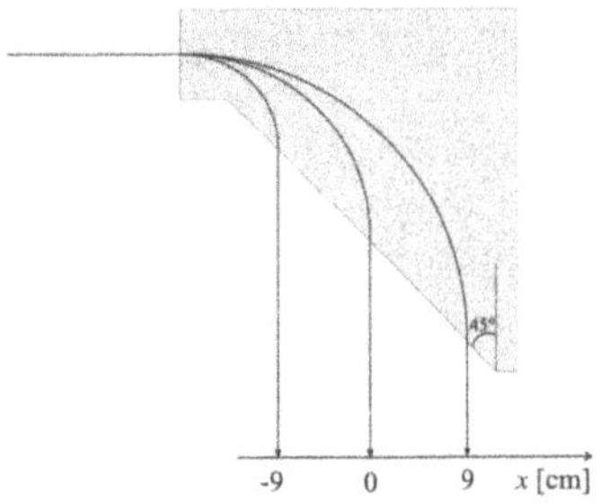


**Figure 2:** Possible magnetic field setup for parallel scanning of the incident electron beam.

## Results and discussion

Figure 3 shows the photon intensity at 100 cm SAD behind a collimator with square holes in comparison to the uncollimated beam. The collimator was assumed as tungsten with a thickness of 10 cm. The hole size $R$ was 0.8 mm and the distance $D$ was 2.4 mm. The effectice photon source was Gaussian distributed with a FWHM of 5 cm and an energy distribution corresponding to the bremsstrahlung spectrum of 20 MeV electrons behind a thin beryllium target. In the Monte Carlo simulation, the scoring plane 100 cm below the source was divided into $0.2 \times 0.2$ mm pixels and the energy fluence in air of the particles intersecting the plane was detected. Due to the small bins a large number of primary photons was necessary in order to obtain sufficient statistics. Besides only a small fraction of the photon lobe is transmitted by the collimator, since it was the objective to eliminate the contribution at larger angles. The intensity in the forward direction is not reduced (cf. figure 3). Simulation of $1 \times 10^6$ primary photons took 12 min on a 500 MHz Alpha with Dec Unix. The resulting photon spot size $a$ at isocenter is about 3 mm. The transmission through the neighbouring holes is less than 3%.

To cover the whole radiation field, the photon beam is aimed at the different holes for a length of time corresponding to the desired intensity matrix. Figure 4 shows a homogeneous field built from $5 \times 5$ scan positions for the collimator resolution as described above. The pixel size was changed to $1 \times 1$ mm in order to decrease the statistical fluctuations. Coverage of the radiation field and a sufficient fluence homogeneity in air are obtained.

By changing the values of $R$ and $D$, the resolution of the collimator can be changed to suit the clinical application. However, it should be noted that a collimator with a higher resolution prolongs the irradiation time as the number of required scan positions increases. Figure 5 shows the simulated fluence profile of a clinical case in the head-and-neck region. In this case a collimator resolution of $a = 1.5$ mm was chosen, corresponding to $2R = 0.38$ mm and $D = 0.87$ mm (simulation with $5 \times 10^7$ primary photons for one beam position).

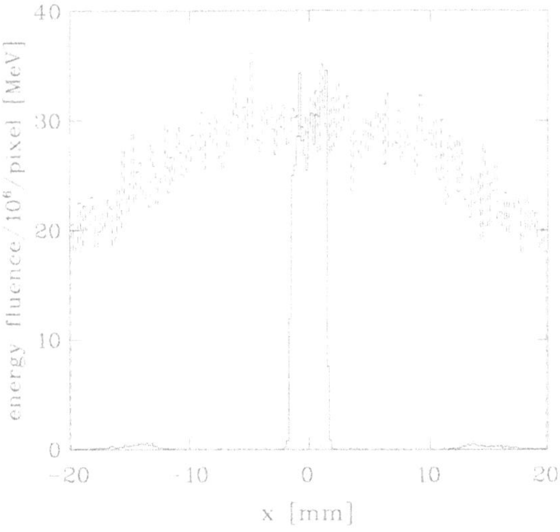


**Figure 3:** Photon beam profile at $y = 0$ and 100 cm SAD (coordinate system as in figure refkolli). The dashed line shows the uncollimated profile, whereas the solid line is the result behind the square-hole collimator. The energy fluence was normalized to $10^6$ primary photons. The simulation included $9 \times 10^7$ primary photons with a pixel size of $0.2 \times 0.2$ mm at 100 cm distance from the source (GEANT with AUTO=1).

## Conclusion

The scanned photon beam technique is an elegant method for the realization of intensity modulated fields. Since radiation is produced only near the radiation field, the problem of leakage radiation does not occur.

With a fixed collimator of the type described above, lateral resolutions of 3 mm and less may be realized for the scanned photon beam technique. The beam penumbra behind the collimator is very small (less than 1 mm for the above examples). This is due to the hole shape and the characteristics of the bremsstrahlung beam above the collimator. For thin targets the source is almost point-like and without a flattening filter the number of scattered photons is small. The resolution is comparable with multileaf collimators and well suited for IMRT. The collimator could in principle also be realized with hexagonal holes. Since the collimator is a fixed plate that is inserted into e.g. the accessory tray, the method is cost-efficient. The only additional demand when using a fixed collimator instead of the uncollimated scanned beam or the combination with a multileaf collimator, is the more complex scanning technique.

The use of such a collimator eliminates all mechanical movement. Beam scanning is much faster than mechanical leaf movement. This gain in time has to be compared with the required number of scan spots and the use of a thin bremsstrahlung target, which results in a lower yield.

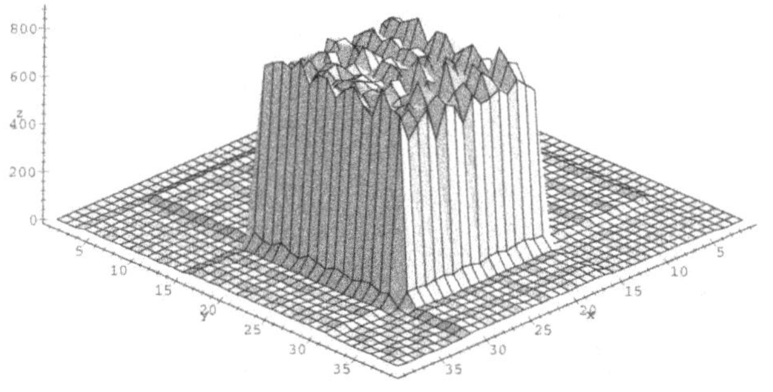


**Figure 4:** A homogeneous radiation field produced by superimposing 5 × 5 photon spots. The grid size at 100 cm SAD was changed to 1 × 1 mm.

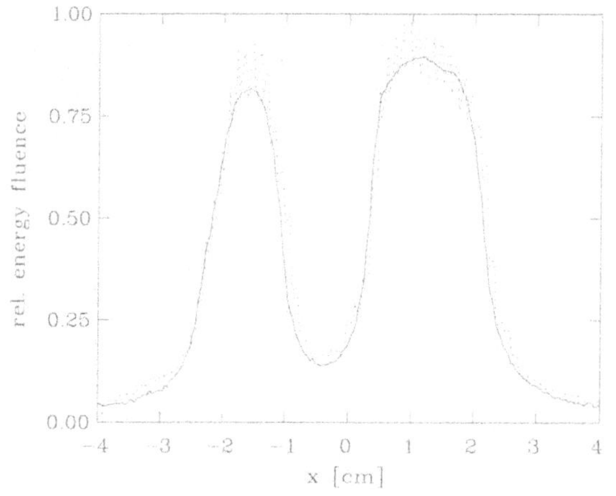


**Figure 5:** Energy fluence profile from superimposed scan spots for a clinical case and a collimator resolution of 1.5 mm. The solid curve represents the desired fluence profile, whereas the dotted lines corresponds to the fluence obtained by superimposing 80 scan spots.

## References


[1] Svensson R and Brahme A 1996 Effective source size, yield and beam profile from multi-layered bremsstrahlung targets *Phys. Med. Biol.* **41** 1353–1379

[2] Svensson R, Åsell M, Näfstadius P and Brahme A 1998 Target, purging magnet and electron collector design for scanned high-energy photon beams *Phys. Med. Biol.* **43** 1–22

[3] Svensson R, Lind B and Brahme A 1998 Beam characteristics and clinical possibilities of a new compact treatment unit design combining narrow pencil beam scanning and segmental multileaf collimation *Med. Phys.* **25** 2358–2369

[4] Küster G 1999 Monte Carlo Studies for the Optimisation of Hardware Used in Conformal Radiation Therapy *PhD Thesis, Universität Heidelberg*

[5] CERN 1994 GEANT - Detector description and simulation tool *CERN Program Library Long Writeup* W5013

[6] Nordell B and Brahme A 1984 Angular distribution and yield from bremsstrahlung targets *Phys. Med. Biol.* **29** 797–810

# Slide and Shoot: A new method for MLC delivery of IMRT.

**Andrew W Beavis[1],Paul S Ganney[1], Viv J Whiton[1]and Lei Xing[2]**

[1] Radiation Physics Department and University of Hull, Princess Royal Hospital, Kingston Upon Hull, HU8 9HE. England, UK, and [2]Department of Radiation Oncology, Stanford University School of Medicine, Stanford, CA 94305, USA

## Introduction

Multileaf collimators (MLC) can be used to produce Intensity Modulated Radiotherapy (IMRT) beams. Currently there are two methods available: 1) Step and Shoot method and 2) Dynamic method. Each offers both advantages and disadvantages in producing the intensity modulation. The Step and Shoot [1] method is simple and intuitive in its approach. Here superposition of a series of discrete multiple sub-fields, each within the beam portal, form the intensity modulation. It produces an exact match when the intensity profiles has zero or infinite gradients. That is in sections over which the intensity is held constant or where there are sudden changes in the profile. The dynamic method [2] is inherently more efficient since the beam is left switched on during leaf repositioning in defining the sub-fields. This produces more accurate approximations of profiles with finite gradients. Flat sections (zero gradients) cannot be produced in the profile since infinite leaf speed would be required. This problem also arises in the production of multiple peaks within profiles. To produce infinite gradients the leaf must remain stationary which is considered inefficient.

We have produced a leaf sequencing algorithm which approximates a 1-D intensity profile to a high degree of agreement whilst retaining the efficiency associated with dynamic motion of the leaves. This combination mode or hybrid approach is called *Slide and Shoot.* The principle is that the leaves move dynamically unless accuracy would be compromised then the beam is switched off during repositioning.

## Material and methods

### Optimised Step and Shoot method

It is common in the Step-and-Shoot method to divide the intensity profile *a priori* into regularly spaced step widths and use a fixed number of regularly incremented intensity levels. We have developed a scheme to optimise the delivery by Step-and-Shoot which increases the accuracy of the delivered beam. This is effected by allowing optimal, non-uniform, incremented steps and intensity levels in the leaf sequence and is described below. To implement this we had to develop a new leaf sequencing algorithm since standard ones rely on equally incremented intensity levels.

Beam profiles are considered as a set of 1-D profiles, each of which is associated with a single leaf pair of the MLC. These are input to the algorithm as a pseudo-continuous curve described by a series of 101 points, representing a profile width, W (nominally 10 cm).

The profile is divided into N steps, where N≤50 and is defined by the user. These have optimal, uneven, widths or may be constrained to be equal. In the general case, the individual widths are selected by ensuring the deviation between the minimum and maximum value of the intensity curve remains within an adaptive tolerance. The tolerance starts at unity and is increased until N steps are found. In the case where N steps cannot be produced the widest is split.

Within each step an optimal intensity level is chosen to approximate the curve within them. The mean value of the original pseudo-curve within each step is taken, resulting in a set of N intensity levels ($I_j$) with uneven, non-uniform, increments. If required, they may be constrained onto equal incremented values by rounding to the nearest one (say 5% or 10%) as defined by the user.

We note that the scheme using equal step size and/or equally incremented intensity levels are special cases of our more general algorithm and they can be generated by selection of appropriate parameters. The reasoning behind making the constrained scheme available was in order to use standard leaf sequences if desired.

The leaf sequencing algorithm [3] converts the representation of the intensity profile developed above into a series of instructions: leaf pair co-ordinates and associated monitor units, the MLC controller can execute to produce the intensity modulated field. That is converting the above representation into segments. The $i^{th}$ segment has an intensity ($\Delta I_i = I_i - I_{i-1}$) and the set of N segments superpose to produce the intensity modulated beam. Standard leaf sequencing algorithms require equally incremented intensity levels. We have produced our own algorithm for our more general scheme of dividing up the intensity profile. In this algorithm the leaf pair begins fully open. The widest (non-zero) level is delivered, the beam is switched off and the leaf ends repositioned to delivered the next widest segment. This is repeated until all the intensity levels have been delivered or the bases of multiple peaks are detected. In the later case fragmented segments are delivered in an optimised order which requires the minimum leaf movements. The leaf sequence can be described by a set of co-ordinates ($x_i^A$, $x_i^B$, $\Delta I_i$) which are transferred to the MLC controller. Between segments the beam is switched off.

### Slide and Shoot method

In order to utilise the benefits afforded by dynamic methods the algorithm described above was extended to allow the beam to remain on during leaf repositioning.

Since, these extra contributions to the profile are always additive, whilst attempting to maintain a high degree of accuracy we elected to always undertreat the profile. To achieve this the minimum intensity value in each step was chosen as the required intensity level.

The philosophy adopted was to allow the leaves to move continuously unless accuracy would be compromised, in these situations the beam is switched off whilst the leaves are repositioned. Once the leaves are at a suitable 'restart' position the beam is switched back on and the motion is continued. These conditions occur when: 1) the profile has multiple peaks, 2) a plateau exists or 3) an inflection exisits within one (or more ) of the steps generated in our division scheme. They are detected during the creation of the leaf sequence using simple numerical methods that measure the profile gradient. Two boolean parameters $b_i$ and $p_i$ are defined for each segment. The first, $b_i$, determines whether the beam should be switched off between delivery of the (i-1)$^{th}$ segment and the i$^{th}$ . The second, $p_i$, determines whether this segment is a peak. From the segment description, ($x_i^A$, $x_i^B$, $\Delta I_i$, $b_i$, $p_i$), the leaf positions, number of monitor units and beam on/off status is passed to the MLC controller.

In order to maintain efficiency it is necessary to prevent the leaf being stationary whilst the beam is on. This may occur due to the fact that the minimum intensity value is used in each step during the optimisation process and presents if the profile gradient at one segment end is much steeper than at the other. The original Step and Shoot segment end points are reduced to a set of control points [($x_j^A$ , $I_j^A$), ($x_k^B$ , $I_k^B$)] where each of the $x_j^\theta$ are unique in value ($\theta$ = leaf A or leaf B), in effect, removing redundant points. In general there will be a different number for the A and B leaves, making this reduced set inappropriate for producing the control file for the MLC controller. Therefore a leaf A position is calculated for every leaf B position where none exists due to the point reduction and similarly for missing leaf B positions. Essentially this results in a small number of the original segment end points being interpolated to new more efficient positions. The new set of control points ($X_i^A$, $X_i^B$, $\Delta I_i$, $b_i$, $p_i$) describe both the dynamic and discrete components of this Slide and Shoot approach (as before $1 \leq i \leq N$).

In order to perform comparisons between different schemes we have implemented a calculation of the delivery time. All beam-on and leaf movement times are summed, assuming a constant dose rate of 300 MU/min and a leaf speed of 1.5 cm/s. In the intensity profile 100% is taken to be 100MU. Only leaf reposition when the beam is switched off is included, the other contributions to the total time are determined by the number of Monitor Units required during the beam on. We have also implemented the Bortfeld (step and shoot) algorithm as a comparison tool.

A simple error, the square of the difference between the original curve and that produced at each point describing the pseudo-continuous profile: $\Sigma_\alpha \{I_\alpha^{cts} - I_\alpha^{delivered}\}^2$, is computed.

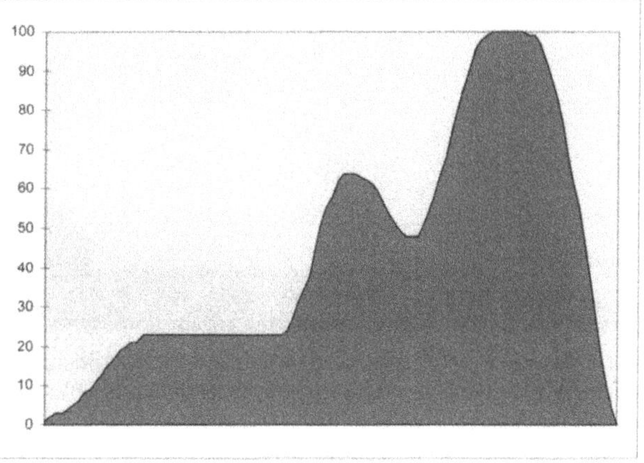


**Figure 1:** A 1-D intensity profile used in the calculation of the results given here to illustrate the optimisation and Slide and Shoot algorithms.

## Results and discussion

We have used the 1-D intensity profile shown in figure 1 as a test curve to illustrate the algorithms presented here.

In the first instance we consider Step and Shoot modes. Using the common division scheme of 10 steps equal in width and intensity level increment (10%) yielded an error of 9908 and execution time of 30.1 s. Increasing to 20 steps (5% increments) reduced the error to 2733 and increased the time to 31.5s.

This result is expected, since we increased the sampling of the curve.

Allowing the step widths to be optimally selected (leaving the increments fixed) gave errors and times of (3848, 25.5s) for 10 steps (N=10) and (853, 30.8s) for N=20. Since the intensity level increment remained fixed we can apply the Bortfeld leaf sequence here which yielded the same errors but times of 30.7s and 32.8s respectively for N=10 and N=20.

Again, increase in curve sampling explains the increased accuracy and time overhead.

Table 1 shows the comparison data when we allow optimisation of both intensity levels (non-uniform increments) and step width in the generation of the leaf sequence. We see how the agreement is increased with increased sampling up to N=30. After that no real benefit is obtained, however no extra time penalty is incurred.

Figure 2 depicts the intesity profile obtained for our 1-D example using the Slide and Shoot algorithm using N=20, non-equal intensity level increments and optimal step widths in the leaf sequence generation.

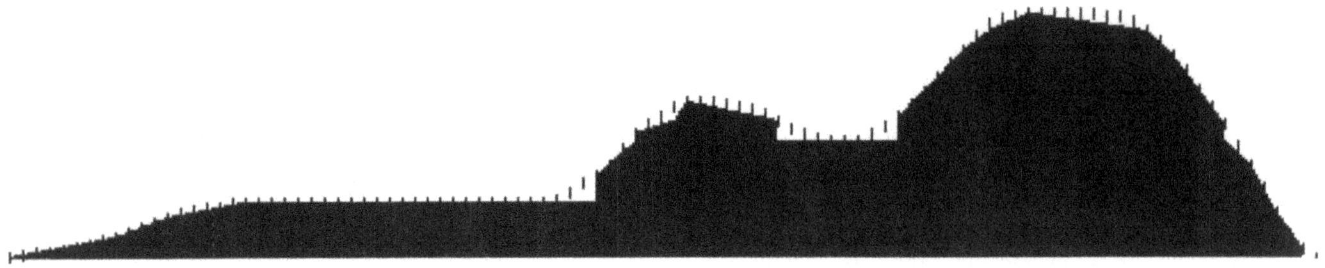

**Figure 2:** A 1-D intensity profile produced using our Slide and Shoot algorithm. Note the obvious discontinuities in the otherwise smooth profile approximation introduced where the beam was switched off to allow leaf repositioning. The marks represent the 101 points defining the input pseudo-continuous 'ideal' profile.

| | error | time |
|---|---|---|
| N=10 | 2784 | 28.1s |
| N=15 | 1061 | 30.7s |
| N=20 | 647 | 31.0s |
| N=25 | 482 | 31.9s |
| N=30 | 345 | 32.6s |
| N=35 | 313 | 33.3s |
| N=40 | 313 | 33.3s |
| N=45 | 310 | 33.7s |
| N=50 | 308 | 33.7s |

**Table 1:** The reduction in the agreement between the continuous curve shown in figure 1 and the intensity map, produced under our optimised step and shoot scheme, as a function of the number of steps used in the generation of the leaf sequence.

We note the excellent agreement to the input profile obtained in the finite gradient sections of the curve. The effect of a beam switch-off and leaf reposition (static component) is obvious just to the right of the plateau. The corresponding segment end of the right hand side of the profile maintains its 'smooth-finite gradient' since the leaf was held at its position until the beam was switched back on. Characteristic 'kinks' are seen in the otherwise smooth profile at the points were beam switch-offs occur due to the requirement of producing multiple peaks.

With Slide and Shoot we get an error and time of (373, 29.6s), (274, 29.5s) and (111, 29.9s) for N=20, 25 and 50 respectively. These results can be interpreted and compared in two ways:

Firstly, for the same delivery time overhead as required with the 'standard' Step and Shoot method, the error in agreement is reduced by a factor of 90 when allowing Slide and Shoot with N=50 as opposed to the standard equal-increment (N=10, 10% levels) division scheme for Step and Shoot. Furthermore, in the Slide and Shoot produced profiles the occurances of over-treatment of the original profile are greatly reduced as a result of the adopted principle. By definition, as we select the mean intensity value within each step as the intensity level for Step and Shoot, part of the area within each and every step is overdosed and the rest is underdosed. Though these overdosed areas may be small, they will occur in all the beams required by the treatment plan and may add significantly.

Secondly, we obtain an error similar in magnitude to those given in Table 1 for N>20, however the delivery time overhead is less. This is because in the majority of the profile creation leaf repositioning is performed as part of the contributary segments. A further advantage of the Slide and Shoot, combination mode, is seen when considering 2-D clinical beam profiles; Since, the optimised Step and Shoot beams require a large number of low monitor unit segments it becomes somewhat problematical to efficiently collate segments across the MLC leaf banks. This will result in a reduction in the potential accuracy gain from fully optimised Step and Shoot and an increase in the delivery time, a reduction in efficiency.

We continue to work on this method, such as improving the process of 'closing' the tops of the peaks and an 'adaptive' restart of dynamic segments to remove the 'kinks' visable in figure 2.

## Conclusion

We have presented a new leaf sequence algorithm, it uses a combination of dynamic and Step and Shoot methods. In the Slide and Shoot method a dynamic sequence is prefered unless contra-indicating feaures are present in the profile. These are the existance of multiple peaks, plateaus or inflections within one (or more) of the steps generated in the creation of the leaf sequence. If any of these conditions occur within each step then the whole delivery is Step and Shoot. Conversely if none are present the entire delivery is dynamic. So Step and shoot and a truly dynamic method are both special cases of our more general algorithm.

## References

[1] Bortfeld T, Boyer AL, Schlegel W, Kahler DL, Waldron TJ. Realization and verification of three-dimensional conformation radiotherapy with modulated fields. 1994 *IJROBP* **30** 899-908.

[2] Spirou S. and Chui C.S., Generation of Arbitrary Intensity Profiles by Dynamic Jaws of Multileaf Collimators. 1994 *Med. Phys.* **21** 1031-1041.

[3] Convery DJ and Rosenbloom ME. The generation of intensity-modulated fields for conformal radiotherapy by dynamic collimation. 1992 PMB **37** 1359-1374

# Applicator-Guided Intensity Modulated Radiation Therapy: A New Approach to Treating Cervical Cancer

**Daniel A. Low, James F. Dempsey, Jerry Markman, Sasa Mutic, Jeffrey F. Williamson and James A. Purdy**

Radiation Oncology Center, Mallinckrodt Institute of Radiology, Washington University School of Medicine, St. Louis, MO USA

## Introduction

We are developing a novel radiation therapy modality, applicator-guided intensity modulated radiation therapy (AGIMRT), for gynecological cancers that provides highly conformal and accurately localized therapy. External beam therapy localized by an intracavitary applicator substitute will replace existing high-dose rate brachytherapy treatments, and the dose distributions will be generated using IMRT dose optimization. An applicator substitute will be inserted into the patient's vagina and uterus and a three-dimensional (3D) image study acquired using magnetic resonance (MR) imaging. The applicator substitute will remain implanted between imaging and treatment to spatially register the tumor and internal organs for both treatment planning and delivery and will either be rigidly attached to the couch or actively monitored. After the treatment plan is calculated the patient will be aligned to the accelerator using the applicator substitute, and after treatment delivery, the applicator substitute will be removed. The fundamental hypothesis of this modality is that the tumor and internal organ positions are spatially constrained to the applicator substitute so that when the dose distribution is aligned with the applicator substitute, it is also aligned with the tumor and critical organs.

Brachytherapy is currently used to treat locally advanced gynecological malignancies when radiation therapy is prescribed. Intracavitary brachytherapy has been relatively successful in part due to the close coupling of the dose distribution to the tumor because of the placement of radioactive sources within the vagina and uterus (1). However, critical structures can easily be overdosed because of their proximity to the radioactive sources and the rapid increase in dose rate as a function of decreased distance from each source. Flexibility in the optimization of intracavitary implant dose distributions is limited by the spatial positioning of the applicators and the inverse-square law. This fundamental limitation exists even if the spatial locations of target and critical structures can be determined exactly, e.g., using 3D imaging and treatment planning. Chao *et al.* (2) investigated the consequences of uterosacral space involvement in patients with stage IIIb cervical cancer. They concluded that the combination of intracavitary brachytherapy and external beam pelvis irradiation did not deliver an adequate dose to tumor in the uterosacral space, and that an improved dose delivery regimen should be investigated.

Conformal radiation therapy (CRT) is not currently employed as a modality for gynecological cancer treatments. It has been found that the tumor-laden tissues move relative to bony anatomy (3). Therefore, portal image-based verification (4-6), a technique widely used in CRT, may not be applicable to this tumor site. Without accurate determination of the tumor and surrounding critical structure positions, a conformal dose distribution cannot be delivered. The development of a procedure for accurate localization of the tumor and critical structures enables the use of CRT, and specifically AGIMRT, for the treatment of gynecological malignancies.

## Materials and methods

Treatment planning simulations were conducted on patients with locally advanced cervical cancer to examine the possibility of substituting IMRT for brachytherapy. The patients were implanted using a CT-compatible Fletcher-Suit applicator and three-dimensional CT scan studies were acquired using 3 mm thick transverse slices. For these preliminary studies, the brachytherapy dose distributions were assumed to be delivered using 3M cesium tubes, with the individual source dose distributions computed using Monte Carlo simulation. Rectal and bladder shields were not modeled in this study, and previous studies indicate they reduce the dose to the bladder and rectum by less than approximately 10% (7). Poor soft tissue contrast made definition of the target volume difficult, so the target volume was defined as the brachytherapy point A isodose surface (8). Physician-defined target volumes based on the MR scan studies will be used in future clinical studies.

The Corvus (NOMOS Corporation, V 1.0) treatment planning system was used to compute the IMRT dose distributions. Serial tomotherapy was used in these examples. Because of poor tissue differentiation using CT, the point-A brachytherapy isodose surface was used as the target volume. The target volume was delineated using the superimposed target isodose lines. For these examples, the treatment plan was optimized to deliver 3800 cGy to target, and limit the bladder and rectum dose to no more than 3800 cGy. The whole-pelvis external beam doses were not modeled in this simulation.

## Results and discussion

Two treatment plans were conducted for each patient to illustrate the flexibility of IMRT. Plan 1 was optimized to provide the maximum target coverage in preference to critical structure avoidance, while the opposite was done for plan 2. Both the brachytherapy and the IMRT treatment plans were normalized to cover 90% of the target volume with the prescription isodose. Figure 1 compares brachytherapy and IMRT isodoses and Figure 2 shows the corresponding cumulative dose-volume histograms (DVHs) of the target and bladder. The target brachytherapy DVH has a shape characteristic of the high dose regions caused by the inverse-square law, while the IMRT dose distributions yields relatively homogeneous target coverage. The doses to the bladder in plan 1 are similar to those in the brachytherapy plan. However, with relatively little variation in the target volume dose, plan 2 demonstrates a marked decrease in the bladder dose. Similar results are seen with the rectum. We anticipate this type of treatment planning flexibility will highlight this new modality. One of the patients had a uterus that wrapped superiorly around the bladder. To illustrate the capabilities of IMRT to deliver a conformal dose distribution, the entire uterus was selected as the target volume. In this case, the brachytherapy dose distribution was normalized to cover the point-A isodose surface while the IMRT dose distribution was optimized to cover 90% of the contoured target volume. Examples of the dose distributions are shown in Figure 3. The axial CT scans project through two sections of the target, as evidenced by the IMRT dose distribution. Because the tandem lies in only one portion of the target, the anterior target is inadequately treated. The DVHs for the target volume are also shown in Figure 3. For this case, the IMRT dose distribution provides superior target coverage to brachytherapy.

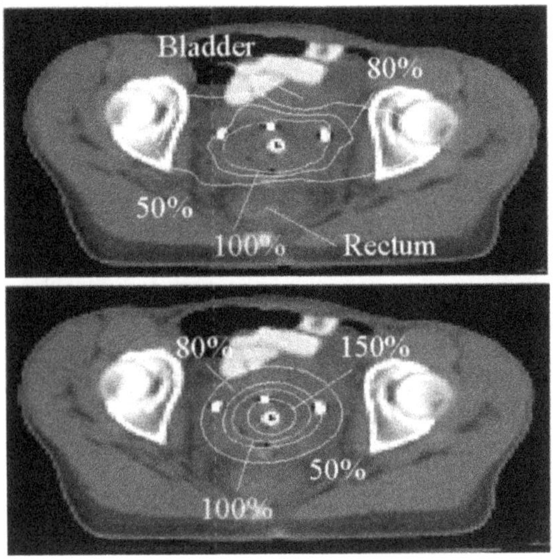


- a)

- b)

**Figure 1:** Isodose distributions for transverse plane passing superior to the cervical os. Doses are shown as percentages of the prescription isodose. a) IMRT isodose distribution 2. b) Brachytherapy isodose distribution

To address some of the concerns regarding the soft tissue following the applicator, serial CT scans of patients with CT-compatible tandems and colpostats were analyzed. The scans were obtained prior to sequential low-dose rate brachytherapy implants scanned 4 to 6 weeks apart. Because the imaging modality was CT, only the bladder and rectum were evaluated and the spatial registration precision analysis was confined to the colpostats. The surfaces of the bladder and rectum, as well as the colpostats, were delineated by a dosimetrist and the contour vertex positions downloaded to a workstation. Two scans for each of three patients were downloaded. AGIMRT will utilize the applicator substitute for dose distribution localization, the coordinate systems of the scan datasets were positioned relative to the colpostats. The coordinate system origin was placed at the mean position of the colpostat centers-of-mass. The coordinate system orientations were aligned relative to the horizontal and vertical axes, completing the scan registration process. To quantify the degree of localization precision of the bladder and rectum using the colpostats, a geometric analysis of the bladder and rectal surfaces was conducted. The contour vertex positions were transformed to the registered coordinate systems and the posterior bladder and anterior rectum positions compared between the two scan datasets. To quantify the bladder surface, the contour vertices were fit to polynomial surfaces and the root-mean square difference of the anteroposterior positions of the surfaces of both scans determined. A similar analysis was conducted for the rectal contours lying between 2.0 cm superior and 2.0 cm inferior to the colpostat centers-of-mass. Table 1 shows the root-mean square differences between the two CT scan studies. The posterior bladder and anterior rectal surfaces were localized using the colpostats to within 1.3 cm and 0.6 cm, respectively. A custom-fabricated applicator substitute may provide more precise organ localization (9) and we anticipate that future studies will compare custom versus standard applicator substitutes for AGIMRT.

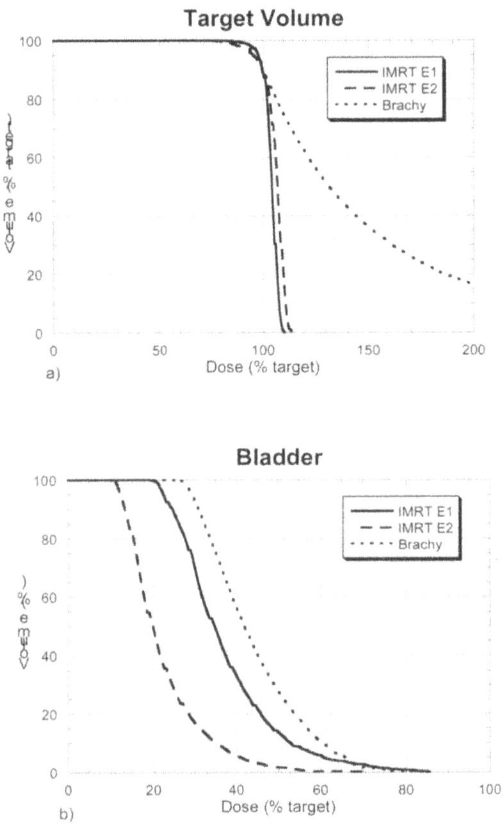


a)

b)

**Figure 2:** Cumulative dose-volume histograms (DVHs) comparing brachytherapy and IMRT dose distributions for the patient shown in Figure 2. a) Target volume DVH. b) Bladder DVH.

| Patient | Bladder | Rectum |
|---|---|---|
| 1 | 0.62 | 0.64 |
| 2 | 0.92 | 0.37 |
| 3 | 1.29 | 0.53 |

**Table 1:** Root-mean square deviation (cm) of posterior bladder and anterior rectal surface positions between two sequential implant procedures. The coordinate systems of the two scan datasets were aligned using the respective colpostat positions.

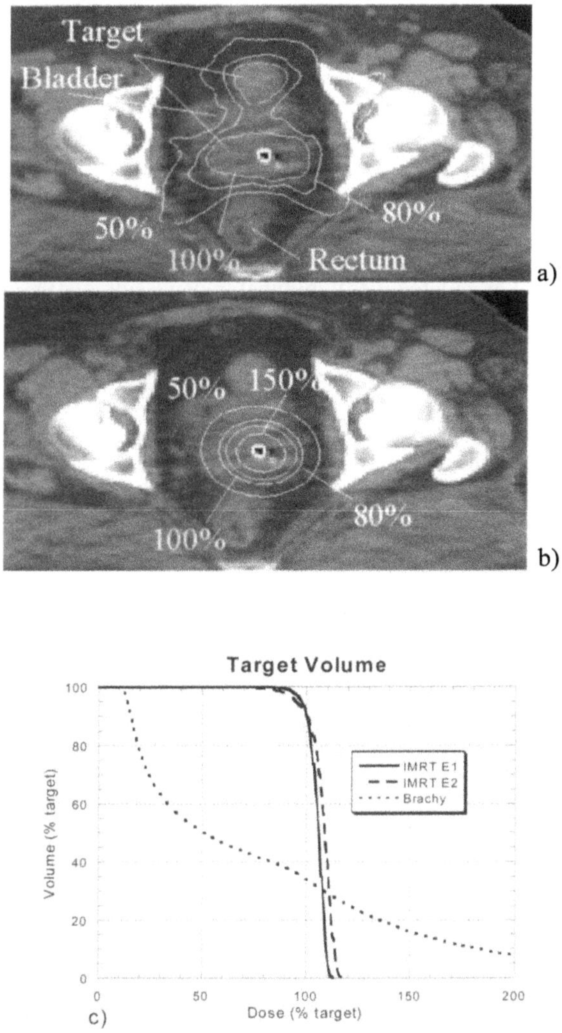


**Figure 3:** Isodose distributions for transverse plane passing superior to the cervical os. Doses are shown as percentages of the prescription isodose. a) IMRT isodose distribution 2. b) Brachytherapy isodose distribution. c) Target DVH.

## Conclusion

AGIMRT shows promise in providing an alternative to, and possible improvement for, HDR brachytherapy for gynecological cancer treatments. Unlike HDR, the dose distribution can be customized to the patient's anatomy. In direct comparison studies (where the target volume was defined by the brachytherapy isodose surface), similar target volume coverage was possible with improved critical structure avoidance. When the target was anatomically delineated, the AGIMRT provided improved target volume coverage.

## References

[1] Corn B, Galvin J, Soffen E, Henze G and Schwaibold F 1993 Positional stability of sources during low-dose-rate brachytherapy for cervical carcinoma, *Int. J. Radiat. Oncol. Biol. Phys.* **26** 513-518

[2] Chao K S, Williamson J F, Grigsby P W and Perez C A 1998 Uterosacral space involvement in locally advanced carcinoma of the uterine cervix, *Int J Radiat Oncol Biol Phys* **40** 397-403

[3] Grigsby P W, Georgiou A, Williamson J F and Perez C A 1993 Anatomic variation of gynecological brachytherapy prescription points, *Int. J. Radiat. Oncol. Biol. Phys.* **20** 725-729

[4] Boyer A L, Antonuk L, Fenster A, Van Herk M, Meertens H, Munro P, Reinstein L E and Wong J 1992 A review of electronic portal imaging devices (EPIDs), *Med Phys* **19** 1-16

[5] Wong J W, Gerber R L, Michalski J M, Graham M L, Halverson K J, Cheng A Y, Grigsby P, Renna M, Sawyer P and Perez C A 1993 On-line image verification in radiation therapy: an early USA experience, *Med Prog Technol* **19** 43-54

[6] Verhey L J, Goitein M, McNulty P, Munzenrider J E and Suit H D 1982 Precise positioning of patients for radiation therapy, *Int J Radiat Oncol Biol Phys* **8** 289-94

[7] Steggerda M J, Moonen L M, Damen E M and Lebesque J V 1997 An analysis of the effect of ovoid shields in a selectron-LDR cervical applicator on dose distributions in rectum and bladder, *Int J Radiat Oncol Biol Phys* **39** 237-45

[8] Perez C A, "Uterine Cervix," in *Principles and Practice of Radiation Oncology, 2nd Edition*, edited by C. A. Perez and L. W. Brady (J.B. Lippincott, Philadelphia, 1992).

[9] Lichter A S, Dillon M B, Rosenshein N B and Order S E 1978 The use of custom molds for intracavitary treatment of carcinoma of the cervix, *International Journal Of Radiation Oncology, Biology, Physics* **4** 873-9

This work supported in part by a grant from the American Cancer Society grant number IRG-58-101-42 and the NOMOS Corporation.

# Application of modifiers for intensity modulated photon fields

**Thorsten Frenzel[1], Rainer Schmidt[1], and Wolfgang Scobel[2]**

[1]Universitäts-Krankenhaus Eppendorf, Radiologische Klinik, Abt. für Strahlentherapie und Radioonkologie, Martinistraße 52, 20246 Hamburg, Germany, and [2]Universität Hamburg, I. Institut für Experimentalphysik, Luruper Chaussee 149, 22761 Hamburg, Germany

## Introduction

The most important goal of radiation oncology is to kill all tumor cells without causing severe damage in the surrounding healthy tissue. For this reason the three-dimensional dose distribution has to be adapted to the geometrical shape of the planning target volume. The use of intensity modulated photon fields is one way of generating high conformal dose distributions that can help to reduce the dose given to organs at risk and to apply a high dose to the planning target volume. Especially for irregularly shaped tumors that surround organs at risk intensity modulated photon fields can help to optimize the dose distribution [1].

Intensity modulated photon fields can be generated with the use of multileaf collimators (MLC), scanning photon beams or modifiers. But before these irradiation techniques can be applied to patients in clinical routine methods for quality assurance have to be developed.

For this reason an intensity modulated treatment plan was created for an Alderson-Rando phantom. The intensity modulated photon fields were generated with modifiers which underwent a dosimetric check before they were used for the irradiation of 198 TLD inside the Alderson-Rando phantom.

## Material and methods

The intensity modulated photon fields were generated using modifiers which were mounted on a perspex plate that can be inserted in the accessory holder of a linear accelerator. A modifier consisted of a negative form inside a 8 cm thick styrodur block which is filled afterwards with a steel granulate from Par Scientific (Odense, Denmark) with a grain size between 0,15 mm and 0,40 mm and a density of 4,63 g/cm³ (Table 1). To allow the use of these modifiers under arbitrary gantry angles perspex plates were mounted on top of the modifiers.

| Component | Fe | Cr | Ni | C |
|---|---|---|---|---|
| % | 73 - 76 | 16 - 18 | 8 - 9 | 0,3 max. |

**Table 1**: Components of the steel granulate

The negative forms were created with computer controlled milling machines. A milling machine "ACD 5" form Par Scientific and a milling machine called "CNC-Flachbettanlage GFM 4433" from Isel-Automation (Eiterfeld, Germany) were used for this purpose. A software was developed for the Isel milling machine to allow full control of the milling process.

To calculate the required thickness of the modifiers the physical attenuation coefficient of the used steel granulate was measured for different field sizes for 6 MV photons of a Siemens Mevatron MDX 2 linear accelerator.

As the steel granulate gives a minimal transmission of 19% at a 5 cm by 5 cm radiation field additional materials had to be used to generate irregular forms of the radiation field. An MLC could be used to generate these contours but even without an MLC the same results can be achieved with a conventional shielding block out of MCP 96 surrounding the modifier (Figure 1). The steel granulate had to be compressed to remove air from inside to modifier. For this purpose a rubber hammer was used. Figure 2 shows a ready made modifier.

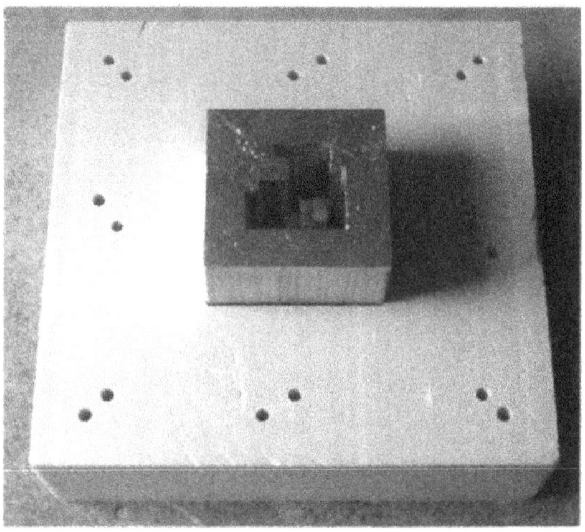

**Figure 1:** Modifier combined with a shielding block

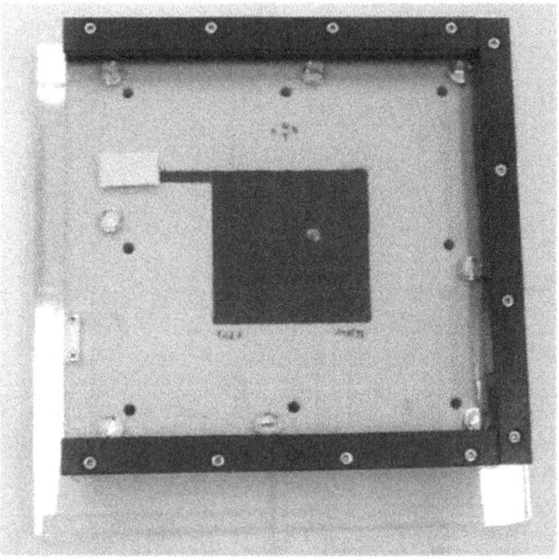

**Figure 2:** Ready made modifier

The irradiation of a squamous cell carcinoma inside the nose between the eyes was simulated for an Alderson-Rando phantom according to an existing patient. An intensity modulated treatment plan with five fields was applied using the "KonRad" treatment planning system developed at the DKFZ (Heidelberg, Germany) and is now sold by the company MRC Systems (Heidelberg, Germany). To verify the accuracy of the dose calculation the treatment plan has been recalculated with "VOXEL-PLAN", a treatment planning system which has also been developed at the DKFZ but has a slightly different dose calculation algorithm.

For the intensity maps a grid size of 1 cm by 1 cm in the isocenter was chosen (analogous to the size of a standard MLC). The dose calculation with KonRad delivers ASCII-files which contain the intensity matrices to be used with an MLC. For this reason a software was developed to convert these files into control data files for the milling machines.

The fluence maps of the intensity modulated photon fields were checked using the fluoroscopic megavoltage imaging system BIS 710 manufactured by Wellhöfer Dosimetrie (Schwarzenbruck, Germany) [2, 3]. The imaging system was 100 cm apart form the focus for all measurements.

A software called "MVI-program" was developed for the comparison of measured and calculated fluence distributions [4]. This software allowed to generate reference images in the Wellhöfer file format from the KonRad fluence ASCII-files. The pixel size and the distance of the imaging system from the focus of the radiation source were taken into account. With this software the measured fluence map could be subtracted from the calculated reference image. The resulting image showed differences at a glance. The whole fluence map could be verified and critical deviations could be seen easily. Also a numerical evaluation was possible by selecting an arbitrary row or column of the subtraction image and transferring the data to a calculation program like Microsoft Excel ®.

The use of reference images also allowed to check the correct alignment of the modifiers. Therefore the position of the BIS 710 had to be aligned with the reference at the isocenter. Misalignments during the fabrication procedure of the modifiers could be determined by measuring the contours of the modifier in relation to the isocenter.

After the verification of the fluence profiles the resultant dose distribution of every radiation field could be measured with film (CEA TVS), IC 10 ionization chamber and the prototype megavoltage imaging system "ADAS" (manufactured by Wellhöfer Dosimetrie), which has a sensitive layer out of amorphous silicon [5]. All measurements were executed in a stack of perspex slabs (2 cm buildup material and 20 cm backscatter material). For two dimensional scans with the IC 10 ionization chamber one of the perspex slabs could be moved with a computer controlled device similar to that used for an ionization chamber inside a water phantom. For the evaluation of the CEA films a VXR 12 scanner (Vidar Corporation, Herndon VA, USA) was calibrated to dose. The measured dose distributions could be compared using the previously described MVI-program.

After checking the modifiers the Alderson-Rando phantom was prepared for the irradiation by inserting 198 TLD 100 (LiF) in one disc of the phantom to get a narrow grid of dose measurements. The phantom was positioned using a vacuum cushion for proper alignment. Afterwards the irradiation was executed with 6 MV photons from a Siemens Mevatron MDX 2 linear accelerator.

The TLD were evaluated followed by an individual calibration with a dose of 1 Gy. Measured and calculated dose values were compared.

## Results and discussion

The attenuation coefficient of the steel granulated was measured for three different field sizes (Table 2).

| Field size in cm x cm | 2 x 2 | 5 x 5 | 10 x 10 |
|---|---|---|---|
| μ in 1/cm | 0,2108 | 0,2089 | 0,2052 |
| $\sigma_\mu$ in 1/cm | 0,0026 | 0,0024 | 0,0026 |

**Table 2:** Measured attenuation coefficients

With the data from Table 2 the required thickness of the modifiers could be calculated from the desired fluence matrix using the exponential attenuation law.

The dose volume histograms calculated with KonRad and VOXEL-PLAN were in good agreement. The shape of the curves did not show any significant deviation. After this control data files were calculated for the milling machines.

The modifiers created with the Par Scientific milling machine showed some artifacts due to a smoothing function in the Par Scientific software that created rounded and not squared intensity grids. With a self developed software and the Isel milling machine these artifacts did not occur. The additional shielding blocks made of MCP 96 were created by standard techniques used in clinical routine. It took approximately 40 minutes to mill one modifier and an additional 20 minutes to assemble it.

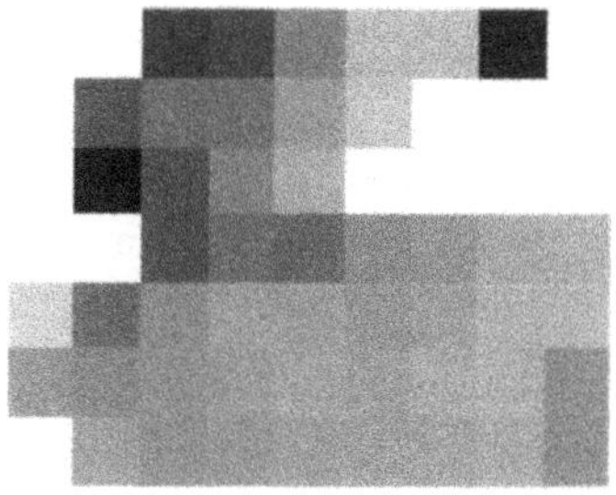

**Figure 3:** Calculated fluence map (KonRad)

The calculated fluence (KonRad) for one radiation field is given in Figure 3. The measured fluence map (BIS 710) is shown in Figure 4 and the subtraction image in Figure 5.

**Figure 4:** Measured fluence map (BIS 710)

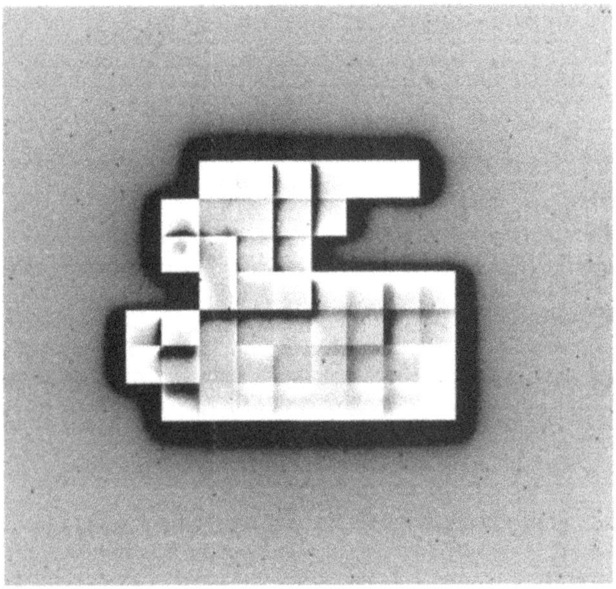

**Figure 5:** Subtraction image

An ideal agreement between a measured and a calculated fluence map should result in a subtraction image that shows a homogenous grey. Figure 5 indicates some differences at steep dose gradients, especially at the edge of the radiation field. Darker colors indicate a higher fluence (e.g. caused by scattered radiation at the edge of the modifier) and brighter colors a lower fluence profile. A numerical analysis showed differences up to 80% for single pixel values but most pixels do not deviate from calculated values by more than 5%. The positioning of the modifiers was accurate within 1.5 mm for all modifiers except for one that had a maximum shift of 2.4 mm in one direction.

The dosimetric analysis of the modifiers proved that films have the most accurate resolution to measure the dose distribution and ionization chambers the worst because of their comparable large sensitive volume which "smears out" steep gradients. With a proper calibration the dose distribution can also be measured with the ADAS which is the fastest method.

The evaluation of the TLD measurements caused some problems due to the steep dose gradients inside the irradiated area. KonRad calculated a dose distribution that reveals inhomogeneities up to 20% of the value of the prescribed dose for the target volume. With these steep gradients a shift of the phantom by one mm could result in a dose that is significantly lower or higher. Therefor minimum and maximum dose values in neighboring voxels were determined to define a confidence interval for each calculated point dose value. More than 50% of the measured dose values were inside these intervals. But also larger differences appeared that were difficult to interpret because of the vicinity of steep dose gradients.

## Conclusion

The application of intensity modulated photon fields is possible without an MLC by the use of modifiers. The fluence map of the modifiers can be verified with the fluoroscopic megavoltage imaging system BIS 710 in an easy way. Also the dosimetric verification is possible with the a-Si megavoltage imaging system ADAS or film.

The interpretation of the measured dose distributions may be the most difficult problem. Due to intended steep dose gradients inside the radiation field deviations between measured and calculated dose are very difficult to interpret. If there is a deviation it will be very hard to find out which component of which radiation field has caused this deviation.

## References

[1] Sternick ES (Ed.) 1997 *The theory and practice of intensity modulated radiation therapy*. Madison: Advanced Medical publishing

[2] Ma L, Geis PB, Boyer AL 1997 Quality assurance for dynamic multileaf collimator modulated fields using a fast beam imaging system. *Medical Physics* **24(8)** 1213-1220

[3] Hesse BM, Spies L, Groh, BA 1998 Tomotherapeutic portal imaging for radiation treatment verification. *Phys. Med. Biol.* **43** 3607-3616

[4] Frenzel T, Schmidt R, Platz V, Kraus KH, Scobel W 1997 Qualitätssicherung bei der Verwendung von Hochenergie-Bildsystemen. *Zeitschrift für Medizinische Physik* **7** 52-58

[5] Frenzel T, Gärtner W, Block T, Platz V, Kraus H, Schmidt R 1998 Performance of a prototype amorphous Si-detector. In: *EPI 98: 5th International Workshop on Electronic Portal Imaging, October 29 – 31, Phoenix, Arizona.* Phoenix, Arizona 148-149

# Delivery of Multiple IMRT Fields Using a Single Physical Attenuator

**Richard Popple and Isaac Rosen**
The University of Texas M. D. Anderson Cancer Center, Houston, TX, USA

## Introduction

Intensity modulated radiotherapy (IMRT) can deliver improved dose distributions compared to conventional radiotherapy. IMRT treatments are delivered using either a multileaf collimator (MLC) or a physical attenuator, the more general case of a missing tissue compensator. There are two important issues that must be addressed when choosing an IMRT delivery method, delivery efficiency and quality assurance.

Delivery with an MLC, either dynamic or step-and-shoot, requires minimal preparation prior to treatment. The desired intensity map is converted to MLC leaf settings and the treatment can be delivered under computer control. However, the treatment time is longer than conventional radiotherapy and is related to the accuracy with which the desired intensity map is delivered.[1] Quality assurance procedures for dynamic MLC delivery of IMRT are still evolving, but it is clear that they are more complex and time consuming than conventional QA and less definitive. [2][3]

Delivery of IMRT with physical attenuators requires significant advance preparation. The desired intensity map is converted into attenuator material thickness. The attenuator is fabricated using a computer controlled milling machine. Fabrication time depends on the milling machine and the control software, but is on the order of 30 minutes to an hour. Treatment time is comparable to conventional radiotherapy, but the treatment cannot be delivered under computer control because of the need to enter the room to change attenuators between beams. On the positive side, quality assurance procedures are similiar to those used for missing tissue compensators and thus are well understood.[4]

We present a method of IMRT delivery that uses a single physical attenuator for multiple beams. The collimator is rotated following each field, using a different region of the attenuator to provide intensity modulation. Because only one attenuator must be fabricated, verified, and used for treatment, IMRT is simplified. The treatment can be delivered under computer control, with the treatment room being entered at most one time to rotate the attenuator (a typical accelerator collimator only rotates through 180 degrees). A 5 beam treatment of a prostate tumor is used to demonstrate this approach.

## Material and methods

### Theory

Consider a tumor volume to be treated with $N$ intensity modulated (IM) beams of length $L$ and width $W$. All $N$ IM beams can be delivered using a single physical attenuator by distributing the regions in a circular pattern about the center of the attenuator as shown in figure 1. The rotational isocenter of the attenuator is shifted from the center of each treatment beam by

$$\Delta = \frac{W}{2\tan(\frac{\pi}{N})} + \frac{L}{2} \tag{1}$$

The total size of the attenuator is given by

$$F = 2\sqrt{\frac{D^2}{4} + (\frac{L}{2} + \Delta)^2} \tag{2}$$

The rotational isocenter shift $\Delta$ and the required physical attenuator size $F$ are shown as functions of square IM beams in figures 2 and 3 for 3, 5, 7, and 9 beams per attenuator. Up to five $10\times10$ cm$^2$ beams and up to seven $9\times9$ cm$^2$ beams can be delivered with a single $40\times40$ cm$^2$ attenuator.

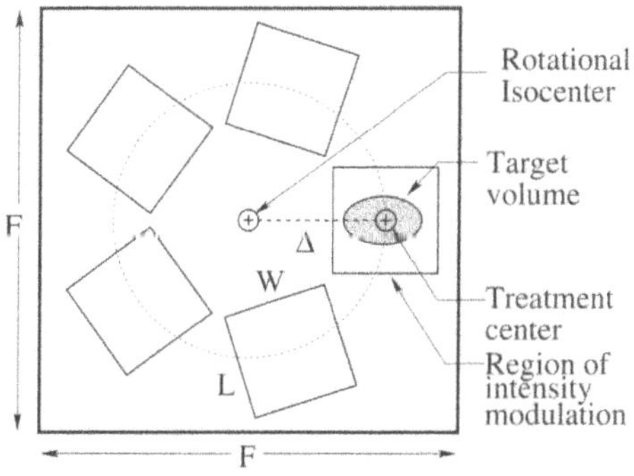


**Figure 1:** Treatment of five intensity modulated fields using a single attenuator. The area outside of the intensity modulated regions is blocked using a combination of the secondary collimating jaws and a MLC.

### Treatment Planning

Treatment plans are developed using inverse planning software, OPTIMA (Optimization Planning Tools for Intensity Modulating Attenuators), which has been developed for IMRT optimization research at The University of Texas M. D. Anderson Cancer Center. OPTIMA is modular in

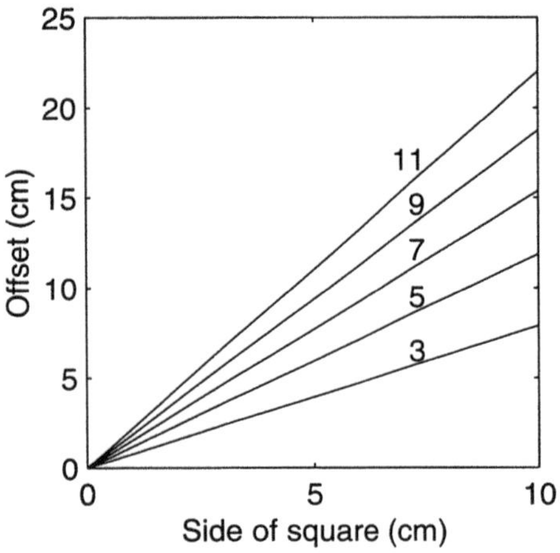


**Figure 2:** Rotational isocenter offset vs. size of square IM beam.

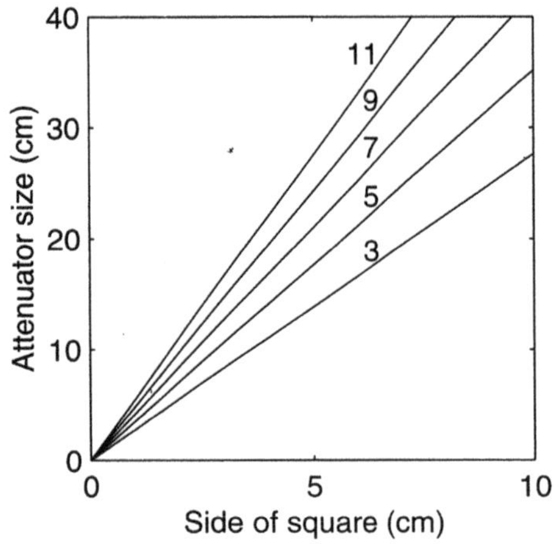


**Figure 3:** Physical attenuator size vs. size of square IM beam.

design for simple implementation of arbitrary cost functions, constraints, and new treatment strategies such as the one described here. The dose model is a Clarkson sector summation algorithm reformulated into Cartesian coordinates to provide geometric conformity to rectangular pencil beams.[5] Primary and scattered dose to each point from each pencil beam is calculated prior to optimization. The model is relatively simple and thus is fast; calculation time on a 266 MHz Pentium II is 30 microseconds per point per pencil beam. The model does not presently account for heterogeneities. Optimum weights based on clinical goals are computed for all of the pencil beams using constrained simulated annealing.[6] OPTIMA is used as an adjunct to a commercial 3-D treatment planning system (3DTPS).[7] Prior to optimization, patient anatomy information and, if necessary, the dose distribution of a prior or concomitant treatment is imported from the 3DTPS. Following optimization, the resultant dose distribution is exported to the 3DTPS for display. Beam transmission maps may be exported to the 3DTPS and used for dose calculation within the 3DTPS.

### Plan Optimization

To produce a multiple field, single attenuator IMRT plan, all beams are divided into the same number of pencil beams. The rotational isocenter is shifted from the treatment isocenter by $\Delta$, given in equation 1. The pencil beam weights are optimized based on the clinical goals using OPTIMA. Following optimization, the pencil beam weights are overlaid to produce a composite transmission map for the single attenuator. Beam weights for pencil beams which do not pass through the target volume are set to a minimum transmission value, typically 5%. The collimating jaw positions are set to define the target volume. The transmission map is exported to the 3DTPS for final dose calculation and display.

## Results and discussion

A transverse section containing the treatment center of a prostate tumor to be treated with five IM beams is displayed in figure 4. The optimization goal was to maximize the minimum dose to the target volume. Dose volume constraints were applied to the bladder, rectum, and femoral heads. These constraints are shown in Table 1. The rotational isocenter was shifted from the treatment center by 11.9 cm. The transmission map of the composite attenuator is shown in figure 5. The final dose calculation was performed using the 3DTPS. The DVHs of the treatment are shown in figure 6.

| | Constraint 1 | Constraint 2 | Maximum dose |
|---|---|---|---|
| Rectum | 25% > 60 Gy | 20% > 70 Gy | 85 Gy |
| Bladder | 30% > 60 Gy | 20% > 70 Gy | 85 Gy |
| Femoral heads | 15% > 45 Gy | 5% > 50 Gy | 55 Gy |

**Table 1:** Dose volume constraints for optimization of prostate treatment. Each constraint gives the volume of organ allowed to exceed the specified dose.

## Conclusion

The example demonstrates the potential of using a single physical attenuator for delivery of multiple intensity modulated beams. This technique overcomes the disadvantages of IMRT delivery using attenuators while retaining the advantages. Only one attenuator must be fabricated, verified, and used for treatment. The treatment room must be entered at most once to rotate the attenuator. However, this approach is limited to about 7 fields for typical target volumes.

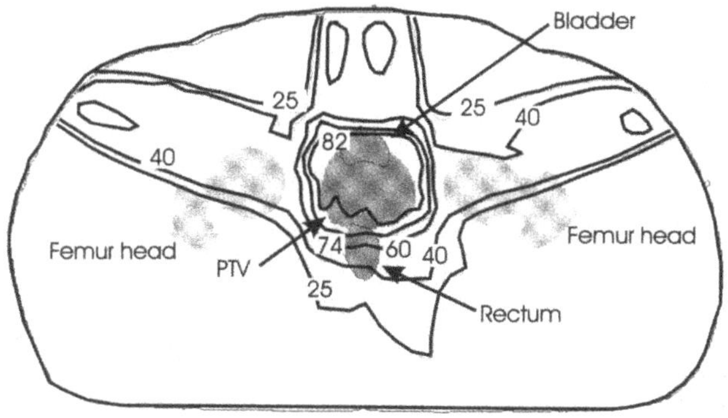


**Figure 4:** Five beam IM treatment of a prostate tumor. The minimum dose to the PTV is 71 Gy. The optimization constraints result in the two posterior beams delivering very little dose.

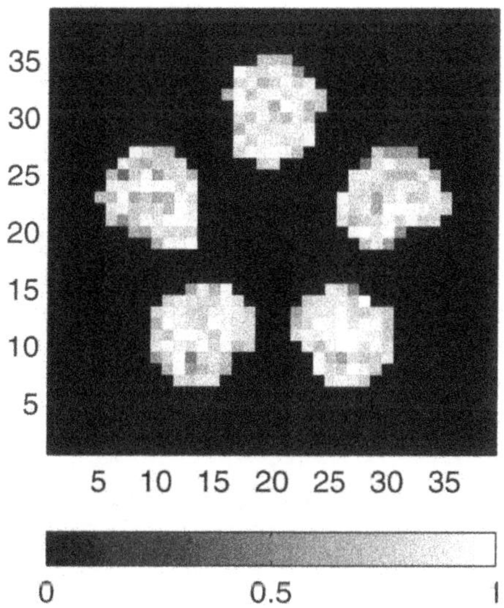


**Figure 5:** Transmission map.

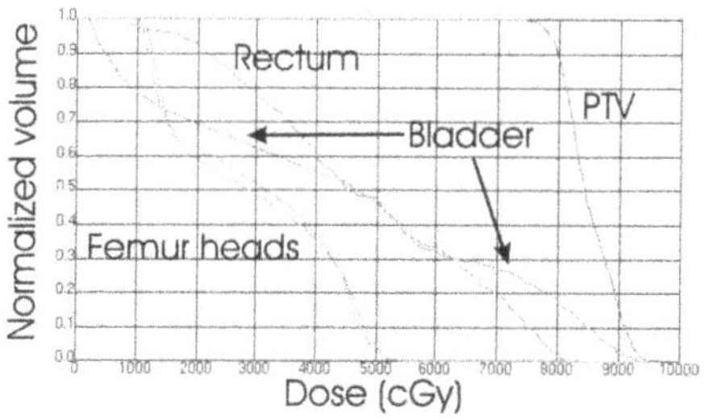


**Figure 6:** Dose volume histogram.

# References


[1] J. Stein, K. Hartwig, S. Levegrün, G. Zhang, K. Preiser, B. Rhein, J. Debus, and T. Bortfeld, in *XIIth International Conference on the Use of Computers in Radiation Therapy, Salt Lake City, Utah, 1997*, edited by D.D. Leavitt and G. Starkschall (Medical Physics Publishing Madison, Wisconsin, 1997), p.338

[2] J. Wong, M. Sharpe, D. Yan, Y. Wu, B. Miller, D. Brabbins, and A. Martinez, in *3-D Conformal Radiation Therapy and Intensity-Modulated Radiation Therapy in the New Millenium, Houston, Texas, 1999*

[3] C. Burman, C. Chui, G. Kutcher, S. Leibel, M. Zelefsky, T. LoSasso, S. Spirou, Q. Wu, J. Yang, J. Stein, R. Mohan, Z. Fuks, and C.C. Ling, "Planning, delivery, and quality assurance of intensity-modulated radiotherapy using dynamic multileaf collimator: A strategy for large scale implementation for the treatment of carcinoma of the prostate," Int. J. Radiation Oncology Biol. Phys. **39**, 863–873 (1997)

[4] D.A. Low, Z. Li, and E.E. Klein "Verification of milled two-dimensional photon compensating filters using an electronic portal imaging device," Med. Phys. **23**, 929–938 (1996)

[5] J.R. Cunningham, "Scatter-Air ratios," Phys. Med. Biol. **17**, 42–51 (1972)

[6] S.M. Morrill, R.G. Lane, and I.I. Rosen, "Constrained simulated annealing for optimized radiation therapy treatment planning," Comput. Programs Biomed. **33**, 135–144 (1990)

[7] ADAC Pinnacle$^3$, ADAC Laboratories, Milipitas, California

# Application of Enhanced Dynamic Wedge to Stereotactic Radiotherapy

**Gordon A. Watson, Dennis D. Leavitt, Matthew Tobler, David K. Gaffney, and Frederic A. Gibbs, Jr.**

Department of Radiation Oncology, University of Utah School of Medicine, Salt Lake City, UT 84132 USA

## Introduction

Linear accelerator based stereotactic radiotherapy systems have traditionally utilized rotational arcs with small circular collimators to create relatively conformal dose distributions within a target volume [1,2]. Large or irregularly shaped targets require multiple isocenters to achieve conformality at the expense of dose inhomogeneity within the target volume. The micro-multileaf (MLC) collimator is a recent innovation specifically designed for small-field stereotactic radiotherapy that has improved the conformality of dose delivery to irregularly shaped targets [3-8]. This is accomplished by movement of the narrow-leaf collimators to conform to the shape of the target as seen through a "beams-eye-view" projection during arc rotation. However, neighboring critical structures and physical constraints imposed by patient fixation devices often limit the beam trajectories and geometries available for dose delivery. Dose delivery through limited numbers of fixed fields may be optimal in these situations. However, it is often difficult to achieve a uniform dose distribution using uncompensated or non-intensity modified beams. The micro-MLC collimators are attached to the linear accelerator as an accessory device, though, and there is no provision for beam intensity modifiers such as physical compensators or wedges. Modification of beam intensity can only be accomplished by dynamic motion of the micro-MLC collimator (intensity modulation) [9] or by dynamic motion of collimators upstream from the micro-MLC collimator (dynamic wedge) [10]. We examined the dose distribution achievable by the addition of dynamic wedge capabilities to fixed conformal fields using the micro-MLC collimator. Data is presented on two reference cases with severe clinical and geometric constraints to treatment delivery due to target shape and proximity of critical structures.

## Material and methods

The BrainLAB™ micro-MLC collimator was used attached as an accessory to a Varian Clinac 2100 CD™ accelerator. Planning CT data was recorded using the BrainLAB™ and RAHD™ treatment planning systems. Target and internal structure volumes were defined and reconstructed in three dimensions using the BrainLAB™ treatment planning system. Beams-eye-views were used to define micro- MLC beam shapes with appropriate margin around the target. Beam trajectories were constrained to exclude or minimize dose to nearby critical structures. The data set was then transported to the RAHD™ treatment planning system as the BrainLAB™ software does not currently support wedge-induced dose modification. Enhanced Dynamic Wedge (EDW) modulation was applied to one or more fixed beams to attempt to improve dose homogeniety throughout the defined target. Dose distributions for non-EDW and EDW-modified treatment plans were recorded and compared for maximum dose within the target and overall dose-volume histogram (DVH) of both the target and any neighboring critical structures.

## Results and discussion

The first example presents a post-resection tumor bed of a low grade leimyosarcoma in the paranasal sinuses located immediately between the eyes. Six MV photons were used to deliver 64 Gy total to the 98% isodose line (IDL) at 2 Gy per fraction. The dimensions of this long, wide, shallow target volume were 43 mm long, 24 mm wide, and 12 mm high encompassing a volume of 8.7 cc. The location of the tumor directly between the eyes constrained beam trajectories to a single sagittal plane. Initially, an orthogonal wedge pair (anterior and vertex) was evaluated and found unacceptable due to the large volume of normal frontal lobe included in the high dose region ($\geq$ 90%). Therefore, three fields were assigned at gantry angles of 90 degrees (vertex field), 125 degrees (anterior superior oblique field), and 180 degrees (direct anterior field). For each field, the micromultileaf collimator encompassed the beams eye view cross section plus a 5 mm margin. The target and beam arrangements (and EDW palcement for the micro-MLC EDW plan) are illustrated in figure 1, which emphasizes the close proximity of the beam paths to the eyes.

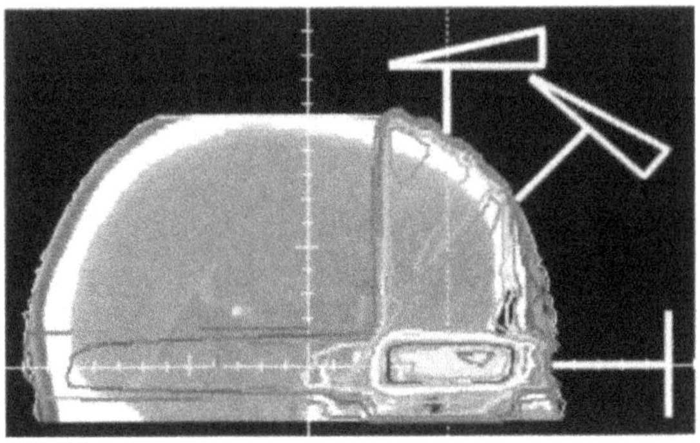

**Figure 1:** Sagittal view with beam and wedge orientation.

The application of these three fields without wedges introduced a dose variation throughout the target volume of +/- 10%. These calculations were then repeated with the application of Enhanced Dynamic Wedge to the fields, and the dose variation was reduced to +/- 4%. This is illustrated in figure 2, which compares the isodose distributions side-by-side for unwedged vs. wedge added treatment plans. Note that no wedge is applied in the anterior field, while the tip of the wedges for the anterior oblique and vertex fields is oriented superiorly. The placement and orientation of the wedge fields enhances the dose to the posterior aspects of the tumor volume, thereby improving the dose uniformity throughout the entire volume.

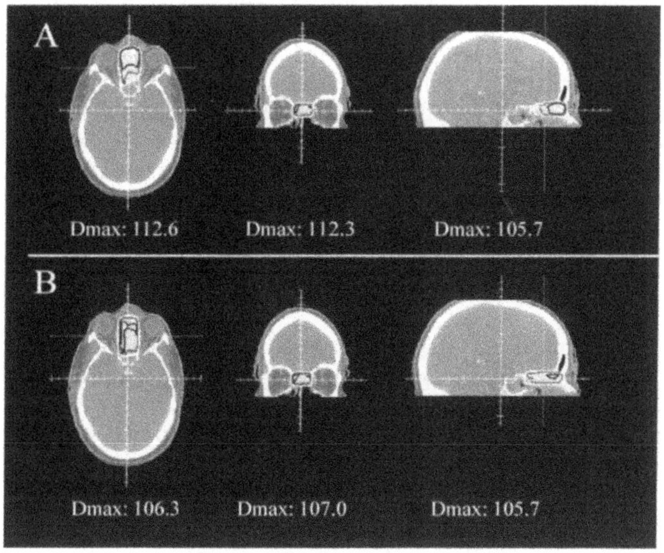


**Figure 2:** Comparison of Dmax values and dose distribution for micro-MLC (A) *vs.* micro-MLC with EDW (B). IDL's: inner white (110%); black (105%); grey (100%); outer white (95%).

The dose-volume histogram in figure 3 demonstrates, quantitatively, the improved dose distribution to the target using the micro-MLC with EDW with relative sparing of the eyes.

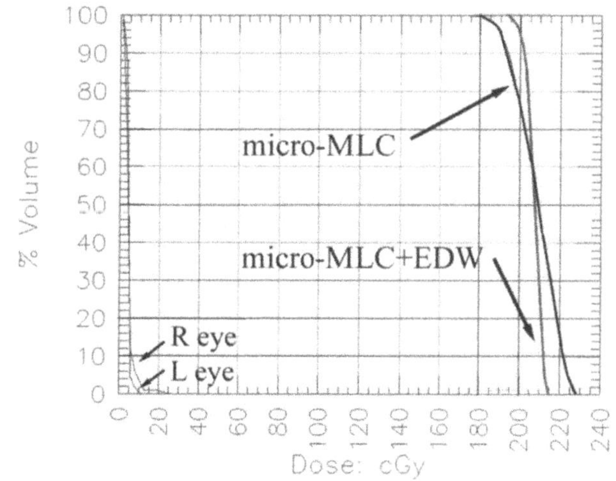


**Figure 3:** Dose-volume histogram of target volume comparing the micro-MLC and micro-MLC with EDW.

The second example presents a recurrent meningioma of complex shape. Tumor was present along the cavernous sinus, sphenoid wing, and retro-orbital space. Six MV photons were used to deliver 50.4 Gy to the 95% IDL at 1.8 Gy per fraction. The radiation fields were designed to encompass the target volume while minimizing dose to the eyes. The dimensions of this target volume were 65 mm long, 56 mm wide, and 55 mm high with a volume of 55 cc. Four conformal coplanar fields were applied to this target. Each field included a 5 mm margin. The target and beam orientations are illustrated in figure 4. The application of these four fields without wedges introduced a dose variation throughout the target volume of +/- 15%.

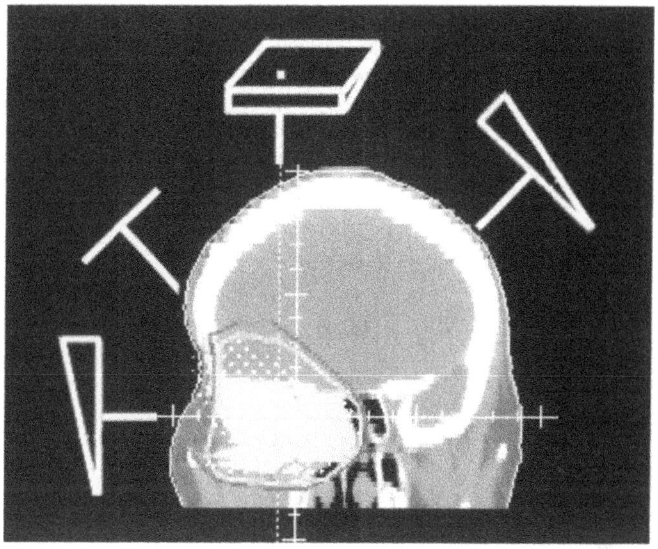

**Figure 4:** Coronal view of beam and wedge orientation.

When EDW was added to 2 fields, the dose uniformity improved to +/- 4%. The high dose region of the radiated volume moved from the frontal lobe of the brain into the target volume, sparing significant normal tissue. Additionally, with the non-EDW plan, it is clear from the coronal view that even the 95% IDL does not completely cover the target volume. This is demonstrated in figure 5.

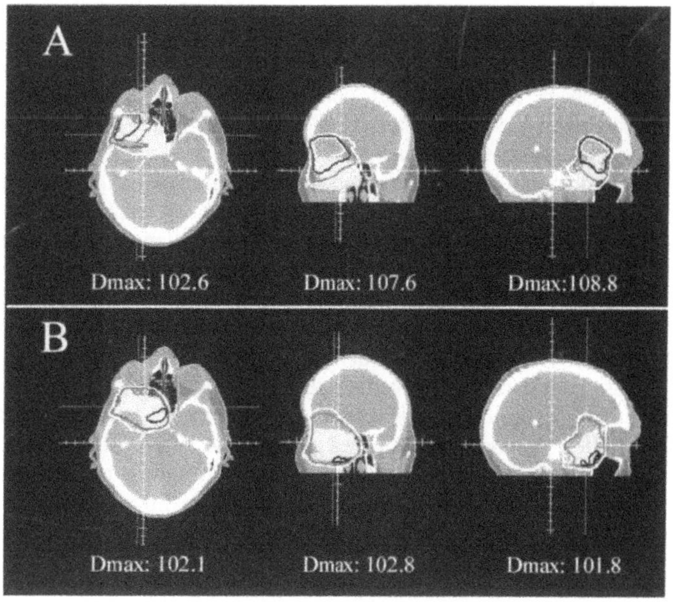


**Figure 5:** Comparison of Dmax values and dose distribution for micro-MLC (A) *vs.* micro-MLC with EDW (B). IDL's: inner white (104%); black (101%); grey (98%); outer white (95%).

The micro-MLC with EDW plan provides coverage of the entire tumor volume at the 95% IDL plus spares a significant volume of neighboring normal tissue, including brain, optic chiasm and eyes. This is shown by the DVH in figure 6 which compares the micro-MLC and the micro-MLC-EDW plans. Importantly, the DVH demonstrates that with standard micro-MLC, the target is encompassed only by the 80% IDL. Treatment at this IDL would result in shifting of the dose 15% higher for all volumes compared to the micro-MLC-EDW plan (which covers target at the 95% IDL). Thus, with standard micro-MLC plan, normal tissues (optic chiasm, eyes and brain) received doses significantly higher than with the micro-MLC-EDW plan.

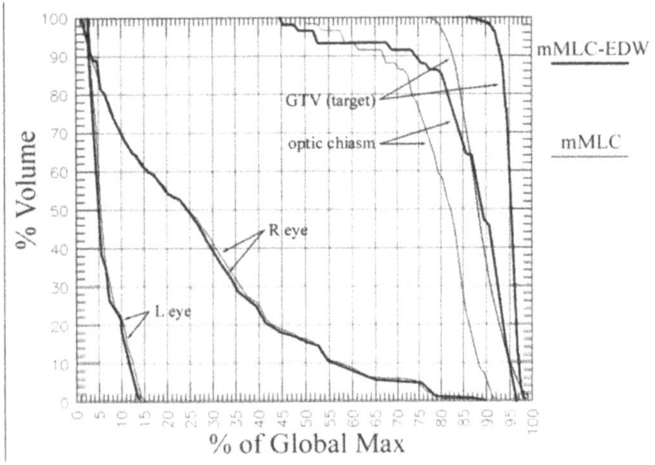


**Figure 6:** Dose-volume histogram of target, optic chiasm and eyes comparing the micro-MLC and micro-MLC with EDW.

## Conclusion

Small field stereotactic radiotherapy using micro-MLC technology and beams-eye-view planning systems has greatly increased the degree of conformality as well as ease of radiation treatment delivery. However, when faced with complex target volumes and/or severe constraints on beam geometry and trajectory, non-intensity modulated plans, even with micro-MLC collimation, can result in significant dose inhomogeneities and unacceptable radiation dose to neighboring critical structures. The application of Enhanced Dynamic Wedge to fixed fields shaped by an accessory micro-MLC allows for modification of beam intensity. This form of intensity modulation, as demonstrated in the preceeding two cases, greatly improved both dose homogeneity through complex target shapes and dose profiles to nearby critical structures. Dose inhomogeneity within the target was decreased by 60-75% with the EDW. Dose to critical structures was below normal tissue tolerance levels while allowing definitive treatment of the target. Thus, this technique has immediate clinical applications.

Currently, the use of micro-MLC with EDW is a "forward planning process" which utilizes a choice of fixed EDW profiles and allows relative weighting of the fields to visually optimize the dose distribution. Beam geometries and trajectories are also chosen via beams-eye-view planning and forward iteration for dose optimization. Attempts to improve upon this technology using inverse planning models are currently being evaluated. Additionally, automated selection of optimal beam geometries and trajectories would likely improve upon both dose homogeneity and allow for avoidance of critical structures and normal tissues. Algorithms for selection of wedge angles and orientation could be added for further optimization. Until these technologies are applicable, though, the use of EDW with the micro-MLC provides a significant improvement in dose delivery for complex structures in critical areas.

## References

[1] Lutz W, Winston K R and Maleki N 1988 A system for stereotactic radiosurgery with a linear accelerator *Int. J. Radiat. Oncol. Biol. Phys.* **14**:373-381

[2] Kooy H M, Bellerive M R and Loeffler J S 1996 Stereotactic Radiotherapy in Teletherapy: Present and Future Mackie R T, Palta J R editors Madison, WI. Advanced Medical Publishing 681-722

[3] Kubo H D, Pappas C T E and Wilder R B 1997 A comparison of arc-based and static mini-multileaf collimator-based radiosurgery plans *Radiother. Oncol.* **45**:89-93

[4] Leavitt D D, Gibbs F A, Heilbrun M P, Moeller J H, and Takach G A 1991 Dynamic field shaping to optimize stereotactic radiosurgery *Int. J. Radiat. Oncol. Biol. Phys.* **21**:1247-1255

[5] Haedinger U, Kubesch R, Neumann M, Richter J and Schlegel W 1997 Development of a micro computer based control system for a dynamic multileaf collimator Proceedings of XII ICCR, ed. Leavitt D D & Starkschall G Medical Physics Publishing 354-356

[6] Schlegel W, Pastyr O, Kubesch R, Stein J, Diemer T, Hover K H and Rhein 1997 A computer controlled micro-multileaf-collimator for stereotactic conformal radiotherapy Proceedings of XII ICCR, ed. Leavitt D D & Starkschall G Medical Physics Publishing 79-82

[7] Shiu A S, Wong J, Ewton J E, Rittichier H E, Tung S S and Long L 1997 Computer-controlled miniature multileaf collimator Proceedings of XII ICCR, ed. Leavitt D D & Starkschall G Medical Physics Publishing 83-85

[8] Leavitt D D 1998 Beam shaping for SRT/SRS *Med. Dosim.* **23**:229-236

[9] Grant W III and Cain R B 1998 Intensity modulated conformal therapy for intracranial lesions *Med. Dosim.* **23**:237-241

[10] Edlund T, Leavitt D D and Gibbs F A Jr 1999 Dosimetric advantages of enhanced dynamic wedge in small field irradiation for the treatment of macular degeneration *Med. Dosim.* **24**:21-26

# An improved technique for tangential breast irradiation applying MLC field shaping and inverse planning

**B. van Asselen, C.P.J. Raaijmakers, P. Hofman and J.J.W. Lagendijk**

[1]Radiotherapy Department, University Medical Center Utrecht, Heidelberglaan 100, 3584 CX Utrecht, The Netherlands

## Introduction

Treatment planning for conventional tangential breast irradiation is generally performed using a 2-D contour of the breast through the central plane. Optimisation of the dose distribution in this plane is performed by manual interactive optimisation of the wedge angle that compensates for the varying contour of the breast. Studies using 3-D CT data sets indicate that the 3-D dose homogeneity is not optimal and that the dose in the target volume may vary by approximately 10-15% [1, 2].
In our institution a standard technique is used for all tangential breast irradiations [3]. Patients are positioned on a wedged breast-board in order to obtain a vertical match plane between the tangential fields and the supraclavicular and axial fields in case of multiple field irradiations. Patients on a breast-board are difficult to position inside a CT scanner due to the limited size of the bore of the scanner. In order to facilitate the positioning of these patients in a CT scanner the concept of breast-board has to be abandoned.
The match of the tangential field to the parasternal field is performed in the central plane. Due to the curvature of the thorax, however, the optimal match is not maintained along the whole length of the field and using a rectangular field setting under-dosage or over-dosage is almost unavoidable.
It was the purpose of this work to develop a new technique for tangential breast irradiation which avoids the above mentioned problems. This technique should fulfil the following criteria: 1) maintain a vertical match plane between the tangential fields and the supraclavicular and axial fields without using a breast-board in order to facilitate the positioning of patients in a CT scanner; 2) have the possibility to match the parasternal field to the tangential field with the same overlap over the whole length of the field and 3) improve dose homogeneity. Since breast irradiation is the most commonly applied technique in our institution the new technique should be relatively simple, reliable and efficient.

## Material and methods

### Patient positioning

Positioning without breast board while avoiding excessive lung irradiation demands the appliance of complicated shielding techniques. A vertical match plane can, however, be obtained by applying MLC field shaping (Fig 1). The use of MLC field shaping also creates the possibility of shaping the medial parasternal entrance of the tangential field in order to match it dosimetrically with the parasternal field along the whole length of the field. On the other hand the use of MLC shaping of the tangential fields implies that wedges cannot be used to optimise the dose distribution since in our linear accelerators (Elekta Oncology Systems, UK) the wedge direction is opposite to the leave direction. Therefore, an IMRT technique had to be developed. The use of MLC field shaping and the 3-D optimisation of the dose distribution implies further that a complete 3D CT data set of the patient has to be available.
Five patients underwent a planning CT scan. Before CT-scanning the conventional field borders were marked under X-ray examination by tiny lead markers on the patients skin in order to visualise the conventional field borders on the CT scan. The patients were positioned supine on a foam breast board with both arms above their head following our conventional technique. In order to analyse the 3-D dose distribution a clinical target volume (CTV) was drawn in by the radiation oncologist. The planning target volume (PTV) was obtained by adding a 1-cm margin to the CTV. The lung and the skin were excluded from the PTV.

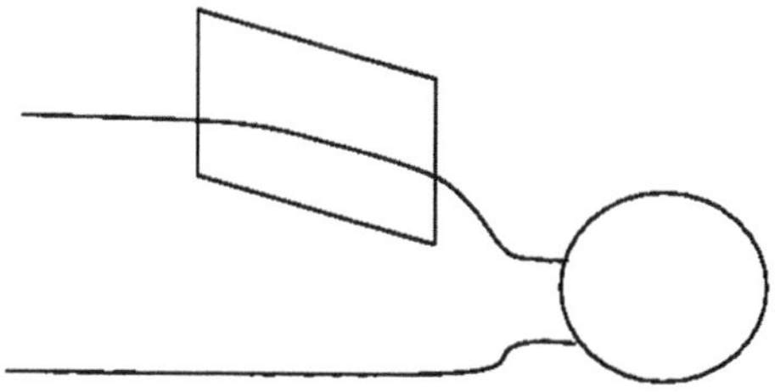

**Figure 1:** Tangential breast irradiation using MLC field shaping. The leave direction is vertical.

### Treatment planning

Various methods were evaluated to optimise the 3-D dose distribution in the PTV without using a conventional wedge. These methods included mimicking a wedge profile by several intensity-modulated fields, optimisation of the dose distribution in the central plane by applying reduced beam intensity to the lung tissue and the use of a prototype inverse planning system. The general problem appeared to be the determination of the shape of the MLC field segments. These segments should be relatively easy to deduce from the patient geometry and must be relatively simple to implement clinically. Eventually a method was developed based on the division of the irradiated volume in segments with a similar equivalent path length.
In first approximation when ignoring scatter effects, the equivalent path length along a ray line from the focus through the breast is proportional to the dose delivered at a specific depth. In case of two opposed tangential fields, ray lines with an equal equivalent path length should approximately have the same beam intensity to obtain a homogeneous dose distribution. To test this approach, 2D equivalent path length maps were generated from the CT data set using software developed in our institution. Ray tracing from the focus through the CT data generated equivalent path length maps (EPM). Differences in tissue composition were taken into

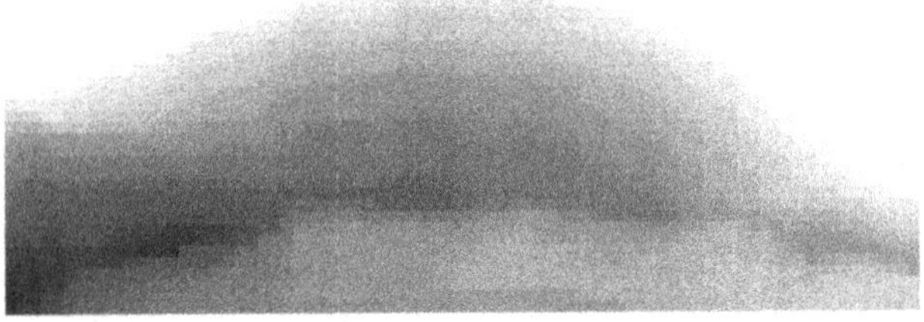

**Figure 2:** Equivalent path length map for a tangential breast irradiation. A low grey value indicates a short path length.

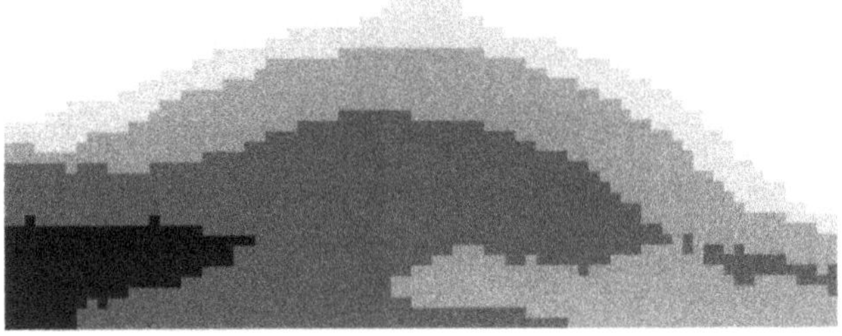

**Figure 3:** Equivalent path length map for a tangential breast irradiation divided into four discrete pathlength segments.

account using a table that transfers hounsfield units to relative electron density (Fig. 2). The translation of such a 2D map into MLC field settings and intensity levels is a complex problem. In first approximation we divided the EPM in four intensity steps (Fig 2). The MLC settings deduced from these maps were entered into a 3-D planning system (PLATO RTS version 2.2, Nucletron Ltd, The Netherlands) and the 3-D dose distribution was calculated applying inhomogeneity correction. Weighting of the various segments was performed in a point centrally in the highest intensity level. Approximately 90% of the dose delivered to this point was delivered by the large open field covering the whole breast. The remaining 10% were equally divided over the other segments. Normalisation of the plans was performed at the isocenter. Dose volume histograms (DVHs) for the IMRT technique were compared to DVHs for the conventional wedge plans. Furthermore, the mean dose for the ipsilateral lung was calculated for each plan.

## Results and discussion

A comparison between the target volume drawn in the CT data and the field setting as derived from conventional X-ray guided localisation yielded that in some cases the field settings had to be adjusted to obtain a complete covering of the target volume.
As expected, the EPMs showed gradual changes in path length over the target volume (Fig 2). Starting from the ventral side, the path length gradually increases until the region is reached were lung tissue is involved. Due to the low relative electron density of the lung compared to breast tissue, the equivalent path length in this area is smaller than that of the adjacent breast tissue. For all patients, the largest path length was obtained in the cranial part of the target volume. In the conventional treatment plans, the dose in these areas was approximately 5-10% lower than the dose at the isocenter. Applying the IMRT technique resulted in an increased dose in these cranial areas and significantly improved DVHs were obtained for four out of five patients (Fig 4). For one patient the DVH for the IMRT plan was comparable to that of the conventional plan. For this patient the conventional plan was, however, already near optimal.
In conventional treatment plans using a wedge, the highest beam intensity is delivered to the part of the irradiated volume that contains lung tissue. When the IMRT technique is used, reduced beam intensity is applied to this area Consequently, a reduction of the mean lung dose was obtained applying the IMRT technique compared to the conventional technique. This reduction amounted to approximately 10-20%.

In this work the patients were positioned on a breast board following our conventional technique. The new technique, however, uses MLC field shaping to shield the lung and can, therefore, also be applied without using the breast board.
Several aspects of the IMRT technique need to be further investigated. The deduction of MLC settings from the EPM was done in this study by eye, ignoring relatively small areas with a slightly different path length. Procedures will be developed to generate MLC settings automatically from the EPM. The number of intensity levels was chosen to be four. This choice was rather arbitrary and needs to be further investigated and quantified. The proportion of the various fields (approximately 90% for the largest field and 10% for the remaining three smaller segments) was also based on experience and not on geometrical patient information alone. This aspect needs to be further optimised. When these various problems are solved a true inverse planning method will be developed for tangential breast irradiation, i.e. a treatment planning method based solely on geometrical information.

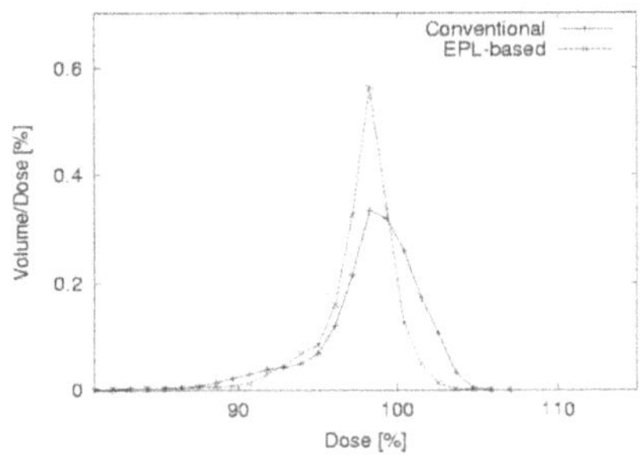


**Figure 4:** DVH of the PTV for a conventional tangential breast irradiation compared with a DVH for the IMRT technique for one patient.

## Conclusion

A new technique has been developed for tangential breast irradiation. This technique uses an equivalent path length map calculated from CT data to deduce MLC field settings, in combination with empirical rules for the beam weights of the various segments. Compared with the conventional wedge plan, increased dose homogeneity over the PTV and a reduction of the mean lung dose by approximately 10-20 % was obtained. The technique allows patient positioning without breast board which facilitates the positioning of the patient in the CT scanner and allows MLC shaping of the tangential fields in order to obtain an optimal match with the parasternal field over the whole length of the field.

## References

[1] Carruthers L J, Redpath A T and Kunkler I H 1999 The use of compensators to optimise the three dimensional dose distribution in radiotherapy of the intact breast *Radiother Oncol* **50** 291-300

[2] Hong L, Hunt M S, Chui C *et al* 1999 Intensity-modulated tangential beam irradiation of the intact breast *Int J Radiat Oncol Biol Phys* **44** 1155-1164

[3] Lagendijk J J W and Hofman P 1992 A standardised multifield irradiation technique for breast tumours using asymmetrical collimators and beam angulation *British Journal of Radiology* **65** 56-62

## Acknowledgements

This work was financially supported by the Dutch Cancer Society (NKB Grant UU 99-1863).

# Eliminating Complex Treatment Setup for Intact Breast or Postmastectomy Treatment with Intensity Modulated Radiation Therapy

**Lijun Ma, Michael Haas, Timothy Holmes, Maria Jacobs, Mohan Suntharalingam, and Cedric Yu**

Department of Radiation Oncology, University of Maryland School of Medicine, Baltimore, MD, USA 21201

## Introduction

Intensity Modulation Radiation Therapy (IMRT) for intact breast or chest wall treatments has been controversial based on the results of recent studies. One study indicates that IMRT significantly reduces normal tissue dose and improves target dose distribution [1] while another suggests that IMRT offers no dosimetric advantages over existing three-dimensional treatment techniques [2]. However, these IMRT studies only considered tangential photon beam modulations for intact breast or chest wall treatment without taking into account the need to treat supraclavicular lymph nodes (SLN) and axillary lymph nodes (ALN). We carried out composite treatment plan comparisons between the standard conformal techniques and IMRT for the full-course treatments of intact breast (IB) or postmastectomy (PM) patients specifically to evaluate this issue.

In order to avoid any underdose or overdose caused by the tangential photon beam divergence or overlapping, it is essential to have proper beam arrangement and reproducible patient setup for standard conformal treatments. A variety of treatment techniques have been developed to accomplish this task. The most common techniques include using rotational half-beam block, independent collimator, couch or collimator rotation, etc.[3-5]. Since IMRT intrinsically compensates for any underdose or overdose caused by the beam divergence or overlapping with the inverse treatment planning optimization, it is plausible to apply IMRT so as to eliminate any complex setups associated with standard three-dimensional treatment techniques. Therefore, it is our goal in this study to investigate the feasibility and the efficiency of IMRT for IB and PM treatment without complex treatment setups.

## Material and methods

Seven patients with clinical indications for radiation therapy were selected for full CT scans that encompassed the primary lesion and supraclavicular and axillary lymph nodes. The primary target site (either intact breast or chest wall) together with the lymph nodes was defined for treatment planning purposes. These target contours were first outlined on a three-dimensional treatment planning system (RederPlan 3D, Elekta Oncology System, GA), and then hand traced onto an IMRT inverse planning system (CORVUS, NOMOS Corporation, PA) by radiation oncologists based on the patient anatomy using the same CT data set. Treatment plans were generated using consistent prescriptions and dose-volume constraints:

For standard three-dimensional conformal treatment planning, composite treatment plans were generated using two tangential photon beams and one anterior-posterior field for lymph node irradiation. A posterior axillary boost (PAB) field was included if it was prescribed for the treatment. The treatment was generated using three-field single-isocenter technique with half-beam blocking plus any necessary couch and collimator rotations [3]. For comparison purpose, 45 Gy was prescribed for all cases to the primary target site that covered the entire planning target volume (PTV), and 50 Gy was prescribed to a fixed point at the depth of 3 cm for lymph node irradiation.

For IMRT treatment planning, two opposed tangential beams and two anterior-posterior oblique beams were used. A schematic of the beam arrangement is shown in Figure 1. The couch angle was fixed at zero degree (IEC) and the collimator was fixed at a single angle for all beams. The dose-volume prescriptions for inverse planning were set to 45 Gy for at least 80% coverage of the target volume and 50 Gy for at least 80% coverage of lymph nodes. We allowed only 15% of normal structures (such as the heart or lung) to receive tolerance doses. The optimization routine typically runs for 15-20 minutes until the plan is ready for analysis. Comparison between the standard conformal treatment plans and IMRT plans was carried out using dose-volume histograms (DVH) and conformity index (CI) for target volumes.

The dose distribution at the junction of the tangential and supraclavicular fields for standard conformal and IMRT treatment plans were measured using ion-chambers in an anthropomorphous rando-phantom. The exact beam configuration for the three-dimensional conformal and IMRT treatment plans were duplicated and recomputed for the rando-phantom. The dose values at the field junction were determined from the calculation to compare with the ion-chamber measurements.

## Results and discussion

A typical plan comparison between the composite isodose distributions for a standard conformal plan and an IMRT plan is shown in Figure 2. The DVH comparison for the same patient is shown in Figure 3. From the results of the DVH and CI comparisons, the IMRT plan provided equivalent dose distribution and coverage for both the IB and PM volumes.

However, significant dose variation was observed in the lymph node region for the standard conformal plans (Figure 3). Only approximately 40% of the lymph node volume received 50 Gy in the standard conformal treatment as compared with 95% in the IMRT treatment. This is primarily caused by the single field irradiation with the dose prescribed to a fixed point at 3 cm in depth. As shown in Figures 2-3, IMRT provides better and more uniform dose coverage for the lymph nodes and also dramatically reduces the dose "hot-spots" in the heart and the lung.

Our phantom measurements show that IMRT provides uniform junction dose for lymph node irradiation. Dose uniformity at the field junction was found to be comparable (within 3%) to standard conformal delivery.

## Conclusion

IMRT is a new modality for improving dose distribution with some reduction in delivery efficiency. In this study, we found IMRT to be more efficient as compared to the standard conformal techniques for IB or PM cancer treatments. Our results demonstrated that IMRT could effectively eliminate complex treatment setups or lengthy simulation processes associated with standard conformal treatment. With simplified treatment setup, IMRT is capable of providing improved composite dose distribution for both the primary lesion and the potentially involved lymph nodes with dramatically reduced hot-spots in the adjoining normal structures such as the heart and the lung.

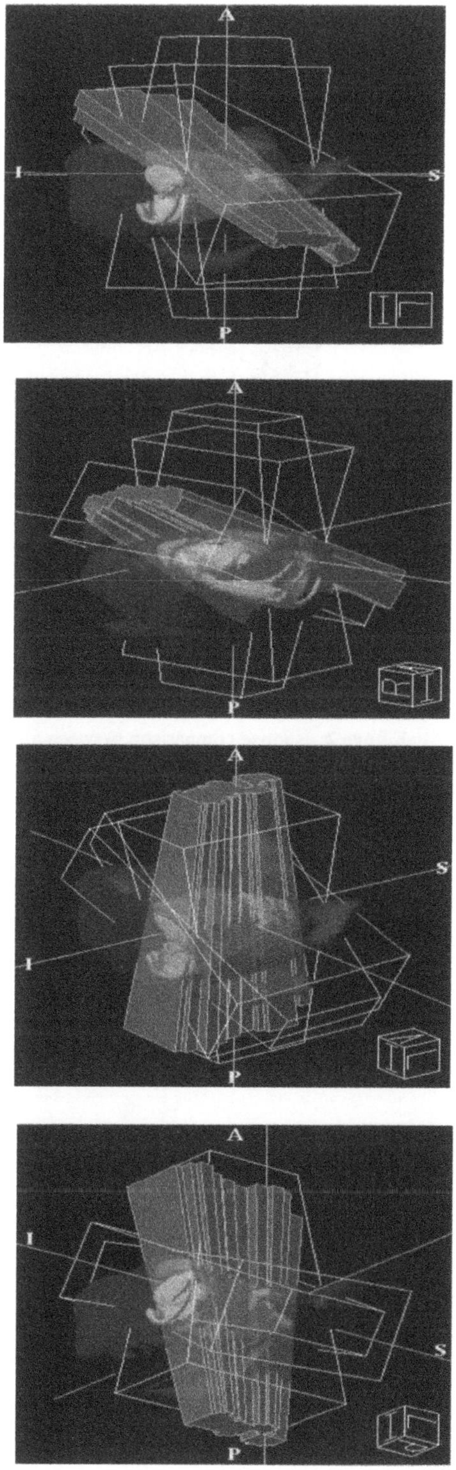

**Figure 1:** Four-field IMRT beam arrangements

## References


[1] Hong L, Hunt M, Chui C, Spirou S, Forster K, Lee H, Yahalom J, Kutcher G J, and McCormick B 1999 Intensity-modulated tangential beam irradiation of the intact breast *Int. J. Radiat. Oncol. Biol. Phys.* **44** No. 5, 1155-1164

[2] Meeks S L, Buatti J M, Bova F J, Friedman W A, Mendenhall W M and Zlotecki R A 1998 Potential clinical Efficacy of Intensity modulated Conformal Therapy *Int. J. Radiat. Oncol. Biol. Phys.* **40** No. 2, 483-495

[3] Siddon R L, Tonnesen G L,Sevensson G K 1981 Three-field technique for breast treatment using a rotatable half-beam block *Int. J. Radiat. Oncol. Biol. Phys.* **7**, 1473-1477

[4] Lichter A S, Sandler H M, Robertson J M, Lawrence T S, Ten Haken R K, McShan D L, Fraass B A 1992 Clinical experience with three-dimensional treatment planning *Sem. Radiat Oncol.* **2**, 274-289

[5] Kutcher GJ, Smith AR, Fowble BL, Owen JB, Hanlon A, Wallace M, Hanks GE 1996 Treatment planning for primary breast cancer: a patterns of care study *Int. J. Radiat. Oncol. Biol. Phys.* **36**, 731-737

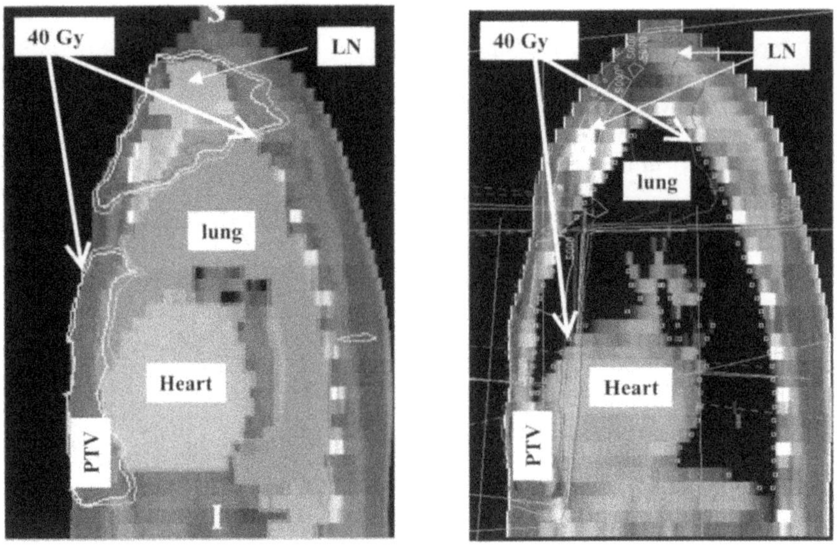


(a) (b)

**Figure 2:** Isodose comparison between an IMRT plan (a) and a standard three-field conformal treatment plan (b) for irradiation of the chest wall (PM) and supraclavicular and axillary lymph nodes of a stage III cancer patient

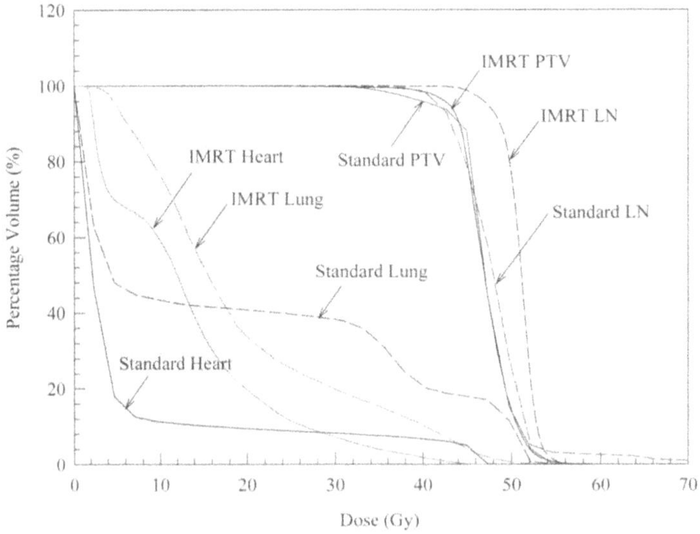


**Figure 3:** A comparison of dose-volume histograms (DVH) between standard three-field irradiation and four-field IMRT

# Clinical implementation of intensity modulated radiotherapy for customised compensation using dynamic multileaf collimation

**Geoffrey J Budgell, Judith H L Mott and Alan R Hounsell**

North Western Medical Physics, Christie Hospital NHS Trust, Withington, Manchester, M20 4BX, UK

## Introduction

The technique of dynamic multileaf collimation (MLC) to deliver intensity modulated radiation therapy (IMRT) has been implemented clinically at our centre since April 1999. Here we describe the planning, delivery and verification methods used to ensure accurate and reliable IMRT treatments. Our initial aim is to provide customised compensation for patient shape in four-field conformal bladder treatments. The clinical intent is to improve dose homogeneity within the planning target volume (PTV) and correct for dose fall-off in the margins of the PTV due to loss of scatter at the beam edge. This is a straightforward adaptation of our current static MLC bladder technique, and acts as a first step towards the introduction of more complex IMRT techniques into the clinic with the potential for shaping dose distributions in the transverse plane [1,2].

## Material and methods

The overall process in shown in figure 1. Firstly, patients are planned for a conventional static MLC conformal treatment.

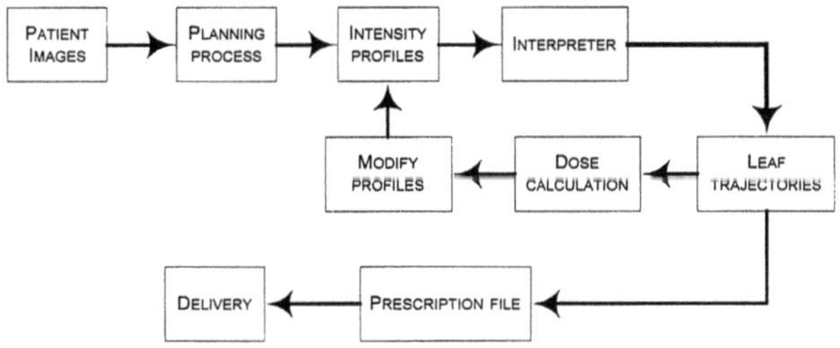


**Figure 1:** Flow chart of the IMRT planning & delivery process

Next, intensity profiles to custom compensate for the patient shape are calculated [3]. This is achieved within the defined PTV by measuring the depth of the isocentric plane below the patient surface from CT images. Primary intensity is calculated from exponential attenuation accounting for radial variation in beam flatness and energy. The inverse of the primary calculation is used as a weighting for patient scatter and head scatter calculations [4]. Primary and scatter contributions are combined to give the final intensity. A typical compensating intensity modulation for a lateral beam is shown in figure 2. The calculated intensities are converted to dynamic leaf and jaw trajectories via leaf sequencing software which accounts for manufacturer specific MLC design constraints using a variation of the 'sliding window' technique [5].

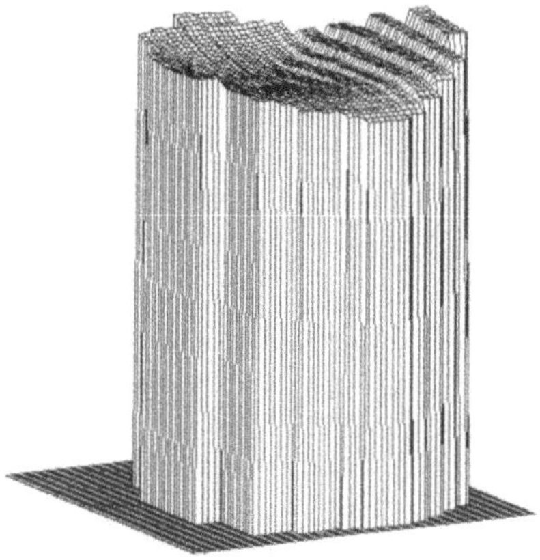

**Figure 2:** Typical lateral beam intensity modulation

A full dose calculation is performed based on the actual dynamic leaf and jaw motion which fully accounts for transmission and tongue and groove effects. Any discrepancy between planned and calculated dose can be accounted for by iteratively correcting the input intensities. In practice, this iterative step has not been found necessary for bladder treatments.

Dynamic prescriptions are delivered using research software on an Elekta SL15 accelerator and dedicated MLC. Dose rate in the research release is limited to 100 monitor units/min and maximum leaf speed to 5 mm/s to avoid temporary beam interrupts. Prescriptions consist of 25 control points, defining all leaf and jaw positions at equal monitor unit increments.

Before a patient begins treatment, doses within a water or solid water phantom using the planned beams for that patient are measured using an ionisation chamber and checked to be within 2% of calculated dose to the phantom. This 'dummy run' of the delivery ensures the prescriptions are deliverable and acts as an independent monitor unit check of the treatment plan.

At treatment, the MLC leaves are initially set to the outer field edges, as for a static field treatment. This allows beams to be checked using paper templates laid on the treatment couch and permits the patient to be set-up as for normal treatments. It also enables a portal image to be performed, as required, before the leaves move across the field to their start positions for dynamic delivery. Dose delivered to the starting beam shape is subtracted from the dynamic delivery dose. During delivery, real-time verification of the leaf positions is achieved using an electronic portal imaging device (EPID). A custom-built circuit monitors the delivered dose and triggers the EPID to acquire a series of snap-shot images showing the positions of the leaves at regular monitor unit intervals during the delivery [6]. A digital template of expected leaf positions is immediately overlaid on the images (figure 3). Leaf positions can therefore be monitored during the treatment and interrupted should a gross error occur. In addition, absolute doses are verified *in vivo* using diode measurements. Entrance dose measurements are compared to those expected after corrections for patient surface temperature, field size and focus to surface distance have been applied. Diode measurements are required to be within 5% of the prescribed dose.

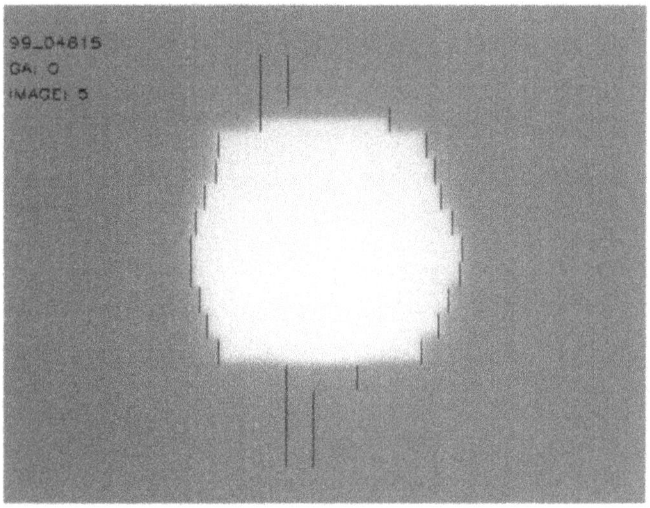

**Figure 3:** Digital template of prescribed leaf positions (in black) overlaid on a snapshot EPI acquired during dynamic MLC delivery.

## Results and discussion

To the end of November 1999, 7 patients have been treated using dynamic MLC for four out of their twenty fractions. The results of the compensation procedure are demonstrated in figures 4 & 5. Figure 4 shows the dose distribution for an example patient at the isocentric slice for a conventional static MLC treatment and with IMRT compensation. The maximum hotspot is reduced from 106% to 102%. Figure 5 shows the improvement in dose homogeneity in the most superior target slice for the same patient. This region is known to suffer dose reduction due to the effects of combined beam penumbrae [7]. The compensation code automatically corrects for this and sharpens the beam penumbrae since scatter is taken into account in the calculation. Hence the homogeneity improvement in figure 5(b).

Delivery efficiency, expressed as inefficiency factors (delivered mu / maximum mu in intensity profile), varied between 1.37 - 1.71. This compares favourably with, for instance, the 20° wedge factor of 1.51 for the same machine at the same energy. Typical treatment times are 20-25 minutes from the patient entering to leaving the room. Beam-on time varies between 5 and 6 minutes, which could be reduced to 1-1.5 minutes at a normal clinical dose rate.

(a)

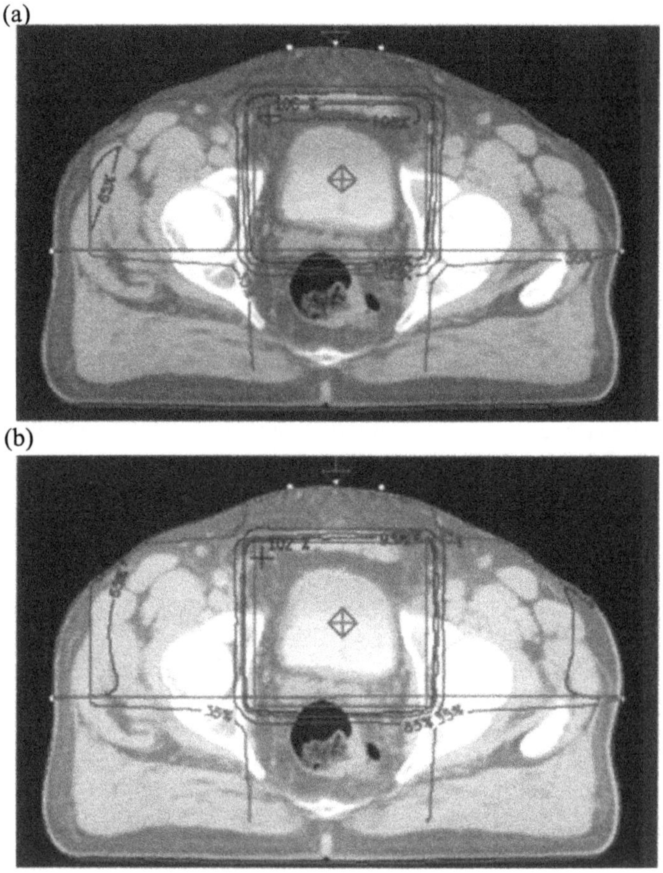

(b)

**Figure 4:** Comparison of (a) static and (b) IMRT compensated dose distributions for the isocentric slice of an example patient.

On one occasion a beam which terminated abnormally during delivery was finished using the beam finish facility provided by the software, whereby the remaining monitor units are entered and a prescription is created to deliver the remaining control points.

The total time required to prepare and deliver IMRT treatments in addition to the time taken in preparing the standard static MLC delivery is given in Table 1. As IMRT treatments become more routine this time will be much reduced, for instance by reduction in the amount of in vivo dosimetry and more efficient planning algorithms.

| Activity | Time (hours) |
|---|---|
| Planning & clinician check of plan | 1 |
| Prepare & transfer of prescriptions and templates | 0.5 |
| Dummy run verification | 2 |
| Physics attendance at treatments | 2 |
| In vivo dosimetry | 1-2 |
| Miscellaneous | 0.5 |
| Total additional time: | 7-8 |

**Table 1:** Additional time per patient required for planning and delivery of IMRT treatments using the current research system.

(a)

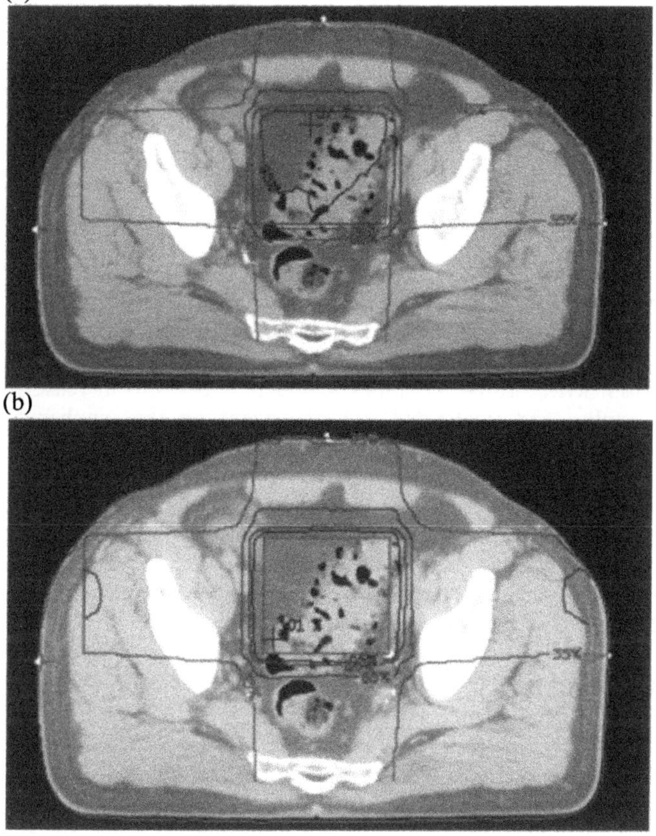

Figure 5: Comparison of (a) static and (b) IMRT compensated dose distributions for the superior slice of an example patient.

## Conclusion

IMRT using the dynamic MLC technique has been successfully introduced with minimal disruption into an extremely busy clinic by application to a relatively simple problem. Thorough treatment verification is increasing confidence in the technique. This methodology paves the way for the introduction of more complex and clinically beneficial IMRT techniques.

## References

[1] Burman C, Chui C-S, Kutcher G, Leibel S, Zelefsky M, LoSasso T, Spirou S, Wu Q, Yang J Y, Stein J, Mohan R, Fuks Z and Ling C C 1997 Planning, delivery, and quality assurance of intensity-modulated radiotherapy using dynamic multileaf collimator: a strategy for large-scale implementation for the treatment of carcinoma of the prostate *Int. J. Radiat. Oncol. Biol. Phys.* **39** 863-873

[2] De Neve W, De Gersem W, Derycke S, De Meerleer G, Moerman M, Bate M, Van Duyse B, Vakaet L, De Deene Y, Mersseman B, De Wagter C 1999 Clinical delivery of intensity modulated conformal radiotherapy for relapsed or second-primary head and neck cancer using a multileaf collimator with dynamic control *Radioth. Oncol.* **50** 301-314

[3] Mott J H L, Hounsell A R, Budgell G J, Wilkinson J M and Williams P C 1999 Customised compensation using intensity modulated beams delivered by dynamic multileaf collimation *Radiother. Oncol.* **53** 57-63

[4] Hounsell A R and Wilkinson J M 1997 Head scatter modelling for irregular field shaping and beam intensity modulation *Phys. Med. Biol.* **42** 1737-1749

[5] Budgell G J, Sykes J R and Wilkinson J M 1998 Rectangular edge synchronization for intensity modulated radiation therapy with dynamic multileaf collimation. *Phys. Med. Biol.* **43** 2769-2784

[6] James H V, Atherton S, Budgell G J, Kirby M C and Williams P C 2000 Verification of dynamic multileaf collimation using an electronic portal imaging device. *Phys. Med. Biol.* (In press)

[7] Dirkx M L P, Heijmen B J M, Korevaar G A, van Os M J H, Stroom J C, Koper P C M and Levendag P C 1997 Field margin reduction using intensity-modulated x-ray beams formed with a multileaf collimator *Int. J. Radiat. Oncol. Biol. Phys.* **38** 1123-129

# Assessment of Treatment Techniques and Collimation in Conformal Stereotactic Radiosurgery and Radiotherapy

Julia Ahlswede[1], Mathias Pfaender[1], Gerhard Grebe[2], Dirk Böhmer[1], Jörg Bohsung[1], Jens Groll[1], Andreas Kaiser[1], Lorenz Schlenger[1], Brit Sommer[1], Dirk Scheffler[1], Martin Stuschke[1], Volker Budach[1], Reinhard Wurm[1]

[1]Klinik für Strahlentherapie, Charité CCM, Universitätsklinikum der Humbold Universität zu Berlin, Schumannstrasse 20/21, 10117 Berlin.
[2]Technische Fachhochschule Berlin, FB II, Medizinische Physik, Luxemburger Str. 10, 13353 Berlin.

## Introduction

In radiation oncology more and more effort is taken to include the dose conformity to the target as well as the dose sparing of risk organs (OAR) and healthy tissue to the treatment planing. Conformal stereotactic radiosurgery and radiotherapy (CSRS and CSRT) offer the potential to optimise these parameters according to the demands of the physician and the physicist. The study compares treatment plans using different techniques for dose delivery as static beams, arcs or multiple isocentres. Also different beam shaping devices for CSRS and CSRT as conformal blocks, circular cones or multileaf collimators have been considered.

## Material and methods

In this study 15 patients with irregular shaped targets were planned using static beams, dynamic arcs and arc techniques with multiple isocentres.
As beam shaping devices 4 multileaf collimators (MLC), conformal blocks and circular collimators were used. The leaf size of the MLC was 10 mm, 5 mm, 1.7 mm and one MLC with 3 different leaf sizes of 3 mm, 4.5 mm and 5.5 mm. The sizes of the circular collimators was between 4 mm and 40 mm, in 2 mm increments.
The planning target volume (PTV) and relevant organs at risk (OAR) were assessed comparing dose statistics, dose–volume histograms (DVH), and the Radiation Therapy Oncology Group (RTOG) stereotactic radiosurgery criteria. The individual assessed objects were copied into each plan to ensure that results are comparable.
The plans were calculated on a BrainScan™ planning station.

## Results and discussion

The sizes of the planning target volumes were calculated to be between 0.5 ccm and 89 ccm.
The plan evaluation showed for the different target sizes examined that the 5 mm and the 10 mm leaf-width MLCs treat, on average, 14 % and 17 % more normal brain, compared to the other MLCs and blocks, respectively. No differences were seen when the 1.7 mm and 3-5.5 mm MLC were compared to blocks. The differences in PTV doses for targets smaller than 4 ccm between the 1.7 mm and 3-5.5 mm leaf-width MLC were 2% ± 1.8 % (minimum PTV), and 0.1% ± 1.9 % (maximum PTV), respectively.
Dynamic treatment delivery with the 3-5.5 mm leaf-width MLC compensated these differences and resulted in improved conformity for lower isodoses.
Multiple isocentre arc plans and careful consideration of collimator size and beam weighting allowed dose distributions close to those achieved with the 1.7 mm and 3-5.5 mm leaf-width MLC. However, this resulted in a 2-3 fold increase in planning and treatment time dependent on the number of isocentres.
The RTOG guidelines showed, the 1.7 mm and 3-5.5 mm leaf-width MLC, as well as blocks and multiple isocentre arc plans provided acceptable PTV coverage with an acceptable homogeneity and comparable conformity index between 1-2. Major coverage deviations were only seen compared to the 5 mm and 10 mm leaf-width MLC.

## Conclusion

The 1.7 mm and 3-5.5 mm leaf-width MLC provided improved PTV coverage with OAR doses within the clinically defined threshold and reduced at the same time substantially planning and treatment times compared to multiple isocentre arc and conformal block plans. Further improvements may be expected using dynamic treatment delivery techniques that do not limit the treatment delivery to static beams or multiple isocentre arc plans.

# General Anatomy Based Segmentation for Intensity Modulated Radiotherapy of Head and Neck Cancer

**W. De Gersem, Ir., F. Claus, MD., L. Vakaet, MD., PhD., V. Remouchamps, MD., I. Vanhoutte, MD., B. Van Duyse, Ir., S. Vermael, Lic. Phys., C. De Wagter, Ir., PhD., and W. De Neve, MD., PhD.**

Division of Radiotherapy, Ghent University Hospital

## Introduction

In head and neck cancer, intensity modulated radiotherapy (IMRT) allows to generate concave dose distributions to match the shape of the planning target volume (PTV). In our department, IMRT is delivered by multiple static convergent beams, that consist of superposition of unmodulated segments. The segment shapes were obtained from the beam's eye view (BEV) projection of PTV(s) and organs at risk (OARs). By making the shape of segments also a function of the patient's outlines (skin surface), a substantial refinement was obtained.

## Material and methods

A concave dose distribution component is obtained by a twelve step procedure.
Steps 1-4 define the BEV projected area inside which all segments must be created. This area includes the PTV projection(s) with a defined margin, however with exclusion of the OAR projection(s).
Step 5 ensures that the number of overlapping segments increases in the vicinity of OAR projections.
Steps 6-7 ensure that the number of overlapping segments increases with the physical pathlength that the rays have to travel from their entrance at the skin to reach the PTV(s). The physical pathlength has an influence on the shapes and the number of segments.
Steps 8-12 involve a transform of the segment outlines to MLC geometries and adaptations to make the shapes executable by an Elekta-MLC (this involves collimator angle optimization if necessary).
Finally the segment weights are obtained by an optimization using a biophysical objective function including TCP-values for the target-volumes and NTCP-values for OARs.

## Results and discussion

This general segmentation tool was used to obtain an intensity modulated radiotherapy plan for patients (n=4) which were treated at the Ghent University Hospital during the 6 week period between the first clinical release of the software and the writing of the abstract. Generation of 50-100 segments for 6-7 beam incidences takes less than 10 minutes, user interaction included. After the optimization of monitor units, 25-40 segments are retained for clinical delivery. Due to the incorporation of skin-target pathlengths as well as the distance of critical organs to values of the segmentation grid, this tool was able to provide the base for intensity modulated treatments with good sparing of organs at risk, with an acceptable dose homogeneity, and with a number of segments that keeps treatment delivery time below 15 minutes (patient positioning with portal imaging included), even for those situations with large differences in pathlengths (i.e. treated regions extending from the base of skull to the upper mediastinum).

## Conclusion

Unlike anatomy based segmentation tools that were previously developed at our department [1], this tool is able to handle multiple and complex target-volumes and organs at risk and inherently includes missing tissue compensation. Due to the high precision of leaf-positioning and the alignment of subsegment-boundaries, high dose-gradients can be obtained between critical organs and target-volumes, resulting in high dose differences between these relevant volumes.

## References

[1] De Neve W, De Gersem W, Derycke S, De Meerleer G, Bate M-T, Van Duyse B, Vakaet L, De Deene Y, Mersseman B and De Wagter C 1999 Clinical delivery of intensity modulated conformal radiotherapy for relapsed or second-primary head and neck cancer using a multileaf collimator with dynamic control *Radiotherapy and Oncology* **50** 301-314

## Acknowledgement

The project "Conformal Radiotherapy U.Z. Gent" is supported by the Vereniging voor Kankerbestrijding and by grants from the Fonds voor Wetenschappelijk Onderzoek Vlaanderen (grants FWO G.0049.98 and G.0039.97), the Ghent University (Verkennend Europees Onderzoek), the Sportvereniging tegen Kanker and the Centrum voor Studie en Behandeling van Gezwelziekten. R-UZG is member of the Elekta IMRT consortium.

# The Use of Compensators and Multiple Static Fields for IMRT of the Breast

**Philip M Evans[1], Natalie Bleackley[1], David J Convery[1], Ellen M Donovan[1], Vibeke N Hansen[1], Mike Partridge[1], Stephanie Reise[1], J Richard N Symonds-Tayler[1] and John R Yarnold[2]**

[1]Joint Physics Department and [2]Department of Radiotherapy, Institute of Cancer Research and Royal Marsden NHS Trust, Downs Road, Sutton, Surrey, SM2 5PT, UK

## Introduction

External beam radiotherapy of the breast has been shown to lead to a significant reduction in the incidence of local recurrence [1]. Unfortunately these gains are partially offset by side effects, such as ischaemic heart disease, arm lymphoedema, brachial plexopathy, breast pain, poor cosmesis and pneumonitis. A major contributing factor to these complications is believed to be the inhomogeneity of the dose distribution from tangential irradiation which often exceeds the figure of 10% considered to be acceptable.

We have developed a method of using transit dosimetry information from electronic portal imaging (EPI) to design intensity modulated beams (IMBs) for tangential breast irradiation [2]. The purpose of the IMBs is to reduce the dose non-uniformity within the breast volume, such that it is within 10%. This is expected to have positive consequences for cosmesis [3].

The effects on cosmesis of improving dose inhomogeneity in the breast, using this method, are currently being evaluated in a clinical trial. 300 patients are being randomised between the standard treatment using wedges as compensators and a customised IMRT treatment. Initially the IMRT treatment was delivered using physical compensators. We have recently commissioned the use of an MLC to deliver a set of multiple static fields (MSFs) as an alternative delivery method.

## Material and methods

### Generation of Ideal IMBs

In this method, an electronic portal image is taken of each tangential field. Each image is calibrated as a map of radiological thickness. From this an estimated set of outlines of breast and lung are generated. These outlines are then used with a TMR based planning system to design the ideal IMBs needed to reduce the volume of tissue outside 95-105% dose – the accepted limits used at this centre. 'Ideal' is used to mean the beams have high spatial and intensity resolution and are not subject to any delivery constraints.

### Generation of Compensators

Once the ideal IMBs have been designed they must be made deliverable. For compensator design, the intensity map of the IMB is turned into a thickness map using measured attenuation coefficients [4]. This thickness map is then used to make a compensator using an automatic compensator cutter (ADC3, QADOS, Sandhurst, UK). In addition, high transmission blocks are sent to our treatment planning system (TPS) (Target, Prism Microsystems, Radlett, UK), which is used to verify the treatment.

### Generation of Multiple Static Fields

To make the ideal IMBs deliverable by the MLC, firstly, the beams are resampled to have 1 cm spatial resolution in the direction orthogonal to leaf travel. Then they are digitised in intensity to have four levels from each side, corresponding to four field components. The first component is like a standard field. It is rectangular in shape and has a universal wedge to provide basic compensation. It delivers typically 85% dose. The three other field components are equal in magnitude and constitute typically 5% dose [5]. They are shaped using the MLC to provide the residual compensation needed, particularly in the superior-inferior direction.

Once the field intensities have been chosen a delivery filter is applied to make them deliverable by the MLC using a close-in technique. The close-in technique was chosen because this allows verification imaging using the first field component, furthermore the tangential beam maps required minimal filtering to fit the close-in paradigm. The constraints on MLC delivery for our system (MLCi, Elekta Oncology Systems, Crawley, UK) are:

1) That there can only be one open region for each field.
2) That opposite and opposite adjacent leaves may not by less than 1 cm apart.
3) That the backup collimators perpendicular to the leaf travel direction may not cross the mid-line.

### Dosimetric evaluation

Both compensator and MSF techniques were evaluated using dosimetric measurements and using our TPS to compare them with the standard, wedged treatment.

For a test patient, compensated and MSF treatments were designed. Our TPS was used to calculate the dose delivered, from these IMBs, at 5 cm depth to a uniform, homogeneous phantom. These calculations were then compared with film measurements to verify relative dosimetry. Ion chamber measurements at the isocentre were used to verify absolute dosimetry.

For a set of 6 patients, both types of IMRT treatment were designed and planned. The volume outside the dose range 95%-105% was determined from dose volume histogram

(DVH) analysis and compared with the corresponding values for the standard treatment.

## Results and discussion

Figure 1 shows a verification image of one of the shaped fields from an MSF treatment. The field is shaped to the breast contour and the chest wall.

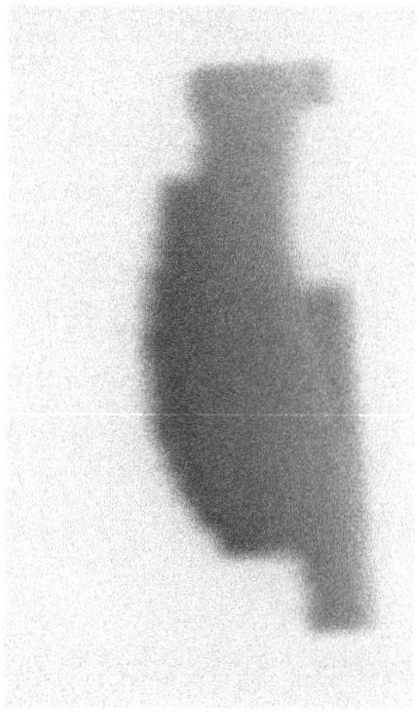

**Figure 1:** Verification image of left medial MSF treatment.

The effects of the delivery filter were found to be minimal, producing a change in the intensity of few points within any given IMB. Furthermore the change in intensity at any point in any IMB was no more than a few percent. This does not significantly affect the advantage of using the MSF close-in technique.

### Dosimetric measurement

For relative dosimetry measurement, the films were scanned through the line of the isocentre in the AB and GT directions and normalised at the isocentre point. The agreement between the two delivery modes was 1% or better. The corresponding TPS calculation also predicted 1% agreement. The measurements and TPS results agreed to with 2% for most regions, with a maximal discrepancy of 4%, immediately superior and inferior to the midline.

The absolute dosimetry measurements with the ion chamber all agreed to within 1%.

### TPS comparisons

The results of the DVH analysis for the six test patients are summarised in table 1. A perfect treatment would have 0% volume in all columns. These results show that the effect of the IMRT is to reduce slightly the volume below 95% dose and to reduce significantly the volume of the high dose region.

The volume of breast outside the dose range 95-105% has been reduced by typically 9% by the use of either IMRT technique.

| | Vol < 95% | Vol > 105% | Sum |
|---|---|---|---|
| Standard | 4.3 | 7.2 | 11.5 |
| Compensator | 1.4 | 0.8 | 2.2 |
| MSF | 2.3 | 0.4 | 2.7 |

**Table 1:** Average percentage volume in each dose range for the three treatment methods. Sum denotes the total volume outside the 95-105% range.

## Conclusion

A method has been developed for using electronic portal imaging to design IMBs to improve the dosimetry of tangential breast irradiation. These IMBs may be delivered as either physical compensators or MSFs.

Measurements show the two delivery techniques to be very similar dosimetrically and to be reasonably well described by the TPS.

A planning study shows the two IMRT methods to yield a significant reduction in the volume of breast outside the 95-105% dose range over the standard treatment. The planning study also predicted the two IMRT methods to yield similar dosimetric improvements.

**Acknowledgements**
This work is supported by the Cancer Research Campaign [CRC], The South Thames Regional Health Authority, and Eletka Oncology Systems.

## References

[1] Overgaard M, Hansen PS, Overgaard J *et al.* 1997 Postoperative radiotherapy in high-risk premenopausal women with breast cancer who receive adjuvant chemotherapy *New Eng J Med* **337** 949-955.
[2] Evans PM, Donovan EM, Fenton N, *et al.* 1998 Practical implementation of compensators in breast radiotherapy *Radiothcr Oncol* **49** 255 265.
[3] Moody AM, Mayles WPM, Bliss JM, *et al.* 1994 The influence of breast size on late radiation effects and association with radiotherapy dose inhomogeneity *Radiother Oncol* **33** 106-112.
[4] Boyer AL 1982 Compensating filters for high energy x rays *Med Phys* **9** 429-433.
[5] Evans PM, Hansen VN and Swindell W 1997 The optimum intensities for multiple static multileaf collimator field compensation *Med Phys* **24** 1147-1156.

# A mixed integer programming approach to the multileaf collimator problem

**Horst W. Hamacher, Frank Lenzen**

University of Kaiserslautern, Dept. of Mathematics, and Institut für Techno- und Wirtschaftsmathematik (ITWM), Kaiserslautern, P.O. Box 3049, D-67653 Kaiserslautern, Germany

## Introduction

In the Multileaf Collimator (MLC) problem one faces the task to generate a 2 dimensional intensity modulated beam using a sequence of shape matrices formed by MLCs. We use (0,1) variables to characterize the set of all MLC setups in which interleaf motion and tongue-and-groove effects are avoided. Among the various options of finding a "good" MLC setup we show, how a mixed integer programming formulation can be used to minimize the treatment time. An optimal solution is obtained using column generation techniques. A reformulation of the problem allows the use of procedures for the partitioning problem.

## Material and methods

### Mathematical modelling

Given an intensity matrix $I$ with $m$ rows and $n$ columns and integer entries, Xia and Verhey (cf. [4]) have described the problem as follows: decompose $I$ into shape matrices $M_t$ such that $\sum_t \lambda_t M_t = I$, where $M_t(i,j) \in \{0,1\}$, $\lambda_t \in R$. Each $M_t$ represents a static field which can be shaped by the MLC. A "1" entry corresponds to an irradiated field whereas a "0" entry in the shape matrix indicates that this cell of the MLC will be blocked by a leaf. In order to minimize the treatment time our aim is to minimize the sum of *beam-on time* and *setup-time*. The beam-on time represents the irradiation-time, i.e. the time when the beam is switched on. The setup-time reflects the time which is needed to build all MLC shapes but the first. Each shape matrix has to fulfill certain properties in order to be deliverable by a commercially available MLC. The most important one is that the "1" entries in a row appear consecutively, i.e. the area of irradiation in a single channel of the MLC is connected and thus can be shaped by the leaf pair, which defines the channel. Two additional constraints are discussed frequently: the *interleaf motion constraint* and the *tongue-and-groove constraint*. The interleaf motion constraint basically prohibits that a left leaf moves further to the right than any of its opposing right leaves in adjacent channels. The tongue-and-groove constraint ensures that two neighbouring cells in adjacent channels are not blocked and irradiated alternately.

Siochi [3] observed that a good approximation of the above objective is obtained by simply minimizing the beam-on time. We follow this approach, but represent the shape matrices as vectors, i.e. we consider the linear program

$$\begin{array}{lrcl} min & \underline{1}^T x & & \\ s.t. & \mathcal{U}x & = & \hat{I} \\ & x & \geq & 0 \end{array} \tag{1}$$

where each column of the matrix $\mathcal{U}$ represents a shape matrix and $\underline{1}$ is the vector of ones. Therefore $\mathcal{U} \in \{0,1\}^{mn \times k}$, where $k$ is the total number of shape matrices. Note that $\hat{I}$ represents $I$ written as a vector columnwise. $x_i > 0$ can be interpreted as the irradiation time of the shape matrix represented by column $i$.

### A column generation approach

Looking at the model presented above we observe a drawback, namely its exponentially large number of columns $k$. Note that $k$ can easily be of the order $10^{20}$, as this is approximately the number of existing shape matrices when $n = m = 10$. Thus even storing or creating the whole matrix $\mathcal{U}$ is prohibitive. But by using the revised simplex method to obtain a solution of the above LP only the basis matrix $\mathcal{U}_B \in \{0,1\}^{mn \times mn}$ has to be computed . In each iteration of the simplex method we are then looking for a column $j$ with reduced costs $\overline{c_j} < 0$ of $\mathcal{U}$ which, when entering the basis, would improve the objective value. So in each iteration we are solving

$$\begin{array}{ll} min & \overline{c_j} \\ s.t. & j \text{ is a column of } \mathcal{U} \end{array} \tag{2}$$

This problem is called the subproblem while the original LP in (1) is the master problem. As is well-known from the theory of linear programming, the master problem's basis is optimal if and only if the optimal objective value of the subproblem is greater than or equal to zero [1].

We do now give a formulation which makes it possible to describe the set of all shape matrices by a set of constraints. Introducing these and the definition of the reduced costs into (2) then yield a mixed integer programming problem of moderate size as a subproblem. Defining

$$L_{i,j} = \begin{cases} 1 & \text{if the left leaf in channel } i \text{ is positioned} \\ & \text{left of column } j \\ 0 & \text{otherwise} \end{cases}$$

[1] For an overview on the column generation technique to solve large scale linear programming problems, see, e.g., [1].

$$R_{i,j} = \begin{cases} 1 & \text{if the right leaf in channel } i \text{ is positioned left of column } j \\ 0 & \text{otherwise} \end{cases}$$

$$\hat{x}_{i,j} = \begin{cases} 1 & \text{if the cell in channel } i \text{ and column } j \text{ is irradiated} \\ 0 & \text{otherwise} \end{cases}$$

Then the subproblem becomes

$$\min \underline{\mathbf{1}}_B^T \mathcal{U}_B^{-1} \hat{x}$$

$$\sum_{j=0}^{N_{Co}+1} L_{i,j} = 1 \ , \ \sum_{j=0}^{N_{Co}+1} R_{i,j} = 1 \quad \forall\, i \in \mathcal{H}$$

$$\sum_{j=0}^{N_{Co}+1} jL_{i,j} \leq \sum_{j=0}^{N_{Co}+1} jR_{k,j} \quad \forall\, i \in \mathcal{H},\ k \in \{i-1, i, i+1\} \cap \mathcal{H}$$

$$\sum_{j=0}^{N_{Co}+1} jL_{i,j} \geq 1 \quad \forall\, i \in \mathcal{H}$$

$$\sum_{j=0}^{N_{Co}+1} jR_{i,j} \leq N_{Co}+1 \quad \forall\, i \in \mathcal{H}$$

$$\hat{x}_{(i-1)N_{Co}+1} \leq L_{i,1} \quad \forall\, i \in \mathcal{H}$$

$$\hat{x}_{(i-1)N_{Co}+j} - \hat{x}_{(i-1)N_{Co}+j-1} \leq L_{i,j} \quad \forall\, i \in \mathcal{H},\ \forall\, j \in \mathcal{K} \setminus \{1\}$$

$$\hat{x}_{(i-1)N_{Co}+j-1} - \hat{x}_{(i-1)N_{Co}+j} \leq R_{i,j} \quad \forall\, i \in \mathcal{H},\ \forall\, j \in \mathcal{K} \setminus \{1\}$$

$$\hat{x}_{(i-1)N_{Co}+N_{Co}} \leq R_{i,N_{Co}+1} \quad \forall\, i \in \mathcal{H}$$

$$\hat{x}_{(i-1)N_{Co}+j} \geq L_{i,j} - R_{i,j} \quad \forall\, i \in \mathcal{H}, j \in \mathcal{K}$$

$$\hat{x}_{(i-1)N_{Co}+j} \geq R_{i,j+1} - L_{i,j+1} \quad \forall\, i \in \mathcal{H}, j \in \mathcal{K}$$

$$L_{i,j}, R_{i,j} \in \{0,1\} \quad \forall\, i \in \mathcal{H},\ \forall\, j \in \mathcal{K} \cup \{0, N_{Co}+1\}$$

$$\hat{x}_{(i-1)N_{Co}+j} \in \{0,1\} \quad \forall\, i \in \mathcal{H}, j \in \mathcal{K}$$

where we denote the set of channels $i$ by $\mathcal{H} := \{1, \ldots, N_{Ch}\}$ (numbered top down), the set of columns $j$ of the intensity matrix $I$ by $\mathcal{K} := \{1, \ldots, N_{Co}\}$ (numbered from left to right). The inequalities characterize the left and right leaf positions and make sure that no interleaf motion occurs. The first of the inequalities is, for instance, equivalent to the condition that the positioning of the left leaf in channel $i$ at position $j$ (i.e. $L_{i,j} = 0$) excludes any right leaf placement in positions $j' < j$ (i.e. $R_{k,j} = 0$ for all $j' < j$ and $k \in \{i-1, -, i+1\}$). Hence, this condition excludes interleaf motion. Due to space constraints, the interpretation of the other inequalities can not be given here, but will be described in the presentation at the conference. In order to solve the subproblem an integer program has to be solved. The next result shows that this can be done in a more structured way than just using standard linear programming algorithms.

**Theorem:** Subproblem 2 can be written as a minimum cost flow problem with 2 unit flows and an additional set of constraints to exclude interleaf motion.

## Handling the tongue-and-groove problem

We introduce a variable $\hat{y}_{(i-1)N_{Co}+j}$, $i \in \mathcal{H} \setminus \{N_{Ch}\}$, $j \in \mathcal{K}$ for each grid line between two neighbouring cells in adjacent channels such that

$$\hat{y}_{(i-1)N_{Co}+j} := \begin{cases} 0 & \text{if } \hat{x}_{(i-1)N_{Co}+j} = \hat{x}_{iN_{Co}+j} = 0 \\ 1 & \text{otherwise} \end{cases}$$

The grid line between two neighbouring cells is irradiated whenever at least one of the cells is irradiated. In order to remove the tongue-and-groove effect completely we can claim and have proven that the grid line and the adjacent cell with the greater intensity requirement have to revceive an equal number of monitor units of irradiation. Therefore we extend each column of $\mathcal{U}$ by $(N_{Ch}-1) * N_{Co}$ rows, such that the column which is obtained from the subproblem, say the q-th column of $\mathcal{U}$, looks as follows $\mathcal{U}_{.q} = \begin{pmatrix} \hat{x} \\ \hat{y} \end{pmatrix}$.

We get a new matrix $\hat{\mathcal{U}}$, which has the same number of columns as $\mathcal{U}$. The right hand side of the master problem has to be extended as well. We transform $\hat{I}$ to $\hat{\underline{I}}$ by adding $(N_{Ch}-1) * N_{Co}$ rows where

$$\hat{\underline{I}}_k = \hat{I}_k,\ k \in \{1, \ldots, N_{Co} * N_{Ch}\}$$

$$\hat{\underline{I}}_{[(N_{Co})(N_{Ch})]+(i-1)*N_{Co}+j} = max\left\{\hat{I}_{(i-1)N_{Co}+j}, \hat{I}_{iN_{Co}+j}\right\} \quad \forall\, i \in \mathcal{H} \setminus \{N_{Ch}\}, j \in \mathcal{K}$$

The new master problem is

$$\begin{array}{lrcl} min & \underline{\mathbf{1}}^T x & & \\ s.t. & \hat{\mathcal{U}} x & = & \hat{\underline{I}} \\ & x & \geq & 0 \end{array} \tag{3}$$

**Theorem:** The tongue-and-groove effect does not occur between the two neighbouring cells in column j and row i and i-1, respectively, if and only if

$$\sum_q \mathcal{U}_{N_{Co}*N_{Ch}+(i-1)*N_{Ch}+j,q} x_q = \hat{\underline{I}}_{N_{Co}*N_{Ch}+(i-1)N_{Ch}+j}.$$

The last result ensures that no tongue-and-groove effect will occur in any solution of the master problem.

## Improving Heuristics

The MLC problem (1) which we tackled in the previous section by a mixed integer programming and column generation approach can also be used to improve existing heuristics , e.g. the one given by Xia and Verhey [4] – known as the reducing level technique. This technique computes a priori a decreasing intensity sequence $(d_k)_k$ based on the maximum intensity level in $I$ and then decomposes the problem into several smaller instances. The latter are then solved sequentially in order to minimize the number of segments. In each step of the procedure the input is a residual intensity matrix $\tilde{I}_k \in Z^{m \times n}$ and it extracts a matrix

$D_k \in \{0,1\}^{m \times n}$ by the following rule:

$$D_k(i,j) := \begin{cases} 1 & \text{if } \tilde{I}_k(i,j) \geq d_k \\ 0 & \text{otherwise} \end{cases}$$

The matrix $\tilde{I}_k - d_k D_k$ is input of the next iterative step. In general, $D_k$ is itself not deliverable and thus is now decomposed again into valid shape matrices $L_k^{(m)} \in \{0,1\}$ such that $\sum_m L_k^{(m)} = D_k$. Each of the problems of decomposing $D_k$ can mathematically be formulated as a partitioning problem using formulation (1). The right hand side of (1) is then a vector containing only zeros and ones. We can thus remove all those constraints with a "0" right hand side and remove those columns $\mathcal{U}_{.j}$ of $\mathcal{U}$ which have a "1" entry in this row and obtain $\overline{\mathcal{U}}$. Finally we change the restriction on $x$ being $x \geq 0$ in (1) to $x \in \{0,1\}^{mn-l}$, where $l$ is the number of removed columns in $\mathcal{U}$. We have obtained the following problem

$$\begin{array}{lrcl} min & \underline{\mathbf{1}}^T x & & \\ s.t. & \overline{\mathcal{U}} x & = & \underline{\mathbf{1}} \\ & x & \in & \{0,1\}^{mn-l} \end{array} \qquad (4)$$

Existing heuristics can be applied to solve each of the partitioning problems.

## Results and discussion

So far, the proposed approach has not been tested in clinical examples. In the presentation during the conference we will in particular address problem in dealing with the inherent degeneracy of master polyhedron which is described by the set $\{x : \mathcal{U}x = \hat{I}, x \geq 0\}$. The degeneracy can be concluded from the fact that the basis has size $n*m$, while the number of segments needed in order to minimize the treatment time is usually much less then $n*m$. Thus most entries in the solution vector $x$ will be 0.

## Conclusion

We have presented a mixed integer programming approach to the MLC problem which can be used to solve the problem exactly as well as approximately using suitable heuristics. The latter approach seems particularly promising, since the problem is thus transformed to a sequence of partitioning problems for which a variety of solution techniques are available. Computational results which show the potential of the proposed approach will be presented during the conference.

Although not much computational work has been done the approach looks rewarding in such a way that we can base our work on an already developed theory which has been applied successfully in many applications.

Further details of the approach can be found in the forthcoming thesis of Lenzen [2]. A joint paper of the authors of this extended abstract on the subjects discussed above is in preparation.

## References

[1] Lasdon L S 1970 Optimization Theory for Large Systems *MacMillan Publishing Co., Inc., New York*, Chap. 1, 3 & 4

[2] Lenzen F 2000, Modeling Multileaf Collimators using Large Scale Mixed Integer Programs *Diploma Thesis, Fachbereich Mathematik, Universität Kaiserslautern*

[3] Siochi R A C 1999 Minimizing Static Intensity Modulation Delivery Time Using an Intensity Solid Paradigm *International Journal of Radiation Oncology Biology Physics* **43** 671–680

[4] Xia P, Verhey L J 1998 Multileaf Collimator leaf sequencing algorithm for intensity modulated beams with multiple static segments *Medical Physics* **25** 1424–1434

# Comparison of Leaf Sequencing Techniques: Dynamic vs. Multiple Static Segments

**H. Gőrkem Kuterdem[1], Paul S. Cho[1,2], Robert J Marks II[1], Mark H Phillips[2] and Homayoon Parsaei [2]**
[1]Department of Electrical Engineering, University of Washington, Seattle, WA 98195-2500, USA and [2]Department of Radiation Oncology, University of Washington, Seattle, WA 98195-6043, USA

## Introduction

Static and dynamic multileaf collimation have been so far identified as two fundementally different methods of intensity modulation in radiotherapy. In multiple static collimation, the desired fluence is deposited using two steps: In the first step, the leaves (and the backup diaphragms if available) are moved to create the desired field, but no radiation is delivered in this step. In the second step, the beam is turned on, but no leaf motion occurs. This process is repeated for each static field until the desired fluence deposition has been obtained. This type of delivery has been chiefly used for the delivery of plans with constant fluence levels over several contiguous bixels.

In dynamic multileaf collimation, the beam is turned on in the beginning of the delivery, and is turned off once the desired fluence profile is obtained, the leaves and the diaphragms being in motion during the delivery. This method has the obvious advantage of increased speed of delivery, in addition to the ability to create smoother gradients along directions of leaf travel. This method, by its very nature, lends itself to be used for the delivery of fluence profiles with rapid changes of intensity, and when the intensity levels do not remain constant over successive bixels or when the bixel sizes are small with respect to the MLC gap constraints. Convery and Webb [1] have also used this method to deliver fields with constant fluence levels.

At the University of Washington, software has been developed that can translate either kind of fluence profile, namely, smoothly varying or discrete. At the current iteration of the software, both types of profiles can be directly translated, or can be preprocessed with such tools as intensity level quantization, spatial subsampling with averaging, spatial oversampling with interpolation and then translated. The translations were designed to minimize tongue-and-groove underdosages [2] and honor the minimum gap constraints of the Elekta MLC (Elekta Oncology Systems, Crawley, UK).

The purpose of this work is to compare the above mentioned techniques of delivery in terms of such factors as efficiency of delivery, total expected time for delivery, total number of segments, tongue-and-groove underdosage, and RMS error (as calculated in delivery simulation).

## Materials and Methods

The following software was developed to handle the different translation needs for the Elekta SL20 MLC for different fluence profiles. Both the dynamic and the static collimation translators have been designed with the MLC constraints (such as minimum gap requirements, leaf velocities, allowable dose rates etc.) in mind, while trying to reduce the delivery error, decrease the total delivery time and facilitate verification.

### Dynamic Multileaf Collimation

Translation of fluence to MLC time-position sequence is performed through the use of *XYLate-D* program which has been developed in house [3]. The fluence profile is input to the software, which then sets the velocities of the left and right bank leaves in accordance with the slope of the fluence profile at a given point [4] and then synchronizes the leaves to minimize tongue-and-groove underdosages [2] and minimum gap constraint violations [3][5]. Furthermore, the backup diaphragms are extensively used to overcome the limitations imposed by the minimum gap constraints.

This method requires preprocessing to be able to cope with prescriptions which have coarse bixel widths comparable to the minimum gap requirements of the MLC. These profiles are characterized with isolated points of large gradients and large regions of zero gradient, which make it difficult to set the leaf velocities efficiently. This problem is overcome with the usage of a preprocessor which spatially interpolates the given profile.

### Static Multileaf Collimation

Another software named *XYLate-S* was developed in house to provide the static multileaf collimation translation services. The software first separates the fluence profile along each track into its components. The algorithm then assembles the components into control points to be sequenced, avoiding assembling components which would violate the minimum gap constraints into the same control point. The control point that outlines the fluence profile is scheduled first, to allow for portal imaging and verification of the dose. The remaining control points are then optimized such that the total leaf travel is minimized. Tongue-and-groove underdosages are minimized through the original control point assembly process, it is not possible to completely eliminate tongue-and-groove artifacts in static delivery using only the MLC leaves[6].

There are two other optional features of *XYLate-S*: Intensity level quantization and spatial subsampling with averaging. At the user's discretion, the fluence profile that was input to the translator can be quantized to any desired number of levels, which decreases the number of segments at the expense of increased delivery error. The quantization method chosen is a uniform quantization scheme, with the maximum intensity of the given profile and the zero intensity level being two of the chosen levels, with the remaining levels chosen in equally spaced intervals between these two extreme values.

Spatial subsampling can be used to merge the bixels of the fluence profile, to make the profile easier to translate, especially if the subsampling level is such that the resulting bixel width that is larger than the minimum gap requirements of the MLC. The subsampling level is user specified and accomplished by merging the bixels and assigning the average of the intensity levels of the merged bixels as the intensity level of the newly created bixel.

### Delivery Simulation

In-air fluence due to primary radiation passing through the MLC opening was calculated by the *vdel* program. For dynamic sequencing the program accounts for the motion of the leaves and diaphragms to accurately simulate the accumulation of photon fluence. The program compares the simulated in-air profile with the prescription and computes RMS errors, maximum underdosage, maximum overdosage, delivery efficiency, and RMS tongue-and-groove underdosage. Delivery efficiency is given by

$$E_{ff} = \frac{\text{Max peak MU}}{\text{Total MU required for delivery}} \qquad (1)$$

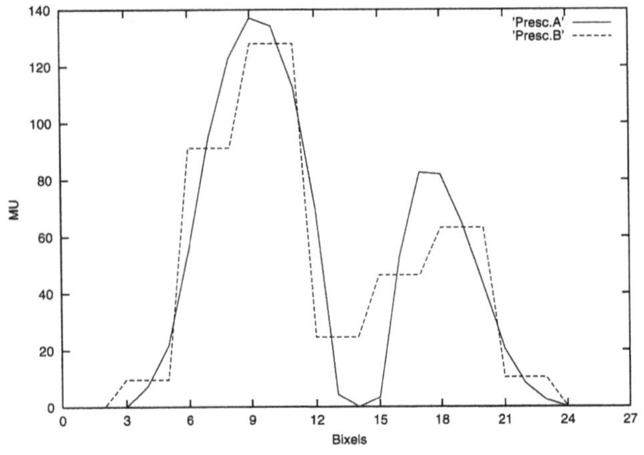


**Figure 1:** Third track of the test prescriptions

## Results and discussion

To compare the merits of various translation strategies, two test prescriptions consisting of 6 MLC tracks were used. Test prescription A has a bixel width of 0.33 cm which is less than the current minimum gap requirement of the Elekta MLC (1.0 cm). The maximum fluence value was 144 MU. Test prescription B has a bixel width of 1 cm, with a maximum fluence value of 136 MU. Figure 1 shows the third track of these test prescriptions. Test prescription A was translated both dynamically and statically (Translation 1 and 2, respectively). Test prescription B was then translated dynamically, with and without interpolation, and statically (Translations 3, 4, and 5, respectively). The parameters of each translation are listed in Table 1.

The machine-related translation parameters were dose rate of 400 MU/min, 1 cm/s maximum leaf and diaphragm velocities, and 1 cm minimum gap requirement. X diaphragm (the one that moves perpendicular to the MLC) pauses were allowed for the dynamic mode. An average beam pause duration of 7 seconds was assumed in estimation of total delivery time.

The results of performance comparison are presented in Tables 2 and 3. Comparison of dynamic and static translation of a profile with fine bixel resolution (Translation 1 and 2) indicates that the dynamic translation scheme achieves low RMS errors with few beam pauses and moderate efficiency, while the multiple static segments can achieve even lower RMS errors if efficiency could be sacrificed. However, the total MU and delivery time required are prohibitively high, thus rendering the static method virtually impractical in this case.

As expected, the dynamic translation algorithm used cannot efficiently cope with prescriptions with large bixel widths without interpolation (Translation 4). In this case, the distance between the bixels is too large for the algorithm to set the leaf velocities with the required precision. When coupled with oversampling, however, the dynamic translation can achieve a high level of performance as seen in the statistics for Translation 3. It is important to note that the static collimation scheme outperforms the dynamic collimation in this case, by presenting a much lower RMS error value without significant efficiency penalties. However, in comparing Translations 3 and 5, we note that while the two translations have the same total beam-on time, the total time required for Translation 5 is almost six times that of Translation 3 due to the number of pauses required to create the static fields. It is expected that, in the next iteration of the MLC control hardware and software, the time for the MLC to recover from a beam pause will be less than one second, in which case the static collimation should also be comparable to the dynamic collimation in terms of total delivery time.

No significant tongue-and-groove underdosages were observed for any of the translations, except for a small residual underdosage in the static translations.

## Conclusions

While, in general, the multiple static collimation method yielded lower RMS errors for a given prescription, the gain in error reduction over the dynamic sequencing may not be clinically significant. If this is true, then clearly the dynamic delivery would be the more efficient method of the two. On the other hand, for coarsely quantized modulation the multiple static scheme may be just as efficient, especially if the duration of beam on/off cycle is made near instantaneous.

## Acknowledgement

This work was supported in part by a grant from the Whitaker Foundation.

## References

[1] Convery D J and Webb S 1998 Generation of discrete beam intensity modulation by dynamic multileaf collimation under minimum leaf seperation constraints *Phys. Med. Biol.* **39** 231–251

[2] van Santvoort J P C and Heijmen B J M 1996 Dynamic multileaf collimation without 'tongue-and-groove' underdosage effects *Phys. Med. Biol.* **41** 2091–2105

[3] Kuterdem H, Cho P and Marks II R 1999 Dynamic multileaf-diaphragm sequencing with adjacency gap constraints *Med. Phys.* **26** 1136

[4] Boyer A L and Strait J P 1997 Delivery of intensity-modulated treatments with dynamic multileaf collimator in *Proceedings of the XIIth ICCR* 13–15

[5] Budgell G J, Sykes J R and Wilkinson J M 1998 Rectangular edge synchronization for intensity modulated radiation radiation therapy with dynamic multileaf collimation *Phys. Med. Biol.* **43** 2769–2784

[6] Xia P and Verhey L J 1998 Multileaf leaf sequencing algorithm for intensity modulated beams with multiple static segments *Med. Phys.* **25** 1424–1434

| Trans. | Presc. | Input bixel width (cm) | Trans. bixel width (cm) | Trans. type |
|---|---|---|---|---|
| 1 | A | 0.33 | 0.33 | Dynamic |
| 2 | A | 0.33 | 0.33 | Static |
| 3 | B | 1.00 | 0.10 | Dynamic |
| 4 | B | 1.00 | 1.00 | Dynamic |
| 5 | B | 1.00 | 1.00 | Static |

**Table 1:** Translation parameters

| Trans. # | # of ctrl. pts | RMS Error (MU) | TG (MU) underdosage | Eff. |
|---|---|---|---|---|
| 1 | 100 | 2.16 | 0.0 | 0.38 |
| 2 | 246 | 0.94 | 0.3 | 0.05 |
| 3 | 159 | 2.51 | 0.0 | 0.44 |
| 4 | 48 | 20.38 | 0.0 | 0.44 |
| 5 | 92 | 0.18 | 0.4 | 0.45 |

**Table 2:** Translation results

| Trans. # | # of pauses | Tot. MU | Beam-on time (sec) | Time to deliv (sec) |
|---|---|---|---|---|
| 1 | 5 | 378 | 57 | 92 |
| 2 | 123 | 2976 | 446 | 1061 |
| 3 | 3 | 306 | 46 | 67 |
| 4 | 0 | 306 | 46 | 46 |
| 5 | 46 | 304 | 46 | 368 |

**Table 3:** Translation results (cont.)

# Evaluation and quality control of a compensation system for intensity-modulated radiotherapy

**Henning Salz, Tilo Wiezorek, Marcel Scheithauer, René Müller and Thomas Wendt**
Klinikum der Friedrich-Schiller-Universität Jena, Radiologische Klinik

## Introduction

Since their introduction, compensators have been mostly used to generate a uniform dose distribution on a specified plane inside of the patient. For this missing tissue or internal tissue inhomogeneities have been taken into account for the calculation of the compensator design [1-3] . In contrast, in intensity-modulated radiotherapy (IMRT) a compensator is used as a beam intensity modifier[4,5].
For the use of compensators for IMRT we have developed a compensator design consisting of a mixture of tin granulate and wax. The goal of this work is the quality assurance of the system: Is there an acceptable constancy of the mechanical properties of the compensator? Is the dosimetric accuracy of the system acceptable for the application of compensation filters? Does the calculated dose distribution show a sufficient agreement with the real distribution?
In this work the mechanical and dosimetrical accuracy of the compensating system and the results of treatment planning for IMRT are discussed.

## Material and methods

### Treatment planning

For the therapy planning we use the 3D treatment planning system Helax TMS [V4.0, MDS Nordion Europe, HELAX AB, Uppsala, Sweden]. This system allows the calculation of fluence profiles for missing tissue compensation and considers tissue inhomogeneities for single fields[4]. Importing a given fluence profile, the system generates a compensator design as a finely spaced matrix of thickness values[6]. A tool for optimisation of fluence profiles for IMRT is in a more recent version. To produce and show fluence matrices, we use a self-developed software tool ("In-Fluence").

### Compensator manufactoring

The thickness value matrix is entered into a programmable milling machine ("Autimo 3D", HEK Lübeck). This machine cuts the shape of the compensation filter in a styrofoam block mounted in the milling unit. For accurate positioning of the block three additional holes have been drilled. Finally, the cavity in the foam is filled with a tin granulate-wax-mixture and shaken to get a homogeneous density. We prefer tin granulate-wax-mixture (density appr. 4.8 g/cm³) because of the lower density than cerrobend[7] or lead. Thus, we can get a higher dosimetric accuracy using the same compensator setup. Furthermore it has been shown[8], that there are only small changes in the energy spectra of photons (Siemens KD2, 6 and 15MV). A disadvantage is the limitation of the higher minimal photon transmission.

### Verification of fabrication of compensators

We checked the following parameters for the quality assurance of the fabricated compensation filters:
- compensator thickness
- orientation and position of the compensator
- material homogeneity
- dosimetric constancy of fabrication

Compensator thickness, orientation and position of the compensator were verified on the milled-out foam block before the filling of the cavity. We accept deviations of less than 1mm in the thickness and 0.5mm for the position (=1.2mm in isocentre). Material homogeneity checks were performed with film (Kodak X-Omat V).
For dosimetric quality control we measured the dose in air with a build-up cap (brass, 5mm) on the central axis and at points on a 10x10cm-grid at the isocentre.

### Quality control of the dose calculation

In the planning system a set of four phantoms was constructed (mostly according to a validation protocol) and compensator calculations were performed. The associated modulation matrix was exported, re-imported and applied to a standard water phantom. The results of the new calculations had been compared with results of real phantom measurements. The following measurements were included: depth dose measurements, profiles and output factor measurements at different field shapes.
In addition tests were performed to validate the proper handling of compensating filters in the planning system.

## Results and discussion

During compensator manufacturing we observed no apparent inaccuracy in compensator thickness, orientation and position, i.e. the inaccuracies are smaller than 0.5mm.
For the quality check of material homogeneity, the use of a film is highly recommended. To simulate homogeneity perturbations we stirred some spheres consisting of wood with diameters between 1 and 4mm into the tin granulate-wax-mixture. Then we checked if we could determine the perturbations of the material homogeneity. Using a film immediately behind a compensator, we could detect all positions of the spheres. On the other hand we could not see any other local inhomogeneities in more than 20 compensators. So we conclude that in well-shaken tin granulate-wax-mixture local density disturbances are to small for detection and without importance. Independent of this, a film check should be performed of every compensator.

For quality control of the homogeneity we also used other methods like Beam Imaging Systems and portal imaging, but we found that they are not satisfactory for suitable quality control.
The verification of the dose treatment planning showed that Helax TMS can be used for the treatment planning with compensators. The depth dose curves showed a good agreement between measured and calculated data. The deviations of the output factor (OF) is in all cases smaller than 4% ( $[OF_{meas}-OF_{calc}]/OF_{meas}$=-0.3%+/-1.8% ). Figure 1 shows an example of profiles of measured and calculated data. The results show sufficient accuracy (<3% inside the beam size) between measurements and calculations. Errors may occur in the case of the constant-dose-plane-method, if there is more than one beam and if the plane is not fully inside the patient surface. Furthermore, it is notable, that the planning system uses a modulation matrix consisting of steps. In contrast to this, the milling machine takes the shortest milling approach from the middle of one pixel to the next, just like an interpolation. So the user should employ milling heads with a small diameter (3mm) to reduce any perturbations.

Lastly, the dosimetric properties of the compensators were studied on eight compensators with the same thickness matrix (depths between several up to 20mm) The ratios of the measured doses at the point of the matrix to the measured mean values of every compensator showed a standard deviation of 0.6%, the maximal deviation amounts 1.4%. So it is shown that the fabrication of compensators occurs with high constancy.

## Conclusion

In this work it is shown that the treatment planning with Helax TMS and the compensator design consisting on tin granulate-wax mixture allows high accuracy for the application of intensity modulated radiotherapy. The dose deviations are expected to be smaller than 4% inside of the field size. In spite of the acceptable and reliable results of quality checks we recommend the following steps for quality checks for every compensator:

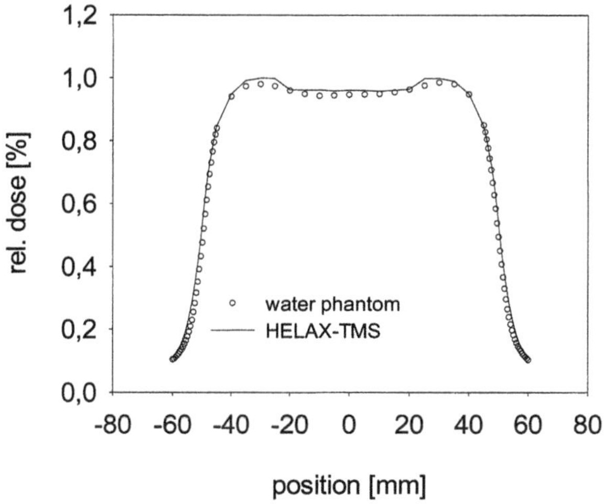


**Figure 1:** Profile of a calculated vs. a measured dose distribution

- simple check of compensator thickness, orientation and position of the compensator
- homogeneity of the filter material (film)
- dose in air (build-up cap) at the central axis or another point (not at high dose gradients)

These checks are easy to handle and do not take a lot of time.

This presentation briefly describes a fabrication method for compensators, the accuracy of the fabrication and the treatment planning. A final test with a phantom and thermoluminescent detectors is intended to be done.
Parallel to it the first treatment plans for IMRT are prepared at present with manual (software "In-Fluence") created fluence profiles. In near future with a tool for the treatment planning optimisation.

## References

[1] Ellis F, Hall E J and Oliver R 1959 A compensator for variations in tissue thickness for high energy beams *Brit J Radiol* **32** 421-422

[2] Mageras G S, Radhe Mohan, Burman C, Barest G D and Kutcher G J 1991 Compensatots for three-dimensional treatment planning *Med. Phys.* **18(2)**, 133 – 140

[3] Jiang S B and Ayyangar K M 1998 On compensator design for photon beam intensity-modulated conformal therapy *Med Phys* **25(5)** 668-675

[4] Basran P S, Ansbacher W, Field G C and Murray B R 1998 Evaluation of optimized compensators on a 3D planning system *Med Phys* **25(10)** 1837-1844

[5] Preiser K, Bortfeld Th, Hartwig K, Schlegel W, Stein J 1998 Inverse Strahlentherapieplanung für intensitäts-modulierte Photonenfelder *Radiologe* **38** 228-234

[6] Ahnesjö A, Weber L, Nilsson P 1995 Modeling transmission and scatter for photon beam attenuators *Med Phys* **22** 1711-1720

[7] Mejaddem Y, Lax Ingmar and Adakkai S K 1997 Procedure for accurate fabrication of tissue compensators with high-density material *Phys Med Biol* **42** 415-421

[8] Scheithauer M, Wiezorek T, Wolf U, Salz H, Keller A, Harder D 1999 Änderung des Bremsstrahlungsspektrums eines medizinischen Linearbeschleunigers durch intensitäts-modulierende Elemente *Gfirtner H. (editor) Medizinische Physik 1999*, DGMP, Passau

# IMRT in routine – experiences from a feasibility study

[1]WFO Schmidt, [1]W Nespor, [1]P Wirth, [1]F Büchler, [1]R Hawliczek

[1]Inst f Radiooncology, Donauspital Vienna, A – 1220 Vienna, Langobardenstr. 122, Austria

## Introduction

1991 the Donauspital, a completely new hospital in a fast growing district of Vienna was opened. The radiological department, a pilot project of the Township of Vienna and SIEMENS, was designed for completely filmless radiography; in Feb. 1996 a new radiooncology institute was integrated into these structures.

It is equipped with a MEVATRON KD2 (SIEMENS), Portal-Imaging and a SIMVIEW 3000 simulator („films" are either storage foils or digitized by a framegrabber). Images are transferred to the network (SIENET, SIEMENS) and held online up to 0.5y. Later they are still available on CD-ROMs in minutes to hours. Up to 1000 images per day are transferred to the institutes MAGICVIEW-station (storage foils, CT, MR,...) and evaluated there.

Management of and working with electronic images and their transfer are in routine since years at our hospital. Images can also be handled on normal PCs with the MAGICVIEW PC-software. All PCs are connected to the intranet of the Donauspital and furthermore to the city-network of the Township of Vienna, enabling data and image transfer between all common hospitals in Vienna.

In spring 1999 hardware and software were updated; at the linac a MLC was installed (together with PRIMEVIEW and SIMTEC as parts of the operating system) and the verification system (LANTIS 4.0) was updated. So IMRT at the linac became possible technically; a feasibility study was started.

## Material and methods

In Aug ′99 the IMRT-planning system CORVUS (NOMOS) was installed. The system, firstly developed for treatment planning with the PEACOCK applicator now also offers the possibility to plan IMRT at linacs with normal MLCs with a "step and shoot"- technique and was integrated into image network and verification system.

Basic data were measured with the MP3 water phantom (PTW) and transferred to the planning system. Verification measurements were performed with different means: Reproducibility with a water phantom (30*30*20ccm) and a FARMER chamber (UNIDOS, PTW). Dose distributions were measured by films (KODAK XOMATV) and evaluated with FIPS densitometer and MEPHYSTO software (PTW). Absolute and relative dose measurements were controlled by point dose measurements with TLDs.

## Results and discussion

Installation and integration of the system into the existing environment was quite simple. Image transfer from SIENET to the system was a "plug-and-plan-game" !

Verification of the planning results at the linac were more time consuming than basic data measurements. Absolute dose measurements in the water phantom were reproducible <2%.

For standard phantom plans film measurements were performed and evaluated. Difficulties arose from absolute calibration of the films (dependent on development as well as densitometer) and are estimated to be accurate within 5%. Isodose lines were compared to planning results and agreed within the limits resulting from absolute calibration. TLD-measurements agreed within 3% at the mean; at sites of high dose gradients maximum deviations up to 15% were measured.

Up to now (Dec. 99) 6 patients were irradiated (Table 1). Mean planning time per patient was ~8h. After verification of the treatment plan by physicians CORVUS calculates dose and dose distribution with the patient′s gantry angles and field segments for a phantom and so offers an easy way of verification. Measurements in this phantom were carried out for all patients with chamber, TLD and film; mean time for measurements (and comparison with planning results) was ~8h. Chamber measurements at a reference point were within 3%, TLD-measurements within 10%. Absolute dose evaluation of the films was not regarded as useful. Main difficulties came from positioning and resulting inaccuracies.

**Table 1: Patients up to Dec. 10, 1999**

| Nr | Diagnosis | Dose (Gy) | Gantry-angles | Segm. | Irrad. (min) |
|---|---|---|---|---|---|
| 1 | Head&Neck | 60/2 | 5 | 45 | 25 |
| 2 | Head&Neck | 60/2 | 3 | 16 | 10 |
| 3 | Cerv. Spinal Cord | 15/3 | 4 | 35 | 20 |
| 4 | Lung | 21/3+12/2 | 3 | 29 | 20 |
| 5 | Head&Neck | 60/2 | 4 | 41 | 25 |
| 6 | Sacrum | 50/2 | 5 | 55 | 20 |
| 7 | Small pelvis | 10/2 | 5 | 45 | --- |

## Conclusions

Since Sep. 9$^{th}$ 6 patients have been treated. The number of routine treatments (up to 70 pat/day) at the linac has not decreased, so only 2 IMRT-cases can be treated at the same time. Nevertheless IMRT treatments have proved to be possible in routine; time necessary for planning and verification can be reduced with rising experience. Difficulties during planning arose because TCP- and NTCP-data are still missing; "class solutions" for different treatment sites could be helpful, also when comparing results with other centers.

Although better agreement between planning and verification is desirable, the largest inaccuracies seem to result from patient positioning in routine; main effort should be directed to it.

# An optimized convolution/superposition based algorithm for dose calculation with photon beams

**Nikos Papanikolaou[1], Rock Mackie[2]**

[1]Dept of Radiation Medicine, University of Kentucky, Lexington, KY, 40536 USA , and [2]Dept of Medical Physics, University of Wisconsin, Madison, Wisconsin 53706 USA

## Introduction

In clinical treatment planning for radiation therapy, the goal is to accurately compute the dose for a given treatment geometry, thus accounting correctly for the patient contour and the inhomogeneities in the treatment volume. Convolution/Superposition based algorithms have emerged as the most accurate methods, besides Monte Carlo, to accomplish that goal for photon beams. By means of a density scaling of the dose deposition kernels and by performing the ray-tracing in radiological space (g/cm$^2$), superposition algorithms can accurately describe the effects of inhomogeneities for regions of atomic number similar to that of water. We have extended the method, to include the effects for higher atomic number (Z>8) inhomogeneities that can be encountered in clinical situations.

## Material and methods

The convolution kernels used in the convolution/superposition dose computation algorithms contain a description of the dose deposition pattern from the transport of primary generated charged particles and photons produced when primary photons interact at a point. The medium specific kernels were generated using an EGS4 version of the Monte Carlo algorithm SCASPH. Energy deposition kernels were computed for a series of photon energies for different materials such as carbon, aluminum, calcium, iron and lead, as well as bone (Figure 1). The kernels were used to compute dose with an enhanced superposition algorithm that implements a ray-tracing in radiological space while maintaining an indexing of the medium along the ray-trace, so that the appropriate kernel is invoked in the calculation. The equations before and after the indexing are shown below.
Ray-tracing based on single water kernel:

$$D(\vec{r}) = \int \frac{\mu(\vec{r} - \vec{r}')}{\rho} \Psi(\vec{r} - \vec{r}') A(\rho \cdot 1(\vec{r}'), \vec{\omega}) d^3\vec{r}'$$

Ray-tracing based on medium specific kernel:

$$D(\vec{r}) = \int \frac{\mu(\vec{r} - \vec{r}')}{\rho} \Psi(\vec{r} - \vec{r}') A(\rho \cdot 1(\vec{r}'), \vec{\omega}, l(\vec{r}')) d^3\vec{r}'$$

When the scatter raytrace crosses a region of different density, the corresponding kernel is now used in the calculation of scatter. The distance from the origin of the kernel that is needed to compute the scatter dose to that point is the cummulative radiological distance from the primary interaction site to the dose deposition site[4]. The algorithm can be coupled with an optimization routine where the fluence or TERMA are optimized to yield dosimetrically conformal distributions to the target volumes

## Results and discussion

The need for medium-specific kernels arises from the inability to use the density-scaled water kernels for high energies and for media with atomic number different than water. The new energy deposition kernels are consistent with their expected physical behavior; namely, the kernels become more forward peaked with the increase in energy but exhibit more lateral scatter at higher atomic numbers (Figure 1). The new algorithm was tested for geometric phantoms (slab like and cube like inhomogeneities) and clinical cases for energies ranging from 1.25-20 MeV. The results are in good agreement with Monte Carlo computations for the same geometries (Figures 2,3).

## Conclusion

A Monte Carlo code was used to generate a number of dose deposition kernels for different energies and atomic numbers. A good agreement in computed depth-doses, profiles and relative dose distributions was obtained between the convolution/superposition algorithm, and the Monte Carlo computations.

## References

[1] N. Papanikolaou, T.R. Mackie, C. Wells, M. Gehring, P. Reckwerdt, "*Investigation of the Convolution Method for Polyenergetic Spectra*,"Med. Phys., **20**(5), 1993

[2] N. Papanikolaou, T.R. Mackie, "*A new Convolution Approach for the Generation of Polyenergetic Photon Beam Dose Distributions*," Med. Phys., **19**(3), 1992

[3] N. Papanikolaou, T.R. Mackie, "*Generation of Photon Convolution Kernels using a Monte Carlo Code for use in Radiotherapy Treatment Planning and Cavity Theory*," Med. Phys., **20**(3), 1993

[4] N. Papanikolaou, T.R. Mackie, "*Extension of the Convolution/Superposition Based Algorithms to Include Atomic Number Effects*," Med. Phys., **22**(6), 1995

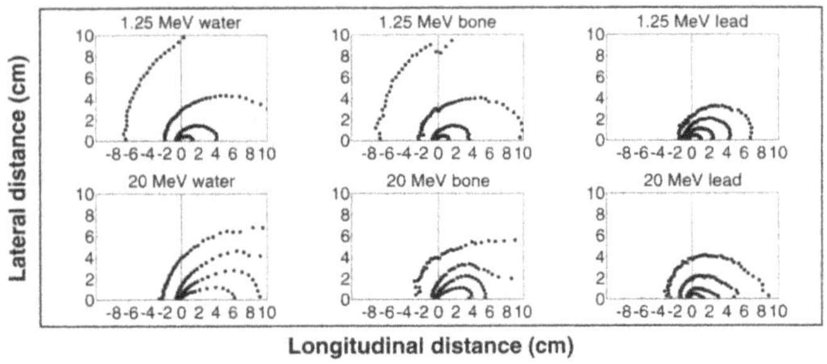


**Figure 1:** Dose deposition kernels for water,bone and lead

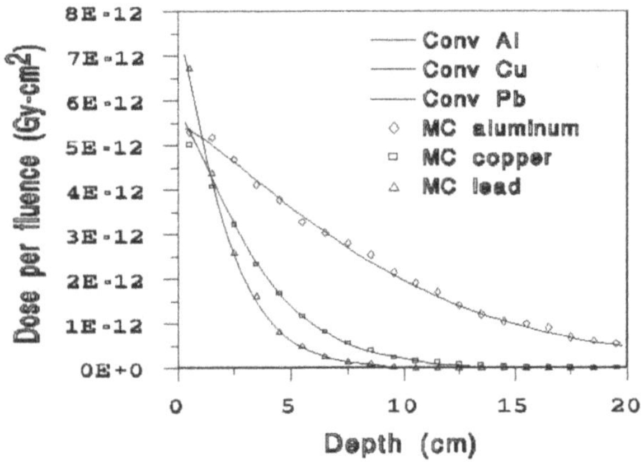


**Figure 2:** Depth dose curves in homogeneous media for 1.25 MeV

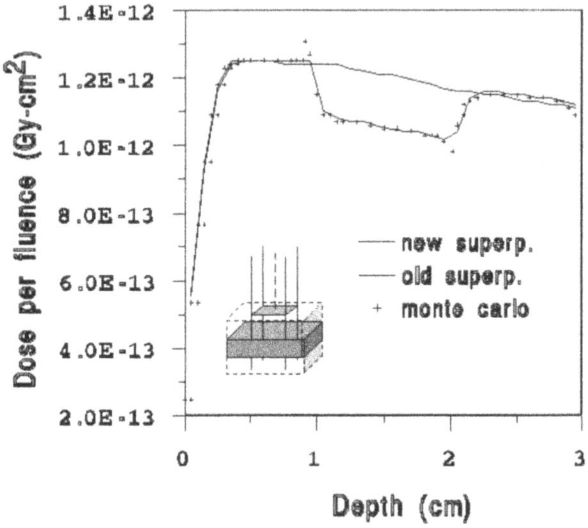


**Figure 3:** 1.25 MeV Depth dose distribution through an Al slab

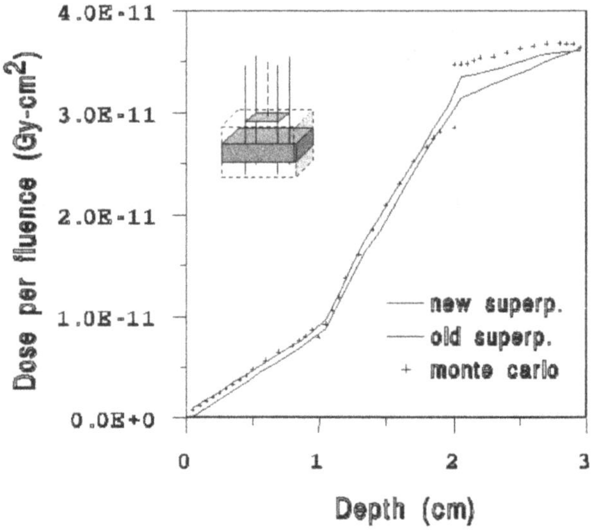


**Figure 4:** 20 MeV depth dose distribution through an Al slab

# A multigrid method for accelerating superposition dose calculations

**Mark Wiesmeyer, Moyed Miften and Suzanne Monthofer**

Computerized Medical Systems, Inc., St. Louis, Missouri, USA.

## Introduction

Current clinical practice relies on the superposition method of photon dose calculations for accurate results in heterogeneous tissues. We introduce a variable resolution, or *multigrid,* method for superposition calculations that is guided by *a priori* knowledge to improve efficiency. In this method, dose is calculated at full resolution in regions where large dose changes are expected. Dose is calculated at half resolution where small dose changes are expected, and interpolation is used to estimate intermediate points in these regions.

Niemierko and Goitein presented an acceleration method that used adaptive iteration, and the relationships between sparsely calculated dose points to determine whether to calculate or to interpolate intermediate points [1]. Large differences between dose values indicated the need to calculate intermediate points; small differences indicated the need to interpolate. Speedups of about 16 times for three-dimensional calculations with little effect on accuracy were reported for large spacings between initially calculated points. Niemierko and Goitein pointed out that it might be possible to miss significant dose changes between widely spaced initial points; thus, leading to inaccurate calculations. Results were only shown for homogeneous calculations.

We present multigrid superposition results for homogeneous and heterogeneous test cases.

## Material and methods

The superposition algorithm that forms the basis of our work is a modified collapsed cone algorithm [2] based on the Mackie's method of superposition calculation [3]. Unique aspects of the algorithm include a kernel hardening correction [4], computation of TERMA in fan coordinates with each fan maintaining its own spectrum, and a number of speed optimizations, including separate primary and scatter dose calculations. There are two versions of our superposition algorithm: Fast superposition uses 8 azimuth and 6 zenith angles for a total of 48 ray traces per dose point; standard superposition uses 8 azimuth and 20 zenith angles. Standard superposition, whose results are reported in this paper, is slightly more accurate (1-2%) than fast superposition, mostly at beam edges. Electron contamination dose for both versions of the algorithm is modeled separately from photon dose.

The multigrid idea is simple: calculate superposition dose at full resolution in regions of high dose gradient derivatives. At all other locations calculate dose at half that resolution, and then use interpolation to estimate intermediate points in these regions. Calculation masks, as shown in Figure 1, determine the points that are calculated using superposition and the points that are interpolated. All lighter colored points are calculated using superposition; spaces representing points between them are interpolated. Since there are separate primary dose and scatter dose calculations, each calculation must have its own calculation mask.

As shown in Figure 1, the multigrid approach limits the number of superposition calculations by: 1) calculating every other dose point outside of the beam; 2) calculating every other point inside the beam, except in a surface buildup region and where there are tissue interfaces; and 3) calculating every point on a beam edge.

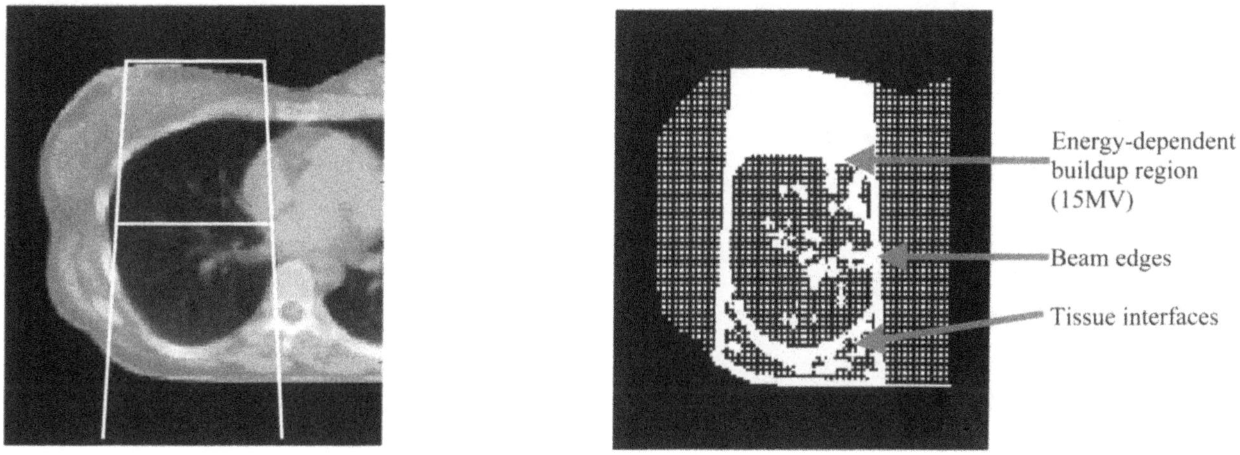


**Figure 1:** Electron densities with superimposed beam (left), and corresponding calculation mask (right).

For linear accelerators, the surface buildup region depth is 4 times the machine's maximum spectrum energy in millimeters. This allows it to completely cover the buildup region for any beam. For cobalt machines, the surface region depth is 1.6cm.

Fast Fourier Transform (FFT) convolution is used to efficiently find tissue interfaces. In this process, electron densities are convolved with a three-dimensional Laplacian kernel, represented mathematically below, which identifies second derivatives.

$$\nabla^2 = \frac{\partial^2}{\partial x^2} + \frac{\partial^2}{\partial y^2} + \frac{\partial^2}{\partial z^2}$$

Laplacian operators are typically used in image analysis software to find the edges of objects to be identified, as in scene recognition [5].

The result of the convolution is real-valued tissue edges. To form a complete calculation mask, thresholding is used to convert the real-valued tissue edges to a binary edge mask. Edges in the mask outside of the beam are then removed. Beam edges, the surface region, and half-resolution points are then calculated using simple geometric methods, and added to the tissue edge mask.

There is essentially no visible difference between a non-optimized calculation and a calculation using the multigrid approach for a 15MV, 10x10 beam, as shown in Figure 2. Other beam sizes and energies showed similar results.

## Results and discussion

### Calculation Speed

The time required for the creation of calculation masks and the interpolation of superposition doses must be a small part of overall calculation time for the multigrid superposition approach to have value. In the current implementation, the mask calculation and interpolation steps require 6 - 24% of the total dose calculation time. Small percentages are for larger fields, and large percentages are for smaller fields. So, for example, for a larger field calculation at a higher dose resolution that takes 120 seconds, about 7 seconds would be needed for multigrid overhead. For a smaller field calculation at lower dose resolution that takes 20 seconds, about 5 seconds would be needed for multigrid overhead. This behavior occurs, since increases in the number of points to be calculated have less of an effect for FFT convolution than they do for superposition.

Using an "every other point strategy" has an upper-bound reduction factor of up to 8 times (one-half cubed is one-eighth). In the current implementation of multigrid superposition, speed improvements of only about 3 times have been observed, due to large constant factors, especially the TERMA and electron dose contamination calculations. Acceleration methods like multigrid tend to work better when point calculation times are much greater than supporting constant time calculations.

### Calculation Accuracy

Multigrid superposition was tested for a variety of beam setups (bolus, physical and dynamic wedges, ports, MLC), machines and energies (Varian 6 & 18MV, Siemens 6 & 15MV, Philips 25MV) using water tank measurements. Results were good: 97% of points for low-energy beams, and 95% of points for high-energy beams passed a 3%/3mm criterion. That is, passing calculated points were either within 3% of measurements, or a matching measured dose could be found within 3mm of the calculated dose point. Points with dose values less than 0.5% of the maximum dose values were not considered in this analysis.

Multigrid superposition doses were compared to EGS4 Monte Carlo calculated doses for lung, lung-bone, bone-lung, two-lung, and lung gap phantoms [6], as shown in Figure 3. Calculations were done in 30x30x30cm phantoms, with the distance to the initial non-water density object being dependent upon the machine energy. This insured that buildup was completed in water-density material, and facilitated

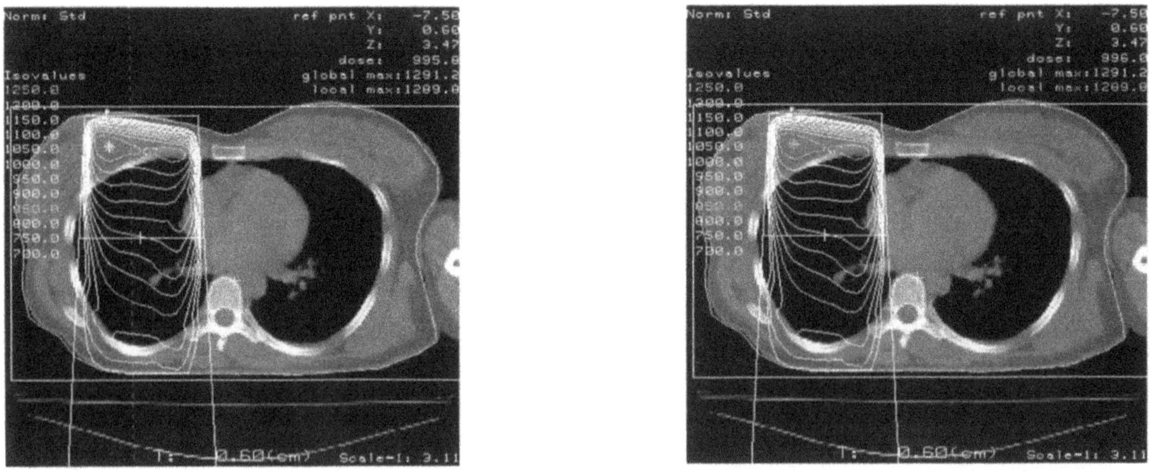

**Figure 2:** 15MV open field calculation - superposition without multigrid (left), and superposition with multigrid (right).

normalization and comparison of superposition and Monte Carlo doses. Lung densities were set to 0.2 or 0.31g/cc, and bone densities were set to 2.40g/cc.

As with measured dose comparisons, a high percentage, 98.6%, of points passed the 3%/3mm criterion. The limits of the multigrid superposition accuracy were tested by tightening the passing criterion to 2%/2mm, 1%/1mm, and finally to 0.5%/0.5mm. The average percentage of points passing were 95.9%, 83.2%, and 54.9%, respectively. Figure 4 shows results broken down on a case-by-case basis. Characteristic errors in these superposition calculations are shown in Figure 5---builddown is underestimated due to the over-simple scaling of water-equivalent dose deposition kernels that does not account for differences in electron densities. These types of errors show up in most superposition algorithms.

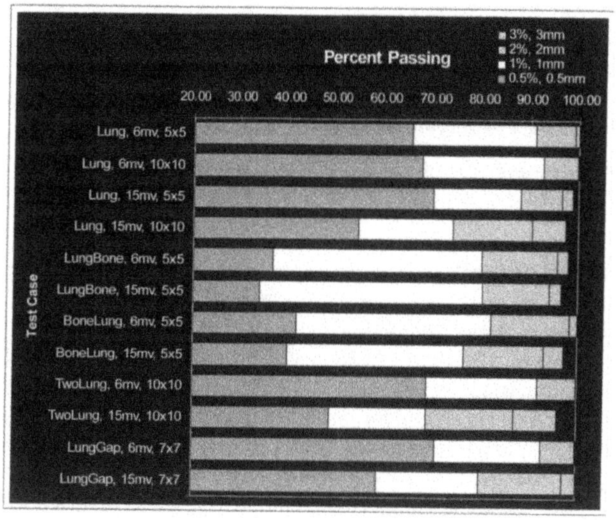


**Figure 4:** Results of Monte Carlo dose comparisons

## Conclusion

Multigrid superposition produces fast and accurate dose calculations. Increasing acceleration requires more spacing between superposition-calculated points in low gradient regions of the beam. Greater point spacing could have been used, but we were conservative in our approach since accurate dose calculations were our goal. The multigrid approach should be applicable to similar types of calculations where gradient information can be estimated prior to point calculations.

## Acknowledgements

Many thanks to Charlie Ma and Ajay Kapur for their Monte Carlo dose calculations.

## References

[1] Niemierko A and Goitein M 1989 The use of variable grid spacing to accelerate dose calculations *Med. Phys.* **16** 357-366

[2] Ahnesjo A 1989 Collapsed cone convolution of radiant energy for photon dose calculation in heterogeneous media *Phys. Med. Biol.* **36** 973-985

[3] Mackie T R, Reckwerdt P J, Gehring M A, Holmes T W, Kusbad S S, Tomadsen B R, Sanders C A, Paliwal B R, and Kinsella, T J 1990 Clinical implementation of the convolution/superposition method, in *The Use of Computers in Radiation Therapy: Proceedings of the 10th Conference*, edited by S. Hukku and P.S. Iyer (Lucknow) 20-23

[4] Hoban P W 1995 Accounting for the variation in collision kerma-to-terma ratio on polyenergetic photon beam convolution *Med. Phys* **22** 2035-2044

[5] Ballard D H and Brown C M 1982 Computer Vision *Prentice Hall, Inc* Englewood Cliffs 76-79

[6] Rice R K, Mijnheer B J and Chin L M 1988 Benchmark measurements for lung dose corrections for x-ray *beams Int. J. Rad. Onc. Biol. Phys.* **15** 399-409

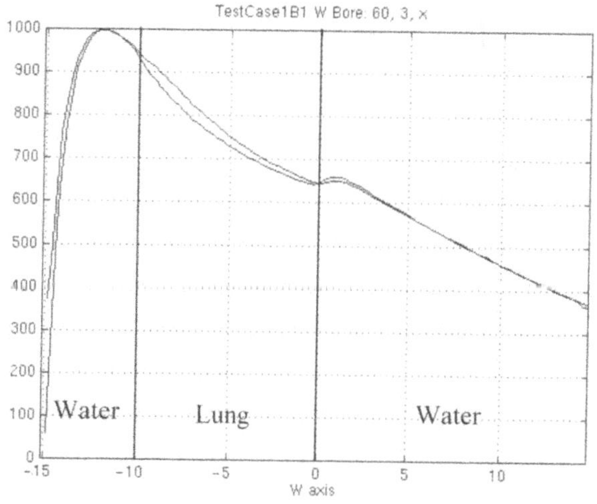


**Figure 5:** Relative dose vs. depth in cm for lung phantom and a 15MV 5x5 beam - Superposition (upper) vs. Monte Carlo (lower)

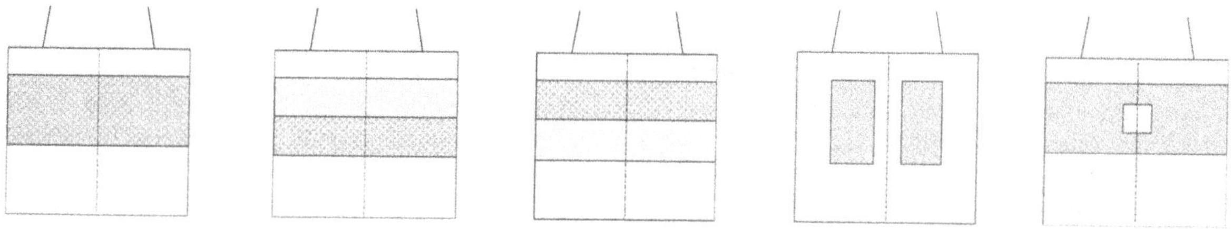

**Figure 3:** Schematics of Monte Carlo test phantoms and beams: lung, lung-bone, bone-lung, two lung, lung gap (left to right).

# Use of Collapsed Cone Convolution for an Initial Investigation of Portal Dose Image Prediction

**Christina Vallhagen Dahlgren[1,2] and Anders Ahnesjö[1]**

[1]MDS Nordion Therapy Systems, Uppsala, Sweden and [2]Dept. of Oncology, Radiology and Clinical Immunology, Section of Biomedical Radiation Sciences, Uppsala University, Uppsala, Sweden

## Introduction

Electronic Portal Imaging Devices (EPIDs) are important for verification of patient position during radiotherapy. Their use for dosimetrical verification is likely to increase in the future with increasing treatment complexity and improved detectors. The term portal dose image (PDI) usually refers to a predicted image, independent of the detector technique. The prediction may use different models and methods [1, 2]. In this work we investigate PDI prediction with the collapsed cone convolution/superposition method [3] as it is formulated in the treatment planning system Helax-TMS (MDS Nordion Therapy Systems).

## Material and methods

### Calculation method

The dose calculation starts with an initial ray-trace of the applied beam through the volume of interest, to determine total energy release per mass (TERMA) separated into a kinetic part (collision KERMA) and a scatter part (SCERMA = TERMA - collision KERMA). The collapsed cone convolution/superposition uses polyenergetic energy deposition kernels superposed from Monte Carlo simulated monoenergetic kernels. Polyenergetic kernels can be analytically well described by

$$h_{\omega}(r,\theta)=(A_{\theta}e^{-a_{\theta}r}+B_{\theta}e^{-b_{\theta}r})/r^{2} \qquad (1)$$

where the parameters $A_\theta$, $B_\theta$, $a_\theta$ and $b_\theta$ depend on the scattering angle $\theta$ and $r$ is the radiological distance from the point of energy release. The first term models the transport of primary released kinetic energy (collision KERMA) while the second term models the scatter energy transport. The parameterized polyenergetic kernel is discretized into cones covering the whole sphere. In the collapsed cone approximation all energy is transported along the cone axes. This enables an efficient recursive energy transport and deposition along each cone axis for fast calculations.

The dose calculation for the simulated EPID has been divided into two parts. First KERMA and SCERMA distributions are calculated by a ray-trace through the phantom/ patient where the transmisson depends on density and tissue composition, including effects due to beam hardening and off axis softening. The dose is calculated with collapsed cone convolution over the detector volume. This dose is referred to as Detector Energy Released dose, **DER**. Secondly, the energy released in the irradiated phantom (or patient) contributes with scattered photons and charged particles hitting the detector. It is referred to as Phantom from Energy Released dose, **PER**. The kernel discretization used for PER dose calculation is chosen with a high resolution in the forward direction. The PER dose is calculated with the recursive energy transport through the phantom for all angles, attenuation in air and dose deposition in the detector. Thus the dose at a point in the detector is calculated as

$$D_{\mathrm{det}}(\mathbf{r})=D_{\mathrm{DER}}(\mathbf{r})+D_{\mathrm{PER}}(\mathbf{r}) \qquad (2)$$

where

$$\begin{aligned} D_{\mathrm{DER}}(\mathbf{r}) &= \iiint_{V_d} P(\mathbf{s})\hat{h}_{p,1}(\mathbf{r}-\mathbf{s})d^3s + \iiint_{V_d} S(\mathbf{s})\hat{h}_{s,1}(\mathbf{r}-\mathbf{s})d^3s \\ D_{\mathrm{PER}}(\mathbf{r}) &= \iiint_{V_p} P(\mathbf{s})\hat{h}_{p,2}(\mathbf{r}-\mathbf{s})d^3s + \iiint_{V_p} S(\mathbf{s})\hat{h}_{s,2}(\mathbf{r}-\mathbf{s})d^3s \end{aligned} \qquad (3)$$

where $\hat{h}_{p,i}$ and $\hat{h}_{s,i}$ are polyenergetic kernels for primary and scatter energy transport with selected discretization $i$, $P(\mathbf{s})$ and $S(\mathbf{s})$ describes the KERMA and SCERMA distributions, and the integration is performed over the volumes of the detector $V_d$ and the phantom $V_p$ respectively.

### Collapsed Cone calculations

The calculations were performed on an object oriented environment developed in C++. The code enables easy manipulation in material, size and position of phantom and detector objects. Homogeneous or modulated fields can be defined. The initial ray-trace is performed for parallel or diverging beams. Different kernels (eventually tilted for divergence) can be selected for convolution within the detector, within the phantom and for energy transported from the phantom to the detector. The primary, scatter and total dose distributions can be output separately for further analysis.

All calculations were done for 6MV with spectra from Mohan et al. [4] and ray-trace parameters were calculated consistent with cross sections in EGS4. Patient phantom and detector phantom objects were created in water with a voxel side of 0.2 cm. KERMA and SCERMA distributions were calculated for parallel fields of various sizes with a simple cutoff at the field edges. The phantom thickness ranged from 5 to 20 cm and the air gap was fixed at 30 cm. The detector was modelled with a 12 cm thick water slab. The kernel for calculating the DER dose was a polyhedron with 106 transport directions which is the current default choice in the treatment planning system Helax-TMS. For the PER dose a separate kernel was obtained using a discretization of $7\times7$ squares with 52.5 cm side at 50 cm distance. The central $5\times5$ squares were subdivided into $25\times25$ squares giving 649 transport directions. The calculated dose is normalized per incident energy fluence enabling direct comparison with Monte Carlo data. It should be noted that the ratio of PER dose to DER dose for parallel beams is much lower than the scatter to primary ratio for diverging beams, at the detector distance.

**Monte Carlo calculations**

Monoenergetic pencil beam kernels have been simulated with the EGS4 code run on Windows NT [5]. The simulation geometry consisted of a homogeneous water phantom of thickness ranging from 5 to 20 cm, a 30 cm air gap and a downstream water volume simulating an EPID. The energy deposit per incident energy fluence was scored in cylindrical voxels with thickness $\Delta z$, an inner cylinder with diameter $\Delta r$ and coaxial rings with radial increment $\Delta r$, with $\Delta r$ and $\Delta z$ equal to 0.2 cm. The scoring included the volumes down to the first 10 cm of the detector depth. Primary energy deposit (from charged particles generated at the interaction of the primary photon), first scatter (from charged particles from first scattered photons) and multiple scatter were scored separately. DER dose and PER dose deposits were scored separately. The simulations were set up with an electron cutoff energy of 0.1 MeV and a photon cutoff of 0.01 MeV. Depth dose curves and profiles for broad beams were calculated using polyenergetic pencil kernels.

## Results and discussion

Dose calculated with the collapsed cone convolution is compared with Monte Carlo simulations for various field sizes in table 1. The evaluation depth is at 1.7 cm in the detector phantom (close to dose maximum). It is shown that the total predicted dose is overestimated by less than 1%. The relative differences for separated dose fractions are larger especially for the PER dose.

| Dose Category | | $D/\Psi$ [cm²/kg] 5×5 | 10×10 | 15×15 | 20×20 |
|---|---|---|---|---|---|
| DER | CC | 9.391 | 9.558 | 9.662 | 9.734 |
| | MC | 9.295 | 9.423 | 9.507 | 9.580 |
| PER | CC | 0.078 | 0.301 | 0.606 | 0.997 |
| | MC | 0.101 | 0.370 | 0.715 | 1.138 |
| Total | CC | 9.469 | 9.859 | 10.27 | 10.73 |
| | MC | 9.396 | 9.793 | 10.22 | 10.72 |
| Total CC /MC | | +0.8% | +0.7% | +0.5% | +0.1% |

**Table 1:** Dose per Incident Energy Fluence for separated DER and PER for 6MV x-rays. The detector phantom evaluation depth is 1.7 cm. Comparisons of EGS4 (MC) and Collapsed Cone (CC) for patient phantom thickness 20 cm and field sizes 5×5, 10×10,15×15 and 20×20 cm² are listed.

In figure 1, depth dose curves for the detector phantom are shown for patient phantom thicknesses from 5 to 20 cm for a 10×10 cm² field. The graph shows an accurate prediction of the buildup region for these thicknesses. Figure 2 shows a detailed view over PER dose for 10 and 20 cm patient phantom thickness.

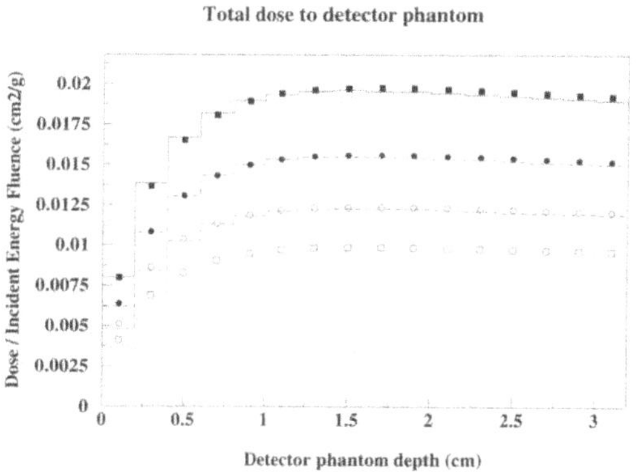


**Figure 1:** Depth doses for detector phantom and a field of 10x10 cm² with EGS4 simulations (histograms) shown versus collapsed cone calculations (markers). From the top of the figure 5, 10, 15, and 20 cm patient phantom thickness is shown for a 30 cm air gap.

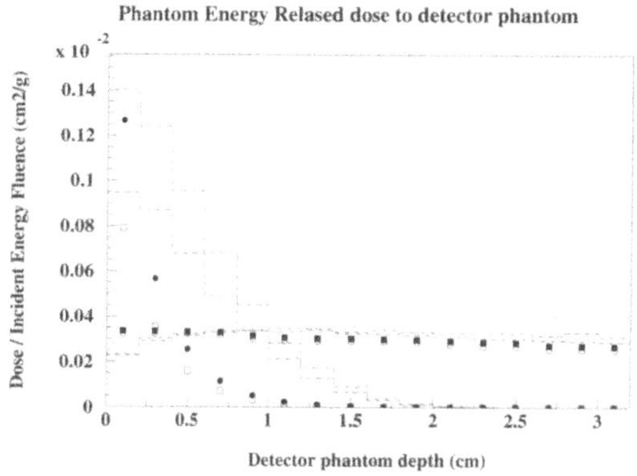


**Figure 2:** PER dose to the detector phantom for EGS4 simulations (histograms) and collapsed cone calculations (markers). The primary and scattered contributions are separated. Patient phantom thicknesses are 10 cm (solid and circles) and 20 cm (dashed and squares). The field size was 10x10 cm².

It is seen in figure 2 that the rectilinear scaling of the primary energy transport neglecting multiple scattering, yields an underestimated PER primary dose near the air/water interface [6, 7]. The predicted scatter dose is slightly underestimated. The magnitude of the scatter dose is almost constant for 10 and 20 cm patient phantom thickness in agreement with Jaffray et al. [8]. PER scatter dose profiles are compared for field sizes 10×10 cm² and 20×20 cm² at a depth of 1.7 cm in figure 3. The collapsed cone calculation is lower compared with Monte Carlo calculations. While the PER dose is only a fraction of the total dose the error is estimated to 1-2% for a clinical beam.

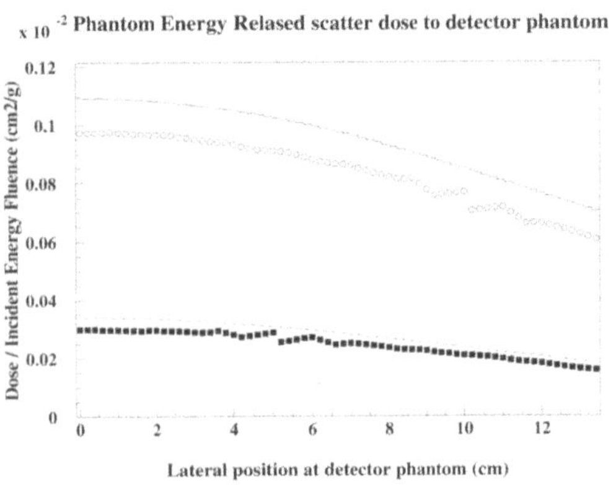


**Figure 3:** Profile at 1.7 cm depth in detector phantom with collapsed cone (markers) versus EGS4 simulations shown. PER scatter dose for 20 cm patient phantom thickness and field size 20x20 $cm^2$ (top) and 10x10 $cm^2$ (bottom) is shown.

## Conclusions

Comparisons between Monte Carlo generated depth dose distributions and collapsed cone convolution show good overall agreement for homogeneous objects and parallel beams. The rectilinear scaling of electron transport through air yields an underestimated primary dose near the surface. There is also an underestimation of the scatter dose from the patient phantom. The influence of these limitations will be analyzed, together with calculations for clinical beams and corresponding measurements for further refinement of the models.

## Acknowledgements

This project is partly financed by the Swedish Research Council for Engineering Sciences.

## References

[1]McNutt T R, Mackie T R, Reckwerdt P, Paliwal B R 1996 Calculation of portal dose using the convolution/superposition method *Medical Physics* **23** 527-535

[2]Pasma K L, Kroonwijk M., de Boer J C J, Visser A G and Heijmen B J M 1998 Portal dose image (PDI) prediction for dosimetric treatment verification in radiotherapy. 1. an algorithm for open beams *Medical Physics* **25** 830-840

[3]Ahnesjö, A 1989 Collapsed cone convolution of radiant energy for photon dose calculation in heterogeneous media. *Medical Physics* **16** 577-92

[4]Mohan R and Chen C 1985 Energy and angular distributions of photons from medical linear accelerators *Medical Physics* **12** 592-597

[5]Nelson W R, Hirayama H and Rogers D W O 1985 The EGS4 code system *Stanford Linear Accelerator Report*, SLAC 265

[6]Woo M K and Cunningham J R 1990 The validity of the density scaling method in primary electron transport for photon and electron beam. *Medical Physics* **17** 187-94

[7]Keall P and Hogan P 1995 Accounting for primary electron scatter in x-ray beam convolution calculations *Medical Physics* **22** 1413-18

[8]Jaffray D A., Battista J J, Fenster A and Munro P 1994 X-ray scatter in megavoltage transmission radiography: physical characteristics and influence on image quality. *Medical Physics* **21** 45-60

# Modelling of photon beam spectral variations

**Anders Ahnesjö, Mikael Saxner and Ingvar Thorslund**

MDS Nordion Therapy Systems, Klostergatan 12, Box 1704, 751 47 Uppsala, Sweden

## Introduction

Accurate dose calculations are a necessity for improvement of radiation therapy through treatment with optimized dose distributions. The radiation leaving the treatment machine must be correctly described and the radiation transport and energy deposition in the patient must be modelled to an extent that accurate dose is achieved. The most explicit description of a beam is provided through Monte Carlo simulations of the treatment head, resulting in extensive phase space data listing energy, location and directions for literally millions of particles exiting the machine. However, accurate dose results can be achieved by using parameterized distributions derived from measured, machine specific dose distributions and known geometric properties. Use of measured data is especially important as to assure quality and self consistency of reconstructed dose results. In this work the modelling of off axis spectral softening in photon beams is studied based on measured attenuation coefficients. We also investigate spectral changes induced by hard wedges, which is modelled based on variation of the ratio of collision kerma and terma per modulated fluence as compared to open beams. We have developed correction methods for dose "engines" using collapsed cone point kernel methods, but the result can in principle also be applied to construct phase space sampling schemes for Monte Carlo dose calculations.

## Theory

### General

Point kernel methods for dose calculation starts by calculating the energy released by the primary beam, i.e. the terma. The terma can be divided into two parts, one being the collision kerma $P$ (to be transported and deposited as *primary dose*), and one describing "scerma" $S$ (the difference between terma and collision kerma; to be transported and deposited as *scatter dose*) [1]. The variation of collision kerma with depth $z$ in a narrow photon beam can be described as

$$P(z)=\sum_{i\in \text{spectrum}} \Psi_{\Delta E_i} \frac{\mu_{en}}{\mu}(E_i)\, e^{-\frac{\mu}{\rho}(E_i)\rho z} \qquad (1)$$

where $\Psi_{\Delta E_i}$ is the energy fluence content of energy bin $E_i$. It is easy to verify that, for typical spectra, the summation over the spectrum can be replaced by a single exponential

$$P(z)=P_0\, e^{-\mu_P(1-\kappa_P\cdot z)\, z} \qquad (2)$$

where $P_0$, $\mu_P$ and $\kappa_P$ are fitting parameters. The parameter $\mu_P$ is equivalent to the narrow beam attenuation coefficient. Analogous, the scerma can be described as

$$S(z)=S_0\, e^{-\mu_S(1-\kappa_S\cdot z)\, z} \qquad (3)$$

where $S_0$, $\mu_S$ and $\kappa_S$ are fitting parameters.

Several workers have measured and analyzed narrow beam attenuation coefficients, see e.g. [2], who also provided a generic parameterization of its lateral variation. Since variations in $\mu_P$ is the most direct way to express the impact from off axis variations of the beam spectrum, it is natural to use the local value of $\mu_P$ as the independent variable for construction of methods to model clinical dosimetric effects from off axis softening.

### Released energy calculations

The distributions of energy, $P(\mathbf{r})$ and $S(\mathbf{r})$, released by the primary beam is transported by secondary particle until deposited as dose. The effects of spectral shift are directly included in $P(\mathbf{r})$ either by using the laterally varying $\mu_P$, given by the Tailor et. al. relation [2] or measured for each machine individually. By comparing data for several spectra and monoenergetic interaction coefficients, simple relations were found to scale the variations of the parameters in eq. (2) and (3) with $\mu_P$, se Table 1. When a hard wedge is inserted into the beam, the spectral shift caused by the wedge can be modelled [3] by modulation dependent quality factors $k_{PQ}$ and $k_{SQ}$ such that

$$\begin{aligned} P_{\text{wed}}(\mathbf{r}) &= \eta k_{PQ} P_{\text{open}}(\mathbf{r}) \\ S_{\text{wed}}(\mathbf{r}) &= \eta k_{SQ} S_{\text{open}}(\mathbf{r}) \end{aligned} \qquad (4)$$

where $\eta$ is the fluence modulation induced by the wedge.

| Parameter | Scaling Relation | |
|---|---|---|
| $P_0$ | Biased into the energy fluence | |
| $S_0$ | $\frac{S_0(\delta)}{P(\delta)}=\frac{S_0(0)}{P_0(0)}+b\cdot(\mu_P(\delta)-\mu_P(0))$ | $b = 18.6037\ \mathrm{cm}^2\cdot\mathrm{g}^{-1}$ |
| $\frac{\mu_S}{\rho}$ | $\frac{\mu_S}{\mu_P}=B_1+B_2\frac{\mu_P}{\rho}\cdot U^{B_3}$ | $B_1 = 0.8566$<br>$B_2 = 1.8082\ \mathrm{g}\cdot\mathrm{cm}^{-2}\ \mathrm{MV}^{[illegible]}$<br>$B_3 = 0.5849$ |
| $\frac{\kappa_P}{\rho}, \frac{\kappa_S}{\rho}$ | only minor variations | |

**Table 1:** Scaling of released energy parameters with the narrow beam attenuation coefficient $\mu_P=\mu_P(\delta)$ where $\delta$ is off axis angle.

### Secondary particle transport

The lower energy of the primary photons at the peripheral parts of the beam induce a slight change in shape of the scatter kernel at these positions. As the scatter kernel is well described by an exponential function [1],

$$\hat{h}_S(r,\theta)=\frac{\hat{B}_\theta\, e^{-b_\theta r}}{r^2} \qquad (5)$$

where $\widehat{B}_\theta$ and $b_\theta$ are parameters depending on scattering angle $\theta$, shape changes due to spectral changes can be modelled through variations of $\widehat{B}_\theta$ and $b_\theta$, i.e.

$$\widehat{B}_\theta(\delta) = \widehat{B}_\theta + \frac{d\widehat{B}_\theta}{d\delta}\delta \qquad (6)$$

which can be coupled to the changes in attenuation through

$$\frac{d\widehat{B}_\theta}{d\delta} = \frac{d\widehat{B}_\theta}{d\mu_P}\frac{d\mu_P}{d\delta} \qquad (7)$$

and similarly for $b_\theta$. The values of $d\widehat{B}_\theta/d\mu_P$ (and $db_\theta/d\mu_P$) were derived from monoenergetic kernels (using $\mu_{en}$ instead of $\mu_P$).

## Methods

The methods were implemented into the Helax-TMS treatment planning system. Spectrum, head scatter parameters and energy fluence distributions were iteratively varied until a good match with measured depth doses, profiles and output factors was achieved. The off axis change of $\mu_P$ was modelled according to the relation from Tailor *et al* [2]. Calculations with and without the spectral corrections were made to illustrate their impact on calculated dose.

## Results and discussion

**Dose kernel methods**
The most important spectral changes are for wedges at low energies, as illustrated in figure 1. This is to a large extent depth dose changes determined by $k_{PQ}$ and $k_{SQ}$. At higher energies $k_{PQ}$ and $k_{SQ}$ have less influence. Instead, changes in off axis kernel shape have an impact on output.

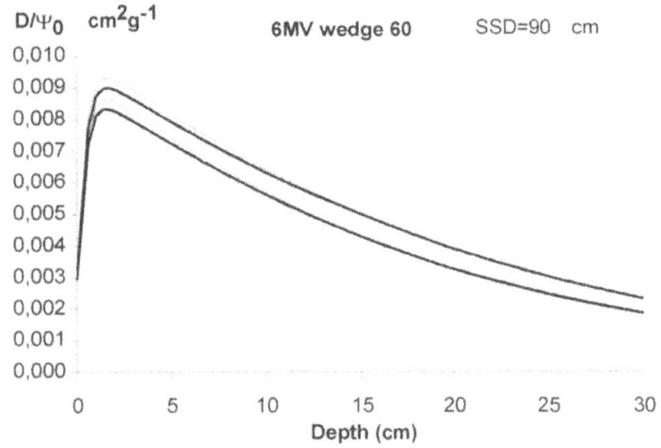


**Figure 1:** The effect of turning spectral corrections off (thin lines) as compared to full modelling (thick lines) for 10x10 cm$^2$ and 20x20 cm$^2$ fields with 60 degree wedge.

The change in kernel shape was calculated separately for a point kernel representative of 18 MV at central axis and at 10° off axis position, as shown in fig. 2. The impact on calculated relative distributions was small but for a wedged, 20x20 cm$^2$, the output was underestimated with 2.5% when kernel changes were neglected.

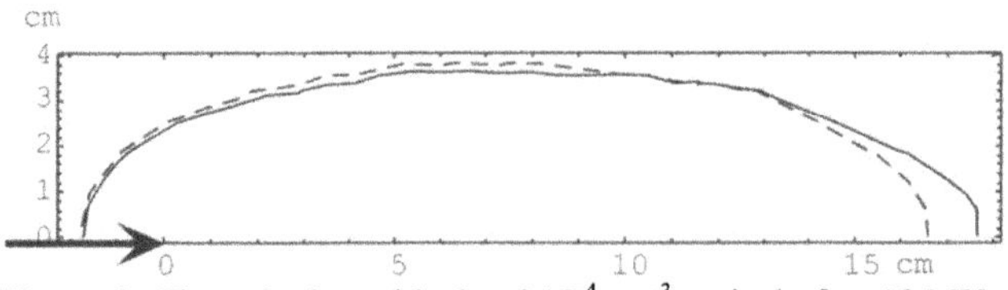


**Figure 2:** The point kernel isolevel 10$^{-4}$ cm$^{-3}$ typical of an 18 MV beam at beam axis (full line) and at a 10 degree off axis position (hatched). The primary photon incidents from left with the interaction point at the origin.

Since a generic description of the narrow beam attenuation coefficient for several machines is published [2], beam commissioning does not necessarily need to involve explicit attenuation measurements provided satisfactory dose result is obtained by using published data.

**Monte Carlo phase space sampling**
The lateral variation of the narrow beam attenuation coefficient may also be applied to generate phase space sampling for Monte Carlo dose calculations. Essentially, what is needed is an "energy shifter" such that a photon sampled from an open beam spectrum at the central axis gets its energy shifted to a lower value by a distribution that is consistent with the change in attenuation parameters.

## Conclusions

Methods for modelling several secondary order effects related to beam quality changes in photon beams has been developed and demonstrated in a point kernel implementation. The only input data needed to describe the off axis change in beam quality is the narrow beam attenuation coefficient which is experimentally accessible by simple means and also published for the most common treatment machines. For wedges, only modulation and material specification is needed to model effects from spectral changes.

## References

[1] Ahnesjö A and Aspradakis M M 1999 Dose calculations for external photon beams in radiotherapy *Phys. Med. Biol.* **44** R99-R155
[2] Tailor R C *et al* 1998 A generic off-axis energy correction for linac photon beam dosimetry *Med. Phys.* **25** 662-667
[3] Ahnesjö A, Weber L and Nilsson P 1995 Modeling transmission and scatter for photon beam attenuators *Med. Phys.* **22** 1711-1720

# Obtaining Realistic Spectra of Photon and Electron Beams

**MD Altschuler, P Bloch, BE Bjarngard, A Kassaee, and J McDonough**

Department of Radiation Oncology, University of Pennsylvania, Philadelphia PA 19104

## Introduction

Modern dose calculation algorithms for high-energy photon and electron beams usually require knowledge of the spectrum of each beam in order to generate a dose kernel. Because the spectrum of a high-energy beam is difficult to obtain by measurement, indirect methods have been used.

In this paper we describe a method that can obtain *realistic* photon and electron spectra for clinical beams from depth dose measurements. Because the problem is ill conditioned, that is, many spectra can fit a set of beam measurements quite well, we need to impose some constraint to ensure that a physically realistic spectrum is obtained. For photon beams, the analysis of depth dose at shallow depths, where the range of Compton-generated electrons increases rapidly with photon energy, is used to obtain information about the incident photon spectrum. Our discussion will describe the mathematical technique to ensure extraction of a realistic spectrum.

## Material and methods

### Photons

For photons, we computed by MonteCarlo the depth doses for $6 \times 6$ cm$^2$ monoenergetic beams for each integral value of MeV from 1 to 20 MeV, and for 0.5, 1.5, and 25 MeV, to obtain a total of 23 basis functions. Ten million primary photon histories were followed to ensure a statistical variation of less than 1% in the mean energy deposited along the central ray. Further reduction in statistical noise for depths exceeding 1 cm was achieved by smoothing with a running average over five depth increments of the 2-mm grid. The calculated depth dose distributions were normalized to value 100 at depth 101 mm (the midpoint of a grid step). Depth dose was sampled every 2 mm between depths 1 and 119 mm, every 10 mm between 125 and 155 mm, and every 50 mm between 200 and 300 mm, for a total of 67 depths. The measured depth dose of 6 and 15 MV photon beams of SSD 100 cm and $6 \times 6$ cm$^2$ field size were used as the data from which spectra were extracted. The small field size minimizes the contribution of contaminating electrons and achieves lateral charged particle equilibrium for clinical photon energies.

The shapes of the normalized basis functions (percent depth dose vs depth), become nearly parallel beyond 6 cm depth. At shallower depths the range of the Compton-generated electrons increases rapidly with photon energy, so that the monoenergetic basis functions are distinguishable and the problem less ill conditioned. Expanding a function as a series of nearly parallel basis functions is a very ill conditioned procedure. Without additional constraints on the solution of the fitting (matrix) equation, some coefficients of such an expansion may become negative. Even with constraints, restriction of the solution to non-negative coefficients can lead to zero values and a jagged rather than smooth spectrum. Consequently, including depth dose values for the deeper depths in the expansion provides little spectral information and leads to ill conditioning. By including only data from depths less than say 11 cm, we can keep information relevant to the spectrum.

The basis functions and measured depth dose for the same geometry are used with the Cimmino feasibility algorithm to extract the spectra of clinical beams. The constraints, corresponding to measured depth dose values at different depths, can be broadened to include a tolerance domain $\varepsilon$ about each measured value (that is, an allowed margin between the measured and derived percent depth dose values). The problem then transforms from solving a matrix equation (for an intersection of hyperplanes) to that of satisfying matrix inequalities (for an intersection of hyperslabs). The convergent Cimmino feasibility algorithm can handle the hyperslab problem. The thickness $\varepsilon$ of the hyperslab is a single parameter that can be varied. If the hyperslab is too thick, the resulting spectrum will be too smooth, and information will be lost. If the hyperslab is too thin, the resulting spectrum will usually be jagged, with zero and peak values, and the resulting spectrum will be unrealistic.

It should be noted that mathematically (by least squares or minmax methods) the best fit to the measured depth dose is almost always given by the thinnest hyperslabs, thus a jagged spectrum. However, the ill-conditioned problem is such that a reasonable hyperslab thickness $\varepsilon$ provides a physically realistic spectrum with very little increase in fitting error.

Suppose we start with a jagged spectrum (of spectral amplitude vs energy) and increase the hyperslab thickness $\varepsilon$ for the constraints. How do we know which $\varepsilon$ to choose? By solving the hyperslab fitting problem for different values of $\varepsilon$, we can plot as a function of $\varepsilon$ both (1) the maximum absolute deviation of the calculated from measured depth dose, and (2) the integral of the absolute curvature of the derived spectrum. The latter function decreases rapidly with increasing $\varepsilon$ to a plateau that corresponds to a smooth spectrum with the correct peak energy. The former function increases with $\varepsilon$ but encounters a local minimum just above the $\varepsilon$ at which the integral of the absolute curvature of the spectrum reaches its minimum plateau. By choosing the hyperslab thickness to correspond to the value of the local minimum (of maximum absolute deviation of calculated from measured depth dose) we can obtain spectra which are realistic.

## Electrons

For electrons, we use MonteCarlo-derived monoenergetic depth dose basis functions at every energy integral value from 1 to 25 MeV calculated for 15 × 15-cm$^2$ fields and 100 cm SSD. Both the measured depth dose (by solid state diode) of a clinical beam and the calculated depth doses of the monoenergetic basis functions are sampled at 2 mm depths from 1 to 147 mm and normalized at depth 3 mm. The same procedure described above for photons can then be carried out. The basis functions for electrons are less ill conditioned than those for photons because the range of the electron is a unique function of the energy of the electron.

A MonteCarlo-derived depth dose basis function was also generated for the bremmsstrahlung component. In the simulation, the target for bremmsstrahlung production was tungsten located at the typical position of the scattering foil about 90 cm from isocenter. The thickness of the tungsten target was the range of a monoenergetic electron possessing the nominal energy of the electron beam. To obtain the energy fluence spectrum at isocenter, the Cimmino-derived spectral weights for the monoenergetic electron depth dose basis functions were weighted by the energy deposition at the normalization depth.

For electron beams, the criterion for a realistic spectrum is not as clear. The electron beam spectrum should clearly peak sharply near its nominal energy. But the spectrum may also include lower-energy scattered electrons (thus being bimodal) and a small bremmsstrahlung component.

## Results and discussion

The photon spectra for the 6 and 15 MV clinical photon beams were derived by the Cimmino algorithm from depth dose values sampled at shallow depths. The smallest value of $\varepsilon$ for which the spectral weights (of the higher energy components) were monotonically decreasing was found to be between 0.9 and 1.2 %. The value of $\varepsilon$ corresponding to these realistic spectra were determined by finding (1) the maximum fractional discrepancy between measured and calculated depth doses at any depth and (2) the domain where the integral of the absolute curvature of the spectrum over energy was small. Thus a linear combination of monoenergetic depth doses (basis vectors) weighted by the Cimmino-derived weights gave calculated depth dose values within about 1% of the measured depth dose for all depths. The Cimmino-derived spectra required no *a priori* assumptions about the maximum photon energy of the beam. The derived energy fluence spectrum for the 6 and 15 MV photon beams agreed well with previously obtained Monte-Carlo-derived spectra [1,2].

The electron spectra were derived from measured depth doses for electron beams from a Varian 2100C/D accelerator. Figure 1 shows the Cimmino-derived energy fluence spectra in air for the nominal 6 and 15 MeV clinical electron beams. The depth dose values calculated from these spectra were within 1% of the measured values

## Conclusion

Realistic spectra for clinical photon and electron beams can be readily obtained with the Cimmino feasibility algorithm if depth dose measurements together with a small tolerance margin are used as constraints.

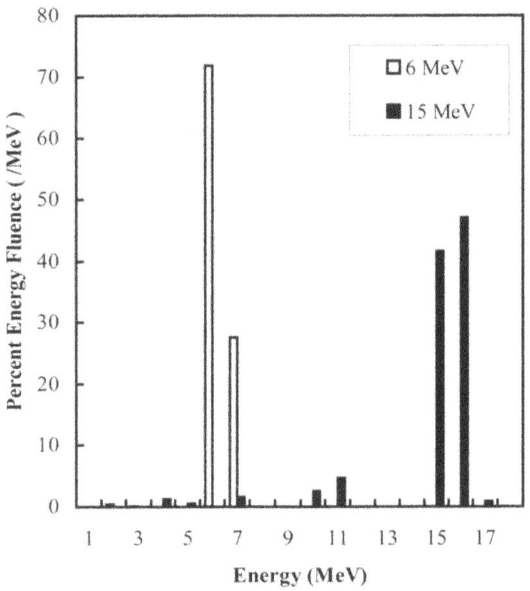


**Figure 1:** Cimmino-derived electron spectra for 6 and 15 MeV clinical beams from measured depth dose and a constraint tolerance.

## References

[1] Altschuler MD, Bloch P, Buhle EL, Ayyalasomayajula S 1992 3D dose calculations for electron and photon beams *Phys Med Biol* **37** 391-411

[2] Bloch P, Altschuler MD, Bjarngard BE, Kassaee A, and McDonough J 2000 Determining clinical photon beam spectra from measured depth dose with the Cimmino algorithm Phys Med Biol **45** 171-183

# A Measured Data Set for Evaluating Electron Beam Dose Algorithms

**Robert Boyd and Kenneth R. Hogstrom**

Department of Radiation Physics, The University of Texas M.D. Anderson Cancer Center, 1515 Holcombe Blvd., Houston, TX, USA

## Introduction

The accuracy of an electron beam dose algorithm as implemented in a teatment planning system should be verified using measured data representative of patient anatomy and treatment beams. The Electron Collaborative Working Group (ECWG) Electron Beam Dose Algorithm Verificaton Data [1] has been the standard for such evaluations the past several years; however, it contains inconsistencies [2] and possible systematic errors [3] resulting from data collection or post-processing. It is our belief that some of the measured data in the ECWG data set is insufficiently accurate for evaluating the accuracy of an electron beam dose algorithm. An improved measured data set utilizing strict quality control was developed, and its accuracy was verified using Monte Carlo techniques.

## Material and methods

### Measured data set

A measured data set to be used to evaluate the accuracy of dose calculated by an electron beam dose algorithm was developed using geometric configurations similar to those of the ECWG data set. Table 1 lists the configuration of the phantoms used in the measured data set. A low (9 MeV) and a high (20 MeV) energy electron beam, similar to the ECWG data set, were selected to evaluate any energy-dependent defeciency in an electron beam dose algorithm. All measurements were done using a single Varian Clinac 2100C (Varian Oncology Systems, Palo Alto, CA) to minimize any errors in consistency that could occur from using different machines (e.g. differences in electron beam energy).

| Experiment # | Phantom Geometry |
|---|---|
| 1-4 | Homogeneous Water (100- and 110-cm SSD) |
| 5,6 | Horizontal air slab |
| 7 | Vertical air slab (20 MeV only) |
| 8,9 | Horizontal bone slab |
| 10 | Vertical bone slab (20 MeV only) |
| 11,12 | 2-cm stepped surface |
| 13,14 | Nose surface |

**Table 1:** Phantom geometries of measured data set.

Dose was measured in water using two p-Si diode electron field detectors (Scanditronix Medical AB, Uppsala, Sweden) in conjunction with a Wellhöfer dosimetry system (Wellhöfer Dosimetrie, Schwarzenbruk, Germany). The Wellhöfer system allows for continuous scanning when one detector is used as a reference and the other is used for point measurements. The effective detection diameter of the diode detector is 2.5 mm, which allows for high spatial resolution in regions of electron disequilibrium.

Two slabs, one consisting of SR4 bone substitute ($\rho$ = 1.585) to model hard bone and one consisting of styrofoam ($\rho$ = 0.0265) to simulate air, were used for the internal inhomogeneity experiments. The dimensions of each slab were 1 cm x 3 cm x 18 cm with the long axis placed perpendicular to the measurement plane, which is a transverse plane in the water phantom that contains central axis. An acrylic clamping device, attachable to the walls of water phantom, was used to hold the ends of the long axis of the slab in place inside the water phantom during measurements. The device allowed the slab to be localized and oriented at the desired depth. The slab was positioned such that its proximal end was 1 cm from the water surface. Each slab was oriented with its 3-cm width placed both perpendicular (horizontal) and parallel (vertical) to the beam axis. Only the 20-MeV beam was used for experiments involving a vertically oriented slab, while both energies were used for a horizontally oriented slab. The source-to-surface distance (SSD) in each experiment was 100 cm.

Styrofoam blocks were used for experiments involving water phantoms with irregular surfaces. The styrofoam blocks were abutted to the distal end of the electron applicator and partially submerged in the water phantom, which displaced water into the desired surface shape. Figure 1 shows the configuration of the 2-cm stepped surface experiment and Figure 2 shows the configuration of the nose surface experiment. The source-to-surface distance in each experiment was 102 cm. The styrofoam block used for the nose surface experiment had a pit drilled into the center such that the displaced water formed a right triangular cylinder (2-cm base, 3-cm high, 4-cm long) identical to the dimensions of the acrylic triangular cylinder used in experiment #9 of the ECWG data set. Trapped air bubbles were removed from the styrofoam/water interface before measurements were performed.

Before each experiment cental-axis depth dose was measured in water at 100 cm SSD. The slab or styrofoam block was then placed and centered along the beam central axis using several profile scans. Once the experimental geometry was properly configured another depth dose, used to normalize the measured profiles, was measured 5 cm lateral to central axis in order to minimize the effects of high dose gradients distal to the heterogeneity along the central axis. Dose profiles were then scanned in the central-axis transverse plane 5 mm below the slab or water surface at incremental depths of 2.5 mm to a depth where the maximum dose was less than 5% relative to the maximum in water.

During post processing the measured depth-dose curves and dose profiles were smoothed using Wellhöfer software tools. Once the data was smoothed a 2D dose distribution was constructed from the measured dose profiles and depth-dose curve. All data was normalized to the maximum dose on central axis in homogeneous water. Finally, an average dose distribution was determined for each experiment from measurements and post processing performed on three separate occasions. Typical data precision was approximately 1% for the standard deviation of the mean in areas of uniform dose.

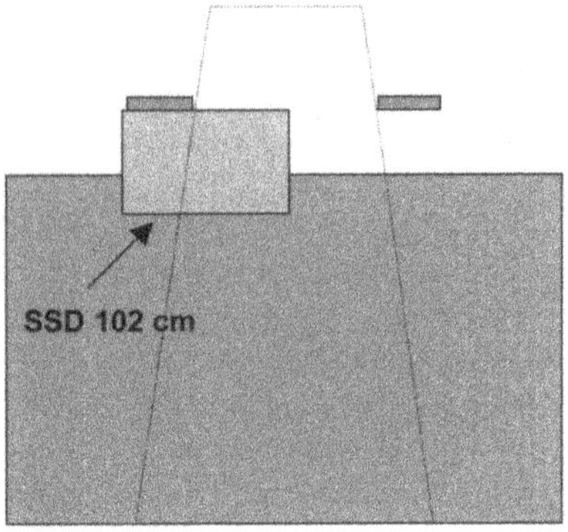


**Figure 1:** Schematic of the stepped surface experiment. The electron beam field is shown (dotted line) with styrofoam block abutted to the applicator and patially immersed in water to create desired surface.

### Monte Carlo verification

Confidence in the accuracy and consistency of the measured data set was gained by comparison with Monte Carlo (MC) calculated dose distributions. The MC software package BEAM [4] was used to model the Clinac 2100 accelerator and to collect a phase space at the distal end of the collimator. To model the sharp irregular surface of the nose experiment another BEAM module was added and a phase space collected at 102 cm SSD. The MC program DOSXYZ was then used to calculate the dose distribution in the transverse plane containing the central axis for comparison with measurements.

The physical characteristics of the accelerator head were modeled with component modules of the BEAM system using information supplied by Varian Oncology Systems under a non-disclosure agreement [5]. An electron source with a Gaussian spatial distribution (1.5-mm full-width at half maximum) was utilized in the BEAM system. The incident energy at the exit window of the accelerator was assumed to be monoenergetic and was determined by manually adjusting the energy until the calculated and measured central-axis depth of 50% dose in water matched. The maximum calculated dose on the central axis in water was used to normalize susequent dose calculations using heterogeneous phantoms.

The EGS4 run parameters were set for both collection of the phase space and subsequent dose calculation as follows: AE = PCUT = 0.70 MeV and AP = PCUT = 0.10 MeV. Approximately $10^9$ histories were simulated for both the normalization factor and the dose distributions in order to achieve <1.0% standard deviation of the mean dose using a 2.5x2.5x2.0-mm$^3$ grid spacing.

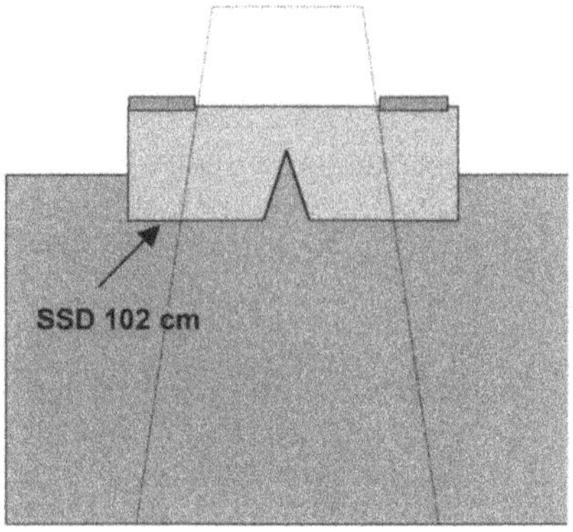


**Figure 2:** Schematic of the irregular nose surface experiment. The electron beam field is shown (dotted line) with styrofoam block abutted to the applicator and patially immersed in water to create desired surface.

## Results and discussion

For this discussion only data from the 20-MeV vertical air slab and nose surface experiments will be compared to MC calculations. The remainder of the data set showed comparable results. Isodose contours in the dose distribution comparisons are shown at 10% intervals, starting at the 10% contour (relative to the central-axis maximum dose in water). Regions on the isodose plot where the difference between the measured and calculated dose is greater than 2% (relative to maximum dose in water) are shaded grey; light grey where the distance-to-agreement (DTA) is within 2 mm and dark grey otherwise. A cumulative dose difference – fractional area histogram is also calculated for the central region plotted in the isodose comparisons.

Figure 3 shows the comparison between the measured and MC-calculated dose distributions for the vertical air slab experiment. Only a few points show dose differences greater than 2% and are located in the high gradient dose region near the distal end of the styrofoam slab. Figure 4 shows the comparison between the measured and MC-calculated dose distributions for the nose surface experiment. Again only a few points show dose differences greater than 2% and are located in the high gradient dose region near the surface.

Figure 5 shows a comparison of the dose difference – fractional area histograms for the 20-MeV homogeneous water, vertical air slab, and nose surface experiment. At 1.0% dose difference the fractional area was 7.5% for the homogeneous water experiment, 17.6% for the vertical air slab experiment, and 11.1% for the nose surface experiment. At 2.0% dose difference the fractional area was 0.0% for the homogeneous water experiment, 0.9% for the vertical air slab experiment, and 1.1% for the nose surface experiment.

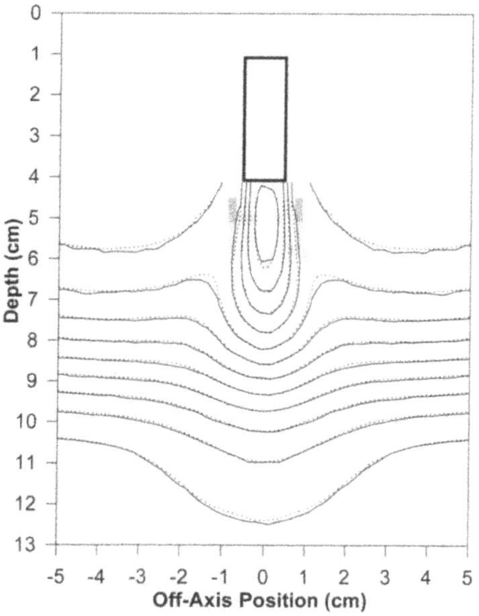


**Figure 3:** 20-MeV vertical air slab experiment. Central region isodose comparison of measured dose (dashed) and MC-calculated dose (solid). Position of styrofoam slab is shown with thick solid line. Points with dose differences > 2% are shaded light gray and points with dose differences > 2% and DTA > 2 mm are shaded dark gray.

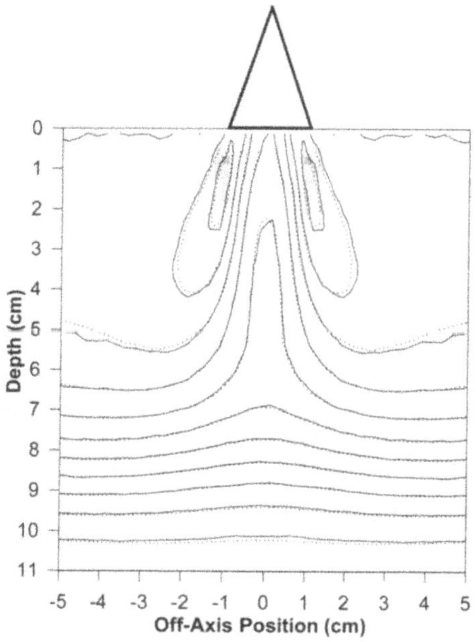


**Figure 4:** 20-MeV nose surface experiment. Central region isodose comparison of measured dose (dashed) and MC-calculated dose (solid). Position of styrofoam slab is shown with thick solid line. Points with dose differences > 2% are shaded light gray and points with dose differences > 2% and DTA > 2 mm are shaded dark gray.

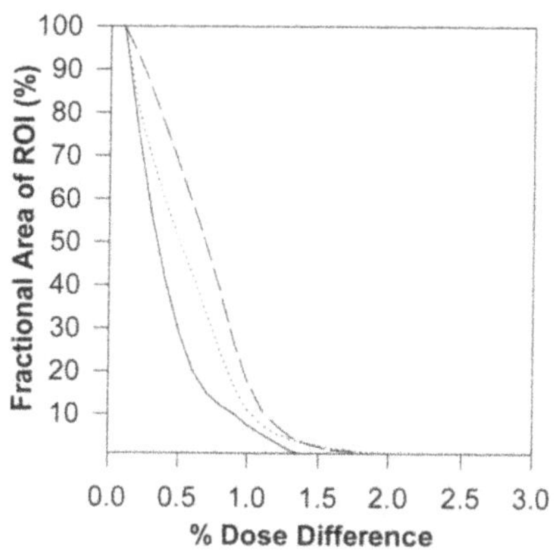


**Figure 5:** Cumulative dose difference-fractional area histogram of the central region (-5.0 to 5.0 cm off-axis position) for the 20-MeV homogeneous water (solid line), vertical air slab (dotted line), and the nose surface (dashed line) experiment.

## Conclusion

The measured data set showed good precision (<1%), and its agreement with MC-calculated dose gives a high degree of confidence in its accuracy. Hence, the quality of these data is superior to that of ECWG and should allow for better evaluation of the accuracy of an electron beam dose algorithm. Also, the benchmarking of the MC should allow it to be used to produce dose distributions in actual patients that can be used to verify analytical algorithms such as the pencil-beam redefinition algorithm.

## References

[1] Shiu A S, Tung S, Hogstrom K R, Wong J W, Gerber R L, Harms W B, Purdy J A, Ten Haken P K, McShan D L, and Fraass B A 1992 Verification data for electron beam dose algorithms *Med Phys* **19** 623-636

[2] Fippel M, Kawrakow I, and Friedrich K 1997 Electron beam dose calculations with the VMC algorithm and the verification data of the NCI working group *Phys Med Biol* **42** 501-520

[3] Boyd R A 1997 The effect of using an initial polyenergetic spectrum with the electron pencil-beam redefinition algorithm *M.S. Thesis, The University of Texas Health Science Center-Houston, Graduate School of Biomedical Sciences*

[4] Rogers D W O, Faddegon B A, Ding G X, Ma C M, We J, and Mackie T R 1995 BEAM: A Monte Carlo code to simulate radiotherapy treatment units *Med Phys* **22** 503-525

[5] Bieda M R 1999 A Monte Carlo method for commissioning electron beams *M.S. Thesis, The University of Texas Health Science Center-Houston, Graduate School of Biomedical Sciences*

# The importance of the dose calculation model on plan evaluation for IMRT

**Moyed Miften**

Computerized Medical System, Inc., St. Louis, MO 63132, USA

## Introduction

The aim of Intensity Modulation Radiation Therapy (IMRT) is to deliver a relatively homogeneous dose to a regular or irregular shaped target while sparing the surrounding normal structures. This can be achieved, regardless of the planning and delivery techniques, by varying the intensity of beams across the fields of treatment. Many IMRT conformal treatments are characterized by the use of fields with multiple segments incident on a target from many gantry angles in order to achieve uniform dose coverage to the target and spare critical structures.

The problem of calculating accurate dose distributions is of basic importance in 3D conformal radiotherapy and IMRT treatments. Many studies state that it is essential to perform accurate dose calculations using only model-based algorithms.[1] Such algorithms must accurately handle the intensity variation across the field and account for the effect of tissue inhomogeneities on the dose distributions. However, many IMRT implementations employ empirical or semi-empirical dose calculation models (conventional models). The reason for using these conventional models is computational speed since optimization of IMRT treatments may take a long time to compute using accurate model-based algorithms, such as the Superposition algorithm. Therefore, a question arises: *What is the importance of the dose calculation model on plan evaluation for IMRT?*

In this work, we present intensity modulated (IM) plan comparison results for treatments of prostate gland, head and neck, and lung tumors using the measurement-based Clarkson[2] and model-based Multigrid Superposition[3] (MGS) dose calculation algorithms. The plan dose volume histograms (DVHs) for the planning target volume (PTV) and sensitive structures, and normal tissue complication probability (NTCP) and tumor control probability (TCP) were compared for both algorithms. Dose distributions, observed in the lung plan, vary significantly with respect to dose uniformity. Differences in the maximum dose of up to 14% were observed in the PTV and sensitive structures for the lung and head and neck plans. Moreover, a difference in the biological outcomes of up to 14% in the NTCP and 4% in the TCP was noticed.

## Material and methods

The IM plans were derived through forward planning using the FOCUS RTP system (Computerized Medical Systems, St. Louis, MO). The plans were generated using both 6 MV and 18 MV beam energies with multiple multileaf collimator (MLC) segments in each field. Parameters used in the forward planning optimization process are to achieve a conformal uniform dose distribution in the PTV, provided that certain dose limits for sensitive structures are not violated. Prescription dose for each plan PTV was normalized to the 95% isodose surface. The goal was to achieve uniform dose coverage to the 95% isodose surface. The IM plan beam setups were first generated using the MGS model as the reference (benchmark) plan. Then, calculations for the *same plan* beam setups and prescriptions were performed using the Clarkson algorithm.

The volume dependence (n), NTCP versus dose slope (m) and the dose to reference volume leading to 50% complication ($TD_{50}$) parameter values, used to calculate NTCP in this study, are based on the work of Burman et al.[4] The TCP model uses the principles of the linear-quadratic model of cell survival. The TCP model and parameters are based on the work of Webb and Nahum.[5]

In the TCP model, a value of 0.35 $Gy^{-1}$ was used for the mean radiosensitivity of a cell population ($\alpha_{mean}$). The standard deviation ($\sigma_\alpha$), or level of inter patient variability of radiosensitivity, was set to 0.08 $Gy^{-1}$. A value of 1 million/cc for the clonogenic cell density was assumed. The effective doubling time for tumor clonogens ($T_{eff}$) of 14, 5 and 5 days were used in the prostate, head and neck and lung IM plans, respectively. The overall elapsed time (T) of 39 days, over the course of radiotherapy treatment, was used. The time between the first treatment and when tumor proliferation begins (kick-off time, T) was set to 0.

The same parameter values were used to calculate TCP and NTCP in both the Clarkson and MGS based plans.

### Dose calculation models

Tissue inhomogeneities cause the greatest distortion in dose distributions compared with those calculated in water phantom. Tissue inhomogeneities that lay along the primary beam fan lines affect the fluence at each point in the patient. The Clarkson and MGS algorithms account correctly for this variation by performing ray tracing through voxel densities along divergent beam fan lines.

In the MGS algorithm, the dose at a point $\underline{r}$ is calculated by convolving total energy released per unit mass (terma) with a density scaled energy deposition kernel:

$$D(\underline{r}) = \int T(\underline{r}') \frac{\rho(\underline{r}')}{\bar{\rho}} K(\bar{\rho}.l(\underline{r}-\underline{r}'), \underline{r}-\underline{r}')d^3r'^3 \quad (2)$$

where $T$ is the terma at the interaction point $\underline{r}'$, $K$ is the energy deposition kernel, $\bar{\rho}$ is the average density along the path between the interaction and dose deposition sites $l(\underline{r}-\underline{r}')$, $\underline{r}-\underline{r}'$ is the distance between interaction and dose deposition sites and $\rho(\underline{r}')$ is the density of the interaction site. $K$ is distorted by the radiological distance $\bar{\rho}.l(\underline{r}-\underline{r}')$. The density scaling method was used to scale the energy deposition kernels to account for the effect of tissue inohomogeneities on the dose distribution. The terma at the interaction point may be calculated as:

$$T(r') = I_{oc}(x,y)I(x,y)\frac{\mu}{\rho}\exp(-\mu|r' - r_o|) \qquad (3)$$

where $\mu/\rho$ is the mass attenuation coefficient, $\mu$ is the linear attenuation coefficient, $\underline{r}_o$ is a point at the patient surface, $I_{oc}$ is the primary off-center relative beam intensity (relative to photon fluence on central axis) along the beam fan line through the position *(x,y)*, which accounts for beam horns. *I(x,y)* is the intensity map which accounts for the modification in the primary intensity due to field defining elements, such as MLC. Note that the MGS dose calculation model accounts for the intensity variations along the field by modifying the intensity along each beam fan line emanating from the source in the terma calculation.

In the Clarkson algorithm, the dose is calculated at a point *(x,y)* in a plane at depth *d* as the sum of primary and scatter dose:

$$D(x,y,d) = I_{oc}(x,y)\left[I(x,y)TAR(0,d_{eff}) + SAR(x,y,d_{eff})\right] \quad (1)$$

*TAR* is the central-axis tissue to air ratio at the radiological depth $d_{eff}$ extrapolated to zero field size. *SAR* is the scatter to air ratio at $d_{eff}$ for the MLC arrangement at the dose point. Here, the Clarkson algorithm accounts for the intensity variation by modifying the primary dose along each beam fan line. Notice that, unlike the MGS algorithm, the Clarkson algorithm does not model the effect of tissue inhomogeneities on scatter dose

**Treatment plans prescriptions**

IM plans were generated for the treatment of prostate gland, head and neck and lung tumors. The prostate plan PTV was treated to 60 Gy. The PTV in the head and neck plan was treated to 60 Gy. The lung plan PTV was treated to 68 Gy and regional nodes were treated to 45 Gy. A margin of 1 cm was added to the PTV to account for positional differences due to setup errors and organ motion.

## Results and discussion

**Prostate IM plan**

The mean, minimum and maximum doses, received by the target, were generated using the Clarkson and MGS models shown in Table 1, along with the TCP and NTCP values. The mean dose, TCP, rectum NTCP and bladder NTCP values are within 1% using both models. The DVHs for the target and sensitive structures, shown in Figure 1, are almost identical.

(a)

| Calculation algorithm | Mean target dose (Gy) | Min. target dose (Gy) | Max. target dose (Gy) |
|---|---|---|---|
| Clarkson | 63.28 | 59.04 | 64.30 |
| MGS | 62.95 | 59.99 | 63.74 |

(b)

| Calculation algorithm | TCP | NTCP rectum | NTCP bladder |
|---|---|---|---|
| Clarkson | 54.3 | 1.8 | 0.1 |
| MGS | 53.6 | 2.0 | 0.1 |

**Table 1:** Prostate IM plan. (a) Mean, minimum and maximum dose in the PTV for the Clarkson and MGS models; (b) TCP and NTCP values.

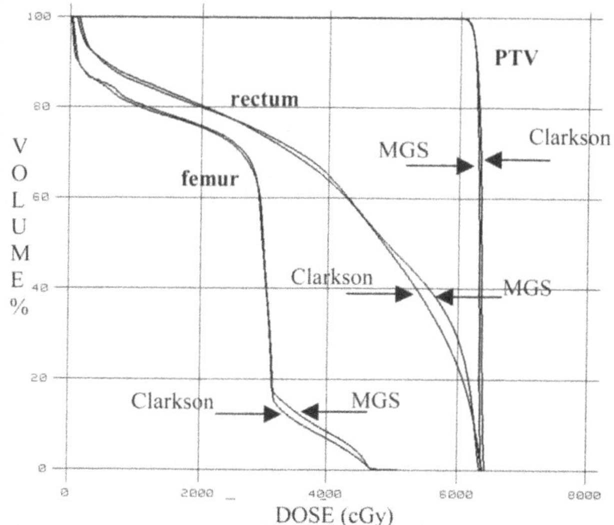


**Figure 1**: Prostate plan PTV, rectum and left femur dose volume histograms for the Clarkson and MGS models.

Results show that the use of conventional models is sufficient for prostate treatments. This is due to the fact that the prostate gland and sensitive structures (rectum, bladder) have densities and properties close to that of water. Those different structures cause little difference in dose compared with dose calculated in water. Therefore, the Clarkson model, which is based on measurements in water, give results close to that of MGS.

**Head and neck IM plan**

The DVH for PTV, right parotid and left parotid are shown in Figure 2 along with TCP and NTCP values in Table 2. The IM conformal plan was created to deliver a high conformal dose to the target on right side of the patient head and neck, spare the left parotid, and minimize the dose to the other critical structures. The mean PTV dose and TCP values are within 1% for both models. However, the Clarkson model *underestimates* the NTCP of the right parotid by 10% compared to MGS. The DVH shows the right Parotid receives a total of 4% less dose using the Clarkson model.

(a)

| Calculation algorithm | Mean target dose (Gy) | Min. target dose (Gy) | Max. target dose (Gy) |
|---|---|---|---|
| Clarkson | 62.25 | 59.34 | 65.71 |
| MGS | 62.40 | 58.55 | 65.35 |

(b)

| Calculation algorithm | TCP | NTCP right parotid | NTCP left parotid | NTCP spinal cord |
|---|---|---|---|---|
| Clarkson | 35.76 | 52.87 | 0 | 0.24 |
| MGS | 36.07 | 62.44 | 0 | 0.35 |

**Table 2:** Head and neck IM plan. (a) Mean, minimum and maximum dose in the PTV for the Clarkson and MGS models; (b) TCP and NTCP values.

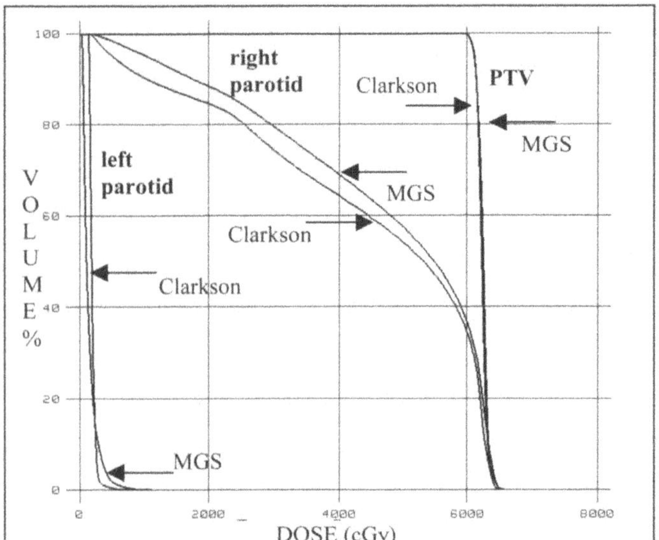

**Figure 2**: Head and neck plan PTV, left parotid and right parotid dose volume histograms for the Clarkson and MGS models.

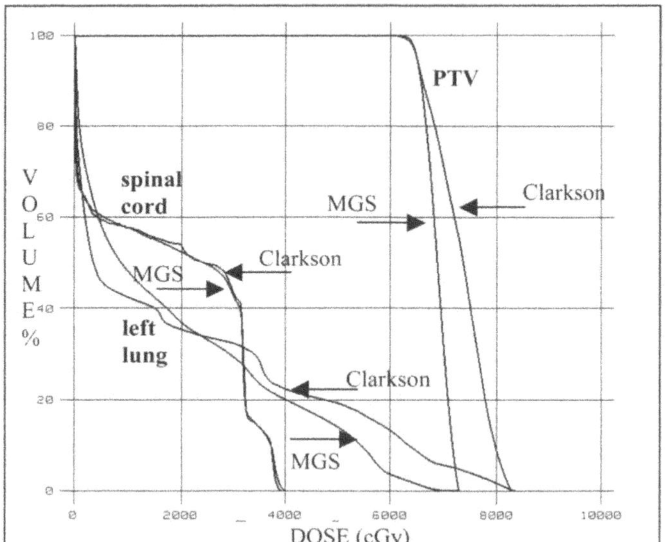

**Figure 3**: Lung plan PTV, left lung and spinal cord dose volume histograms for the Clarkson and MGS models.

The results from the Clarkson model may *incorrectly* point the treatment planner or the inverse planning model to increase dose to the tumor, if a higher NTCP limit for the right parotid was acceptable. Hence, increasing the *already underestimated* dose to the parotid may cause further complications. The Clarkson model generates less accurate doses, and therefore incorrect biological outcomes for the critical structures are predicted. This is mainly due to the effect of not accurately handling tissue inhomogeneities and missing tissue scatter, which dominates head and neck treatments.

**Lung IM plan**

The lung IM conformal plan showed the largest difference between the Clarkson and MGS models. The doses received by the target, TCP and NTCP values are shown in Table 3. The DVH of the plan is shown in Figure 3. The Clarkson model shows the maximum PTV dose is hotter by 14% compared to MGS. In addition, the Clarkson model generates less uniform dose in the PTV and overestimates the TCP by 4% and the left lung NTCP by 12%. Furthermore, the DVH shows that more of the left lung volume, where the tumor resides, is irradiated using the Clarkson algorithm.

(a)

| Calculation algorithm | Mean target dose (Gy) | Min. target dose (Gy) | Max. target dose (Gy) |
|---|---|---|---|
| Clarkson | 73.07 | 61.14 | 83.23 |
| MGS | 68.54 | 59.34 | 72.83 |

(b)

| Calculation algorithm | TCP | NTCP left lung | NTCP esophagus | NTCP spinal cord |
|---|---|---|---|---|
| Clarkson | 49.87 | 32.99 | 7.74 | 0.35 |
| MGS | 45.59 | 18.78 | 7.31 | 0.37 |

**Table 3:** Lung IM plan. (a) Mean, minimum and maximum dose in the PTV for the Clarkson and MGS models; (b) TCP and NTCP values.

The plan clearly shows the limitation of conventional models in lung cases, where tissue inhomogeneities affect dose distributions greatly. The use of models that incorporate simple inohomogeneity corrections can not be used for optimization and IMRT treatments in lung. Such models will generate inaccurate dose distributions and biological expectations in the target and critical structures.

## Conclusions

The IMRT plans clearly indicate the need for accurate dose calculation models to determine the dose in the target and critical structures for lung and head and neck treatments. Biological models were used to evaluate and compare IMRT plans. Results suggest that IMRT optimization algorithms that employ DVH, TCP and NTCP objective functions should not use conventional dose calculation models.

## References

[1] Mohan R 1997 Why Monte Carlo? *Proc. of the XIIth Int. Conf. On the Use of Computers in Radiation Therapy* 16-18

[2] Cunningham J R, Shrivastava P N and Wilkinson 1972 Program IRREG-calculation of dose from irregularly shaped radiation beams *Comp. Prog. Biomed.* **2** 192

[3] Miften M, Wiesmeyer M, Suzanne M and Krippner K 1999 Implementation of FFT convolution and multigrid superposition models in the FOCUS RTP system *Phys. Med. Bio.* (accepted)

[4] Burman C, Kutcher G J, Emami B and Goitein M 1991 Fitting of normal tissue tolerance data to an analytic function *Int. J. Rad. Onc. Bio. Phys.* **21** 123-135

[5] Webb S and Nahum A E 1993 A model calculating tumor control probability in radiotherapy including the effects of inhomogeneous distributions of dose and clonogenic cell density *Phys. Med. Bio.* **38** 653-666

# Biological optimisation including both the normal and tumour tissues in the target volume.

**Lois Jones[1], Peter Hoban[2]**

[1]Department of Radiation Oncology, Liverpool Hospital, Locked Bag 7103, Liverpool BC NSW 1871 Australia , and [2]Department of Radiation Oncology, Prince of Wales Hospital, High st, Randwick NSW 2031 Australia

## Introduction

Intensity Modulated Radiotherapy (IMRT) provides the potential for conformal dose distributions far superior to those achieveable with previous methods. Various optimisation methods and cost functions have been suggested for the required inverse planning techniques. Despite the limitations of biologically based methods, these ideally would provide the basis for any cost function considered. This study has considered biologically based optimisation methods. A fluence changing method based on biological factors and including the complications to normal tissue which may be in the target volume was considered. A tissue weight changing method has also been considered and can also be based both on physical or biological parameters.

## Material and methods

To consider the possiblity of including the normal tissues in the target volume when optimising, a ratio fluence changing method which has been previously discussed (1) was used. The situation of a critical and target volume such as a prostate treatment was assessed. A physical optimisation and two biological optimisation methods one with and one without the normal tissues in the target volume were considered. Thirty-five beams each containing 99 pencil beams were evenly positioned around the prostate being treated and the ratio method used to adjust the fluence of each pencil beam following each iteration. The physical method used was as follows:

$$R_{physj} = 1 + \frac{\sum w_{ij} \Delta D_{ij} / \sum w_{ij}}{\sum D_{ij} / N}$$

Where ΔD is the change in dose for each voxel determined by the difference between the intended dose and the delivered dose, N is the total number of voxels being traversed by the beam and w represents the weights of the relevant tissue.

For the biological ratio the following was used when the normal tissues were included in the target volume:

$$R_{biol1j} = 1 + \frac{\begin{pmatrix} n_t w_t \Delta EUD + n_n w_n \Delta IBED_n + \\ n_t w_{nt} \Delta IBED_{nt} + n_c w_c \Delta IBED_c \end{pmatrix} \Big/ \begin{pmatrix} n_t w_t + n_n w_n + \\ n_t w_{nt} + n_c w_c \end{pmatrix}}{\left(n_t EUD_j + n_c IBED_{cj} + n_n IBED_{nj} + n_t IBED_{ntj}\right)/N}$$

and a similar expression was used when the normal tissues in the target volume were not considered:

$$R_{biol2j} = 1 + \frac{(n_t w_t \Delta EUD + n_n w_n \Delta IBED_n + n_c w_c \Delta IBED_c)/(n_t w_t + n_n w_n + n_c w_c)}{(n_t EUD_j + n_c IBED_{cj} + n_n IBED_{nj})/N}$$

Where IBED is the Integral Biological Effective Dose (2) and EUD is the Equivalent Uniform Dose (3). These values are calculated for each pencil beam and used to change the value of this beam. The tissue weights for all situations have been determined using an iterative weighting method which can also be physically or biologically based and continues to adjust the weights for the individual tissues until a required parameter is met or all weights are changed. The weights for the normal tissues in the target volume when this was considered were not dynamically changed and were maintained as low values compared to the tumour weight. This was to ensure that the dose to the tumour was not significantly reduced in an extreme attempt to minimise the complications to the normal tissues.

## Results and discussion

The results from the optimisation show that the biological optimisation including the normal tissues in the target volume can result in a much flatter dose distribution across the tumour compared to the situation where the normal tissues in the target volume are not considered. Figure 1 shows the dose distribution achieved when the normal tissues in the target volume are not considered and Figure 2 shows the dose distribution achieved when normal tissues in the target volume are considered. The situation where the normal tissues in the target volume are considered results in very similar distributions to those achieved with a physical optimisation. This perhaps provides some biological background for the homogeneous dose distributions which have always been intended with physical optimisation. For the prostate this results in dose distributions which are much more clinically acceptable. Due to the difficulty in postioning the prostate, high doses to the target volume may also result in high target doses to the rectum if the prostate moves slightly. Consequently, homogeneous dose distributions to the prostate may be more acceptable.

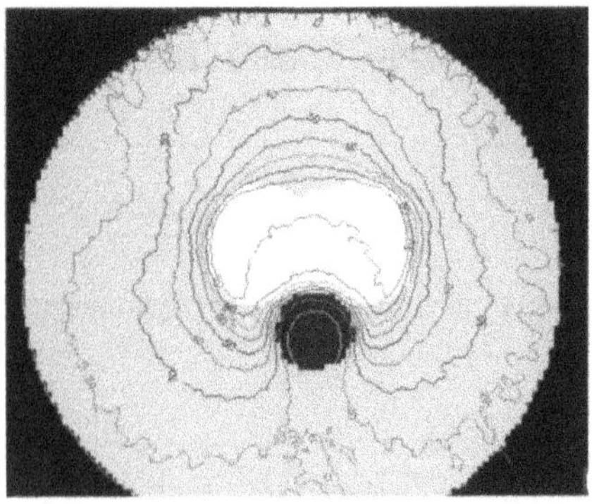

**Figure 1:** Dose distribution achieved using the ratio method with the normal tissues in the target volume considered

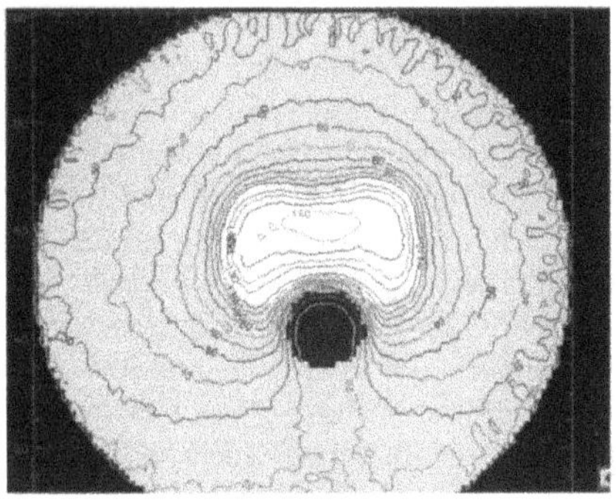

**Figure 2:** Dose distribution achieved using the ratio method without the normal tissues in the target volume considered

## Conclusion

The dose distributions possible by considering the normal tissues in the target volume as well as elsewhere can result in much more homogeneous doses to the prostate. This provides an optimisation technique which achieves a highly conformal dose distribution to the prostate and will hopefully allow for higher doses to be delivered without the impact of high doses to the normal tissues.

## References


[1] L. Jones, P. Hoban, Should intensity modulated Cost functions be Biologically or Physically based?, 41st AAPM annual meeting, Nashville (Med Phys, 1999).

[2] B. G. Clark, et al., The integral biologically effective dose to predict brain stem toxicity of hypofractionated stereotactic radiotherapy*Int J Radiat Oncol Biol Phys* **40**, 667-75 (1998).

[3] A. Niemierko, Reporting and analyzing dose distributions: a concept of equivalent uniform dose *Med Phys* **24**, 103-10 (1997).

# Limitations in using dose-volume histograms for radiotherapy dose optimization

**Vitali Moiseenko[1], Jake Van Dyk[1,2], Jerry Battista[1,2] and Elizabeth Travis[3]**

[1]London Regional Cancer Centre, [2]Department of Oncolology, University of Western Ontario, London, ON, Canada and [3]M.D.Anderson Cancer Center, Houston, TX

Dose-volume histograms (DVH) are commonly used to represent dose variations in organs at risk (OAR). The DVH is then reduced to manageable form and used to predict normal tissue complication probability (NTCP). In this paper we examine two limitations in their applicability to optimizing treatment plans for radiotherapy: (1) the impact of the choice of the DVH reduction scheme and the NTCP biological model on final treatment plan rankings, using human data for liver complications, and (2) the applicability of the DVH concept to partial lung irradiation using two independent sets of rodent data (mice, rats). It is demonstrated that treatment plan rankings depend on the choice of the DVH reduction scheme and NTCP model. Furthermore, lung data for rodents indicate the existence of non-uniform regional effects which will require additional consideration for the absolute location of subvolumes and their interdependent responses.

## Introduction

New technologies of radiation dose delivery, such as 3-D conformal radiation therapy and tomotherapy, allow dose distributions to conform tightly with target volumes. Complications in organs at risk (OAR) will serve as a constraint for dose escalation protocols achievable with these new technologies. A particular problem, which has to be addressed at the treatment planning stage, is the prediction of normal tissue complication probability (NTCP) following highly nonuniform irradiation of normal tissue. Dose-volume histograms are commonly used to represent this dose variation in the OAR.

Ideally, the DVH reduction scheme should preserve complication probability while converting a complicated DVH profile to a "single dose, single volume" step function. The resultant NTCP is expected to reflect biological outcome. Unfortunately, our knowledge of complications in normal tissues following nonuniform or partial volume irradiation is very limited. A comprehensive review and guidelines for tolerance doses following partial volume irradiation acknowledges that dose values for partial volumes are often speculative. For organs in general there is no clear NTCP model of choice due to the difficulty of proving their individual assumptions and distinguishing their overall predictive power.

The applicability of DVH as representative of OAR function has also been questioned. There are suggestions to use organ functional maps instead, such as perfusion in lung. There are also reports of incidents when complications were observed in unirradiated parts of the OAR, for example in the bilateral response of lung following unilateral irradiation. This "out of field" lung effect questions the adequacy of the pure DVH description and any similarly based profile (e.g. dose-function histogram) restricted only to the irradiated part of OAR.

In this paper, we present results of an evaluation of the impact of DVH reduction and NTCP modelling on treatment plan rankings, using liver as a model. We also examine available experimental lung data for lethality and micronuclei production in rodents following partial volume lung irradiation. This latter analysis has the aim of probing for the possible existence of regional effects and "cross-talk" in lung response.

## Material and methods

Four commonly used NTCP models: Schultheiss, Kallman-k, Kallman-s and Lyman model were used to calculate NTCP. The first model is logistic, the next two are Poisson-based and the Lyman model is probit-based. The two Poisson-based models differ in the description of the organ architecture, since the Kallman-s model uses designated parameter (s) to describe the relative seriality of the organ. DVH reduction was carried out by using either the "preferred Lyman" [1] or Kutcher's "effective volume" scheme [2]. Published human data for complications in liver were used to obtain estimates of model parameters. Liver data were used because upon reviewing the available literature on normal tissue tolerance, this human data set was judged to be the most self-consistent. Following fitting of the NTCP models to this data set, the impact of DVH reduction methods and NTCP modelling on treatment plan rankings was examined. A sample treatment plan for liver irradiation has been used to generate a DVH for the reference treatment plan. Following this, compensating hot and cold spots were introduced into the reference DVH to simulate DVHs for competing plans with different dose uniformity but the same mean dose. The two DVH reduction shemes and four NTCP models were applied afterwards to obtain treatment plan rankings according to the calculated complication probability. This resulted in eight possible rankings for competing treatment plans (i.e. two DVH reductions x four NTCP models).

Two sets of radiobiological data for rodent lungs were used to isolate volume effects following partial lung irradiation. Lethality data for mice were obtained at the M.D.Anderson Cancer Center, Houston, TX [3]. Micronuclei production data in lungs of rats, representative of radiation-induced DNA damage, were obtained at the Ontario Cancer Institute, Toronto, Ontario [4]. The latter data showed that irradiation of the lung base yields micronuclei production in the adjoining shielded lung apex. This "out-of-field" effect was not, however, observed for apical irradiation, which suggests the existence of unidirectional "cross-talk" effects. This appears consistent with lethality data in mice, where increased sensitivity to irradiation was observed in the base of lung. Using lethality data, we obtained response curve fits for the Lyman NTCP model using whole volume and the largest available volume to set the model parameters. Model predictions were then extrapolated to smaller volumes to determine compliance with experimental data.

Since micronuclei production is related to chromosome aberrations, this forms a basis to partially account for lethal lesions, as had been observed in mice. We used micronuclei data following partial lung irradiation as an assay for regional "out of field" damage. Using these observations it will be possible to develop NTCP models which incorporate directional parameters. This mathematical development is beyond the scope of this paper. We therefore restrict our attention to identifying the problem rather than providing a solution.

## Results and discussion

### A. Choice of DVH reduction and NTCP models (liver data)

Values obtained for liver $D_{50}$, the dose to the whole volume leading to fifty percent complication probability, were close for three NTCP models (approximately 43 Gy). The Schultheiss model was an exception, yielding a $D_{50}$ of 52.7±3.5 Gy. This model also showed rather shallow dose-complication probability curves for whole and partial liver volumes. The volume effect parameter, n, from the Lyman model was used for DVH reduction using "effective volume" method. The estimated value for this parameter was n=0.52±0.06.

For liver, the Lyman DVH reduction scheme is not sensitive to compensatory hot and cold regions. In fact, by its nature, this scheme leads to a volume-weighted mean dose unless at some stage of DVH reduction, the predicted NTCP *decreases*. The method explicitly applies a constraint to forbid this NTCP reduction. In contrast, the result obtained using the "effective volume" DVH reduction scheme for the same organ was different in its implications for NTCP values.

We first calculated isoeffective curves using of the above NTCP models. An example for $D_5$, the dose leading to five percent complication probability, is shown in Figure 1. The Figure shows a major difference (10 Gy) in the dose values for the volume range of 0.4-0.6, ignoring Schultheiss' model. This means that depending on the choice of a NTCP model a twenty percent dose escalation could be either accepted or rejected because of this variability in the predicted complications.

We also assessed the impact of different dose variations across the liver while maintaining the mean dose value per NTCP model. The reference DVH was first adjusted to yield a matching five percent complication probability for each model. Balancing hot and cold doses were then incorporated in approximately 1/3 of a volume irradiated to high dose so that standard deviation to mean dose ratio was 0.1. The predicted biological response to these hot and cold spots was different for each NTCP model used. Lyman's model did not show any change in predicted NTCP value. The Schulteiss model showed a moderate *increase* of NTCP value. However, the Kallman-s model showed a moderate *decrease* of NTCP. The Kallman-k model predicted a large change of NTCP from five to almost fifteen percent.

The choice of DVH reduction scheme and NTCP model will therefore be a determining factor in ranking of treatment plans. Unfortunately our limited knowledge of response of organs to partial volume irradiation and variation of dose in the organ volume does not presently allow us to determine the method of choice.

### B. Regional out-of-field effects (lung data)

The whole concept of DVH is vulnerable if a response of OAR is governed by other factors which are beyond dose-volume considerations. This limitation has been identified previously and suggestions have been made to incorporate functional mapping of the organ. Furthermore, recent observations of lethality in mice and micronuclei production in rat lung, following partial volume lung irradiation, point to the existense of regional effects in the propagation of lung damage in rodent lung.

Lyman's NTCP model was fit to a whole volume and largest partial volume data sets, separately for the base and apex irradiation. The results of fitting and the predicted curves obtained following extrapolation to a partial volume of 0.7 are shown in Figures 2 and 3. Figure 2 shows that for apex irradiation the volume adequately serves as a good measure of complications. We were able to obtain a good fit for the whole apex data set with common model parameters. However, this is not true for base irradiation (Figure 3) where extrapolated dose-response curves substantially overpredict the dose for the 50% ($D_{50}$) complication probability. To force a betrter fit for smaller volumes, the value of the parameter, n, governing the strength of volume dependence, had to be re-adjusted for every fractional volume data set.

The authors of the mice lethality study [3] explained this effect by assuming that the target cells for radiation pneumonitis are not uniformly distributed in the volume of the lung. In this work, we suggest an alternative explanation based on the results obtained for micronuclei production in rat lung as an assay for lethal lesion production in lung cells. This consequently makes radiation pneumonitis dependent not only on the volume or proportion of target cells irradiated, but also on the location of the irradiated volume.

We have proceeded to develop a variant of the NTCP model which includes killing of "out-of-field" target cells in the *shielded* parts of the lung. The cell survival depends on the dose, the volume, and the location of the irradiated part of the lung. We further assumed that this effect is more pronounced for base irradiation affecting apex reaction, and rather small for apex irradiation affecting base reaction. To be consistent with the rat data set we also allowed for partial volume irradiation effects for "in-field" cell killing.

By allowing for this "out of field" effect we obtained a very good fit to mice lethality data assuming that lethal lesion yield in the apex is of the order of 30 – 40 % of that in the irradiated base part of the lung. This is in a remarkable agreement with micronuclei data obtained in the rat lung. This supports the hypothesis that rodent lung exhibits regional effects. The response to apical irradiation will be different from the response to base irradiation, even if the same fractional volume is involved. If regional effects indeed exist also for the human lung, then DVH profiles alone will no longer be sufficient to predict lung complications since DVH data ignores geometric positional information. Our interpretation of mice lethality data is not intended to supersede the original, cell density hypothesis [3]. Indeed, mathematically the resultant equations can be similar in their form. The interpretation of the model parameters may be that of functional weights, differential cellular sensitivity, or a term needed to include directional effects. Integral radiobiological endpoints, such as lethality, are unlikely to allow one to distinguish between the validity of competing lung response models. Cellular effect studies are required and mechanisms involved in the development of radiation pneumonitis have to be illucidated.

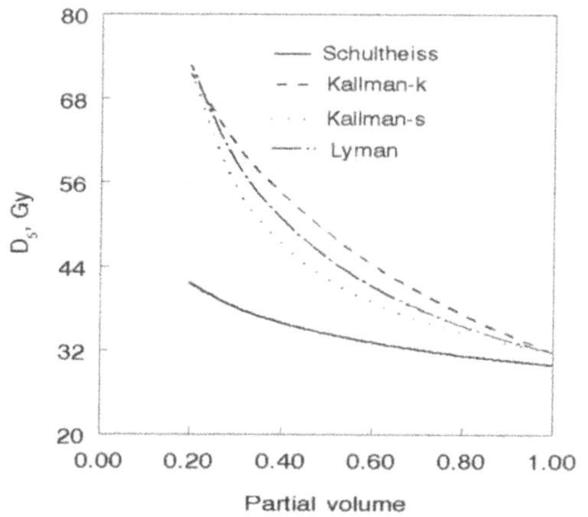


**Figure 1:** Isoeffective curves for five percent complication probability predicted by different models for liver

## Conclusion

There are two serious implications to the work presented here which warrant precautions in the blind use of DHV data for predicting NTCP values for optimization of treatment plans:
(1) The choice of dose-volume histogram reduction method and normal tissue complication probability model influences the ranking of treatment plans, and (2) animal data in rodents for lethality and DNA damage assayed by micronuclei induction following partial volume lung irradiations show that regional effects may exist. This will make the DVH concept insufficient unless geometrical positional information is incorporated.

A joint effort on collecting normal tissue complication data from 3D radiotherapy clinical trails will facilitate our progress in addressing these complex issues.

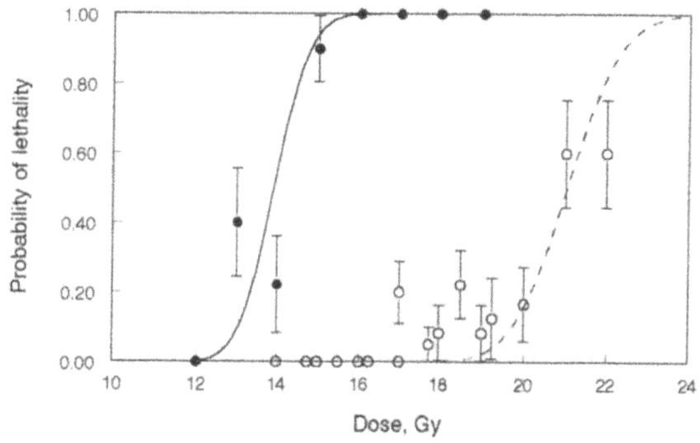


**Figure 2:** Dose-probability of lethality dependence for apex irradiation. Initial fit to whole volume and 94 percent volume data (closed circles, solid line) was extrapolated to 70 percent volume (open circles, dashed line).

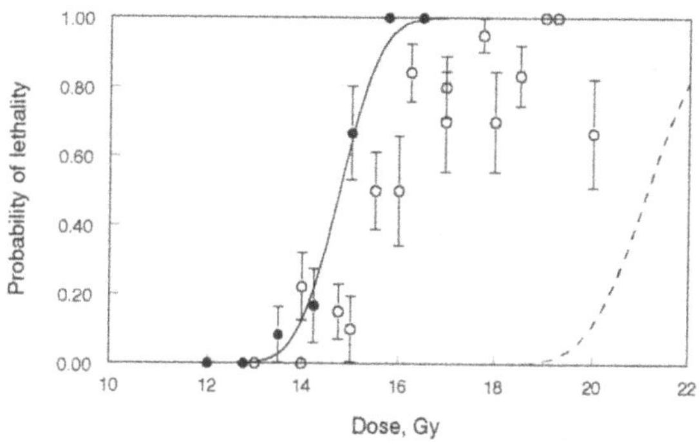


**Figure 3:** Dose-probability of lethality dependence for base irradiation. Initial fit to whole volume and 90 percent volume data (closed circles, solid line) was extrapolated to 70 percent volume (open circles, dashed line).

## Acknowledgements

We acknowledge financial support from the Medical Research Council of Canada.

## References

[1] Lyman JT, Wolbarst AB 1989 Optimization of radiation therapy, IV: a dose-volume histogram reduction algorithm. Int J Radiation Oncology Biol Phys **17** 433-436

[2] Kutcher GJ, Burman C 1989 Calculation of complication probability factors for non-uniform normal tissue irradiation: the effective volume method. Int J Radiation Oncology Biol Phys **16** 1623-1630

[3] Liao Z-X, Travis EL, Tucker SL 1995 Damage and morbidity from pneumonitis after irradiation of partial volumes of mouse lung. Int J Radiat Oncol Biol Phys **32** 1359-1370

[4] Khan MA, Hill RP, Van Dyk J 1998 Partial volume rat lung irradiation: an evaluation of early DNA damage. Int J Radiat Oncol Biol Phys **40** 467-476

# Development of software to calculate the biological effect of different fractionation schedules in model tumours.

**D.E. Wilkins, S. Gupta, J.E. Cygler, G.P. Raaphorst**
Ottawa Regional Cancer Centre, Ottawa, Canada K1H 8L6

## Introduction

Modern treatment planning systems do a reasonably good job of predicting the physical dose as a function of spatial position for a particular treatment. However, the parameter of clinical interest is the biological response of tumour and normal tissue, which is a function of the spatial and temporal distribution of dose (i.e. the fractionation scheme).
Given reasonable models, knowledge of biological parameters, and sufficient computing power, the treatment planning process could be extended into the temporal dimension to predict not just physical dose, but biological effect.
The linear-quadratic (LQ) model of cell survival provides a formalism for predicting the biological effect of radiotherapy on tumors. The BED (biologically effective dose) formalism of the LQ model[1-3] has the advantage of being conceptually simple and easy to apply. However, there is no explicit account of repair in this formalism, i.e. there is an underlying assumption of complete repair of damage between fractions. There is no allowance for the possibility of different rates of repair between normal and tumour tissue, which could be of clinical significance[4-6]. In addition, the simple formulation of the LQ model does account for tumour proliferation during the course of radiotherapy. It would be useful to have available a more general model with explicit account of repair, for application in situations such as hyperfractionation or pulse-dose rate brachytherapy (PDR), and with a realistic account of tumour proliferation, for situations such as treatment interruptions in head and neck and other fast growing tumours.
We have developed a VisualBasic program called Virtual Radiotherapy (VR). This software incorporates a formulation of the LQ model which explicitly accounts for repair, a Gompertzian-exponential model of tumour growth[7] to account for proliferation during the course of radiotherapy, and a database of cellular radiation response and tumour proliferation parameters.

## Material and methods

The Virtual Radiotherapy program calculates the time factor, cell survival, biologically effective dose, and tumor control probability for any arbitrarily spaced fractionation schedule consisting of N fractions of equal dose and dose rate. The software includes a Gompertzian-Exponential model of tumor growth[7], to account for tumor proliferation during radiotherapy. Parallel calculations can be done for tumor, and early and late responding normal tissues. Linked to the software is a database of radiobiological parameters extracted from the literature for 235 cell lines, with references.
The effects of fractionation can be calculated by inclusion of the Lea-Catcheside time factor G [8-9] in the LQ model, which explicitly accounts for repair during the course of protracted radiotherapy.

## Results and discussion

The VR software currently consists of some 4000 lines of code, comprising the calculation algorithms, modules for input of cellular characteristics, error checking modules for reasonableness of input data, a module for input of the fractionation schedule, and preliminary output modules for writing results to the screen or to file for export to spreadsheet or plotting software. The code has been thoroughly tested by reproducing the results of fractionation and tumour proliferation calculations reported in the literature.
The VR software is novel for several reasons. It incorporates a generalized formulation of the Lea-Catcheside time factor G[8-9], allowing for unequal intervals between fractions (generalized from a derivation by Dale[10] for equally spaced fractions, derived independently but identical to Narayama[11]). This formulation is currently restricted to equal dose/fraction, but will be extended to unequal dose/fraction (e.g. to allow for mixed brachytherapy / external beam treatments). The Gompertzian-exponential (with doomed cells) model of tumour proliferation[7] in VR is more sophisticated and realistic than the purely exponential proliferation model typically used in calculations of this type. The Microsoft Access database of cellular radiobiological parameters surveyed from the literature (approximately 150 entries so far, with references linked to the entries) is a unique resource for any type of radiobiology calculations or comparisons. The Visual Basic 5.0 interface of VR is windows-style, menu-driven and intuitive. The interface allows the input of a range of values for any particular parameter, so that the dependence of survival on that parameter can easily be plotted. Extensive help files explain the models and provide explanations of all parameters.
Figure 1 presents an example of one of the screens of the Virtual Radiotherapy program.
This software has been used to investigate the effects of treatment interruptions for tumors of the head and neck, and methods of compensating for missed treatments. Additional fractions delivered BID without increasing overall treatment time results in reduced late normal tissue damage compared with adding extra fractions at the end of the treatment, for the same level of tumor cell kill. However, due to the nature of Gompertzian-Exponential proliferation kinetics, in some circumstances increasing the dose per fraction for the remaining treatments results in lower late normal tissue reactions, due to a reduction in the overall dose required to achieve the same level of tumor cell kill. The VR software can also predict the results of the modelled effect of interruption position, whether early or late in the course of treatment.

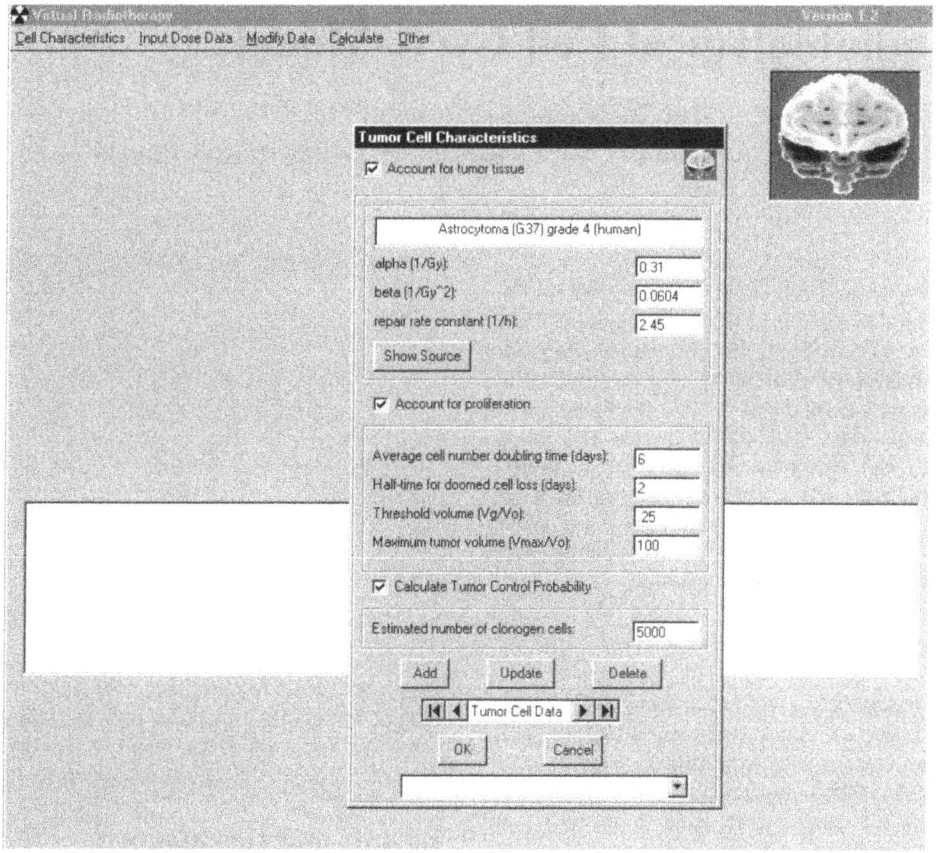


**Figure 1:** Cell characteristics input screen of VR software. The lower part of the screen links to a Microsoft Access database of cell characteristics extracted from the literature. Similar screens exist for the input of the characteristics of early and late responding normal tissues.

## Conclusions

The VR software currently incorporates a reasonably general model of radiation response, a sophisticated model of tumour proliferation, and a database of cellular parameters. Improvements to be made include generalization to unequal dose/fraction, improved search tools for an expanded database, and graphing tools for enhanced output of calculation results. With these improvements, VR will be a valuable tool for including biological response in the treatment planning process.

## References

[1] Barendsen GW 1982 Dose fractionation, dose rate, and iso-effect relationships for normal tissue responses Int J Radiat Oncol Biol Phys **8** 1981-1997

[2] Dale RG 1985 The application of the linear-quadratic dose-effect equation to fractionated and protracted radiotherapy Br J Radiology **58** 515-528

[3] Fowler J 1989 The linear quadratic model and progress in fractionated radiotherapy Br J Radiology **62** 679-94

[4] Fowler JF 1995 Are half-times of repair reliably shorter for tumors than for late normal-tissue effects? Int J Radiat Oncol Biol Phys **31(1)** 189-90

[5] Hall EJ and Brenner DJ 1994 Sublethal damage repair rates – a new tool for improving therapeutic ratios? Int J Radiat Oncol Biol Phys **30** 241-242

[6] Brenner DJ, Armour E, Corry P and Hall EJ 1998 Sublethal damage repair times for a late-responding tissue relevant to brachytherapy (and external-beam radiotherapy): implications for new brachytherapy protocols Int J Radiat Oncol Biol Phys **41** 135-138

[7] O'Donoghue JA 1997 The response of tumours with Gompertzian growth characteristics to fractionated radiotherapy Int J Radiation Biol **72** 325-339

[8] Lea DE and Catcheside DG 1942 The mechanism of the induction by radiation of chromosome aberrations in *tradescantia* J Genetics **44** 216-244

[9] Brenner DJ, Hlatky LR, Hahnfeldt PJ, Huang Y and Sachs RK 1998 The linear-quadratic model and most other common radiobiological models result in similar predictions of time-dose relationships Radiation Res **150** 83-91

[10] Dale RG, Huczkowski J and Trott KR 1988 "Possible dose rate dependence of recovery kinetics as deduced from a preliminary analysis of the effects of fractionated irradiations at varying dose rates" The British Journal of Radiology **61** 153-157

[11] Narayana V 1997 Physical and biological approaches to the improvement of dosimetry and delivery of brachytherapy PhD thesis, Medical Physics Dept. Wayne State University, Detroit

# A Novel Radiobiological Cell Cycle Model

**Rasmus Wegener**[1], **Fridtjof Nüsslin**[2]

[1]Department of Medical Physics, Radiological University Clinic, Hoppe-Seyler-Str. 3, 72076 Tübingen, Germany

## Introduction

We developed a radiobiological cell cycle (RBC) model on the basis of which computer simulations of tissue responses toward irradiation are possible. In a first step the simulations recreate the radiosensitive behavior of individual proliferating cells which in a second step are consolidated to yield the behavior of a whole cell population. The RBC-model unites the latest results of molecular and radiation biology. It is multi-dimensional and non-linear since diverse aspects such as radiation quality, energy and dose, fractionation regimen, DNA damage and repair mechanisms, as well as genetic and molecular biological factors are taken into account.

## Methods

Opposed to conventional models of radiation cell killing which rely on mathematical fits of macroscopically obtained cell survival responses, the strongly interdisciplinary approach of the RBC-model empathizes the comprehensive description and inclusion of the impact of radiation on cells. It mimics cell growth and cellular as well as cell population responses to irradiation in an *ab initio*, molecular-based approach that does not rely on any *a priori* instrumenting of dose response survival curves.

Among the keystones of the RBC-model's workings is the discovery that cellular radiosensitivity is less the result of incomplete repair of the genetic code but rather the consequence of inadequate cell cycle regulation ensuing DNA injury [1]. Lately, the protein p53 has caught widespread attention as playing a central role in the signaling process and the initiation cascades of cellular DNA repair mechanisms. Its concentration in the form of an active chemical complex is simulated in dependence on the type and extent of DNA damage [2]. Furthermore, the RBC-model takes into account the protein's varying impact on cycle control [3, 4] at different stages of the cell cycle.

While, in principle, the RBC-model is applicable to both proliferating as well as non-proliferating cells, our current work is limited to the analysis of proliferating cells. Therefore the careful observation and integration of kinetic processes is especially important. Three types of cell kinetic reactions can be represented by the model: cell death in the form of apoptosis [5] or disintegration, cellular sterility evidenced by a loss of clonogenic activity, and, thirdly, delay of mitotic cell division.

The RBC-model (Fig. 1) is based on two sub-cycles which coexist in any proliferating cell: a cell growth cycle (CGC) and a DNA division cycle (DDC) [6]. The two cycles share a common starting point. The classic intermitotic cell cycle time $T_C$ begins and ends at mitotic events which also mark the end of the DDC but not of the CGC. The familiar cell cycle phases S, $G_2$, and M continue to exist in the model, yet the $G_1$ phase is split into a post-mitotic ($G_1pM$) and a pre-synthesis ($G_1pS$) part. Furthermore, the model possesses checkpoints at which

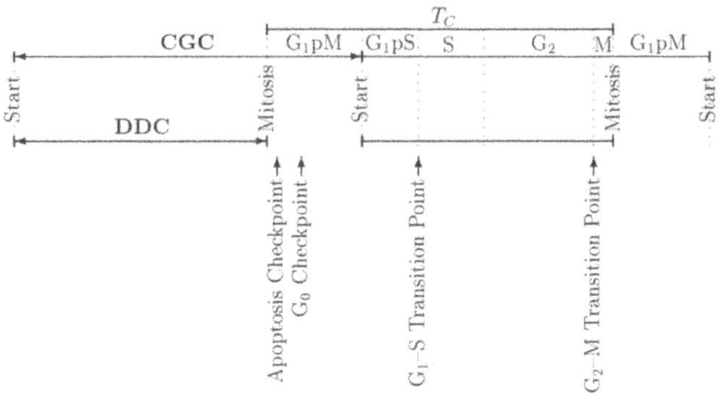


**Figure 1:** The RBC-model.

simulated molecular switches determine a cell's turn towards apoptosis or differentiation. At two transition points (TP) certain molecular concentrations initiate TP stops: the DDC is halted to allow for DNA lesion repair while a cell's CGC and therefore growth continues uninterruptedly [7].

## Results and Discussion

In good agreement with current literature, the RBC-model reproduces diverse cellular phenomena found in real biological systems: cellular radiosensitivity is cycle phase dependent [8], and cells with little or defective p53 show a marked radiation resistance just as is displayed by approximately 50% of all

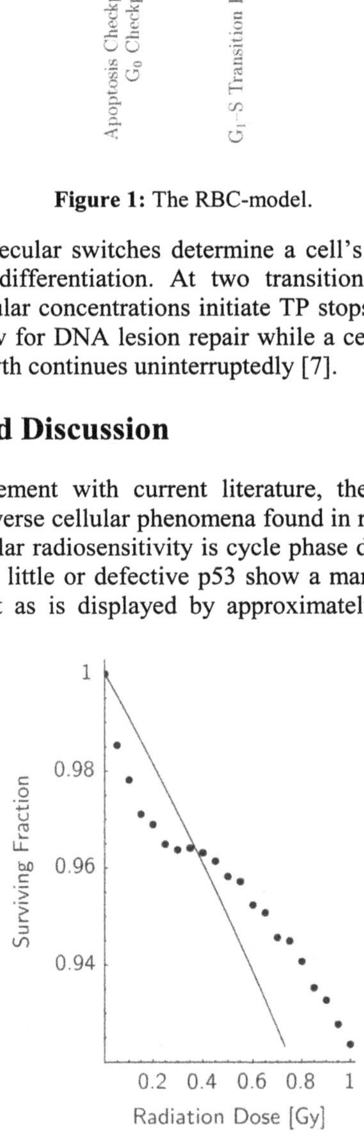


**Figure 2:** Dose response of a simulated cell population at doses below 1 Gy. Dots represent the surviving fraction over radiation dose and illustrate the phenomenon of hypersensitivity to irradiation at small doses ranging from 0 to approximately 0.3 Gy as predicted by the RBC-model. The full curve relates to an extrapolated fit of radiation responses towards doses exceeding 1 Gy employing the common linear-quadratic mode.

human tumor cell strains. Increases in radiosensitivity result from the simulated use of combined radio-chemotherapy or from molecular variations found in, for instance, ataxia telangiectasia patients. High doses lead to long TP stops and consequently to the formation of polyploid cells.
The sum of cellular radiation effects then forms the basis of macroscopic, population-scale effects like growth synchronization within a cell population following irradiation. The biological impact of simulated irradiation also depends on the radiation's linear energy transfer value, the dose applied, and the fractionation schedule.
Phenomena such as the clinically relevant low-dose hypersensitivity [9] become accessible through the RBC-model simulations (Fig. 2).

## Conclusion

With the RBC-model there now is a tool at hand for testing and integrating new and interesting hypotheses concerning the molecular origins and control mechanisms of phenomena related to cellular and tissular radiation sensitivity. Our current work aims at extending the RBC-model to better cover the effects of radiation on non-proliferating cells and to integrate the model into our radiation treatment planning system.

## References

[1] M. Durante, et al. 1994 Radiation-induced chromosomal aberrations in mouse 10T1/2 cells: dependence on the cell-cycle stage at the time of irradiation *Int. J. Radiat. Biol.* **65** 437–447
[2] A. J. Levine 1997 p53, the cellular gatekeeper for growth and division *Cell* **88** 323–331
[3] J. Yarnold 1997 Molecular aspects of cellular responses to radiotherapy *Radiother. Oncol.* **44** 1–7
[4] N. E. A. Crompton 1998 Programmed cellular response to ionizing radiation damage *Acta Oncol.* **37** 129–142
[5] M. Raff, Cell suicide for beginners 1998 *Nature* **396** 119–122
[6] R. Sennerstam and J.-O. Strömberg 1991 Dissociation of cell growth and DNA synthesis and alteration of the nucleo-cytoplasmic ration in growing embryonal carcinoma cells *Dev. Growth Diff.* **33** 353–363
[7] H. M. Rosenberg and E. C. Gregg 1969 Kinetics of cell volume changes of murine lymphoma cells subjected to different agents *in vitro Biophys. J.* **9** 592–606
[8] W. K. Sinclair and R. A. Morton 1995 X-ray and ultraviolet sensitivity of synchronized Chinese hamster cells at various stages of the cell cycle *Biophys. J.* **5** 1–25
[9] Smith, L. G. et al. 1999 Investigation of Hypersensitivity to fraactionated low-dose radiation exposure *Int. J. Radiat. Oncol. Biol. Phys.* **45** 187–191

# Estimation of complication probabilities after radiosurgery of AVM patients using a biological model

**Lan Ton, Sabine Levegrün, Jürgen Debus, Sebastian Swiderski and Wolfgang Schlegel**

German Cancer Research Center, INF 280, 69120 Heidelberg, Germany

## Introduction

For the optimum use of radiotherapy, a precise knowledge of normal tissue tolerance data and complication probabilities is necessary. Mathematical algorithms were developed that attempt to predict the biological response of normal tissues to radiation, based on the physical dose distribution and radiobiological data. These biological models allow the calculation of normal tissue complication probabilities (NTCP). While biological models could potentially provide a valuable means to score and optimize treatment plans, their merit has not been proven yet and the underlying model parameters are affected with large uncertainties. However, studies that actually confront model predictions with clinical data are sparse.

Since it is often difficult to separate the effect of the tumor on the normal tissue reaction, an evaluation of benign tumors like arteriovenous malformations (AVMs) is of particular interest. The purpose of this study was to evaluate the usefulness of current model predictions, using an existing NTCP model with published parameters, to estimate the side effects after radiosurgery of AVM patients, and to investigate dose-response relations.

## Material and methods

In total, 270 AVM patients treated at the German Cancer Research Center up to 1997 using a stereotactic radiosurgery technique with available follow up were studied. Complications after radiosurgery were investigated. This study concentrated on radiation-induced tissue changes like edema, blood-brain barrier (BBB) breakdown, gliosis and brain necrosis, the most serious complication. There are two groups of patients in this collective. Group 1, consisting of 210 AVM patients, was treated with a single fraction radiosurgery using round collimators and a convergent arc technique. 172 of these patients had one target point. Group 2, consisting of 60 patients, was treated between 1994 and 1997 using a micro-multileaf-collimator [MMLC-radiosurgery] with a leaf width of 1,5 mm at isocenter distance. Patients were followed in intervals of 6 months with magnetic resonance imaging and neurological exam and analysed with regard to radiological and clinical effects.

For stereotactic single fraction irradiation [1], the validity of a biological model to predict NTCP after the application of a single high dose fraction was examined. The phenomenological model introduced by Flickinger [2], which is described below, was used for this purpose. This model was specifically developed to predict complication probabilities from stereotactic radiosurgery.

A logistic function [3] is used to describe the probability of a complication occurring after a dose, D, administered to the whole brain:

$$NTCP(D) = 1/\{[NTD_2(D_{50})/NTD_2(D)]^k + 1\}, \qquad (1)$$

where $NTD_2(D_{50})$ is the normalized total dose (NTD) at 2 Gy per fraction (indicated by the subscript 2) administered to the reference volume (whole brain) which would cause a 50% complication probability. $NTD_2(D)$ is the normalized total dose at 2 Gy per fraction administered to the same volume.

When the fractional volume of an organ v is irradiated to dose d, the expression in Eq.2 can be used:

$$NTCP(d,v) = 1 - \{[NTD_2(d)/NTD_2(D_{50})]^k + 1\}^{-v/V}. \qquad (2)$$

V is the total volume of the organ. In the case of an inhomogeneous dose distribution, the complication probability is calculated separately for each dose bin i in the differential dose-volume histogram, and the integrated logistic function is given by:

$$NTCP(d_0, d_1, ..d_n) = 1 - \prod_i \{[NTD_2(d_i)/NTD_2(D_{50})]^k + 1\}^{-v_i/V}. \qquad (3)$$

The high single dose applied in radiosurgery is converted into a total dose biologically equivalent to a standard fractionation scheme (2 Gy fractions) through a linear quadratic formula:

$$NTD_2 = \sum_i n_i (0.1887 d_i^2 + 0.6226 d_i) x_i^{-0.12} \qquad (4)$$

where n is the number of fractions, d is the dose per fraction in Gy, and x is the number of fractions divided by the total time cf the treatment course (in days).

The following model parameters, which were published by Flickinger [2], were used in the integrated logistic formula of the model in the linear quadratic version: $NTD_2(D_{50})$=72,2 Gy, k=18,5.

## Results and discussion

Results of the analysis of radiation-induced brain necrosis are shown in figure 1. The collimator diameter is plotted versus the dose at the target point for group 1. For patients with more than one target point, an equivalent collimator diameter ∅, where the corresponding volume is equal to the total irradiated brain volume, and the maximal target dose were plotted in figure 1. There is a direct correlation between the collimator diameter and the irradiated brain volume. Therefore, one can calculate curves of the same NTCP (isoeffect curves) using the logistic formula and the parameters for brain necrosis (given above).

Necrosis is a serious complication after radiosurgery. In the first patient group, only three patients (1,4%) developed a necrosis. These patients are all in the area of high NTCP, predicted by the biological model (Figure 1).

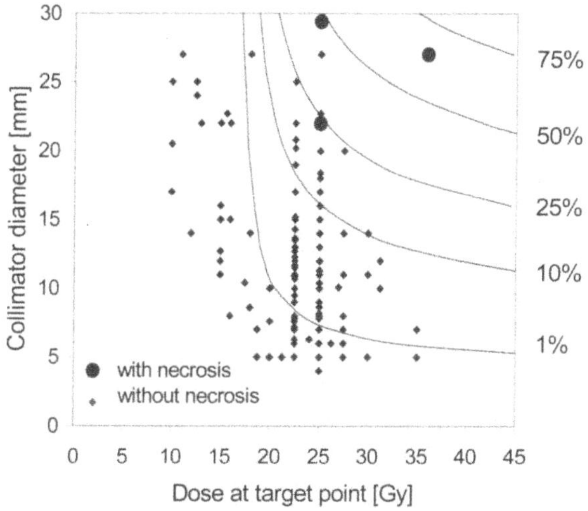


**Figure 1:** Dose-volume isoeffect curves for brain necrosis after radiosurgery predicted by the linear quadratic version of Flickinger's integrated logistic formula. Patients without necrosis are indicated by the squares, patients with necrosis by the circles. The three patients with necrosis are in the area of high NTCP prediction. (Total: 210 patients).

The new technique of MMLC-radiosurgery enables the exact conformation of the delivered dose distribution to AVMs with a complex irregular shape. Dose-volume-histograms of each patient in the second group were used for the NTCP calculation with the Flickinger logistic formula in linear quadratic version to estimate the risk of brain necrosis. For all patients in group 2, the calculated values are smaller than 8%. In fact, none of the patients in group 2 developed a clinically significant radiation necrosis.

Figure 2 shows the relation of collimator diameter versus target dose for patients with and without radiation-induced tissue changes like edema, BBB breakdown, and gliosis in group 1. Comparing the locations of patients with edema, and BBB breakdown in different areas of the diagram, divided by the isoeffect curves for brain necrosis, indicates that the clinical incidence of tissue changes increases with higher NTCP prediction.

Figure 3 shows the incidence of radiologically observed edema and BBB breakdown in patients with one target point for different collimator diameters Ø (indicated by different symbols) as a function of the dose D at the target point. Since the number of patients with the same collimator diameter is relatively small, patients were grouped into ranges of collimator diameters for a proper evaluation. For the collimator diameters 10-12mm and 13-15 mm, a logistic formula

$$NTCP(D) = 1/[1 + (d_{50} / D)^k] \qquad (5)$$

was fit to the clinical data using a maximum-likelihood technique. This allowed an estimation of the dose $d_{50}$, corresponding to NTCP=50%, and of the parameter k characterising the slope at $d_{50}$ of the dose-response curves for edema and BBB breakdown:

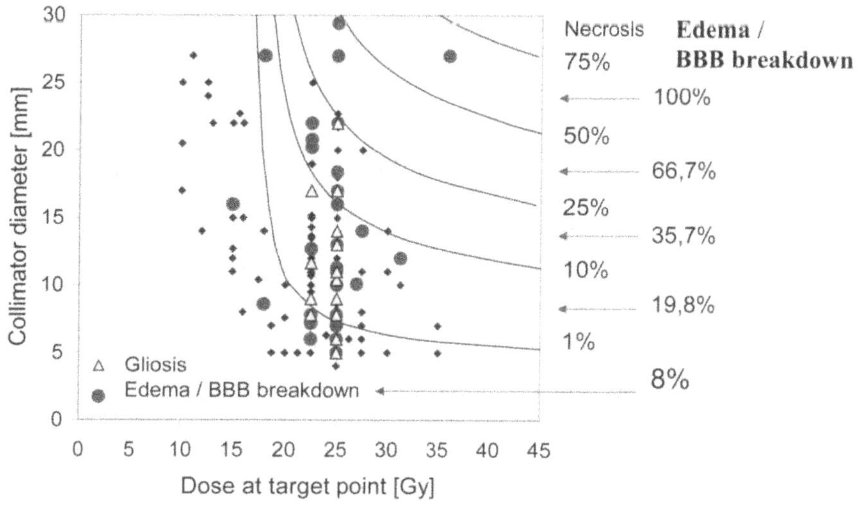


**Figure 2:** Radiation-induced tissue changes in 210 AVM patients after radiosurgery using round collimators. The percent numbers in the right column next to the arrows show the clinical incidence of edema and blood-brain barrier breakdown in different areas. This incidence increases with higher NTCP predictions.

$d_{50} \sim 28{,}5$ Gy ; k~9,9 for $\varnothing = 13\text{-}15$ mm
$d_{50} \sim 30{,}6$ Gy ; k~7,5 for $\varnothing = 10\text{-}12$ mm.

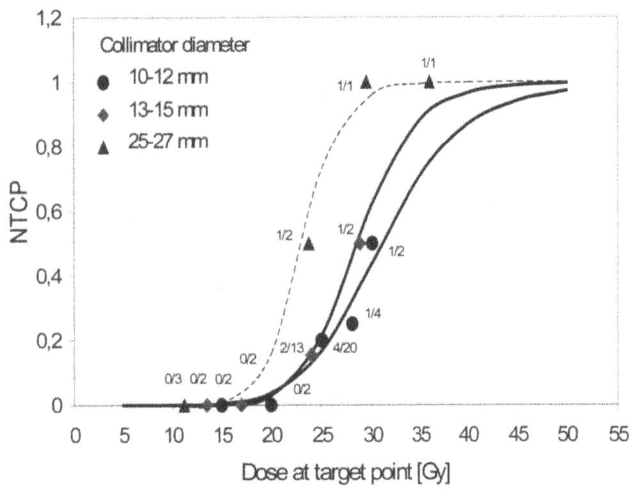


**Figure 3:** Dose-response curves of edema and BBB breakdown after radiosurgery of AVMs for different ranges of collimator diameter for patients with one target point. The numbers next to the symbols show the ratio of patients with complications to all patients at that point.

For the large collimator diameters (25-27mm), too few data were available for a fit. Instead, a dose-response curve was plotted to connect the symbols (without regression fit).

## Conclusion

This study indicates that it may be possible to identify patients that are at a high risk for complications after radiosurgery by means of a biological model to predict NTCP. In the next step, a statistical analysis will be performed to correlate model predictions with clinical outcome data. For certain collimator diameters, dose-response curves for edema and BBB breakdown were derived to estimate the dose $d_{50}$ for these radiation-induced tissue changes. Future investigations will attempt to determine model parameters with a higher precision.

### Acknowledgements

We would like to thank Dr. M.A.Keller-Reichenbecher for his help.

## References

[1] Debus J, Pirzkall A, Schlegel W, Wannenmacher M 1999 Stereotaktische Einzeitbestrahlung (Radiochirurgie) *Strahlenther. Onkol.* **175** 47-56.
[2] Flickinger J C 1989 An integrated logistic formula for prediction of complications from radiosurgery *Int. J. Radiation Oncology Biol. Phys.* **17** 879-885.
[3] Schultheiss T E, Orton C G, Peck R A 1983 Models in radiotherapy: volume effects *Med.Phys.* **10** 410-415.

# Implementation of EvTool, a quantitative and radiobiological evaluation system, in a commercial RTPS.

**Roberto Anselmi[1], Luciano Andreucci[2], Fabrizio Bisi[3], Monica Bevegni[4]**

Biophysics Laboratory, National Cancer Institute, L.go R. Benzi 10, 16132 Genoa, Italy.
E-mail: 1 elwood@hp380.ist.unige.it, 2 luciano@hp380.ist.unige.it, 3 bix@hp380.ist.unige.it, 4 bevegni@hp380.ist.unige.it

## Introduction

The fast evolution of 3D Treatment Planning Systems of last few years, make necessary having available a system of evaluation of RT plans and comparison between them. At now the individuation of the *best plan*, i.e. the more similar to the *optimal one*, present more and more difficulties because of the continuos growing of the techniques' complexity, made available by new hardware and software instrumentation. For this reason an exclusively qualitative evaluation of the plan and comparison between plans is not still adequate, or at least not sufficient, for the purpose of making real 3D treatments. In order to solve this problem, our group at the Biophysics Laboratory of the National Cancer Institute of Genoa developed EvTool, a system that allow the user to have quantitative and/or radiobiological helping to answer to the important question: which is the *best plan*? The author is now implementing EvTool inside the 3DLine RTPS ERGO, to use it as evaluation module for the RT plans of 3DLine Dynamic double-focused MultiLeaf Collimator System.

## Material and methods

EvTool was developed using a Silicon Graphics Indy with OS Irix5.3 and was tested without any problem with SGI Indigo2 and O2 with OS up to Irix6.5. The code is written in C using the standard graphics libraries X, Xt, Xmotif, and is compiled with the C++ compiler. At now we are testing a Linux β-version of EvTool too.
Every time the user make a comparison between rival RT plans the system build an *EvPlan* containing all the information used, such as: number of fractions, reference dose, plans and contours evaluated, $\alpha/\beta$, $TD_{50}$ and so on. Then EvTool is basically composed of two distinct part:

*a)* EvPlan creation from patient and the RT plans data;
*b)* EvPlan evaluation.

The role of this intermediate step (EvPlan) has two main reason: allow the user to re-load previous evaluations and, via a DicomRT import routine scheduled for future releases, make available the comparison between plans coming from different TPS.
EvTool starts from the ERGO PMM (Patient Management Module) and automatically load patient's contours information and the last saved EvPlan. Anyway the user can build a new EvPlan loading RT plans previously made with the RTPS ERGO. No settings of the evaluation parameters is asked to the user at this level.
The second part of EvTool consist of the evaluation of the loaded or just created EvPlan. In this phase the user can use up to 4 different visualisation window, choosing for each one between three different modality:

*a)* Dose-Volume Histograms (cumulative and differential);
*b)* Dose Statistics (mean, max, mean, modal, EUD:Equivalent Uniform Dose);
*c)* Radiobiological TCP/NTCP using Niemierko's models.

DVHs and Statistics modalities are provided either using real fraction-dose than performing the 2Gy/fraction normalisation.
In addition for each window the user can choose between different VOIs selecting them from a list containing the RTPS defined and new user defined VOIs. In fact EvTool allow the user to build new VOIs adding the RTPS defined ones. In this way it is possible, only for evaluation purpose, to build useful VOIs such as the well known OAR (Organs At Risk), PTV, CTV and any other, taking obviously care that the addition has clinical sense. Another aspect of this facility is that it is not necessary to define the target volume at RTPS level, particularly useful in case of boosts or similar situation where sub-target are defined.
For making the use of EvTool easier and more intuitive either Dose Statistics and Radiobiological Models are visualised by Bar-Histograms; in this way the information provided are the same, but the graphical aspect make more evident the comparison between plans.
In conclusion EvTool allow the user to customise its window to better solve particular necessities; in fact it is possible to view at the same time different information for the same VOI (e.g. cumulative DVH + Mean dose + EUD + TCP) or alternatively the same information for different VOI (e.g. differential DVH for 4 different VOI) or every combination of these two limit situations.

## Conclusion

We think EvTool is a powerful system to evaluate and compare RT plans. Its importance grows with the complexity of the RT techniques, and for this reason its use is particularly indicate inside to a system such as ERGO, dedicated to a dynamic MLC i.e. a Linac high technology accessory. In fact we think that without an appropriate quantitative evaluation system, such as EvTool, the Radiotherapy run the risk that the new technologies now available will be strongly underused because of physicists and physicians intuition and clinical experience will be not more sufficient.

## References

[1] R.Anselmi, L.Andreucci "Valutazione quantitativa e radiobiologica dei piani di trattamento 3D" in Proc. of "Procedure operative di misura e Valutazioni Dosimetriche in Radioterapia e Medicina Nucleare", pag. 67-71, S.Miniato (PI), 1-2 July 1999

# Computer-Aided Side Effect Monitoring

**Dieter Fehrentz, Arne Binder**

University of Heidelberg, Department of Clinical Radiology, 69120 Heidelberg, Germany.

## Abstract

On the basis of three-dimensional treatment planning and the actual fractionation data from a verify and recording system (LANTIS) at the accelerators (Mevatrons) an EDP-based determination of side effect probabilities has been installed. The set up parameters of an accelerator are transmitted from a treatment planning system (TMS-Helax) to the accelerator.The dose distributions in the organs are made available in the form of dose-volume histograms.These are converted into effective volumes with the maximum doses, for which the same biological responses are expected as the really given dose distributions. Effective volumes and maximum doses are transferred to a patient treatment file as well as the sequential irradiation data from the verify and recording system.

The side effect probabilities are calculated by a biophysical computer program. It uses a generalized time-dependent formula of the linear quadratic model to calculate biological effects in conection with the sigmoidal dose effect courses and tolerance dose values from the literature. Comparisons of calculations with side effect specifications from the literature turned out to be satisfying in the context of given inaccuracies. The program system was created for a sequential side effect monitoring of the patients with warning notes in case of critical values as well as for queries in individual cases.

# A Deterministic Photon and Electron Transport Algorithm for Radiation Dosimetry

**Albert Mesa and John DeMarco**

200 UCLA Medical Plaza, Radiation Oncology, Suite B265, Los Angeles, CA 90095

## Introduction

The dose calculation algorithm is fundamental to many advances in radiation therapy physics. From simple correction based methods to sophisticated transport methods, the dose calculation algorithm is critical to accurate dose estimation. More sophisticated algorithms also represent a challenge to the speed and memory requirements of even the most modern of computers. For these reasons, the continual development and refinement of the dose calculation algorithm is a necessity.

In an effort to produce a transport method which approaches Monte Carlo in accuracy and surpasses Monte Carlo in speed, a transport algorithm is under development which transports photons and electrons deterministically. This novel transport method borrows from both the stochastic Monte Carlo methods and the deterministic discrete ordinates methods to produce a formidable dose calculation vehicle.

## Material and methods

### Linear Boltzman equation

The basis of all transport methods is rooted in the Boltzman equation.

$$\Omega \bullet \nabla\phi(r,E,\Omega)+\mu(r,E)(r,E,\Omega)$$
$$-\int dE'\int d\Omega'\mu s(r,E'\to E,\Omega'\to\Omega)\phi(r,E',\Omega')-S(r,E,\Omega)=0$$

The Boltzman equation mathematically represents the particle balance throughout space for particles of various energies traveling in various directions. The basic form of the equation represents a continuum in space, energy, and direction. An analytical solution to this equation is obtainable for only the most simple cases. For more realistic problems, numerical methods are applied.

### Discrete ordinates method

The classic numerical solution to the Boltzman equation is the discrete ordinates method[1,2]. Most often applied for neutral particle transport, the method groups the angular variables into a finite number of bins called discrete ordinates. In order to facilitate calculation, the energy and space variables are also discretized. The method then utilizes numerical techniques and an iterative scheme to solve the transport equation.

A shortcoming of the conventional discrete ordinates method is evident when it is used to simulate highly anisotropic scatter (e.g. megavoltage x-rays scatter or electron scatter). Known as the ray effect, the simulation of highly forward peaked scattering results in an artificial pileup of particles in the direction of the discrete ordinates. A possible solution to this dilemma is to increase the order of the discrete ordinates; thus, producing finer directional resolution. However, this solution produces difficulties due to a substantial increase in memory requirements and computation time. For these reasons, the discrete ordinates method has found limited success in the simulation of anisotropic particle scatter.

### Photon transport by a finite differencing technique

For photon transport, our method borrows from the conventional discrete ordinates method to produce a unique finite differencing technique. By eliminating the source-scattering term of the Boltzman equation, one is left with an equation representing first order scatter. By itself, this equation would provide a trivial means to solve for uncollided flux. However, due to the nature of the discrete ordinates method, this method would still suffer from the difficulty of simulating highly anisotropic scatter.

We remedy this difficulty by using a coupled angular discretization technique (figure 1). For a given location in a three dimensional matrix, we couple each lattice element to all the surrounding lattice elements. This allows a fine angular discretization that circumvents many difficulties of simulating photon scatter with conventional discrete ordinates.

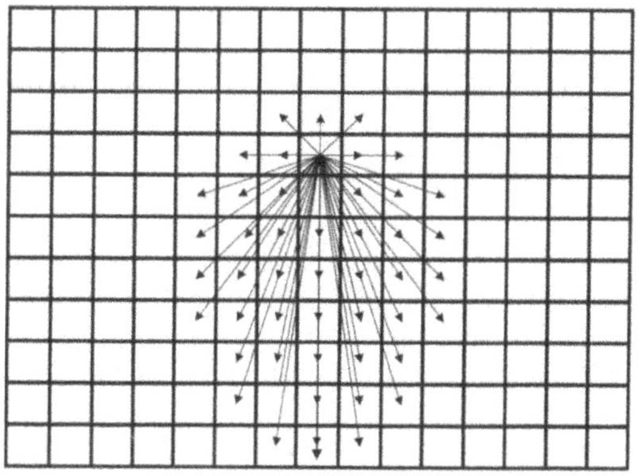

**Figure 1:** Angular discretization based upon lattice to lattice coupling.

Our approach is to apply this method to a three dimensional lattice geometry. For an external photon source, the flux if photons impinging on the lattice surface is determined from an inverse square calculation. This flux is used as boundary values for a finite differencing calculation throughout the inside of the matrix. From the external boundary, the flux is calculated flowing away from the center of divergence. The calculation provides a fast, accurate primary flux calculation. .

For scattered photons, each lattice element is treated as a scattering site. Given the energy and direction of the incident photons, we are able to determine scattering distributions from each lattice element. The primary flux calculation provides the incident photon flux distribution, while the laws of photon scatter provide the scattering distribution. Like the primary photon calculation, the first order scatter photon flux is calculated flowing away from the scattering source. In this case, the flow of photons is calculated separately for each of eight octants. To account for the angular scattering cross sections, the flux to every lattice element is weighted according to the angular cross section and solid angle subtended by that lattice element. Higher orders of scatter follow from successive calculations.

### Electron transport by the Monte Carlo method

Unlike photon interactions which occur on a relatively infrequent basis, electron interactions occur at a far greater frequency. Due to this characteristic of electron interaction, an analogue simulation of electron transport by the Monte Carlo method would be prohibitively time consuming. To circumvent this difficulty a condensed history technique has been adopted to simulate electron transport by the Monte Carlo method[3,4,5]. This technique incorporates the use of multiple scattering theory, secondary particle production and dose deposition in the continuous slowing down approximation (CSDA)[6]. The success of this method has been documented, and we borrow from this method to develop a deterministic electron transport method

### A deterministic electron transport method

Due to the highly anisotropic nature of electron scatter, a prerequisite to deterministic electron transport is a fine angular resolution. Similar to our photon transport scheme, we have adopted a lattice element to lattice element coupled angular discretization scheme. This angular discretization scheme provides adequate angular resolution to simulate electron scatter.

As an example of our electron transport method, we will briefly describe the simulation of an external electron source impinging on a water phantom. The phantom is a uniform three dimensional lattice. The electrons are coupled along raylines to each lattice element, and the electron dose is calculated by the CSDA approximation. In order to simulate multiple scatter, the energy incident upon each voxel is determined by the CSDA approximation. Once this energy is calculated, we treat each voxel as an electron multiple scattering site. Given the energy incident on each voxel, the material composition of each voxel, and the pathlength along a rayline through each voxel we are able to determine the multiple scattering distribution for each element of the lattice. The energy deposition from the scattered electrons is then calculated in the CSDA approximation. The process repeats itself for higher orders of multiple scatter. The effect of ionization electron production and bremsstrahlung production are determined similarly.

## Results and discussion

### Photon KERMA calculations

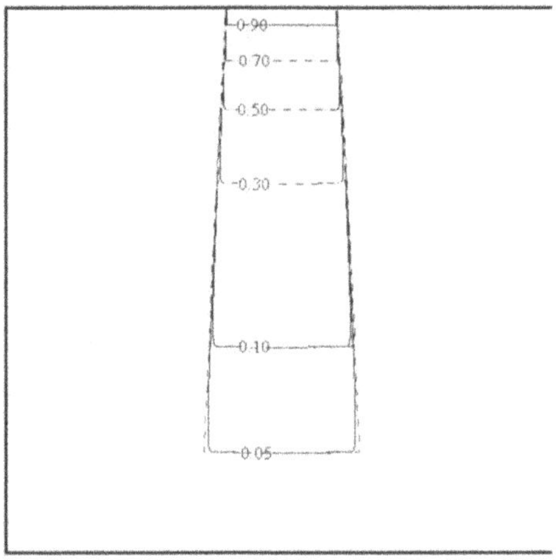


**Figure 2:** Kerma isolines computed from both the Monte Carlo Method and the finite differencing technique.

In order to test the validity of our photon transport algorithm, we performed several photon kerma calculations. Results were benchmarked against Monte Carlo simulations. Figure 2 shows the primary kerma distributions for photons transported through a uniform lattice. As is evident, the distributions are superimposed. Figure 3 shows the primary kerma distribution for photons transported through an inhomogeneous lattice. Once again, the distributions are superimposed.

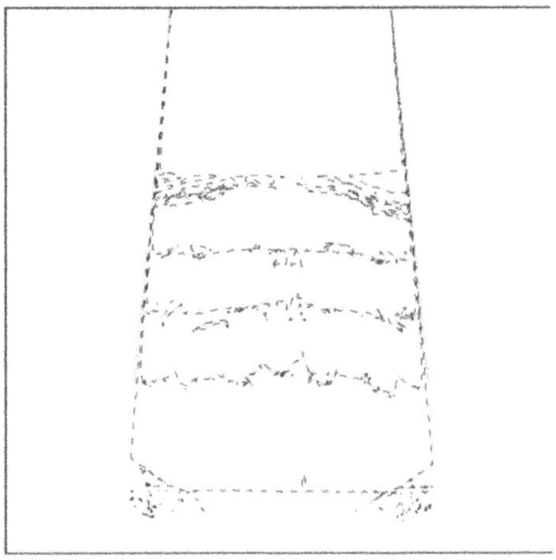

**Figure 3:** Kerma isolines in inhomogeneous media computed from both the Monte Carlo Method and the finite differencing technique.

In order to test the validity of our scattering method, a 20 MeV scatter kernel is generated by our algorithm and compared to a Monte Carlo calculation. The results of this comparison are shown in figure 4. As is evident, the distributions are superimposed with the exception of the inwardly directed peak in the Monte Carlo distribution. The peak is due to the fact that the Monte Carlo calculations incorporate coherent scatter, while our algorithm has yet to incorporate coherent scatter.

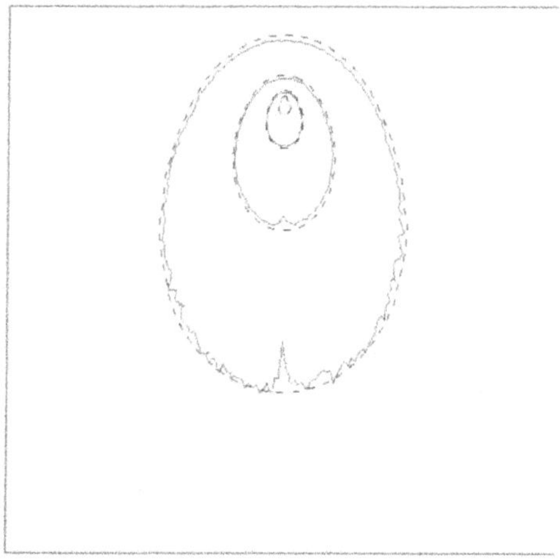

**Figure 4:** First order scattered KERMA distributions calculated from the Monte Carlo method and the finite differencing technique.

**Electron dose calculations**

In order to test the validity of our electron transport algorithm, we performed several electron dose calculations. Results were benchmarked against Monte Carlo simulations. Figures 5-7 show the depth dose distributions for 20 MeV electrons transported through a uniform lattice. Figure 5 shows the effect of modeling only multiple scatter. Figure 6 shows the effect of modeling only ionization interactions. Finally, figure 7 shows the effect of a properly balanced mix of interactions. Each figure shows a comparison with a Monte Carlo simulation.

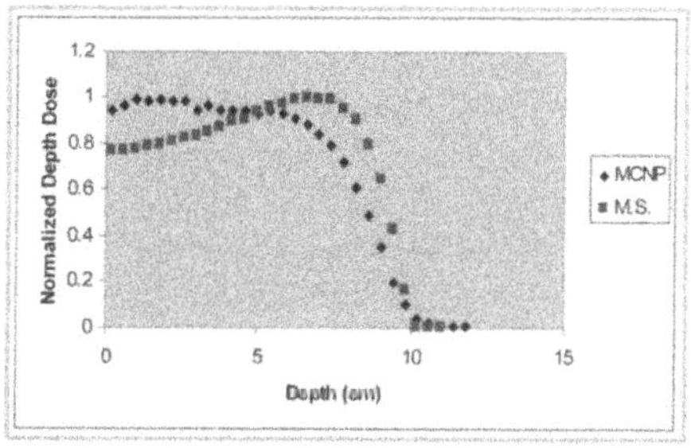


**Figure 5:** 20 MeV depth dose curves computed from Monte Carlo (MCNP) and the deterministic algorithm (MS) modeling only multiple scatter.

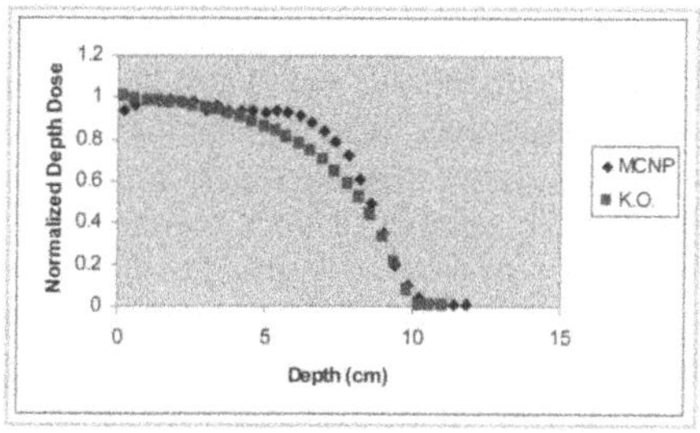


**Figure 6:** 20 MeV depth dose curves computed from Monte Carlo (MCNP) and the deterministic algorithm (KO) modeling only knock-on interactions.

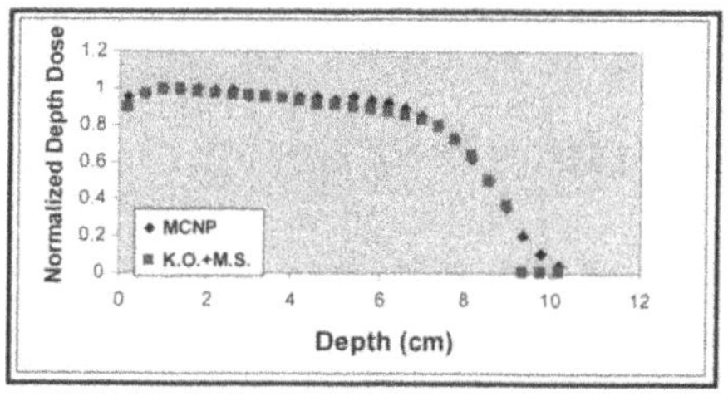


**Figure 7:** 20 MeV depth dose curves computed from Monte Carlo (MCNP) and the deterministic algorithm (KO+MS) modeling both multiple scatter and knock on electron interactions.

## Conclusion

A new photon and electron transport algorithm would provide exciting prospects for radiation therapy. Our algorithm both utilizes the fundamental particle interaction laws and is capable of simulating the effect of individual lattice elements. For these reasons, this algorithm should provide accurate results in inhomogeneous media. The deterministic nature of this algorithm provides for the prospect of decreased calculations times. Since entire distributions are calculated instead of sampling individual particle histories, we believe this will lead to a faster dose determination.

The algorithm can be applied in a multitude of areas. In medical imaging, the photon transport algorithm can be used for image rendering or computed tomography image simulation. In nuclear medicine, the algorithm can be applied for either image simulation or dose determination. In radiation therapy, this method can be used to calculate dose distributions, simulate particle transport in inhomogeneous medial, or the algorithm can be used as a benchmarking tool.

## References

[1] Duderstadt J J and Martin W R 1979 "Transport Theory" Wiley and Sons New York, New York

[2] Bell G I and Glasstone S 1970 "Nuclear Reactor Theory" Robert E. Krieger Publishing, Malabar, Florida

[3] Rogers D W O and Bielajew A F 1990 Monte Carlo techniques of electron and photon transport for radiation dosimetry *The dosimetry of ionizing radiation* **3** 427-536

[4] Berger M J 1963 Monte Carlo calculation of the penetration and diffusion of fast charged particles *Methods in Computational Physics* **1** 135-215

[5] Starodubtsev S V and Romanov A M 1965 "The Passage of Charged Particles through Matter" Israel Program for Scientific Translation, Jerusalem

[6] Goudsmit S and Saunderson J L 1940 Multiple Scattering of Electrons *Physical Review* **57** 24-29

# Siemens Virtual Wedge: A dose calculation model with constraint checking

**Moyed Miften[1], X. Ron Zhu[2], Kaz Takahashi[1], Francesco Lopez[2] and Michael T. Gillin[2]**

[1]Computerized Medical System, Inc., St. Louis, MO 63132, USA and [2]Medical College of Wisconsin, Milwaukee, WI 53226, USA

## Introduction

Radiation therapy treatment planning for many clinical situations requires wedge-shaped isodose distributions. The wedged dose distributions can be generated through the use of physical wedges, motorized wedges, and the synchronization of jaw or multi-leaf collimator (MLC) dynamic motion with accelerator dose output. The Siemens Vritual Wedge (VW) (Siemens Oncology Systems, Concord, CA) delivers wedged shaped dose distributions by combining computer controlled dose delivery with collimator motion. The clinical advantages of using Siemens Virtual Wedges have been discussed in many articles.[1,2]

In this paper, we describe a model to calculate dose for VW using either the Clarkson[3] or Convolution/Superposition[4] algorithms. The VW implementation models the dose generated by VW using the Siemens monitor units (MU) analytic formalism which determines the number of MU required to deliver dose at points across the VW beam. For any treatment setup, the VW algorithm generates a "transmission matrix" that will be used to model the modification of fluence emanating from the source. The transmission (intensity) map is calculated as the ratio of the MU delivered on the axis divided by the monitor units delivered on the central-axis MU(0); MU(0) is also the number of monitor units that is entered at the machine console. The MU analytic formalism used for calculating the intensity matrix (which affects the calculation of dose) may be modified through the fine tuning of the attenuation correction factor *c*.

The VW implementation models the operational constraints due to radiation delivery sequence in the different Siemens linear accelerators. Specifically, for a given VW beam setup, after the dose and MU calculations are performed, the VW model checks the machine dose rate and jaw speed constraints for the delivery of VW.

Agreement within 2% or 2 mm was found between calculated and measured doses, over a large set of test cases, for 15, 30, 45 and 60 degree symmetric and asymmetric VW fields, using the Siemens supplied $\mu$ and $c$ values for each beam.

## Material and methods

The VW model is implemented in the FOCUS radiotherapy treatment planning (RTP) system (Computerized Medical Systems, St. Louis, MO). Calculated dose distributions are compared to measured profiles on Siemens Mevatron MD and Primus accelerators. Profiles for 6, 15 and 23 MV beams were measured at 0.5, *dmax*, 3.0, 5.0, 10.0 and 20.0 cm depths for 15, 30, 45 and 60 degree wedge angles and 10x10, 15x10, 20x20 and 25x25 cm field sizes in a water phantom. Measurements were acquired with a Wellhofer water scanning system using a Wellhofer ion chamber array detector (CA24, Wellhofer Dosimetrie, Schwrazenbruck, Germany). The chamber array has 23 ion chambers spaced 2 cm apart in a linear fashion and an additional reference chamber. Spatial resolution finer than 2 cm is achieved by shifting the chamber array by a specific spacing. Data presented in this study were measured using a spacing of 6.7 mm or 10 mm depending on the field size of the VW field. The isocenter of the accelerator is 100 cm and the surface of the water was placed at 100 cm source to skin distance (SSD). Selected wedge dose profiles measured by the chamber array detector were verified by a diode detector array (Profiler, Sun Nuclear, Melbourne, FL). Point-by-point measurements were also performed using an ion chamber (PTW N23364) in a scanning water phantom to verify the dose profile for a 60 VW beam with the field size of 20x20 cm.

### Intensity map

The delivery of a VW treatment is a simple one-dimensional (1D) intensity modulation. The jaw motion produces a 1D pattern of intensity $g(x)$ across the field that Siemens express by the following analytic formula:

$$g(x) = \exp(c\mu\, x \tan\alpha) \quad (1)$$

where x is the position away from the central-axis, $c$ is a Siemens supplied attenuation correction factor (close to unity) used to accurately specify $\mu$ for the specific beam, $\mu$ is the effective linear attenuation coefficient of the VW for the nominal beam energy, and $\alpha$ is the desired VW angle to be delivered. The wedge angle can be set to any value when treating a patient and can be delivered if beam constraints are not violated.

The accelerator output is represented in MU and therefore Siemens assumes proportionality between dose and MU that can be written as:

$$MU(x) = MU(0)\exp(c\mu\, x \tan\alpha) \quad (2)$$

where MU($x$) is the number of monitor units delivered at a point $x$ and MU(0) is the number of monitor units delivered at central-axis (collimator rotation axis), $x$=0. MU(0) is also the number of monitor units that is entered at the machine console. This results in central-axis cGy/MU calibration factor values for VW that are similar to those of the open field with the same field size because the number of MUs delivered at that position are the same. Therefore, the wedge factor (WF) at the central-axis is close to unity, for all field sizes. Researchers found that the WFs for VW are close to unity with deviations from 1 as large as 4% for large wedge angles and field sizes.[1,2]

### Dose calculations

Two parameters are modulated during the course of the delivery: the jaw positions and the dose rate. Together these modulations produce a fluence profile similar to that generated by physical wedges. Both modulations occur in real time when implemented by a Siemens linear accelerator. The MU formula in (2) specifies the dose delivered for any dynamic collimator position, provided that the dose at the central-axis and the wedge angle are prescribed. Therefore, for any VW treatment, it is possible to calculate the dose delivered to any given dynamic collimator position. The information in equation (2) can be used to generate a transmission matrix. Note that the use of this transmission matrix is different for the Clarkson and Convolution/Superposition algorithms. The transmission matrix is used to modulate primary dose in the Clarkson algorithm and it is used to modulate fluence in the Convolution/Superposition algorithm

Let us consider a point at the surface of a water phantom that is going to be irradiated with VW. The point will be directly exposed to the source for a portion of the total MU delivery. The rest of the time, the moving jaw will be interposed. Thus, the "weight" of any element of the transmission matrix can be constructed as:

$$W(x) = \frac{MU(x)}{MU(0)} = \exp(c\mu\ x \tan\alpha) \qquad (3)$$

Notice that the modulation can be a function of width ($x$ direction) or length ($y$ direction) along four wedge orientations (in, out, right, left). VW is only available in the length ($y$ direction) for Siemens machines with MLC.

The complete transmission matrix used in the dose calculation algorithms, can be constructed for each fluence (Convolution/Superposition) or primary dose (Clarkson) "fan" using the weight ratio defined in (3):

$$T(m,n) = W(x(m,n)) \qquad (4)$$

where the fan at issue is the $m,n^{th}$ fan in the matrix, $x(m,n)$ is the position of the moving jaw when it is coincident upon the $m,n^{th}$ fan in the matrix. The derived transmission matrix is used in the dose calculation, and dose calculation proceeds as for physical wedges. For any clinical beam setup, the VW model determines the WF at the weight point as the ratio of the dose delivered on the axis of the weight point divided by the dose delivered on the central-axis. If the VW beam weight point is at central-axis ($x$=0), then equation (3) indicates a transmission weight factor of 1. For VW fields with wedge factor at the central-axis that deviates from 1, the transmission map is re-scaled to by the measured WF.

**Constraint checking on the delivery of VW in planning**

Since the different Siemens linear accelerators equipped with VW have different dosimetric and mechanical designs, it is critical to know which fields can be delivered during the treatment planning process. The range of combinations of field size, wedge angle, and the number of monitor units at the central-axis MU(0) that can be delivered on a Siemens machine is dependent on the maximum and minimum dose rate and jaw speed for that particular machine.

Once the radiation energy and the wedge angle are selected for planning, the VW model computes the intensity map for VW. A dose and MU calculations then can be performed, respectively. Following the MU calculation, the VW model performs the required physics (dose rate, jaw speed) constraint checking on the delivery of VW. The idea is to prevent the situation that requires modifying the plan after the isodose distributions and MU calculations are complete.

The VW model computes the required jaw speed to deliver a VW beam.[1] Further, the model checks if the jaw speed is less or greater than the minimum or maximum machine jaw speed, then the VW beam can not be delivered. The VW model displays a message indicating the machine constraints have been violated. In order to deliver the VW beam, in the case of *the jaw speed becoming less than the minimum machine jaw speed*, the dose MU(0) (beam weight) must be decreased or the machine maximum dose rate must be increased. On the other hand, in the case of *the jaw speed becoming greater than the maximum machine jaw speed*, the dose MU(0) must be increased or the machine minimum dose rate must be decreased. For both cases, dose rate changes can be performed provided that the machine required dose rate range allows it.

Prior to the delivery of a VW field, the dynamic jaw is moved to the opposing static to leave only a gap of 1 cm. In the VW model, once a VW is used for a treatment, constraint checking is performed for the field size. The Siemens deliverable field size has limitations along the wedged direction. These include the entire width (or length) of the wedged direction, and the positions of the static and moving jaws. The default gap is the minimum gap of 1 cm. When the gap is greater than 1 cm due to the moving jaw travel across central-axis is not far enough, the VW model will display a warning message. The model will still perform the dose calculation, however, a 'plateau' or flat region of dose at the 'toe' region will be generated.

## Results and discussion

We have performed dose calculations for 6, 15, and 23 MV beams, 15, 30, 45 and 60 degree VW angles, symmetric and asymmetric fields using the Clarkson and Convolution/Superposition algorithms. Figures 1 displays measured and Convolution/Superposition calculated dose profiles at depths of *dmax*, 10 and 20 cm for Primus 6 MV, 10x10 cm, 30 and 60 degree VW beams. Figure 2 shows measured and Convolution/Superposition calculated dose profiles at depths of *dmax*, 10 and 20 cm for Mevatron MD 15 MV, 20x20 cm, 15 and 45 degree VW beams. We found good agreement within 2% or 2 mm (distance to agreement) between calculations and measurements for 15, 30, 45 and 60 degree VW angles, and 6 MV, 15 and 23 MV beams, using the Siemens supplied $c$ and $\mu$ values. Similar agreement was observed for asymmetric fields. Also similar results were observed using the Clarkson algorithm for both symmetric and asymmetric fields. The results show that using the Siemens MU formalism with the supplied $c$ and $\mu$ to generate an intensity map yields accurate dose results, without the need for measured data to model VW as a physical filter.

We noticed that the VW model overestimates the dose in the toe region of the wedge by a maximum of 5%, especially for large wedge angles and large field sizes, as shown in Figure 2. One would suspect that possible measurement artifacts using the chamber array detector cause this difference. However, point-by-point measurements with spacing of 2.5 mm for a 60 degree VW in the Primus 6 MV beam using a scanning ion chamber in a water phantom confirm the accuracy of the chamber array detector. The most likely reason for this difference is that VW is delivered initially through a narrow beam strip, e.g., 1x20 cm, for a certain number of monitor

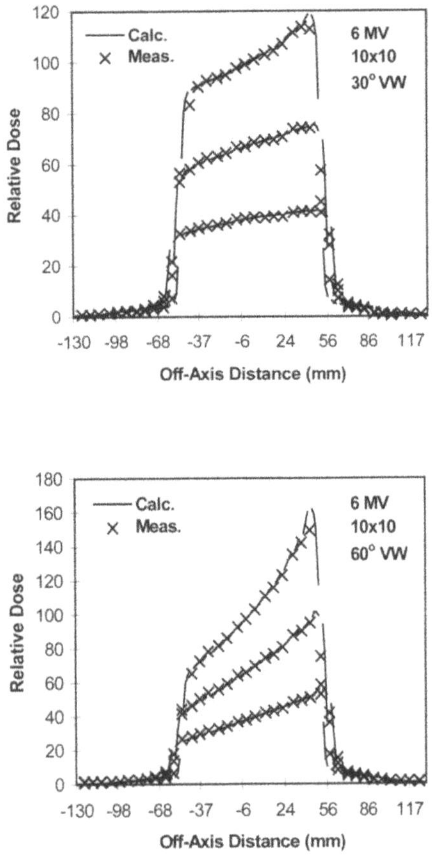


**Figure 1**: Measured and calculated dose profiles at depths of dmax, 10, and 20 cm for 30° and 60°, 10x10 cm Primus 6 MV beams.

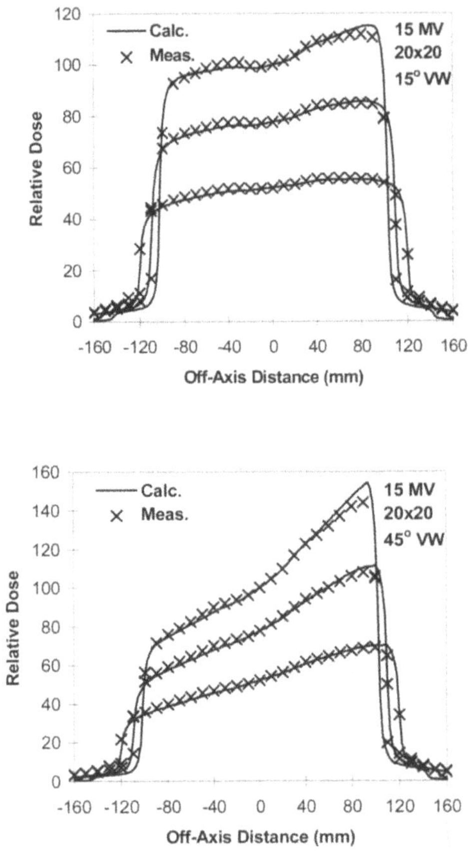


**Figure 2**: Measured and calculated dose profiles at depths of dmax, 10, and 20 cm for 15° and 45°, 20x20 cm Mevatron MD 15 MV beams.

units. The jaw starts to move and the field size in the wedge direction gradually increases. There is a lack of electronic equilibrium for very narrow beams. Consequently, the dose delivered is less than algorithms predict using a broad beam scatter model. Once the moving jaw travels into a more open geometry (more than 1-2 cm along the beam toe), the calculated and measured doses agree better. With smaller wedge angles, smaller field sizes and depths larger than $d_{max}$ the difference in dose is smaller within 2%. The clinical significance of the up to 5% overestimation of the dose in the toe region of the wedge for large wedge angles and large field sizes for the 6 MV beam is modest at best. The calculated dose distribution would show an increased hot spot in dose in the toe region of the wedge.

## Conclusions

The implementation of VW in RTP systems provides clinics with flexible and practical feature for radiotherapy treatment planning. To utilize the clinical advantages of VW, accurate dose calculation and constraint checking are required during the treatment planning process. We have presented a model, which relays on the Siemens monitor unit formalism, to accurately calculate dose. Results show that a transmission matrix calculated from ratio of MU delivered can be used to generate accurate dose calculations. Finally, we demonstrated that it is possible to include the VW beam delivery constraints in treatment planning. The efficiency of the treatment planning process is improved by including constraint checking.

## References

[1] van Santvoort J 1998 Dosimetric evaluation of the Siemens Virtual Wedge *Phys. Med. Bio.* **43** 2651-2663

[2] Desorby G E, Waldron T J and Das I J 1998 Validation of a new virtual wedge model *Med. Phys.* **25** 71-73

[3] Cunningham J R, Shrivastava P N and Wilkinson 1972 Program IRREG-calculation of dose from irregularly shaped radiation beams *Comp. Prog. Biomed.* **2** 192

[4] Miften M, Wiesmeyer M, Suzanne M and Krippner K 1999 Implementation of FFT convolution and multigrid superposition models in the FOCUS RTP system *Phys. Med. Bio.* (accepted)

# Development of On-line Beam Data Acquisition and Treatment Planning Software

**B.Paul Ravindran**

Department of Radiation Oncology, CMC Hospital, Vellore, India 632 004.

## Introduction

This paper describes a 2-D Radiation Field Analyzer (RFA) and an External beam treatment planning software developed in the department and in use for the last few years. A number of commercial treatment planning systems which provide sophisticated methods of patient data transfer to computer, fast computation of dose distribution, color and 3-D display of treatment plans and attractive hardcopy output are available. However most commercial systems have several limitations such as I) the user does not have access to the software to know the accuracy of the dosimetric parameters, the steps and algorithm utilized in arriving at a treatment plan. ii) The TPS may not have facility for all the beam shaping methods that would be needed for successful radiotherapy. In spite of using a sophisticated computer, if the data and algorithms used were poor and inaccurate, then the result would be poor. This situtaion is referred to as the "Ostrich syndrome' (Mould, 1981). Hence a project was undertaken to I) develop a water phantom (Radiation field analyser) for on-line acquisition of Central Axis Depth Dose (CADD) and Beam profiles and ii) to develop a software for external beam treatment planning using the data acquired with the RFA.

## Material and methods

In this project 1. Radiation Field analyzer for On-line data acquisition and 2. Treatment planning software were developed.

**1. Radiation Field Analyzer (RFA):** The development of the RFA for on-line beam data acquisition involves fabrication of a water phantom with X-Y movement of the detector. The X movement of the detector was achieved by using the "Gear and belt" movement system of a dot matrix printer with a stepper motor. To determine the position of the probe a multi-turn potentiometer was fixed in the same 'Gear and Belt' system and a 5 volt DC was applied to the end terminals of the potentiometer. The Voltage at the center-tapping of the potentiometer was calibrated to read the position of the detector. The Y movement was established by using two lead screws which were run by two separate stepper motors. The stepper motors used were of 4 pole type, having torque of 2Kg/cm. A 0.07cc ion chamber of a Capintec dosimeter was used for data acquisition. The analog output of the Model 192 Capintec dosiemeter was amplified with an operational amplifier and fed to a Data acquisition board (A/D converter). A personal computer with a stepper motor controller and a PCL 207 data acquisition board was used to control the movement of the stepper motor (i.e ion chamber) and to acquire the data from the Capintec dosimeter.

A software "SCANBEAM" was developed in QUICK BASIC to obtain the CADD and beam profile data using the water phantom system. This software controls the movement of the detector and its direction using the stepper motor driver. It also acquires the signal from the capintec dosimeter and from the potentiometer through the data acquisition board (Analog to Digital Converter). Once the scan is over the user can store the data in an ASCII file. The software can read the file and display in graphical form. A sub-routine to carryout bspline fit and cubic spline fit to the data has also been developed. The spline fit is used to smoothen the depth dose or the profile curve.

To obtain isodose curves two methods namely the decrement line method (Evans 1959,Orchard 1964) and Fan-line method (Milan, 1975) have been adopted. The ratio of the dose at any point on a transverse plane to the dose at the corresponding depth on the central ray is called the decrement dose or off-axis ratio (OAR) at that point. The points with the same decrement value (or same OAR) at different depths lie on a straight line. This was investigated for $^{60}Co$, 6 and 15 MV X-ray beam and also for electron beams. It was found that the decrement lines do not fall on a straight line for electron beams. Fan-line method represents a radiation beam in a given plane, in terms of three values, namely, the x coordinates, the depth 'd' and the off axis dose, which is the product of OAR and the CADD values at a given depth 'd'. Fortyseven off-axis ratio (OAR) values were determined from the beam profile measurements i.e 23 to the left and 23 to the right and one at the central axis (the value of which by definition will always be unity) for each profile. Data for 4 such profiles would be required for each beam, one measured at Dmax depth.

For the purpose of treatment planning a subroutine has been developed to generate a 'dose matrix' from the fan-line data. For the dose matrix of a given beam of width 'w', a grid with cartesian coordianates system $x_i$, $d_i$ was developed, with x varying from –w to w and d varying from 0 to 30cm with interspacing distance of 1 cm common to both axes. The dose matrices were generated for 4x4, 10 x 10, 15 x 15, 20 x 20 and 30 x 30 $cm^2$. The dose matrices for other field sizes were obtained by linear interpolation

**2. Treatment Planning software:** A treatment planning software that utilizes the data obtained by the above RFA was developed initialy with Quick BASIC and later upgraded with Visual Basic. The software works on lower level Pentium PC's however higher processors would be preferred. This system provides dose distribution on two dimension with provision to obtain dose distribution on off axis slices. The patient contour could be input with a digitizer (presently a Graptec) or from a CT image stored in BMP format. Multiple CT slices could be selected from an image database and the external contour and the contour of the tumour and critical organs could be digitized on each image. These are stored in a file in a separate folder named 'PTDATA'. The user can directly go to the 'Beam modeling' and plan the treatment. In the 'beam modeling' form the user can alter the Technique, Energy / Treatment unit, field size, gantry angle, wedge angle, beam weightage etc. Buttons have been provided on this form to calculate Isodose curves, normalise the dose distribution, obtain point dose, selected isodose curves, save and retrieve the plan and to obtain the Dose Area Histrogram. The software provides Dose Area Histograms for tumour and any selected critical organ. Either cumulative or differential histogram could be obtained.

The dose engine used to calculate the dose distribution uses the 'dose matrix' generated by the RFA software. This dose engine corrects for the surface obliquity using the Tissue air ratio method (ICRU 24, 1976) and equivalent path length method for the organ density. This routine generates a total dose matrix with 5 mm spacing and a contour drawing sub-routine is used to generate the isodose curves. The time taken for calculation of each beam is approximately 2 seconds on a pentium 166 machine.

A separate sub-routine has been provided to calculate the treatment time / monitor units and to store them with the beam parameters in a file. This routine also calculates the radiobiological factors such as the TDF and the ERD values.

## Results and discussion

The Central Axis Depth Dose and the beam profile obtained with the Radiation field analyzer developed was compared with those given in BJR supplimet No. 17. The results were found to match BJR values. The beam profiles obtained were checked for the FWHM (Full Width at Half Maximum). The Full Width at Half Maximum gives the correct field size at the depth. The beam profile obtained for blocked beam (simulating a mantel field) with the RFA for $^{60}$Co beam is given in Figure. 1. The isodose curves generated using the RFA software for these beam profiles is shown in Figure 2.

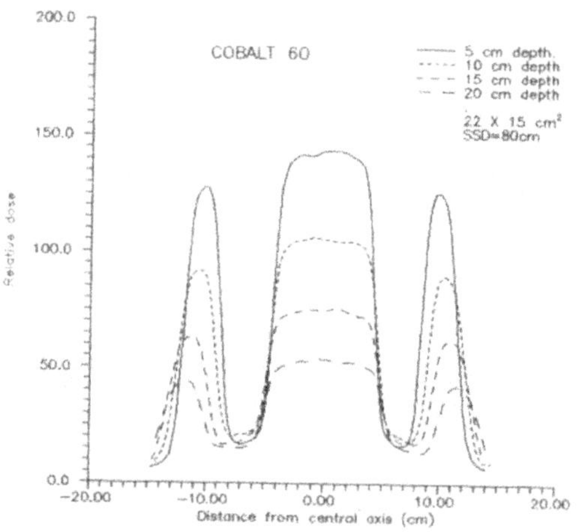


**Figure 1:** Beam profiles for blocked beams obtained with the RFA developed.

The External beam treatment planning software developed provides dose distribution for $^{60}$Co, 6 and 15 MV X-rays and for Electron beams. The results were compared with commercial planning system for cobalt 60. The dose distribution and point doses obtained were comparable. The dose distribution for a 4 field box technique obtained on a CT image is shown in Figure 3.

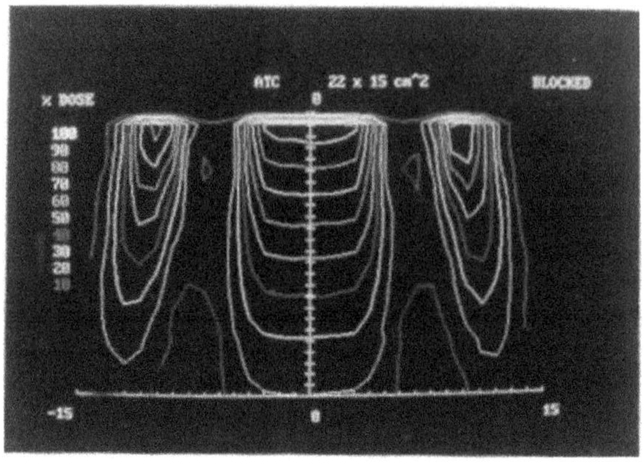


**Figure 2**. Isodose curves generated from the blocked beam profiles using fan line method

## Conclusion

A Radiation Field Analyzer and an External Beam treatment planning software have been developed. The Treament planning software can directly access the data generated by the Radiation Field analyzer. This is achieved either by floppy disk transfer or by netwrok. The Treament planning software is installed on a windows network so that the plan carried out by the physicist could be accessed by the Oncologists in their clinic.

## References

[1] Evans, E. Ann (1959), "A method for construction of isodose charts from minimum experimental data'. Am J Roentgenol. 81, 24

[2] Milan, J and Benteley, R.E., (1974), ' The storage and manipulation of radiation dose data in small digital computer, Br.J.Radiol. 47, 115

[3] Orchard, P.G., (1964), 'Decrement lines: a new persentation of data in cobalt -60 beam dosimetry, Br.J.Radiol, **37**,756

[4] ICRU (1976), "Determination of absorbed dose in a patient irradiated by beams of X or gamma rays in radiotherapy procedures', ICRU, Report 24, (International commission of Radiation Units and Measurements)

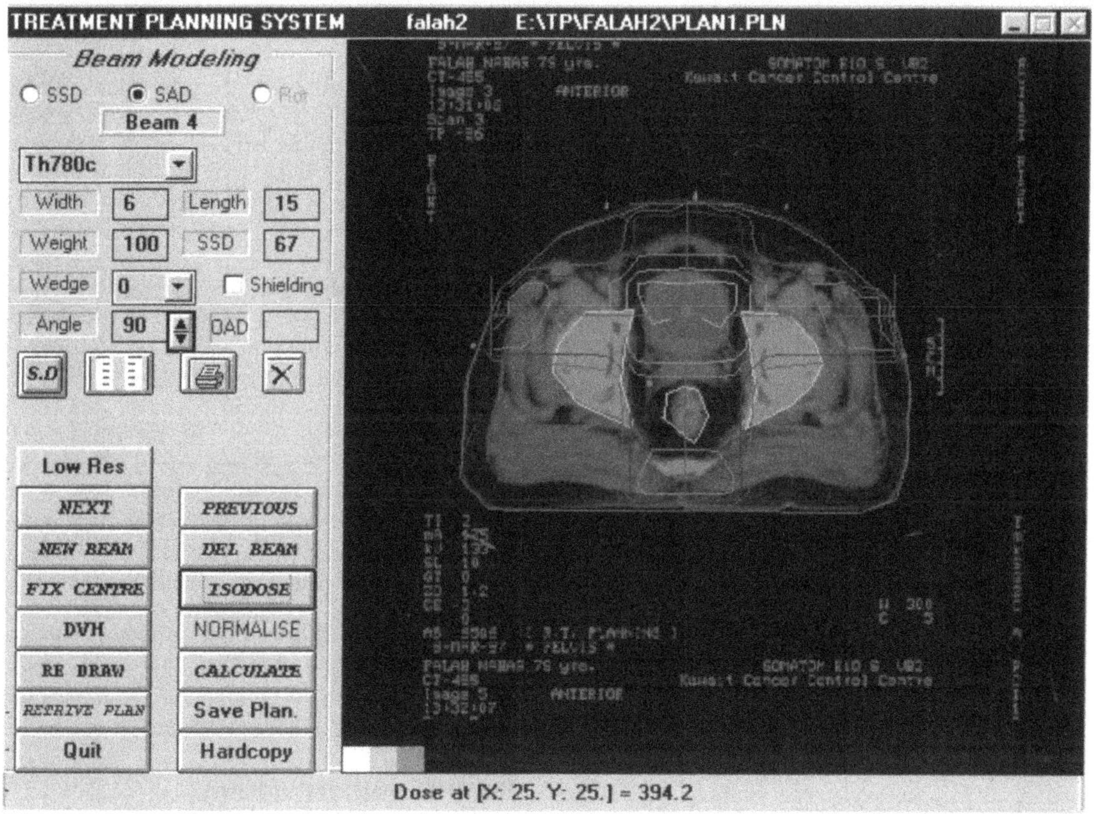


**Figure 3:** 'Beam Modeling' form of the Treatment planning software with Dose distribution on a scanned CT image.

# Influence of the dose response model for normal tissue on the dose distribution in IMRT

**Otto A Sauer**

Universität Würzburg, Klinik für Strahlentherapie, Josef-Schneider-Str. 4, 97080 Würzburg, Germany

## Introduction

In order to model the effect of generally inhomogeneous dose distributions for organs at risk (OARs), a variety of approaches can be found in the literature. Källman et al. [1] developed a model which attributes a relative seriality to each organ. Probability theory leads to a simplistic, but still computational expensive model for the functionality of an organ. The power law model is a popular approach, because clinical data may be easily modeled [2, 3]. Bortfeld et al. added dose-volume constraints as penalty term to a $\chi^2$-type objective function [4]. Generally, the influence of the choice of a model and its parameters is not clear in full detail. In this work, the power law relationship between dose $D$ and effect $E$ is compared with a piecewise linear fit of a sigmoidal dose response relation and a linear relation followed by a plateau at high dose values.

## Material and methods

### Patient and dose calculation model

A cylindrical phantom with a L-shaped target, lung and spinal cord as OARs was used as a simple patient model. Dose calculation was performed by convolution of Monte-Carlo generated energy deposition kernels [5]. The dose distributions of 2 mm wide pencil beams was precalculated. For the examples shown here, 7 beams were used. Starting with 0° at the horizontal from left to right, the gantry angles were equidistantly spaced The intensities of the pencil beams was determined by an optimization algorithm.

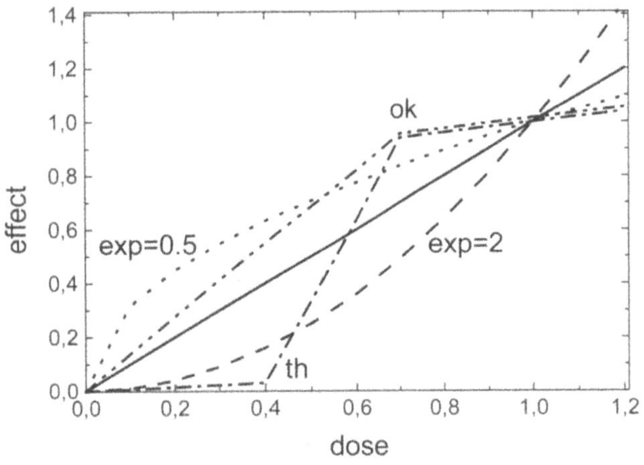


**Figure 1:** Different dose-effect relations applied to lung.

### Optimization models

The optimization followed the principles as published by Sauer et al. [6]: The dose to OARs was minimized subject to target dose being constrained between upper and lower bounds. For an organ of serial type, like the spinal cord, an upper limit constraint was set. A value of 0.5 was applied for all examples shown in this work. It is known, that setting constraints is more efficient than adding penalty terms to the objective function. For organs showing a volume effect, like the lung, we now implemented and tested different dose-effect relations (See Figure 1). A seriality exponent $S$ ($E=D^S$) was varied between 0.5 and 2 (see solid, dashed and dotted curves in Figure 1). For a ramp function the overkill-dose OK was varied between 0.2 and 1. At dose values below OK, the effect was proportional to the dose, while at the plateau above OK the slope was set to 0.1 (dashed-double-dotted curve). For a step function, additionally the threshold dose value was varied between 0.3 and 0.7 (dashed-dotted curve). The step function is close to a sigmoidal dose-response function, as it is expected theoretically.
As optimization engine, the program "fmincon" from the Matlab optimization library version 2 was used [7]. It utilizes sequential quadratic programming i.e. at each iteration step the objective function is approximated as a quadratic subproblem.

## Results and discussion

Figures 2 to 4 show dose distributions achieved with the different methods. The inner circle borders the "lung", the quadrate in the bow of the target "L" on the left hand side of the phantom is the model for the "spinal cord".
In Figure 2, the dose distributions result from different exponents $S$. While the lung dose is more homogeneous for the least squares type of objective function ($S$=2), a high dose region within the lung develops and the dose to the rest of the lung decreases when decreasing the exponent $S$. S=1.2 as used in the middle plot is the value derived by fitting the clinical data from the compilation published by Emami et al. [8]. The upper plot in Figure 5 shows that the mean dose in the lung, and consequently the integral dose, do hardly change, but because the frequency of very high and very low dose values increases, the standard deviation increases with decreasing $S$.
For the calculation of the dose distributions in Figure 3 the dose-response relation is linear, however, beginning at a certain dose, the overkill dose OK, the effect increases only slightly with dose. Due to the normalization of dose to one, for a value greater than one, OK has virtually no effect on the objective function. Therefore the distribution shown left results from a simply linear dose-effect relation. As it should be, the dose distribution is similar to the S=1.2 case in Figure 2. For OK=0.5 the most extreme distribution is achieved. For even

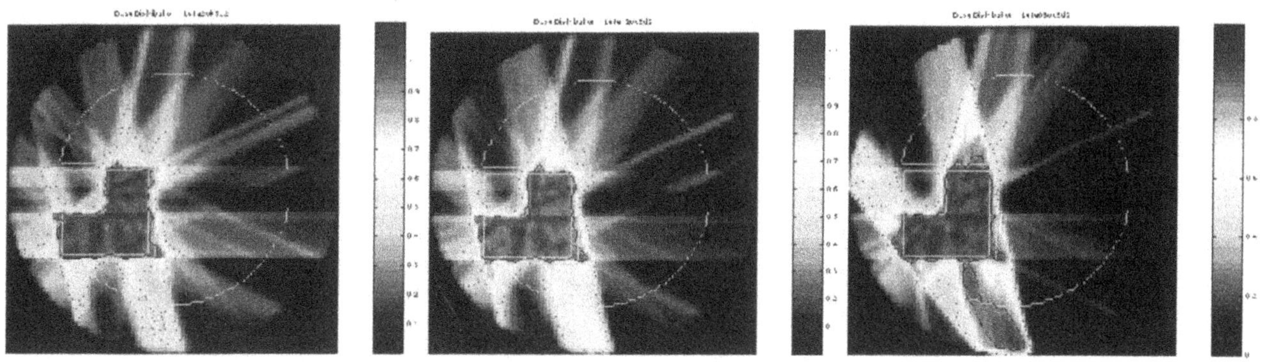

**Figure 2:** Seriality exponent varies from 2 left, over 1.2 middle, to 0.5 at the right picture .

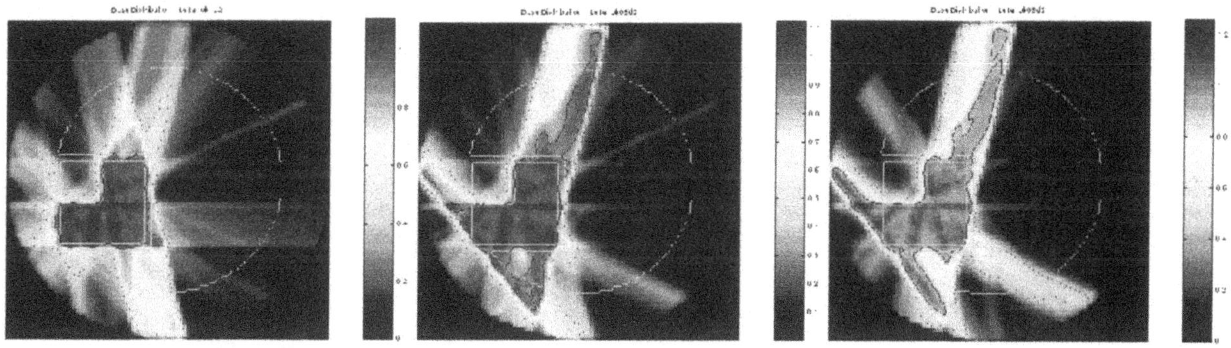

**Figure 3:** Overkill dose (OK) varies from 1 left, over 0.5 middle, to 0.3 at the right picture.

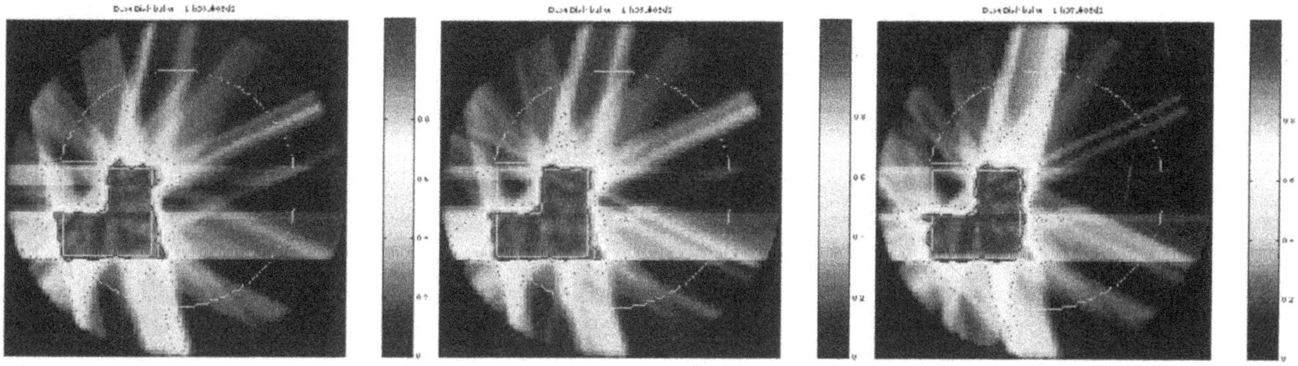

**Figure 4:** Threshold dose varies from 0.3 left, over 0.5 middle, to 0.7 at the right picture; OK is fixed at 0.8.

lower OK values, the magnitude of dose in the high dose region decreases, however, the region still grows in order to further reduce the dose in the low dose region. This behavior is reflected by the decreasing standard deviation of the mean dose for the lung as shown on the middle plot in Figure 5.

The behavior of the dose distribution with varying threshold dose is shown in Figure 4. For these examples, OK was fixed to a value of 0.8. Because now rather medium dose levels experience almost the same penalty in the objective function as the low dose levels, their fraction of the lung volume is higher for this approach. On the other hand, the very hot spots within the lung are avoided. With decreasing threshold dose, the dose-effect relation approaches the more simple ramp function. The resulting dose distribution behaves the same way. Again, the mean dose does not change by varying the parameters.

## Conclusion

We have demonstrated the usability of different dose response functions within the framework of our constrained optimization software. Contradictory input parameters leading to infeasibility of the optimization problem are not possible within this system. Interactive adaptation of parameters is not necessary; the optimization runs without any user interaction. All tested functions result in the same mean dose for the lung. If, as recently proposed [9], the mean dose is the decisive criterion for the prediction of radiation pneumonitis, all results are almost equivalent. However, generally clinicians want the fraction of volume with low probability for side effects as big as possible. This is modeled by all the functions proposed here.

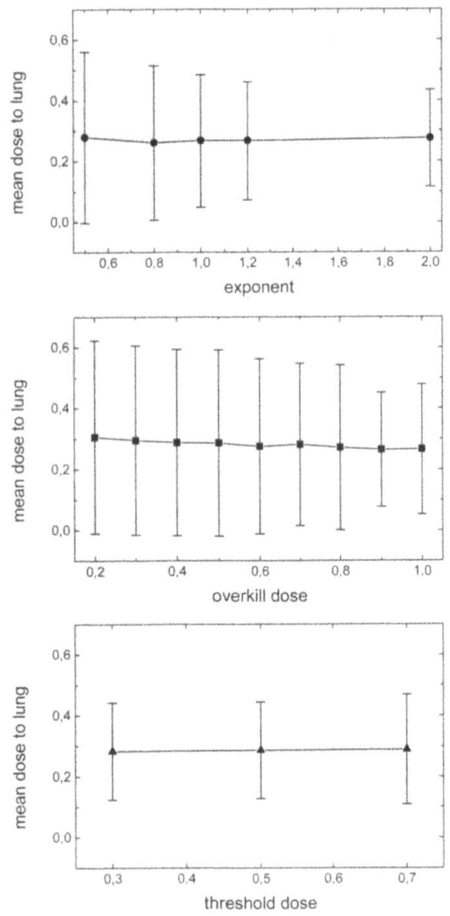


**Figure 5:** Different dose-effect relations applied to lung.

For the choice of the model we would suggest the following criteria: The computational burden. For our examples the CPU-time was highest for the threshold-overkill dose model, but the potential to spare time was not investigated in this work. Decisive should be the clinical applicability. Here, the latter models use dose values known from clinical experience. For the phenomenological power law model, the exponent has to fitted to clinical data. This, however, is not a problem either.

## References

[1] Källman P, Ågren A, Brahme A 1992 Tumour and normal tissue responses to fractionated non-uniform dose delivery *Int. J. Radiat. Biol.* **62** 249-262

[2] Mohan R, Mageras G S, Baldwin B, Brewster L J, Kutcher G J 1992 Clinically relevant optimization of 3-D conformal treatments *Med. Phys.* **19** 933-944

[3] Niemierko A 1999 A unified model of tissue response to Radiation *Med. Phys.* **26** 1100 (Abstract)

[4] Bortfeld T, Stein J, Preiser K 1997 Clinically relevant intensity modulation optimization using physical criteria, In: Proc. XIIth Int. Conference on Computers in Radiation Therapy, Editors: Leavitt D D, Starkschall G, Medical Physics Publishing, Madison Wi., 1-4

[5] Shepard D M, Olivera G, Angelos L, Sauer O A, Reckwerdt P, Mackie T R 1999 A simple model for examining issues in radiotherapy optimization, *Med. Phys.* **26** 1212-1221

[6] Sauer O A, Shepard D M, Mackie T R 1999 Application of constrained optimization to radiotherapy planning, *Med. Phys.* **26** 2359-2366

[7] Coleman T, Branch M A, Grace A 1999 Optimization toolbox for use with MatLab The Mathworks Inc., 24 Prime Park Way, Natick, MA 01760-1500, USA,

[8] Emami B, Lyman J, Brown A, Coia L, Goitein M et al. 1991 Tolerance of normal tissue to therapeutic irradiation *Int. J.Radiat. Oncol. Biol. Phys.* **21** 109-122,

[9] Kwa S L S, Theuws J C M, Wagenaar A, Damen E M F, Boersma L J, Baas P, Muller S H, Lebesque J V, 1998 Evaluation of two dose-volume reduction models for the prediction of radiation pneumonitis *Radiother. Oncol.* **48** 61-69

# Application of Biological Modelling to Facilitate the Transition from Conventional to Intensity Modulated Radiation Therapy Treatment

**Vernon Smith, Barby Pickett, Ping Xia, Andrea Pirzkall, Mack Roach III, and Lynn Verhey**

Department of Radiation Oncology, University of California, San Francisco, CA, 94143-0226, USA

## Introduction

Intensity modulated radiation therapy (IMRT) makes possible new and potentially more powerful treatment techniques, but at the same time carries the risks associated with venturing beyond the realm of clinical experience. A case in point is the use of IMRT to treat prostate cancer differentially such that the whole prostate gland is treated to a minimum dose but a portion, which has been shown to be cancerous by magnetic resonance spectroscopy, is treated to a higher dose. The question then arises as to what dose and fractionation scheme can yield the optimal combination of tumor control and minimal complications. Guidance can be provided through the use of biological models which allow the calculation of tumor control probability (TCP) and normal tissue complication probability (NTCP). We show how these models can provide the basis of selecting a safe and effective treatment scheme.

## Material and methods

The general form of the algorithms used for the NTCP and TCP calculations has previously been described by Smith et al (5). The methodology in brief is as follows. TCP calculations are based on the assumption that the tumor has a parallel structure and can be divided into a number of small volumes in which the dose can be considered to be constant. The overall TCP for inhomogeneous irradiation is given by

$TCP = \Pi_i\ [\ P(D_i, v_i)\ ]$ where $P(D_i, v_i)$ represents the response of the $i^{th}$ fractional volume $v_i$ irradiated to a dose $D_i$. We assumed the Poisson model for P (1) which yields for the response of the fractional volume v,

$P(D,v) = 2 - e^{[e\gamma(1 - D/D_{50}) + \ln v]}$. We have assumed that $\gamma$ has a value of 3, and that $D_{50}$ has a log-linear relationship given by $D_{50} = D_0 \ln(10^7 . V/ 0.693)$, where $N_0$ is the number of clonogens in the tumor, V is the tumor volume, and $D_0$ is the "effective mean lethal dose". We have assumed that $D_0$ has a value of 3.7 which yields $D_{50}$ values of 52.5, 61.0, and 69.5 Gy for volumes of 0.1, 1, and 10 cc respectively. The calculation of NTCP for an inhomogeneously irradiated organ was based on a simple serial model for which Schultheiss has shown (4) that

$NTCP = 1 - \Pi_i\ [1 - P_i(D,1)\ ]^{v}$. Schultheiss has also analyzed late GI and GU complications in the treatment of several hundred patients with prostate cancer (3), and we used his dose response curve for late Grade 2 GI morbidity to generate parameters for the NTCP model.

| | MS3D | Corvus | Peacock |
|---|---|---|---|
| 95% PTV Dose (Gy) | 73.5 | 81.0 | 82.3 |
| 95% DIL Dose (Gy) | 88.2 | 95.8 | 95.7 |
| % NTCP | 2.4 | 1.7 | 1.9 |

**Table 1:** Doses to the Planning Target Volume and the Dominant Intraprostatic Lesion, and the Predicted NTCP for the Rectum, normalized to a TCP of 90% for three different IMRT techniques.

## Results and discussion

As an example of the method, the analysis was performed for a specific prostate patient with a Dominant Intraprostatic Lesion (DIL) which had been localized using Magnetic Resonance Spectroscopy (2). Three different IMRT techniques were investigated. The first, labelled MS3D, was generated using a forward planning system and a small number of field segments. The second, labelled Corvus, was generated using the Nomos Corvus inverse planning system for a conventional Multi-Leaf Collimator (MLC) system, and the third, labelled Peacock, was also generated using the Corvus system but for the MIMIC delivery system. Plans were optimized to provide basic coverage to the PTV for the prostate gland plus a boost to the DIL of about one third higher dose. DVH's were calculated for the PTV and for the rectum, and these histograms were used to calculate NTCP and TCP values for each plan. For each plan the isodose surface enclosing 95% of the PTV was chosen for dose prescription. The dose prescribed to this isodose was adjusted to give a TCP value of 0.9, and then the NTCP value was calculated resulting from this dose presciption. This approach has the advantage that it avoids the pitfalls of combining NTCP and TCP into a single figure of merit, which has been criticized.

## Conclusion

In this particular example the results show that for the same predicted TCP one needs to prescribe quite different doses to the PTV. For the three techniques investigated the predicted NTCP values were not very different, however the dose to 95% of the DIL was less in the case of the MS3D than for the other two techniqes. Even though the prescription dose was chosen in each case to give a TCP of 90%, this was based on the assumption that this probability was uniform throughout the organ, and this is manifestly not the case since for the DIL. So the techniques giving an increased dose to the DIL should be advantageous. The lesson to be gained from this specific example is that without the aid of biological modelling it would be very difficult make treatment decisions for these new and very different techniques.

## References

1. Kallman, P.; Agren, A.; Brahme, A. Tumour and normal tissue responses to fractionated non-uniform dose delivery. Int J Radiat Biol. 62(2):249-62; 1992.
2. Pickett, B.; Vigneault, E.; Kurhanewicz, J.; Verhey, L.; Roach, M. Static field intensity modulation to treat a dominant intra-prostatic lesion to 90 Gy compared to seven field 3-dimensional radiotherapy. Int J Radiat Oncol Biol Phys. 44(4):921-9; 1999.
3. Schultheiss, T. E.; Lee, W. R.; Hunt, M. A.; Hanlon, A. L.; Peter, R. S.; Hanks, G. E. Late GI and GU complications in the treatment of prostate cancer. Int J Radiat Oncol Biol Phys. 37(1):3-11; 1997.
4. Schultheiss, T. E.; Orton, C. G.; Peck, R. A. Models in radiotherapy: volume effects. Med Phys. 10(4):410-5; 1983.
5. Smith, V.; Verhey, L.; Serago, C. F. Comparison of radiosurgery treatment modalities based on complication and control probabilities. Int J Radiat Oncol Biol Phys. 40(2):507-13; 1998.

# Phoenix 2000, A 3D conformal Treatment Planning System

**Luo Zhengming[1], Yang Dailun[1], Wu Zhangwen[1], Bai Sen[2], Fu Yuchuan[1], Hou Qing[1], Wang Yingguan[1], Gou Chengjun[1], Yang Zhiming[1], Wen Xinmin[1], Yang Heli[2],Xia Xingyuan[1] and Shen Guanqing[1]**

[1]The Key Lab. for Radiation Physics and Technology of the Education Ministry of China, and Center for Radiation Physics, INST, Sichuan University, Chengdu, 610064, P.R.China, and [2]Sichuan Tumor Hospital, Chengdu, 610041, P.R.China

## Abstract

Phoenix 2000 is a 3D conformal treatment planning system developed by the center for radiation physics of Sichuan University cooperating with the Sichuan Tumor Hospital. This paper gives a brief account of the system, which meets the needs of modern radiation therapy. In the aspect of medical image technology, the system can reconstruct a stereoscopic display of the anatomy structure and the target volumes directly by means of CT data. And it can conveniently provide users with automatic, semi-automatic or manual-operated way to sketch contour of the target volumes and the anatomy, and with a flexible tool to reconstruct the 3D images of them. The dose algorithms in this system include photon beam algorithm and electron beam algorithm. For the former we use the improved Convolution/ Superposition method, in which the concept of equivalent radiation source is applied to carefully treat the radiation field perturbation induced by bone. For the latter the bipartition model for electron transport, which has been extended from 1D inhomogeneous media to 3D inhomogeneous media, is used. Results obtained by using the above methods are in reasonable agreement with experiment results and Monte Carlo data. The algorithm for electron dose has a high calculating efficiency. For example, it takes less than one minute to calculate the electron dose distribution in a water phantom for a 20 MeV electron beam with 10cm x 10 cm field by using a 166 MHz cpu PC machine. In the aspect of inverse treatment planning and radiotherapeutical optimization, we use a hybrid method, namely the regularization method along with the simulated annealing method and it reduces the calculation time remarkably. The influence of important components and parts such as multi-leaf collimators, wedges, lead blocks and compensators upon photon or electron dose distribution in clinical practice are taken into account. For users' convenience, interactive interface operation has been carefully handled in the system.

# Progress in portal imaging techniques

**Marcel van Herk**

The Netherlands Cancer Institute, Plesmanlaan 121, 1066CX Amsterdam, The Netherlands. E-mail: portal@nki.nl

## Introduction

In this paper, developments in the field of electronic portal imaging for verification of geometric aspects of radiotherapy will be discussed. Portal dosimetry falls outside the scope of this paper. Conformal radiotherapy aims at maximizing tumor control while minimizing damage to the surrounding tissues. To increase the therapeutic range, smaller and smaller margins are being used between the clinical target volume (CTV), and the planning target volume (PTV). To achieve a high precision each step in the conformal radiotherapy procedure is image guided. In its simplest form, conformal radiotherapy consists of the following four steps: 1. External patient marking, usually under simulator image guidance. 2. CT scanning while aligning the patient with lasers to the external patient marks. 3 Treatment planning, delineation the tumor and planning beams relative to the patient marks as visible on the CT scan. 4. Treatment, before which the patient is aligning with lasers on the patient marks.

Figure 1 shows a flow diagram of a typical treatment procedure in radiotherapy. The patient enters the graph on the left. Going to the top of the graph we follow the physical patient: the skin marks are aligned on the lasers, the lasers are aligned with the CT room coordinates. Then the patient is moved to the treatment room, where lasers are used to align the patient's skin marks again. However, the patient's bone may have moved with respect to the skin marks and the tumor may have moved with respect to the bone. Going to the bottom of the graph, we follow the patient's CT scan through the planning process, to beam setup, and beam delivery. The dotted line shows the importance of portal imaging. By verifying the location of the planned relation between bone and beam (on a DRR), against the actual relation between bone and beam during treatment (on the portal image), the majority of the error sources in radiotherapy is verified. Organ motion (movement between bone and tumor), and uncertainties in target volume delineation must be verified separately.

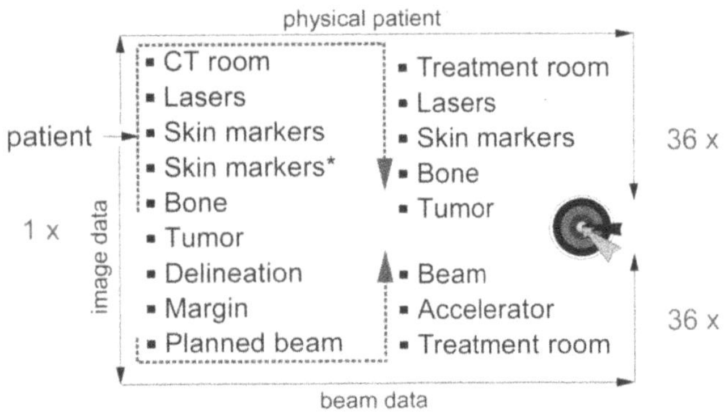


**Figure 1:** Schematic diagram of the radiotherapy procedure. Each step is a small source of uncertainty. The dotted line shows the importance of portal imaging. By verifying the location of the planned relation between bone and beam (on a DRR), compared with the measures relation between bone and beam (on the portal image), the majority of the error sources in radiotherapy is verified. *These skin markers and the object below relate to the virtual patient, i.e., the data as it is processed by the planning system.

To enable the task of portal imaging, a number of items have to be in place: image acquisition equipment, reference images, image analysis software, and decision rules for minimizing setup errors. Each of these items will next be discussed.

## Portal image acquisition

The past few years, a number of improvements have been made to existing EPID systems, leading to increased quantum efficiency. Video based EPID systems have been augmented using high DQE cameras (cooled CCD cameras originally designed for astronomical research) [10], and a high speed liquid ion chamber has been produced [17]. But, undoubtedly, the advent of solid-state flat panel imaging systems (almost all based on a scintillating screen coupled to an amorphous silicon light detector), is the most promising development [1]. A challenge remains, however, to mass produce the solid-state flat panel devices at acceptable prices. What the newer portal imaging devices have in common is that good or acceptable quality portal images can be made with a lower dose as before. This development, and the introduction of smaller and smaller treatment fields has lead to an increased use of (orthogonal) localization images. These larger images, in turn, simplify the analysis of the portal images.

## Reference images

The introduction shows that a DRR (figure 2) is the best reference image for 2-D portal image analysis in conformal radiotherapy. DICOM-RT defines a radiotherapy image object which allows transmission of the DRR and associated beam data from the planning system into a portal imaging system. However, until now, the support of commercial EPID systems for DICOM is limited and only a few planning systems can export DRRs through DICOM at this stage.

## Portal image analysis

Quantitative analysis of portal images is a prerequisite for accurate decision making [20]. The objectives of portal image analysis are: 1) verify that the treatment field has the right shape, 2) verify that the patient is in the correct position. To answer the first question, field edge detection and field edge matching software has been developed. For instance, field edge matching algorithms based on chamfer matching provide a quick and simple calibration of the detector position relative to the treatment beam and at the same time, quantify the misfit between the planned beam shape and the actual field shape expressed in terms of mean, maximum, and/or root mean

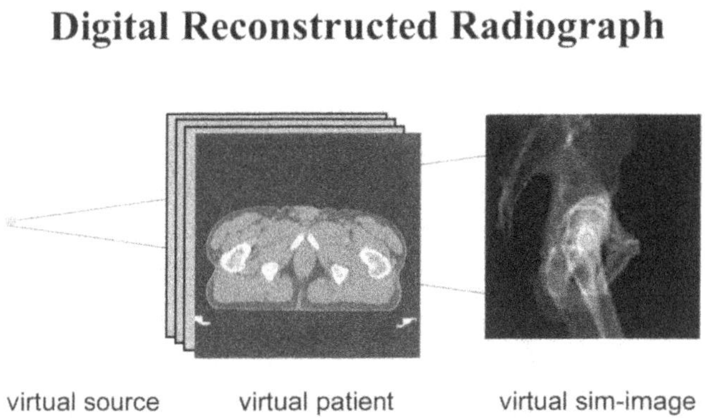


**Figure 2:** The use of a similator image as reference image for portal image analysis is sub-optimal. It is much better to compare the portal image with a DRR, acting as a virtual simulator image.

square deviations [8]. At present, however, a remaining challenge is to perform this analysis for images acquired during dynamic IMRT, in particular using scanning detectors (such as some types of flat panel imagers and the liquid ion chamber) [12,13]. To answer the second question it is customary to register the anatomy in the portal image with the reference image. However, one should be aware that anatomy matching is an ill-posed problem in the presence of rotations or distortions of the anatomy, since there will be no unique solution where all parts of the reference image match with the portal image [9]. In addition, the relatively poor image quality of portal images complicates automated algorithms for anatomy matching. Until now, only image registration algorithms based on segmented images [16] have found clinical application, with mixed success. An interesting development is the use of implanted markers to localize the tumor from day to day [2,18]. This is an example of a technique which not only addresses setup error, but that can be used to measure organ movement as well.

A possible improvement in the portal image analysis algorithms in the near future is to provide automated feature extraction of bony anatomy in the reference images [16]. Gray value matching algorithms, in which all pixels are applied, use more information than segmented images, and can potentially be more accurate [7,11]. However, clinical validation of these techniques is limited so far.

A well posed solution to measure rigid body motion (of bone) from portal images is 3D/2D analysis (figure 3). Such a technique [9] has been implemented in our institution (figure 3), and it has been proven useful, accurate and reliable for pelvis and head and neck treatments in medium scale clinical studies [15]. A challenge remain for the manufacturers to incorporate 3D/2D techniques in commercial product. Especially for 3D-2D registration, full communication between the treatment planning system and the portal imaging system is required. DICOM will play an important role here as well.

## Decision rules

After quantitative analysis of a set of portal images, the next step is to decide how to use the obtained information clinically. First of all, it is important to combine the 2D analysis information from multiple portal images taken during a single

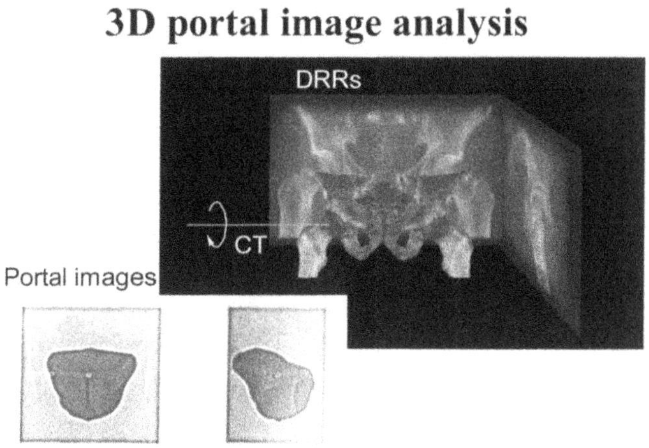


**Figure 3:** 2D registration of a single portal image with a DRR is an ill-posed problem in the presence of rotations. To solve this problem, 2D-3D image registration algorithms have been developed which analyze the motion of rigid anatomy with six degrees of freedom by registering the CT data with a pair of portal images.

fraction. Bel et al describe this problem can be solved universally, in an appendix to an article about setup errors in the parotid region [4]. Their method is based on estimates of the uncertainties in the measurement process, correct coordinate transformations and weighted averaging based on covariance matrices. The 3-D setup error data must next be processed by a decision protocol. It is important to realize that, for a single patient, systematic errors introduced during the preparation stage of radiotherapy have a much larger impact on the dose delivered to the CTV compared to random day to day variation during treatment execution. For this reason, the most used protocols are off-line, aimed at correcting systematic errors with a limited workload. On-line protocols also address day to day variation in patient setup, but do so at a considerable cost in workload [6]. The most widely used protocol was developed by Bel et al [3]. This protocol has been tested in thousands of patients (prostate cancer and others) in a Dutch cooperative study [5]. This protocol was designed to truncate the error distribution at a certain 3D vector length and has been proven to be very effective, even when corrections are performed in a crude way, such as by redrawing isocenter markers on the skin. Using computer controlled treatment tables with digital readout, the effectiveness of these protocols can be increased because the uncertainty in the corrections is limited. One should keep in mind, however, that additional workload is required to keep these protocols inherently safe. For instance, it is always a good idea to re-measure the patient setup after a correction has been made, to reduce the possibility of mistreatment due to operator or software errors. When the software become more efficient, it becomes possible to accept a higher workload in terms of number of measurements and corrections, and even further improve the accuracy. For instance, Yan et al have developed a technique called adaptive radiotherapy, in which the margin is adjusted to the attainable precision on a patient by patient basis [19]. Note that reduction of treatment margins is only safe when other uncertainties in the radiotherapy procedure are known and reduced. In particular, one should be aware of the large uncertainty in the delineation of the target volume [14]. Again, commercial implementation of decision rules is lagging behind considerably compared to research implementation.

## Future developments

An important development is verification of soft tissue position during treatment. For lung radiotherapy, it is often possible to see the tumor and evaluate its motion directly from portal images. For other sites, implanted markers have been used successfully [2, 18]. Megavoltage (MV) CT has some promise to localize soft tissue without markers. However, with MV CT it is extremely difficult to obtain sufficient contrast resolution to recognize tissues other than air or bone. Because the localization of bone in 3D can be done in other ways using orthogonal images, the additional value of MV CT is therefore limited. For this reason, on-line kilovoltage CT on the treatment machine is being pursued [10].

## Conclusion

Electronic portal imaging is becoming mature: all elements are in place to implement EPI and automatic image analysis. However, user friendly implementation in commercial products, in particular of the image analysis software and decision rules, remains to be done. For this reason, it is still a major undertaking to fully implement portal imaging in clinical practice. It is a sign of the importance of EPI as a quality control tool that so many groups have invested in this development.

## References

[1]Antonuk LE, Yorkston J, Huang W, Sandler H, Siewerdsen JH and el-Mohri Y. 1996 Megavoltage imaging with a large-area, flat-panel, amorphous silicon imager. *Int J Radiat Oncol Biol Phys* **36(3)** 661-672

[2]Balter JM, Lam KL, Sandler HM, Littles JF, Bree RL, Ten Haken RK 1995 Automated localization of the prostate at the time of treatment using implanted radiopaque markers: technical feasibility. *Int J Radiat Oncol Biol Phys* **33(5)** 1281-1286

[3]Bel A, van Herk M, Bartelink H, Lebesque JV 1993 A verification procedure to improve patient set-up accuracy using portal images. *Radiother Oncol* **29(2)** 253-260

[4]Bel A, Keus R, Vijlbrief RE and Lebesque JV 1995 Setup deviations in wedged pair irradiation of parotid gland and tonsillar tumors, measured with an electronic portal imaging device. *Radiother Oncol* **37(2)** 153-159

[5]Bel A, Vos PH, Rodrigus PT, Creutzberg CL, Visser AG, Stroom JC, Lebesque JV 1996 High-precision prostate cancer irradiation by clinical application of an offline patient setup verification procedure, using portal imaging. *Int J Radiat Oncol Biol Phys* **35(2)** 321-332

[6]De Neve W, Van den Heuvel F, Coghe M, Verellen D, De Beukeleer M, Roelstraete A, De Roover P, Thon L and Storme G 1993 Interactive use of on-line portal imaging in pelvic radiation. *Int J Radiat Oncol Biol Phys* **25(3)** 517-524

[7]Eilertsen K, Skretting A and TennvassDs TL 1994 Methods for fully automated verification of patient set-up in external beam radiotherapy with polygon shaped fields. *Phys Med Biol* **39** 993-1012

[8]Gilhuijs KGA and van Herk M 1993 Automatic on-line inspection of patient setup in radiation therapy using digital portal images. *Med Phys* **20** 667-671

[9]Gilhuijs KG, van de Ven PJ and van Herk M 1996 Automatic three-dimensional inspection of patient setup in radiation therapy using portal images, simulator images, and computed tomography data. *Med Phys* **23(3)** 389-399

[10]Jaffray DA, Drake DG, Moreau M, Martinez AA, Wong JW 1999 A radiographic and tomographic imaging system integrated into a medical linear accelerator for localization of bone and soft-tissue targets. *Int J Radiat Oncol Biol Phys* **45(3)** 773-789

[11]Moseley J and Munro P 1994 A semiautomatic method for registration of portal images. *Med Phys* **21(4)** 551-558

[12]Partridge M, Evans PM, Mosleh-Shirazi A, Convery D 1998 Independent verification using portal imaging of intensity-modulated beam delivery by the dynamic MLC technique. *Med Phys* **25(10)** 1872-1879

[13]Ploeger LS, van Herk M, Gilhuijs KGA, de Boer RW 1998 Static and dynamic properties of a liquid-filled EPID. *in: Proc. EPI98 (Phoenix, USA)* 106-107

[14]Rasch C, Barillot I, Remeijer P, Touw A, van Herk M and Lebesque JV. 1999 Definition of the prostate in CT and MRI: a multi-observer study. *Int J Radiat Oncol Biol Phys* **43** 57-66

[15]Remeijer P, Geerlof E, Ploeger L, Gilhuijs KGA, van Herk M, Lebesque JV 2000 3-D portal image analysis in clinical practice: an evaluation of 2-D and 3-D analysis techniques as applied to 30 prostate cancer patients *Int J Radiat Oncol Biol Phys* **in press**

[16]van Herk M, Bel A, Gilhuijs KG, Vijlbrief RE 1993 A comprehensive system for the analysis of portal images *Radiother Oncol 29(2)* 221-229

[17]van Herk M, Ploeger LS 1998 MTF and DQE of a liquid-filled matrix ionization chamber EPID. *in: Proc. EPI98 (Phoenix, USA)* 108-109

[18]Vigneault E, Pouliot J, Laverdiere J, Roy J, Dorion M 1997 Electronic portal imaging device detection of radioopaque markers for the evaluation of prostate position during megavoltage irradiation: a clinical study. *Int J Radiat Oncol Biol Phys* **37(1)** 205-312

[19]Yan D, Wong J, Vicini F, Michalski J, Pan C, Frazier A, Horwitz E, and Martinez A 1997 Adaptive modification of treatment planning to minimize the deleterious effects of treatment setup errors. *Int J Radiat Oncol Biol Phys* **38(1)** 197-206

[20]Yin FF, Rubin P, Schell MC, Wynn R, Raubertas RF, Uschold G, Sandhu A and Nelson DF 1996 An observer study for direct comparison of clinical efficacy of electronic to film portal images. *Int J Radiat Oncol Biol Phys* **35(5)** 985-991

# On the use of electronic portal imaging for treatment verification

**John Wong**

Department of Radiation Oncology, William Beaumont Hospital, Royal Oak, Michigan, USA

## Introduction

Treatment verification provides the important link between a desired treatment for the patient and the one that is actually delivered. There are many aspects to treatment verification, from concerns of machine stability to patient setup. Because patient re-positioning is often more variable than machine performance, treatment verification has mostly focussed on ensuring geometric accuracy of the patient setup. It follows then that portal imaging would play a key role in treatment verification as it provides a direct measurement, albeit in the form of a 2D projection, of the geometric relationship between the radiation beam and the anatomy of patient.
With the advent of increasingly complex treatment methods, such as intensity modulation, treatment verification becomes ever so critical. It would be worthwhile to re-examine the use of portal imaging for treatment verification.

## Components of treatment verification

It is important to remind ourselves that treatment verification is performed because we believe that setup errors, or excursions that are larger than acceptable, will occur. What constitutes an unacceptable setup error is implicitly defined by the margin that we set when prescribing the planning target volume (PTV). The desire for dose escalation reduces our tolerance, or margin, for setup error and therefore increases the probability that a particular setup would be considered erroneous. Given that, it must also be stressed that there are 3 components to treatment verification. They are the detection, analysis and correction of a setup error. Detecting a setup error is by far the simplest component of treatment verification. With portal imaging, the task has been made even easier with the availability of new film technology (i.e. the ECL film from Kodak) that can accommodate a wider range of radiation exposure, and the development of electronic portal imaging devices (EPIDs). But the remaining 2 tasks of analyzing and correcting a detected setup error are more germane to the ensurance of setup accuracy, and far more complex. With treatment methods that increasingly emphasize the 3D nature of the problem, conventional approaches such as simple translational adjustment of the patient, may no longer suffice.

## Treatment verification with portal images

In treatment verification, one needs to address the variation in patient setup, and also the resultant variation in dose delivered to the patient. Ignoring machine output variation for the moment, patient dosimetry is a dependent variable of treatment geometry. But interestingly, the geometric and dosimetric problems are considered independently at present, as evident in the study of the field placement errors and portal dose images as a surrogate for "in vivo" dosimetry.

### Setup Verification

When using portal images to verify patient setup, it is critical to first establish a correction model and an action level. The choice of correction model will directly impact on the clinical workload and therefore should be reasonable for the desired goal of the treatment. It has become apparent that much of the demise of (or the lack of) EPID acceptance in North America stems from the lack of a properly defined correction model. On the other hand, a properly defined correction model, such as the decision rule model implemented in the Netherlands [1], clearly demonstrates that electronic portal imaging can be highly effective in reducing systematic setup error.
An implicit and imperative requirement in adapting a correction model and defining an action level, is an understanding of the level of setup accuracy that can be achieved. Rigid phantoms can be used to evaluate the correction models, and typically excellent setup accuarcy, of the order of 2 mm, can be achieved. However, phantom results obtained in the idealized laboratory setting cannot be used to infer performance in the clinic. For a patient whose setup would likely include some degree of anatomic rotation and distortion [2,3,4] Dr. Van Herk has already pointed out that the matching of bony anatomy in portal images would lead to ambiguous determination of setup error. It is possible to reduce some of the ambiguity by using more imaging information, such as in the CT-based 3D/2D technique developed at the Netherlands Cancer Institute to measure rigid motion of bony structures in the pelvic and head and neck regions [5]. But in most cases, treatment verification using portal images only provide a perceived error. At present, it is difficult to estimate how close is our preceived setup error from the true setup error, since the latter is seldom measurable in the clinical setting.
In summary, the user is reminded that appreciable residual uncertainties remain when using portal images for treatment verification. As also mentioned by Dr. Van Herk earlier, the use of bony landmark for error determination cannot always be used to infer target position. It is important for the user to have a knowledge of the residual uncertainties and to include them in the design of the correction model.

### Dosimetric Verification

The ultimate goal of treatment verification is of course to ensure that the patient is treated with the correct dose (or dose distribution). A portal image contains both anatomic and dosimetric information and would, in theory, allow some degree of dosimetric verification. The concept of using a portal dose image (PDI) [6,7] as a surrogate for in vivo dosimetry has attracted some interest in Europe where the latter is traditionally measured as part of treatment QA [8,9]. Certainly, a PDI can be used to verify patient positioning and certain straight-forward irradiation parameters, such as the orientation of a wedge.

However, the fact that a PDI contains both anatomic and transmitted fluence information also compromises its effectiveness to resolve a detected treatment error. The evaluation of a PDI requires a very accurate dose calculation algorithm that can resolve the effects of setup changes on the scatter dose measured with a PDI. One can avoid the difficult scatter calculation by acquiring a PDI at extended distance. But then, such a PDI would be insensitive to SSD error, or any anatomic variation in the direction of the beam axis. The effectiveness of PDI verification also diminishes with more advanced treatment techniques. For conformal treatment, the lack of anatomic information reduces the sensitivity of a PDI for error detection. For intensity modulated treatment, it would be hard to determine whether an observed discrepancy in transmitted fluence is due to variation in patient position or radiation output.

The author is of the opinion that the use of a single projection PDI to infer in vivo (or mid-plane) patient dosimetry, is an approach that is susceptiable to large uncertainty. In vivo dosimetry as currently practised is not a measured quantity, but merely an estimation. The necessary assumptions render the estimation no more, if not less, accurate than a plan recalculation. (It is confusing to the author why the measured intensity in a PDI cannot be used as quantity to verify the constancy of the beam output). Often, many of the ambiguities encountered when analyzing a single projection PDI can be resolved by having more imaging information from other projection angles. Such observation simply emphasizes that geometric or anatomic information is fundamental to the problem of treatment verification. Indeed, in the present era where computer control has greatly improved the reproducibility of machine perfermance, such as the placement of a MLC field, patient geometry can be, and should be, verified independent of machine performance. If comprehensive 3D data can be acquired, such as with the use of on-board CT capability [10,11,12] then treatment verification would allow unambiguous determination of the 3D dosimetry delivered to the patient.

## Discussion

It is clear that with the advances made in treatment optimization and delivery, the task of treatment verification would be more demanding. The role of portal imaging needs to be re-examined so that it can be used effectively. At present, there are residual errors that have not been quantified and it is unclear as to how accurate we can setup a patient using portal imaging. On the other hand, not all treatment goals require the use of a minimal margin. It is imperative that all treatment personnel has a clear understanding of the treatment goal, action level and correction model. With the present state of technology, the verification of patient setup and machine performance can be considered independently. It is no longer necessary to require that a portal or localization, image, be acquired in the same geometry of the treatment beam --- an unrealistic requirement for techniques such as tomotherapy or stereotactic radiotherapy. On the other hand, more imaging information would allow more effective treatment verification, setup correction and determination of patient dosimetry. Taking note that traditional use of bony landmark for setup verification cannot guarantee accurate irradiation of the clinical target volume, it seems inevitable that the next milestone in treatment verification would be based on tomographic imaging. Tomographic images acquired at the time of treatment will show the true setup that is not possible with portal imaging. Clearly, technology and methodology to do so are already available. However, the author would like to end with a note that tomographic imaging will not be the end all to treatment verification. Ultimately, biological status of the disease must also be addressed in treatment verification.

## References


[1] Bel A., Vos P.H., Rodrigus P.T.R., Creutzberg C.L., Visser A.G., Stroom J.C., Lebesque J.V. (1996). High precision prostate cancer irradiation by a clinical application of an offline patient setup verification procedure using portal imaging. Int J Radiat Oncol Biol Phys, 35: 321-332.

[2] Hanley J, Magras GS, Sun J. et al (1993). The effects of out-of-plane rotations on two dimensional portal image registration in conformal radiotherapy of the prostate. Int J Radiat Oncol Biol Phys, 33:1331-1343.

[3] Remeijer P, Geerlof E, Ploeger L, Gilhuijs KGA, van Herk M, Lebesque JV (2000). 3-D portal image analysis in clinical practice: an evaluation of 2-D and 3-D analysis techniques as applied to 30 prostate cancer patients Int J Radiat Oncol Biol Phys *in press*

[4] Pisani L.J., Lockman D., Jaffray D., Yan D., Martinez A., Wong J. (1999) Factor limiting the accuracy of on-line setup correction using electronic localization radiographs. Int J Radiat Oncol Biol Phys, *submitted for publication.*

[5] Gilhuijs KG, van de Ven PJ and van Herk M (1996). Automatic three-dimensional inspection of patient setup in radiation therapy using portal images, simulator images, and computed tomography data. Med Phys 23:389-399.

[6] Wong JW, Slessinger ED, Hermes RE, Offutt CJ, Roy T, Vannier MW (1990). Portal dose images I: Quantitative treatment plan verification. Int J Radiat Oncol Biol Phys, 18:1455-1463.

[7] Ying X, Geer LY, Wong JW (1990). Portal dose images II: Patient dose estimation. Int J Radiat Oncol Biol Phys, 18: 1465-1475.

[8] Boellaard R (April 1998). In vivo dosimetry with a liquid-filled electronic portal imaging device. PhD thesis, Free University, Amsterdam.

[9] Pasma KL (September 1999). Dosimetry with a fluoroscopicelectronic portal imaging device. PhD thesis, Erasmus Universiteit Rotterdam.

[10] Mackie T.R., Holmes T., Swerdloff S., Reckwerdt P., Deasy J.O., Yang J., Paliwal B., Kinsella T. (1993). Tomotherapy: a new concept for the delivery of dynamic conformal therapy. Med Phys, 20: 1709-1719.

[11] Jaffray D.A., Drake D.G., Moreau M., et.al. (1999). Radiographic and tomographic localization of bone and soft-tissue targets on a clinical accelerator. Int J Radiat Oncol Biol Phys, 45:773-789.

[12] Jaffray D.A., Siewerdsen J. H., Drake D. G. (1999). Performance of a volumetric CT scanner based upon a flat-panel imager. SPIE Physics of Medical Imaging Vol. 3659, *in press*.

# Computational methods for treatment verification: the Full Monte Carlo contribution.

**F. Sánchez-Doblado[1,2], M. Perucha[1], A. Leal[1], M. Rincón[1], R. Arráns[2], L. Núñez[3], J. Roselló[3], E. Carrasco[1], G. Martín[1], J.C. Medrano[3], L. Errazquin[2], J. A. Sánchez-Calzado[2]**

[1]Dpto. de Fisiología Médica y Biofísica. Facultad de Medicina. Univ. Sevilla. Spain, [2]Hosp. Univ. Virgen Macarena. Servicio de Oncología Radioterápica. Sevilla. Spain and [3]Clínica Puerta de Hierro. Madrid. Spain

## Introduction

The aim of Radiophysics is, within the frame of Radiotherapy, the precise knowledge of the dose distribution inside the human body due to the energy delivery coming from a radiation beam, either from a particle accelerator or from a radioactive source. The planning systems are mainly devoted to this purpose. These pieces of software, which run usually on powerful computers, simulate the process by means of experimental data and specially suited algorithms. Although the precision of these systems, some uncertainties still remain mainly regarding scattering effects and inhomogeneities. This is so because the calculations are not made generally in true 3D and on the other hand, inhomogeneities are not accounted for in detail. In standard Radiotherapy these uncertainties are may be small, but in the case of special techniques or situations, the accurate knowledge of the dose becomes more critical[1,2,3,4,5,6]. The new codes simulating the particle transport using the Monte Carlo method are an appropriate alternative as they seem to be the only tool allowing a whole and accurate knowledge of the beam characteristics, spectral and spatial distribution[7]. This is because it takes into account every single tissue and medium crossed by the beam which may contribute to the delivered dose. The main drawback of this method is the time of calculation which is being decreasing with the new computers[8].
The objectives of our work have therefore been three-folded: first, the optimisation of CPU time by means of process distribution. Second, Dosimetric data verification and together with clinical cases evaluation by comparison with experimental data and commercial planning systems, respectively.

## Material and method

Most simulations have been performed for a Philips SL-18 and a Siemens Mevatron 74. The Monte Carlo code used was the EGS4 under OMEGA-BEAM code, developed by Dave Rogers and collaborators at the National Research Council of Canada (NRCC)[9]. The phase space (reference plane at any relevant position, where the particle transport has been stopped and stored in a file containing its type, position, incidence angle and energy) has been calculated by means of the BEAM code[10]. This calculation includes, not only the linac head simulation, but every specific equipment needed for special techniques (additional collimators in radiosurgery, multileaves or blocks in conformal therapy, etc). With the DOSXYZ code the calculation on either heterogeneous phantoms or patients has been performed[11]. In this last case, the geometric data has been obtained from a CT Toshiba X-speed II or a Siemens Somaton DRH. For this purpose, some experiments have been performed and a software tool has been developed to convert the CT information to the Monte Carlo requirements (geometry, medium and density). The most complex geometry has been used for radiosurgery, where 60 to 80 CT slices with 512x512 pixels resolution have been converted to 256x256 pixels, leading to a resolution of about 1mm[12].
Concerning computing facilities, at a first instance two SGI (Octane dual processor MIPS R-10000 with 384 MB and a O2 R-5000 processor with 96 MB), as well as a cluster of four PC Pentium III (500 MHz and 256 x 4 MB), have been utilised. The main use of this equipment has been the fieldwork, the previous simulations and the graphic display of the images. We have priority access to a supercomputer (HP X-class SPP 2000 with 2 GB and 24 processors type PA-RISK 8000)[13]. For PC based distribution process, we can make use of some sixty PC (Pentium II or III with 64 MB minimum). These configurations allows to obtain results between 20 minutes and less than 1 hour in most situations. In the figure 1 we can observe the ratio for different configurations in comparison with our supercomputer.

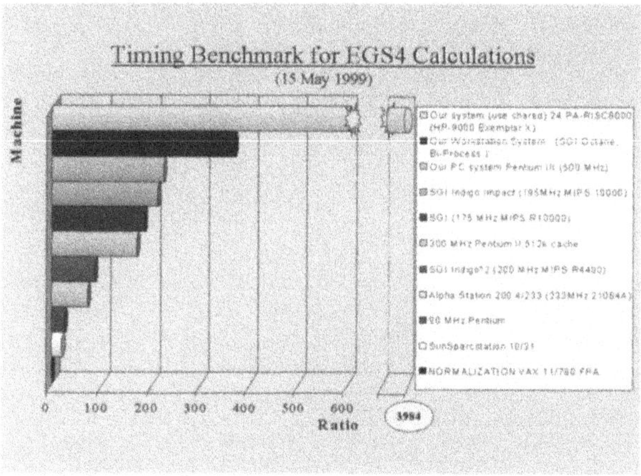


**Figure 1:** Ratio for our supercomputer configuration.

For dosimetric verification, the experimental data obtained with different detectors (either for standard or special fields) have been compared to the Monte Carlo calculations. The values that have been compared are the ones usually handled by the planning systems (PDD, TPR, OAR and OF). The energy spectrum has also been studied, in special situations, to estimate the stopping power needed for absolute dose calculations[14].

A large number of clinical cases with different situations and complexities have been studied. Commercial planning system calculations (Nucletron Plato, Levinger Fisher and Focus) have been compared with the Monte Carlo results[15]. Differences in dose at a point of interest and distances between isodose lines have been estimated. Furthermore, comparison of the whole 3D dose distributions by means of Dose Volume Histograms (DVH) as well as estimates of the impact of these differences upon the Normal Tissue Complication Probabilities (NTCP) and Tumour Control Probability (TCP) have been carried out[16].

## Results

In most dosimetrical studies there is a good agreement between empirical and simulated data. Nevertheless, larger discrepancies have been found when dealing with small (see Figure 2) and irregular fields in photon and electron beams. Analogously, the planning system calculation matches the Monte Carlo calculations in the majority of the standard cases. However, they show disagreements of up to 30% in some isodose curves when inhomogeneities, complex or critical situations are considered. Figure 3 shows an example of this discrepancies for a radiosurgery treatment.

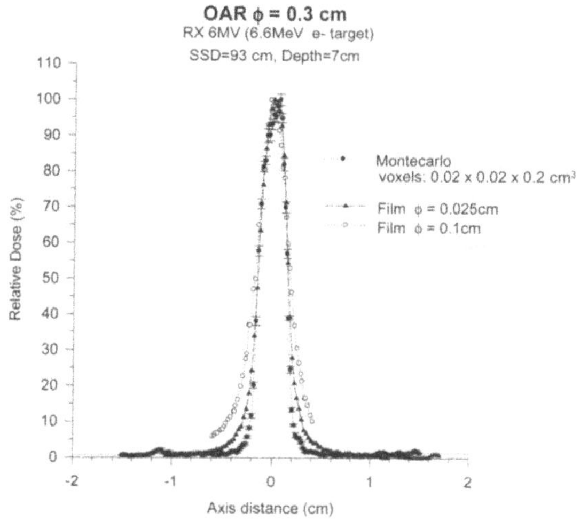


**Figure 2:** Spatial resolution effect.

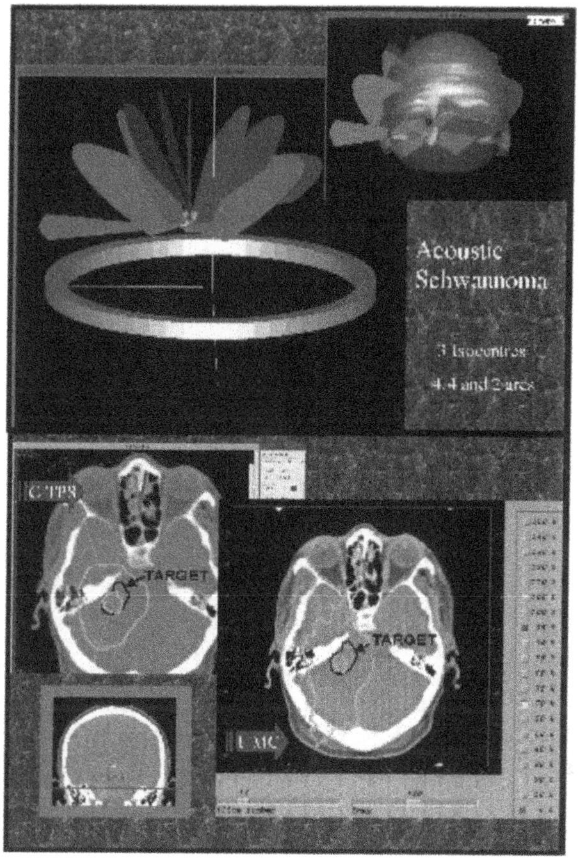


**Figure 3:** Isodoses (70 and 5%) differences between Monte Carlo (F MC) and a conventional planing system (C TPS).

## Conclusions

Some distribution processes (Supercomputer and PC-based network) calculation tools for Full Monte Carlo (FMC) have been implemented. Although the CPU times have not been reduced when compared with conventional treatment planning systems, they are short enough to be used as an alternative method of verification.

Monte Carlo is a powerful tool to calculate reliable dose distribution, especially in those cases when conventional detectors are not trustworthy.

Full Monte Carlo planning highlights the need of improvement of the conventional algorithms used in radiosurgery. Nevertheless, the availability of an alternative method for verification is an invaluable tool for quality assurance of treatments.

## References

[1] Sánchez-Doblado F, Arráns R, Terrón J A., Sánchez-Nieto B and Errazquin L 1994 Computerized semiconductor probe based system for in vivo dosimetry of patients undergoing high energy radiotherapy *Medical & Biological Engineering & Computing* **32**(5) 588-592

[2] Sánchez Doblado F, Terrón J A., Arráns R, Sánchez-Nieto B , Errazquin L, Biggs D, Lee C, Núñez L, Delgado A and Muñiz J L 1995 Verification of an on line and in vivo semiconductor dosimetry system for TBI with two TLD procedures *Radiotherapy and Oncology* **34** 73-77

[3] Sánchez Doblado F, Quast U, Arráns R, Errazquin L, Sánchez-Nieto, B and Terrón, JA. 1995 Total Body Irradiation prior to Bone Marrow Transplantation *EBMT* ISBN: 84-605-3132-5

[4] Nuñez L and Sánchez-Doblado F 1999 Small field dosimetry in Radiosurgery *Dynarad* ISBN: 84-605-7911-5

[5] Nuñez L, Sánchez-Doblado F, Gallardo M, Cutanda F, Muñiz J L and Delgado A 1999 Dosimetric verification in radiosurgery whith linac non-coplanar arc beams *Radiation Protection Dosimetry* **85** 409-412

[6] Nuñez L, Sánchez-Doblado F, Muñiz J L, Ispizua M C, Medrano J C, Gallardo M and Delgado A 1999 Comparison of Dosimetric Detectors in Radiosurgery Planning *Radiation Protection Dosimetry* **85** 405-408

[7] Ma C-M, Mok E, Kapur A, Pawlicki T, Findley D, Brain S, Forster K and Boyer A L 1999 Clinical implementation of a Monte Carlo treatment planning system *Medical Physics* **26** (10) 2133-2143

[8] Ma C-M, Jiang S B 1999 Monte Carlo modelling of electron beams from medical accelerators *Physics in Medicine and Biology* **44** 157-189

[9] Rogers D W O, Faddegon B A, Ding G X, Ma C-M and We J 1995 BEAM: A Monte Carlo code to simulate radiotherapy treatment units *Medical Physics* **22** (5) 503-524

[10] Ma C-M, Reckwerdt P, Holmes M, Rogers D W O, Geiser B and Walters B 1998 BEAM Users Manual *NRCC report* PIRS-0509B(revC) Ottawa

[11] Ma C-M, Reckwerdt P, Holmes M, Rogers D W O, Geiser B and Walters B 1998 DOSXYZ Users Manual *NRCC report* PIRS-0509B(revC) Ottawa

[12] Sánchez-Doblado F, Perucha M, Núñez L, Leal A, Rincón M, Arráns R, Carrasco E, Roselló J, Errazquin L, Sánchez-Calzado J A 1999 To what extend does Full Monte Carlo make sense in Radiosurgery? *Physica Medica*, **XV**(3) 188

[13] Leal A, Sánchez-Doblado F, Rincón M, Perucha M, Camacho I, Sierra M, Arráns R, Carrasco E, Sánchez-Calzado J A, Errazquin L 1999 Parallel processing for Full Monte Carlo time optimisation *Physica Medica* **XV**(3) 187

[14] Perucha M, Sánchez-Doblado F, Leal A, Rincón M, Nuñez L, Roselló J, Arráns R, Carrasco E, Errazquin L, Sánchez-Calzado J A 1999 Monte Carlo as a tool to evaluate radiosurgery dosimetric data and treatment planning *Physica Medica* **XV**(3) 188

[15] Sánchez-Doblado F, Arráns R, Leal A, Rincón M, Perucha M, Carrasco E, Sánchez-Calzado J A, Errazquin L, Salmerón J, Glez del Corral M 1999 Telematic implementation for the verification of treatment planning by Monte Carlo techniques. *Physica Medica* **XV**(3) 175

[16] Sánchez-Nieto B and Nahum A E 1999 The ΔTCP concept: a clinically useful measure of tumour control probability *International Journal of Radiation Oncology Biology and Physics* **44** (2) 369-380

## Acknowledgements

The authors wish to thank Dr. Beatriz Sánchez-Nieto (Institute of Cancer Research, Royal Marsden Hospital, U.K.) for this valuable comments and criticism. This work has been possible thanks to the "Health Research Grant"(FIS) as well as to the L.R.U. contract between the University of Seville and the Andalusian Health Service (SAS).

# Quality Management in Conformal Radiotherapy

**Fridtjof Nüsslin**

Abt.Medizinische Physik, Universitätsklinikum Tübingen, Germany

## Introduction

Any quality management system in radiotherapy aims at three key issues, (i) state of the art treatment, (ii) accuracy of dose delivery and (iii) safety for the patient, staff and public. Furthermore, cost effectiveness and motivation of the entire staff is expected to emanate from an adequate and properly designed QMS. This paper reviews the principle of a QMS and ways to get it implemented into clinical routine concomitantly adressing some specific aspects of relevant to conformal radiotherapy.

## Principle of a Quality Management System

According to the definitions introduced by the ISO 9000 standards [1] a quality system comprises the entire organisational structure, procedures, processes and resources of the radiotherapy institution. The consistency and flexibility of a QMS is achieved simply by the requirement that the institution itself defines the quality system, and it is its responsibility to manage all processes necessary to ensure that the `product', i.e. the treatment conforms to the patients requirements (fig.1).

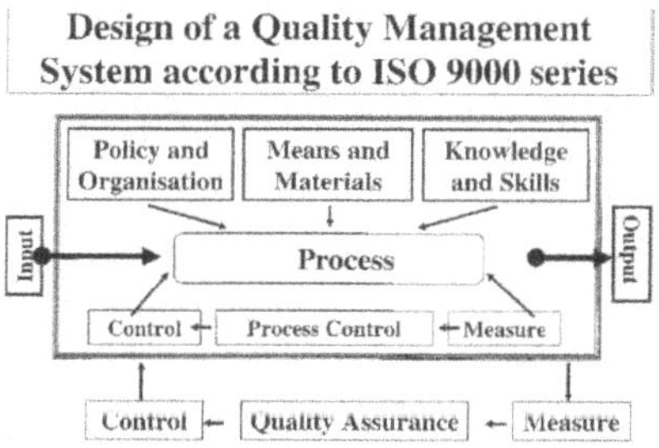


**Figure 1:** Quality Management System.

The 'product/service' realization is subject to a process loop, the QMS which includes measurements, analysis and continuing improvement of the whole treatment process. Following a suitable quality policy the institution is responsible to provide all means, materials and well trained and skilled staff required for an adequate and state of the art treatment. The key modules of a QMS include, (i) measurements of accuracy and precision of equipment used for QA, (ii) same for equipment for planning, delivering and verification of treatment, (iii) documentation, regular review and analysis of QA tests, and (iv) adjustment of the QMS by means of a proper feedback mechanism considering the test results, errors, malfunctions, staff training, new methods and technical progress.

## Design of a QMS in Conformal Radiotherapy

Quality management in radiotherapy has been recommended by the WHO [2] and in particular by the later ESTRO initiatives which set a widely accepted standard in most institutions. With the progress of radiotherapy towards conformal treatments these guidelines can easily be adapted to the specific needs of the related processes.

The following requirements on a QMS can be identified:

1. *Aims and structure of the institution*: CRT requires sophisticated equipment. It is not least cost effectiveness which challenges the institution to clearly define it's role within a regional network, the breadth of expertise and the match of CRT to local resources and pattern of patient transferral. A well organised structure with clear description of everybodies role, responsibility and duties is essential when providing CRT.
2. *Means and materials*: CRT requires utmost accuracy. Therefore, a QA programme based on standards and consensus reports has to be established for any equipment to ensure performance and safety standards throughout its lifetime.
3. *Process control*: This is the most extensive part of a QMS, and within the EU there are specific requirements to be considered (EC-Directive 43/97/Euratom). Process control may be structured according to the procedural steps in clinical routine. Considering the patient data (identification, recording, storing) there are no greater differences to conventional radiotherapy, standards such as ICRU-50 could be easily extended to CRT, in particular in dose specification. Application of treatment protocols ensure local consistency and state of the art treatment. Treatment prescription, localisation and planning should refer to national/international standards. Tayloring a 3-dimensional dose distribution precisely to the shape of the PTV provokes even more the risk of geometrical miss if no proper margins are added to the CTV. The ICRU-50 supplement [3] is adressing this problem. Computerized methods for optimizing margins have been suggested by several authors [4]. Since CRT is more than any conventional radiotherapy based on volume dose planning, all imaging systems (CT, MR, PET, etc.) must be included in a QA programme. Furthermore, all data processing and transport, and most importantly the treatment planning system needs careful tests of all components (HW & SW). It is interesting to note for instance the fluence matrix optimised for a given field when comparing different IMRT-approaches [fig.2]. Other critical items in CRT dose calculation are related to inhomogeneities, outputfactor for small fields and multileaf collimators. As more clinicians are using DVH for comparing alternative plans this and other tools for plan evaluation should be subject to QA. [5]. Special multi-purpose phantoms have been designed for testing non-dosimetric features of 3D-treatment

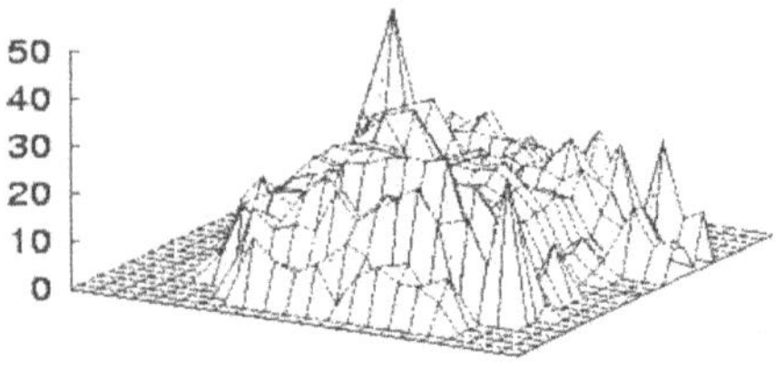


**Figure 2:** IMRT Fluence matrix calculated with *KONRAD*.

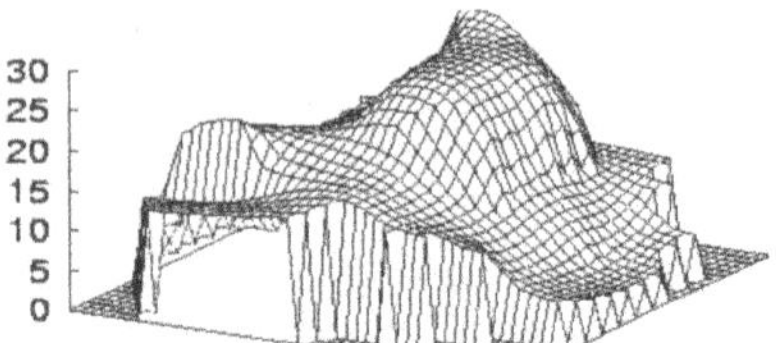


**Figure 3:** IMRT Fluence matrix calculated with *HYPERION*.

planning system and CT-simulator [6]. Numerous investigations have been performed to experimentally verify dose calculation algorithms. Recently, Monte-Carlo simulation turned out to be another verification method which may be prefered when measurement uncertainty is significant [7]. Most critical in CRT is the treatment delivery itself which includes dosimetry and performance tolerances of the equipment (treatment unit, accessories, aids for positioning and immobilisation of the patient, manufacturing of compensators, recording etc.). In IMRT often small fields or fields with a few monitor units only are applied which not too rarely represent boarderline cases of specifications. In particular, when using MLC for field shaping or fluence modulation regular tests of leaf positioning and velocity is essential. Static and dynamic techniques of MLC-based IMRT need comprehensive checks. Patient immobilisation or more precisely tracking of the PTV in space and time is crucial in CRT and is currently the most challenging part of the process. Various innovative approaches are investigated such as image-guided tracking or electromagnetic field localisation technique etc. Treatment verification, for instance by means of EPID, needs test procedures specifically designed for the equipment used. As the final step of the process control, quality auditing should be incorporated into the quality system. This comprises internal measures (interdisciplinary collaboration, dummy runs etc.) and external auditing like multicenter studies, visiting teams, intercomparison actions of dosimetry, planning systems and treatment units etc.). The need for not only focusing on physical issues is emphasized. Medical decisions like contouring, definition of CTV, dose prescription, fractionation schemes, treatment evaluation etc. are subject to quality assurance.

4. *Knowledge and skill*: In particular, the specialised techniques of CRT challenge for providing adequate training of all staff groups.
5. *Control of the quality system*: Procedures have to be established which allow to control the quality system itself. Measures have to be taken to regularly review and improve the entire system.

## Implementation of a Quality Management System

When preparing a quality system the most simple approach is to start writing down a *quality manual* which describes the pace of the different steps of the radiotherapy process. Such a manual has both an external and internal function providing a platform for collaboration and for further improvement and development of existing or new techniques, respectively. The quality manual adresses two questions, (i) what is the standard required, and (ii) how to meet that standard. It is decisive for the success of the entire quality system how it is implemented. The implementation can be structured into three phases, (i) a training phase which should consist of short but repeated sessions on a few items of practical relevance in daily routine, (ii) a validation phase aiming at testing the appropriateness, feasibility and proper adjustment of the procedures, and (iii) a consolidation phase preferably performed by quality auditing. The consolidation phase is based on a formal system review. Helpful examples are to be found in the recent *Practical Guidelines of the ESTRO Quality Assurance Committee.*

## Conclusion

A quality system is the right answer to the request of the patient for a safe and up to date treatment. It is the only way to provide in the rapidly progressing development of modern treatment techniques such as IMRT a high standard and cost effective treatment quality.

## References

[1] ISO 9000 1999 Quality Management Systems *ISO/TC 176/SC 2/N*

[2] WHO 1988 Quality assurance in radiotherapy *WHO publications*

[3] International Commission on Radiation Units and Measurements 1999 Prescribing, recording and reporting photon beam therapy (supplement to ICRU Report 50) *ICRU report 62*

[4] Mageras G S, Fuks Z, Leibel S A, Ling C C, Zelefsky M J, Kooy H M, van Herk M and Kutcher G J 1999 Computerized design of target margins for treatment uncertainties in conformal radiotherapy *Int. J. Radiation Oncology Biol. Phys* **43 (2)** 437-445

[5] Panitsa E, Rosenwald J C and Kappas C 1998 Quality control of dose volume histogram computation characteristics of 3D treatment planning systems *Phys. Med. Biol.* **43** 2807-2816

[6] Craig T, Brochu D and van Dyk J 1999 A quality assurance phantom for three-dimensional radiation treatment planning *Int. J. Radiation Oncology Biol. Phys.* **44 (4),** 955-966

[7] Laub W, Alber M, Birkner M and Nüsslin F 1999 Monte-Carlo dose calculation for IMRT optimisation. Submitted to *Phys. Med. Biol.*

# Improving dosimetric accuracy of a dynamic MLC technique

**David J Convery, Vivian P Cosgrove and Steve Webb**

Joint Department of Physics, Institute of Cancer Research & Royal Marsden NHS Trust, Sutton, Surrey, SM2 5PT, UK

## Introduction

Work has been undertaken to commission the commercial NOMOS Corvus inverse treatment planning system for treatment delivery by dynamic multileaf collimation using an Elekta MLC at the Royal Marsden NHS Trust, Sutton. This paper describes corrections applied to the raw Corvus output to improve agreement between calculated and measured dose distributions.

## Material and methods

In the currently-installed version of Corvus (v3.0) at the Royal Marsden, Sutton, support for the Elekta dynamic MLC is provided indirectly. "Ideal" beam intensity modulations derived by the inverse-planning phase of Corvus are exported as raw monitor unit (MU) distribution files (typically using a discrete 1cm × 1cm beam element resolution) from which the dynamic MLC delivery sequence is then derived using software (an "interpreter") developed at the Royal Marsden [1]. In addition to the actual MU distribution for the beams these files also contain some patient demographics (name, hospital ID, plan ID, etc) and beam orientation information (gantry, collimator and couch isocentric rotations). These export files are generated from within Corvus and exported to an external computer system (e.g. PC) for processing via a choice of NFS, FTP or simple floppy disk transfer.

Once transferred to the external computer system, dynamic MLC delivery sequences are derived using the Corvus-exported MU distribution files as input. An Elekta-MLC-specific algorithm has been developed in-house [1] to derive deliverable dynamic sequences to generate the often very highly modulated discrete intensity distributions determined by Corvus. In this algorithm, full account is taken of MLC-specific constraints such as minimum leaf and diaphragm separations and the prevention of leaf interdigitation, and the MLC's backup diaphragms are also employed in addition to the MLC leaves themselves. Full correction to prevent tongue-and-groove underexposure [2] is performed. Details of the algorithm are provided in [1].

This derivation of the MLC delivery sequence is done assuming a primary-only beam model. It was next necessary to perform corrections to account for the additional transmission and head-scattered radiation that will be present on actual delivery. This was achieved by employing an iterative correction scheme [3]. Using the MLC delivery sequence derived from the Corvus-generated monitor unit distributions, the distributions of transmitted and head-scattered radiation were then calculated. (The head scatter model used is based on an integration over the "visible" portion of the head scatter source during the dynamic delivery. The source of the head-scattered radiation is assumed to be an area source located at the level of the flattening filter, and its spatial distribution is represented as a sum of Gaussians terms; this model and its application has previously been described in [3])).

It should be noted that the dose model used in the current version of Corvus does not use the actual MLC delivery sequence as its input, rather instead it uses the "ideal" beam intensity distributions derived by its inverse-planning routine. Therefore, the aim of the correction process described above (schematically illustrated in Figure 1) has been to achieve as good agreement as possible between the MU distributions derived by Corvus and the total delivery (primary, transmission and head-scatter) calculated in the iterative loop. This in turn corresponds to deriving modified MU distributions and dynamic MLC delivery sequences such that the delivered 3D dose distribution matches as closely as possible that calculated with Corvus.

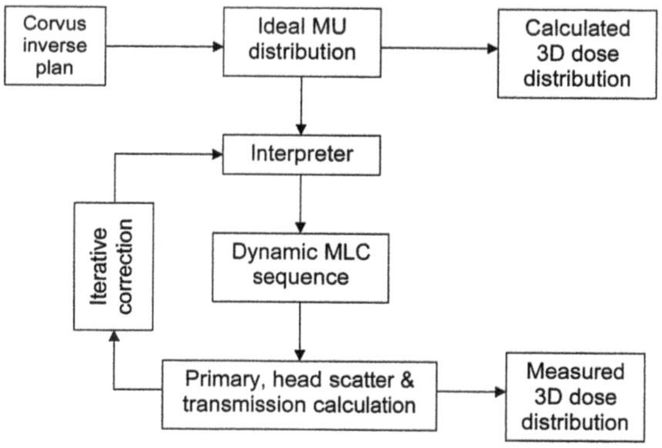


**Figure 1:** Overview of iterative correction applied.

## Results and discussion

The above process – matching the MU distributions derived by Corvus with the total calculated in the iterative loop – relies on two implicit assumptions: that the Corvus calculations of the relative dose distribution and the in-house calculations of the transmission and head-scatter distributions are each accurate in their own right. Work has therefore been done to evaluate each separately.

The accuracy of the basic Corvus calculation was been assessed for a number of regularly- and irregularly-shaped static MLC fields. A number of test modulated fields have also been studied.

For both regular and irregular static fields, good agreement between Corvus-calculated and measured dose distributions has been found, generally of the order of 1-2% for central axis percentage depth dose and ~2mm for isodose line position agreement in the beam penumbra. This indicates that the basic dose model is correct and that the integration of phantom scatter within the irradiated area is performed adequately.

One case where this has not been found to hold true, however, is for complex irregular fields such as those that might be found during dynamic MLC delivery. One such case is shown in Figure 2(a), where the left backup is used to provide shielding whilst maintaining the minimum 1cm MLC leaf (and opposite adjacent leaf) separation criteria. The measured dose distribution (measured at $d_{max}$ at isocentre, 6MV beam) is shown in Figure 2(b). The dose arising outside of the geometrical field from the extra transmission component can be clearly seen. Since the Corvus dose model does not take the actual field delivery sequence into account in its calculation, the resulting dose distribution calculated is that in Figure 2(c). Providing Corvus with details of the extra transmission component gives the significantly improved distribution in 2(d), and illustrates the need to calculate and correct for these terms in a dynamic (or step-and-shoot) delivery.

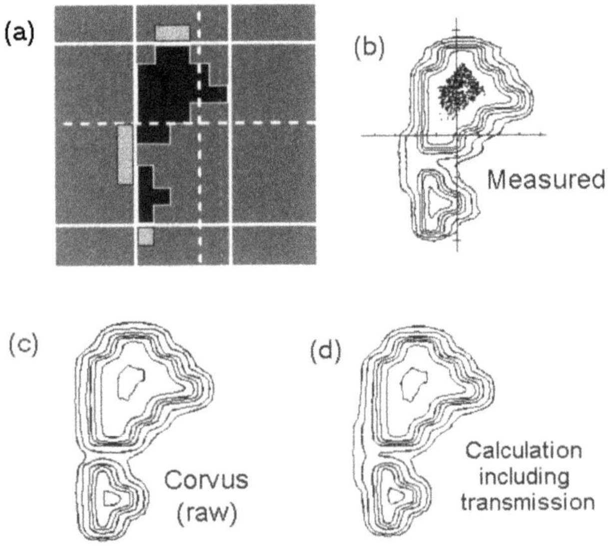


**Figure 2:** (a) Complex irregular MLC field, typical of dynamic delivery. (b) Measured relative dose distribution. (c) Basic Corvus calculation, and (d) modified calculation with the extra transmission component included.

Accuracy of the in-house corrections for transmission and head-scattered radiation was evaluated by performing in-air measurements (made using a small-volume ion chamber fitted with an aluminium build-up cap), as this separates these calculations from any uncertainty or inaccuracy associated with the in-phantom scatter integration and dose calculation performed in Corvus. Typically, the accuracy of in-air measured output factors for complex Corvus-generated dynamic fields has been found to be approximately 1-2%. An example is shown in Figure 3.

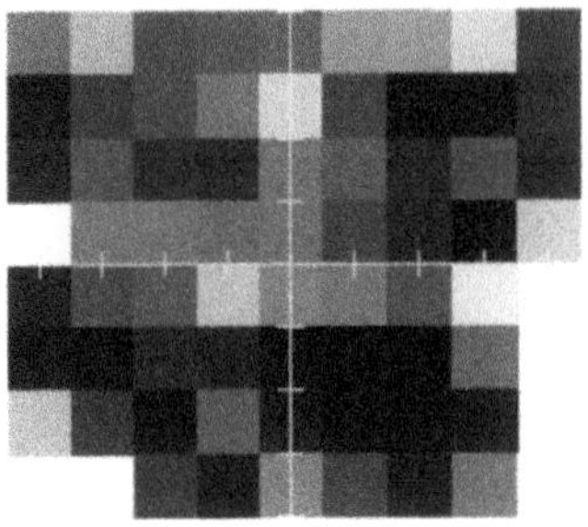

**Figure 3:** Corvus-generated IMRT field. Calculated in-air output factor (OPF) at isocentre = 0.191, measured OPF = 0.189 (dynamic MLC delivery)

The overall accuracy of the application of this correction scheme is illustrated in Figure 4, where 4(a) shows the Corvus calculation and 4(b) the measured distribution following application of the iterative correction scheme described above for transmission and head-scattered radiation, generating modified MU distributions and field shapes. A five-field coplanar plan was used, with 72 degree separation between each of the field directions. Delivery was by dynamic MLC, with a maximum leaf speed of 1cm/sec. It should be noted that these are *absolute* dose distributions, rather than renormalised relative dose distributions. Measurements were performed with Kodak X-Omat V film sandwiched in an elliptical perspex (PMMA) phantom, with corrections applied for film optical density *vs* dose non-linearity. The treatment plan prescription dose of 200cGy was rescaled for the actual delivery to 50cGy to avoid saturating the film. The same four-fold reduction in the set beam monitor units and delivery dose rate was used to ensure that the dynamic MLC motion for the delivery of 50cGy to the film was the same as for delivery of 200cGy to a patient.

Studies of the delivered dose distributions in three dimensions using polymer gel dosimetry is also under evaluation [4].

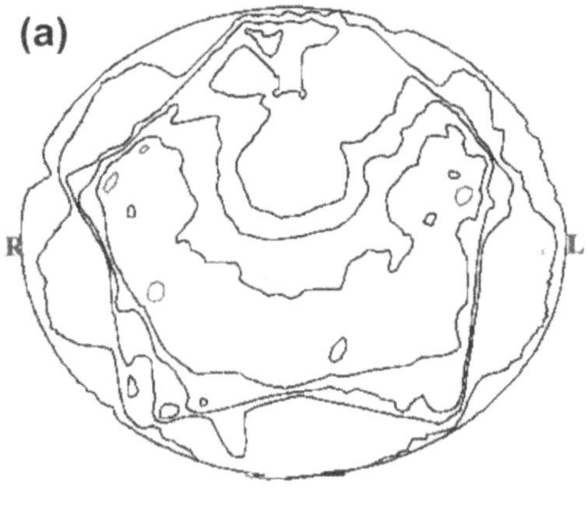

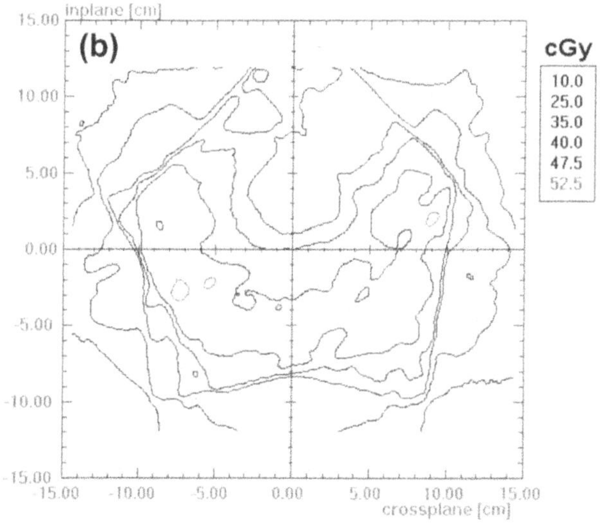


**Figure 4:** (a) Calculated and (b) measured dose distribution (five field inverse plan, equispaced fields). Absolute isodoses are plotted at 10, 25, 35, 40, 47.5 and 52.5 cGy (corresponding to 20, 50, 70, 80, 95 and 105% of the 50cGy prescription dose).

It is emphasised that the only corrections to the MU used in the above work are those derived from the iterative correction scheme described. In particular, the Corvus "Treatment Unit Calibration Factor" – a multiplicative correction factor that can be used to improve agreement between set MU and the doses actually measured – has been set to unity, *i.e.* it is not applied here.

Whilst such a multiplicative calibration factor can improve agreement of the delivered dose to the prescription point in the target, it is necessarily only an average factor, being the average correction derived from measurements made over a sample of test plans ranging from simple to complex treatments and geometries. It does not correct optimally on a plan-by-plan basis. Additionally, as it is a simple scaling factor, its applicability and validity will be different in high and low intensity parts of a beam and of a plan.

An additional problem that can be identified with the basic Corvus dose model as it is currently implemented is that regions within or around a beam that are assigned zero weight by the inverse planning process are assumed to have zero fluence in the dose calculation. No direct account is taken of the actual transmitted or head-scattered radiation reaching these regions, although the in-phantom scattered radiation to such points is integrated. This problem was previously illustrated in Figure 2. This can affect, in particular, the calculated dose distribution outside of the target volume (which it may therefore underestimate) and consequently also affect the validity of dose-volume histogram statistics for organs at risk.

An improved approach would be to incorporate the recalculated MU (intensity) distributions based on the actual delivery sequence – derived, for example, from the iterative correction scheme described above – back into Corvus for recalculation of the final dose distribution. This should then further improve the agreement between calculated and measured distributions (although it may then violate the inverse planning goals) and also eliminate the potential need for any "planning system calibration factor". Work is currently under way to incorporate this last step into the system at Sutton.

## Conclusion

Improvements to the accuracy of the basic Corvus inverse planning system's dose calculation to take into account the details of the actual dynamic MLC delivery have been described and measured data presented. Potential further improvements by using this final corrected data within the Corvus system are suggested and are currently being investigated.

Although the corrections discussed and applied here have been described within the context of dynamic MLC delivery, they are equally applicable to step-and-shoot (multiple static MLC field) delivery.

The authors would like to acknowledge the support of NOMOS in this development work, and in particular Rob Hill for the development of the Elekta interface used.

This work has been carried out in conjunction with the Elekta International IMRT Consortium (Royal Marsden, Sutton, UK; Christie Hospital, UK; William Beaumont Hospital, USA; University of Gent, Belgium; University of Washington, Seattle, USA; NKI, Amsterdam; University of Maryland, USA; Thomas Jefferson University, Philadelphia, USA). Numerous discussions with members of each of these sites and with the development team at Elekta are acknowledged.

## References

[1] Convery D J and Webb S 1998 Generation of discrete beam intensity modulation by dynamic multileaf collimation under minimum leaf separation constraints *Phys. Med. Biol.* **43** 2521-2538

[2] van Santvoort J P C and Heijmen B J M 1996 Dynamic multileaf collimation without 'tongue-and-groove' underdosage effects *Phys. Med. Biol.* **41** 2091-2105

[3] Convery D J and Webb S 1997 Calculation of the distribution of head-scattered radiation in dynamically-collimated MLC fields *Proc 12th Int. Conf. Computers in Radiotherapy (ICCR) (Salt Lake City, Utah, USA)* ed D D Leavitt and G Starkschall, 350-353

[4] Cosgrove V P, Convery D J, Murphy P S, Nutting C M and Webb S 2000 Dynamic MLC delivered IMRT: verification using Polyacrylamide gel dosimetry *Submitted to 13th Int. Conf. Computers in Radiotherapy (ICCR), Heidelberg*

# Dynamic multileaf collimation and three-dimensional verification in IMRT

**Nzhde Agazaryan, Timothy D. Solberg, Alonso R. Arellano, Timothy J. Paul**

Department of Radiation Oncology, University of California Los Angeles School of Medicine

## Introduction

We have developed software for constructing the leaf sequences necessary for IMRT delivery using a multileaf collimator. The algorithm used is an enhancement of the sliding window technique and supports several accelerator/MLC combinations [1,2]. Several factors are addressed in this application. The user specifies the RMS difference between the desired profile and the profile obtained with translated MLC motion. Tolerance of leaf positioning is also a user input. Transmission through MLC leaves is corrected using an iterative method. Leakage between opposing and neighboring leaves is minimized. Individual leaves are synchronized to reduce tongue and grove effect by varying their relative starting and ending times. The application supports fixed gantry step-and-shoot, fixed gantry dynamic, and fixed gantry optimized modes. During fixed gantry optimized mode, the delivery is dynamic, but switches to step-and-shoot mode in instances where MLC leaves cannot meet tolerance specification. Verifications have been performed using film dosimetry and amorphous Silicon (a-Si:H) 2D array detector acquisitions [3]. Output factor correction for small fields is found to be the most challenging phenomena for dosimetry. For IMRT verification, a cylindrical phantom is constructed for three-dimensional dosimetric verification. The phantom has 15 cylindrical inserts holding diode detectors. Each detector is connected to Sun Nuclear's IVD (In Vivo Dosimeter) system and then fed to computer with specialized software. The readings of each detector can be recorded at 2 second intervals.

## Material and methods

Measurements were performed on a Novalis linear accelerator (BrainLab, Heimstetten Germany) equipped with an $m_3$ micro-multileaf collimator, consisting of fifty-two individually motorized tungsten leaves that shape a treatment field of up to 10x10 $cm^2$. The leaves range from 3.0 mm at the center of the field to 5.5 mm at the edge of the field. There are fourteen pairs of 3mm wide, three pairs of 4.5 mm wide, and three pairs of 5.5 mm wide leaves. The front faces of the leaves are curved to minimize the penumbra variations as a function of position.

There are several MLC characteristics that effect the IMRT implementation. These characteristics include, but are not limited, to leaf width, leaf height, maximum travel over centerline, maximum retract position, and maximum leaf spread. BrainLab and Varian MLC parameters respectively are: maximum distance over centerline - 5.0cm and 16.0cm, maximum retract distance - 5.0cm and 20.1cm, and maximum leaf spread - 10.0cm and 14.5cm.

Some other MLC parameters that are investigated for IMRT are penumbra, intraleaf leakage, interleaf leakage, and tongue and groove effect. These parameters are taken into account in leaf sequencing portion of IMRT implementation.

Treatment specifications for the MLC are given to the Linac in ASCII text files called DMLC field files. The output of our leaf sequencing software is a DMLC file for each gantry angle. These files contain a series of leaf positions and an index numbers associated with those positions indicating the fraction of commulative MU delivered until that step. DMLC files contain no information about how MLC leaves move except the discrete positions and MU fractions. The MLC control application determines the details of movement.

The translated DMLC leaf sequence can be viewed using the Varian MLC Shaper program, the GUI of which is presented in figure 1. This program allows manual DMLC file creation, visualization, film simulation, movement simulation, CRC generation, and some error checking. In the future this DMLC file generation will be a part of the treatment planning system and detailed knowledge of its structure may become less critical. However, familiarity with this structure gives valuable insight into MLC control and operation. To investigate the interleaf leakage, intraleaf leakage, and transmission characteristics of the MLC and accelerator combination, 400MU were delivered with a closed MLC field. Leaf pair #1 has a small gap opened as in figure 1, since the MLC control system does not allow completely closed field delivery.

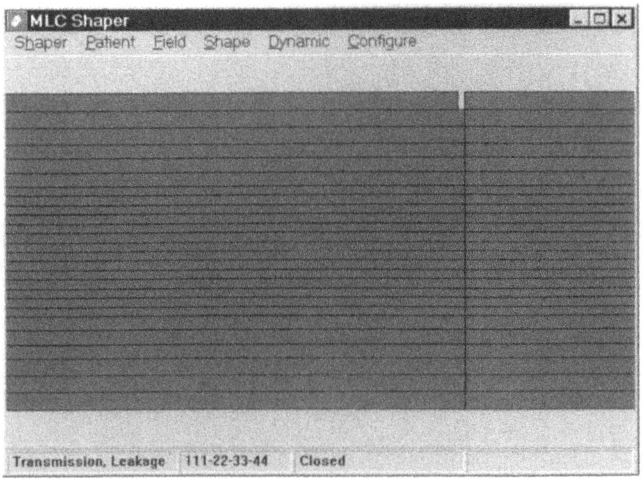


**Figure 1:** A closed field snopshot of MLC shaper.

The measurement of complex dose distributions created with IMRT requires a dosimeter that can integrate the dose during a complete treatment. Integrating dosimeter devices generally are capable of measuring only dose at small, point-like volumes. Film dosimetry is capable of measuring planar dose distribution. For fixed gantry modes, film dosimetry is a good

way of verifying each plane of delivery. However, error propagation uncertainties call for efficient and accurate three-dimensional verification. IMRT verification calls for a dosimeter that can record and display a 3D dose distribution or at least the dose at certain points in a chosen volume. BANG-gel has been used at our institution for three-dimensional dosimetry but this method also has well known drawbacks. The use of multiple diodes is more efficient and real time.
We have constructed IMRT verification phantom which allows real time verification at distributed points of treatment volume. A photograph of the system is presented in figure 2. The phantom is cylindrical (25cm diameter) with small cylindrical inserts (~1cm). The phantom is constructed from Dry Water™. The inserts have ISORAD-p diodes embedded into them and are free to move in axial direction. The inserts have several fixed positions in longitudinal direction that they can occupy by simply rotating the phantom. The phantom fabrication is conducted by Radiology Support Devices, Inc.

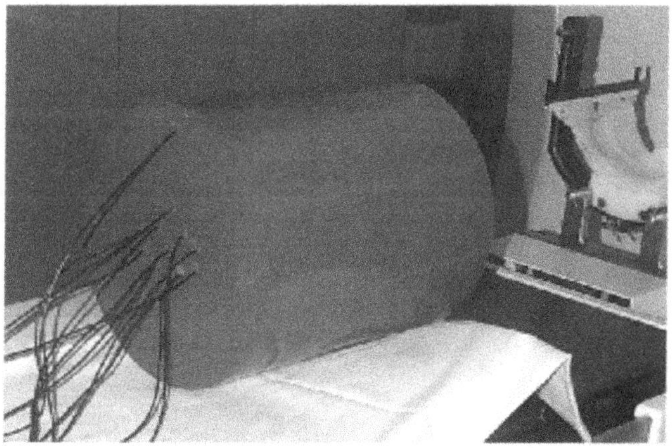

**Figure 2:** The photograph of IMRT phantom.

Inversely calculated profiles are applied to the phantom by doing forward calculation with 3D-calculation engine. On the other hand, the same profiles are translated using the leaf-sequencing algorithm and delivered to the phantom. The measured dose at points where the diodes are positioned are compared to the forward calculation.
The CT scan of the phantom presented in figure 3 includes

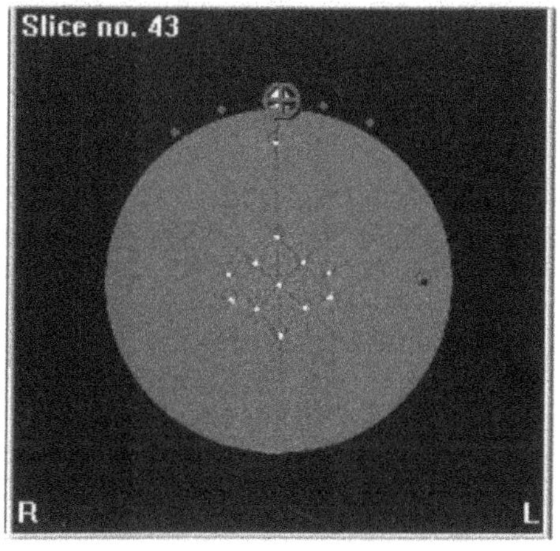


**Figure 3:** CT scan of the IMRT phantom.

infrared external markers. Infrared external markers allow accurate positioning using the BrainLab ExacTrac infrared positioning system.

## Results and discussion

The BrainLab $m_3$ MLC characteristics have been investigated for leaf sequencing software development. In addition to leaf width, leaf height, maximum travel over centerline, maximum retract position, and maximum leaf spread presented in previous section, 400MU were delivered with a closed MLC field (Leaf pair #1 slightly opened, see figure 1). Film dosimetry was performed in a water equivalent phantom at the depth of maximum dose and analyzed using a commercial film dosimetry system (RIT 113, Version 3.06, Radiological Imaging Technology, Inc.) Figure 4 shows a closed film data set presented as a Transform GUI snapshot.

| | |
|---|---|
| **Interleaf leakage** (leakage between neighboring leaves) | |
| Interleaf leakage in central region: | 2.10% |
| Interleaf leakage in peripheral region: | 1.53% |
| **Intraleaf leakage** (leakage between opposing leaves) | |
| Intraleaf leakage: | 3.56% |
| **Transmission** (transmitted radiation trough the leaves) | |
| Transmission in central region: | 1.74% |
| Transmission in peripheral region: | 1.51% |

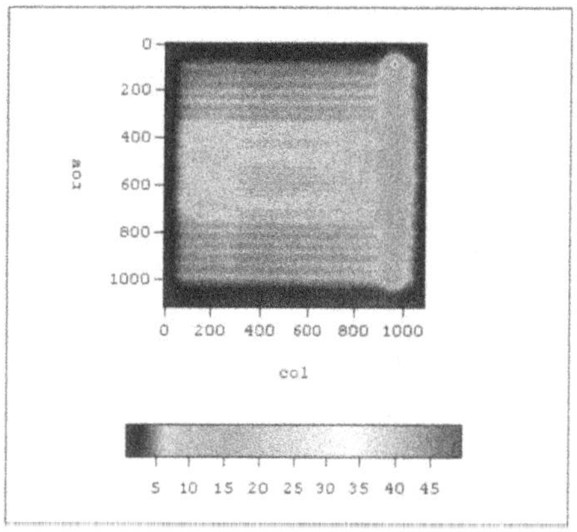


**Figure 4:** Leakage and Transmission Data.

Several key factors are addressed in *MLC_Trans* leaf sequencing software.
**RMS**: A calculated difference between the desired profile obtained from inverse planning and the profile obtained with translated leaf movements before applying the transmission correction. A small RMS allows finer dosimetric resolution without increasing delivery time. **Tolerance**: The limit in cm above which the accelerator will modulate the radiation rate allowing the leaves to catch-up. This is a parameter that determines how close the actual leaf positions must be to the prescribed positions. The tolerance is the allowed error at the isocenter. **Transmission Correction**: Corrects for transmission through the leaves. **Dynamic Mode**: Fixed Beam Dynamic delivery has multiple segments per beam and the beam is activated between segments. **Step and Shoot Mode**: Fixed Beam Step-and-Shoot delivery has multiple segments per beam, and the beam is off between segments. **Optimized Mode**: Hybrid technique where the delivery is dynamic but

switches to step-and-shoot technique to avoid the reduction of the dose rate at instances where the leaves do not have enough time to meet the set tolerance. **Synchronization**: It is still possible to synchronize leaf movements and still deliver with sliding window algorithm. This is due to fact that not all leaves go through the same number of segments, and it is possible to manipulate relative starting and ending times of the leaves. In our sequencing software, synchronization with a factor of 0 means that all leaves start together and those that are done with delivery earlier move out of field under the backup jaws until others finish with delivery. On the other hand, synchronization with a factor of 100 means that the leaves with less segments to deliver wait outside of the field, under the backup jaw, and start later resulting in all the leaves finishing their delivery together. Synchronization in time space can be set to any factor between 0 and 100. As illustrated in figure 5, it can have a dramatic effect on tongue and groove effect.
**Auto Synchronization**: This routine determines a synchronization factor depending on the profile and synchronizes accordingly.
An experiment with leaf synchronization proves that relative starting and ending times do have significant effect on tongue and groove effect. This idea is implemented in manual and automatic synchronization options of the software.

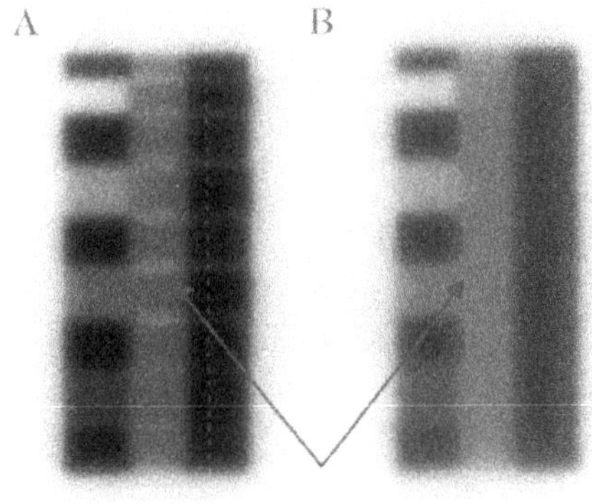


**Figure 5:** The same TG study test pattern is obtained: A. without synchronization and B. with synchronization factor of 100.

With this synchronization, the delivery is still done with the sliding window algorithm, and thus leakage between opposing and neighboring leaves is minimized.
Many other DMLC field files are constructed, delivered, and dosimetric measurements performed using the film dosimetry

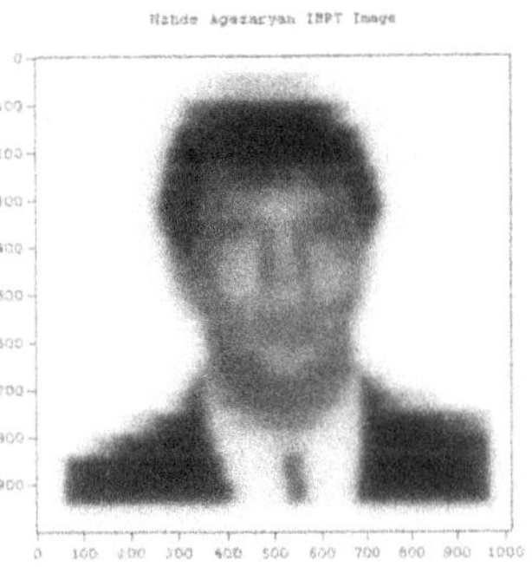

**Figure 6:** IMRT Portrait.

system. For comparison, the same profile has been obtained with a different delivery technique, transmission correction, tolerance, and RMS.
The input format of the sequencing software is flexible. Besides the output of inverse planning software, it is also capable of translating the ordinary image files to leaf sequences. Figure 6 is an example of such sequencing and delivery.

## Conclusion

The UCLA leaf sequencing software successfully implemented step-and-shoot, dynamic, and optimized (hybrid) modes. The issues of transmission, leakage, tolerance, and leaf synchronization have been satisfactory addressed.
The output factor changes for small fields present the most dosimetric challenge for IMRT delivery and are under close investigation at our institution. These output factor changes are primarily due to the lack of lateral electronic equilibrium in small segments and off-axis output variations.
The complete system of IMRT phantom and data acquisition has been constructed. Figure 7 is a photograph of that system.

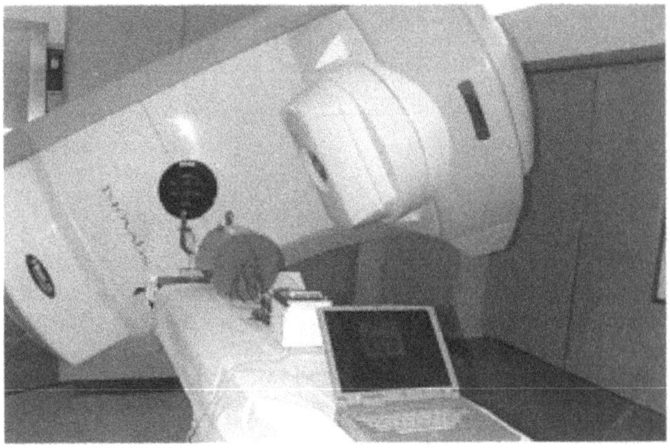

**Figure 7:** Photograph of cylindrical phantom and data acquisition

## References

[1] Bortfeld T, Boyer A L, Schlegel W, Kahler D L, Waldron T J 1994 Realization and verification of three-dimensional conformal radiotherapy with modulated fields *International Journal of Radiation Oncology, Biology, Physics* **30** 899-908.

[2] Ma L, Boyer L A, Xing L and Ma C-M 1998 An optimized leaf-setting algorithm for beam intensity modulation using dynamic multileaf collimator *Physics in Medicine and Biology* **43** 1629-1643

[3] Paul T, Solberg T, Leu M, Rosemark P, Smathers J, Mollenhauer U, Agazaryan N Independent, Real-Time Verification of Dynamically Shaped Intensity Modulated Radiotherapy (IMRT) using an Amorphous Silicon (a-Si:H) 1999 Medical Physics **26** 1065

# Delivery and Dosimetry Verification in IMRT

**Homayoon Parsaei, M.Sc.[1,2], Mark H. Phillips, Ph.D.[1], Paul S. Cho, Ph.D.[1], Görkem H. Kuterdem, M.Sc.[1,3], Hege Kippenes, DVM[4], and Pat Gavin, Ph.D., DVM[4]**
[1]University of Washington, Department of Radiation Oncology, Seattle, WA, USA
[2]University of British Columbia, Department of Physics, Vancouver, BC, Canada
[3]University of Washington, Department of Electrical Engineering, Seattle, WA, USA
[4]Washington State University, School of Veterinary Medicine, Pullman, WA, USA

## Introduction

Dose distribution delivered in multiple complex field irradiations can often be improved significantly by modulation of the 2-D intensity profiles of each beam [?, ?]. Intensity modulated radiation therapy (IMRT) delivered with dynamic multileaf collimators (MLC) promises increased local control of certain tumors by providing improved dose localization within the target volume and minimal damage to surrounding tissues with low tolerance to ionizing radiation. With this irradiation technique, the tumor dose can be substantially escalated, thereby improving the probability of tumor control [?].

One class of tumor is likely to benefit from this approach is one in close proximity to critical structures, such as the spinal cord.

This paper presents a comprehensive study of planning, delivery, and dosimetry verification of intensity modulated beams delivered to subject beagle dogs with tumor volumes adjacent to the spinal cord. 3-D dose distributions for each beam are calculated using a macro pencil beam (MPB) model [?], and the optimum beam intensity distributions are calculated using an inverse planning algorithm that is developed based on the technique of projections onto convex sets (POCS) [?]. The validity of our inverse planning algorithm, dose calculation model, and dosimetry verification techniques were investigated and compared with in-phantom measurements.

This project is a collaboration between the Department of Radiation Oncology of the University of Washington Medical Center (UWMC) and the Department of Clinical Veterinary Sciences at Washington State University (WSU). Both institutions share common equipment for the delivery of IMRT.

## Material and methods

Measurements were carried out on an Elekta SL20 series linear accelerator[1] equipped with a multileaf collimator. Research software was provided by Elekta that provided IMRT capability on the linac. The physical measurements were performed in phantom, deceased dogs, and live subject canines that were bred for the treatment of non-tumor target volumes. In addition, dogs presenting with spontaneous head and neck tumors were used for the delivery of IMRT. Theremoluminescent dosimeters (TLDs), films[2], and diodes[3] were used for the measurements.

### Planning

Each dog began the treatment process by being fitted into an immobilization device (see Figure 1), consisting of an inflatable-pillow and a bite-block, attached to a ring used for patient localization and image correlation. CT scans were taken for the purpose of treatment planning and contours were drawn on each set of CT scans to outline the target volume and the critical structures to be avoided in delivery of the beams. The shape of the target in each case was determined mainly to allow assessment of variation of dose gradients and misdeliveries.

All contouring, beam setup, and dose calculations were performed using our treatment planning system, Prism [?]. Seven equidistance gantry angles were used to design the beam portals defining the MLC shapes that conformed to the shape of the target.

Pre-optimization dose arrays for each beam portal were calculated using the MPB model. The algorithm calculates the dose matrix due to the contribution from each dose point in a coordinate grid, defined in the anatomy. Each beam is then divided into beam elements and the algorithm computes the dose to that point in the dose grid. The execution time for dose computation for each plan, depending on the desired dose grid resolution, varied from 1-2 hours on a 266 MHz Alpha workstation.

The inverse planning algorithm, POCS, was used to calculate the optimized dose profiles, given a set of user defined constraints such as uniform dose distribution in the target and what the maximum dose should be in the spine. The optimized fluence profiles for each beam were then translated and output to a file, specifying the position of the MLC leaves for each control segment using a translator program [?]. The translated file was then read by Prism and the MPB algorithm was then used to calculate the dose distributions for all control points in phantom or patient geometry. The files were then converted into machine readable binary format and transferred via network protocols to MLC computers.

The monitor unit (MU) settings needed for the delivery of each beam was determined using the MPB model and

[1]Elekta Oncology Systems

[2]Kodak Ready-Pack, X-OmatV

[3]Profiler, Sun Nuclear Corp.

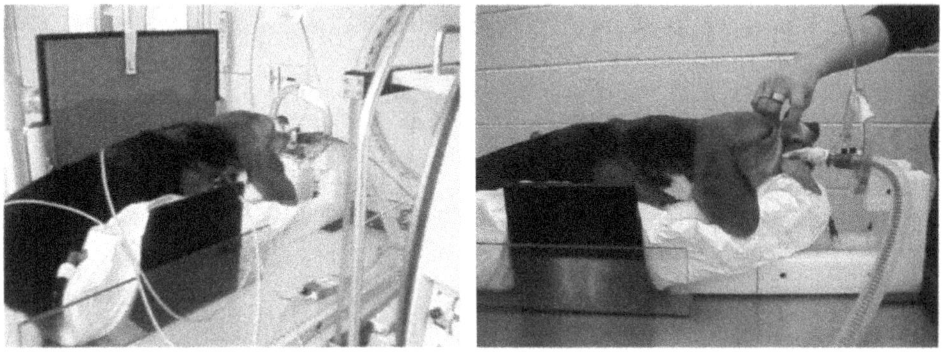

**Figure 1:** The immobilization bed with the bite-block in place used both for planning and treatment.

checked with in-phantom measurements for any further adjustments, if needed.

### Dose Delivery and Verification

Measurements were carried out with calibrated TLDs, films and diodes. TLDs were calibrated individually to obtain consistent and accurate readings in dosimetrically meaningful units. Likewise, films were calibrated under known radiation field settings to generate optical density to dose conversion curves. The linear portion of the characteristic curves was used in the conversion of optical density to dose. Diodes were also calibrated to obtain sensitivity factors for each detector which was applied to the measured output of a detector to convert the collected signal into absolute dose.

The treatment delivery scheme was 20 fractions of 400 cGy per fraction. As a quality assurance task, in order to check the accuracy of the dose calculation and inverse planning algorithms, the optimized plans were first transferred to a cylindrical phantom, and various dosimeters (TLDs, films and diodes) were used to measure the one-dimensional and planar dose distribution along a leaf motion and compared with the calculated dose points. Furthermore, prior to the treatment, a set of TLDs (typically between 40-50 TLDs, each 1x2 mm in size) was used to measure the dose to the esophagus during treatment and compared with dose point calculations from Prism.

### Patient Positioning

Port films were taken daily and used to adjust the patient position. In addition, possible errors involved in setup and organ motion were investigated by correlating pre-treat CT images with post-treatment images using an image registration program (See related paper, Phillips *et al.*).

## Results and discussion

The two dimensional dose distribution for in-phantom measurement for one clinical case is shown in Figure 2. A film

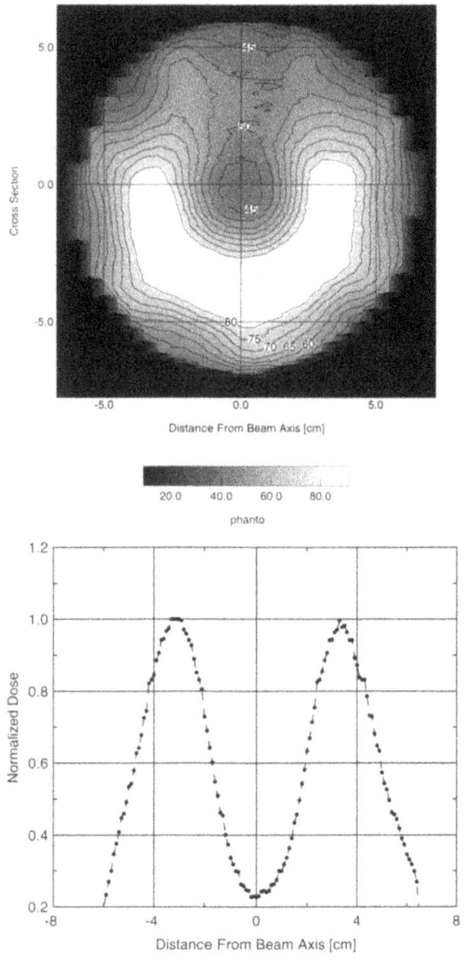


**Figure 2:** 2-D dose distribution in phantom (top) and dose profile along the track of one MLC leaf sweep (bottom) as measured with film .

was placed in the phantom, in a plane parallel to the central axis of the beam, along one of the MLC leaf tracks. A constraint on optimization was to limit the dose to the spine to 50% of the total dose. The results show the sparing of the spine, which was chosen so that the center of the spine would be at isocenter. The bottom figure illustrates a scan through the film in the direction normal to the beam axis. Doses were normalized to 1.

Figure 3 shows the comparison of MPB calculations and the measurements for one beam along the direction of the MLC for track number 20 corresponding to a position 0.5 cm superior to the beam axis. The results show good agreement between the simulated dose as calculated by the MPB model and that of measurements.

For the purpose of comparison in our dosimetry techniques, Figure 4 shows a dose profile for a beam at a different angle.

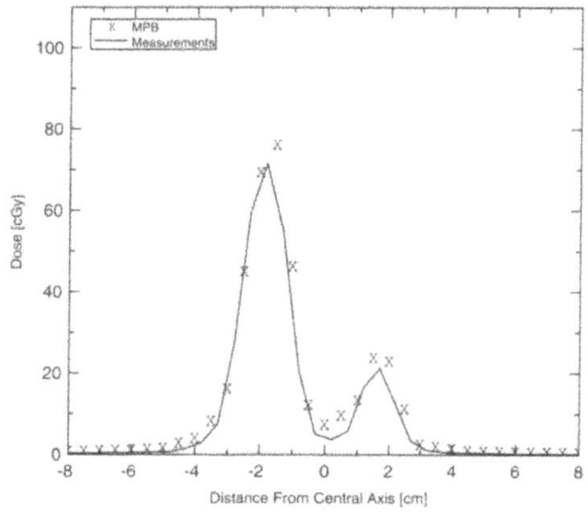


**Figure 3:** Comparison of dose profile obtained with measurements and calculations for one MLC track and a given beam angle.

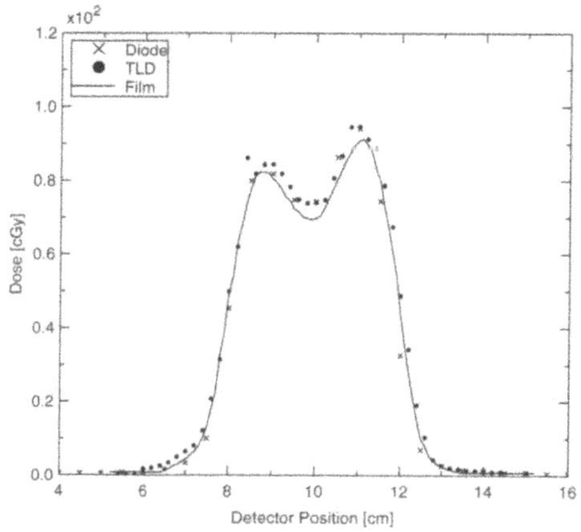


**Figure 4:** Measurements of dose profiles measured with various dosimeters for MLC track and a given beam angle.

# Conclusion

The dosimetric verification of dynamic intensity modulated plans is a critical prerequisite to clinical implementation of this technique. The objective of this study was to assess the degree to which IMRT technique can deliver highly localized dose distributions in the regions of head and neck. It was found that IMRT dose distributions delivered were sufficiently accurate and highly conformal. Dosimetric verification provided significant support to our inverse planning algorithm and 3-D dose calculation model. In addition, these studies are being followed and the effects of radiation to the spine,, esophagus, and surrounding normal tissues will be measured using clinical measures and pathology reviews.

# Acknowledgements

This work was supported in part by grants from Elekta Oncology Systems and the Whitaker Foundation.

# Dosimetry of Gated Intensity Modulated Radiotherapy

**Timothy D. Solberg[1,3], Timothy J. Paul[1], Nzhde N. Agazaryan[1], Ted Urmanita,[2] Alonso R. Arellano[1], Jorge Llacer[4], Rex A. Boone[1], Randi Fogg[1], John J. DeMarco[1,3], Indrin Chetty[1] and James B. Smathers[1,3]**

[1]Department of Radiation Oncology, [2]Department of Clinical Engineering and [3]Jonsson Comprehensive cancer Center, 200 UCLA Medical Plaza, suite B265, Los Angeles, CA 90095-6951 USA, [4]EC Engineering Consultants LLC Los Gatos, CA, USA

## Introduction

Recent years have seen the development of sophisticated delivery technologies designed to enhance the efficacy of clinical radiotherapy through the escalation of tumor dose. Key among these is the use of intensity modulated x-ray beams now becoming widely available through innovations in multileaf collimator (MLC) technology. Yet the successful delivery of intensity modulated radiotherapy (IMRT) depends on additional factors beyond the techniques for radiation delivery. In particular, fundamental problems associated with the practical issues of patient positioning, setup reproducibility and organ motion have yet to be adequately addressed. Of particular interest are techniques designed to compensate for breathing motion associated with respiration, i.e., respiratory gating. In this work we have investigated an initial implementation of gated IMRT with regard to dosimetric issues. Dosimetry was compared for gated and non-gated irradiation conditions for the following field configurations: open rectangular fields, irregular fields, and wedged and arbitrarily modulated fields delivered by dynamic MLC. Gating was facilitated through a clinical gating interface provided by the linac manufacturer. Gating frequency was varied from 0.2 to 1.0 Hz and monitor units were varied from 25 to 200. In this manner gating effects could be studied for a wide range of leaf speeds. Two-dimensional dose maps were obtained using an amorphous-silicon detector. Standard dosimetric parameters of regular fields such as flatness and symmetry were essentially unaffected by gating. Differences of up to 18 % were observed between gated and non-gated dynamic wedge fields. The largest differences corresponded to small numbers of monitor units, resulting from fast leaf motion. At 100 monitor units and above no variations exceeded 3.5%. Variations averaged over the entire field were less than 3.5% in all cases and less then 1% at 100 monitor units and above. Differences relative to gating frequency were observed only for low numbers (< 100) of monitor units. Similar results were obtained for arbitrary IMRT fields such as those encountered in inverse planning. At UCLA, inverse planning is performed using a variant of the dynamically penalized likelihood (DPL) method [1].

## Material and methods

Radiation was delivered using the UCLA Novalis, a 6MV electron linear accerelator with an integrated micro-multileaf collimator (mMLC). Initially intended primarily as a neurosurgical tool, the Novalis is capable of conventional arc radiosurgery, conformal radiotherapy using multiple static shaped beams, dynamic arc radiotherapy, in which arc delivery is combined with dynamic field shaping, and IMRT. Leaves vary in width from 3 to 5.5 mm projected at isocenter for a maximum field size of 10 x 10 $cm^2$. Several features make the Novalis ideally suited to IMRT and/or gated delivery. These include: high output (1200 mu/min in clinical mode), dynamic capabilities, and the ability to monitor radiation to within 0.01 monitor unit.

Recently a commercial respiratory gating interface was installed on the Novalis. The gating interface consists of a 25-pin connector inserted between the dynamic MLC (dMLC) cable and the console backplane. A 3-pin connector provides access for a 12 volt DC signal to the MHOLDOFF/status bit on the console backplane. A beam inhibit is triggered whenever this bit is low. Gating is controlled through a switching device connected between pins 1 and 2 of the 3-pin connector. An open switch generates an *initial position* (IPSN) interlock on the accelerator controller. For dynamic treatments, absense of an IPSN interlock ensures that neither the dose nor collimator position vary more than 0.2 monitor units and 0.2 cm respectively [2]. Thus this interlock halts both radiation and leaf motion and is cleared immediately upon closure of the switch. A description of the radiation delay mechanism is provided by Ramsey et al [3].

All measurements were made using an amorphous-silicon imaging system (Scanditronix Medical / Wellhöfer Dosimetrie, Uppsala, Sweden). The system consists of a 256 x 256 flat panel array coupled to a personal computer. The size of individual detector elements is 0.8 mm per pixel. Calibration runs were performed to determine and correct for the sensitivity of each detector element. All images were also corrected for dark signal. Frames were acquired every 80 milliseconds and integrated to obtain an absolute dose map. Dosimetric properties of an earlier generation device have been described previously [4].

Gating was controlled by a simple signal generator; a future implementation facilitating a computer controlled signal generated by a respiratory gating system is presently under development. Gating frequency was varied from 0.2 to 1.0 Hz. The lower end of this range corresponds approximately to that of the human respiratory cycle.

For regular beams, FWHM, flatness and symmetry as well as absolute dose were evaluated as a function of gating frequency. Leaf sequencing for dynamic wedges and arbitrary intensity profiles was performed using a modified Bortfeld algorithm that accounts for leakage and transmission and minimizes tongue-and-groove effect [5,6]. Modulated treatments were delivered in a dynamic fashion on the Novalis unit, with the beam on continually while the leaves were moving. It was felt that dynamic delivery technique presented a greater challenge for the system with regard to gated dosimetric reproducibility, thus a step-and-shoot delivery approach has yet to be evaluated. Measurements were repeated for monitor units ranging from 25 to 200 with no gating and at the gating frequencies between 0.2 to 1.0 Hz. Each image was corrected for pixel sensitivity and the dark signal was removed appropriately based on the number of acquired frames. At each MU and gating frequency level, non-gated images were subtracted from gated to facilitate analysis.

## Results and discussion

Figure 1 shows normalized profiles obtained for a 10 x 10 $cm^2$ square field non-gated and at 3 gating frequencies. Measured field size (FWHM), flatness and symmetry are listed in *Table 1*. Results are reported for 100 monitor units but are essentially constant throughout the rance between 25 and 200 MU These observations are in agreement with those of Ramsey et al [3].

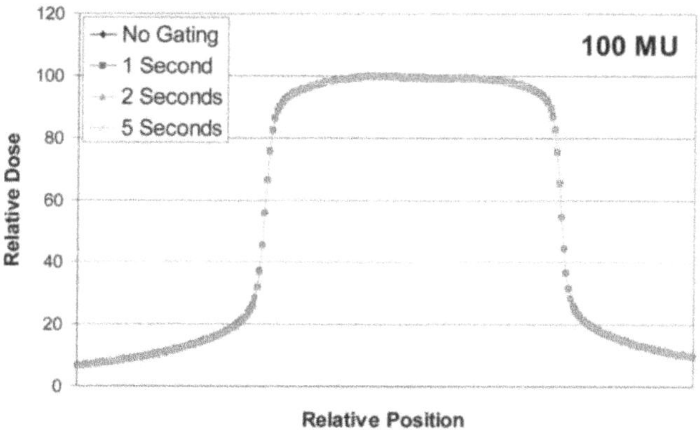


**Figure 1:** Normalized profiles from a 10 x 10 $cm^2$ square field. Two dimensional data was measured using the amorphous silicon device. 4 gating frequencies (non-gated and 0.2, 0.5 and 1.0 Hz) were used.

| Gating Frequency (Hz) | FWHM (mm) | Flatness (%) | Symmetry (%) |
|---|---|---|---|
| Non-gated | 99.13 | 2.64 | 1.92 |
| 0.2 | 99.13 | 2.56 | 1.94 |
| 0.5 | 99.13 | 2.65 | 1.95 |
| 1.0 | 99.11 | 2.68 | 1.94 |

**Table 1:** Field size (FWHM), flatness and symmetry for a 9.8 x 9.8 $cm^2$ square field given 100 monitor units.

Figure 2 shows 2-dimensional dosimetry maps of two dynamically wedged fields given 25 monitor units with no gating and a gating frequency of 1.0 Hz. Profiles along the central axis are shown in Figure 3 for both 25 and 200 monitor units. Small differences can be observed in the 25 MU data while that at 200 MU is esentially constant as a function of gating frequency. Dose linearity of the detector is also apparent from the two graphs. In Figure 4 these difference have been quantified by determining the average and maximum differences, calculated from:

$$\frac{1}{NxN}\sum_{i,j}^{NxN}\frac{(Gated)_{i,j}-(NonGated)_{i,j}}{(NonGated)_{i,j}}$$

and

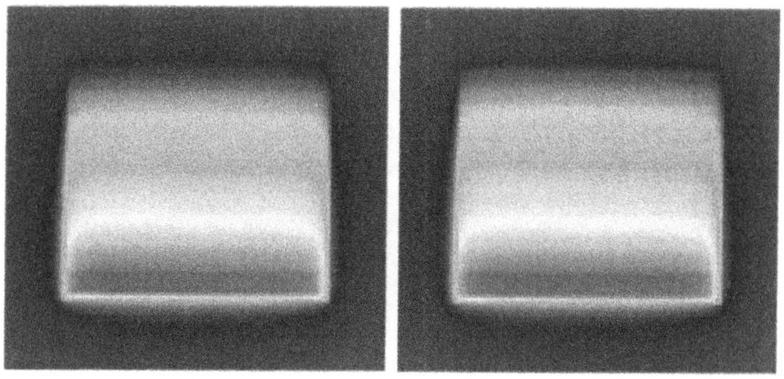

**Figure 2:** 10 x 10 $cm^2$ dynamically wedged fields non-gated (left) and gated at a frequency of 1.0 Hz (right). 25 monitor units were delivered to the detector placed beneath 10 cm of solid water.

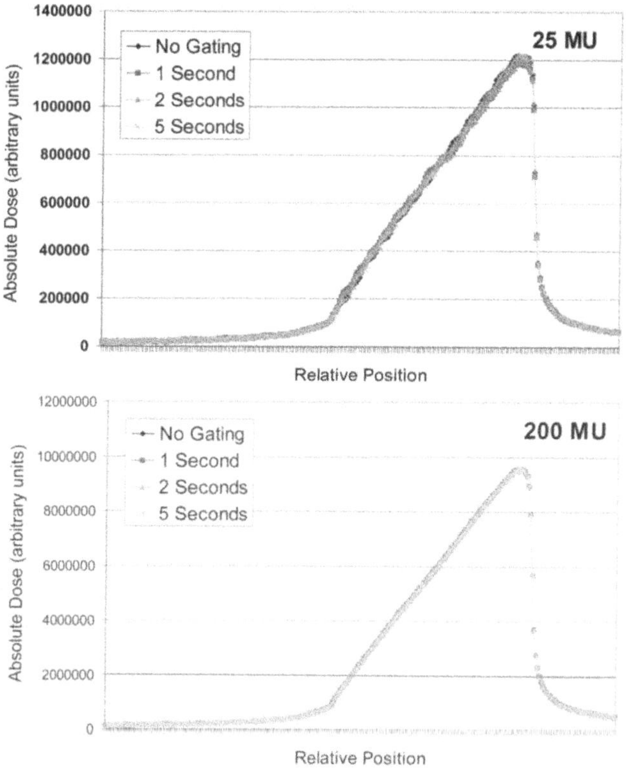


**Figure 3:** Wedge profiles for dynamically wedged fields given 25 (top) and 200 (bottom) monitor units. Fields were gated frequencies ranging from 0.2 to 1.0 Hz. Data is plotted on an absolute scale to facilitate direct comparison.

$$\max\left\{\frac{(Gated)_{i,j}-(NonGated)_{i,j}}{(NonGated)_{i,j}}\right\}$$

Fourier analysis performed on the subtracted images demonstrated small effects attributable to gating. As in Figure 4, the magnitude of these effects increases with gating frequency.

Finally, an arbitrary intensity pattern is shown in Figure 5 with the corresponding non-gated and gated dose maps. For the IMRT delivery the intensity pattern was broken into 14 levels. With a desired RMS of 1% this produced 29 segments. Radiation was delivered in a continuous fashion; interpolation of the individual segments to a continuous motion was facilitated by the Novalis MLC controller. Figure 6 shows profiles through the center column of the images at gating periods of 1, 2 and 5 seconds. Average and maximum differences between gated and non-gated images are of the same magnitude as those for the dynamic wedge.

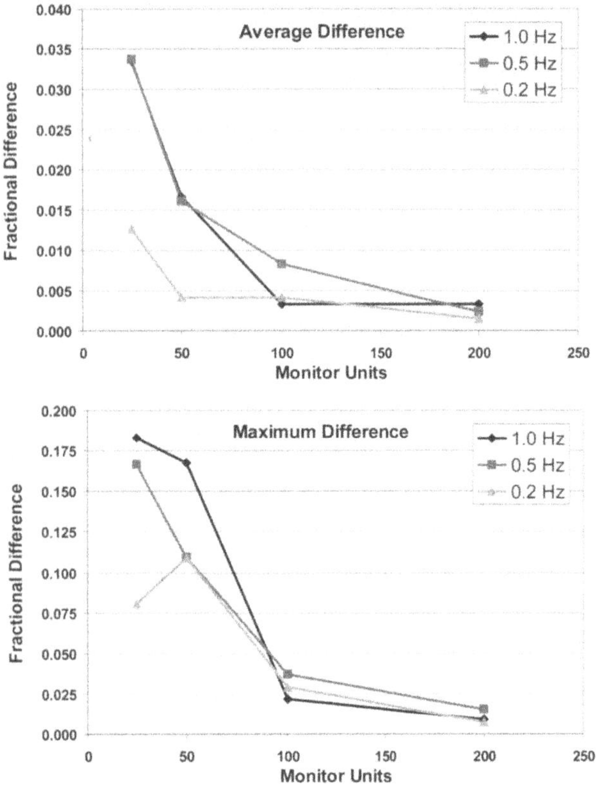


**Figure 4:** Average and maximum fractional difference in absolute dose as a function of monitor units and gating frequency.

## Conclusion

The effect of gating frequencies consistent with respiratory motion was investigated for dynamically delivered IMRT fields using monitor units appropriate for IMRT delivery. Dose reproducibility is maintained under gating conditions except at very low monitor units and high gating frequencies. Dosimetric

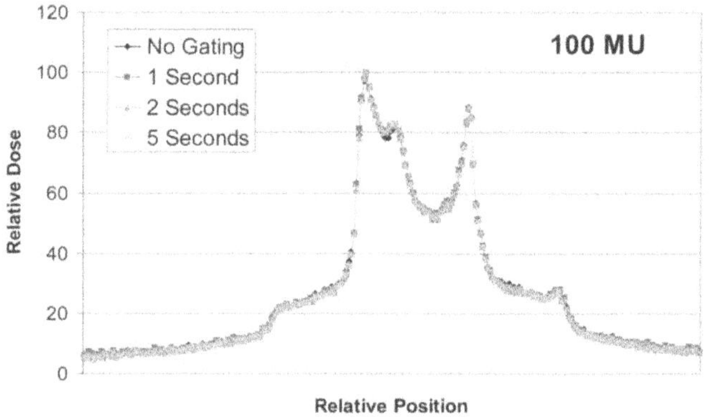


**Figure 6:** Normalized profiles for an arbirtary intensity pattern (Figure 5) delivered under gated and non-gated conditions.

capabilities of the Novalis device are consistent with delivery of respiratory gated IMRT.

## References


[1] Llacer, J. Inverse Radiation Treatment Planning using the Dynamically Penalized Likelihood Method 1997 *Medical Physics* **24** 1751-64

[2] Enhanced Dynamic Wedge Implementation Guide 1996 *Varian Oncology Systems publication* #1103580-01

[3] Ramsey C R, Cordrel I L and Oliver A L 1999 A comparison of beam characteristics for gated and nongated clinical x-ray beams *Medical Physics* **26** 2086-2091

[4] Paul T J, Solberg T D, Leu MY, Rosemark PJ, Smathers JB. Independent Real-Time Verification of Dynamically Shaped Intensity Modulated Radiotherapy (IMRT) using an Amorphous Silicon (a-Si:H) Detector Array 1999 *Medical Physics* **26** 1065

[5] Bortfeld T R, Kahler D L, Waldron T J, Boyer A L. X-ray field compensation with multileaf collimators 1994 *International Journal of Radiation Oncology Biology Physics* **28** 723-730

[6] Agazaryan N, Solberg T D, Arellano A R, Paul T J. Leaf Sequencing for Fluence Modulated Radiation Therapy 1999 *Medical Physics* **26** 1139


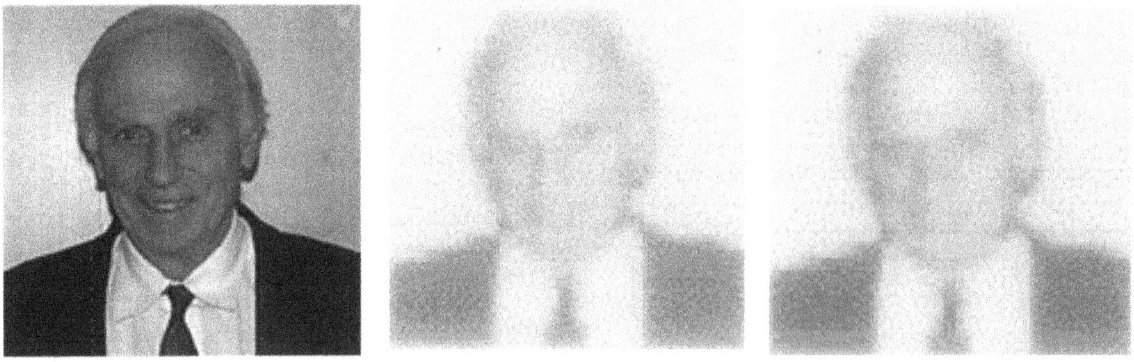

**Figure 5:** Original intensity profile (left) shown with resulting dose maps for non-gated IMRT (middle) and IMRT gated with a frequency of 1.0 Hz (right).

# The Dosimetric Consequences of Patient Movement on Three Classes of Intensity-Modulated Delivery Techniques in Breast Radiotherapy

**Charlotte L. Hector, Philip M. Evans and Steve Webb**

Joint Department of Physics, Institute of Cancer Research and Royal Marsden NHS Trust, Downs Road, Sutton, Surrey, SM2 5PT.

## Introduction

It has long been realised that irradiation of the breast using an opposed wedged tangential pair causes a large dose inhomogeneity within the breast (the so called conventional technique). It has been demonstrated that this dose inhomogeneity exceeds the figure of 10% normally considered acceptable. This large dose heterogeneity is suspected of being one of the main contributing factors to poor cosmesis.

The use of compensators in breast radiotherapy has been shown to reduce this dose inhomogeneity. The compensators shape the treatment to take into account the contour of the breast and are the simplest method to create the intensity-modulated beams required. However, as the treatment is shaped to take account of the contours of the breast, patient movement may cause errors in the dose distribution that could result in a treatment that is suspected of being inferior to the conventional technique.

Instead of using a physical compensator, a multileaf collimator (MLC) could be used to deliver the treatment. The intensity-modulated beam is then created as a series of field components. The main potential advantage is that the MLC could be used adaptively to redesign a patient's treatment on each day thus removing the problem of patient movement.

The study reported here investigated the MLC technique and evaluated whether an improvement can be achieved by designing the patient's treatment each imaged fraction using either a multiple-static-field (MSF) MLC technique or a dynamic multileaf collimator (DMLC) technique. The MLC dose-plans were compared with the compensated technique currently used in our institution where the compensators are designed based on the first day of treatment and then reused at each subsequent occasion. These compensated dose-plans were also compared to dose-plans delivered by compensators which were designed on each available imaged fraction. This was used to provide a benchmark with which to compare the MLC treatments. Two MSF techniques were evaluated, each designed with a different number of field components. Finally a DMLC technique was investigated to evaluate the improvement that could be gained over the MSF techniques.

## Material and methods

The study was performed on a group of six post-menopausal patients who underwent conventional breast irradiation as part of their breast-conserving therapy. A series of electronic portal images (5-8, mean 6) were obtained at various intervals during their treatments using a portal imaging system developed at this Institute. Estimated CT-sets were created from the lateral portal image for each patient using the methods described in [1]. Each of the compensators were designed in conjunction with a wedge to reduce the intensity-modulation required. The method used to design the intensity-modulated beams is described in [1]. Both compensators and MLC were modelled as transmission maps and planning was carried out on the VOXELPLAN 3D treatment-planning system [2].

Compensators were simulated as a series of 0.5mm thick sheets of lead. Two different delivery techniques were investigated. The first uses the images taken on day 1 only to design a set of compensators. This set of compensators was then reused to create the plans for the subsequent available images. This is the main method currently used in our Institution. In the second method a set of compensators is designed from each of the portal images available. This would be the 'ideal' treatment in which the intensity-modulation is adapted throughout the course of treatment, but is impractical as it would not be possible to fabricate a set of compensators for each day of treatment.

Two different multiple-static-field (MSF) MLC techniques were investigated and were simulated as delivered by the Elekta MLC. The first is a 4-field MSF-MLC technique that consists of an open and wedged pair and 3 'top-up' fields. This technique has just been commissioned in our Institution. The second technique is a 'quantised' MSF-MLC technique; so called because the quantisation between each of the field components is equal to the change in intensity (2.4%) that corresponds to the attenuation through a 0.5mm thick sheet of lead used in designing the compensators. This method was chosen to investigate the magnitude of improvement gained over the 4-field method.

The beam parameters (isocentre, wedge, gantry and collimator angles) were the same as those used when setting up the compensated plans. Initially the fluence profiles were designed using the same method used to design the compensators. The fluence profiles were then rescaled in the superior-inferior direction to create the 1cm leaf widths. Once the ideal intensity-modulated beam had been designed they were passed through an 'interpreter' to check they were deliverable with the Elekta MLC. A close-in delivery method was used as in general the intensity profiles only contain one maximum, which is usually at the thickest part of the breast.

Finally a DMLC technique was investigated. This technique was simulated by taking the fluence map created for compensated method and setting the spatial resolution in the superior-inferior direction to correspond to the 1cm leaf widths of the MLC.

To investigate the potential improvements that could be achieved with the techniques described above a number of comparisons were made. Below are the 4 cases investigated:

Case 1. A comparison of compensated dose-plans designed for each imaged fraction with compensated dose-plans designed on day 1 only.

Case 2. A comparison of MSF-MLC dose-plans designed with an intensity interval of 2.4% between fields ('quantised' MLC plans) for each imaged fraction with the compensated dose-plans designed on day 1 only.

Case 3. A comparison of 4-field-components MLC dose-plans designed for each imaged fraction with compensated dose-plans designed on day 1 only.

Case 4. A comparison of DMLC designed for each imaged fraction with compensated dose-plans designed on day 1 only.

The mean and standard deviation of the breast volume was calculated for the volume less than 95% dose, volume greater than 105% dose and volume outside the dose range 95-105% for each of the 5 techniques. Each of the cases discussed above were assessed by means of a paired, two-tailed t-test in which the volume outside the dose range 95-105% was used.

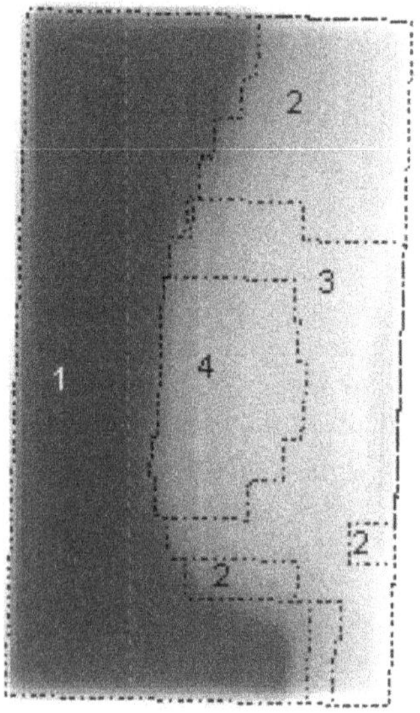


**Figure 1:** Example of a 4-field mutiple-static-field arrangement superimposed onto the original portal image.

## Results and discussion

Figure 1. illustrates a multiple-static-field arrangement superimposed over the original portal image to demonstrate a typical 4-field component arrangment.

The weighted mean and standard deviation were also calculated for the pooled patient group for the following parameters; breast volume less than 95% dose, breast volume greater than 105% dose and the breast volume outside the dose range 95-105%. The results of these calculations are shown in table 1.

| | Weighted mean volume <95% dose (SD) | Weighted mean volume >105% dose (SD) | Weighted mean volume outside 95-105% dose (SD) |
|---|---|---|---|
| Compensator (designed on day 1 only) | 2.61 (4.19) | 2.45 (5.66) | 5.06 (5.08) |
| Compensator (designed on each imaged fraction) | 1.71 (1.17) | 1.12 (1.08) | 2.83 (3.56) |
| 4-field MLC (designed on each imaged fraction) | 2.82 (4.4) | 1.65 (5.11) | 4.47 (11.97) |
| 'quantised' MLC (designed on each imaged fraction) | 1.69 (0.84) | 2.39 (7.83) | 4.08 (11.07) |
| DMLC (designed on each imaged fraction) | 2.22 (2.14) | 0.90 (0.84) | 3.12 (4.61) |

**Table 1:** Summary of the dose-volume statistics for all patients.

The data show that designing the compensators for each imaged fraction results in a reduction in the volume outside the range 95-105% dose of 2.23% compared to designing the compensators on day 1 only. This reduction is reduced to 0.98% when the 'quantised' MLC is used. Examination of the volume outside the dose range 95-105% for the 4-field-component technique shows that there is little difference between this method and the technique where the compensators are designed on day 1 only. The DMLC technique shows an improvement of 1.94% in the volume outside 95-105% dose when compared to the compensators designed on day 1 only and is an improvement over the 'quantised' MSF-MLC technique.

Examining the results from the t-test (table 2) reveals in case 1, a statistically significant change in the volume outside 95-105% dose is achieved ($p$=0.0045). For case 2 a reduction in the volume outside 95-105% dose is not achieved to the 95% confidence level by using this technique ($p$=0.32). The comparison between the 4-field MLC technique and the technique in which the compensators are designed on day 1 only also show no statistically significant reduction in the volume outside 95-105% dose ($p$=0.55). Finally for case 4, where the DMLC technique is compared to the compensated technique in which the compensators are designed on day 1 only, a statistically significant reduction in the volume outside 95-105% is achieved ($p$=0.024).

| | Breast Volume <95% dose | Breast volume >105% dose | Breast volume outside 95-105% dose |
|---|---|---|---|
| Case 1 | $p$=0.088 | $p$=0.097 | $p$=0.0045 |
| Case 2 | $p$=0.12 | $p$=0.95 | $p$=0.32 |
| Case 3 | $p$=0.66 | $p$=0.31 | $p$=0.55 |
| Case 4 | $p$=0.5 | $p$=0.054 | $p$=0.024 |

**Table 2:** Summary of the p-values calculated for each of the 4 cases.

## Conclusion

In conclusion, the results show that designing the treatment using a 'quantised' set of MLC fields for each treatment fraction does not significantly reduce the volume outside 95-105% when compared to the technique where the compensators are designed on day 1 only. Therefore, it would not be feasible to warrant the large amount of resources that would be required to design a treatment for each fraction. The results from the DMLC do however show a statistically significant reduction in the volume outside 95-105% ($p$=0.024). Therefore it would be a feasible technique to use if an adaptive approach to treatment design were to be undertaken. To make this technique feasible an 'action level' is required for both setup error and for any changes in breast volume that may occur during treatment above which intervention is required. These parameters are currently under investigation.

## References

[1] Evans P M, Hansen V N, Mayles W P M, Swindell W, Torr M, and Yarnold J R 1995 Design of compensators for breast radiotherapy using electronic portal imaging *Radiotherapy and Oncology* **37** 43-54.

[2]Bendl R, Pross J, Keller M A and Schlegel W. 1994 VIRTUOS: A program for virtual simulation and verification In: Hounsell AR, Wilkinson JM, Williams PC. editors. *Proceedings of the 11th Conference on the use of Computers in Radiation therapy*, Manchester, 226.

# Monitor Units Verification Calculation in IMRT as a Patient Specific Dosimetry QA.

**Jong H. Kung[1], Ph.D; George T. Y. Chen[2], Ph.D**

[1,2]Massachusetts General Hospital /[2]Harvard University/[1]Harvard Medical School
[1]jkung@patners.org, [2]gchen@partners.org

## Introduction

In standard teletherapy, a treatment plan with isodoses and monitor units (MU) for each field is calculated by a treatment planning computer system. In clinical practice, it is common to verify the MU's with an independent MU verification calculation (MUVC). A MUVC uses look up tables of beam data and information about each treatment field (e.g., equivalent square, jaw dimensions, depth in tissue, accessories and wedge, and dose contribution by each field) to calculate the required MU for each field. The MUVC essentially verified that a point in a target volume will receive the dose as calculated by a treatment planning system.

In IMRT, with its non-uniform fluences, the concept of an equivalent square is not well defined, and therefore there is a technical difficulty of performing a MUVC. We propose an accurate dose calculation algorithm applicable for a non-uniform fluence, which is simple enough to be implemented on a desktop computer as a MUVC in IMRT. In analogy to the MUVC in standard teletherapy, the algorithm uses look up table of beam data and information about each IMRT treatment field (e.g., jaw dimensions, depth in tissue, DMLC file, MU for each field) to calculate a dose contribution by each field to a dose point of interest.

## Materials and Methods

### I. A Modified Clarkson Integration (MCI) for IMRT.

Consider the problem of calculating dose when tissue is irradiated with a non-uniform fluence. We first consider an idealized problem of calculating dose at a depth along the central axis (CAX) in a homogeneous water equivalent medium with a flat tissue contour. In IMRT, each field is composed of many MLC subfields called segments. Each segment delivers some fraction of the total MU of the field. Figure 1 shows an intensity map in air for an IMRT field. Mathematically, the intensity map is a sum of all MLC subfield apertures weighted by monitor units delivered with each subfield, i.e., MU(x,y). Corrections to the intensity map from a (1-2)% MLC transmission can be calculated and incorporated into MU(x,y)[1].

Because of azimuthal scattering symmetry, a dose along the central axis is unchanged when the intensity MU(x,y) is replaced by its azimuthal average (Figure 1), i.e.,

$$MU(r) \equiv \frac{1}{2\pi} \int_{\text{circle}} MU(x,y) d\phi \qquad (1)$$

The dose along the CAX can now be readily calculated as shown in equation 2 (see next page).

The first and the second terms represent primary and scattered dose, respectively. This is a variation of the Clarkson integration in which fluence is first averaged along the CAX and than a scatter dose contribution is summed over annular sectors instead of pie sectors.

### II. Implementation of the MCI algorithm on a desktop computer for a MUVC in IMRT

We wrote code to implement the MCI algorithm. The code was written in Mathematica. To test the algorithm, five CORVUS IMRT plans (6MV, 1cmx1cm, step and shoot) were generated for pelvis, brain, and a Lucite phantom. The code reads in a DMLC file of a treatment field created by CORVUS, converts fluence MU(x,y) into its azimuthal averages MU(r)'s, and performs the MCI. The code uses beam data (Sc, Sp, TPR) and requires user input for jaw dimensions, SSD and depth along CAX to a dose point of interest. We used r=1cm beam data for the calculation of the primary dose. On a 266MHZ desktop computer, the code takes less than 15 seconds to calculate a dose at a single point. Finally, the doses calculated with the MCI were compared with the doses that were calculated by CORVUS.

## Results and discussion

Table I shows that the doses calculated with the MCI agree with the doses calculated by CORVUS to within +/- 3%. The MCI algorithm includes scatter factors, radiation field offset, and MLC transmission.

The present version of the code allows dose calculation only along the CAX. The code also assumes a flat tissue contour and a homogeneous medium. A future project will investigate the general case.

## References

[1] J. H. Kung and G. T. Y. Chen, "A Hand Calculation of Monitor Units in IMRT as a Dosimetry QA," submitted to Med. Phys.

[2] A. Boyer, L. Xing, C. M. Ma, B. Curran, et al., "Theoretical Considerations of Monitor Unit Calculations for Intensity Modulated Beam Treatment Planning," Med. Phys. 26, 187-195 (1999).

[3] L. Xing, Y. Chen, G. Luxton, J. G. Li, and A. L. Boyer, " Monitor Unit Calculation for Intensity Modulated Photon Field," Stanford University preprint.

$$D(d) = S_c\left(\frac{D}{MU}\right)_{ref}\left(MU(0)S_p(0)TPR(0) + \sum_r MU(r)\left(S_p(r+\Delta r)TPR(r+\Delta r,d) - S_p(r)TPR(r,d)\right)\right)$$

Sc(r)= collimator scatter factor
Sp(r)= phantom scatter factor
TPR(r,d)=tissue phantom ratio
(D/MU)ref=reference dose rate
d=depth in tissue along CAX

**Equation 2**

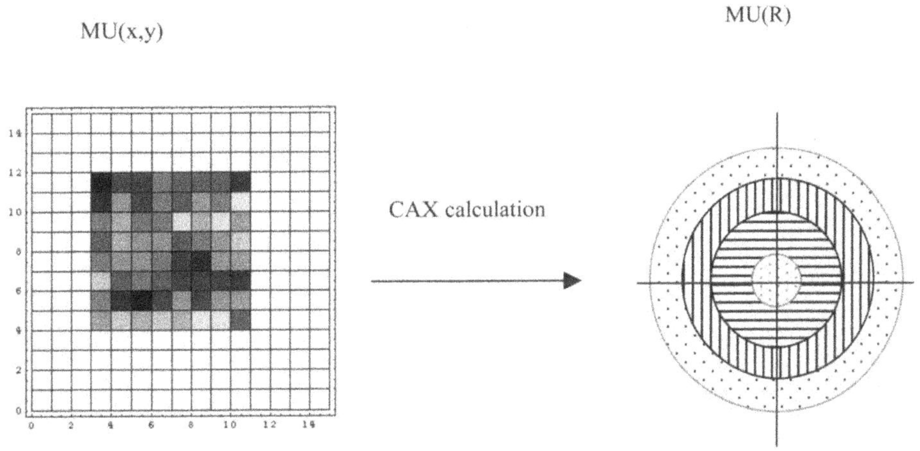


**Figure 1.** Dose alone the CAX is unchanged when incident fluence is replaced by its azimuthal average

| Testing the MCI algorithm | | | | |
|---|---|---|---|---|
| 6MV<br>Inhomogeneity correction was not used in either CORVUS or in the MCI algorithm<br>2.5% MLC transmission was used by both CORVUS and the MCI algorithm | | | | |
| Site | Comment | number of fields | Dose point | D(MCI)/D(CORVUS) |
| Pancreas | Patient CT | 9 flds | 1cm superior from isocenter | 99% |
| Pancreas boost | Patient CT | 9 flds | at isocenter | 101% |
| Pituitary | Patient CT | 9 flds | 1.5cm superior from Isocenter | 97% |
| U shaped target | Cylinder phantom* | 7 flds | .5cm superior from isocenter | 102% |
| Convex target | Cylinder Phantom* | 5 flds | .8cm inferior from isocenter | 103% |
| *Cylinder was a 8.8cm diameter Lucite phantom | | | | |

**Table I.** A comparison of the doses calculated with the MCI algorithm and the doses calculated by CORVUS.

# Database Energy Fluence Verification and the Importance of On-Board CT Imaging in Dose Reconstruction

**JM Kapatoes[1], GH Olivera[1,2], KJ Ruchala[2], PJ Reckwerdt[2], JB Smilowitz[1], JP Balog[2], DW Pearson[1,2], and TR Mackie[1,2]**

[1]University of Wisconsin – Madison, 1300 University Ave., Madison, Wisconsin, USA, 53706, and [2]TomoTherapy, Inc., 2228 Evergreen Rd., Middleton, Wisconsin, USA, 53562

## Introduction

Helical tomotherapy is a radiation therapy technique that utilizes a rotating fan beam of intensity-modulated radiation to deliver dose. The integration of the accelerator, multi-leaf collimator (MLC), and a computed tomography (CT) detector on a single ring gantry allows for dose reconstruction, in which the full 3D dose delivered to the patient is reconstructed[1]. The incident energy fluence computed using the detected signal[2] and a CT image in the treatment position are the inputs for any model-based dose computation algorithm such as convolution/superposition (C/S) or Monte Carlo (MC).

To obtain the incident energy fluence using the exit signal, a transfer matrix is needed for each beam angle used. To avoid having to measure this matrix[2], it was devised that a database of signal profiles as a function of radiological pathlength and patient-to-detector distance (PDD) could be used in conjunction with a CT in the treatment position to compute the transfer matrix. This method was tested in the head region of a dog cadaver.

Using the transfer matrix, energy fluence values were obtained and the dose reconstructed using a CT at the time of treatment. Reconstructed dose results will be shown for the dog treatment. Moreover, the impact of delivery errors associated with positioning and the role of the CT image in detection of such errors will also be illustrated.

## Material and methods

**Benchtop**

For all measurements and deliveries, the UW Tomotherapy Workbench was used. This includes a 4 MV General Electric (Buc, France) ORION accelerator (avg. energy = 1.37 MV), a NOMOS (Sewickly, PA) MIMiC MLC (top row used only, thus 20 leaves), a Parker Hannifin (Rohnert Park, CA) rotation/translation table, and a General Electric (Milwaukee, WI) CT detector with xenon as the main filling gas. All signal profiles from the detector used for dose reconstruction must be corrected for two phenomena: leakage and transmission, and tongue-and-groove/penumbra effects[2].

**Canine Nasopharygeal Treatment**

In conjunction with the University of Wisconsin – Madison Veterinary School, a nasopharygeal treatment was planned on a dog cadaver. A kVCT of the head region was taken at the UW-Hospital, contours drawn using the image, and an optimised treatment plan created[3]. The dog cadaver was treated on the Benchtop, with MVCT data acquired in the treatment position. The delivery covered 34 slices and the tumour region extended over 32 slices (12.2 cm). Regions of interest (ROI's) are resented for three slices (Figure 1). Slice 14 (Fig. 1a) lies in the snout of the dog, while slice 21 (Fig. b) is located in the sinus area, and slice 29 (Figs. 1c) is in the head proper. There are no sensitive structures present in slice 14, but the tumour region is split by the oral cavity (internal contour). Of interest in slice 21 is the presence of low density (0.2-0.4 g/cm$^3$) regions within the tumour. Lastly, the tumour is surrounded by normal ROI's in slice 29. Regarding the extent of the sensitive structures, the left and right eyes spanned slices 25-30 (2.3 cm total), while the brain was present in slices 29-39 (4.2 cm total). The nose (not pictured) was in slices 1-3 (1.1 cm).

The ROI's in Figure 1 will be correct provided the dog was in the same position for the treatment as the kVCT. In fact, this was not the case as the Benchtop table and system were asynchronous for this delivery. This resulted in a rotational offset of 8.7$^{\circ}$. Thus these ROI's, which were used for the optimisation, were not congruent with the actual treatment position.

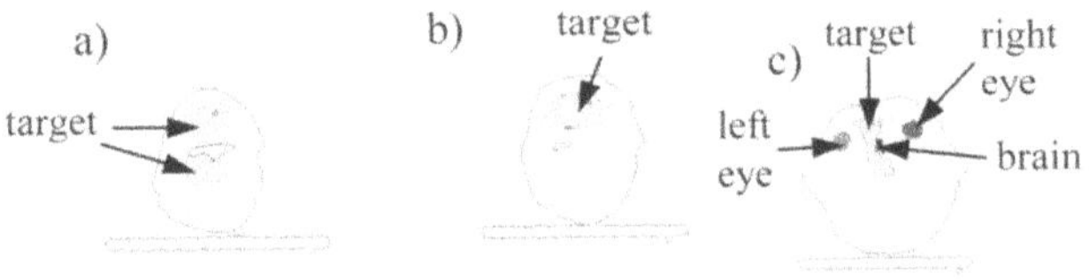


**Figure 1:** Regions of interest (ROI's) of three representative slices from the dog treatment; slice 14(a), 21(b) and 29(c).

**Transfer Matrix Measurement**

The transfer matrix was measured upon completion of the treatment. The measurement involved opening each leaf individually, and rotating the head using the same pitch and starting position as the treatment[2]. Each leaf measurement represents a column of the transfer matrix. The rows correspond to the projections (or beam angles) at which the optimisation software delivered dose.

**Database Measurement**

The database of signal profiles was measured by placing a known amount of solid water on the Benchtop table at a fixed distance from the detector; and then opening the leaves one-at-a-time. Once the signal for each leaf was recorded, the amount of material and/or distance from the detector was changed, and the process repeated. The measured set of radiological pathlengths and phantom-to-detector distances (PDD) ranged from 0.0 to 34.1 cm, and 12.0 to 34.0 cm, respectively.

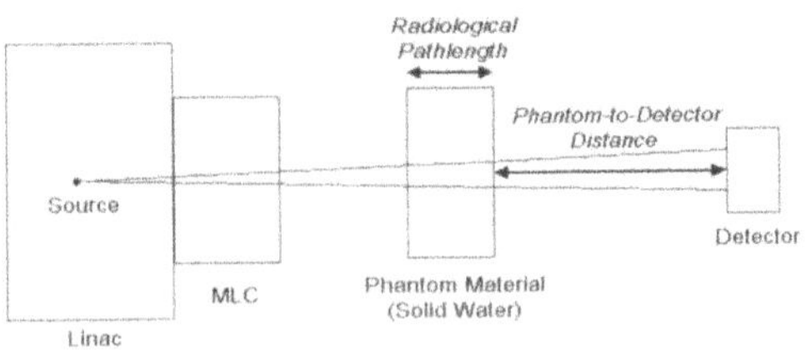


**Figure 2:** Set-up used for measurement of the database.

**Transfer Matrix Computation**
The transfer matrix was computed using the MVCT and measured database. For each projection (beam angle) used in the optimisation process, the radiological pathlength and PDD was calculated for each leaf from the MVCT. These values were used to access the database and derive the signal profile for all leaves over all projections. In turn, this filled all the columns and rows of the transfer matrix and completed the process.

**Energy Fluence and Dose Computation**
Once a transfer matrix was obtained, it was inverted and multiplied by the pulse-by-pulse detector signal to yield the actual pulse-by-pulse energy fluence for each leaf. This fluence sinogram was averaged over projections. The projection-by-projection energy fluence and the MVCT were used to compute by C/S the dose actually delivered.

## Results and discussion

Energy fluence sinograms for the entire treatment are shown in Figure 3. The columns represent the leaf number and the rows represent the projection. There are a total of 1683 rows (33 slices x 51 projections per slice) in each sinogram. The

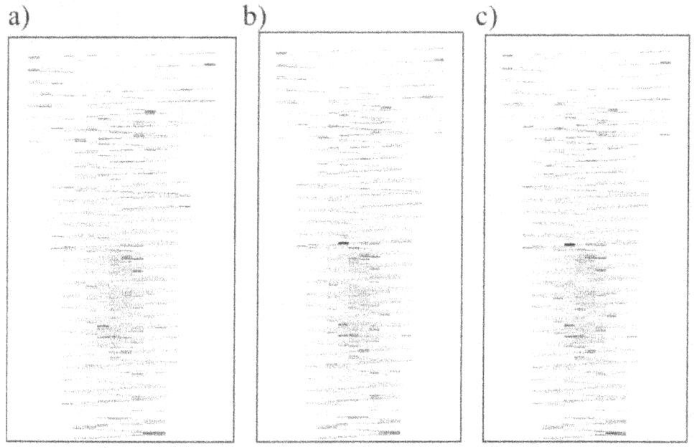


**Figure 3:** Energy fluence sinograms. (a) The optimized or planned sinogram. (b) The verification sinogram using the measured tranfer matrix. (b) The verification sinogram using the database-derived transfer matrix.

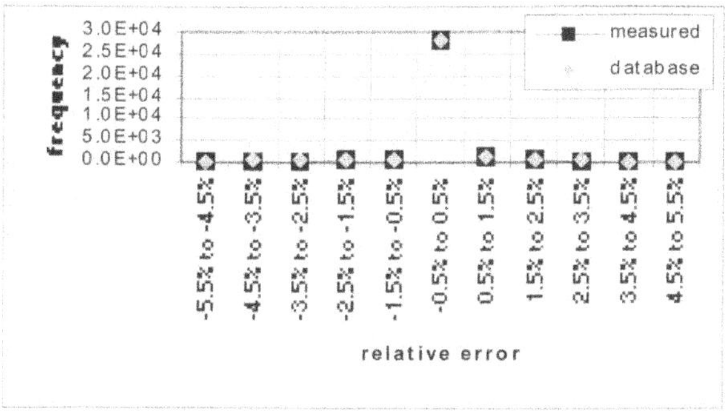


**Figure 4:** Histogram of relative error for both verification sinograms in Figure 3 (b and c). The difference values between the verification sinograms and the planned energy fluence sinogram (Fig. 3a) were normalized to the mean planned energy fluence value to yield the relative error values.

optimised sinogram (Figure 3a), the verification sinogram calculated using the measured transfer matrix (Figure 3b), and the verification sinogram calculated using the database transfer matrix appear qualitatively identical. This is confirmed in Figure 4. The difference between the optimised sinogram and the two verification sinograms was taken and a histogram of these difference values is shown. The histograms are indeed very similar. Moreover, the majority of the values fall in the –0.5% to +0.5% bin, confirming the overall success of the delivery with regards to the linac and MLC.

Dose was computed for four cases. Their designations and descriptions are as follows:

1. *Reconstructed dose*: verification sinogram (Fig. 3c) convolved with the MVCT (actual dog position)
2. *Optimised dose*: optimised sinogram (Fig. 3a) convolved with the kVCT (planning position).
3. *Estimated optimal dose*: optimised sinogram convolved with the MVCT. This is an estimated optimal dose since the MVCT was in the actual position and not necessarily in the position of the planning kVCT.
4. *Estimated reconstructed dose*: verification sinogram, computed using a transfer matrix based on the kVCT, convolved with the kVCT. This is an estimate because the planning kVCT is used for the entire process, thus assuming that the treatment position is exactly the same as that of the planning kVCT.

Reconstructed dose images with contours representing the ROI's from Figure 1 are presented in Figure 5. The rotational error discussed previously is present as large portions of the high dose regions lie outside the tumour contour. This is supported in Figure 6. MVCT images are displayed for slice 29 in Figure 6 with the 30, 50 and 90% isodose lines superimposed. The reconstructed dose is common to all figures and is compared to the optimised dose (Fig. 6a), the

a) b) c)

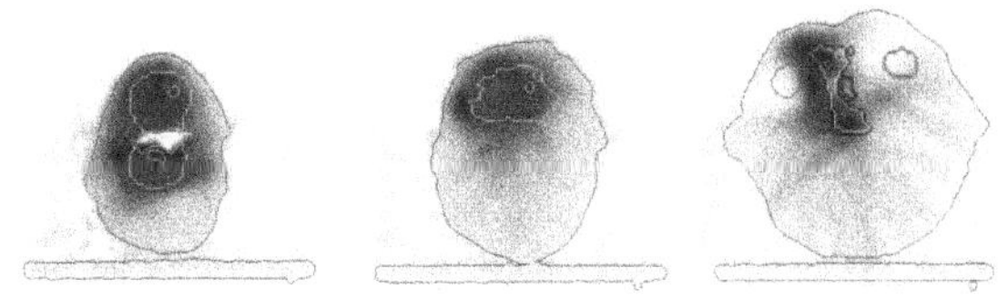

**Figure 5:** Reconstructed dose images with ROI contours. Pictured are slices 14 (a, b), 21 (c, d) and 29(e, f). Large portions of the high dose areas are outside of the tumour contour due to the rotational error in the position of the dog.

a) b) c)

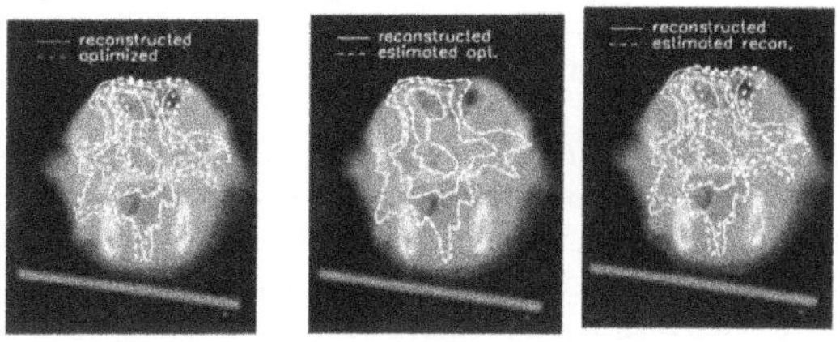


**Figure 6:** CT with the 30, 50 and 90% isodoses for slice 29. The reconstructed distribution is compared with three other distributions (see text for description) to find out the importance of certain factors in dose reconstruction.

a) b) c)

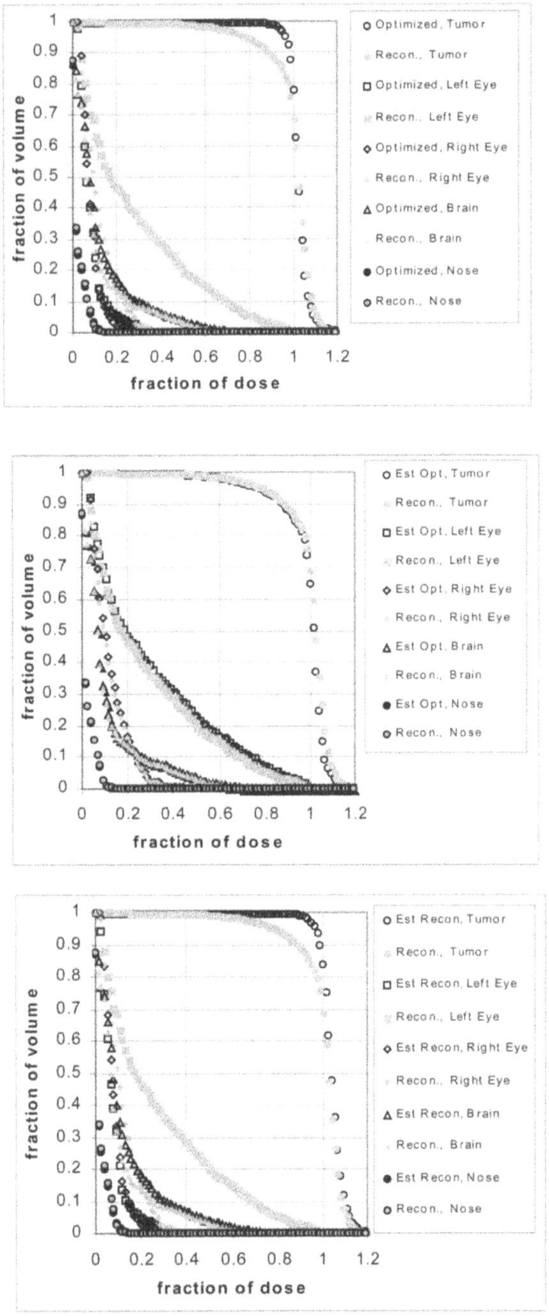


**Figure 7:** Dose volume histogram comparison. For (a)-(c), the grey DVH is for the reconstructed distribution computed using the energy fluence in Fig. 3c and the MVCT in the actual position. The other DVH's are from: (a) the optimized distribution created using the energy fluence in Fig. 3a and the MVCT in the actual position (Figs 5a, c, e). (b) the optimized distribution created using the energy fluence in Fig. 3a and the CT in the non-rotated, planning position (not shown). (c) the reconstructed distribution created using the CT in the non-rotated position (not shown) for both the energy fluence and dose computations. Case (c) is analogous to using a CT from treatment planning for dose reconstruction. Notice the error easily seen in the grey DVH is not revealed, underscoring the importance of a CT in the actual treatment position.

estimated optimal dose (Fig. 6b), and the estimated reconstructed dose (Fig. 6c). The discrepancy between the reconstructed and the optimised dose (Fig. 6a) is startling. The same applies for the reconstructed versus the estimated reconstructed dose (Fig 6c) but not the reconstructed versus the estimated optimal dose (Fig 6b).

Looking at quantitative results, dose volume histograms (DVH's) are provided in Figure 7 for the same three qualitative comparisons made in Figure 6. The contrast between the optimised and reconstructed DVH (Fig 7a) clearly displays that there was a problem in the delivery. There are two glaring differences: the tumour dose was much lower for a large fraction of the volume, and the right eye received a huge dose relative to the planned dose. This is a direct result of the dog being positioned incorrectly.

Figure 7b is a confirmation that dose reconstruction does indeed work since the same CT image is used to compute dose in both cases (removing positional errors), and the actual energy fluence is used for the reconstructed dose.

The comparison in Figure 7c is synonymous to using the original treatment planning CT to perform dose reconstruction for any given fraction. The effect of the rotational offset is not seen. Thus, although an incorrect transfer matrix was applied to the actual treatment sinogram, the true effects on the dose remain hidden. The full error will only be revealed if dose is computed with a CT in the actual treatment position.

## Conclusion

Dose reconstruction was performed using the Tomotherapy Workbench. Results using a transfer matrix derived from a database of signal profiles were nearly identical to those using a measured matrix. Both approaches agreed very well with the planned parameters in energy fluence and dose. Such results validate the concept of a database-derived transfer matrix and make energy fluence verification without extra table time or patient dose a reality.

The effects of positioning errors were investigated. It was found that without a CT image of the true position during treatment, dose errors were not exposed. This could lead to a severe over- or under-dosage of one or many structures. With a CT in the treatment position such problems will be detected, allowing for adaptive radiotherapy.

## References

[1] McNutt T R, Mackie T R, and Paliwal B R 1997 Analysis and convergence of the iterative convolution/superposition dose reconstruction technique for multiple treatment beams and tomotherapy *Med. Phys.* **24** 1465-1476.

[2] Kapatoes J K, Olivera G H, Reckwerdt P J, Fitchard E E, Schloesser E A, and Mackie T R 1999 Delivery verification in sequential and helical tomotherapy *Phys. Med. Biol.* **44** 1815-1841.

[3] Shepard D M, Olivera G H, and Mackie T R 2000 Iterative approaches to dose optimisation in tomotherapy *Phys. Med. Biol.* **45** 69-90.

# Delivery Modification as an Alternative to Patient Repositioning in Tomotherapy

G.H. Olivera[1,2], E.E. Fitchard[2], P.J.Reckwerdt[2], K.Ruchala[2] and T.R.Mackie[1,2]

[1]Deparment of Medical Physics University of Wisconsin-Madison 1300 University Av. Madison WI 53705, USA, and [2]Tomotherapy Inc. 2228 Evergreen Road, Middleton WI, (53562-4241), USA.

## Introduction

Tomotherapy is an Intensity Modulated Radiotherapy (IMRT) technique that has a set of processes completing a closed loop for planning, delivery and verification in radiotherapy[1].

In tomotherapy, patient positioning can be accomplished in two ways:

a) using the computed tomographic capabilities[2] in order to produce CT images of the patient at a reference position which will be registered with another CT image obtained during the fraction to compute the offset between both patient's position.
b) using registration in projection space[3, 4] i.e. by taking a loose helical sinogram at a reference position which can be compared with another loose helical sinogram taken during the fraction to obtain the six parameters (three rotational, three translational) offset without need to reconstruct the image and performing a registration between two-dimensional images.

Once that the patient's offset was computed for a particular fraction, there are in principle two possible ways to accommodate the patient accordingly to the geometry of the optimized treatment plan:

1) Shift the patient manually in order to account or the patient offset. This may be, however, an error prone methodology.
2) Use a couch with three-dimensional movement capabilities to account for the patient's shift. However, with this kind of couch, accounting for patient's offset such as pitch, jaw and roll is extremelly difficult.

A more appealing approach will be maintain the patient in the same position at the couch and modify the treatment delivery accordingly to the patient's offset. The method must be fast enough to be performed with the patient on the couch. A technique will be presented that will be referred to as *delivery modification* (DM) and is a first step toward this goal. Specifically, delivery modification is the set of transformations applied to the planned energy fluence sinogram to account for the patient offset technique and will be the topic of this manuscript.

## Material and methods

The result of the optimized treatment planning in tomotherapy is a sinogram called the *planned energy fluence sinogram*. This is a two-dimensional array containing the information about the energy fluence that should be delivered to the patient. The rows represent projection angles and the columns represent different leaves. Therefore it contains information about where and how long every leaf should be open.

This energy fluence sinogram can be delivered if the patient is in the same position that the treatment was optimized. However, when the patient is positioned on the couch in a particular fraction, there may be an offset with respect to the position where the treatment was optimized.

A flow diagram of the delivery modification processes is presented in figure 1. The inputs are the planned energy fluence sinogram and the six parameter offset of the patient provided for instance from registration in projection space. The planned energy fluence sinogram is modified using a set of transformations that will produce a new energy fluence sinogram (delivery modified sinogram) that accounts for the patient's offset.

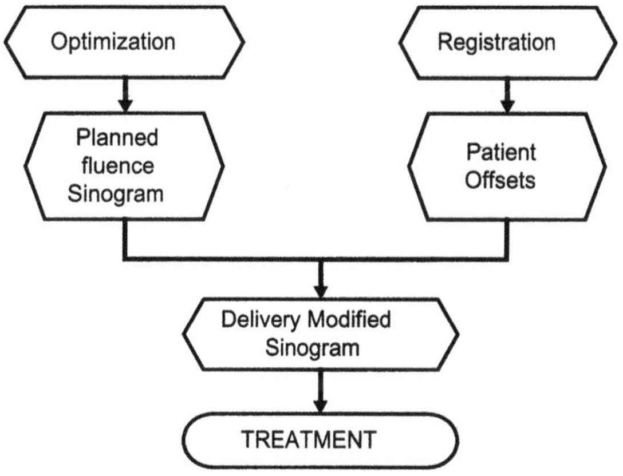


**Figure 1:** Flow diagram of the delivery verification processes

When a patient has an offset in the z direction (with the z-axis parallel to the inferior superior direction) or a roll offset, the sinogram is shifted by enough rows in order to account for this offset.

Offsets in the x or y direction are little more involved because the planned fluence sinogram is intented for a fan beam. In principle, modifications accounting for x-y offsets geometry can be applied to this sinogram, but in practice is easier to resample this sinogram to a parallel ray sinogram.

In this parallel ray sinogram, it is only necesary to account for the perpendicular component to the pencil beam of the x-y offset. Therefore, for every projection, the x-y offset will be corrected by shifting the sinogram columns by an amount corresponding to the perpendicular x-y offset in that projection. This column shift will involve interpolations with respect to the fluence between neighboring leaves. Different interpolations have been tested including, linear, spline and half leaf decision. A more effective approach to perform the interpolation is in Fourier space as proposed by Fitchard[5] using the shift theorem. This proves that when one function is the translation of another, their Fourier transforms differ only by a phase factor,

$$F(f(x-\alpha, y-\beta)) = F(u,v)e^{-i2\pi(u\alpha+v\beta)} \quad (1)$$

where F denotes the Fourier transform, $\alpha$ and $\beta$ are the translation parameters, $u$ and $v$ are the Fourier conjugated variables and $f$ is the function considered.

The pitch and yaw offsets can be accounted by modifying the sinograms in x and y with the corresponding x-y offsets for each of regions in the inferior superior direction.

It should be mentioned that this set of transforms for this method assumes that the patient moves as a rigid body.

Figure 2 presents the planned delivery fluence for a prostate treatment that will be described in the next section and the corresponding delivery modified sinogram that accounts for an offset of 1 cm in the x-direction.

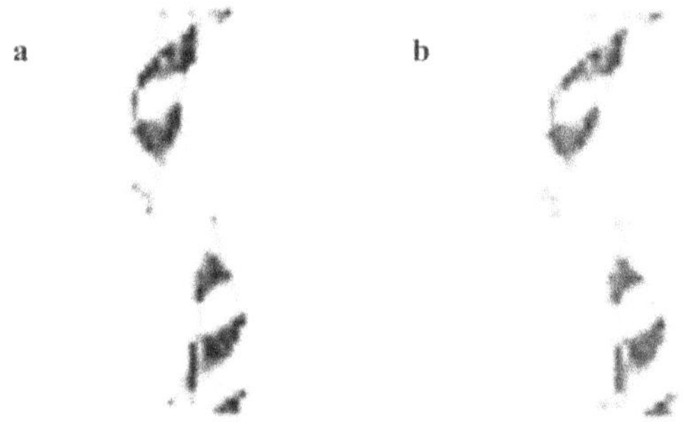


**Figure 2: a )**Planned energy fluence sinogram for a prostate treatment; **b)** delivery modified energy fluence sinogram for a prostate tretament accounting for an offset of 1 cm in the x-direction.

## Results and discussion

Results will be presented for a conformal and a conformal avoidance case. The optimization was performed using the tomotherapy optimization technique described elsewhere[1, 6]. The delivery in both cases was axial, optimized for 51 projections and with 64 leaves of size 0.625 x 1 $cm^2$ at 93 cm isocenter. The beam was 4 MV and the dose was computed using the convolution-superposition method, therefore, including inhomogeneity corrections.

The conformal case is a prostate treatment. The cumulative DVH is presented in figure 3.

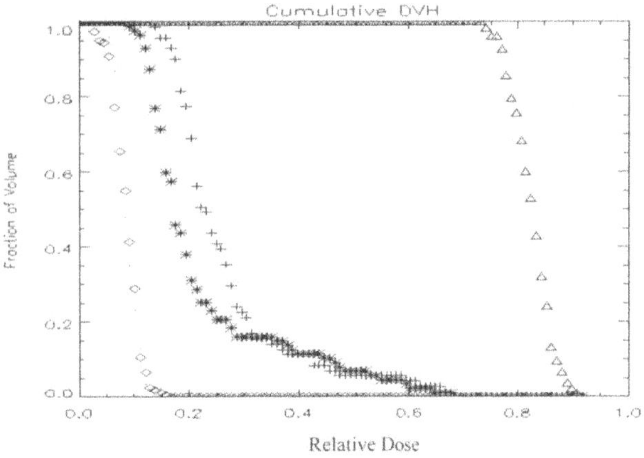


**Figure 3:** Cumulative DVH histogram for the prostate treatment: triangle, prostate; cross, bladder; asterisk, rectum; dot, right femur; diamond, left femur.

The prescription was for a relative dose of 0.75 to the prostate and that no more than 20 % of the rectum and bladder receive no more than 0.3 relative dose.

Figure 4 a and b are the isodose curves for the optimized plan plot over the CT and the Regions of Interest (ROI). As can be observed a good conformity is achieved and even when 51 projections where used during the optimization, and all of them contribute, the radiation is largely incident from four angular sectors that resemble a four field oblique standard treatment. The figures show that there are overlap between tumor and bladder and rectum. Therefore, high gradient regions are present at the intersection between structures.

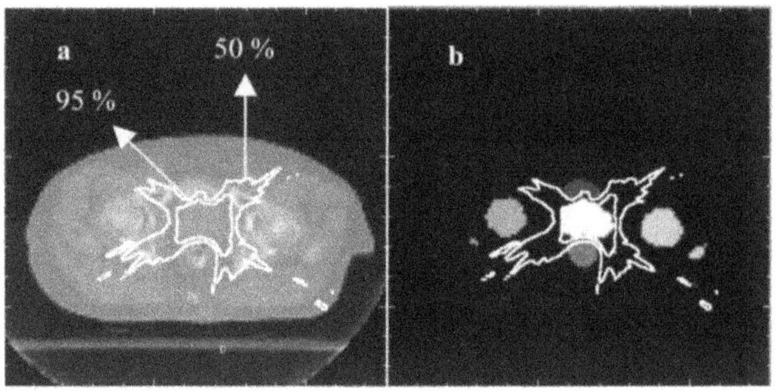


**Figure 4: a)** and **b)** Isodoses for the optimized prostate treatment plan ovelap with the CT and the ROI's respectively: 50 % isodose line, and 95 % isodose lines.

Figure 5 a and b show the dose distribution obtained by a delivery modification of the planned energy fluence sinogram accounting for a 1 cm offset in the x direction. As can be observed, the conformity of the dose distribution around the tumor is very good, however can be seen that the lower isodose line is more spread in the delivery modified case. However, the avoidance of the structures is still good. This behavior is in part due to the finite size of the MLC leaves and the number of projections used in the optimization.

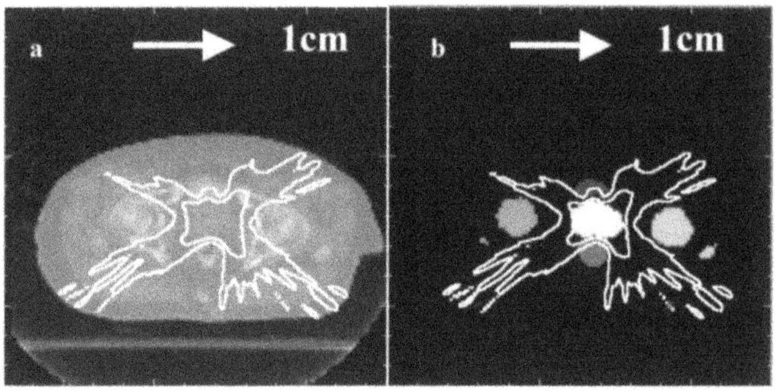


**Figure 5: a)** and **b)** Isodoses for the delivery modified prostate treatment plan ovelap with the CT and the ROI's respectively: 50 % isodose line, and 95 % isodose lines (captions as in figure 4).

The method has been tested for several offsets and it was found that the technique is independent of the magnitude and direction of the applied offset. Figure 6 presents results for the same treatment as figure 4 but in this case for an offset in the x and y direction of 1 cm each respectively. The isodoses present the same behavior as in the previous case, both in the tumor and regions at risk respectively.

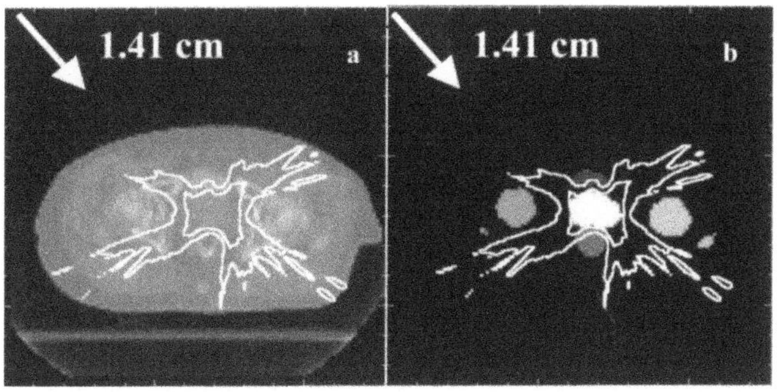


**Figure 6: a)** and **b)** Isodoses for the delivery modified prostate treatment plan ovelap with the CT and the ROI's respectively: 50 % isodose line, and 95 % isodose lines (captions as in figure 4).

Finally, a conformal avoidance nasopharingeal treatment is also presented. The goal in this case was to spare the parotid glands while providing enough uniformity and dose coverage in the nodal region. This case is in some ways more difficult due to the big extent of the tumor. Figure 7 shows the optimized and delivery modified isodose curves. The sparing of the sensitive structure is very good and the dose in the tumor even though not identical, can be considered as acceptable except for a few voxels on the upper right corner of the 80 % delivery modified isodose line.

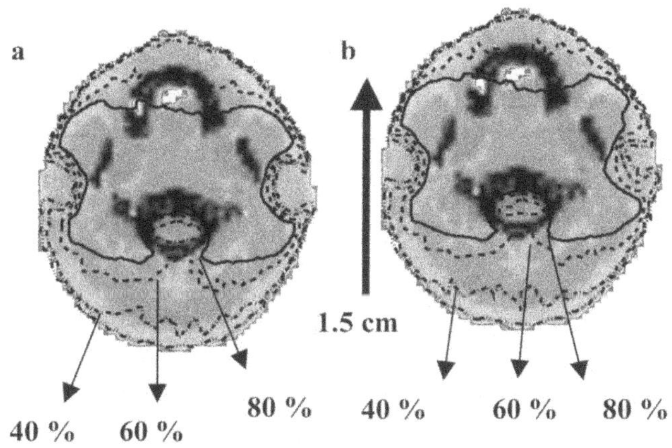


**Figure 7: a)** Isodoses for the optimized prostate treatment plan ovelap with the CT, **b)** Isodoses for the delivery modified prostate treatment plan ovelap wit the CT accountion for an offset of 1.5 cm.

This technique as described still needs some development in order to be used clinically. When this technique becomes operational, however, new perspectives will become visible. Up until now, we are able to account for rigid body movement only but uniform scaling can also be included relatively simply. Delivery modification can be performed very quickly, and tomotherapy also has a fast technique to know patient's offsets with very limited information[3]. Therefore, for those movements that can be considered or approximated as rigid body movements the delivery can be modified on-the-fly during treatment. Therefore, DM will enable an adaptive radiotherapy within the same fraction. Moreover, this technique may also serve as a basis for more elaborated methods of accounting for patient movement during delivery. Another possible application is to create templates of first-guess planned energy fluence sinograms that can be shifted and scaled for each particular case to speed up treatment planning optimization.

## Conclusion

A delivery modification technique was presented. Results were shown in a conformal and conformal avoidance treatment. The technique has the capability to modify the treatment in few seconds without need for re-optimizing the treatment. This technique assumes that the patient is offset as a rigid body. The big advantage is that the patient does not need to be re-positioned for every fraction if there is has an offset relative to the reference position. This, in principle will increase the patient throughput. The technique needs some improvements before being applied clinically, but will open new opportunities that may even include, for some treatments, a method for adaptive radiotherapy during each fraction.

## References


[1] Olivera, G.H., D.M. Shepard, K. Ruchala, J.S. Aldridge, J.M. Kapatoes, E.E. Fitchard, P.J. Reckwerdt, G. Fang, J. Balog, J. Zachman and T.R. Mackie, *Tomotherapy*, in *Modern Technology of Radiation Oncology*, J. Van Dyk, Editor. 1999, Medical Physics Publishing: Madison. p. 521-587.

[2] Ruchala, K.J., G.H. Olivera, E.A. Schloesser and T.R. Mackie, *Megavoltage CT on a tomotherapy system.* Phys. In Med. and Biol., 1999. **44**: p. 2597-2621.

[3] Lu, W., E.E. Fitchard, G.H. Olivera, J.S. Aldridge, J. You, K. Ruchala, J.S. Aldridge and T.R. Mackie, *Image/patient registration from (partial) projection data by fourier phase matching method.* Phys. in Med. and Biol., 1999. **44**: p. 2029--2048.

[4] Fitchard, E.E., J.S. Aldridge, K. Ruchala, G. Fang, J.P. Balog, D.W. Pearson, G.H. Olivera, E.A. Schloesser, D. Wenman, P.J. Reckwerdt and T.R. Mackie, *Registration using tomographic projection files.* Phys. Med. Biol., 1999. **44**: p. 495-507.

[5] Fitchard, E.E., *Personal comunication.* 1998.

[6] Shepard, D.M., G.H. Olivera, P. Reckwerdt and T.R. Mackie, *Iterative approaches to dose optimization in tomotherapy.* Phys. Med. Biol., 2000. **45**: p. 69-90.

# Optimized Decomposition of Virtual Micro Intensity Maps

**R. Alfredo C. Siochi**

Siemens Medical Systems, Apex, North Carolina 27502, USA

## Introduction

Virtual Micro-Intensity Modulated Radiation Therapy (VMIMRT) is a technique that uses a 10 mm leaf width multi-leaf collimator (MLC) to deliver treatments with 5 mm x 5 mm beamlets. The virtual micro intensity map (VMIM), *I(i,j)*, has to be decomposed into two orthogonal intensity maps. The map with the zero offset in collimator angle, *Z(i,j)*, has 10 mm x 5 mm beamlets while the one with a ninety degree offset, *N(i,j)*, has 5 mm x 10 mm beamlets. Figure 1 shows an example of the decomposition for a single 10 mm x 10 mm macrobeam (a group of four 5 mm x 5 mm beamlets that can be covered by a leaf pair in either collimator angle). In this example, there is only one way to perform the decomposition. However, in addition to a local gradient, *G(i,j)*, there can be a nonzero component, *U(i,j)*, that is locally uniform over each macrobeam. In such cases, one needs to decide how to apportion the uniform component between *Z(i,j)* and *N(i,j)* for each macrobeam. This becomes an optimization problem with as many parameters as there are macrobeams with nonzero uniform components in *I(i,j)*, since an appropriately chosen set of parameters will minimize the total beam on time to deliver *I(i,j)*.

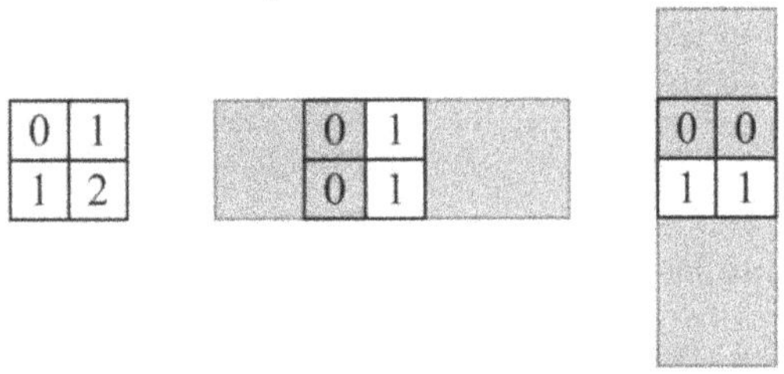


**Figure 1:** Decomposition of *I(i,j)* into *Z(i,j) + N(i,j)*

## Material and methods

The VMIM, *I(i,j)*, is a specific type of matrix for which $I(i,j) - I(i,j+1) = I(i+1,j) - I(i+1,j+1)$ and $I(i,j) - I(i+1,j) = I(i,j+1) - I(i+1,j+1)$ for all macrobeams in the matrix, and all elements are integers. It can be represented with the following equations:

$$I(i,j) = Z(i,j) + N(i,j) \quad (1)$$
$$I(i,j) = G(i,j) + U(i,j) \quad (2)$$
$$G(i,j) = G_z(i,j) + G_n(i,j) \quad (3)$$
$$U(i,j) = U_z(i,j) + U_n(i,j) \quad (4)$$
$$Z(i,j) = U_z(i,j) + G_z(i,j) \quad (5)$$
$$N(i,j) = U_n(i,j) + G_n(i,j) \quad (6)$$

Here, *U(i,j)* is the locally uniform component determined by the following equation:

$$U(i,j) = Min(I(i,j), I(i+1,j), I(i,j+1), I(i+1,j+1)),$$
$$U(i+1,j) = U(i,j+1) = U(i+1,j+1) = U(i,j),$$
$$i, j = 0, 2, 4, \ldots\ldots \quad (7)$$

The function *Min* takes the minimum of its arguments, and all the matrices are positioned such that the gridlines above the even numbered rows coincide with the zero offset MLC leaf edges (parallel to the leaf motion direction) and the gridlines to the left of the even numbered columns coincide with the ninety degree rotated MLC leaf edges.

After obtaining *U*, we can determine *G* with equation 2. Using this value of *G*, we can solve for $G_z$ and $G_n$ from the following equations:

$$G_z(i,j) = G_z(i+1,j) = Min(G(i,j), G(i+1,j))$$
$$G_z(i,j+1) = G_z(i+1,j+1) = Min(G(i,j+1), G(i+1,j+1))$$
$$G_n(i,j) = G_n(i,j+1) = Min(G(i,j), G(i,j+1))$$
$$G_n(i+1,j) = G_n(i+1,j+1) = Min(G(i+1,j), G(i+1,j+1)) \quad (8)$$

While the determination of $G_z$ and $G_n$ is fixed by equation 8, the determination of $U_z$ and $U_n$ is variable. If we define a parameter matrix *P(k,l)* such that $k = i \ div\ 2$ and $l = j \ div\ 2$ (where *div* returns an integer result), the elements of this matrix can take on the following values:

$$P(k,l) = \{ 0, \ldots, U(i,j) \} \quad (9)$$

Once a parameter matrix is formed by picking one value from the set for each matrix element, then we can determine $U_z$ and $U_n$ from equations 5 and 9 as follows:

$$U_z(i,j) = U_z(i+1,j) = U_z(i,j+1) = U_z(i+1,j+1) = P(k,l)$$
$$U_n(i,j) = U_n(i+1,j) = U_n(i,j+1) = U_n(i+1,j+1) = U(i,j) - P(k,l) \quad (10)$$

Finally, from equations 5, 6, 8, 9, and 10 we can determine *Z(i,j)* and *N(i,j)*. These matrices can then be segmented into MLC shapes. The number of segments produced and the treatment time for step and shoot IMRT will depend on the maximum values and the number of peaks and valleys in these matrices. A good single measure of this complexity for a given intensity map is the maximum sum of the positive gradients along the leaf motion direction. This value will be directly affected by the choice of P(k,l) in equation 9. In order to minimize the treatment time for VMIMRT, the parameter matrix must be varied to minimize the sum of the quantities

$$Max\left\{ i, \sum_j S_z(i,j)\Delta Z(i,j) \right\} \quad (11a)$$

$$Max\left\{ j, \sum_i S_n(i,j)\Delta N(i,j) \right\} \quad (11b)$$

where the function *Max* takes the maximum value among the values generated by evaluating the second argument for all possible values of the first argument and the functions $\Delta Z$, $\Delta N$, $S_z$, and $S_n$, are defined as follows:

$$\Delta Z(i,j)=\begin{cases} Z(i,j)-Z(i,j-1), & j>0 \\ Z(i,j), & j=0 \end{cases} \quad (12a)$$

$$\Delta N(i,j)=\begin{cases} N(i,j)-N(i-1,j) & i>0 \\ N(i,j) & i=0 \end{cases} \quad (12b)$$

$$S_z(i,j)=\begin{cases} 1, & \Delta Z(i,j)>0 \\ 0, & \Delta Z(i,j)\le 0 \end{cases} \quad (13a)$$

$$S_n(i,j)=\begin{cases} 1, & \Delta N(i,j)>0 \\ 0, & \Delta N(i,j)\le 0 \end{cases} \quad (13b)$$

Since the gradients within each macrobeam can not be changed by varying P, the only gradients that will change in equations 12a and b are those gradients for which *i* and *j* are even numbers. Also, varying $P(k,l)$ changes the gradients $\Delta Z(i,j)$, $\Delta Z(i, j+2)$, $\Delta N(i,j)$ and $\Delta N(i+2,j)$. (Since rows *i* and *i+1* are identical in Z, and columns *j* and *j+1* are identical in *N*, we only need to analyze the even numbered rows in *Z* and the even numbered columns in *N*. We will omit the odd numbered index expressions henceforth.) Consequently, minimizing the sum of 11a and 11b involves minimizing the expressions

$$|\Delta Z_P(i,j)| \quad (14a)$$
$$|\Delta N_p(i,j)| \quad (14b)$$

where

$$\Delta Z_P(i,j) = \Delta Z(i,j) - \Delta Z(i, j+2) \quad (15a)$$
$$\Delta N_p(i,j) = \Delta N(i,j) - \Delta N(i+2, j). \quad (15b)$$

we use the following procedure:

*Loop until the limit of non-improving configuratons is reached*

1. *Look for the row or column corresponding to the maximum between 11a and b.*
2. *Look for the maximum of expressions 14a (if in a row) or b (if in a column) only among indices for which P(k,l) has not been changed in this round*
3. *Change P(k,l) by a fourth of 15a (row) or 15b (column) in order to reduce 14a (row) or 14b (column). Limit P(k,l) to the allowed values in equation 9.*
4. *Evaluate 11a + 11b.*
5. *If this is less than the current best value, record the set of parameters and reset the number of non-improving configurations to zero; otherwise increase the number of non-improving configurations.*
6. *Increment the round when all P(k,l) have been changed exactly once.*

As with all optimization routines, the final result could be affected by the initial set of parameters. Three different initial sets were used. In one set, AllZ, $P(k,l) = U(i,j)$. In a second set, AllN, $P(k,l) = 0$. In the final set, Shared, $P(k,l) = Ceil(U(i,j)/2)$ where *Ceil* rounds its argument upwards.

Two test intensity maps were studied. Case I is shown in figure 2 while Case II is shown in figure 3. Four decomposition methods were studied, three of them were the initial configurations previously described, while the other one was the optimization routine using the Shared initial configuration. For each of these methods, the resulting orthogonal intensity maps *Z* and *N* were segmented using the sweeping window method [1] and the IMFAST algorithm [2] for three different MLC constraints: interdigitating, non-interdigitating (collision), tongue and groove elimination (tongue and groove). A comparison of the number of segments was done to determine the effectiveness of the optimization routine.

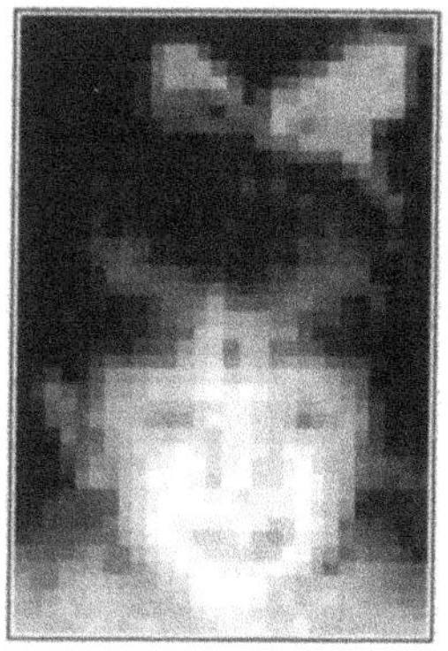

**Figure 2** The virtual micro intensity map of case I. It consists of 42 rows by 28 columns, and it has a maximum of 16 levels.

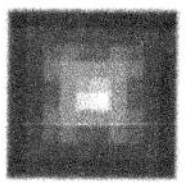

**Figure 3** The virtual micro intensity map of case II. It consists of 10 rows by 10 columns, and it has a maximum of 9 levels.

## Results and discussion

Figure 4 shows the convergence of the optimization routine for three different initial configurations for Case I. Regardless of the initial configuration, very similar final values for the merit function were obtained. The shared configuration converged to a slightly lower value than the others, reaching the same final value at a much earlier point. This suggests that the optimization routine found a near-global minimum, since the initial configurations represent extreme sets of parameters

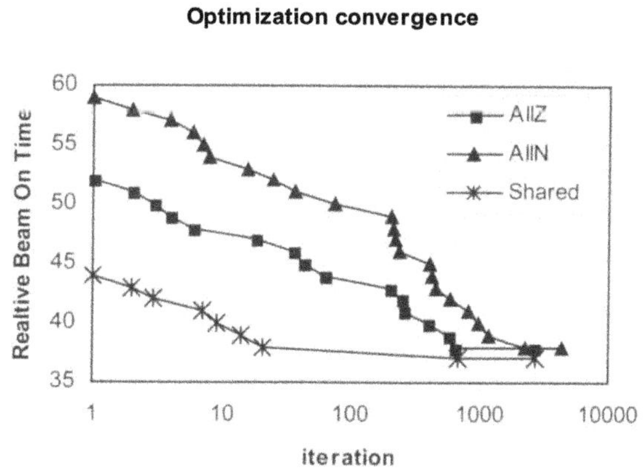


**Figure 4** Convergence of the decomposition optimization process. The merit function is graphed against the iteration at which the value was achieved.

| Decomposition | | Interdigitating | | Collision | | Tongue and Groove | | |
|---|---|---|---|---|---|---|---|---|
| Initial | Optimized | IMFAST | Sweep | IMFAST | Sweep | IMFAST | Sweep | Average |
| Shared | Yes | 35 | 37 | 43 | 45 | 54 | 54 | 44.67 |
| Shared | No | 37 | 43 | 44 | 47 | 58 | 58 | 47.83 |
| AllZ | No | 38 | 50 | 63 | 72 | 71 | 75 | 61.50 |
| AllN | No | 42 | 58 | 65 | 79 | 77 | 83 | 67.33 |

**Table I**. The number of segments produced by various segmentation algorithms under diferent constraints. The results are for Case I.

| Decomposition | | Interdigitating | | Collision | | Tongue and Groove | | |
|---|---|---|---|---|---|---|---|---|
| Initial | Optimized | IMFAST | Sweep | IMFAST | Sweep | IMFAST | Sweep | Average |
| Shared | Yes | 8 | 9 | 8 | 9 | 8 | 9 | 8.50 |
| Shared | No | 9 | 10 | 9 | 10 | 10 | 10 | 9.67 |
| AllZ | No | 12 | 13 | 13 | 13 | 13 | 13 | 12.83 |
| AllN | No | 12 | 14 | 13 | 14 | 13 | 14 | 13.33 |

**Table II**. The same comparison as in Table I, except that the results are for Case II.

(AllN or AllZ) and a midpoint set of parameters (Shared). The test above was repeated with a slight modification to step 5 of the optimization; the set of parameters were recorded as long as the merit function was less than or equal to the current best value. The final values for the merit function were exactly the same, again indicating that a near global minimum was found.

Since the optimization performed slightly better with the Shared configuration, the comparisons for the segmentation were done using this initial configuration for the optimization. Table I shows the resulting number of segments for the 4 decomposition methods (Shared Optimized, Shared, AllN and AllZ) for Case I, while table II shows the results for Case II. The average column shows that regardless of the constraint or the segmentation algorithm, the Shared Optimized decomposition method produces the least number of segments. A quick look through the individual columns also confirms this to be true. Of particular interest is the number of segments produced by the interdigitating sweep algorithm for the optimized decomposition. Here, each segment received one level, so the beam on time was identical to the number of segments. This value turned out to be the same as the merit function used in the optimization.

The ability of IMFAST to reduce the number of segments as compared to the sweep method increases with increasing complexity in the intensity map [2]. This is consistent with the results in the table, showing the most reduction in the number of segments coming from the AllN method. This is because for case 1, this put almost all the levels into the $N$ matrix, and that required the leaves to travel over longer distances with many peaks and valleys. In the Shared method, the number of levels in each map was split into about half that of the original map, making each piece less complex, so there were not too many segments to be reduced by using IMFAST. In the Shared Optimized method, the least gains are realized by using IMFAST, indicating that the goal of minimizing the number and magnitude of the peaks and valleys was realized. This is because step 3 of the procedure tends to flatten out the peaks and fill in the valleys. Figure 5 shows the resulting orthogonal maps for the VMIM of Case I, using the Shared Optimized method.

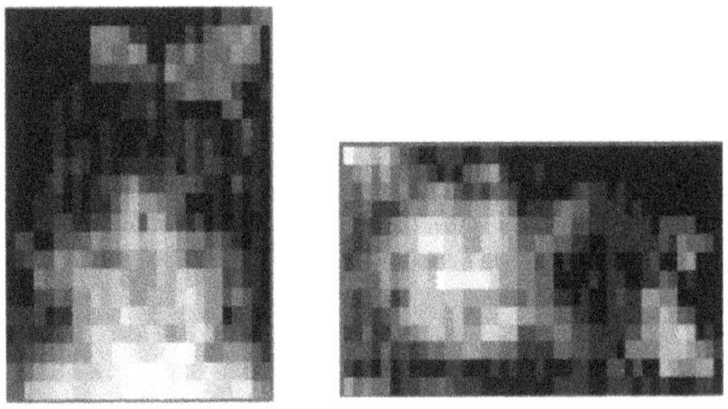

**Figure 5** The orthogonal maps for the VMIM of Case I. The images are oriented with the MLC leaves moving from left to right. $Z$ is on the left, $N$ is on the right. $N$ is delivered at a 90 degree collimator offset relative to $Z$.

## Conclusion

The Optimizaton method developed here is important to use when decomposing a VMIM into its orthogonal field components. It reduces the number of segments regardless of MLC constraint and segmentation algorithm; hence it reduces the total treatment time. For step and shoot IMRT, this is significant. This allows users with 1 cm leaf width MLCs to treat with a resolution of 5 mm x 5 mm in the least amount of time.

## References

[1] Bortfeld T, Kahler DL, Waldron TJ, et al. X-ray Field compensation with multileaf collimators. Int J Radiat Oncol Biol Phys; 28:723-730, 1994.

[2] Siochi R A C. Minimizing static intensity modulation delivery time using an intensity solid paradigm. Int J Radiat Oncol Biol Phys; 43:671-680, 1999.

# Fluence segmentation for micro intensity modulated radiotherapy with a miniature multileaf collimator

**Martin Bues[1], Hanne M. Kooy[1] and Peter Hoban[2]**

[1] Massachusetts General Hospital, Department of Radiation Oncology, Harvard Medical School, Boston, MA USA, and [2] Radiation Oncology Department, Prince of Wales Hospital, Randwick NSW 2031 Australia

## Introduction

Micro-IMRT has recently been shown to be a highly effective technique for the stereotactic radiotherapy of intracranial tumors [1-2]. Figure 1 shows the eminent advantage of micro-IMRT compared to the other treatment techniques considered. The data is shown in the form of a boxplot comparing the ranges of target volume ratios (TVRs) in an 11 patient study presented at the 1999 ASTRO meeting [2]. TVR, which is defined as the treated volume divided by the planning target volume, serves as a standard indicator of the conformality of a stereotactic radiotherapy plan.

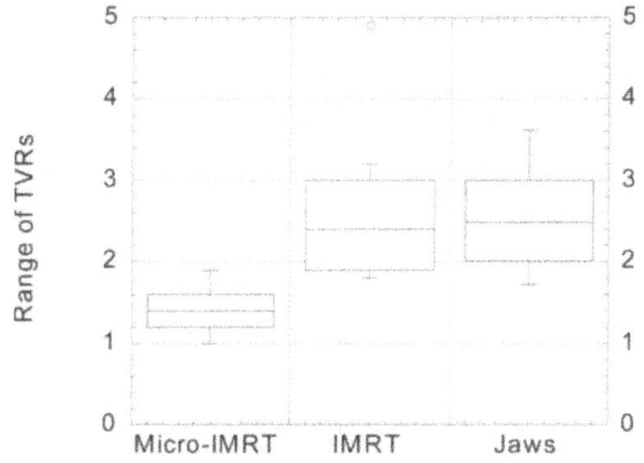


**Figure 1:** Range of TVRs for 11 patients planned with micro-IMRT (4mm bixel size), IMRT (10mm bixel size) and circular collimated arcs with additional jaw collimation.

A central problem in the delivery of micro intensity modulated radiotherapy is, given an opening density and a segmentation, to accurately predict the corresponding photon fluence in air in the isocenter plane. Measurements taken using the Radionics miniature multileaf collimator suggest that the conventional approach of obtaining fluences from opening densities by convolving with a kernel breaks down if the fluence pattern is composed of bixels four millimeters in size. This is because a linear convolution map can no longer describe the map from the space of opening densities to the space of fluences. Rather the map crucially depends on the segmentation chosen to prepare the opening density. It therefor becomes necessary to consider the physics of the delivery device at each segmentation step.

## Material and methods

We present an explicit two-dimensional map from the space of segmented opening densities to the space of fluences, which accurately accounts for the non-linear physics of the delivery device. This map models the finite size of the radiation source, collimator scatter, penumbra of the MMLC leaves both parallel and perpendicular to the direction of leaf motion and finite transmission through the MMLC leaves. The parameters characterizing the map are easily extracted from basic measurements. We have implemented a segmentation algorithm first proposed by Xia and Verhey [3] and a discretized version of the sliding window technique [4-6] suitable for the step and shoot approach to intensity modulated radiotherapy. Utilizing the map described above we compute the delivered fluence at each step of the segmentation process and iteratively adjust the segmented opening densities in order to closely approximate the desired fluence computed by an inverse planning system. Figure 2 shows the comparison of predicted and planned fluence at an intermediate iteration step. The implementation of two segmentation strategies allows for a realistic comparison of the advantages and disadvantages of the two segmentation strategies for micro-IMRT under realistic circumstance.

## Results and discussion

We find a discrepancy of up to 20% between fluence maps calculated using the linear convolution map and our map on the space of segmented opening densities. Film measurements show that given a segmented opening density we are able to compute the delivered fluence within an accuracy greater than 3%.

While the segmentation algorithm of Xia and Verhey performs superiorly under the simplified assumptions of a linear relation between opening density and fluence, i.e. under the assumption that it is sufficient to segment the opening densities, this advantage vanishes when iterative corrections are applied to faithfully reproduce a desired fluence.

## Conclusion

We successfully address a key problem in the implementation of micro-IMRT using a miniature multileaf collimator with a projected leaf width smaller than four millimeters in the isocenter plane. This allows us to implement segmentation algorithms, which faithfully prepare any desired fluence. These implementations allow for a comparison of the algorithms under conditions relevant for the clinical implementation of micro-IMRT

## References


[1] Bues M, Kooy HM, Hacker FL, Tarbell NJ, Chapman P, Loeffler JS. Micro intensity-modulated radiotherapy - a case study. Radiosurgery 1999; 3:(to appear).

[2] Bues M, Kooy HM, Hacker FL, Tarbell NJ, Chapman P, Loeffler JS. Micro-IMRT for stereotactic radiotherapy of intracranial tumors, American Society for therapeutic radiology and oncology 41st annual meeting, San Antonio Texas, 1999. Elsevier Science Inc.

[3] Xia P, Verhey LJ. Multileaf collimator leaf sequencing algorithm for intensity modulated beams with multiple static segments. Medical Physics 1998; 25:1424-34.

[4] Spirou SV, Chui CS. Generation of arbitrary intensity profiles by dynamic jaws or multileaf collimators. Medical Physics 1994; 21:1031-41.

[5] Stein J, Bortfeld T, Dorschel B, Schlegel W. Dynamic X-ray compensation for conformal radiotherapy by means of multi-leaf collimation. Radiotherapy & Oncology 1994; 32:163-73.

[6] Svensson R, Kallman P, Brahme A. An analytical solution for the dynamic control of multileaf collimators. Physics in Medicine & Biology 1994; 39:37-61.


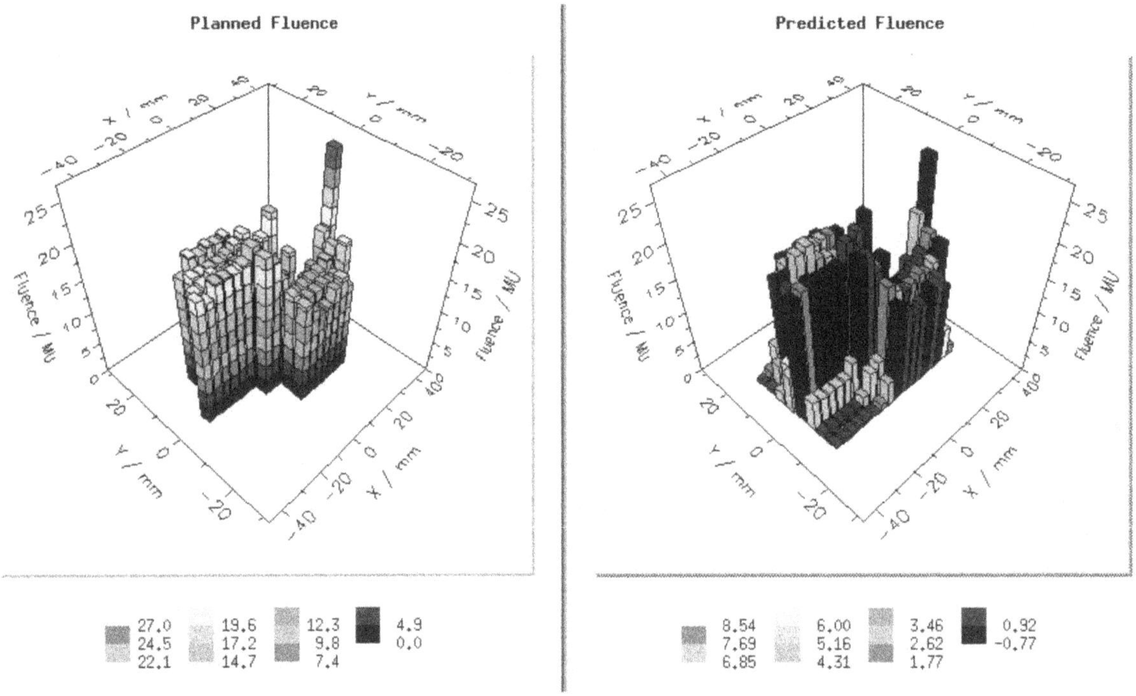


**Figure 2:** Comparison of predicted to planned flunece. Colors in the planned fluence pannel correspond to absolute monitor unit values. Colors in the predicted fluence pannel correspond to the difference between planned and predicted fluence.

# The effects of beamlet size on IMRT optimization

**B. Yi[2], Y. Chen[1], A. Boyer[1]**

[1]Radiation Oncology Department, Stanford University School of Medicine, Stanford, CA 94305, USA, and [2]Asan Medical Center, University of Ulsan, College of Medicine, Seoul, 138-736,Korea

## Introduction

Intensity modulated radiation therapy (IMRT) has been implemented using multileaf collimators (MLCs) whose leaves project to a 1-cm width at isocenter using a 1-cm step size for a "step-and-shoot" leaf sequences [1]. It is well known that the smaller leaf width generates better shielding effects for the unmodulated beam. Althouh intuitive notion, that smaller beamlet size generates better intensity modulation effects, seems to be valid, we can hardly find the report which supports that this is the fact.
This study explored the clinical usefulness of smaller beamlet sizes for IMRT produced by smaller step sizes and thinner leaf widths.

## Material and methods

The Corvus (NOMOS Inc. Sewickley, Pennsylvania) planning system was used to compute inverse plans using beamlet sizes for 10x10($mm^2$), 5x10($mm^2$), 5x5($mm^2$). The beamlet size 5x10 means that 5mm-step MLC movement with 10mm-thickness of MLC leaf. The beamlet sizes for 2x10($mm^2$) and 2x5($mm^2$) are used as well.

### 1. Case selection

Three cases were selected for this study. The first case was the brain tumor which is in cranium close to the orbits, the optic nerves, the optic chiasm, and the brain stem. A prostate cancer site was chosen for the second case, for which bladder, rectum and the small intestine were regarded as the critical organs. A lymphoma was chosen for the last case, for which the lungs, the spinal cord were considered as the organs to be preserved.

| | Limiting Dose(%) | Volume above LD(%) | Maximum Dose(%) |
|---|---|---|---|
| Optic Nerve* | 50 | 7 | 53 |
| Eye* | 44 | 10 | 69 |
| Optic Chiasm | 50 | 5 | 61 |
| Brain Stem | 56 | 5 | 67 |

* ipsilateral site

**Table 1:** The prescription dose (limiting dose) of the plan optimization for brain case.

### 2. Plan comparison

The coplanar nine IMRT fields were spaced at angles from 20° to 340° at 40° intervals. Same optimization procedures are repeated for all of the each beamlet size plans. Table 1 shows that the prescription of the optimization. Three to eleven odd-numbered beam directions were used for these plans as well, in order to investigate the number of beam directions dependency on beamlet sizes. With these results, the effects of step sizes of 10mm and 5mm for a 10-mm wide and for a 5-mm wide MLC leaf were analyzed (10x10, 5x10, and 5x5$mm^2$), while no changes to the input parameters were made. The computation was repeated for 15-MV, 6-MV and 4-MV photon beams in order to investigate energy dependencies. All plans were normalized to the isodose line that covered 95% of target volume. For 10x10 $mm^2$ beamlet size optimizations, the position of the isocenter might influence the optimized result since it is the biggest beamlet size among those beamlets. The isocenter was moved to 5mm (to the direction of up, anterior, and right lateral) and the optimization results are compared to those from the original isocenter.

## Results and discussion

Figure 1 shows the optimized dose distribution from each beamlet sizes. Figure 2 shows that the DVH's of the target and the critical organs. Fig. 2-(a) shows the DVH's of the target volume, Fig. 2-(b) shows those of the ipsilateral eye and the ipsilateral optic nerve. Fig. 2-(c-d) show those of the optic chiasm and the brain stem, respectively. As we can see explicitly, smaller beamlet size generates better results. Smaller beamlet generates better homogenous target dose distribution and less dose to the critical organs. We could always achieve the results close to the prescription with 5x5, but not always with 10x10. Better plan was expected to be obtained by finding the best isocenter position of the plan. But, Fig. 3 shows that smaller beamlet generates superior plan even we could find the best isocenter position. The plan result from 5x5 beamlet is always than better any other plans from 10x10 beamlets with various isocenter positions. Figure 4 shows the volume which receives higher dose than the presription dose shown in Table 1. Figure 4 indicates that the beamlet size is more sensitive factor in an optimization for smaller number of beam directions. The beamlet size dependency tends to be smaller for the larger number of fields. For 10x10 beamlet size optimization, the number of portals is important factor. But, for 5x5 beamlet size optimization we could achieve similar resuts no matter how the number of portals for most of the organs[2]. Figure 5 confirms that the smaller beamlet size generates better results for other sites as well. But, as we can see in Figure 5, the beamlet size dependency for a large field is not as distinct as we can found for brain case of which field size is relatively small. Especially, the DVH's for spinal cord Fig. 5(d) shows that the 5x5-beamlet generates worse result than others.

A MLC generates a scalloped penumbra. It is believed that this effect may lead to a larger dose to critical organs or a smaller dose to a target volume. One would expect better results to be obtained with the smaller leaf width. This investigation showed that a smaller beamlet size produced better target dose homogeneity. And the results for normal structures also were consistent. This tendency is emphasized for the case of the smaller number of fields. This might arise from multiple beam effects that diffuse the scalloped penumbra. The phrase, 'the smaller the better' is not always valid. Table 2 shows that the beamlet size smaller than 5x5 sometimes generates worse results. This might arise from two reasons.

| Beamlet size | Volume above Limiting Dose | | | |
|---|---|---|---|---|
| | Optic nerve* | Eye* | Optic Chiasam | Brain Stem |
| 10×10 | 43.5 | 12.5 | 6.3 | 11.7 |
| 5×10 | 31.4 | 3.4 | 8.8 | 16.4 |
| 5×5 | 13.6 | 0.1 | 2.1 | 7.9 |
| 2×10 | 25.9 | 0.9 | 10.9 | 11.8 |
| 2×5 | 21.7 | 4.7 | 5.0 | 12.2 |

* ipsilateral site

**Table 2.** The critical volume which receive the dose above the limiting dose for nine ports(brain Case)

One is from the optimization procedure and the other is from the photon attenuation through the MLC. If we assume that the beam fluence patterns from the optimization are same no matter which beamlet size we use, then the treatment monitor units should be almost similar to each beamlet size, and the number of the segments of the IMRT fields should be close to proportional to the ratio of the beamlet sizes. Figure 6 shows that we have much more segments than we expect for small beamlet size. Rapid increase of the number of the segments for smaller beamlet size than 5x5. This implies that the optimized beam fluence patterns are completely different between the beamlet size bigger than 5x5 and smaller than 5x5. The beam attenuation through the MLC leaf is about 1.5% for Vaian MLC. For the plans from the beamlet size 10x10 – 5x5, total monitor units are less than 3 times of the non-modulated beam monitor units. This means that additive dose from the MLC attenuation to the critical organs due to larger monitor units is less than 5%. But, we need to irradiate almost 15 times more monitor units for the plan optimized by 2x5 beamlet size. By considering this factor, the critical organs shielded by MLC leaf will be exposed more than 20% of the target dose only from the beam attenuation by the MLC. It will definitely reduce the optimizing power during the optimization procedure. So, the optimization procedure from the beam fluence pattern may not function properly because of high dose given to the critical organs. This implies that there is an optimum beamlet size for the IMRT optimization, which should be bigger than 2mm and probably around 5mm.

In the Corvus system, optimization for smaller beamlet sizes requires longer calculation times. However, as faster computers become available, the significance of longer and more complex computations is lessened relative to gains in improved dose distributions.

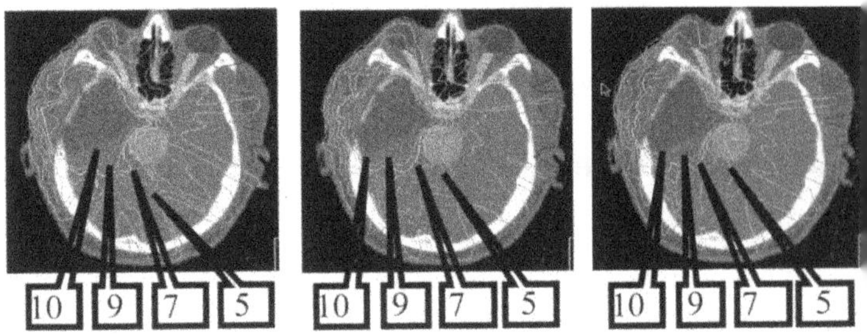


**Figure 1 :** Optimized dose distribution from various beamlet size, (a) 10×10 mm$^2$, (b) 5×10 mm$^2$, (c) 5×10 mm$^2$

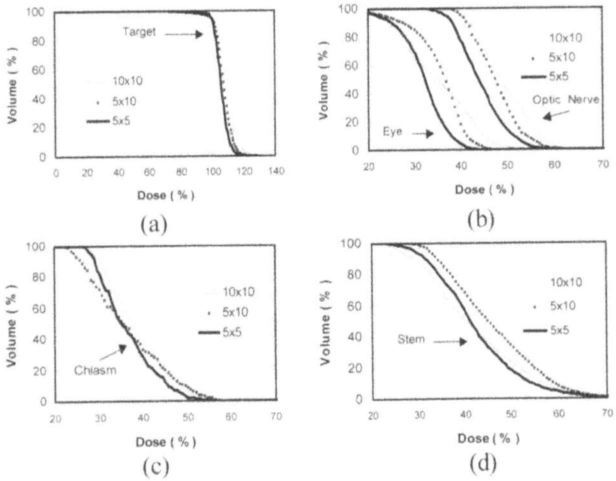


**Figure 2:** DVH's for the target and the critical organs with various beamlet sizes, (a) target, (b) ipsilateral eye and ipsilateral optic nerve, (c) optic chiasm and (d) brain stem.

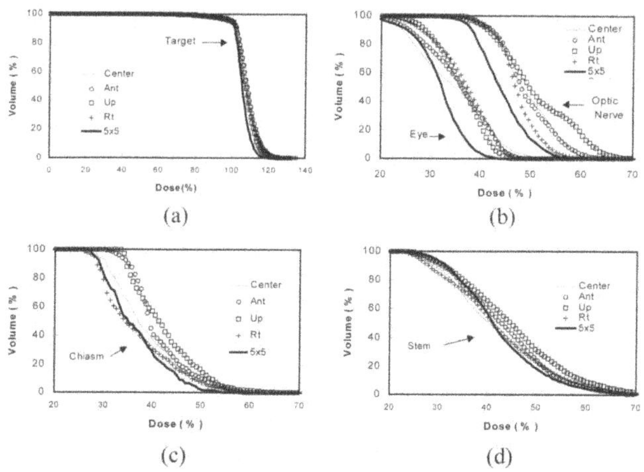


**Figure 3 :** The isocenter position effects on the optimization, (a) target, (b) ipsilateral eye, (c) ipsilateral optic nerve, (d) brain stem. Four plans from various isocenter with 10×10 beamlet soze show different result. But 5×5 generates always the best result

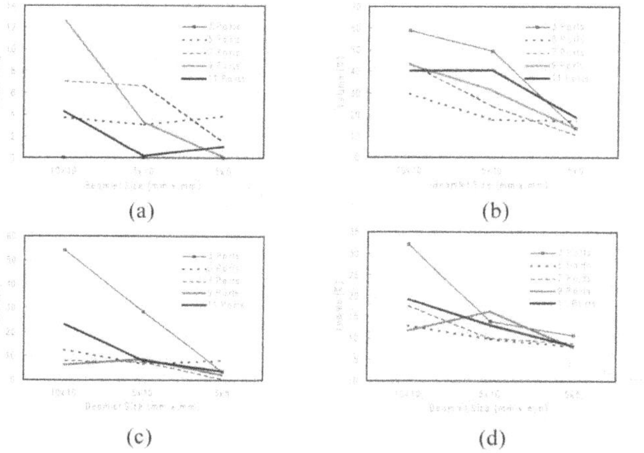


**Figure 4:** The critical organ volume which receive. The dose above the limiting dose brain case, (a) ipsilateral eye, (b) ipsilateral nerve, (c) optic chiasm, (d) brain stem. Stronger beamlet size dependency was found for smaller number of the fields. We could achieve similar results for 5×5 beamlet no matter how many fields.

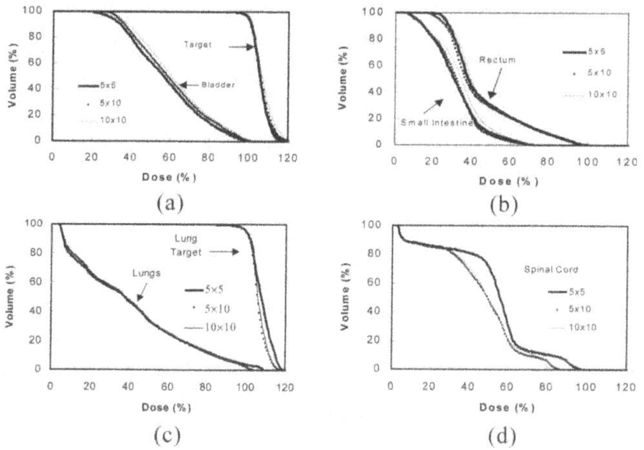


**Figure 5 :** DVH,s for the target and the critical organs with various beamlet size for the lymphoma(a, b) and the prostate(c, d) cases.

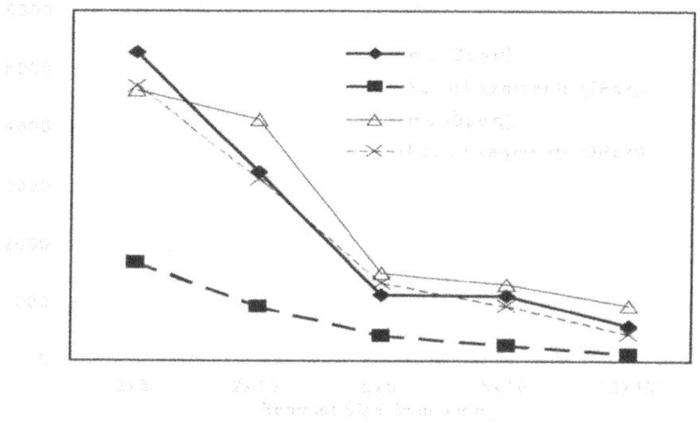

**Figure 6 :** Beamlet size versus monitor units and number of segments

## Conclusion

Smaller beamlet always generated better plan results for all of the cases under testing for the beamlet sizes of 10x10(mm$^2$), 5x10(mm$^2$), and 5x5(mm$^2$). Smaller number of beam directions generated more beamlet size dependencies on the treatment optimization. These results support the intuitive notion that smaller beamlets associated with thinner MLC leaf widths and smaller step sizes will, for the most part, produce superior optimized IMRT treatment planning results for the beamlet size down to 5mm. But, it was hard to find any evidences that the plans from 2x10 or 2x5 generate better results. It showed that it is impractical to use such a small beamlet size for an IMRT optimization. This implies that there might be an optimum beamlet size for the best optimization probably around 5mm. But, the plan results from 2-mm beamlet size showed that it is not always true that the smaller beamlet size the better plan results.

## References

[1] Boyer AL, Yu CX, Intensity–modulated radiation therapy with dynamic multileaf collimators. Seminars in radiation Oncology 1999 : 9(1). 48-59

[2] Lasasso T., Chui cs., Kutcher GJ., Leibel SA., Fuks Z. and Ling CC. The use of a multi-leaf collimator for conformal radiotherapy of carcinomas of the prostate and nasopharynx. Int. J. Radiation Oncology Biol. Phys. 1993 : 25. 161-170

# Reduction of Treatment Time in IMRT Step and Shoot Irradiations by Means of a Changed Fractionation Scheme

**Karl-Heinz Grosser**

German Cancer Research Center (DKFZ), Department of Medical Physics,Im Neuenheimer Feld 280, D-69120 Heidelberg

## Introduction

In the summer 1998 we started IMRT treatments with the step and shoot approach, using KONRAD inverse treatment planning system and a sequencer tool that has been developed at DKFZ [1]. Compared to conventional multiple field irradiation techniques the treatment time is longer in IMRT step and shoot treatments. Using a SIEMENS accelerator and a SIEMENS MLC the treatment time is in complex cases up to 50 minutes. Therefore the number of patients per day who can be treated is restricted to a small number.

In addition a long treatment time must tolerated by the patients. The treatment time is determined by the number of field components of a given beam arrangement. Several approches have been published to find solutions with a lower number of field components [2,3,4,5]. It is possible to reduce the number of field components to a certain extend using intelligent sequencer solutions [2,3,4,5]. Beyond this lower limit there is no further reduction possible with conventional methods. Therefore a method is proposed to reduce treatment time performing a new fractionation scheme.

## Material and methods

In conventional IMRT the same absolute dose will be given every treatment day and identical relative dose distribution will be generated.

To reduce the treatment time by reducing the number of field components, the fractionation scheme will be changed in the following way:

- The relative dose distributions and the absolute dose distributions of the original and the changed scheme are equal.
- The sum of the relative dose distribution and the absolute dose values of two succsessive fractions of the changed scheme is equal to the sum of two fractions of the original scheme.
- To deliver an odd total number of fractions, one must divide the total number of fractions into an even number of fractions, delivered according to the changed fractionating scheme, and one remaining conventional fraction

| Mo | Tu | We | Thu | Fr | Sa | So | Mo | Tu | We | Thu | Fr | Sa | ••• |
|---|---|---|---|---|---|---|---|---|---|---|---|---|---|

Original fractionation scheme

| Mo | Tu | We | Thu | Fr | Sa | So | Mo | Tu | We | Thu | Fr | Sa | ••• |
|---|---|---|---|---|---|---|---|---|---|---|---|---|---|

Changed fractionation scheme

- In order to reduce the number of field components per fraction each intensity map gets double dose and is divided into two parts.

This procedure is illustrated in the following sketch. A certain intensity map $I_n$ is cutted into layers. Then all slices with an even number will build a new intensity map called '$e_n$' (even), and all slices with an odd number will also composed as a new intensity map called '$o_n$' (odd).

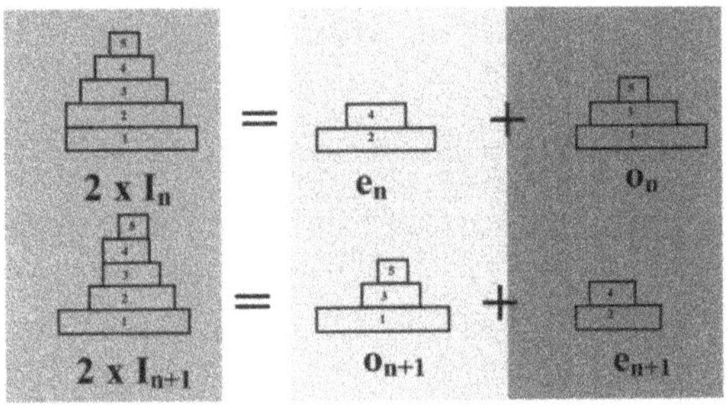


The next intensity map $I_{n+1}$ that belongs to the same beam arrangement will also divided into two parts, but now the 'even' part and the 'odd' part are exchanged. The reason for that procedure is to generate dose distributions that are only slightly different from the original dose distribution. All intensity maps will be divided in this way. As a result of this procedure one get two new beam arrangements. In the following the first arrangement is called 'even' and the second is called 'odd'.

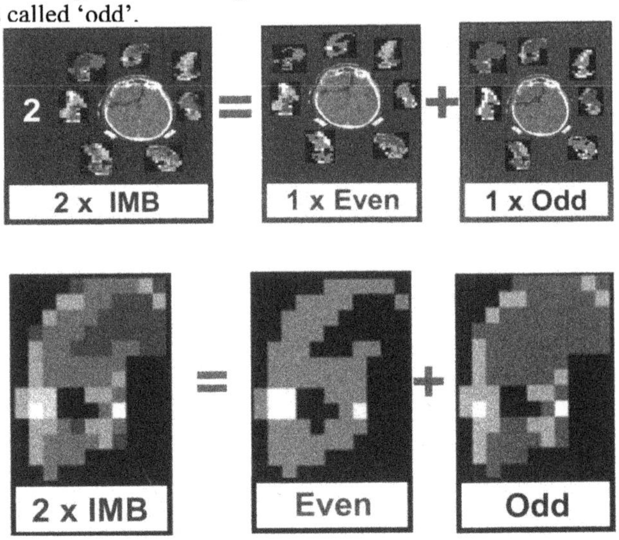


**Figure 1:** Illustration of the procedure to change the fractionation scheme.

Even and odd will then be decomposed. This method reduces the number of field components per fraction by about 50%.Figure 1 shows an example of a beam arrangement with seven intensity modulated beams. The intensity maps have five discrete intensity levels. As a result of the proposed procedure we get two new beam arrangements shown in the picture.

## Results and discussion

**Case studies:**
Inverse treatment planning was performed with KONRAD program, which was developed at DKFZ. A sequencer tool has been developed, which seeks specifically to minimize matchline artifacts and is linked to the KONRAD programe. This sequencer has been modified in order to perform the changed decomposition procedure. Then we applied the proposed method to IMRT patient cases.

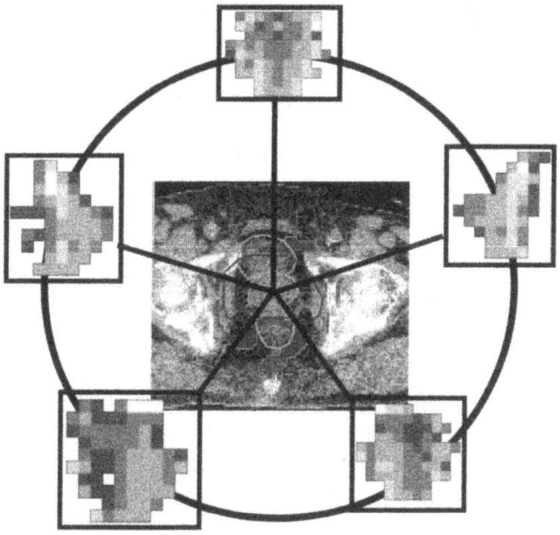

**Figure 2:** Beam arrangement of a prostate case used to test the 'odd-even' procedure. Five intensity levels have been chosen. The target volume, the rectum and the bladder is drawn in.

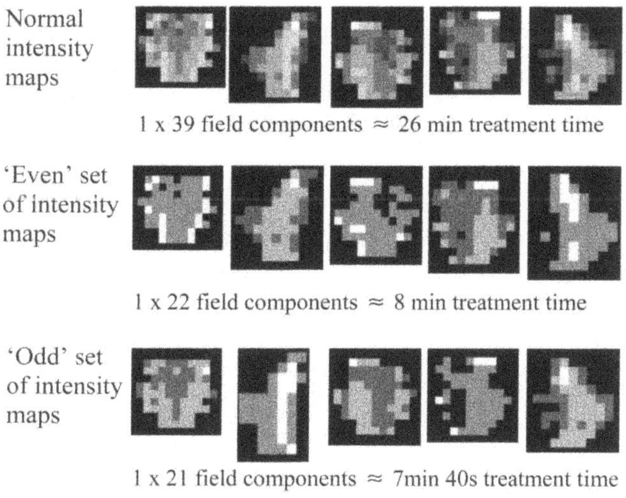


**Figure 3:** The three sets of intensity maps. The row on top represents the original intensity maps, the lower two rows show the 'even' and 'odd' distribution as a result of the proposed method.

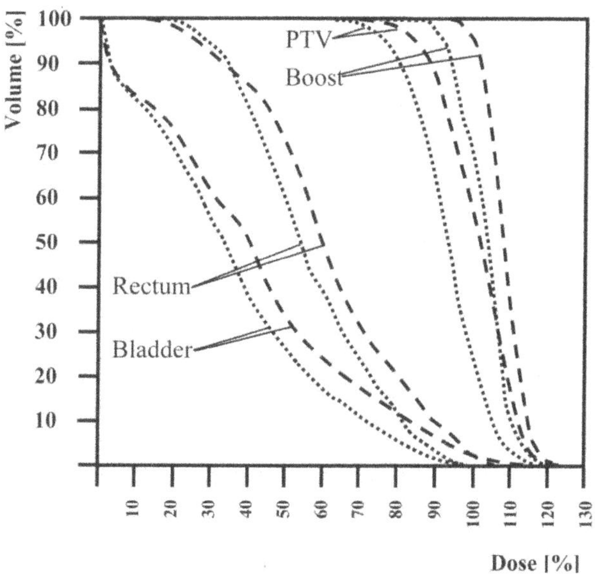


**Figure 4:** DVH of the two resulting dose distributions 'odd' – – and 'even' ······· . Considered are the blader, the rectum, PTV and a boost volume. The DVHs are normalized to the median dose in PTV of the original unchanged dose distribution.

| | Norm | Even | Odd |
|---|---|---|---|
| **Max. dose PTV** | 2.11 | 2.17 | 2.26 |
| **Min. dose PTV** | 1.19 | **0.96** | 1.05 |
| **Mean dose PTV** | 1.80 | 1.69 | 1.91 |
| **Max. dose boost** | 2.11 | 2.17 | 2.26 |
| **Min. dose boost** | 1.72 | 1.55 | 1.66 |
| **Mean dose boost** | 1.96 | 1.86 | 2.06 |
| **Max. dose rectum** | 1.98 | 1.88 | 2.16 |
| **Min. dose rectum** | 0.25 | **0.20** | 0.23 |
| **Mean dose rectum** | 1.10 | 1.02 | 1.18 |
| **Max. dose bladder** | 1.98 | 1.86 | 2.11 |
| **Min. dose bladder** | 0.02 | 0.02 | 0.02 |
| **Mean dose bladder** | 0.73 | **0.65** | 0.81 |

**Table 1:** The table shows maximum, minimum and mean dose values of the normal dose distribution, the even and the odd dose distributions. Dose values of 'even' and 'odd' that differ by more than 10% of the dose values of the normal plan are highlighted.

Figure 2 shows a typical beam confirugation of a prostate cancer case with the original intensity maps drawn in. Figure 3 shows the result of the splitted intensity maps 'even' and 'odd'. Based on these intensity maps, we calculated the new dose distributions. Figure 4 shows the DVHs of the two plans 'even' and 'odd' and table 1 gives characteristic dose values belonging to the dose dostributions. With the changed fractionation schedule the daily treatment time is reduced by about five minutes.

As another class of examples we calculated dose distributions of meningioma cases. As a standard beam arrangement we take seven equally spaced beams and five intensity levels.

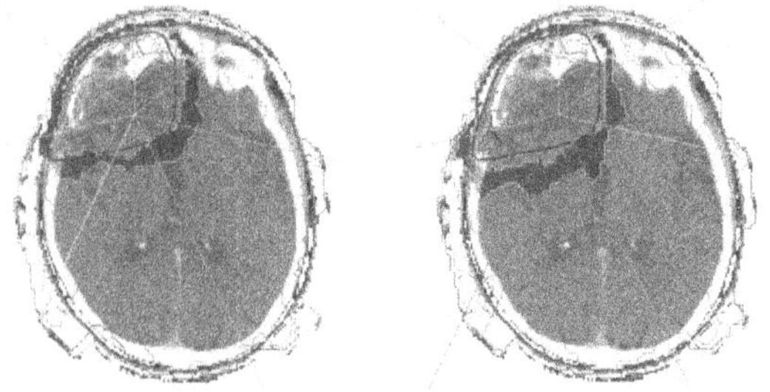


**Figure 5:** Dose distributions of the two plans 'even' and 'odd' shown in the transversal target point slice.

Because this kind of patients get a more complicated beam arrangement, the treatment time is higher compared to the prostate cases.

Figure 5 shows the dose distribution of the two changed plans 'even' and 'odd' for a meningiom case. The plans are usually normalized to the median dose value in the target volume of the unchanged dose distribution. On the first sight, one can see only a slight difference of the isodose pattern. The following table summarizes the gain of time, if the changed fractionation scheme will be applied.

| | Field components | Treatment time |
|---|---|---|
| **Original Plan:** | 70 | 24 min |
| **Even:** | 34 | 13 min |
| **Odd:** | 38 | 14 min |
| **Overall saving of treatment time:** | | |
| **Per fraction (averaged):** | | 10.5 min |
| **Whole treatment (32 fractions):** | | 5.6 h |

The mean daily treatment time per fraction could be reduced to 13.5 min. That is 44% less time needed.

**Technical feasibility**

The new procedure is technically feasible, if the accelerator controlling and documentation procedures were modified. Up to now it is not possible yet to manage a fractionation scheme with treatment modalities that are changing daily. One have to define two completely separate treatment plans.

The effort for verification procedure is slightly higher compared to standard fractionation scheme, because one must evaluate two dose distributions. On the other hand, this is justified by the lower treatment time.

**Radiobiological aspects:**

Another subject of further investigations is the question, whether there are differences in the radiobiological effects between the original and the changed fractionation scheme. The day to day dose changes are in the most organs at risk and in the target volumes smaller than 10%. Every second day the overall dose of the new fractionation scheme is equal to the original scheme. Hence we expect only very low differences of the radiobiological effects. Anyhow one must evaluate these difference.

**Matchlines**

The fractionation scheme is modified in such a way that no matchlines between two fractions can occur. The preliminary results of a case study has shown that the dose distributions of the new fractionation scheme are not more sensitive for setup errors and patient movements than the original dose distributions.

## Conclusion

The proposed method offers a way to cut down the number of field components in IMRT step and shoot approach by 50% down to a half. The changed fractionation scheme is technically feasible, and if the linac control procedures and patient documentation procedures will be adapted to the new method, there is no additional effort necessary to perform this treatment scheme.

However radiobiological investigations have to be performed to evaluate the radiobiological differences between the two treatment modalities.

## References

[1] Bortfeld T, Kahler D L, Waldron T J, Boyer A L 1994 X-ray field compensation with multileaf collimators. *Int J Rad Oncol Biol Phys* **32** 163-173.

[2] Xia P, Verhey L J 1998 Multileaf collimator leaf sequencing algorithm for intensity modulated beams with multiple static segments. *Med Phys* **25** 1424-1434

[3] Galvin J M, Chen X G, Smith R M 1993 Combining multileaf field to modulate fluence distributions. *Int J Rad Oncol Biol Phys* **27** 97-705.

[4] Que W 1999 Comparison of algorithms for multileaf collimator field segmentation. *Med Phys* **26** 2390-2396

[5] Siochi. R A C Minimizing static intensity modulation delivery time using an intensity solid paradigm. 1999 *Int J Rad Oncol Biol Phys* **43** 671-680.

# Dynamic MLC delivered IMRT: verification using Polyacrylamide gel dosimetry

**Vivian P. Cosgrove[1], David J. Convery[1], Philip S. Murphy[1, 2], Christopher M. Nutting[3] and Steve Webb[1]**

[1]Joint Dept. of Physics, [2]CRC Clinical MR Research Group, [3]Dept. Radiotherapy, The Institute of Cancer Research and The Royal Marsden NHS Trust, Downs Road, Sutton, Surrey, SM2 5PT, United Kingdom.

## Introduction

A programme is underway to commission for clinical use a Corvus v3.0 IMRT inverse planning system to use in conjunction with an Elekta MLC operating in dynamic mode. As part of this programme treatment dosimetry and verification have been carried out using Polyacrylamide gels. The gels, manufactured on-site, are a useful adjunct to conventional dosimeters such as ionisation chambers and film. They allow a versatile means of measuring dose distributions in multiple 2D slices positioned in any arbitrary plane and, ultimately, can provide full 3D volumetric dosimetry of an irradiation.

This work presents the first experimentation using the dosimeters for this unique application.

## Material and methods

### Phantom design

A phantom was designed and constructed specifically for high-precision, intra-cranial treatment applications. It has a 15.5cm diameter cylindrical Perspex outer shell with 3mm thick walls and a hemi-spherical base (see figure 1). Within this is located a glass flask with 3mm thick walls, a 9.6cm diameter spherical body and a 5cm diameter, 10cm long neck. Gel can be poured into the flask and then sealed by means of a compression cap and rubber O-ring. This ensures that air will not contaminate the gel once sealed, as oxygen inhibits gel polymerisation. The space between the glass flask and the outer phantom walls is filled with water. Screw fittings on the phantom casing allow precise attachment to a couch-mount used for patient immobilisation. The treatment isocentre is marked on the outer-surface of the phantom to facilitate positioning using the treatment room lasers.

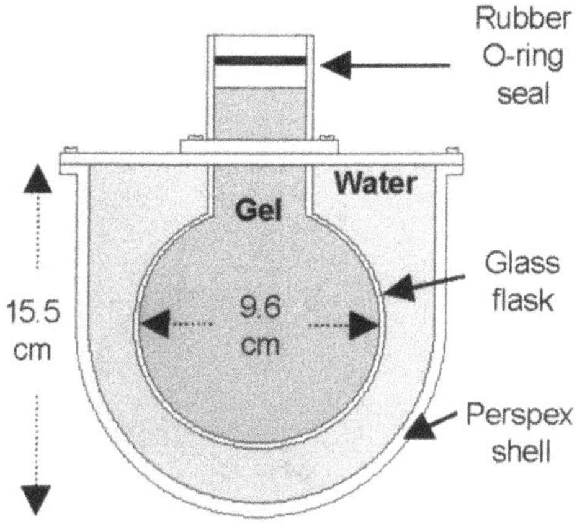


**Figure 1:** The Polyacrylamide gel phantom

### Gel preparation

A BANG-1 formulation gel [1] was manufactured following the experimental procedure described previously [2]. In summary, gels were prepared in a sealed glove-box with a nitrogen atmosphere. Oxygen levels were maintained below 0.1% and were continuously monitored with an $O_2$ meter (Neotox-XL meter, Zellweger Analytics Ltd, UK). 5% w/v gelatin (300-Bloom), 3% w/v acrylamide and 3% w/v N, N'-methylene-bis-acrylamide (all electrophoresis grade) were dissolved in heated, distilled water that had been degassed with nitrogen for approximately 1 hour. The phantom and nine smaller calibration vessels (30ml volume, 2.5cm diameter circular body, 7cm length, 1mm thick glass walls) were filled with gel within the glove-box. Once sealed the gels were transferred to a refrigerator and left to set for 24 hours prior to irradiation. Gel preparation was completed in approximately 3 hours.

### Planning and irradiation

The gel phantom was CT scanned with a slice thickness and spacing of 3mm. The data were transferred to the Corvus planning system and an arbitrary, "U"-shaped target (~ 6 x 4cm) was drawn onto the central slice. This was copied onto 10 slices above and below, producing a 6cm long volume. Five, co-planar treatment fields were then positioned around the target volume at 72° intervals and an intensity modulated treatment plan was calculated by inverse techniques [3]. The monitor unit maps of the resulting intensity modulated fields were transferred via floppy disk to a separate PC so that they could be interpreted into dynamic MLC delivery sequences. An Elekta MLC specific algorithm has been previously developed to derive these delivery sequences, taking into account minimum leaf separation constraints and correcting for tongue-and-groove under-exposure [4].

Irradiations were carried out on an Elekta SL25 linear accelerator using 6MV photons and a dose-rate of 100MU/min. A total dose of 6Gy was delivered to the 100% isodose point. To calibrate the phantom dose distributions the smaller gel vessels were separately positioned in the centre of a Perspex, water filled phantom and irradiated along their length with 10 x 10 $cm^2$ fields (gantry angle = $180^0$, SSD = 100 cm) to doses of between 1 and 8 Gy at $d_{max}$, with a vessel left unirradiated to define a background reading [2].

### Imaging

$T_2$ relaxation imaging was performed on all the gels using a 1.5 Tesla Siemens Vision MR scanner. Gel samples were placed in the climate controlled magnet room at least 12 hours

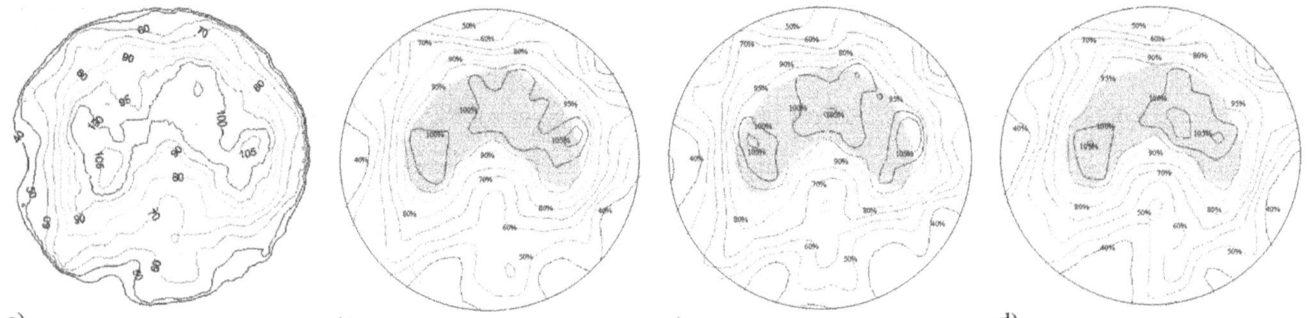

a) b) c) d)

**Figure 2**: Dose distributions in the transverse plane a) Gel measurement, b) Corvus calculation, c) calculation in a plane 2mm inferior to b) and d) calculation in a plane 2mm anterior to b).

prior to measurement, to ensure temperature equilibrium. Imaging was undertaken within 4 days of irradiation. A standard, multiple spin-echo sequence was used with a sixteen-echo train length. Images were acquired with an initial echo-time ($T_E$) of 50ms, with further 50ms increments, and a repetition-time ($T_R$) of 2s, field-of-view (FOV) 256mm and a 256 x 256 matrix size. In-plane image resolution was 1mm. With an image slice thickness of 5mm, transverse, coronal and sagittal $T_2$ relaxation maps were generated with the Siemens' system software. Each slice acquisition required 8½ minutes scanning time.

The measured changes in relaxation rate $R_2$ (defined as $1/T_2$) with depth in the calibration vessels were plotted against measured depth-dose distributions to produce a characteristic $R_2$ versus dose curve. A third-order polynomial curve was fitted to the data and this was used to convert the two-dimensional $R_2$ images of the phantoms into absorbed dose maps.

## Results and discussion

Figure 2a illustrates the gel measurement in the transverse plane and 2b the Corvus dose calculation. The gel distributions are normalized to the 100% dose region. Also shown are the calculations in the planes 2mm below and 2mm above this slice (2c and 2d, respectively). It is observed that the dose distribution can change quite significantly in this short distance. The measurement in gel, being 5mm thick, should, therefore, represent a mean of these distributions. To aid a more quantitative comparison between the distributions dose-area histograms were calculated for all these planes. These are plotted in Figure 3.

A systematic shift was observed between the measured and calculated dose distributions that could not be attributed to the variations noted between the 2mm shifted planes. This was also seen in the Coronal and Sagittal planes (figures 4 and 5). In general, good agreement was seen between the ≥90% isodose areas, although larger areas are enclosed by the < 90% isodoses in the gel measurements relative to those calculated on Corvus. It is, as yet uncertain as to why these deviations exist. Repeat measurements are currently underway to determine whether these results are reproducible.

Using conventional dosimetry techniques (ionisation chamber and film) it has been established that some deviations between the Corvus calculations and the dose delivery can occur [5]. The current version of the software does not use the actual MLC delivery sequence in the final dose calculation. Therefore, the effects of leaf and primary jaw transmission and head-scattered radiation in the actual delivery are not included in the dose calculation. An iterative technique to correct for these effects is under investigation [5]. However, it is not believed that the differences observed here can be fully accounted for by the limitations in the dose calculation algorithm, as measurements with film have not revealed comparable variations.

Other experiments at the Royal Marsden using Polyacrylamide gel manufactured in an identical way have shown the relative dosimetry to be reproducible and spatially matches dose calculations, produced by conventional radiotherapy planning systems, to within a few millimetres [6]. Absolute dosimetry, however, has proved to be problematic, with the calibrated dose measured in the phantom gel being consistently higher than that delivered. The 100% dose measured in phantom in this work was 6.9 ± 0.09Gy, 15 ±1.5% higher than that delivered. There are a number of factors that can influence the absolute dose measurements, including gel temperature changes during MR scanning, oxygen contamination of the gel and artefacts in the $T_2$ imaging related to RF field inhomogeneity. Differences in structural and/or polymerisation reactions between the calibration and phantom gels are also being investigated as a potential source of error.

The dose distributions calculated and measured in the Sagittal plane are illustrated in figure 6.

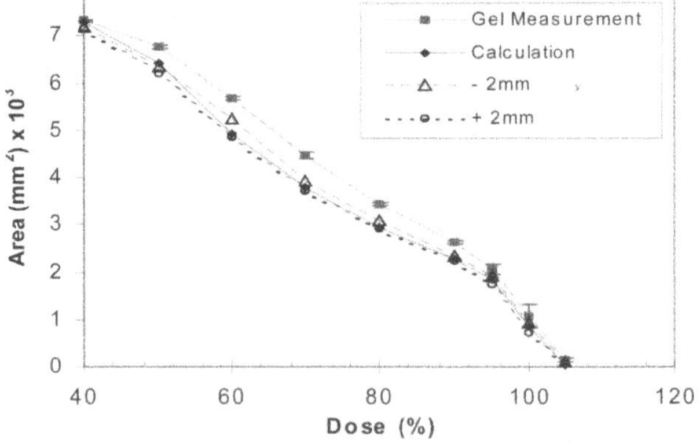


**Figure 3**: Dose-Area histograms in the transverse plane.

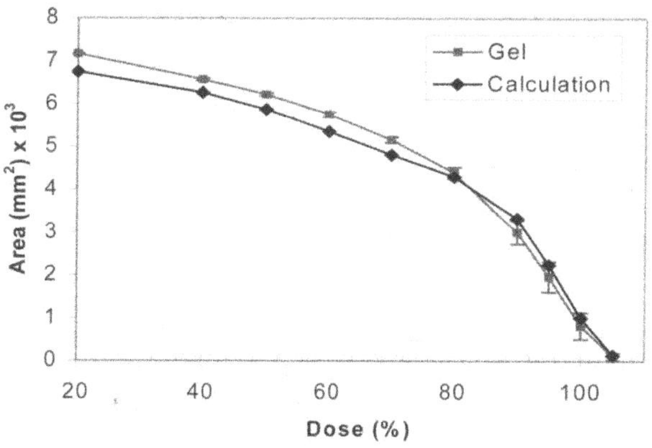

**Figure 4**: Dose-Area histograms in the Coronal plane.

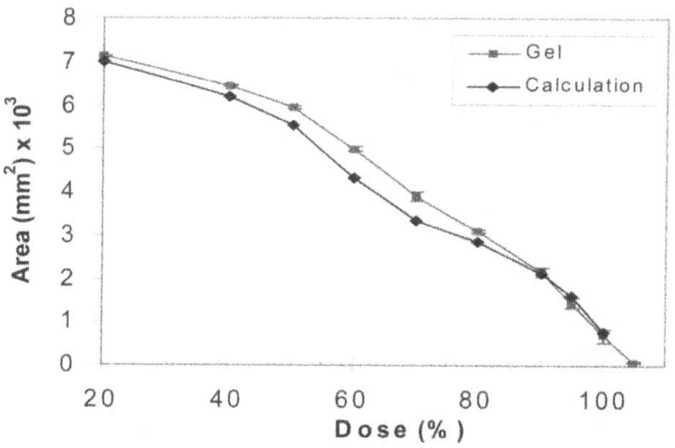

**Figure 5**: Dose-Area histograms in the Sagittal plane.

## Conclusions

Although the gel dosimetry technique can be problematic, is labour intensive and requires access to a MR scanner, the volumetric dosimetry information that can be obtained from an irradiated gel is invaluable when verifying complex radiotherapy applications. Investigations are currently underway to improve the accuracy of the absolute dosimetry with our gels. However, absolute doses can be measured with a high accuracy in-phantom at single points using conventional ionisation chambers and TLDs. Gel dosimeters, however, are the only method available that allow complete visualization of a complex irradiation geometry in three dimensions. Therefore, these complementary dosimetry techniques will be used together during commissioning and clinical verification of our Corvus planning system and Elekta dynamic MLC. More direct ways of measuring and calibrating the gel polymerisation densities will be sought that are less sensitive to the factors known to affect standard MR relaxation time imaging. Further characterization of the polymer gel is also underway to understand more completely the dynamics of gel polymerization following irradiation.

When comparing measurements with calculations it would obviously be advantageous to reduce the thickness of the MR scan so that it is comparable with the calculation matrix. This is of particular relevance here as the dose distributions are seen to vary in planes only a few millimetres apart. However, this requires additional imaging time to get adequate signal-to-noise discrimination. The multiple-echo imaging sequence used here requires 8½ minutes per 5mm thick scan. Compromises on the minimum scan thickness used are sometimes necessary due to limitations on the availability of the MR scanner.

## Acknowledgements

We would like to thank the Cancer Research Campaign (SP2311/0102, SP1780/0103) and the EPSRC (EPS003-GR/L 26780) for financial assistance. VP Cosgrove and DJ Convery are supported by Elekta Oncology Systems.

## References


[1] Maryanski MJ, Schultz RJ, Ibbott GS, Gatenby JC, Xie J, Horton D and Gore JC 1994 Magnetic resonance imaging of radiation dose distributions using a polymer-gel dosimeter *Phys. Med. Biol.* **39** 1437-55

[2] Oldham M, McJury M, Baustert I, Webb S, and Leach MO 1998 Improving calibration accuracy in gel dosimetry. *Phys. Med. Biol.* **43** 2709-20

[3] Webb S. 1994 Optimizing the planning of intensity modulated radiotherapy *Phys. Med. Biol.* **39** 2229-46

[4] Convery DJ and Webb S 1998 Generation of discrete beam intensity modulation by dynamic multileaf collimation under minimum leaf separation constraints *Phys. Med. Biol.* **43** 2521-38

[5] Convery DJ Cosgrove VP Webb S 1999 Improving dosimetric accuracy of a dynamic MLC technique (*Submitted to XIII ICCR*).

[6] Cosgrove VP Murphy PS McJury M Adams EJ Warrington AP Leach MO Webb S 1999 The reproducibility of Polyacrylamide gel dosimetry applied to stereotactic conformal radiotherapy (*Submitted to Phys. Med. Biol.*).


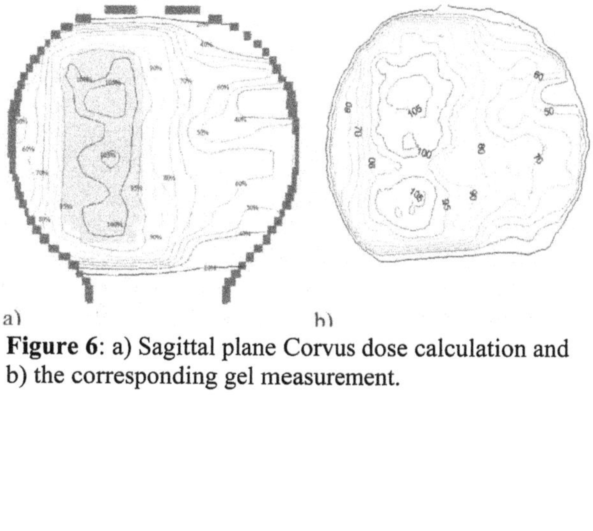

a) b)

**Figure 6**: a) Sagittal plane Corvus dose calculation and b) the corresponding gel measurement.

# Tomographic Verification of Tomotherapy -- Before, During, and After Treatment

**KJ Ruchala[1], GH Olivera[1,2], JM Kapatoes[2], JB Smilowitz[2], EA Schloesser[1], DW Pearson[1,2], JP Balog[1], PJ Reckwerdt[1] and TR Mackie[1,2]**

[1]TomoTherapy Inc., 2228 Evergreen Rd, Middleton, WI 53562, and [2]University of Wisconsin - Madison, Department of Medical Physics, 1300 University Ave, Madison, WI 53706

## Introduction

Many improvements in conformal radiotherapy have allowed for increased precision in treatment delivery, and the goal of tomotherapy is to carry these improvements further. However, the ability to deliver highly conformal radiation therapy treatments is only useful to the extent that the patient's position and anatomy are known. Certainly, it is important to set-up the patient correctly, but ideally, one should also verify that a patient's internal organs are correctly positioned and that they have not changed in size or shape. This verification can be achieved through the integration of tomographic imaging capabilities. Tomotherapy systems will feature such tomographic verification, initally through megavoltage CT (MVCT), and potentially with on-board kilovoltage CT (kVCT) in future implementations. In addition to being important to treatments, tomographic images are also necessary for *dose reconstruction* to verify the treatment delivery [1,2].

One tomographic option is to collect MVCT images immediately before or after a tomotherapeutic treatment. This was performed for a treatment to a German shepherd's head on the University of Wisconsin Tomotherapy Benchtop. These images are compared to kVCT images taken on a separate, commercial system.

It is also possible to reduce time and/or dose by collecting the MVCT images during the treatment itself. Two different methods of generating MVCT images during treatment are investigated, namely *treatment modification* and *leakage imaging*.

## Material and methods

### Imaging Before and After Treatment

A tomotherapeutic treatment was delivered to a German shepherd's head using the University of Wisconsin Tomotherapy Benchtop. This system features a stationary, 4 MV Orion linac (General Electric, Buc, France) that can deliver treatments to objects situated on a rotating and translating table. The linac beam is temporally modulated using a Nomos MIMiC (Sewickley, PA) multi-leaf collimator (MLC). Finally, a 738-channel xenon detector (General Electric, Milwaukee, WI) is placed opposite the linac to allow for the collection of transmission data.

Prior to the treatment, the dog's head was scanned on a Siemens' Hi-Q axial scanner. This data set was rendered using Pinnacle (ADAC Laboratories, Milpitas, CA), and the rendering is shown in Figure 1, along with two transverse slices.

The head was also scanned helically using the Tomotherapy Benchtop MVCT system, immediately prior to the treatment. This scan had a pitch of 1 and a 4 mm slice thickness. The dose for these images, shown in Figure 2, was 7 cGy. While these images are noisier than the kVCT images, they do clearly show the dog's external boundary and the high contrasts (i.e. bone and air) inside the head. Soft tissue contrasts of better than 1% can also be seen with a 7 cGy MVCT scan [3], although this dog head was largely devoid of soft tissue contrast.

The main benefit of MVCT, performed in this way, is that it can provide tomographic images of the patient in the treatment position, without the additional cost and complication of on-

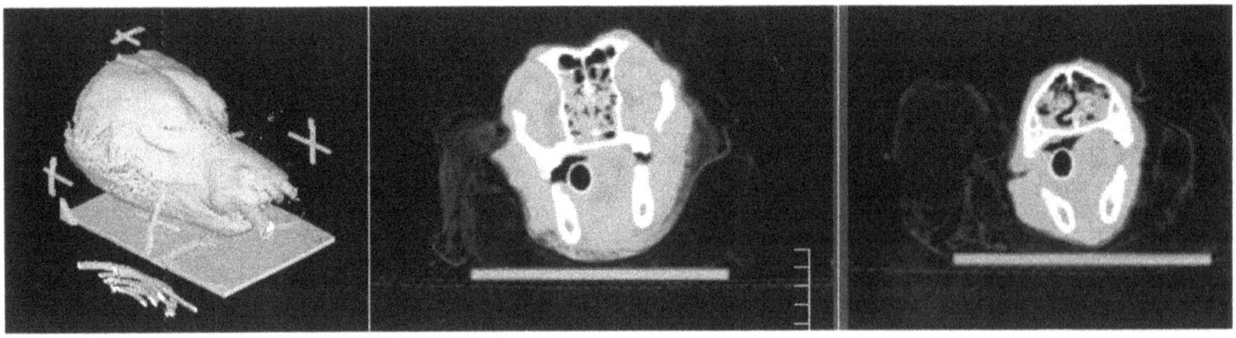

**Figure 1:** Kilovoltage CT of the German shepherd head

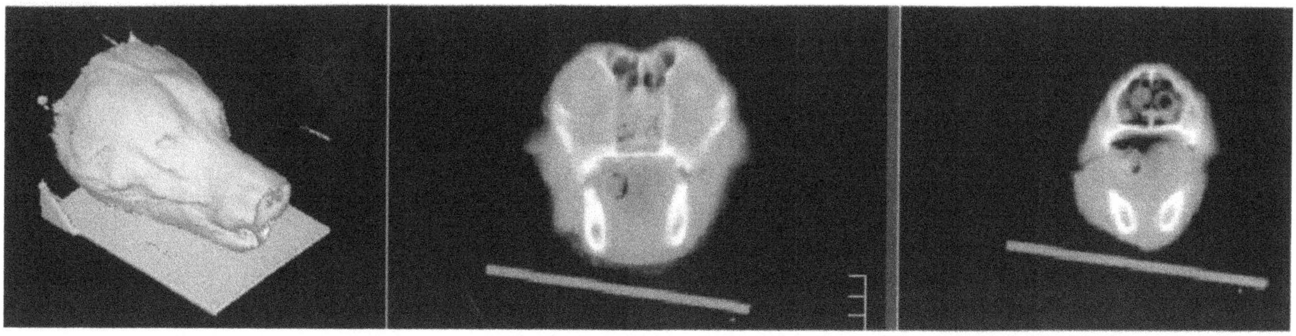

**Figure 2:** Megavoltage CT of the German shepherd head from the Tomotherapy Benchtop (7 cGy)

board kVCT. Similarly, if the patient is believed to have moved during the treatment, an MVCT can be taken after the treatment to further verify a patient's position. It has also been shown that for high atomic number materials, MVCT is less subject to beam hardening artifacts than kVCT, and the reconstructed values exhibit better linearity with electron density [4].

**Imaging During Treatment**

Another option for MVCT imaging is to collect the tomograms during the treatment itself. Ideally, this will allow for reduced patient table time and correspondingly increased patient throughput. In addition, if one can utilize dose that is already being delivered to the patient, it may be possible to reduce additional imaging dose. A reduction in dose may enable the more frequent collection of MVCT images, such that daily tomographic verification may ultimately be possible.

Two methods of MVCT reconstruction during treatment delivery were investigated, specifically treatment modification and leakage imaging. Treatment modification is based on the premise that the MLC is modulated to optimize the dose to the tumor, while minimizing dose to healthy tissue. Nonetheless, it is feasible that the MLC modulations could be modestly adjusted, if doing so conferred benefits that compensated for the additional dose.

Presently, Tomotherapy delivery plans are quantized into a number of *projections,* and the times during treatment when the most leaves are open is in the middle of each projection. Thus, one potential treatment modification is to "flash" all of the leaves open at the middle of some projections. Since many of the leaves are already open at these times, this process would not significantly disrupt the treatment. Yet, the benefit is that it would allow for a number of complete views of data to be collected and normalized, and these complete views could be reconstructed into a crude image of the patient.

The other option is to generate MVCT images using MLC leakage. That is, it has been found that the NOMOS MIMiC MLC leaks and transmits radiation. This leakage signal, as measured directly behind the closed leaves of the MLC, is approximately 0.3% of the signal measured with the leaves open. This signal, while unintended and otherwise undesirable, can potentially be used for image reconstruction.

In general, these leakage signals are small, and are easily lost amongst scatter if other leaves are open. However, when all of the leaves are closed, the use of these signals is more feasible. In this context, it should be noted that the present method of Tomotherapy delivery results in all of the MLC leaves being briefly closed between each projection. Thus, even without any treatment modification, there are a number of occassions during each treatment when complete views of tomographic data are collected for the patient. Nonetheless, it should be noted that these leakage views are very low dose and irregular, by nature of passing through the MLC jaws.

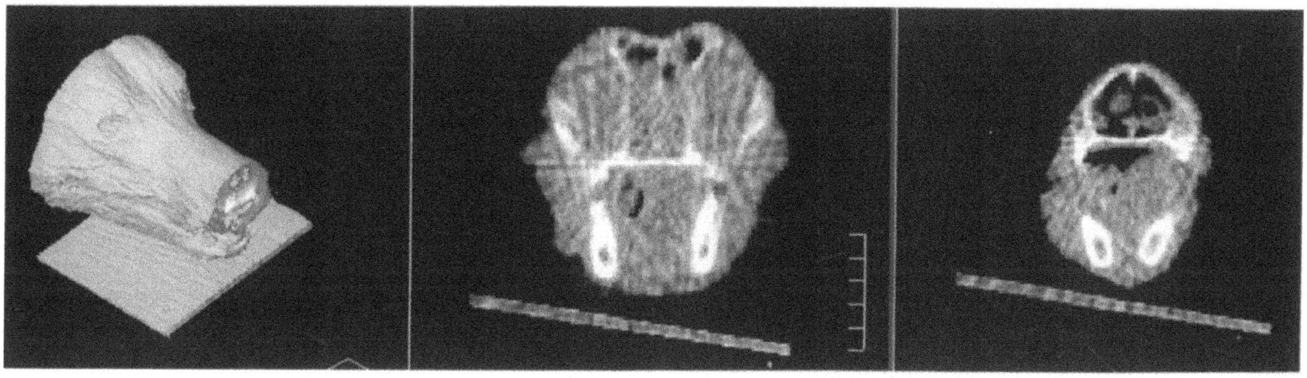

**Figure 3:** MVCT using only 51 "flash"-views per reconstructed slice, collected during treatment

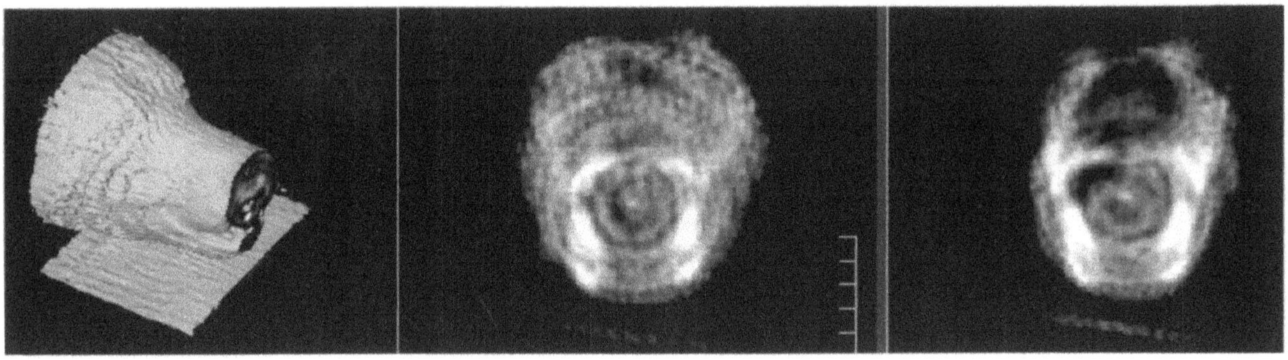

**Figure 4:** MVCT using only the leakage through the NOMOS MIMiC MLC, collected during the treatment

## Results and discussion

The treatment delivered to the dog's head was composed of 51 projections per rotation and delivered with a pitch of 0.5. A leaf flash was performed at the center of every other projection, and the data from every 51 flashes was reconstructed. The imaging dose for this flash data is approximately 2.5 cGy. A rendering of these reconstructed slices, as well as two transverse slices, can be seen in Figure 3. The main limitation of these images is that the reduced number of views results in significant streak artifacting. Nonetheless, these images do allow the bones, air, and patient boundaries to be seen. This can help determine whether the patient is properly situated during the actual treatment and flag whether additional tomographic information should be collected. In phantoms with more low-contrast tissue, contrasts on the order of 5% can be detected [4] using this method.

The additional dose incurred by using this technique depends on the leaf speed, the linac output rate, and the number of flashes used. Ideally, the linac will have a gridded-gun, such that there will be no wasted dose during the delivery of the flashes; otherwise, dose will be delivered as the leaves open and close, yet this dose will not be useful for imaging. The Tomotherapy Prototype is expected to have a gridded-gun, but at present, there are no such controls on the Orion, and combined with the motion time of the NOMOS leaves, the delivered dose for these flashes was closer to 10 cGy. The Tomotherapy Prototype is also anticipated to have faster leaves, which will allow for a greater number of flashes, and a corresponding reduction of streak artifacts.

Finally, the leakage images are shown in Figure 4. These images are the poorest in quality, but that is because these images require **no additional dose** and **no additional scan time**. Instead, these leakage images are purely a by-product of MLC leakage. Since the leakage signals are very small and irregular, these images are necessarily poor. However, the benefit is that these images are effectively "free", and can provide crude images of the patient at the time of treatment. The information provided by such leakage images can help determine if it the collection of higher quality images is warranted, and those could be taken immediately following the treatment, with the the patient still in the treatment position.

## Conclusion

Tomotherapy is designed to improve upon the delivery of conformal radiation. Yet, key to this goal is ensuring that knowledge of the patient's position and anatomy is congruous with the ability to control the radiation delivery. This verification goal can be achieved tomographically, and megavoltage computed tomography is believed to be adequate for this task while reducing cost and complexity as compared to kilovoltage CT.

The best MVCT images are collected analogously to kVCT – using a full field-of-view and a large number of view angles. This can be done before or after the treatment, and with a dose between 5 and 10 cGy.

However, it is also possible to collect MVCT images entirely during the treatment. One option is to modestly alter the treatment delivery such that complete views can be collected. At present, the main limitation is the additional delivered dose (~10 cGy) and the small number of views, but both of these problems are potentially remediable with a gridded-gun linac and faster MLC leaves, expected improvements for the Tomotherapy Prototype. The other option is to collect treatment images using only MLC leakage. These images are quite limited, as they utilize the unintended dose to the patient, but they are perhaps sufficient to provide a crude sense of patient positioning, and determine whether higher quality tomographic imaging is justified.

## References


[1] Kapatoes, JM, *et al.,* Delivery Verification in Sequential and Helical Tomotherapy, *Phys. Med. Biol.* **44** 1815-1841

[2] Olivera, GH, *et al.,* Tomotherapy, in The Modern Technology of Radiation Oncology, Jacob Van Dyk ed., Medical Physics Publishing, Madison, WI, 1999, 521-587

[3] Ruchala, KJ, *et al.*, Megavoltage CT on a Tomotherapy System. *Phys. Med. Biol.* **44** 2597-2621

[4] Ruchala, KJ, Megavoltage Computed Tomography for Tomotherapeutic Verification, *Ph. D. Thesis,*University of Wisconsin-Madison, 1999

# Computer Simulated Patient Motion and Setup Uncertainties in Intensity Modulated Radiotherapy

**Ping Xia, Cynthia Chaung, Felix Nguyen-Tan, Karen K. Fu, Lynn J. Verhey**

University of California at San Francisco, San Francisco CA 94143, U.S.A.

## Introduction

The advent of intensity modulated radiotherapy (IMRT) has enhanced our ability to tailor radiation dose distribution highly conformal to tumor target shape three dimensionally, and thus minimize radiation damage to the surrounding normal tissues. Taking the advantage of high conformality in IMRT plans, the prescribed dose to the tumor target is often escalated while keeping the critical normal tissue within tolerance. It is anticipated that IMRT will increase uncomplicated local tumor control, and improve cancer patient survival. To realize this high expectation, it is essential to deliver IMRT plans accurately and precisely. Much effort and research have been focused on how to improve mechanical precision in linear accelerators, and how to improve dose calculation accuracy by using Monte Carlo method[1-3]. Little research has been done on how uncertainties in patient positioning and immobilization can affect the IMRT plans[4, 5]. The purpose of this paper is to investigate this issue.

## Methods and Materials

A group of five patients with nasopharyngeal carcinoma treated with IMRT plans in our institution were selected for this study. All these patients received a full course of IMRT treatment. These patients were immobilized with thermal plastic head masks, similar to that used for conventional radiotherapy. The IMRT plans for these patients were produced with a commercial inverse treatment planning system (Corvus 3.0, NOMOS), using a multi-vane collimator (MIMIC, NOMOS) delivered with sequential multiple arcs. In these plans, the dose distributions were highly conformal to the primary nasopharyngeal region and matched to the upper neck fields treated with conventional lateral opposing beams. Depending on the extension of the gross tumor, the nasopharyngeal tumors are often adjacent to numerous critical structures, such as spinal cord, brain stem, optic structures, and parotid glands. The treatment goal was to deliver a minimum of 70 Gy to more than 95% of the gross tumor volume (GTV), and a minimum of 60 Gy to more than 95 % of the clinical tumor volume (CTV). The dose constraint to 1% volume of the sensitive structures brain stem, optical chiasm, spinal cord was limited to 50 Gy, 45 Gy, and 45 Gy respectively. The dose constraint to 50% volumes of parotid glands was limited to 30 Gy. Our previous study[6] showed that this treatment goal is achievable if using inversely planned IMRT plans even for advanced nasopharyngeal carcinoma with intracranial extension.

Previous studies and clinical observations have shown that for patients immobilized with the head mask the most likely head motion is rotation with the chin up or down. It is estimated that the average magnitude of motion was about 1-3 mm [7, 8]. To truly simulate possible patient head rotation with the current planning systems is difficult, because it requires rotation of the patient's entire CT data set, which is not feasible in any of our current treatment planning systems. A simple approximate method of simulating such rotations is shifting the iso-center superiorly and posteriorly for the chin up motion, and inferiorly and anteriorly for the chin down motion, while keeping the original field shapes the same. Using this iso-center shifting method to simulate patient's motion and setup errors is trivial for a manually designed (forward) plan. This method, however, becomes non-trivial for an inverse plan, because shifting iso-center may also change the final optimized plan. To keep the plan with shifted iso-center the same as the original optimized plan, a tool called creating phantom plan provided in the inverse planning system is very useful. Using this tool, one is able to apply the original plan directly to any phantom geometry with an associated iso-center. The dose distribution for the phantom plan is calculated based on the phantom geometry and iso-center location, but using the beam configuration of the patient's plan. This tool was originally designed for verifying patient plan using a regular shaped phantom. We extended the usage of this tool to simulate iso-center shifting. First, a patient plan is copied and the plan status was changed to a phantom plan, and then through the procedure of creating the phantom plan, the original patient plan was directly applied to the phantom plan with the patient's anatomical geometry but with a new iso-center location. To simulate patient's head rotation for chin up, we shifted the original iso-center 3 mm posterior and 3 mm superior simultaneously. For the chin down rotation, we shifted the iso-center 3 mm anterior and 3 mm inferior simultaneously.

## Results and Discussions

Fig. 1 shows the percentage of the GTV receiving a minimum dose of 70 Gy when patients were positioned in the following three positions: (1) normal iso-center; (2) iso-center shifted 3 mm posterior and superior; (3) iso-center shifted 3 mm anterior and inferior. Except for patient #2, the GTV volume receiving a minimum dose of 70 Gy was reduced in average about 5%, assuming the patient positioning in these three positions is random. Fig. 2 shows the percentage of the CTV receiving a minimum dose of 60 Gy for the five patients at these three positions. For all five patients, the CTV volume covered by the prescribed dose was reduced in average about 3%. From these data, we found that the dose coverage of both the GTV and the CTV are not significantly affected by the setup uncertainties within a magnitude of 3 mm.

Fig. 3 shows the maximum dose received by 1% of the brain stem volume for these five patients in the three different positions. The maximum dose received by 1% of the brain stem was below the tolerance dose of 50 Gy in all five original plans. Patient head rotation along the superior and posterior direction increased the maximum dose to the brain stem, but the motion along the anterior and inferior rotation tended to decrease the dose to the brain stem.

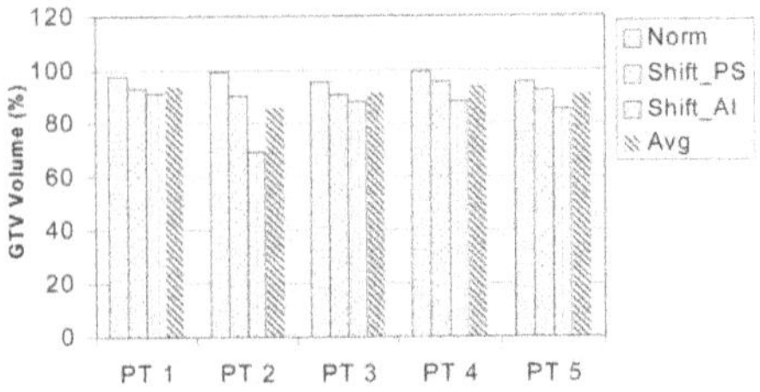


**Figure 1:** The percentage of the GTV volume receiving ≥70 Gy.

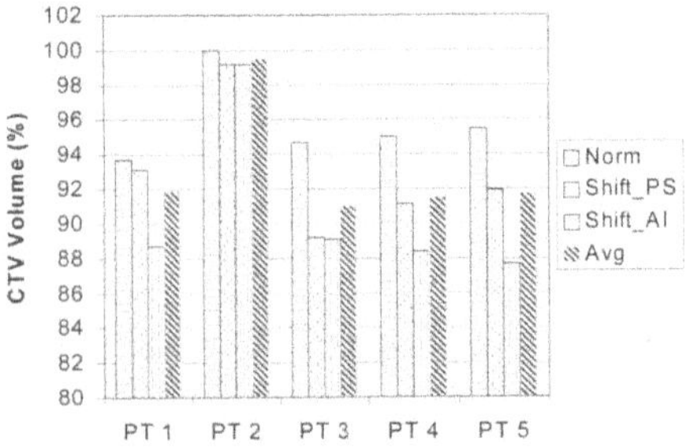


**Figure 2:** The percentage of the CTV volume receiving ≥ 60 Gy.

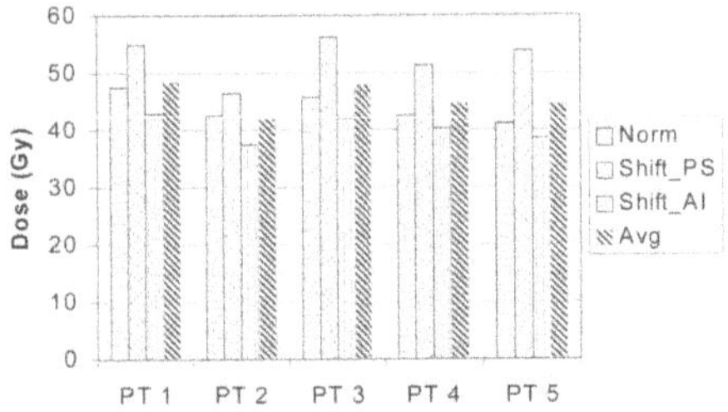


**Figure 3:** The Maximum dose received by 1% of the barin stem

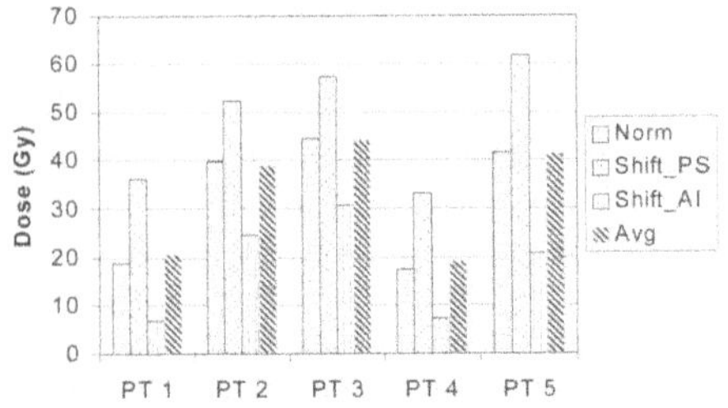


**Figure 4:** The maximum dose received by 1% of the chiasm.

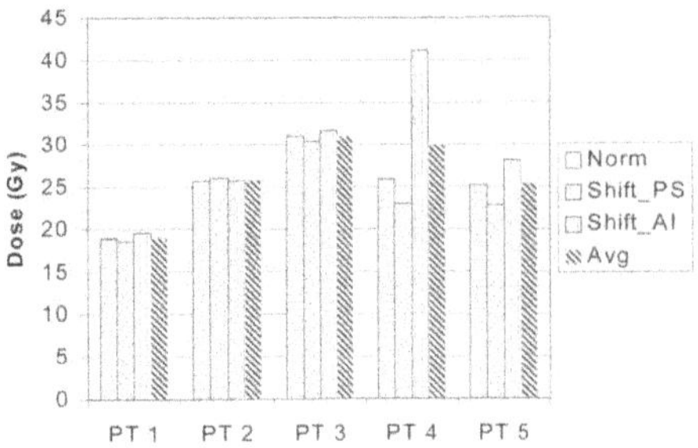


**Figure 5:** The dose to 50% of ipsilateral parotid gland

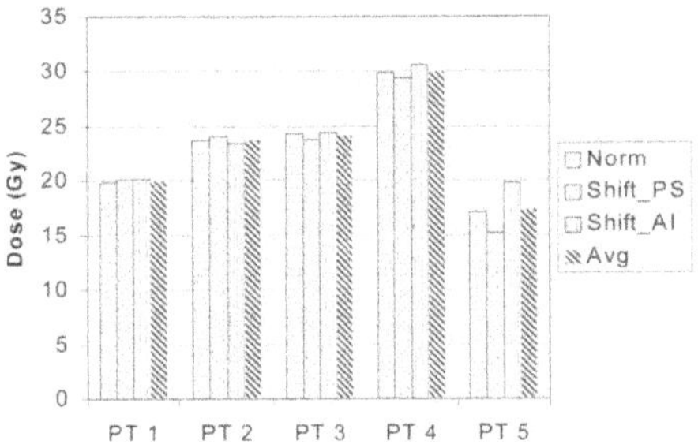


**Figure 6:** The dose to 50% of contralateral parotid gland

If we assume the patient positioning in these three positions was random, the average maximum dose to the brain stem was still below the tolerance. Similar trends were observed for changes in the maximum dose received by 1% of the chiasm, as shown in Fig. 4. It should be noted that the patient's head consistently rotated toward chin up, the maximum dose to the brain stem and the chiasm will increase by about 20% and 35%, respectively. In order to separate the treatment of the neck node from the primary tumor, most patients were positioned in a hyper-extended head position. The most likely head rotation in this setup is chin moved down. In this position, the maximum dose to the brain stem and the chiasm for four out of five will be decreased without significantly reducing dose to the tumor volume. For patient #2, 69% of the GTV instead of 99 % of GTV will receive a minimum dose of 70 Gy in the chin down motion. In this position, the CTV coverage will be reduced but not significantly. Fig. 5 and Fig. 6 show the dose received by 50% of the ipsilateral parotid gland and the contralateral parotid gland in these three positions for the same group of patients. The observed changes in parotid glands were insignificant for both the chin up and chin down positions.

## Conclusions

Our preliminary results based on five nasopharyngeal cases demonstrate that for IMRT plans changes in dose coverage to both the GTV and the CTV are not very sensitive to the random patient motion and setup error up to 3 mm. Under this circumstance, the average changes in dose to sensitive structures are also not significant. However, consistent setup error such as chin up motion can introduce significant change in dose to sensitive structures as the brain stem and the chiasm. Further research on this subject is needed to include more patients, as well as other critical structures.

## References


1. van Santvoort, J.P. and B.J. Heijmen, *Dynamic multileaf collimation without 'tongue-and-groove' underdosage effects.* Phys Med Biol, 1996. **41**(10): p. 2091-105.
2. Xing, L., *et al.*, *Dosimetric verification of a commercial inverse treatment planning system.* Phys Med Biol, 1999. **44**(2): p. 463-78.
3. Low, D., *et al.*, *Quality assurance of serial tomotherapy for head and neck patient treatments.* Int. J. Radiation Oncology Biol. Phys., 1998. **42**(3): p. 681-692.
4. Tsai, J.S., *et al.*, *A non-invasive immobilization system and related quality assurance for dynamic intensity modulated radiation therapy of intracranial and head and neck disease.* Int J Radiat Oncol Biol Phys, 1999. **43**(2): p. 455-67.
5. Verellen, D., *et al.*, *Initial experience with intensity-modulated conformal radiation therapy for treatment of the head and neck region.* Int J Radiat Oncol Biol Phys, 1997. **39**(1): p. 99-114.
6. Xia, P., *et al.*, *Comparison of treatment plans involving intensity modulated radiotherapy for Nasopharyngeal Carcinoma.* Int. J. Radiat. Oncol. Biol. Phys. In Press, 1999.
7. Verhey, L.J., *et al.*, *Precise positioning of patients for radiation therapy.* Int J Radiat Oncol Biol Phys, 1982. **8**(2): p. 289-94.
8. Leibel, S.A., *et al.*, *Improved dose distributions for 3D conformal boost treatments in carcinoma of the nasopharynx.* Int J Radiat Oncol Biol Phys, 1991. **20**(4): p. 823-33.

# Intensity modulated proton therapy: A first clinical example.

**A J Lomax, T Boehringer, A Coray, E Egger, G Goitein, M Grossmann, P Juelke, S Lin, E Pedroni, B Rohrer, W Roser, B Rossi, B Siegenthaler, O Stadelmann, H Stauble, C Vetter, L Wisser.**

Division of Radiation Medicine, The Paul Scherrer Institute, 5232 Villigen-PSI, Switzerland.

## Introduction.

By the end of 1999, over 40 patients will have been treated at the Paul Scherrer Institute with protons using the spot scanning technique [1]. For each of these treatments, an optimisation process has been used to calculate the weights of the many thousands of individually applied proton pencil beams which typically make up a single treatment port [2,3]. For the majority of these treatments however, the optimisation procedure has been applied on a field-by-field basis only, and in such a way as to ensure that a homogenous dose is applied across the target volume from each individual field.

Here we report on the first treatment of a patient using fully automated 3D intensity modulated proton therapy (IMPT). By 3D IMPT, we refer to the calculation and delivery of multiple ports for which the optimisation process has been applied to all three dimensionally distributed proton Bragg peaks from all fields simultaneously. This results in a set of individually *in-homogenous* fields which nevertheless combine to deliver a homogenous resultant dose across the target volume. From the delivery point of view, this change is exactly analogous to the change from static photon delivery techniques to photon IMRT, a process in which homogenous or linearly varying photon fluences have been replaced by highly inhomogenous fluences.

## Materials and methods.

A 34 year old man was referred for proton therapy with a Chondrosarcoma in the posterior portion of the seventh and eighth thoracic vertebrae. The defined target volume was prescribed a dose of 72Gy and was found to wrap partially around the spinal cord creating a 'classic' treatment planning problem (figure 1). The spinal cord was assigned a maximum tolerance dose of 60Gy. The planning problem in this case was accentuated by two additional physical constraints. Firstly, beams through the heart and lung were to be avoided due to errors in the delivered dose that could result from motion of these organs. Secondly, the delivery of highly weighted Bragg peaks deposited directly against the spinal cord were to be avoided, due to the risk of dose 'overshoot' into the spinal cord and possible RBE effects in the distal edge of the Bragg peaks.

In order to avoid these problems, a three field, patched technique was adopted, with Bragg peaks from all three fields being optimised using the 3D IMPT method described by Lomax [4]. However, as for all treatment plans there is a relatively large probability that the dose delivered to the patient will differ in a number of regards from that which has been computed, a detailed analysis of the plan, and in particular the Bragg peak positions and weights, was additionally performed. Three independent assessments of the sensitivity of the calculated plan to potential delivery and calculation errors were used; 1) range error analysis, 2) patient set-up error analysis and 3) Monte Carlo verification of the analytic dose calculation.

For the range error analysis, the plan was recalculated with a 10% reduction of all values in the patient's CT data, thus simulating the effects of a 10% overshoot of proton range for all fields. Patient positioning errors were simulated by recalculating the dose repeatedly in a number of translated versions of the patients CT set, with each version being offset in relation to the nominal position by 5mm along one of the major anatomical axes (right and left lateral, cranial and caudal, anterior and posterior). As an additional check, the magnitude of organ motion in the region of the target volume was assessed through the acquisition of inhalation and exhalation CT slices during the course of the treatment and, as is performed for all our treatments, prior to the first fraction, detailed dose verifications were made in water for each field using orthogonal ionisation chamber profile measurements and film stack dosimetry.

## Results.

### The plan.

Figure 1 shows the optimised dose distributions of the individual fields planned for this case. Three fields were defined; right posterior oblique (figure 1a), posterior (figure 1b) and left posterior oblique (figure 1c). In order to avoid directing proton pencil beams directly at the spinal cord, both the RPO and LPO fields were designed such as to only cover the left and right lobes of the target volume respectively (figure 1a and 1c).

With the RPO and LPO beams alone, it is impossible to achieve a homogenous dose across the full target volume due to the combined plateau doses in the middle-posterior portion of the target volume (the portion immediately posterior to the spinal cord). The third, posterior beam was therefore introduced. This beam was designed to deliver proton Bragg peaks throughout the full target volume but with the main objective of increasing the dose in the two lateral lobes. As a result of the raised dose in the RPO-LPO overlap region, and in order to obtain a homogenous resultant dose, the multiple field optimisation process necessarily reduces beam weights in the central portion of the posterior beam (see figure 1b). Due to the geometry of the patched field arrangement, these beams are also the ones that are incident on the spinal cord. Thus, after optimisation, the posterior field delivers only Bragg peaks of a relatively low weight against the spinal cord.

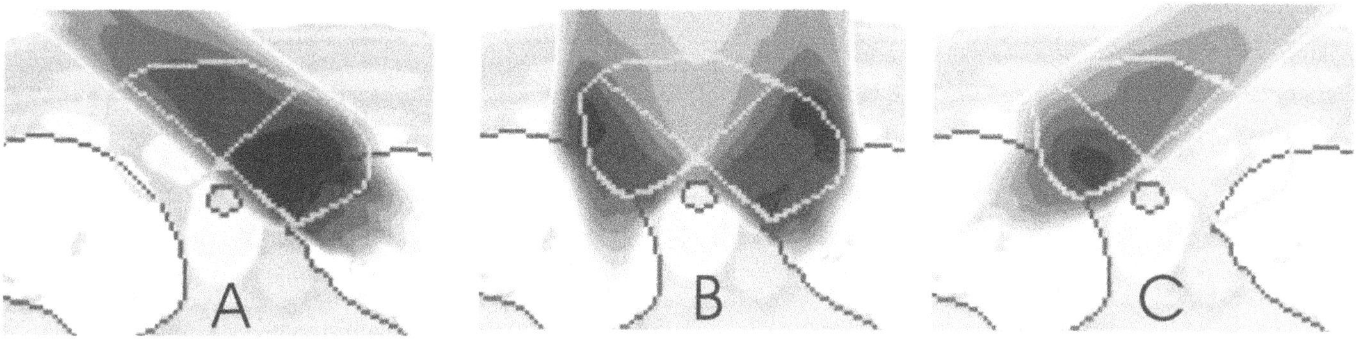


**Figure 1:** RPO (A), posterior (B) and LPO (C) fields for the optimised 3D IMPT plan. Note the clearly reduced dose in the central portion of the posterior field (the portion incident on the spinal cord) and the patched arrangement of the RPO and LPO fields.

The resultant dose distribution for all fields together is shown in figure 2a. Through the use of three patched fields (none of which pass through the thorax) and 3D IMPT, a high degree of conformity could be achieved with almost complete sparing of both the lungs and heart and with no high weighted Bragg peaks being directed at the spinal cord.

**Error analysis.**

The recalculated dose distribution with 10% reduced CT values is shown in figure 2b. Although an overshoot of dose from the RPO and LPO beams into the lungs is clearly seen, no similar effect is evident in the region of the spinal cord, indicating that the plan is relatively insensitive to range errors in this region. Indeed, comparison of the nominal and overshoot spinal cord DVHs showed that although the mean dose to the cord would be increased in the case of such an error in range, the maximum dose would remain the same (58Gy in both cases).

Figure 2c shows a composite, or 'worst case', dose distribution derived from the six error dose distributions resulting from the set-up error analysis (one for each of the offsets along the major anatomical axes). This 'worst case' distribution is constructed by taking, on a point by point basis, the *minimum* dose from these six distributions for each dose grid point that is *within* the target volume, and the *maximum* dose for each point that is *outside* of the target volume. Although the resultant dose distribution is clearly unphysical, it provides one sided error-bands for the nominal calculated doses and a succinct format by which target coverage and normal tissue dose can be viewed and assessed in the light of the potential errors associated with fractionated radiotherapy.

The 'worst case' distribution clearly shows the possibility of cold regions in the target volume as the result of positioning errors (figure 2c). Further analysis revealed that these areas would result from offsets of the patients positioning in the AP direction in particular. This information was subsequently used to guide the radiographers performing the daily treatment set-ups such that systematic offsets of the patient along this axis could be avoided. That this could be achieved successfully is indicated by the post-treatment analysis of the patients positioning, assessed from the orthogonal scout images acquired routinely prior to the delivery of each fraction. Although day to day variations of the order +/- 4mm (2SD) were observed, the mean offset over all fractions in the AP direction was found to be only 0.1mm.

Of the other checks performed, the Monte Carlo calculation did not differ significantly from the analytical dose calculation and the measured dose in water was accurate to 2% for all the fields. An example profile from the verification of this plan in water is shown in figure 3.

Due to the site of the lesion and the dynamic nature of the treatment method, it was also considered necessary to assess the magnitude of the organ motion in the region of the target volume. To this purpose, representative inhalation and exhalation CT slices were acquired twice through the course of the treatment. Both checks indicated that motion in the

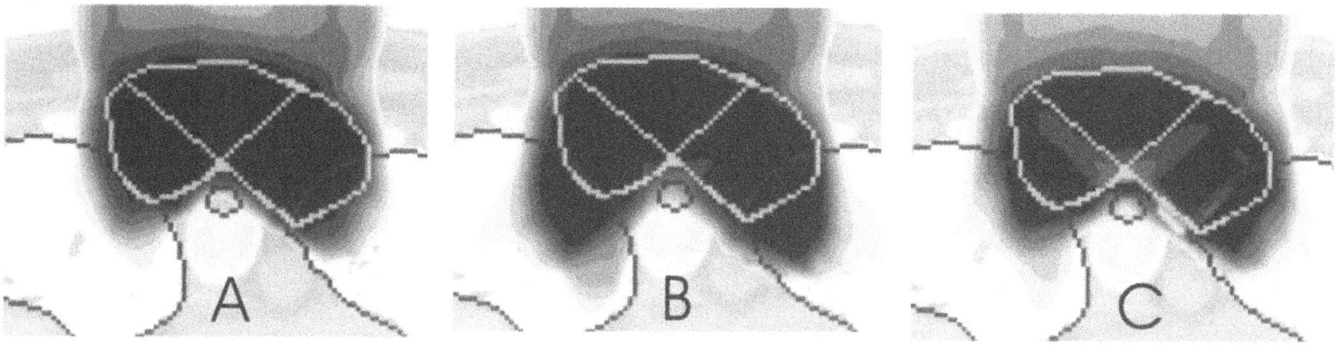


**Figure 2:** The nominal (A), 10% overshoot (B) and worst case (C ) 3 field IMPT plans. Note degree of conformation achieved by the nominal plan (A), the sparing of the spinal cord even when considering large range uncertainties (B) and the potential cold areas (< 95% of PTV dose) along the patch lines that could result from positioning errors of 5mm in the AP direction.

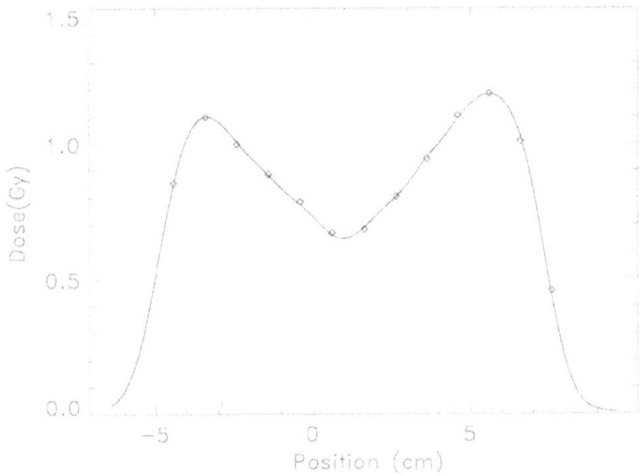


**Figure 3:** Predicted profile in water (solid line) and ionisation chamber meaurements (crosses) for the posterior field delivered in water.

region of the target was minimal (of the order of 1mm), even though motion in the thorax (away from the target volume) could be quite considerable.

## Discussion.

The close proximity of a high dose target to the spinal cord, coupled with the site of the lesion, in which many geometrically useful field directions were not useable due to the problems of treating through dynamically varying organs such as the heart and lungs, made this case particularly challenging. Through field patching and 3D IMPT, a high degree of conformity has been achieved with the use of only three field directions, resulting in a relatively short treatment time (typical delivery times per field of 1-2 minutes). In addition, by choosing three fields that all come from the posterior aspect of the patient, minimal dose is delivered to the heart and lungs and overall integral dose has also been significantly reduced.

The main advantage of this approach however, is the inherently safer set of Bragg peak positions and weights that result. That this is the case has been shown by the error analysis applied to this case. The range error analysis presented here has been calculated assuming a 10% underestimate of the CT (proton stopping power) values in treatment planning. In fact, this figure is something of a worst case value. Direct measurements of proton stopping powers for biological tissues indicate that these can be estimated from our CT with an accuracy of about 1% in soft tissues and 2% in bone [5]. However, as this patient was relatively large, we took a value of 10% for this case to also allow for day to day variations in the amount of soft tissue that may lie posteriorly to the target volume. Even with this relatively large error, the spinal cord was found to be well protected using this treatment technique. Although other effects were observed when assessing potential positioning errors, these could be predicted *a priori* and could to a certain extent be controlled through careful assessment, and if necessary correction, of the patients position before each fraction was delivered.

Although the dose distributions delivered for each field for this case are quite different to those normally delivered to patients at our facility, it should be noted that this patient could nevertheless be treated with *no* modifications to our existing delivery hardware. As our treatments anyway consist of the delivery of many thousands of individually weighted Bragg peaks, whether these weights are calculated such as to deliver a homogenous or an in-homogenous dose across the target volume plays no role from the point of view of their delivery. As such, the resultant fields were verified and delivered in an identical way to our normal treatments. Indeed, the fields themselves, although essentially in-homogenous, are relatively smoothly varying (see figure 3), in contrast to what may be expected for multiple field IM X-ray plans.

## Conclusions.

3D IMPT has been clinically applied for the first time. Detailed error analysis of the plan has demonstrated that the treatment can be applied safely (indeed this was the main impetus to apply IMPT methods in this case) and that highly conformal plans can be constructed using small numbers of fields in a challenging treatment site.

## References.

[1] L.Wisser, G.Goitein, 1999 Protonentherapie am Paul Scherrer Institut - Erfahrungen der ersten drei Jahre Gantry Strahlenther Onkol S1,126

[2] Pedroni E, Bacher R, Blattmann H, Boehringer T, Coray A, Lomax A, Lin S, Munkel G, Scheib S, Schneider U, Tourovsky A 1995 The 200 MeV proton therapy project at PSI: Conceptual design and practical realisation *Med. Phys.* **22** 37-53.

[3] Lomax A, Pedroni E, Schaffner B, Scheib S, Schneider U, Tourovsky A 1996 3D treatment planning for conformal proton therapy by spot scanning *Proc. 19th L H Gray Conference, (BIR publishing, London)* 67-71

[4] Lomax A 1999 Intensity modulation methods for proton radiotherapy *Phys. Med. Biol.* **44** 185-205.

[5] Schaffner B, Pedroni E 1998 The precision of proton range calculations in proton treatment planning: experimental verification of the relation between CT-HU and proton stopping power *Phys. Med. Biol.* **43** 1579-1592

# Physical and Biological Dose Distribution Due to Primary Protons and Secondary Particles From Nuclear Interactions

**Harald Paganetti and Michael Goitein**

Department of Radiation Oncology, Massachusetts General Hospital, Boston, MA 02114, USA

## Introduction

Protons offer dose-shaping advantages over photons by virtue of their Bragg peak dose distributions. The challenge for physics is to develop proton treatment planning and delivery that takes full advantage of the physical superiority of protons over photons.
There are uncertainties in delivering radiation therapy, no matter what the modality; some of these are attributable to the dose calculation algorithm. We know that there are "error bars" on dose distributions and that treatment techniques (such as the design of proton beam penetration and compensation) have to take these errors into account. As a corollary, the more accurate the calculational algorithms, the less allowance one need make for algorithmic uncertainty and, in consequence, the better one can conform the dose to the target. We propose to follow the lead of Petti, who has demonstrated the value of Monte Carlo techniques in calculating proton dose in the patient, and has proposed an approach to take advantage of the increased understanding that it can provide [1].
We Have been interested in understanding physical effects in the beam line or patient. Available Monte Carlo codes differ both in the comprehensiveness with which they model the underlying physics and in the generality and ease of definition of the geometries which they can simulate. The choice of code depends a great deal on the problem one wishes to solve. For example, if dose distributions in the patient do not depend on the details of nuclear fragmentation, the burden on the physics is modest, but the representation of the geometries of both the beam delivery system and the patient needs to be very detailed and sophisticated. On the other hand, if one is interested in the radiobiological consequences of a given irradiation, nuclear fragmentation might be very important, while geometric details are likely to be relatively unimportant. Of course, a code which had all the physics and the most general possible geometric capabilities (and would run very fast!) would be the best of all possible choices. In practice, we need to solve different problems with different codes – and solve some problems for the individual patient and others for the general case. With respect to future fast Monte Carlo treatment planning, one goal was to find out the necessary accuracy with respect to the settings of calculation parameters and to the neglection of specific physical or biological effects.
At least three topics require the use of Monte Carlo technique, namely the modeling of beam delivery systems, the investigations on nuclear interaction effects, and the study of RBE effects.

## Material and methods

The beam simulation was done with the Monte Carlo code GEANT [2]. GEANT, although developed for high-energy applications, is well suited for investigations on proton radiation therapy [3, 4]. The particle transport includes electromagnetic and hadronic interactions. The generated particle distributions contain primary and secondary particles, the latter coming from inelastic nuclear interactions.
To estimate the influence of nuclear interactions on dose or biological effect one has to rely on nuclear models implemented in Monte Carlo programs. Recently, an experimental method to check these models at proton therapy energies was introduced measuring the distribution of projected ranges of charged secondaries from nuclear interactions in a stack of insulated copper plates using a 160 MeV proton beam [3]. The method measures charge rather than dose, and primary protons stopping by electromagnetic processes are completely separated. The stack was simulated using GEANT with two nuclear models. FLUKA [5] agrees quite well with the measurement but GHEISHA [6], designed for much higher energies, does not. We therefore suggest the use of the FLUKA nuclear interaction module .
To study the differences between the biologically equivalent dose and the physical dose, biophysical models have to be used. These models require biological parameters, e.g. the size of the cell nucleus and the response to x-ray radiation, as well as physical parameters, e.g. the LET distributions of the particles entering a given volume. The track structure theory [7, 8] was used to calculate the RBE values from the particle energy distributions obtained by the Monte Carlo simulations.

## Results and discussion

We did a Monte Carlo modeling of the beam delivery apparatus of the Northeast Proton Therapy Center (NPTC). Figure 1 shows such a simulation in which protons are followed through the gantry nozzle and the paths of primary and secondary particles are traced. Using this approach we have explored issues of neutron backgrounds and have been able to gain confidence that we are not experiencing a problem (either dosimetrically or radiobiologically) from low energy scattered protons or nuclear interaction products originating from the nozzle elements..
However, in the target volume secondary particles might become more important. The measured dose distribution in charged particle therapy contains the contributions from several different particle types. The total dose is the integral over the fluence and the linear energy transfer for all particle contributions. In proton radiation therapy, a significant contribution to the total dose could be, besides the primary protons, due to secondary protons, alpha particles, deuterons, and tritons originating from nuclear interactions.
The three-dimensional distributions of dose from primary and secondary particles have been calculated for a monoenergetic beam incident on a phantom consisting entirely of water

(Figure 2) and a water phantom containing a bone structure. The dose build-up due to secondary particles is visible and discredit Monte Carlo models where the secondary dose is deposited locally at the interaction point. In addition the particle energy distributions and the yields for different nuclear interaction channels (e.g., (p,p'), (p,n), (p,2p') etc. ) as a function of position in the phantoms were studied. The three-dimensional dose distribution reflects these three-dimensional reaction distributions.

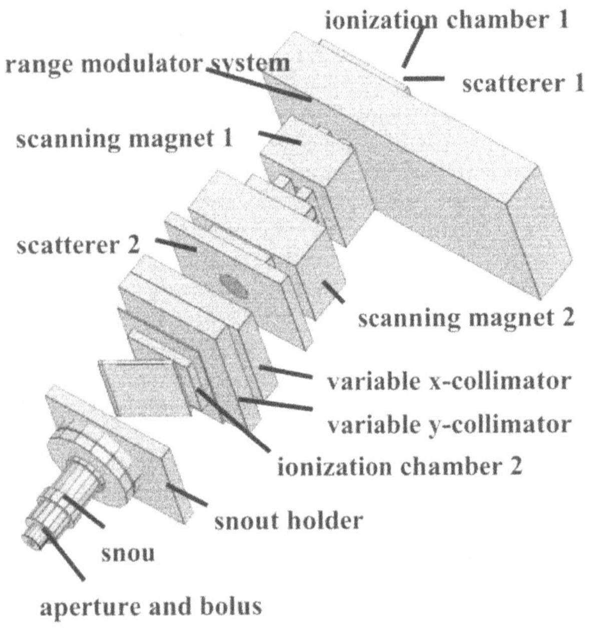


Figure 1: GEANT Monte Carlo simulation of the gantry nozzle at NPTC

There are several remaining technical problems in proton beam therapy such as the explanation of the elevated RBE in even the apparently relatively "low LET" entrance region. The explanations for these effects are likely to depend on details of the nuclear interactions of protons with target nuclei (i.e. species, energy and angular distributions of the nuclear fragments). RBE values have been calculated not only for primary protons but for charged secondaries. We studied the influence of secondaries other than protons in proton therapy in terms of their influence on the total RBE.

## Conclusion

Monte Carlo calculations are a powerful tool to study the influence of scattering effects in beam delivery systems. In addition, the study of nuclear interaction effects are of particular interest. After we tested the nuclear models used in GEANT experimentally, we studied the three-dimensional distribution of reaction channles and dose deposition originating from primary and secondary particles. A dose build-up effect due to nuclear interactions can be clearly seen. Therefore, detailed nuclear interactions models have to be included in Monte Carlo dose calculation engines for proton therapy. However, it remains questionable if the enhanced relative biological effectiveness from secondary particles heavier than protons has to be taken into account in general in proton therapy.

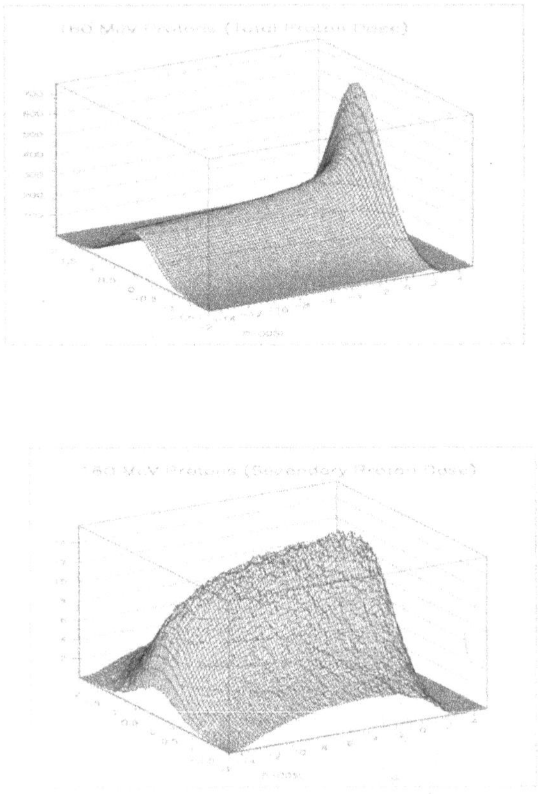

Figure 2: Primary and secondary proton dose distribution for a 160 MeV beam incident on a water phantom.

## References

[1] Petti P L 1996 Evaluation of a pencil-beam dose calculation technique for charged particle radiotherapy. *International Journal of Radiation Oncology, Biology, Physics* **35** 1049-1057

[2] Goosens M, Giani S, Ravndal S 1993 GEANT: detector description and simulation tool. *Technical Report CERN Program Library, long writeup, CERN, Geneva, Switzerland* **W5013**

[3] Gottschalk B, Platais R, Paganetti H 1999 Nuclear interactions of 160 MeV protons stopping in copper: a test of Monte Carlo nuclear models. *Medical Physics* in press

[4] Paganetti H 1998 Monte Carlo method to study the proton fluence for treatment planning. *Medical Physics* **25** 2370-2375

[5] Ferrari A, Sala P R 1997 Intermediate and high energy models in FLUKA: improvements, benchmarks and applications. *Conference Proceedings, Nuclear Data for Science and Technology, Reffo, G.; Ventura, A.; Grandi, C. (Eds.), SIF, Bologna* **59** 247-253

[6] Fesefeldt H C 1985 Simulation of hadronic showers; physics and applications. *Technical Report PITHA, RWTH Aachen* **85-02**

[7] Katz R 1988 Radiobiological Modeling Based On Track Structure. *Quantitative Mathematical Models in Radiation Biology, Edt. J. Kiefer* 57-83

[8] Paganetti H 1998 Calculation of the spatial variation of relative biological effectiveness in a therapeutic proton field for eye treatment. *Physics in Medicine and Biology* **43** 2147-2157

# A new planning tool for IMRT treatments: Implementation and first application for proton beams

**Simeon Nill, Uwe Oelfke and Thomas Bortfeld**
DKFZ-Heidelberg, Department of Medical Physics, Im Neuenheimer Feld 280, 69120 Heidelberg

## Introduction

More and more dedicated clinical hadron facilities will be implemented in the near future. Especially, the use of proton beams is planned on a large scale in the United States. Central aim of these new treatment centers is to demonstrate a clinical advantage of charged particle beams in comparison to state of the art radiation therapy with high energy photons, i.e., in comparison to photon IMRT. While intensity modulated dose delivery techniques can be elegantly realised for hadronic beams with the spot scanning approach [1], currently available treatment planning tools for this costly therapy modality have not yet reached the high standards of IMRT planning tools for photon beams.

The most prominent approach for IMRT planning is based on the concept of inverse planning, where 2-dimensional fluence matrices for a number of pre-selected beam portals are directly derived from the desired 3-D dose distribution. For IMRT with heavy ion or proton beams (IMPT) the inverse planning approach has to be extended in order to account for individual energy variations of each beam spot. The program presented in this paper computes energy and fluence distributions for each specified beam portal with an iterative algorithm, which is adopted from the standard IMRT planning tool *KonRad* developed at the DKFZ [2]. Substantial changes and additions to the existing code were performed to create the basis for a multi-modality IMRT treatment planning system. E.g., a complete reorganization of the optimization loop had to be implemented. Moreover, a first version of a simple proton dose algorithm has been integrated into this experimental platform. In the following the important features of the program with some preliminary results will be described.

## Material and methods

The new program takes advantage of existing data structures (e.g. for CT data), graphic user interfaces, dose display utilities and DVH-analysis tools of the original *KonRad* program. Moreover, the set of available optimization criteria – the basic input for the optimization – process remained unchanged. The most striking changes occur in the reorganisation of the optimisation loop, which for most currently available inverse planning systems is intertwined with the dose calculation engine to reduce the speed of the iterative optimisation. The new *KonRad*-module achieves a clear modularization between the three profound optimization components, i.e., i) the dose calculation, ii) the evaluation of the objective function which ranks the obtained dose distributions and iii) the optimization algorithm (engine) used to find the minimum value of the objective function. The advantage of this concept is that each module can be easily and independently replaced by other optional components. However, to achieve this structural flexibility the program needs a large amount of computer memory (see table:2). The implemented optimization loop and the model for the proton dose calculation algorithm will be explained in the following subsections.

### The optimization loop

For the present implementation of the program standard dose constraints are used for the optimization of the 3-D dose distribution [3]: i) the target dose can be adjusted by thresholds for over- and underdosage and ii) the dose in organs at risk is optimized by the specification of a global tolerance dose or a set of dose-volume histogram constraints. The optimization parameters consist of the weight factors $\{w_j\}$ for the delivery of the pencil beams (or beam spots) $j$. Each pencil beam represents a defined number of particles of energy $E$, which are emitted from a pre-specified direction of incidence. Depending on the chosen technique for the treatment delivery, the number of beam spots and their respective weights can be easily in the order of a few ten-thousand. As an example, we have listed in table 2 the number of pencil beams obtained for the clinical case of a clivus chordoma for the distal edge tracking technique and a full 3D-modulation of beam intensities and energies as described by A. Lomax [4].

To accomplish the iterative solution of an optimisation problem with such an enormous number of degrees of freedom a pre-calculation of the 3-D dose distribution is performed once. The dose fraction $D_{ij}$ from a normalised pencil beam $j$ to the voxel $i$ is stored and used for every step in the iterative search for the optimal set of beam weights $\{w_j\}$. This optimisation strategy naturally requires a vast a mount of RAM for the treatment planning hardware. Some typical numbers for a considered clinical case can be found also in table 2.

Employing the described concept together with a fast gradient algorithm leads to the following iterative optimisation scheme :

i) Calculate the dose distribution and the value of its respective objective function $F(t)$ for a set of weigths $w_j(t)$ at iteration step $t$:

$$F(t) \equiv F(t)[\{d_i = \sum_j D_{ij} w_j(t)\}]$$

with $d_i$ as dose delivered to voxel $i$.

ii) Determine the gradient of $F$ with respect to $w_j$ and calculate the set of weights $w_j(t+1)$ for the next step of the iteration according to:

$$w_j(t+1) = w_j(t) - \alpha(D_{ij}) \frac{\partial F(t)}{\partial w_j(t)} [D_{ij}, w_j(t)]$$

The chosen scaling factor $\alpha$ as well as the partial derivative only depend on the pre-calulated dose matrix $D_{ij}$ and the weights $w_j(t)$.

iii) Go back to step i) of the iteration, i.e., evaluate the new dose distribution and objective function and continue through step ii) until a criterion on the value of the objective function ends the iteration.

### Proton dose calculation

As mentioned before, the dose calculation is done only once by computing the matrix $D_{ij}$. At the moment we have implemented a simple algorithm which employs measured depth dose curves for a broad proton beam as input for the central axis values $D_{\text{CAX}}$. The lateral dose fall-off is modeled by a Gaussian distribution with a depth dependent width $\sigma(l_{ij}^{\text{rad}})$. For any voxel $i$ of the CT-cube the lateral distance $r_{ij}$ to the central axis of pencil beam $j$ and the radiological pathlength $l_{ij}^{\text{rad}}$ are determined by employing the ray tracer of Siddon[5]. The basic geometry of the dose calculation is shown in figure (1).

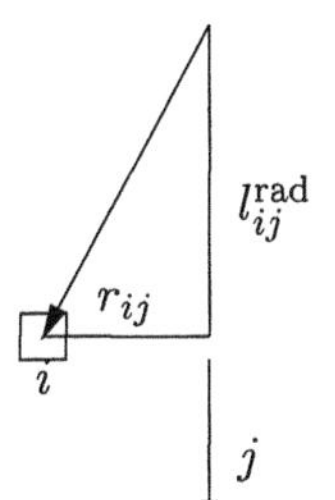


**Figure 1:** Dose calculation

With the given definitions the matrix $D_{ij}$ takes the form:

$$D_{ij} = \frac{1}{2\pi\sigma^2(l_{ij}^{\text{rad}})} * e^{-\frac{(r_{ij})^2}{2*\sigma^2(l_{ij}^{\text{rad}})}} * D_{\text{CAX}}(l_{ij}^{\text{rad}})$$

To increase the speed of the calculation only voxels with a lateral distance less than 3 $\sigma$ are taken into account. Inhomogeneity corrections are considered by one dimensional density scaling of the radiological pathlength along the central axis of the pencil beam. The lateral distribution $\sigma(l^{\text{rad}})$ is interpolated from stored data taken from ref. [6]. Fig. 2 displays a set of dose data for a 160 MeV proton beam 2).

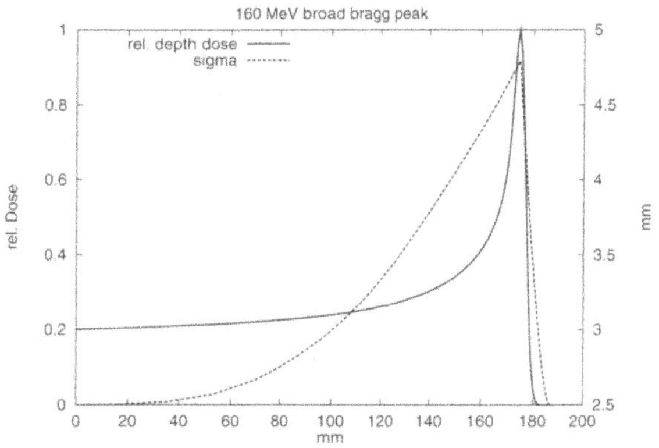


**Figure 2:** Sample of stored dose data

### The determination of the initial set of beam spots

A central issue of the spot scanning technique is the determination of the appropiate spot positions and respective beam energies. Based on the outlined tumor contours the program determines first the maximal beam energy for each spot such that the distal target edge coincides with the Bragg peak of the considered pencil beam. From these positions (denoted as (A) in Fig. 3) new Bragg peak positions are determined on a regular grid along their central axis(see Fig. 3).

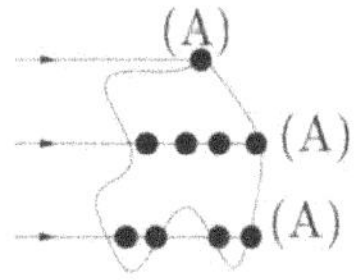


**Figure 3:** Spot positions

## Results and discussion

For a first test of the new platform we considered the clinical case of a clivus chordoma. The chosen target volume wraps directly around the brainstem, the only OAR considered in the optimization process. The organ parameters, which define the relevant dose constraints in our calculation are summarized in table (1). They were taken from a photon-IMRT treatment plan, created in an earlier study with the original *KonRad* system. First, the performance and hardware requirements of the new system were evaluated for the complete 3D spot-scanning technique and dose delivery via distal edge tracking (DET). The resolution of the dose grid was 2.62 $mm^2$ and the proton beam spots were placed on a 3 mm equidistant grid. The calulations were performed on a DEC-$\alpha$ (500 Mhz) with 1.5 GB of RAM.

| | target | brainstem | patient contour |
|---|---|---|---|
| min dose | 68 | 0 | 0 |
| min penalty $s$ | 99 | 0 | 0 |
| max dose | 71.5 | 0 | 70 |
| max penalty $s$ | 20 | 6 | 3 |

**Table 1:** Organ parameter

The number of optimization parameters together with the used RAM and observed calculation times for a treatment with 5 and 7 portals are shown in table 2. For the full 3D-scanning mode and a maximum number of 57200 beam weights the optimization could be done within 4 hours. For our example, the DET technique was approximately faster by a factor of 10 in comparsion to the 3D-technique without compromising the quality of the treatment plan. However, one has to note that observation is made just for this specific clinical case.

| Number of fields | Technique | Number of pencil beams | Memory (MB) | Time (h) |
|---|---|---|---|---|
| 5 | DET | 2720 | 60 | 0.3 |
| 7 | DET | 3807 | 80 | 0.5 |
| 5 | 3D | 40000 | 700 | 3 |
| 7 | 3D | 57200 | 900 | 4 |

**Table 2:** Overview of different techniques

As a second result, we compare a seven beam IMRT plan for 15 MV photons with the proton IMRT obtained for 3D spot scanning. The corresponding dose volume histograms for the target volume and the brainstem are shown in fig. 4. While the dose coverage of the target is identical for photons and protons, a significant dose sparing of the brainstem is achieved by employing proton IMRT. Again, one has to keep in mind that this is only one patient for which the same organ parameters and penalty values in the objective function were used.

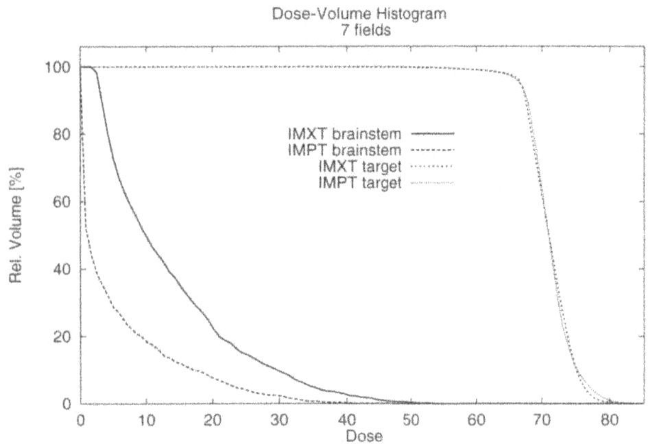


**Figure 4:** DVH comparision of a 7 field plan

## Conclusion

We have presented a first treatment planning platform which conceptually allows the optimization of different beam modalities, dose delivery techniques and optimization concepts. This was achieved by restructuring the software design of the original treatment planning software *KonRad*, currently used for IMRT treatment planning with photons. In order to test the new software for IMRT treatment planning with charged particle beams, a simple proton dose algorithm was integrated in the software package and tested for a first clinical case. Further evaluation and testing of this program is necessary in the future.

### Acknowledgments

We would like to thank MRC Systems Heidelberg – especially Dr. M. A. Keller Reichenbecher – for their support with the *KonRad* program.

## References

[1] Pedroni E et al., The 200 MeV proton therapy project at the PSI: conceptual design and practical realization, *Med. Phys.* **22**, 1995, 37-53

[2] Preiser K, Bortfeld T, Hartwig K, Schlegel W and Stein J, A new program for inverse radiotherapy planning *Procceding of XII Int. Conf on the Use of Computers in Radiation Therapy, Salt Lake City, Utah 1997*, p 425 -428

[3] Bortfeld T, Stein and Preiser K, Clinically relevant intensity modulation optimization using physical constraints *Procceding of XII Int. Conf on the Use of Computers in Radiation Therapy, Salt Lake City, Utah 1997*, p 1 - 4

[4] Lomax J A, Intensity modulation methods for proton radiotherapy *Physics in Medicine and Biology* **44**, 1999, 185–205

[5] Siddon R L, Calculation of the radiological depth *Medical Physics* **12** 84–87

[6] K. U. Gardey, A pencil beam model for proton therapy - treatment planning and experimental results, PhD Thesis, DKFZ Heidelberg, 1996

# OCTOPUS, a planning tool for proton therapy of eye tumours

**Karsten Pfeiffer[1], Barbara Dobler[1], Christoph Rethfeldt[2], Wolfgang Schlegel[1], Rolf Bendl[1]**

[1] Deutsches Krebsforschungszentrum, Abt. Medizinische Physik, INF 280, 69120 Heidelberg, Germany,
[2] Hahn Meitner Institut, Gleinicker Str. 100, 14109 Berlin, Germany

## Introduction

Radiotherapy of eye tumours with proton beams is a successful treatment method established in more than twenty medical proton facilities throughout the world. So far the therapy planning is done with the program *EYEPLAN* [1] that now has been used for 15 years. *EYEPLAN* has several restrictions (e.g.: a simple spherical eye model, no support of modern three-dimensional image sequences). These restrictions may lead to planning uncertainties in about 20% of all treated cases, as experience of radiotherapists at the Hahn-Meitner-Institute (HMI) in Berlin has shown. To guarantee in those cases the necessary therapeutical dose in the target volume, safety margins must be increased. This may increase the side effects of the treatment, since radiosensitive structures near the target volume may suffer from high doses, which would lead to severe impairment or even loss of sight.
These uncertainties in the planning process shall be overcome by our new program *OCTOPUS* (*OCular Tumour Planning UitilitieS*). We hope, that by means of the enhanced precision of this new program side effects of such treatments can be reduced for a markedly number of patients. Furthermore *OCTOPUS* shall allow a more efficient and ergonomic treatment, to arrive at an optimal plan more quickly.
*OCTOPUS* was developed at the German Cancer Research Centre (DKFZ) in collaboration with HMI in Berlin, where it will be used for treatment planning.

## Material and methods

### Treatment Procedure

Because of the anatomy of the eye there are some additional difficulties, in contrast to conventional radiotherapy:

- Distances between target volume and structures at risk in the eye are in the range of mm and sub mm. The required precision in treatment planning, positioning and verification are much higher.
- The eyeball can move freely. An active or passive fixation method is necessary, to reposition the patient exactly between fractions.
- Additional diagnostic input is available and should be considered, (e.g. the tumour can be seen through the lens non invasively).

A detailed description of the standard treatment procedure can be found in [2]. The patient is treated sitting on a movable chair, his head is immobilised with a mask (see figure 1). A mono-energetic proton beam is widened by scattering foils and its energy is decreased by an absorber to fit the maximum depth of the tumour. A dynamic range modulation of the protons is achieved by a spinning wheel of variable thickness that adds extra path length through material and allows the adaptation of the depth of the Spread Out Bragg Peak (SOBP) to the longitudinal size of the tumour. In front of the eye a collimator achieves a tumour-conform *lateral* adaptation of the homogeneous proton beam..
As the proton beam delivery system is stationary in most facilities, the *eye* has to be positioned in a way, that the desired irradiation direction is achieved. This is done by chair translation and (re)positioning of a fixation light that the patient is gazing at. With this procedure alone, a reproducibility of positioning between two fractions of 1 *mm* can be achieved already [3]. To verify the actual position of the tumour, Tantal markers are used, which are sewn on the Sclera around the tumour. The clips can be detected quite well on X-ray images. The clip positions in two ortogonal X-ray images, made in treatment position, are compared with the positions predicted by the therapy planning program. Then the position of treatment chair *and* fixation light are adapted iteratively until the predicted position is reached. In this way the setup precision is better than 0.2 *mm* [3].
To conform the dose better to the tumour's distal end wedges

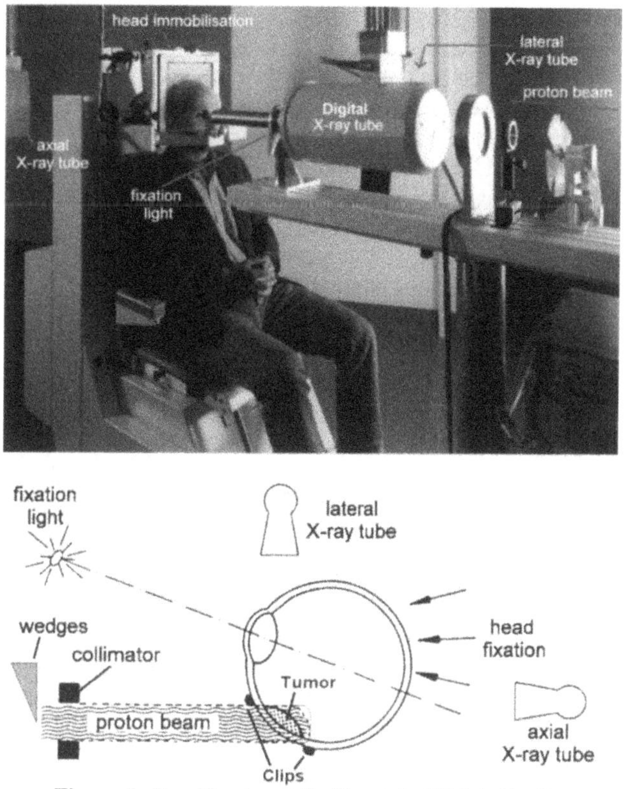


**Figure 1:** Top: Treatment facility at the HMI in Berlin, Bottom: schematic sketch of the treatment process.

can be used. In contrast to radiotherapy with photons, they do not modulate intensity of the beam (number of particles) but the entrance energy of the incoming protons and thus, they only *shift* the dose distribution to a more proximal location.

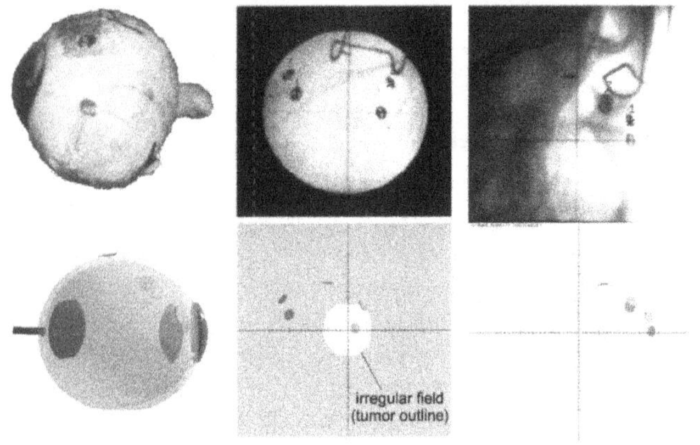


**Figure 2:** Top row: real pictures. Bottom row: program output. Left: pig's eye with Tantal clips sewn on Sclera (top) and model of human eye (bottom). Center: axial X-ray and right column: lateral X-ray of the eye with actual and predicted clip positions (patient not yet positioned exactly)

### Planning Process

As a result of the planning process the program has to provide the maximum depth and width of the SOPB, the form of the collimator, the position of the fixation light, parameters for the wedges and two artificial orthogonal X-ray images, showing the clip positions for iterative positioning of the patient (see figure 2).

The planning process consists of five independent steps:

1. Modelling the patient's eye.
2. Choosing treatment parameters:
   - Position of fixation light = gazing angle
   - Lateral, distal and proximal safety margins
   - Wedges (orientation, inclination, distance to isocenter)
   - Form of patient contour
   - Distance of eyes for calculation of viewing parallax, if fixating eye is not tumour eye
3. Dose calculation with precise algorithm
4. Evaluation of plan and iterative adaptation → step 2.
5. Choosing one of the calculated plans

To make the planning process in *OCTOPUS* more precise, step (1) and (3) were improved in comparison to *EYEPLAN*. The improvement is achieved by a more complex eye model, which can be adapted interactively to CT or MR data sets. They eye is represented by an ellipsoid and not only by a simple sphere. In addition, a pencil beam algorithm was implemented, which is able to consider the density information of CT data sets and beam properties more precisely.
To increase the efficiency step (2) and (4) were fused by means of a real-time dose calculation, that allows a direct evaluation of the current plan, simultaneously to parameter changes. This allows promptly the rejection of sub-optimal parameter sets. Therefore the precise but time consuming pencil beam algorithm must be involved less often. This way, the planning time can be reduced markedly.

## Results and discussion

*OCTOPUS* is a dedicated planning tool for proton therapy of eye tumours. A graphical user interface, that allows a direct evaluation of the selected plan parameters has been implemented. This is achieved by a 3D- real time dose calculation, that was fully integrated into the graphical user interface of *OCTOPUS*. While the user selects therapy parameters as e.g. gazing angles in the Beam's Eye View (see figure 3 upper left) a three dimensional dose distribution is calculated and visualised in the eye model in the Observer's View (see figure 3: bottom row). This dose distribution is an estimation of the deposited dose in the eye for the selected treatment parameters. As speed was given a priority for this kind of calculation, several assumptions have been made:

- The density in the eye is assumed to be homogeneous. This is true for the eye within a few percent.
- The dose calculation considers only one beam, therefore complex geometric overlaps of different beams need not to be calculated. This is no limitation for proton therapy of eye tumours, since for that kind of treatment normally only one beam is used.
- The dose calculation is performed on the eye model ($\approx 10^4$ triangles) and not on the CT cube ($\approx 10^6$ voxels). So the dose distribution becomes sensitive to segmentation artefacts
- The dose is not represented in a dose cube with $10^6$ voxels, but by triangulated surfaces of isodose volumes ($\approx 10^4$ triangles). This restriction to only a few fixed isodose intervals is a loss of information, which cannot be regained.
- These isodose volumes are all modelled as a function of 30 parameters: 10 sampling points each to describe the lateral,

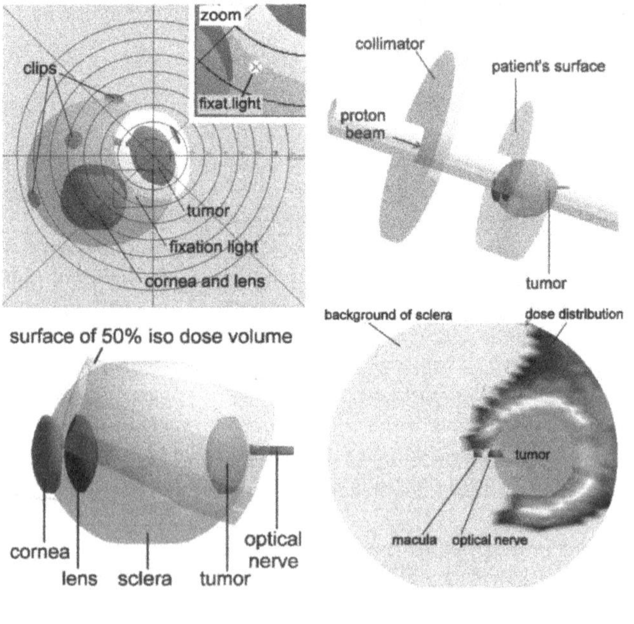


**Figure 3:** Top: 3D eye model in beam's eye view and observers view, Bottom: Dose distribution of real time dose calculation in observer's view and in virtual fundus view

proximal and distal dose drop. These dose drops are assumed to be independent of depth and width of the SOPB, that is size and location of the tumour.

These restrictions lead to a dose distribution where about 65% of the voxels in the dose cube show no difference compared to a dose distribution produced by the pencil beam algorithm (error less than ±5%) [7]. For 30% of the voxels differences of less than 10% were observed. It should be noted however, that the algorithm does not aim to give the correct answer, but to give a first impression of the qualitative dose distribution in relation to the eye structures. It turned out, that it shows the overall topology quite accurate. To do the fine tuning, later on in the planning procedure, the dose distribution should be calculated with a more precise but time consuming algorithm.

**Program Features for higher efficiency**

Once the dose calculation modelled the isodose surfaces, an estimation of the dose for any point in space can be given. This way dose volume histograms (DVHs) can be generated in real-time, too, with the restriction of only 10 dose bins. As the DVHs are monotone functions, a reasonable smooth curve can be achieved by interpolation. Furthermore the dose distribution can be displayed on an artificial Fundus View (2-D projection of the eye's background) or on the surface of any other eye structures in the three dimensional model [6]. All these preliminary dose distributions allow the radiotherapist a direct evaluation of the selected plan parameters *during* the planning process and lead to a new, straight forward approach to treatment planning.

After dose calculation with the implemented, more precise pencil beam algorithm, the resulting dose distributions can be visualised to show different aspects of a plan simultaneously: Dose visualisation in the 3D eye model, on CT slices, on a virtual Fundus View, in dose volume histograms and TCP/NTCP calculations are implemented among others. Furthermore it is possible to load several plans and compare them to each other. Tools are provided, to enhance the differences of these plans, as subtraction of dose volume histograms or dose distributions.

**Program Features for higher precision**

Most eyes can be modelled by a simple geometrical model without problems. But already for patient that suffer from myopia a spherical geometry may not be sufficiently precise to model the eye. Very deformed eyes finally (e.g. after prior operations) lead to unsuperable difficulties in the planning process when constricting the eye model to such a basic geometry. Therefore the model was not restricted to such a fixed geometry.

To make the model as flexible as possible the patient's eye geometry is represented by a model with more parameters. The modelling is done in three steps. First parameters of an *elliptical* eye model (such as eye length and width, cornea radius, distance lens-cornea etc.) can be entered numerically. Then this eye (or a pre-selected eye with standard parameters) can be fitted interactively to CT or MR images. In this procedure the whole eye or only some selected substructures can be transformed independently by translation, rotation and scaling. If by this proceeding the fit of the model to the eye cannot be achieved with the desired precision, all structures may be adapted individually to fit even very deformed eyes in a fourth step. [4].

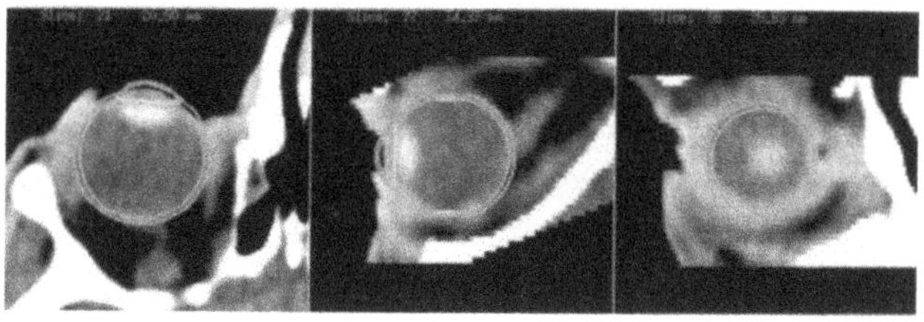

**Figure 4:** Fitting the eye model to a CT cube (transversal, sagittal and frontal view) by rotation, translation and scaling.

As already mentioned a pencil beam algorithm was implemented at the HMI for the calculation of an accurate dose distribution and thus enable the radiotherapist to evaluate the selected parameters for a given plan as precise as possible. To achieve this the calculation takes into account the properties of the HMI proton facility in detail [5] and is based on CT cubes and thus considers the inhomogeneous density in the patient's eye. Furthermore it does not depend on the eye model and so is less sensitive to segmentation artefacts. By this means it can describe the individual dose drops of the SOBP for different tumour depths, forms and sizes and in different patients more accurately.

## Conclusion

With *OCTOPUS* a new treatment planning tool for proton therapy of eye tumours has been implemented, to offer the functionality required for such a treatment planning process. We hope that by the new tools the planning process will become more precise and efficient. *OCTOPUS* has been installed at the HMI in Berlin recently, to test it in a clinical environment.

## References


[1] Goitein M. et al., 1983; Planning proton therapy of the eye; *Med. Phys.* **10** 275

[2] Alberti W.E.,.Sagermann R.H (editors), 1993, Radiotherapy of Intraocular and orbital tumours; *Springer*

[3] Chauvel P. et al., 1997, Clinical and Technical Requirements for Proton Traetment Planning of Ocular Diseases, in T. Wiegel (Hrsg) Radiotherapy of Ocular Disease; *Front. Radiat. Ther. Oncol.* **30** 133

[4] Dobler B., 1999 A new eye model for precise proton therapy of ocular tumours ; *Radioth. Oncol.* **51** s8

[5] Paganetti H., 1998, Monte Carlo method to study the proton fluence for treatment planning, *Med. Phys.* **25** 2370

[6] Pfeiffer K., 1999 A new eye model for precise proton therapy of ocular tumours ; *Radioth. Oncol.* **51** s48

[7] Pfeiffer K., 1999 Implementierung eines Echtzeitdosisberechnungsalgorithmus für die Protonentherapieplanung bei Augentumouren; *PhD Thesis, University Heidelberg.* **51** s48

# Patient set-up for proton radiotherapy using digital X-ray images of implanted fiducials

**Piotr Zygmanski and Stanley Rosenthal**

Department of Radiation Oncology, Massachusetts General Hospital, Boston, MA 02114-2696, USA

## Introduction

Efficient employment of the superior physical characteristics of protons (dose localization in depth as well as in the latteral direction [1]) for fractionated therapy requires high level of patient registration accuracy. For the localization required in proton beam therapy we routinely employ radiographic alignment, using a set of three orthogonal x-ray tubes. Orthogonal x-ray images of the patient are compared with the prescription geometry, which is usually recorded as Digitally Reconstructed Radiographs (DRR) generated by the treatment planning program for each set up. We align to either anatomic landmarks or, in a technique which we introduced [2], implanted fiducial markers. The anatomic landmarks technique has larger localization tolerance than the fiducial markers technique, but it has an advantage of being noninvasive and is a more generally applicable.

To improve speed and accuracy in positioning of proton therapy patients we have developed a semi-automatic stereotactic digital imaging systemcalled DIGIRAD. In developing the system we have been following the criteria of: (i) a translation and rotational accuracy and reproducibility of 0.5 mm and 0.5 deg correspondingly, (ii) fast, reliable and practical (user friendly) computer / image processing tools, (iii) flexibility of the software to include set up based on fiducial markers to be extended to anatomical landmark based set-up.

## Material and methods

Three radio-opaque markers are implanted in the outer table of a patient's skull. The positions of the markers relative to the beam directions and isocenter, determined from treatment planning, constitute a 3-D reference position for the treatment (Figure 1).

In order to determine 3D translation and rotation transformations needed to move patient to the prescribed reference position a pair of orthogonal diagnostic images aligned to isocenter are captured digitally at treatment time. The 3D transformations are calculated in a number of steps: (i) from the two radiographic images 2D image coordinates of the three fiducial markers are obtained, (ii) images are corrected for artifacts of the image capture system (ii) these image coordinates are rescaled to give the respective coordinates of the markers in the two detector planes, (iii) from the knowledge of the coordinates in the detector planes and the position of the detector planes with respect to the isocenter 3D coordinates of the markers in the physical space are determined, (iv) the three markers define a 3D orthogonal system, which is compared to a system defined by the prescribed reference treatment positions of the markers, and (v) the transfromations are found by performing a least-square-fit (LSF) on the ideal and measured coordinates.

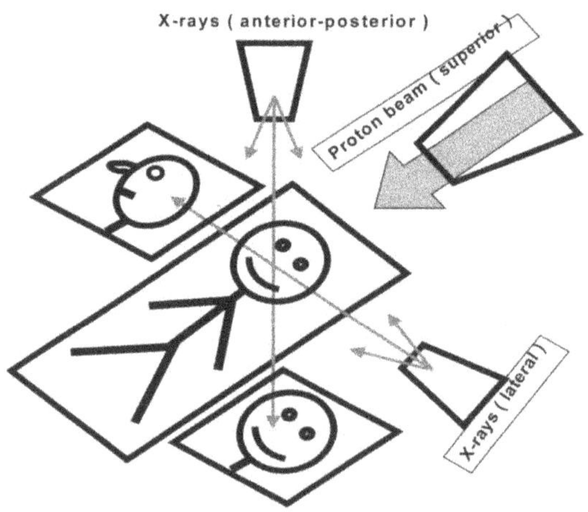


**Figure 1:** Patient set-up for proton treatment.

We have installed two imaging devices consisting of CCD cameras and gadolinium intensifying screens having fields of view of 30 x 30 cm in the treatment room (Figure 2). One of the devices sits below the couch and another at the side of the patient and can be retracted when not in use. The distance to the isocenter is different for each CCD, however, due to their different sizes (512 x 512 and 1024x1024 pixels) the spatial resolution is about 2.0-3.0 line pairs/mm at isocenter. We use scientific grade cooled CCDs of low noise properties manufactured by Tektronics as well as Kodak Lanex Regular intensifying screens. One of the CCDs is incorporated in a camera system by PMIS Photometrics and another by MedOptics. Each camera runs its own vendor supplied software. We have written software to incorporate both these systems and general enough to use other imaging devices.

A program has been developed to provide an easy interface for therapists to capture digital radiography images and rapidly to identify fiducial markers with sub-mm accuracy (Figure 3). The system communicates with the patient positioning system to move the couch and align the patient and greatly speeds up patient setup by eliminating film development, film analysis, and minimizing human errors.

The therapist interface software has been written in IDL and is runs on a PC. An algorithm based on rigid body transformations computes the 3-D realignment motions necessary to bring the patient to the desired position for treatment. The use of a digital imaging system permits automated fiducial marker recognition and localization.

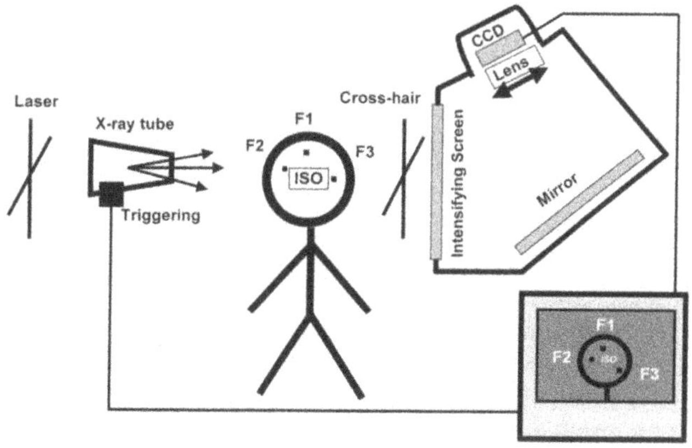


**Figure 2:** Schematic representation of the CCD-intensifying screen system

## Results and discussion

The accuracy of repositioning phantoms using the technique described in [1] in the patient room at the Harvard Cyclotron Laboratory (HCL) is better than 0.5 mm and 0.5 degrees (1 standard deviation). The accuracy in routine positioning of patients is limited to 1 mm and 1 degree due to patient motion and treatment device innaccuracies. These limitations which can be improved as follows. Projected cross wires are used to define isocenter, instead by rigidly fixing the imaging planes we can tie isocenter to a pixel location. The patient positioner couch has a back-lash greater than 1 mm. The prescription is based on the 3D location of markers from a CT scan this contributes up to 1.0 mm uncertainty in the slice direction.

We have found that the inherent precision of the image processing tools that we use in localization of the fiducial markers depends on the marker size. For our 1 mm spherical markers it is better than 1 pixel, which is equivalent to one third of mm. Improving the other set-up devices will allow 0.5 mm / 0.5 deg accuracy for the routine patient localization.

Our experience suggests that it will be possible to perform the image capture and analysis, and program the requisit couch correction moves in less than 15 seconds.

## Conclusion

We have developed a fast and practical digital patient positioning system that uses fiducial markers as the stereotactic frame of reference.

It has been shown that this system, which does not require invasive immobilization devices, has superior accuracy [3,4]. Our future work will include realizing the sub-millimeter accuracy at an upgraded treatment facility now under construction, and the clinical extension of the system to include anatomical landmark set-up. The software tools that we have developed are readily available for such an extension.

## References

[1] Verhey L J and Munzenrider J E 1982 Proton Beam Therapy *Ann. Rev. Biophys. Bioeng.* **11** 331-339

[2] Gall KP, Verhey LJ and Wagner M 1992 Computer-assisted positioning of radiotherapy patients using implanted radiopaque fiducials *Med. Phys.* **20**, 1153-1159

[3] Gilhuijs KGA, van de Ven PJP and van Herk M 1995 Automatic three-dimensional inspection of patient setup in radiation therapy using portal images, simulator images, and computed tomography data *Med. Phys.* **20**, 667-677

[4] Lemieux L, Jagoe R, Fish DR, Kitchen ND and Thomas DGT 1994 A patient-to-computed-tomography image registration method based on digitally reconstructed radiographs *Phys. Med. Biol.* **39**, 1925-1928

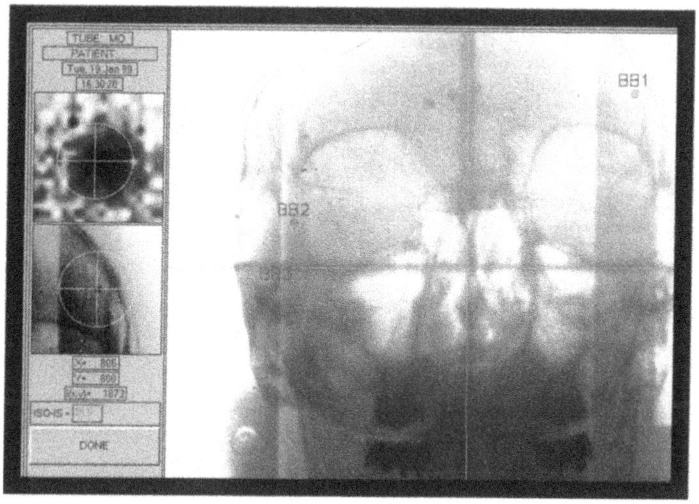


**Figure 3:** Screen from "DIGIRAD" Patient Localization Program

# VolEye - An application for interactive 3D-visualization and treatment planning of intraocular tumors

**T. Holtkämper[1,2,3], M. Bambynek[1,2], U. Quast[2], P. Spilles[2,4], D. Wegener[1]**
[1]Institut für Physik, Universität Dortmund, D-44221 Dortmund, Germany, [2]Klinische Strahlenphysik, Abteilung für Strahlentherapie, Universitätsklinikum, D-45122 Essen, Germany, [3]Institut für Medienkommunikation, GMD - Forschungszentrum Informationstechnik GmbH, D-53754 Sankt Augustin, Germany, and [4]Institut für Informatik, Universität Dortmund, D-44221 Dortmund, Germany

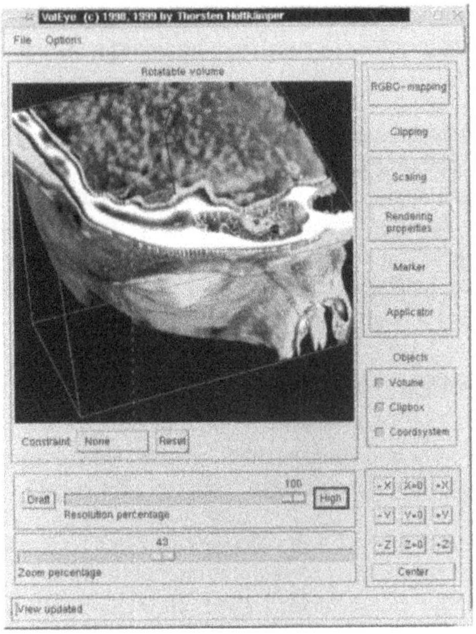


**Figure 1:** The VolEye main window.

## Introduction

Curative brachytherapy of small and medium sized intraocular tumors by applying ophthalmic plaques has been established for years. The clinical experiences indicate that optimal tumor control and the avoidance of normal tissue complications can only be achieved if the location of the tumor and of the structues at risc as well as the spatial distribution of dose in the eye region are exactly known. To reach that goal we developed a computer application called VolEye (fig. 1), which uses 3D-visualizations of tomographic pictures of the affected eye. With VolEye it is possible to localize the tumor within the 3D-visualization of the eye, to insert an individual ophthalmic plaque and to request its dose distribution values at any spatial point.

## Material and methods

The 3D-visualizations of the affected eyes are based on data of CT-scanners installed at Essen University Hospital. It consists of up to 21 slices with a maximum resolution of 512 × 512 pixels. In a preprocessing step we enhanced the picture quality by increasing the number of slices up to 84 by linear interpolation. In addition we converted the different CT-scanner's data formats to a unified, VolEye-readable raw data format.

As visualization technique we used volume rendering, where additionally, artificially generated objects like the ophthalmic plaque or a three-dimensional cursor are modelled as polygon objects and shown within the volume rendering.

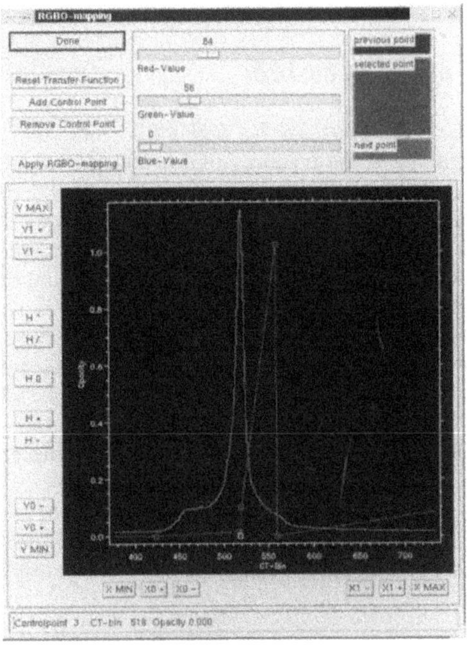


**Figure 2:** The VolEye window for transfer function manipulation. The axis of abscissae represents CT-values, the axis of ordinates opacity values. Color values are assigned to the control points of the transfer function (squares). In the background a CT value histogram is shown.

VolEye is designed as a client/server application: the server process is dedicated to rendering, the client process represents the graphical user interface to access the server's services. The client/server communication is realized through interprocess communication, e. g. named pipes, shared memory or signals. As programming language we used C++ for the server and IDL for the client application. The renderer is based on the multithreading C++ library Volume Graphics Library (VGL) which combines rendering of volumes and OpenGL polygon objects. Vol-

Eye runs on a double Pentium II processor system equipped with 256 MB of memory and driven by the GNU/Linux operating system.

Localization of selected anatomic structures is done by manipulating the transfer function between CT-values and the color and opacity values of the volume rendering. Since the quality of the localization results strongly depends on how accurately this transfer function can be manipulated we laid strong emphasis on the VolEye's user interface (fig. 2).

For the dosimetric part in VolEye we exemplarily measured 3D-distributions of dose of an $^{125}$I-plaque by using a single channel dosemeter system based on plastic scintillator. In order to determine relative dose values at certain spatial points within the CT-visualization, we developed a relation between voxel distances and metric values for the used CT-scanner.

## Results and discussion

The goal of tumor localization was reached. A high quality of the segmentation of the tumor tissue in the eyeball liquid could be accomplished, which fits well to the needs of treatment planning (fig. 3). We have shown that volume rendering based on CT data can efficiently be used as visualization technique to support eye tumor treatment, since, on one hand, it enables displaying transparency effects efficiently, and, on the other hand, the smoothing capablilities of volume rendering generate a realistic impression of the CT data while preserving accurate spatial information necessary for treatment planning.

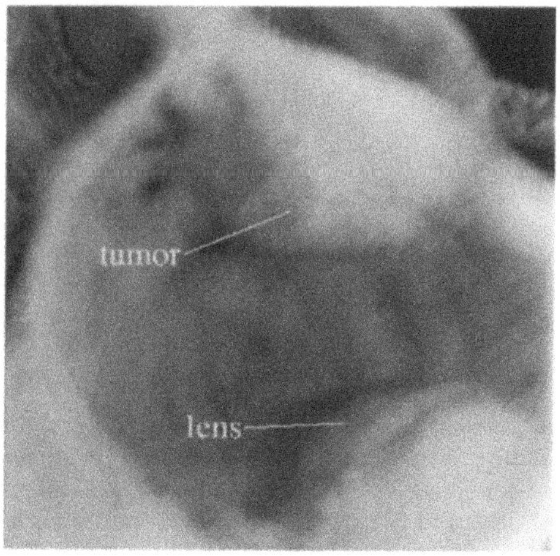


**Figure 3:** A tumor within the eyeball.

The basic dosimetric features in VolEye are implemented and already proofed their usability. Relative dose values in conjunction with metric values can directly be requested within the 3D-visualization (fig. 4). Future work will be the optimization of the 3D-cursor object and the plaque model for individual and non-symmetric plaques.

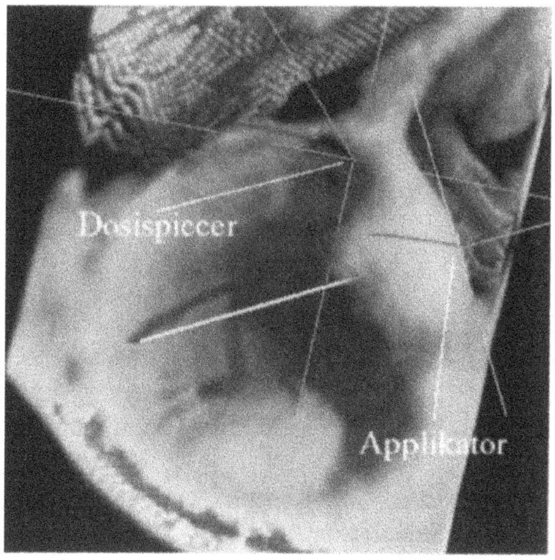


**Figure 4:** The plaque polygon object, the "Applikator", is placed right behind the tumor. The 3D-cursor, the "Dosispiccer", is placed in front of a structure at risc, the optic nerve.

## Acknowledgments

These investigations were partially supported by the Deutsche Forschungsgemeinschaft (DFG), the German Research Foundation, contract number Qu-39/7-1 and -2.

## References

[1] Holtkämper T 1999 Augentumor-Lokalisation und Dosimetrie in 3D-Visualisierungen von CT-Bildern *Diplomarbeit im Fachbereich Physik, Universität Dortmund*

[2] Flühs D, Heintz M, Indenkämpen F, Wieczorek C, Kolanoski H, Quast U 1996 Direct reading measurement of absorbed dose with plastic scintillators - The general concept and applications to ophthalmic plaque dosimetry *Med. Phys.* **23(3)** 427–434

# An improved 3D-Model for a Therapeutic Carbon Beam

**U.Weber[1], D.Schardt[1], P.Heeg[2] and G.Kraft[1]**

[1]GSI Darmstadt [2]DKFZ Heidelberg

## Introduction

The prerequisite for treatment planning with heavy ions and a raster scanner is an accurate beam model that provides the dose distribution, the fluence distribution and energy spectra of the primary carbon ions and secondary fragments in a water absorber [1].

Presently a one-dimensional model and an appropriate code (YIELD) [2] that calculates depth dose distributions $D_{E0}(z)$ and energy spectra for light heavy-ion beams (inclusive the secondary fragments) in dependence from the penetration depth in water are used. This model has been optimized over the years and agrees now very well with precise measurements of depth dose profiles [3]. In order to get a 3D-distribution, the one-dimensional depth dose profile D(z) is simply multiplied with a two-dimensional Gaussian function:

$$D(x,y,z) = D(z) \times \left(2\pi\sigma^2\right)^{-1} \exp\left(-(x^2+y^2)/(2\sigma^2)\right) \quad ,$$

where $\sigma=\sigma(z)$ depends on the penetration depth and the initial beam energy taking into account the beam envelope given by the ion optics and the continuous multiple scattering in a water absorber [4].

However, precise measurements of the transverse dose distribution show a deviation from a gaussian function at large distances ($r>2\sigma$) from the beam axis, especially behind the Bragg peak ($z>z_{peak}$). This can mainly be explained by two arguments:

- The Gaussian function is only an approximation to the Moliere distribution for multiple scattering [5].
- The fraction of the dose deposited by the secondary fragments is much more scattered than that of the primary particles and differs significantly from a Gaussian function [6].

## Material and methods

In order to improve the beam model with respect to these problems, we have developed a new Monte Carlo code that combines the one-dimensional spectra data calculated with the Haberer code (YIELD), the formulas of Moliere [7] for continuous multiple scattering in the absorber material and experimental angular distributions for fragment scattering ($^{12}C$ in water) [6].

The code can handle an initial beam divergence due to the ion optics and accepts any absorber material in any desired order or thickness. The subdivision of the absorbers in sufficiently thin slabs is done automatically. For all slabs i with depth $z_i$ the code produces the following output data for the use in treatment planning:

- The dose distribution $D_{E0}(x,y,z_i)$ of the beam (with initial beam energy $E_0$) and $D_{E0,Z}(x,y,z_i)$ for the fraction of the dose deposited by the fragments ($Z=1,2,\ldots,Z_0-1$) or by the primary particles ($Z=Z_0$).
- The fluence $F_{E0,Z}(x,y,z_i)$ of the particles ($Z=1\ldots Z_0$).

For the verification of these calculated data we measured the radial dose distribution in water of a 270 MeV/u $^{12}C$-beam using a parallel plate ionisation chamber as beam intensity monitor and a small diamond diode as dosimeter that could be moved automatically in x, y and z-direction.

First, the radial dose profile was measured at two different z-positions without water absorber in order to determine the beam divergence as input data for the Monte Carlo code. Then we measured the radial dose profiles in a water phantom (aquarium) in various depths: z=60mm (plateau region), 127mm (just before the Bragg peak) and 154mm (behind the Bragg Peak).

## Results and discussion

Fig 1 compares measured and calculated data where the dose values of the data points are multiplied with the corresponding radius r. This gives a better impression of the deposited energy, since the total energy loss of the beam at a penetration depth z is given by the integral $2\pi \int r \times D(r,z)\, dr$.

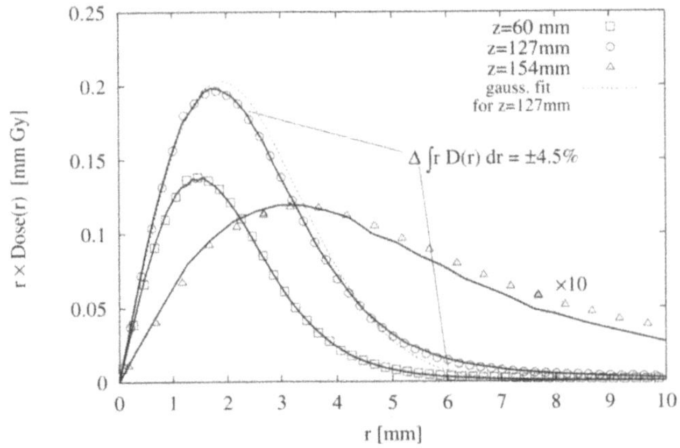


**Figure 1:** Measurement (points) and calculation (solid lines) of the radial dose distribution of a 270 MeV/u $^{12}C$ beam in water at different depths multiplied with the radius r. A Gaussian fit to the measured data of z=127 mm normalized to the same integral dose is shown for comparison. The integral difference $\Delta\int r \times D(r,z)dr$ from r=0 to 4.5mm between the Gaussian fit and the data is +4.5% of the total integral.

The deviation from the fitted Gaussian profile (z=127mm) becomes clearly visible. In the central part the measured dose values are lower and higher in the tail. This behavior is well reproduced by our improved beam model (solid lines) with accurate treatment of the beam scattering and angular distributions of secondary fragments.

As can be seen from the figure, typically 5% of the total deposited energy is shifted from the central part to the tail of the radial dose profile in comparison to the Gaussian approximation with the same integral dose. This makes clear that the Gaussian fit for the radial dose (or fluence) distribution leads to inaccuracies in the treatment planning which can be avoided by using this improved 3D-model.

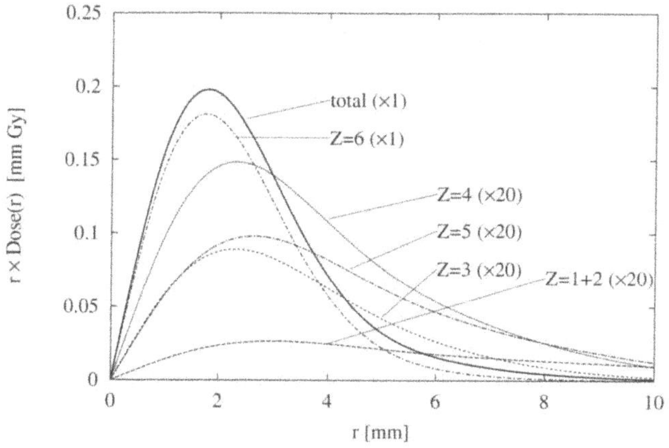


**Figure 2:** Calculated fraction of the dose deposited by the primary particles, the secondary fragments and the total dose.

Fig. 2 shows the calculated individual contributions of the fragments with different nuclear charge Z. It becomes visible that the width of the lateral dose distribution is much larger for the contribution of the light fragments.

## References

[1] Krämer M , Jäckel O 1997 Therapy planning for heavy ion therapy *Advances in Hadrontherapy* (Proc. Int. Week on Hadrontherapy ESI Archamps France (1995) and 2nd Int. Symposium on Hadrontherapy PSI and CERN Switzerland (1996)) (Amsterdam: Elsevier) pp 351-358

[2] Haberer T 1994 Entwicklung eines magnetischen Strahlführungssystems *PHD Thesis* Universität Heidelberg pp 73-93

[3] Schardt D 1993 Bragg curve measurements with ionisations chambers *GSI-Scietific Report 1992* GSI-93-1 p 336

[4] Weber U 1996 Volumenkonforme Bestrahlung mit Kohlenstoff-Ionen PHD Thesis GHK Kassel pp 24-36

[5] Moliere G 1948 Theorie der Streuung schneller geladener Teilchen *Z. Naturforsch.* **3a** 78

[6] Golovkov M et al. 1997 Fragmentation of 270 A MeV carbon ions in water *Advances in Hadrontherapy* (Proc. Int. Week on Hadrontherapy ESI Archamps France (1995) and 2nd Int. Symposium on Hadrontherapy PSI and CERN Switzerland (1996)) (Amsterdam: Elsevier) pp 316-24

[7] Gottschalk B et al. 1993 Multiple Coulomb scattering of 160 MeV protons *Nucl. Instrum. Methods* **B74** 467

# The depth-dose profile analyzer: a dosimetry system for fast measurement of 3D depth-dose profiles in charged-particle tumor therapy with scanning techniques

**C. Brusasco, B. Voss, D. Schardt, M. Krämer and G. Kraft**
GSI, Darmstadt

## Introduction

The verification of patient treatment plans is an extremely important task in radiotherapy; in fact it represents the final check of the correctness of the overall therapy procedure, from the dose optimization in the treatment plan up to the actual release of the irradiation by means of the beam-delivery system. The treatment plans performed at GSI, Darmstadt are characterized by a very high complexity because of the active beam-delivery system utilized. This system [1] shapes the dose distributions by scanning a pencil beam on the transversal shape of the target, while the energy of the beam is actively varied by the accelerator in order to shift the ions stopping-position in depth. As the resulting treatment plans have locally very high instantaneous dose rates, it is important to perform simultaneous measurements at many different points in the irradiation volume.
Two complications arise from the use of $^{12}C$ ions and a active beam-delivery system as far as the dosimetry is concerned:

- due to the fact that the beam sweeps across the target volume, for each measured point it is necessary to integrate the dose for the whole irradiation time (approximately 10 minutes at GSI);
- the dose deposited in the target volume results from the interaction of primary ions and secondary fragments with different energies.

The first point implies the necessity of a detector system with a high spatial granularity, as repeating several time the measurement would be too much time-consuming. The second point excludes the use of solid state detectors, because of their non linear response as a function of the energy and charge of the interacting particles. The use of ionization chambers instead allows measurements of the absolute dose with relative errors of the order of a few percent. However, it provides usually a poor spatial resolution in the target volume, because each detector represents one measured point only. As an example, the system adopted at GSI for the absolute dose measurements makes use of a water tank with 24 thimble ionization chambers, providing a sampling measurement of the dose in 24 isolated points in the target volume, but no full 3D reconstruction of the dose distributions. In order to achieve a 3D reconstruction of the relative depth-dose distributions in a short time, with high granularity and over large volumes, a new detector system was developed in GSI: the depth-dose profile analyzer.

## Material and methods

The principle of functioning of the depth-dose profile analyzer relies on the separation of the 3D dose measurement into two independent measurements, taking advantage of the active beam-delivery system of GSI:

1. the measurement of the one-dimensional depth-dose profile, integrated over the whole transversal area. This measurement is performed in our system by a stack of parallel-plate ionization chambers (IC) with plastic plates interleaved to simulate the patient tissue;
2. the acquisition of the shape of the dose deposition transversal to the beam by means of a Multi Wire Proportional Chamber (MWPC), coupled to a parallel-plate IC placed in front of the ICs-stack.

A sketch of the GSI detection system is shown in Fig. 1. For a fixed energy step, while the beam moves along a pre-

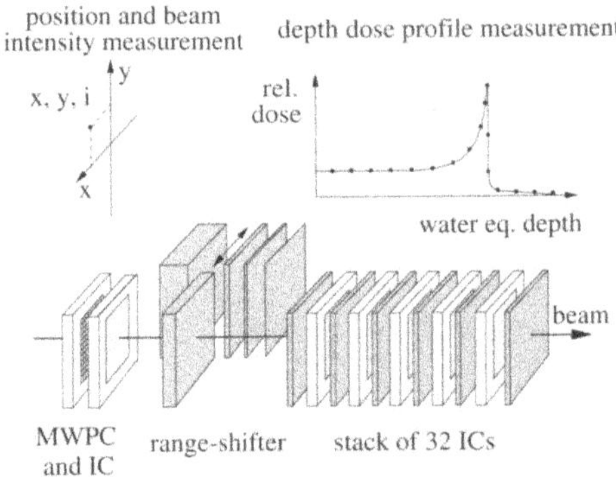


**Figure 1:** Sketch of the depth-dose profile analyzer.

defined pattern to irradiate the target in the transversal direction, the measurement of the transversal dose deposition is performed by the same monitor system that controls on-line the release of the treatment plan [2]. Two MWPCs record the movement of the beam with a sampling time of 150 $\mu$s and a position resolution of about 0.3 mm. Simultaneously, three ICs monitor the beam intensity with a sampling time of 12.5 $\mu$s. The detectors have an active area of (25x25) $cm^2$ and are read-out by a fast digitizing electronics, located on boards close to the chambers [3]. The measurements are processed by Digital Signal Processors placed on VME boards, which evaluate in real time the position, lateral profile and intensity of the beam [4].

The depth-dose profile for each energy step is measured by the stack of 32 ICs sandwiched between 5 mm thick plastic plates, which form the phantom of reference material. Each detector integrates the charge deposited on the whole active area. The convolution of the depth-dose profile with the transversal dose distribution provides a 3D reconstruction of the deposited dose corresponding to one energy step. By summing up the contributions from all the energies of the treatment the complete 3D dose distribution is obtained. The depth offset can be adjusted to the region of interest of a given treatment plan by means of a range shifter device, located in front of the IC stack, with a range from 0.6 to 300 mm of water-equivalent thickness. This device may also be used to increase the number of measured points in the depth-dose profile by shifting the absolute depth of the ICs stack and repeating the measurement. The 3D reconstruction is realized off-line by means of a C program as schematically shown in Fig. 2.

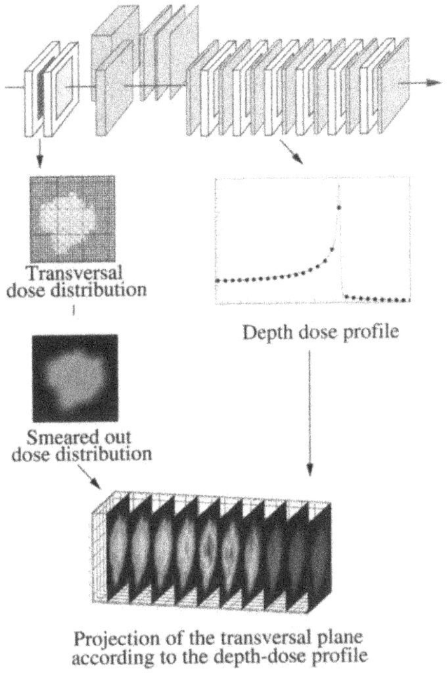


**Figure 2:** Principle of the 3D reconstruction of the treatment plans. The color code for the transversal dose distribution is the same as the one used in Fig. 3.

After the release of a plan, the software accesses the two data files corresponding respectively to the measured transversal dose distribution, acquired by the monitor system, and to its depth-dose profile, acquired by the stack of chambers. For each energy step, the program smears out the transversal dose distribution by reproducing the distribution of the ion density in the beam spot for every recorded position. For this purpose, the integral dose measured by the monitor chamber is distributed according to a two-dimensional gaussian function centered in the position measured by the coupled MWPC, with a FWHM fixed by the focusing setting of the beam. The convolution of the depth-dose profile with the transversal dose distribution provides a 3D reconstruction of the deposited dose, corresponding to one energy step. Then, by accumulating the contributions from all the energies of the treatment, the complete 3D dose distribution is obtained. The granularity in depth is fixed by the thickness of the comb slabs (5.6 mm of water equivalent) if the treatment is measured one time and can be improved by repeating the measurement with the insertion of slabs of the range-shifter. The granularity in the two dimensions orthogonal to the beam direction is defined by overlaying in the program a regular grid to the continuous transversal dose distribution (smeared out by the gaussian distribution of the beam intensity). In order to keep the 3D output file at a reasonable size , the step is normally fixed to 0.5 mm. For the visualization of the reconstruction, the IBM Visualization Data Explorer is used in the version 3.1.4. For the 3D visualization, the package performs an interpolation of the data according to a regular cubic grid. In principle, the 3D reconstruction can also be performed on-line in the time intervals between the spills by integrating the software into the therapy control system. The uncertainty in the dose measurement is the result of several different contributions coming from the leakage current of the ICs, from the non-linearity of the electronics, from the variation of the W value with the ion energy, from the loss of signal due to the recombination and from the poorer collection efficiency at the counter borders. The overall effect of all these contributions gives a asymmetric relative error of +3% and -1% in the measurements in the region corresponding to the target volume and in the plateau. The tail region has a higher relative error of the order of 20% originating from the leakage current contribution; however, since the corresponding dose deposition is very low, the absolute value of this error is negligible.

## Results and discussion

To verify if the program performs a correct 3D reconstruction, we measured a series of standard plans with simple geometrical shapes and with homogeneous or stepped dose depositions. In Fig. 3 the measurement corresponding to a cube of homogeneous dose deposition is shown. A cube with 2 cm edge length was centered at a water-equivalent depth of 12 cm. The beam enters the volume from the left side and the dose deposition is represented by means of a color scale. The 3D volume can be represented by means of slabs oriented in the three different volume planes, where the slabs orthogonal to the beam direction correspond in depth to the positions in water-equivalent of the ICs (plot *a*) in Fig. 3. The interpolation of the data along the beam direction allows the display of the longitudinal planes (plots *b*) and *c*) of Fig. 3. Another way to visualize the volume shape of the treatment plan is to use a representation with isodose surfaces. The volume is clipped by a plane cutting it in the middle and only the lower half is shown to allow a view of the internal structures (plot *d*) of Fig. 3.

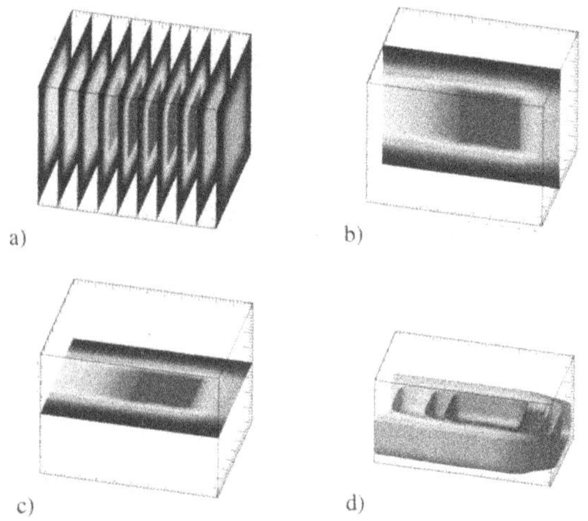


**Figure 3:** 3D measurement corresponding to a cube of homogeneous dose deposition. The dose deposition is represented by means of a color scale from blue to red. The red correspond to 95% of the measured maximum (to allow for a 5% error in the target dose), the blue to zero dose. Plot a) shows the slabs orthogonal to the beam direction and corresponding to 10 ICs of the stack. Plots b) and c) show the central slab of the two planes longitudinal to the beam. Plot d) shows an isosurface representation of the measurement. The dataset is divided in 10 equal intervals and the surfaces connect the isovalues corresponding to the boundaries of the intervals.

The next step was the verification of the patient specific treatment plans. In Fig. 4 a comparison of the measurement with the calculated treatment plan the measurement corresponding to one field of the first patient treatment at GSI in December 1997 is shown. The comparison is performed as the difference between the measured and the planned treatment for a slice positioned in the target volume (at 8 cm water-equivalent depth). As it can be seen the central area corresponding to the target volume shows differences as low as a few percents. At the borders of the treatment field the relative differences reach values of up to 35%, resulting in negligible absolute errors due to the very low dose deposited at the edges.

## Conclusion

With an active beam-delivery system, the principle of combining a position sensitive detector with a stack of ionization chambers and a range shifter represents a realistic way to obtain a 3D reconstruction of the relative depth-dose distributions with a good granularity and a relatively low number of electronics channels. The resolution in the transversal plane is better than 1 mm. Along the beam path, the granularity of the measurement is in average 5.76 mm when the PMMA plates are inserted. The offset in depth can be adjusted by a range-shifter with a range from

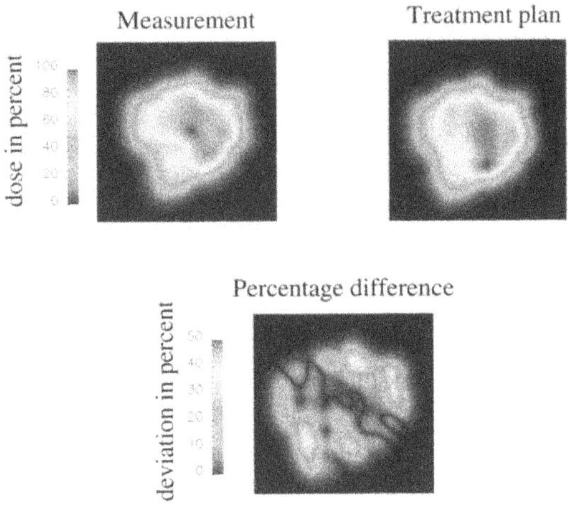


**Figure 4:** Comparison of the measured and the planned treatment of the first patient treatment at GSI for 1 slice positioned in the target volume at 8 cm water-equivalent depth. The color code of the right figure refers to the percentage difference between the measured and the planned treatment.

0.6 to 300 mm of water-equivalent thickness. This device may also be used to increase the number of measured points in the depth-dose profile thus improving the resolution of the measurements along the beam path up to 0.6 mm of water. The error of the dose measurement is +3% and -1% in the region corresponding to the target volume. The water-equivalent positions of the measured points are determined with errors of less than 1%.

## References

[1] Th. Haberer, W. Becher, D. Schardt and G. Kraft, Magnetic scanning system for heavy ion therapy, Nucl. Instr. Meth. A 330 (1993), 296

[2] B. Voss, H. Junk, H, Stelzer, The monitor system of the Therapy Project, GSI-Rep-98-1 (1998), 187

[3] K. Poppensieker et al., ICALEPCS Conf. Proc., Beijing 1997

[4] H. Brand, H. G. Essel, H. Hardel, J. Hoffmann, N. Kurz, W. Ott, M. Richter, Therapy Slow Control System, Data Analysis and Online Monitoring, GSI-Rep-98-1 (1998), 146

# An Integrated Treatment Delivery System for SRS and SRT

**Almon Shiu, Brent Parker, Jin-Song Ye and Jim Lii**

Department of Radiation Physics, Then University of Texas, M. D. Anderson Cancer Center, 1515 Holcombe Blvd., Houston, Texas, 77030, U.S.A.

## Introduction

The current technology of Linac-based stereotactic radiosurgery (SRS) as practiced in most institutions around the world is based on 3-dimensional cross firing of the target by multiple arc beams.[1] This delivers a spherical homogeneous treatment volume with a very rapid fall off in dose. This treatment is best suited for small tumors that resemble spheres. In instances of less ideally shaped tumors, the treatment volume will include a larger proportion of healthy brain. Hence, treatment with a larger circular collimator exposes more normal brain to high dose irradiation. It is for this reason that doses prescribed to be delivered with larger collimators are lower than those are delivered with smaller collimators. Therefore, volumes larger than 4 cm in diameter are not even considered for SRS. To better conform to an irregular tumor volume, 2 or more overlapping isocenters can be used. This leads to hot areas within the overlap region and increased complications.[2] It is clear that brain toxicity can be reduced by conforming the irradiated volume to the target volume and by maintaining the dose distribution within the target as uniformly as possible. This goal can now be achieved with the development of the miniature multileaf collimator[3] (mMLC) in the Radiation Physics department of the University Texas M. D. Anderson Cancer Center (UTMDACC). In 1998, a plan for a dedicated integrated delivery system was approved by our institution. The development of this integrated delivery system is the corporations among Siemens Medical Systems, Inc., Radionics, Inc., and UTMDCC.

## Material and methods

*The Linear Accelerator*: The PRIMART was chosen because it was developed by Siemens as the IMRT machine. Its configuration is easier to integrate the RADIONICS mMLC into this treatment delivery system. In addition, it is compatible to IMPAC data base and information system. Some of specifications for the PRIMART are (1) 6 MV photons, (2) interlock for photon jaw steeting of 12.2 x 14.4 cm when the mMLC is attached to the collimator of PRIMART, (3) Beam flatness and symmetry for 10 x 10 cm field without mMLC is within 2% at 10 cm depth for the area is 2cm inside the geometric field edge.

*The mMLC*: The RADIONICS mMLC is the secondary generation of MDACC prototype mMLC. The original design from the source to the bottom of mMLC leaf distance is 67.5 cm. The plans for this dedicated machine are to extend the stereotactic technique from intracranial lesions to extracranial sites, e.g., head and neck, lung, liver, spinal cord, and prostate. The distance from the source to the bottom of mMLC will reduce to 62.5 cm. With a minor modification, the penumbral and the radiation leakage should be maintained about the same values as the original design. The leaf width at isocenter, (100cm SAD) will increase from 4 mm to 4.32 mm. In addition, the circular collimator shall be able to use for SRS as the option.

*The RADIONICS mMLC/SIEMENS PRIMART integration*: Both geometric field shaping or IMRT that produces the prescribed dose conformal to the target volume is one strategy that can be used to reduce dose to normal tissue while minimizing the dose inhomogeneity within the target volume. As we all know, the treatment settings can be very complicated. It is essential to be able to download all the treatment parameters, including a single leaf setting file and dose prescription from the treatment planning system to the patient database and treatment record and verify system electronically. This approach will greatly reduce the human errors for entering the wrong treatment parameters, especially for IMRT. In addition, after the patient setup is verified, the treatment delivery system shall be capable to deliver a set of treatment fields automatically.

## Results and discussion

The PRIMART (LEXAR) and mMLC were accepted on September 27, 1999. All acceptance measurements were within specifications. Some of the results are (1) radiation isocenter is within 0.5 mm, (2) the depth of maximum dose ($D_{100}$) along the central axis is 1.5 cm and the depth dose at 10 cm is 67.4% of $D_{100}$, and (3) the beam flatness @ 10 cm for cross-plane is +0.1 %/-1.7% and in-plane is +0.2%/-1.3%. Both are normalized with respect to the dose at central axis for the same depth

The penumbra value (80%-20% width) for each mMLC leaf is around 3 mm which is about 0.3 mm wider than the penumbra from the original design. The penumbra value is almost independent of the off-axis position of a leaf. The interleaf leakage (between the leaf and the leaf ends) was found to be 1.4% maximum (1.1% average), while the intraleaf leakage (transmission through the height of the leaves) was 0.9%. The matchlines between the abutting fields were found to be straight and of uniform width less than 0.4 mm and with less than 0.4 mm variation. The leaf position precision was found to be better than 0.6 mm for all the leaves.

The mMLC is integrated as part of PRIMART is shown in Figure 1. The circular collimator housing is attached to the opening window of the mMLC and is shown in Figure 2. The same collimator insert can be used with this new housing. All the circular beam data were measured with photon-jaw setting for 6 x 6 cm. The RPC head phantom was used to evaluate the accuracy of the whole process of SRS treatment. The accuracy of the alignment is within 0.5 mm and the deviation of dose delivery is within 2% of the prescribed dose.

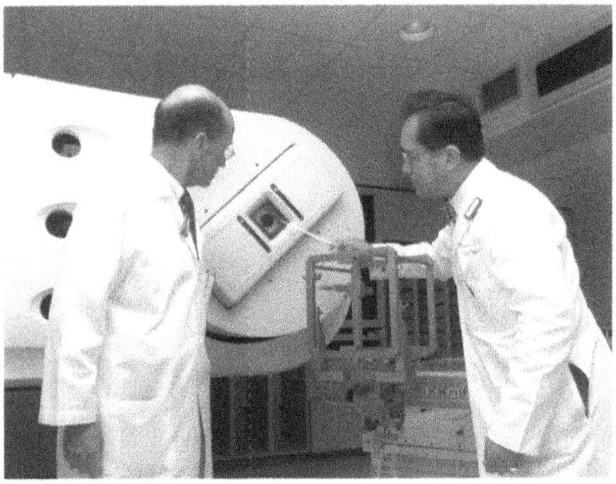

**Figure 1.** The mMLC is part of PRIMART linear accelerator.

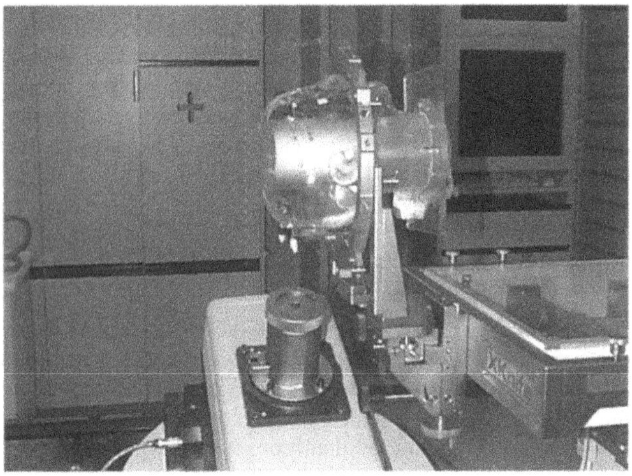

**Figure 2.** The circular collimator housing is attached to the opening window of mMLC.

The integration among Xplan treatment planning system, mMLC and PRIMART linear accelerator has been tested and the integration is achieved with a few minor deficiencies. Figure 3 shows the block diagram to illustrate the flow of data through this integration process. This process is consists of two phases. First is the planning phase: Patient is created in the ACCESS through IMPAC Server and is planned with XPlan treatment planning system. The treatment data file is FTP to the PrimView computer. Then, open the ACCESS and import the treatment data file for that patient. Treatment data file includes mMLC code, filed shape code, Jaw setting not exceed 12.2 x 14.4 cm, MU, gantry position and collimator position, couch positions, setup tolerance, etc. The sequence of the mMLC field, the mMLC leaf positioning with unique mMLC block code specifically for that field, patient name and ID are exported to mMLC controller from Xplan.

Second is the treatment phase: the treatment is downloaded from IMPAC ACCESS via PrimeView into the PRIMART Console. As shown in the diagram, serial communication lines (Digital Mevatron Interface Protocol or DMIP) are monitored by the mMLC PC and alert the mMLC Controller software when a mMLC treatment is to begin. Data on these lines specify the patient and field (within the treatment plan). MMLC controller locates the treatment file and sets the specified field. Subsequent fields for the same patient are set from the same treatment file.

When a field is set successfully, The mMLC controller set a value in the Block Code Interface (BCI) box inside the LINAC. Siemens software reads this value and, if it corresponds to the anticipated value, allows treatment to proceed. At this moment, on the Console displays all treatment-preset parameters match the actual parameters. The user presses Accept driving the system to the Ready State. There is a different value for each field in the treatment. While the mMLC is in the process of setting a field (leaves are moving, correct position not confirmed), a special value is set, this value indicates that the mMLC is "Not Ready." Treatment cannot proceed when this value is set. During the treatment, the power to the motor of each leaf is interrupted till the treatment for this field is completed. After Treatment completion the console will upload treatment parameters.

In case of an IMRT treatment, a group of segments will be created in PrimeView. Each segment will have a specific block code. The Console will be designed to allow during PAUSE beam block changes performed by the mMLC Controller and the block code interface. During PAUSE and while the Block Code is changed and the mMLC leaves are moving the interlock will remain asserted.

The minor deficiencies we have encountered were that the mMLC controller does not monitor collimator, gantry, and couch positions. In the event of an error, the PrimView is only being told that the field was not set successfully. No field label is shown on the mMLC control monitor. Due to the sorting nature of IMPAC ACCESS, the label for each mMLC leaf setting needs to ensure the segments of each IMRT field will not be rearranged when the file is FTP and import to the ACCESS. Acquisition of beam data for treatment planning, calibration, quality assurance procedures and patient alignment procedures were completed and releasd for clinical use on October 23, 1999. Comparison of geometric confirmation and IMRT will be presented.

## Conclusion

A dedicated integrated auto-delivery system has been established at University of Texas, M. D. anderson Cancer center. The un it is capable to deliver conventional SRS and SRT, geometric conformal SRS and SRT. We have expanded the treatment site to head and neck. In the near future, the IMRT technique will be available. Coupled with the need for conformal SRS and SRT or IMRT, the development of an on-line image system is essential. In addition, gating the beam to synchronize the breath cycle of a patient for treating a small lung tumor or a small liver lesion stereotactically.

## References

[1] Kooy H M, Neszi L A, Loffer J S, Alexander E, Cheng C 1991 Treatment planning for stereotactic radiosurgery of intra-cranial lesions. Int. J. Radiat. Oncol. Biol. Phys. 21:683-693.

[2] Nedzi L A, Kooy H M, Alexander E, Gelman R S, Loffler J S 1991 Variables associatee with the development of complications from radiosurgery of intracranial tumors. Int. J. Radiat. Oncol. Biol. Phys. 21:591-599.

[3] Shiu A S, Kooy H M, Ewton J R, Tung S S, Wong J, Antes K, Maor M H 1997 Comparison of miniature multileaf collimation (MMLC) with circular collimation for stereotactic treatment Int. J. Radiat. Oncol. Biol. Phys. 37:679-688.

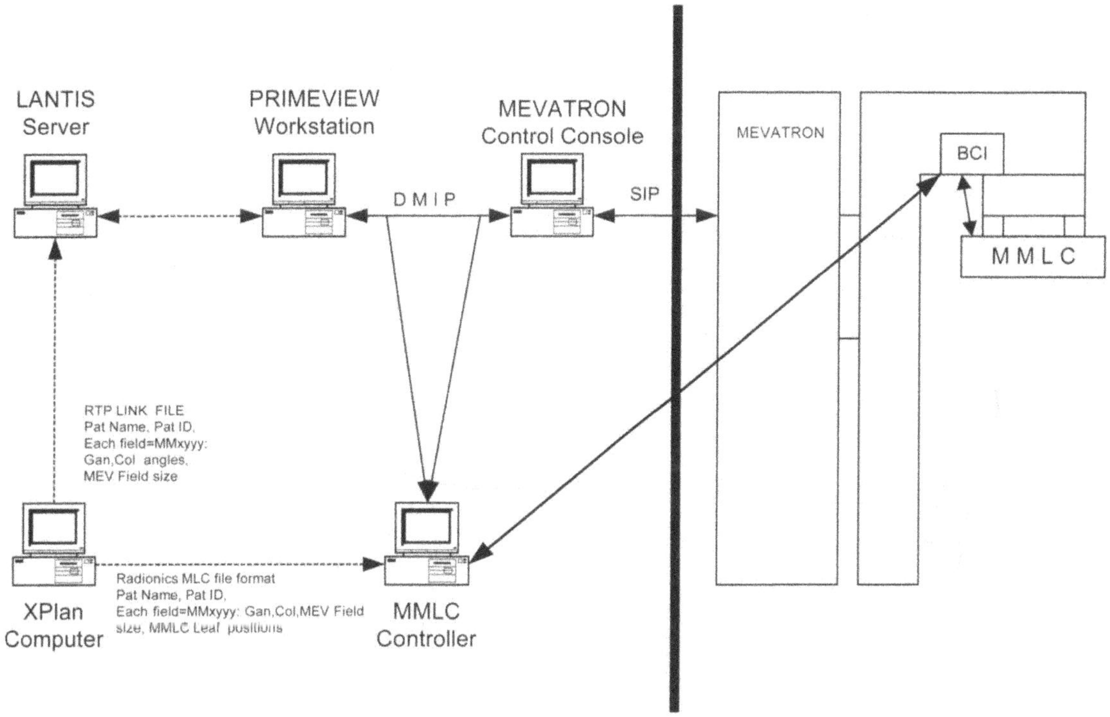


**Figure 3.** The overall system diagram of the Xplan, mMLC and PRIMART integration

# Monte Carlo for the Cyberknife

**Thomas Guerrero, M.D., Ph.D.[1], Todd Pawlicki, Ph.D. [1], Steve B. Jiang, Ph.D. [1], Jenny Hai, Ph.D. [1], Gary Luxton, Ph.D. [1], Cihat Ozhasoglu, Ph.D. [1], John R Adler, Jr., M.D.[2] , and C.-M. Ma, Ph.D. [1]**

[1] Department of Radiation Oncology and [2]Department of Neurosurgery, Stanford University Medical Center, Stanford, CA, USA

## Introduction

The Cyberknife™ is an image guided robot arm mounted linear accelerator capable of frameless stereotactic treatment of both intracranial as well as extracranial sites[1-3]. The Cyberknife utilizes a lightweight 6 MV X-band linear accelerator. The Cyberknife is used clinically for treatment of intracranial, head and neck, and spinal lesions. It is presently being proposed for use in treatment protocol to extracranial sites including the pancreas, lung, and prostate. The goal of this work is to characterize the Cyberknife linac for the development of a Monte Carlo treatment plan verification tool.

### Cyberknife Treatment Planning System

The Cyberknife treatment planning system uses a simple tissue-phantom-ratio dose algorithm[4] given by:

$$D(SAD,d,r,f) = (800/SAD)^2\, DM(f)\, TPR(d,f)\, OCR(d,f)\, MU,$$

where SAD is the source-axis distance, d is the depth in tissue, f is the field size, DM is the collimator Output Factor, TPR is the Tissue Phantom Radio, OCR is the off-center ratio, and MU is the number of monitor units[3]. The monitor unit calibration is defined experimentally to yield one cGy at a depth of 1.5 cm, approximately the $d_{max}$, as measured with a small ionization chamber with an SAD of 80 cm utilizing the 60 mm secondary collimator. In this study the OCR and DM factors are obtained from Monte Carlo simulations and compared with the measured values.

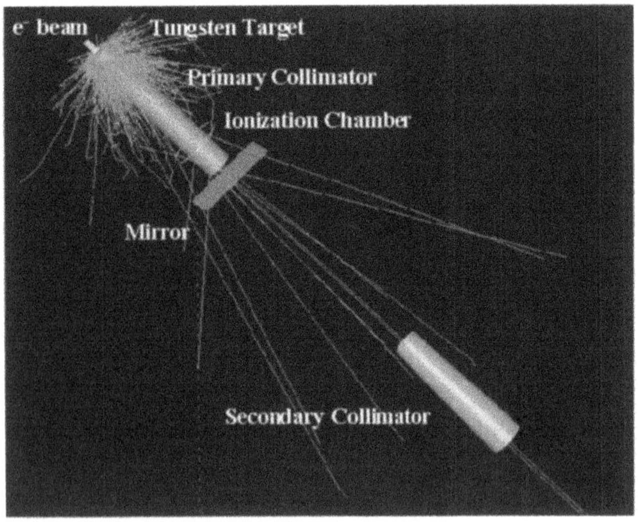


**Figure 1:** Representation of the EGS4/BEAM simulation of the Cyberknife. A monoenergetic electron beam was incident on a tungsten target. The bremsstrahlung photons were followed creating a phase space file at the secondary collimator output.

### Cyberknife Treatment Delivery

Treatments are performed as a series of point and shoot nodes located along predefined paths designed to avoid collisions with the patient or other structures. A typical treatment consist of between 100 and 300 nodes each delivering a variable dose using a variable number of secondary collimator sizes. The secondary collimators produce 5, 7.5, 10, 12.5, 15, 17.5, 20, 25, 30, 40, 50, and 60 mm field sizes at 80 cm SAD. The treatment axis of each node may intersect at differing points throughout the target, without the restriction of an isocenter.

### Monte Carlo Validation using EGS4 /MCDOSE

We have previously reported on the EGS4/MCDOSE dose calculation tool for treatment plan verification[6]. Patient treatment plans generated by clinically used treatment planning systems are recalculated using the Monte Carlo tool. The first phase of this study will generate phase space data characterizing the linac output for each of the secondary collimators for use with EGS4/MCDOSE dose calculation tool.

## Material and methods

Monte Carlo simulations of the Cyberknife's X-band linear accelerator were performed using the EGS4/BEAM code[6,7] to characterize the accelerator. Proprietary accelerator information was obtained from Accuray (Accuray, Sunnyvale, CA). The accelerator components simulated include the bremsstrahlung target, soft x-ray filter, primary collimator, ionization chamber, laser alignment mirror, and range of field defining secondary collimators. Figure 1 illustrates the accelerator geometry used. A monoenergetic electron beam of variable energy and radius incident on the tungsten target produced the primary bremsstrahlung photons.

Depth dose and profile measurements were made for the entire set of collimators at 80 cm SSD using a water phantom and a 6 mm diameter thimble ionization chamber. The depth dose water phantom measurements were simulated with the electron beam energy varied through the range of 5.2 MeV to 7.5 MeV until a match with the measured depth dose characteristics along the central axis was obtained. The incident electron beam diameter was varied from 0.1 mm to 7.5 mm, and the best fit with the measured profile data was obtained. The incident e-beam energy and diameter were set to those characteristic values for all further Monte Carlo simulations.

A large phase space data file was created with 25 million particles at the output of the primary collimator. This was applied to a series of simulations for the range of secondary collimator sizes, producing a phase space file for each collimator. A simulation of a water phantom placed at 80 cm

SSD was made and profile characteristics at 1.5, 5, 10, 20 cm depth obtained. The central 6 mm dose was utilized to obtain collimator output factors, except for the field sizes less than 10 mm where the central 1.5 mm dose was used. The simulations were run to yield a statistical uncertainty of less than one percent. A simulation of the monthly Cyberknife calibration was performed to allow direct calculation of dose via a calibration factor for each phase space data set. The MCDOSE user code was modified to accommodate the unique geometry of the Cyberknife and a simple hypothetical treatment plan calculated.

## Results and discussion

Simulations for incident electron beam energies of 5.1 to 7.5 MeV were performed. The resulting depth dose values along the central axis at 80 cm SSD are shown in figure 2. The best

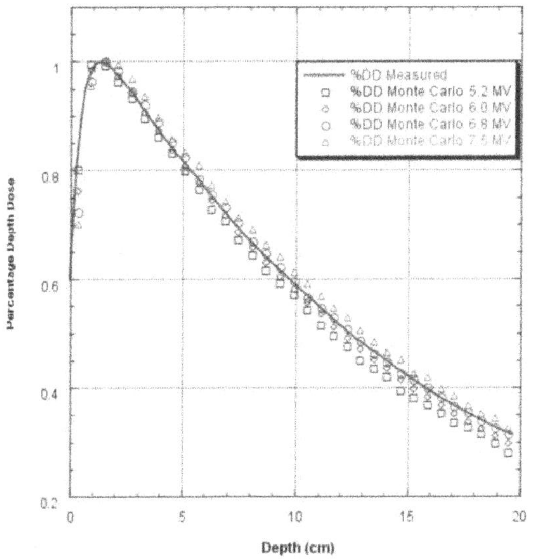


**Figure 2:** Shows a comparison between measured depth dose and Monte Carlo simulation depth dose for 5.2, 6.0, 6.8, and 7.5 MV bremsstrahlung sources.

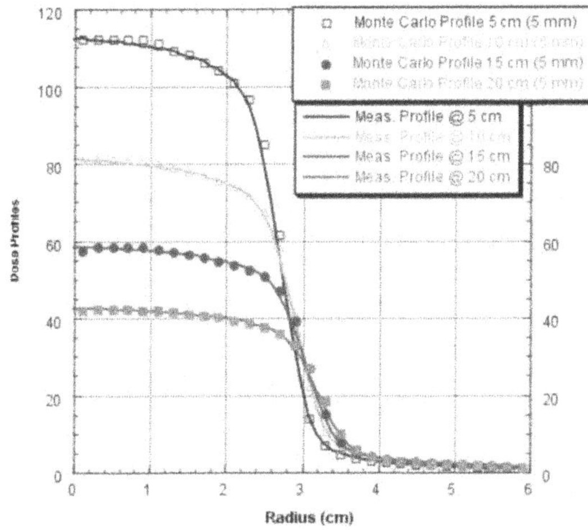


**Figure 4:** Radial profile in a water phantom at 5, 10, 15, & 20 cm depth for primary photon beams of 6.8 MV and 5 mm diameter compared with measurement for a 50 mm secondary collimator.

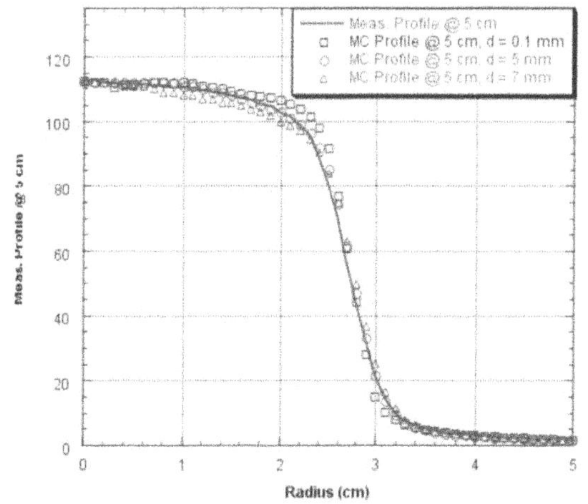


**Figure 3:** Radial dose profile in a water phantom at 5 cm depth for electron beams of 0.1, 5, 7 mm diameter incident on the tungsten target compared with measurement.

fit with the measured depth dose data is obtained for an incident electron beam energy of 6.8 MeV. As expected the depth dose characteristics for beam energies above 6.8 MeV exhibited less attenuation and those with energies below 6.8 MeV exhibited more attenuation with depth.

The beam profiles were calculated in a water phantom with SSD of 80 cm using the 50 mm secondary collimator. The profiles were obtained for 5, 10, 15, 20, and 25 cm depth. A range of electron beam diameters was utilized including 0.1, 5, and 7 mm. The resulting profiles were compared with measured data and are shown in figure 3. Beam diameters greater than 5 mm resulted in excess profile broadening and those with diameters less than 5 mm were excessively sharp. The 5 mm beam diameter best fit the measured profile data and corresponds with the diameter of the linac output region immediately prior to the target.

The 6.8 MeV electron beam. energy and beam diameter of 5 mm were used in subsequent simulations. The radial profiles generated were compared for an 80 cm SSD at depths of 5, 10, 15, 20 cm for the 50 mm collimator. The results in figure 4 show excellent agreement between the measured and simulation data.

A series of phase space data files were generated, one for each of the secondary collimators. These were used as input to a simple simulation of a water phantom at 80 cm SAD and an idealized detector centered at 1.5 cm depth. The resulting dose values obtained in the detector were used to calculate the collimator output factors and are compared with the measured values in Table 1. There is excellent agreement between the measured and simulation values. The percentage differences are all less than three percent. Further experiments using small detectors such as thermoluminescent detectors are planned.

A dose calibration factor of 4.13 x $10^{-16}$ Gy/incident particle was obtained for the 60 mm secondary collimator with an EGS4/BEAM simulation of the calibration set-up. The dose calibration factor will be used to obtain absolute dose calculations in subsequent simulations.

| | Measured | Simulated | % difference |
|---|---|---|---|
| 5 mm | 0.627 | 0.623 | -0.64 % |
| 7.5 | 0.856 | 0.831 | -2.9 |
| 10 | 0.890 | 0.863 | -3.0 |
| 12.5 | 0.929 | 0.913 | -1.7 |
| 15 | 0.951 | 0.943 | -0.84 |
| 20 | 0.970 | 0.953 | -1.8 |
| 25 | 0.978 | 0.960 | -1.8 |
| 30 | 0.984 | 0.977 | -0.71 |
| 40 | 0.991 | 0.990 | -0.10 |
| 50 | 0.997 | 0.996 | -0.10 |
| 60 | 1.000 | 1.000 | - |

**Table 1:** Measured versus EGS4/BEAM simulated collimator output factors DM(f), simulated water phantom dose at 1.5 cm.

The EGS4/MCDOSE software was modified to accommodate the unique geometry of the Cyberknife. A hypothetical case composed of four beams incident on a vertebral body tumor metastasis was calculated and is shown in figure 5 below. Further development to accommodate complex Cyberknife treatment plans is in progress.

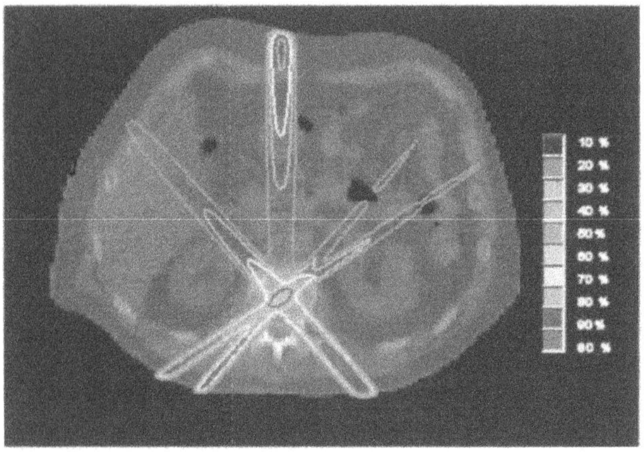

**Figure 5:** Isodose distributions for a simple hypothetical Cyberknife case consisting of four nodes: AP 50 mm, 315 deg 5 mm, 300 deg 10 mm and 45 deg 25 mm secondary collimators.

## Conclusion

The Cyberknife's lightweight 6 MV X-band linear accelerator was modelled and simulations performed with the EGS4/BEAM Monte Carlo package. The simulations were compared with measured values for the depth dose and profiles at various depths allowing the characterization of the accelerator . The collimator output factors were obtained from simulation and compared with measured values. There was excellent agreement between the measured values and the simulations. Phase space data sets were generated for the complete set of secondary collimators. Modifications were made to the MCDOSE user code and a simple hypothetical patient case isodose distribution was calculated. These results will allow the development of a Monte Carlo treatment plan verification tool to investigate the Accuray treatment planning system as indications for the Cyberknife extend to extracranial sites including the pancreas, lung, and prostate

## References

[1] Adler, J.R., Chang, S.D., Murphy, M.J., Doty, J, Geis, P., Hancock, S.L. "The Cyberknife: A Frameless Robotic System for Radiosurgery," *Stereotactic and Functional Neurosurgery*, **69**:124-128, 1997.

[2] Chang, S.D., Murphy, M.J., Geis, P., Martin, D.P., Hancock, S.L., Doty, J.R., and Adler, J.R., "Clinical Experience with Image-guided Robotic Radiosurgery (the Cyberknife) in the Treatment of Brain and Spinal Cord Tumors," *Neurol Med Chir* (Tokyo) **38**:780-783, 1998.

[3] Accuray, Inc, "CyberKnife System for Stereotactic Radiosurgery and Radiotherapy Treatment Planning Technical Manual," Accuray document #71-10597, Rev B, 1999.

[4] Karzmark CJ, Deubert A, Loevinger R (1965) Tissue-phantom ratios – an aid to treatment planning. *Br. J. Radiol.* **38**:158.

[5] Ma C-M, Pawlicki T A, Li J, Jiang S, Deng J, Kapur A, Mok E, Luxton G, and Boyer AL (1999) MCDOSE – A Dose Calculation Tool for Radiotherapy Treatment Planning, *Med. Phys.* **26**(6):1148

[6] Nelson R, Hirayama H and Rogers DWO (1985). The EGS4 code system, Stanford Linear Accelerator Center Report *SLAC-265* (SLAC, Stanford, CA).

[7] Rogers DWO, Faddegon BA, Ding GX, Ma C-M, Wei JS, Mackie TR (1995). BEAM: A Monte Carlo code to simulate radiotherapy treatment units. *Med. Phys.* **22**: 503-25.

[8] Ma C-M, Mok E, Kapur A, Pawlicki T A, Findley D, Brain S, Forster K and Boyer AL (1999) Clinical implementation of a Monte Carlo treatment planning system for radiotherapy, *Med. Phys.* **26**: 2133-43.

[9] Webb, S (1999) Conformal intensity-modulated radiotherapy (IMRT) delivered by robotic linac – testing IMRT to the limit?" *Physics in Medicine & Biology,* **44**:1639-1654.

# Investigations on medical aspects of *CoRA* – A new *Co*balt *R*adiotherapy *A*rrangement (feasibility study)

**Simone Barthold, Wolfgang Schlegel, Otto Pastyr, Gernot Echner**

German Cancer Research Center Heidelberg, Department of Medical Physics, 69120 Heidelberg, INF 280

## Introduction

Linear accelaerators (Linac) are the standard irradiation treatment units in clinical routine for both radiotherapy and radiosurgery. The available infrastructure in developing countries together with technical and economical arguments allow in most cases only the use of isotope units for radiotherapy. On the other side there is a natural interest in modern conformal treatment techniques in these countries. However, the technology of todays gamma teletherapy units and modern treatment methods are mutually exclusive in most cases. Isotope units can not be utilized in combination with multileaf collimators (MLC) due to their large source sizes and the mechanical conditions of these units do not allow stereotactic radiosurgery. Poffenbarger and Podgorsak [1] investigated the viability of an isocentric cobalt unit for stereotactic radiosurgery with respect to its use in developing countries. The Gamma-Knife [2] and the Rotating Gamma Unit [3] exclusively designed for radiosurgical treatments are only applicable for cranial lessons. So in developing countries the postulation for a multifunctional treatment unit is existent based also on financial limitations.

Therefore we developed a new concept of an irradiation system which combines the advantages of the Gamma Knife and the Linac. It allows the delivery of fractionated radiotherapy, usage of MLC for irregular field shaping, simultaneous irradiation form different directions, geometrical accuracy etc.. The unit is designed as an isocentric device. Stereotactic treatment techniques will also be possible. The source holders including the sources are fixed on a swivel-mounted arc in such a way that their beam axes intersect at the isocenter of the unit (see figure 1). The system gives also the possibility to attach beam limiting devices like MLC. For the first time CoRA allows the irradiation of more than one irregular field at the same time for all target positions.

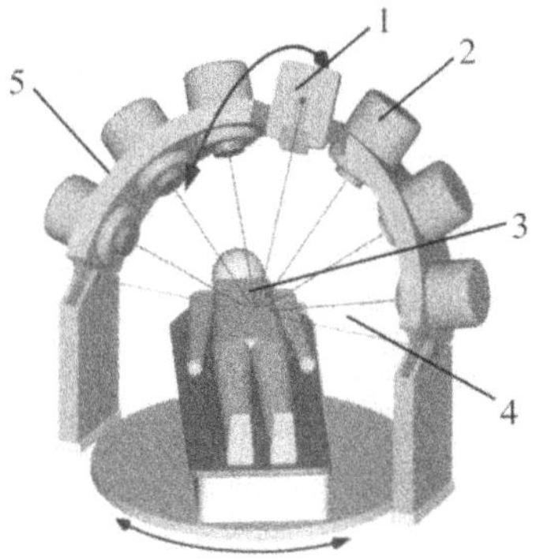


**Figure 1:** Schematic picture of CoRA indicates the components.

The aim of the study is to investigate the viability of CoRA for radiosurgery and radiotherapy by means of various clinical examples. We compared several treatment situations planed under CoRA conditions with treatment plans derived for a standard Linac using the treatment simulation by modul "VIRTUOS" [4].

## Material and methods

Radiotherapy simulations for different treatment situations were performed with the planning tool "VIRTUOS". First we investigated the influence of technical parameters like number of sources, field shaping and field weight and also the influence of swivel angle and couch rotation on the dose distribution. We defined the following start parameters based on this investigations:

- five sources are sufficient
- irregular field shaping if necessary
- optimization using field weighting is profitable
- the swivel angle should be greater than 90°
- depending on the treatment situation a couch rotation will be necessary.

Second we performed therapy simulation for radiotherapy and radiosurgery using the defined parameters.

### Case 1: Liver metastasis

The following treatment techniques were employed:
A: coplanar technique using 6 fields (real treatment situation)
B: 40 irregular single fields using 8 swivel angels and different couch rotations
C: 40 irregular single fields using 8 swivel angels, different couch rotations and weighting of some beam directions.
More Parameters are given in table 1.

| | plan A | plan B | plan C |
|---|---|---|---|
| treatment unit | Linac | CoRA | CoRA |
| radiation type | 15 MV photons | $^{60}$Co | $^{60}$Co |
| no. of irregular fields | 6 | 40 | 40 |
| gantry/ swivel angle | 60°, 90°, 135°, 195°, 290°, 340° | 15°, 30°, -15°, -30°, 135°, 150°, -135°, -150° | 15°, 30°, -15°, -30°, 135°, 150°, -135°, -150° |
| field weighting | 195° double | | single beam directions |

**Table 1:** Therapy simulation parameters for case 1.

### Case 2: Brain metastasis

Moving the swivel-mounted arc constitutes a treatment technique different from the multiple arc technique (see figure 2). The multiple arc technique is a convergent radiosurgery method using the Linac.

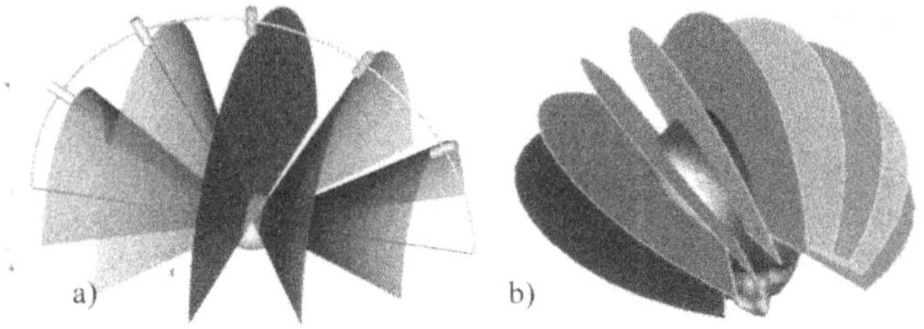


**Figure 2:** Two different treatment techniques: a) CoRA arc technique and b) multiple arc technique.

The so called CoRA arc technique (D) is compared with a clinical treatment plan based on the multiple arc technique (E). Detailed Parameters for the two treatment techniques are given in table 2.

| | plan D | plan E |
|---|---|---|
| treatment unit | Linac | CoRA |
| radiation type | 15 MV photons | $^{60}$Co |
| no. of arcs | 5 | 9 |
| arc lenght | 140° | 140° |

**Table 2:** Therapy simulation parameters for case 2.

For the treatment simulations a dose calculation algorithm is used which is based on pencil beam kernels [5].

## Results and discussion

### Case 1

The result of treatment technique B in comparison with A is shown in figure 3 and 4. The dose application in the PTV, GTV and the organs at risk was investigated using the integral dose volume histogram.

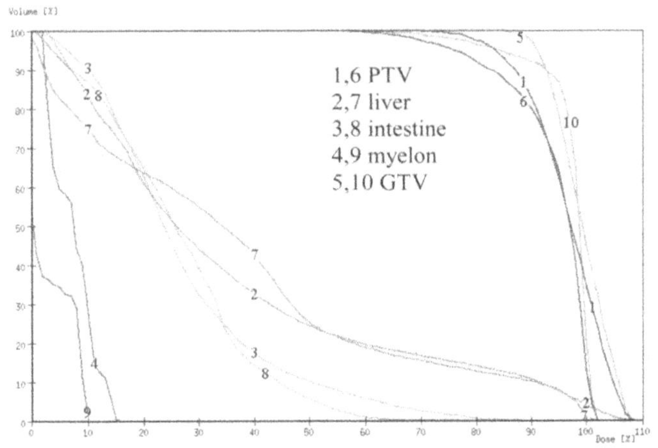


**Figure 4:** Integral dose volume histogram for treatment situations A and B (plan A: curves 6-10, plan B: curves 1-5).

Table 3 lists some special values for the dose volume histogram shown in figure 4.

| dose [%] | PTV volume [%] | | GTV volume [%] | | liver volume [%] | | intestine volume [%] | |
|---|---|---|---|---|---|---|---|---|
| | A | B | A | B | A | B | A | B |
| 100 | 14 | 36 | 26 | 47 | 4 | 4 | 0 | 0 |
| 90 | 82 | 80 | 94 | 92 | 10 | 11 | 0 | 0 |
| 80 | 90 | 97 | 96 | 100 | 13 | 15 | 0 | 1 |
| 60 | 100 | 100 | 100 | 100 | 19 | 22 | 1 | 7 |
| 50 | 100 | 100 | 100 | 100 | 25 | 27 | 7 | 11 |
| 20 | 100 | 100 | 100 | 100 | 64 | 64 | 65 | 60 |
| 10 | 100 | 100 | 100 | 100 | 75 | 82 | 88 | 90 |

**Table 3:** Values of the dose volume histogram.

The Comparison of the dose distribution between the simulated and the real treatment plan show that an acceptable dose can be delivered to the PTV and GTV is possible. Only the differences

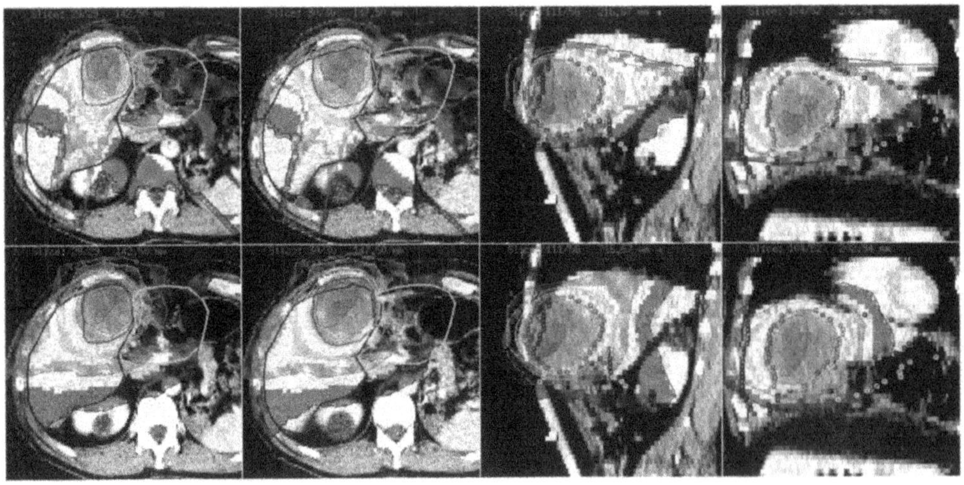

**Figure 3:** Frontal, sagittal and lateral Dose distribution for plan A (row 1) and plan B (row 2).

in the intestine region are not negligible. We tried to optimize this treatment situation based on beam weighting. The result (C) is shown in figure 5.
A minor improvement of the dose delivered to the intestine was possible, but we could not achieve the result of plan A shown in figure 4. We think this will be a problem of the known physical properties of $^{60}$Co-sources and our basis data used for the dose calculation. This data are based on a cobalt source with a large source diameter (20 mm). A better result can be anticipated if a smaller source is used, e.g. 10 mm.

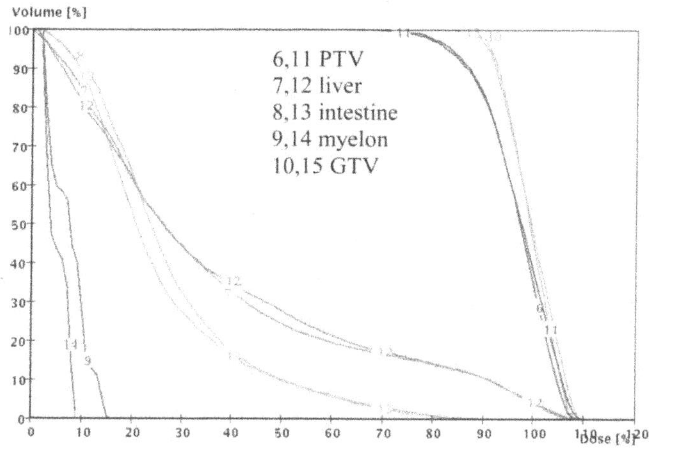


**Figure 5:** Integral dose volume histogram for treatment situations B and C (plan B: curves 6-10, plan C: curves 11-15).

Independent thereof we found that the disadvantage of the lower penetration of radiation from a cobalt source in comparission to a Linac can be counterbalanced by the many beam directions. This will be possible without increasing the delivered dose to the organs at risk.

**Case 2**

In contrast to the large target volume (example 1) we investigated also the dose delivery to a small target volume.
The result of the simulation in comparison to a clinical standard treatment plan is shown in figure 6.

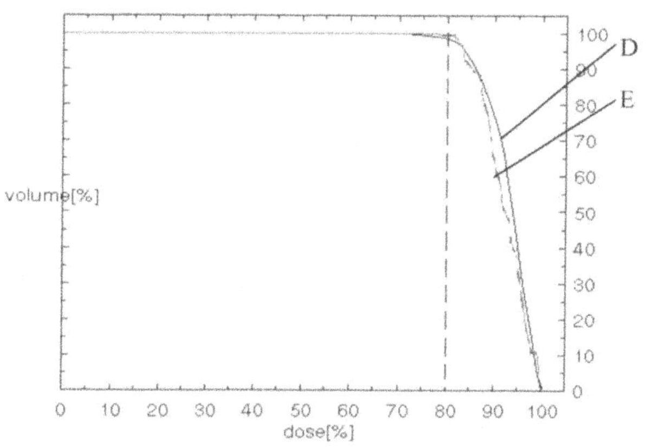


**Figure 6:** Dose volume histogram for treatment situations D and E.

There are no significant differences between the two treatment techniques. In clinical treatment planning using the multiple arc technique the 80% isodose is practised for dosage [6]. In consideration of this aspect we found that both techniques are equivalent. No disadvantages due to the large source diameter and the lower energy of the used cobalt source became visible.

## Conclusion

It was found that the System CoRA and the CoRA arc technique will be suitable for treatments of cranial target volumes (example 2). In comparison with the multiple arc technique no drawback is noticeable due to the reduced number of arcs. The CoRA arc technique has the advantage of simultaneous beam application, e.g. the ability for an optimization of the treatment time.
For extra cranial targets, particular large target volumes, it was shown that an acceptable dose distribution in the PTV and GTV will be realizable. The delivery of higher dose to organs at risk, which are located directly close to the target like the intestine, should be reduced. We think this will be possible if an optimized beam application system due to the utilization of a MLC in combination with better physical properties, e.g. a smaller source, would be used. It is possible that the higher number of single beams can increase the treatment time. If a motorized multileaf collimator is used the treatment time can be optimized through the simultaneous beam application.
The availability and the multifunctional aspects of CoRA can lead to a wide variety of applications. CoRA can contribute to improve the health care especially for centers in developing countries. Today cobalt units, because of their relatively low cost and the beam stability, provide in most cases the only high-energy radiation source for radiotherapy in these countries. These units have to be modified, with respect to their geometric accuracy and the restrictions due to their lower source axis distance of 800 mm, if they should be used for radiosurgery [1].
In the future CoRA perhaps will provide a treatment modality suitable for both radiotherapy and radiosurgery in developing countries.

## References

[1] Poffenbarger B. A. and Podgorsak E. B., 1998, Viability of an isocentric cobalt-60 teletherapy unit for stereotactic radiosurgery. *Med Phys* **25** 1935-1943
[2] Leksell L., 1971; The stereotaxic gamma unit. *In: Stereotaxis and radiosurgery – An operative system; Springfield: Chales C. Thomas Publisher* 5-7
[3] Goetsch S. J., Murphy M. S., Schmidt B. S. et al., 1999, Physics of rotating gamma systems for stereotactic radiosurgery. *Int J Radiat Oncol Biol Phys* **43** 689-696
[4] Bendl R., Pross J., Hoess A. et al., 1994, VIRTUOS – A program for VIRTUal radiOtherapy Simulation and verification. *In: Proc. of the 11th Int. Conf. on the Use of Computers in Radiation Therapy; Ed.:Hounsell A. R. et al.; Manchester: North Western Med. Physics Dept.* 226-227
[5] Bortfeld T., Schlegel W. and Rhein B., 1993, Decomposition of pencil beam kernels for fast dose calculations in three-dimensional treatment planning. *Med Phys* **20** 311-318
[6] Debus J., Pirzkall A., Schlegel W. et al., 1999, Stereotaktische Einzeitbestrahlung (Radiochirurgie). *Strahlenther Onkol* **175** 47-56

# Planning and Optimisation of Stereotactic Laser-Neurosurgery

**Rolf Bendl[1], Jürgen Dams[1], Stefan Fischer[2], Marcus Götz[2]**

[1]Deutsches Krebsforschungszentrum, D-69120 Heidelberg, Germany,
[2]MRC Systems, Heidelberg

## Introduction

We present a new planning, optimisation and monitoring system for a new kind of tumour therapy. Instead of ionising beams we will use a laser beam for removing deep-seated tumour tissue.
In opposite to conventional laser surgery, where laser light is converted into heat and used to coagulate tissue, we will use an ultra short-pulsed laser which has no thermal interaction with tissue, but provides the ability to ablate it.
Similar to radiotherapy we must plan and optimise the access path and laser control preoperatively to minimise damaging of surrounding healthy tissue.

## Material and methods

### Laser Neurosurgery

The use of conventional laser beams in neurosurgery has some important limitations. The laser coagulates tissue but does not remove it. Due to the diffusion of heat into surrounding healthy tissue severe side-effects were observed, and therefore the application areas are very restricted. In addition, the coagulated tissue remains in situ and can cause dangerous necrosis.
Together with the Institute of Applied Physics of the University of Heidelberg and the Clinic for Stereotactic and Functional Neurosurgery of the University in Cologne we develop a new therapeutical approach to remove deep-seated tumours with minimal irritation of the surrounding healthy tissue, by using an ultra short-pulsed laser (Nd:YLF). The interaction mode of ultra short laser pulses with tissue is called plasma-mediated. Because mechanical effects dominate this interaction mechanism and because ultra short pulse duration does not allow conduction of heat to the surrounding tissue, there is no thermal injury of sensible structures close to the target volume [1]. In-vitro studies with calf brain have shown the possibility to ablate tissue with an extremely high precision without histopathological damages to adjacent structures [2].

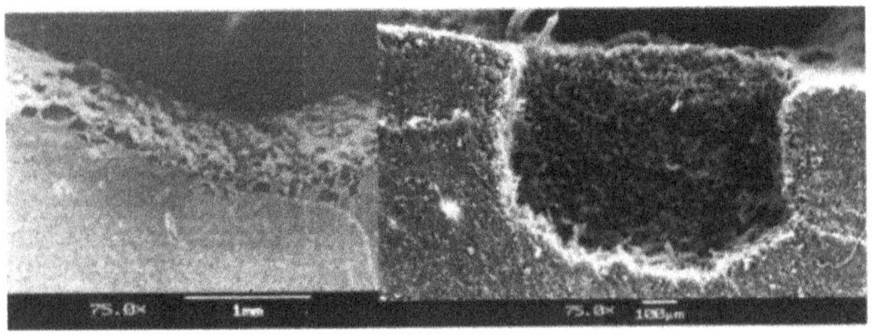

**Fig. 1:** microscopic images of laser/tissue interaction, left: coagulation produced with a conventional $CO_2$ laser, right: ablation with ultra short-pulsed laser

Because of the high energy densities of the laser, glass fibres are unsuitable for transmission of laser pulses into the operation field. Therefore a rigid stereotactic probe with a diameter of 5.5 mm was constructed (Fig. 2), where the laser is transmitted by small deflecting mirrors. The probe is a three tube system, where the single tubes can be moved and rotated by step motors [3]. By moving the tube up and down and rotating it, the target volume can be ablated in cylinders from inside to outside.

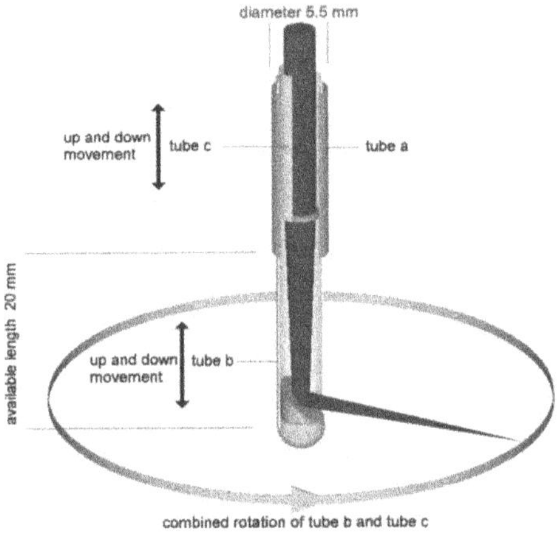


**Figure 2:** Laser Probe.

Due to the high precision of tissue ablation the therapeutic intervention will be very time consuming and must be planned and optimised preoperatively.
By means of a pressure-controlled irrigation/aspiration system the ablated tissue fragments (debris) will be removed out of the operation cavity. The irrigation/aspiration system should control and preserve the intra-cranial pressure and the anatomical relations in the operation area. Nevertheless, a monitoring system is required, to observe the operation field and to detect possible tissue displacements.
We prefer ablation of tumour tissue instead of coagulation. Yet, if there are vessels in the operation field, coagulation is still needed. Otherwise the ablation laser might cause dangerous bleedings. Therefore an additional coagulation laser is integrated inside the probe. An important task of the planning system is the pre- and intra-operative optimisation of the laser control, to switch between the different laser modes.

### Planning System

The planning system consists of three components. An interactive planning tool, for the definition and optimisation of the laser probe's trajectory. A calculation module for computing the ablation sequence and a monitoring module to observe the operation area.

To plan the trajectory of the laser probe, the surgeon needs interactive tools similar to those, used for planning other stereotactic interventions. Depending on the location and size of the tumour, the surgeon must define trajectories without any risk of damaging vessels or important neurological structures.
Interactive tools, comparable to those, already used in radiotherapy planning support this difficult task. Because there are a series of restrictions, additional information must be visualised.
The laser probe has a limited ablation range. To position the probe in a way, that the tumour is completely enclosed by the possible ablation volume, the ablation range must be visualised, too. The intervention should be controlled either by an interventional MR or by 3D ultrasound. The possible monitoring devices must be considered during the planning step, too. If MR is used for monitoring, the size of the MR tube limits the number of possible trajectories. Because of the size of the laser probe, it cannot be applied from arbitrary directions inside of the tube. Ultrasound transducers have only a limited image field, therefore the position and direction of the US transducer must be optimised preoperatively in dependence of the selected trajectory of the laser probe. Fig. 3 presents an Observer's View, where the possible ablation area and the image field of an US transducer are displayed.

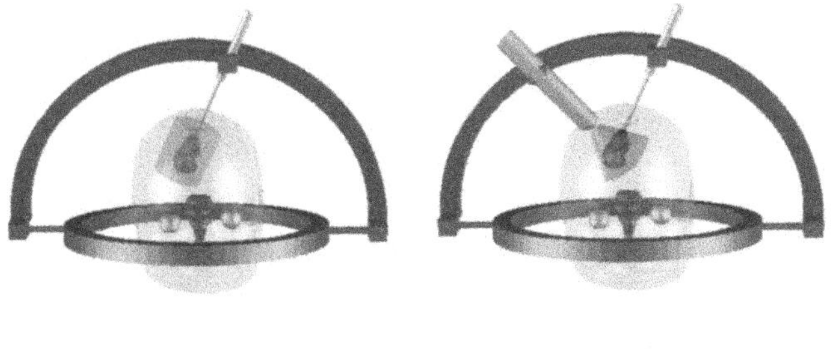

**Fig. 3:** Observer's View, left: maximal ablation volume, right: image field of US transducer

The Probe's Eye View, similar to the Beam's Eye View in radiotherapy planning shows, which structures will be penetrated by the probe itself. The Spherical View, which has only limited benefit in radiotherapy, because it cannot take into account the necessary portal size, can be a valuable tool to avoid penetration of important vessels by the laser probe. Since the diameter of the laser probe is very small, the Spherical View shows appropriate trajectories very reliably (Fig. 4a). An additional help to avoid the penetration of vessels is the generation of maximum intensity projections (MIPs) of the image sequence from the position of the probe (Fig. 4b).

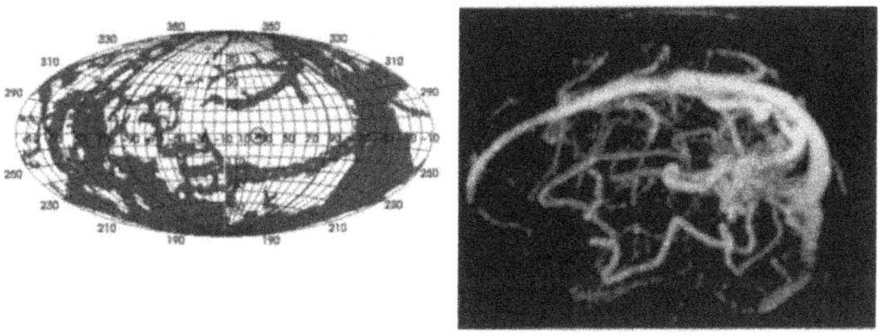

**Fig. 4a:** Spherical View with vessel tree
**4b:** corresponding MIP of CT angiography

**Optimisation of Laser Control**

Opposite to normal neurosurgical interventions the surgeon must not only consider the spatial positions of important anatomical structures, but some technical constraints, too. As already mentioned, the tumour must be completely enclosed by the possible ablation volume, and the selected trajectory must allow intra-operative imaging with MR or US.
In order to speed up and optimise the ablation process, the target volume has to be split into several sub-volumes: one which can be ablated fast and roughly after initial tissue coagulation (the inner part of the target volume, away from critical structures), and other ones, where the tumour tissue must be ablated very precisely without damaging the surrounding tissue.
The ablation planes are perpendicular to the main axis of the probe and the target volume will be ablated in cylindrical slices. As long as the ablation cylinder is completely inside of the tumour, the laser control is simple. If the ablation spot would be inside of healthy tissue, the laser must be switched off. These "inactive" periods will increase the overall intervention time. To minimise the intervention time, one additional optimisation task is the selection of trajectories where the volume, which can be ablated without switching the laser on and off, will be maximal.
Since interactive consideration of the last two constraints is difficult, an optimisation module was designed which pre-calculates the different partial volumes and the expectable ablation time. The colour-coded result of that calculation can be projected onto the surface of the three-dimensional model of the patient's anatomy. This information can then be used by the surgeon, when he selects the trajectory. This way he is able to consider not only anatomical constraints, but the more technical ones, too.

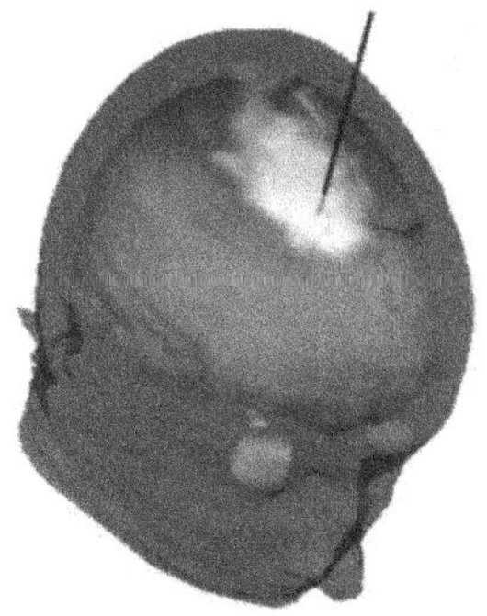

**Fig. 5:** Result of optimisation procedure, to minimise ablation time trajectories in brighter areas should be preferred

**Pre-calculation of the Laser Control**

Based on extensive examinations of the laser/tissue interactions [2] the calculation module produces a detailed protocol, describing the number of ablation planes and cylinders, describing when the laser must be switched off and when it is necessary to switch into the coagulation mode.

**Monitoring of the Intervention**

The exact planning and optimisation of the ablation strategy is an important prerequisite to speed up the intervention. But the pre-calculation of the laser control assumes static spatial

relations between the anatomic structures. Even if the irrigation/aspiration system could preserve the intra-cranial pressure, it might be possible, that the ablation process will result in a spatial displacement of tumour and brain tissue. Therefore it is necessary to monitor the intervention in real-time.
Since US is an inexpensive intra-operative imaging modality and widely used, we have first investigated US for monitoring the intervention. Depending on the histology intra-cranial tumours can be delineated quite well in US images. The transducer will be applied through an additional bore-hole. In most cases ablation slices will not have the same orientation as the image plane of a 2D US transducer. Therefore we have examined several 3D US systems [4]. 3D sequences have the additional advantage, to allow monitoring of the whole ablation volume, this is an important prerequisite to detect tissue displacements promptly. Alternatively the usage of an interventional MR scanner is evaluated. Here work is still in progress.

## Results and discussion

The initial prototype of the laser has had not enough power, to ablate larger volumes in an acceptable time. Since end of 1999 a more powerful laser is available, which is currently examined in animal trials. After successful evaluation it is planned to start with the first patient treatment in summer 2000.
The development of the planning module is nearly finished. For defining an optimal trajectory a connection to an anatomical atlas is desirably, to visualise important brain structures, which cannot be delineated in conventional CT and MR data sets.
Additional work must be spent on the image registration sub-module, besides of stereotactic and landmark based methods an algorithm based on the maximisation of mutual information was integrated, which should allow matching of multi-modal image sequences [5]. This method has the advantage that no external reference system is necessary and no landmarks must be defined. Both restrictions are important when using US images, there the position of external markers are not available and the determination of corresponding landmarks is often difficult, because of the limited image field. First examinations have shown, that the matcher produces sufficient results when matching MR against CT data sets, but our implementation of the algorithm needs additional fine-tuning to use it in combination with arbitrarily orientated US sequences.
A series of US systems (Aloka, HP, Kretz, Siemens, Volumetrics) were evaluated in phantom studies and in conventional neurosurgical operations. Acceptable registration with other modalities seems to be possible (Fig. 6). Additional work must be spent, to do this routinely in a robust and automatic fashion.

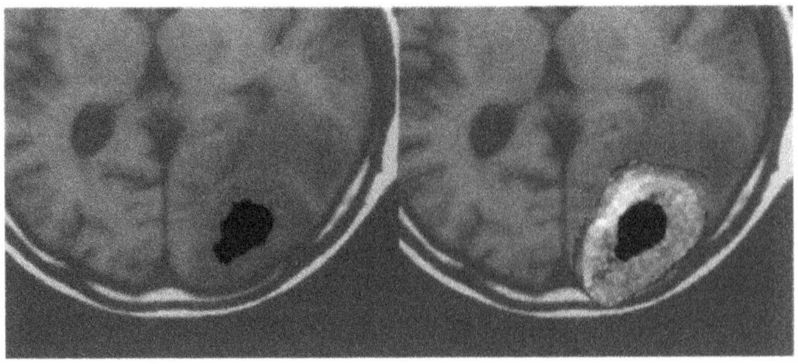

**Fig. 6:** Result of a manual match between intra-operatively acquired MR and US images. Left: MR, Right: MR with overlay of US image. US image acquired with Siemens Siescape

While nearly all examined systems have acquired single images with sufficient quality, non of the systems was able to meet all demands for our special application completely. Either the penetration depth was not sufficient, or the acquisition time was not acceptable, or the three-dimensional reconstruction has shown geometrical distortions or the overall handling was to complex, to use the system for continuous monitoring in a time-consuming intervention. Therefore we focus our efforts at the moment on the usage of images acquired with an interventional MR scanner. Nevertheless we are convinced, that 3D US imaging will prove its abilities for intra-operative imaging in neurosurgical interventions in future.
Work on a comprehensive and dedicated monitoring module is still in progress and should be finished in Summer 2000.

## References

[1] Isner JM and Clarke RH 1987, The paradox of thermal ablation without thermal injury *Lasers Med Sci* **2**, 165 - 173
[2] Suhm N et al. 1996 In vitro ablation of nervous tissue with short pulsed laser: Histopathological examination of the lesions *Acta Neurochir* **138**, 346-349
[3] Goetz MH et al. 1999 Computer-guided laser probe for ablation of brain tumours with ultra-short laser pulses *Phys. Med. Biol.* **44,** N119-N127
[4] Suhm N et al. 1998 Limitations for Three-Dimensional Ultrasound Imaging Through a Bore-Hole Trepanation *Ultrasound in Medicine and Biology* **24** 5 663 - 671
[5] Maes F et al. 1997 Multimodality Image Registration by Maximization of Mutual Information *IEEE Transactions on Medical Imaging* **16** 2, 187 - 197

# Automated Analysis of Film Checks for QA of Stereotactic Treatment Setup

**Markus Buchgeister[1], Gerd Becker[2], André Mondry[1], Mattias Birkner[1], Michael Bamberg[2] and Fridtjof Nüsslin[1]**

[1]Abteilung für Medizinische Physik and [2]Abteilung für Strahlentherapie, Universitätsklinikum Tübingen, D-72076 Tübingen, Germany

## Introduction

Stereotactic radiotherapy with high doses per treatment strongly depends among other factors on the mechanical accuracy of the setup of the patient at the linear accelerator. A commonly used quality assurance tool for radiosurgery with circular collimators is a film check introduced by Winston and Lutz [1] to evaluate the positional accuracy of the gantry and couch rotation around a radiopaque target ball that is positioned in the isocenter by means of the stereotactic setup. There are different manual methods to determine the shift between the center of the exposures of the circular collimator and the sometimes hardly recognizable target ball on the film that naturally depend on the individual skills of the analyzing person to estimate the appropriate centers. Since stereotactic radiotherapy as well as radiosurgery steadily gain importance in cancer treatment, an automated tool to speed up and standardize the analysis of Winston-Lutz film QA checks would be very helpful.

## Material and methods

Film checks for 6 couch–gantry angle combinations for a given isocenter are evaluated by manual reading and automated fit of a scanned BMP-file.

At our site the manual offset reading of a Winston-Lutz film check is performed by first centering a circle of the approximate diameter of the collimator printed on a transparency to the collimator spot on the check film and then centering a second circle of the approximate diameter of the target ball printed on a separate transparency to the corresponding spot on the check film. The second transparency also shows an identical circle of the collimator concentrically to the target ball circle such that after fixation of both transparencies the offset can be optically determined from the maximal difference of the two collimator circles with the help of a precision 10x scale magnifier (ESCHENBACH, Nürnberg, Germany). The minimal measurable separation with this magnifier is 0.1 mm.

For the automatic offset fit the film is digitized with the help of a standard commercial desktop scanner with transparency option (Hewlett-Packard, HP ScanJet 4c) and a resolution of 100 dpi into uncompressed BMP file format with 256 gray levels (see Figure 1).

The fit routine determines the 50% gray level for the collimator spot from minimal and maximal gray levels of a histogram of the BMP file to be independent of the individual film's background gray level and exposure conditions. A circle is fitted by a gradient algorithm to pixels found for the corresponding gray level with the parameters x_collimator, y_collimator and radius_collimator. Pixels of a distance greater than a definable value of the collimator radius are eliminated by a filter routine until a predefined convergence limit is reached. A similar procedure is performed for the target ball fit with the parameters x_ball, y_ball and radius_ball for pixels within a square centered inside the collimator circle. The offset as determined from the center coordinates of collimator and target ball and the known pixel scale of the BMP file is displayed as well as a check BMP file with the fitted collimator and target ball circles as white pixels and is saved for optical checks of the fit result (see Figure 2).

## Results and discussion

The numerical results of the offset between collimator and target ball for 6 couch-gantry angle combinations as determined by manual and automated analysis of a sample case are listed in Table 1. The maximal observed difference is 0.16 mm for the couch-gantry angles 270°/320°. Generally, the fit results are slightly lower than the manual results as also reflected by the average over all six film checks for the example given. The standard deviation is almost identical as

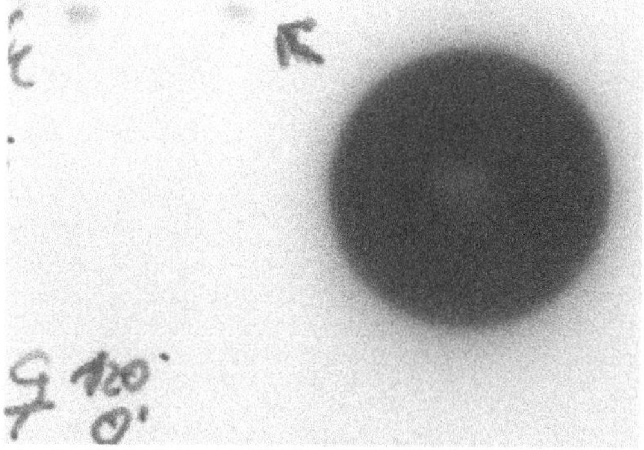

**Figure 1:** Single Winston-Lutz film check for 0° couch and 120° gantry angle as scanned with 100 dpi, 256 gray levels.

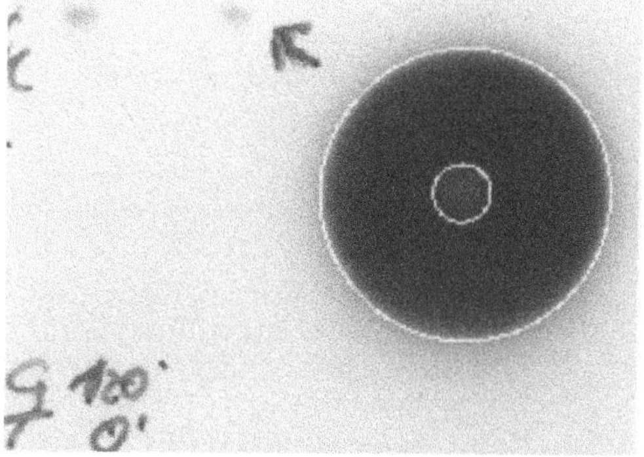

**Figure 2:** Winston-Lutz film check of Figure 1 with automatically fitted circles for collimator and target ball.

the observed differences between the two methods are within the resolution of the optical scale of the used magnifier.
The manual analysis has been performed by an experienced person, so that the close match of the results between manual and automated analysis can be taken as proof for the accuracy of the implemented algorithm.

| Couch / gantry angle | Manual offset reading [mm] | Automated offset fit [mm] |
|---|---|---|
| 0° / 240° | 0.6 | 0.56 |
| 315° / 270° | 0.7 | 0.76 |
| 270° / 320° | 0.9 | 0.74 |
| 90° / 40° | 1.2 | 1.13 |
| 45° / 90° | 0.6 | 0.55 |
| 0° / 120° | 0.5 | 0.49 |
| Average: | 0.75 ± 0.26 | 0.71 ± 0.24 |

**Table 1:** Collimator-target ball offset in mm as determined by manual and automated analysis.

## Conclusion

The analysis of Winston-Lutz film checks can be standardized to be independent of individual skills of the analyzing person with the help of an automated analysis as presented in this paper. Additionally, depending on the quality of the scanning device, even hard to recognize exposures of the target ball can be analyzed avoiding the need to repeat the series of film checks. The scan resolution of 100 dpi is rather moderate, thus the good fit results prove even more the robustness of this automated analysis. With the help of such a computer program the time of the analysis of the film check can be speeded up as well.

## References

[1] Winston K A and Lutz W 1988 Linear Accelerator as a Neurosurgical Tool for Stereotactic Radiosurgery *Neurosurgery* **22** 454-464

# Treatment planning for ion radiotherapy

**M.Krämer**[1], **O. Jäkel**[2]
[1]GSI Darmstadt,[2]DKFZ Heidelberg

## Introduction

One of the main objectives in radiotherapy is the conformal delivery of the prescribed dose to the target volume, whereas the surrounding healthy tissue and critical structures should be spared as much as possible. Compared to photon beams, therapeutic ion beams in general offer the advantage of a depth dose profile with a pronounced maximum (Bragg peak) at large penetration depth. Heavier ions like $^{12}C$ offer further advantages over protons or other lighter charged particles. Their lateral scattering in tissue is reduced and they show an increased relative biological effectiveness (RBE), especially in the stopping region at the Bragg peak. These particular properties make carbon ion beams an ideal candidate to be combined with the evolving techniques of intensity modulated radiotherapy (IMRT).

## Material and methods

Several radiotherapy facilities around the world already exploit the advantages of the inverted dose profile of heavy charged particles. Most of them, however, use patient specific hardware like collimators, compensators and ridge filters to match the tumor in beams eye view. Such techniques are used e.g. at NIRS [1], the only other facility besides GSI which currently uses carbon ion beams for tumor therapy. The next step to better exploit the advantages of ion beams is to use magnetic deflection of narrow beams to cover cross sections of the target volume. Energy variation of the ion beams allows coverage of different slices at different depths, resulting in an excellent dose conformation not only at the distal, but also at the proximal end of the target volume. So far two facilities have implemented this method for clinical use: PSI with their proton spot scanning [2] and GSI with the raster scan device for heavier ions. The unique GSI scanner is the first one to combine magnetic lateral deflection of ion beams with active energy variation. The scanning technique implies the handling and control of a huge set of parameters for both, the treatment planning as well as the patient irradiation. Obviously this requires the development and usage of dedicated software. Typical tumor sizes require several ten thousands of single beam positions and particle fluences to be determined. This task can only be solved by means of automated inverse planning.

A physical as well as a radiobiological beam model has been developed to describe the characteristics of ion beams. The physical beam model is designed to generate depth dose profiles for given primary ion energies. The model takes into account the fragmentation of projectiles based on semi-empirical cross sections. The knowledge of particle charge and energy distributions is a prerequisite for the calculation of radiobiological effects as well as detector responses.

The radiobiological properties of ion radiation are described using the model of Scholz [3]. It allows to compute RBE and biologically effective dose over a wide range of ion species and energies.

Several algorithms are used to optimize the ion beam fluences with respect to the resultant biologically effective dose. Dose distributions are calculated not only for the target volume but for the entire irradiation region taking into account the different radiosensitivity of the different tissues. For multiport treatments the nonlinear superposition of biological dose is taken into account.

## Results and discussion

The newly developed software package TRiP has incorporated all relevant aspects of irradiation with scanned ion beams [4]. The TRiP system standalone as well as in combination with Voxelplan is in use since 1995 for the planning of numerous irradiation experiments including inhomogeneous phantoms, cell and animal experiments such as mini-pig lungs and the central nervous system of rats. It is in clinical use for patient treatment since 1997. So far $\approx$ 50 patients have been planned and treated with carbon ions, most of them with at least two opposing fields. Good target conformation and sparing of healthy tissued could be achieved. Fast tumor remission and only minor side effects like erythema have been observed, in accordance with the biological dose level.

## Conclusion

At the GSI radiotherapy project the first treatment planning system is in clinical use which fully supports the active 3D field shaping techniques together with the radiobiological properties of ion beams.

## References

[1] Kanai T, Kawachi K, Tsujii H and Morita K 1996 *J. Jpn. Soc. Ther. Radiol. Oncol.* **8** 231–238

[2] Pedroni E, Bacher R, Blattmann H, Böhringer T, Coray A at al. 1995 *Med. Phys.* **22** 37–53

[3] Scholz M, Kellerer A M, Kraft-Weyrather W, Kraft G 1997 *Rad. Environ. Biophysics* **36** 59–66

[4] Jäkel O, Krämer M 1998 *Physica Medica* **XIV/1** 53–62

# Determination of dose-volumes parameters to characterise the conformity of stereotactic treatment plans

**Dimitri Lefkopoulos, Catherine Dejean, Hanna El-Balaa, Kalliopi Platoni, Pascal Grandjean, Jean-Noël Foulquier and Michel Schlienger**

Medical Physics Unit, Radiation Oncology Department, Tenon Hospital, 4 rue de la Chine, 75 020 PARIS
email: dimitri.lefkopoulos@tnn.ap-hop-paris.fr

## Introduction

The intracranial stereotactic irradiations are an excellent example of conformal radiotherapy[1].
The aim of this study is to determine DVH indices which will permit to quantitatively evaluate the conformity of treatment plans. RTOG has already determined some parameters to address the above. We try to complete this RTOG protocol [2] by determining other parameters based on the underdosed lesion factor (ULF) and the overdosed healthy tissues (HT) factor (OHTF). Moreover, we determined as quality of a given treatment plan the standard deviation of the corresponding differential DVH of the lesion. We quantified the conformity of a treatment plan by an index equal to the sum of the ULF and OHTF.
The validation and the relationship between the determined parameters were studied through a series of 408 arteriovenous malformations (AVMs) already planned by our SALT group (Sainte-Anne, Lariboisiere, Tenon Hospitals). The RTOG parameters were also studied as function of the plan quality as determined by our group.

## Material and methods

### The studied series

The studied series concern 408 AVMs treated in one fraction: 223 are mono-isocentric, 185 multi-isocentric (2 isocentres : 106 cases; 3 isocenters : 35 cases; 4 isocenters : 38 cases; 5 isocenters : 6 cases).
The irradiation was performed with a 15 MV linear accelerator with additional circular collimators [3] (diameters ranging from 6 to 20 mm). A Betti movable chair and a Talairach stereotactic were used. Anatomical data are obtained from stereotactic angiography, CT and MRI imaging and are incorporated in our computerised dosimetric TPS ARTEMIS-3D/Dosigray [4].
The irradiation parameters of the studied plans were empirically determined taking into account clinical considerations. The prescription isodose is usually ranged between 50% and 80%.

### DVH

Dose volume histograms (DVH) graphically summarised the dose distribution in the lesion and in the healthy tissues. The sampling of the isodose range of the differential DVH (DDVH) is of 1%. The dose is computed in voxels of 1x1x1 $mm^3$ spaced 1 mm apart in a 100x100x100 $mm^3$ matrix. The maximum isodose is normalised to 100%.

### Methodology of SALT group

Standard deviation of lesion DDVH (sd)

This sd index is used to classify the plans according their quality.

$$sd = \sqrt{\frac{\sum_{j=1}^{LV}(D(j) - \bar{D})^2}{LV}}$$

D(j): relative dose in the lesion voxel j
$\bar{D}$ : mean relative dose in the lesion
LV: lesion volume

When the plan quality deteriorates, sd increases. The sd could characterise the dose homogeneity in the lesion.

Underdosed lesion factor (ULF)

$$ULF = \frac{\text{volume of lesion receiving isodoses} \prec PI}{\text{lesion volume}}$$

Overdosed healthy tissues factor (OHTF)

$$OHTF = \frac{\text{volume of healthy tissues receiving isodoses} \geq PI}{\text{lesion volume}}$$

Geometric conformity factor (g) [5]

$$g = ULF + OHTF$$

The best geometric conformity is achieved when g is minimum since g represents the tridimensionnal geometric difference between two surfaces (lesion surface, prescription isodose surface).

### RTOG indices

We use the definition concerning the radiosurgery quality assurance guidelines [2].

Coverage index (CI)

$$CI = \frac{\text{minimum isodose in the lesion}}{\text{prescription isodose}}$$

Homogeneity index (MDPD)

$$MDPD = \frac{\text{maximum isodose in the lesion}}{\text{prescription isodose}} = \frac{100}{IP}$$

because the maximum isodose is located in the lesion and is normalised at 100%.

Conformity index (PITV)

$$PITV = \frac{\text{volume of the prescription isodose surface}}{\text{target volume}}$$

RTOG Indices classification

| Index | Interval | Classification |
|---|---|---|
| | $0.9 \leq CI \leq 1$ | PP |
| Coverage | $0.8 \leq CI < 0.9$ | MD |
| Index | $CI < 0.8$ | MAD |
| | $MDPD \leq 2$ | PP |
| Homogeneity | $2 < MDPD \leq 2.5$ | MD |
| Index | $MDPD \geq 2.5$ | MAD |
| | $PITV > 2.5$ | MAD |
| | $2 < PITV \leq 2.5$ | MD |
| Conformity | $1 \leq PITV \leq 2$ | PP |
| Index | $0.9 \leq PITV < 1$ | MD |
| | $PITV < 0.9$ | MAD |

**Table 1** : RTOG indices classification : PP per protocol, MD minor deviation and MAD major acceptable deviation.

## Results

**SALT group**

<u>Standard deviation index (s.d.)</u>

Two classes of sd have been arbitrarily defined:

- s.d. ≤ 12%, good quality of planning,
- otherwise, cases are classified of deteriorated quality

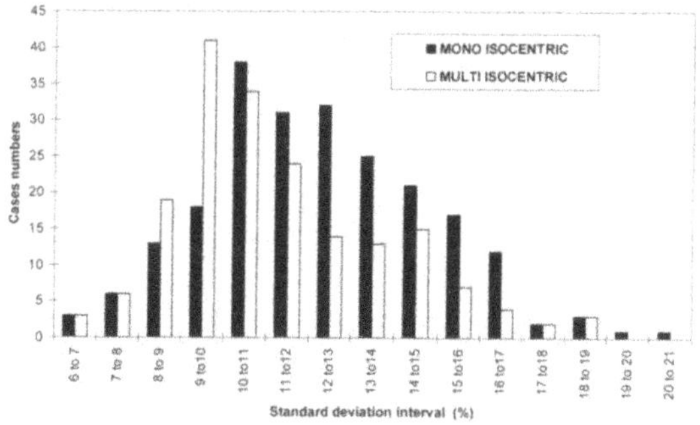


**Figure 1** : Classification of treatment plans as function of sd.

68,6% of the multi-isocentric and 48,9% of the mono-isocentric cases are classified with a good quality of planning .

<u>ULF and OHTF</u>

These two factors depend on the prescription isodose and their variations are opposed. Our results show that the lesion underdosage increases with the sd following respectively the equation ULF = 2,61sd - 0,15 ($R^2$=0,46, i.e. significant results) for the mono-isocentric and ULF = 2,9sd - 0,13 ($R^2$=0,36, i.e. significant results) for the multi-isocentric cases.

The results concerning OHTF show a general downward trend but the results are spread around the linear regression line; there is less correlation between the sd and the overdosed healthy tissues.

<u>Geometric conformity factor</u>

The g factor is the sum of the ULF and OHTF, the results show a stability of this factor (figure 2). It means that whatever the difficulty of the planning, the expert manages to keep a relatively constant geometric conformity index.

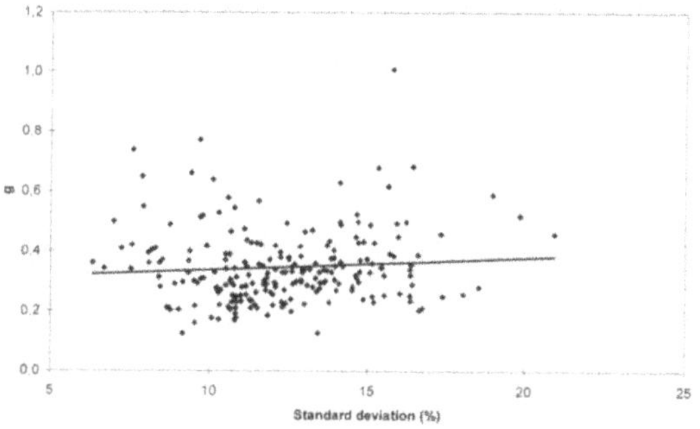


**Figure 2** : Geometric conformity factor function of the lesion DDVH standard deviation, concerning the mono isocentric cases

**RTOG**

<u>RTOG Coverage index</u>

As the minimum isodose in the lesion decreases when the sd increases, the RTOG conformity index decreases with a slope equal to 3,95 for the mono-isocentric, 3,62 for the multi-isocentric cases.

RTOG recommends choosing a prescription isodose close to the minimum isodose in the lesion. The majority of the cases are classified "major acceptable deviation" (table 2) as we do not follow that statement in our methodology.

<u>RTOG Homogeneity index</u>

This index is equivalent to the inverse of the prescription isodose (PI). To be considered per protocol, we have to choose PI superior to 50% which is always the case in our methodology (table 2).

<u>RTOG Conformity index</u>

PITV is the only RTOG volumetric index. We observe that PITV is decreasing when the sd increases, with an important slope of 4,8 for mono-isocentric (figure 3) and 4,5 for multi-isocentric cases..

48,5% of the mono-isocentric and 50,8% of the multi-isocentric cases were classified 'per protocol'.

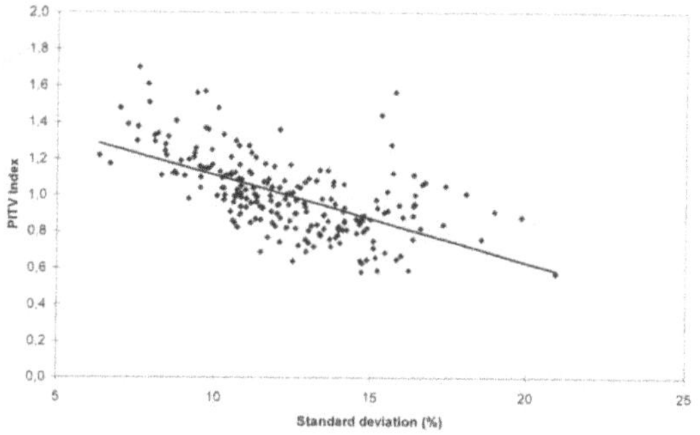


**Figure 3** : RTOG conformity index function of the lesion DDVH standard deviation, concerning the mono isocentric cases

| Coverage Index CI | | Mono isocentric Number of cases | Percentage | Multi isocentric Number of cases | Percentage |
|---|---|---|---|---|---|
| **0,9 ≤ CI ≤ 1** | PP | 6 | 2,7% | 3 | 1,6% |
| **0,8 ≤ CI < 0,9** | MD | 30 | 13,4% | 18 | 9,7% |
| **CI < 0,8** | MAD | 187 | 83,9% | 164 | 88,7% |
| **Homogeneity Index HI** | | | | | |
| **MDPD ≤ 2** | PP | 223 | 100% | 185 | 100% |
| **2 < MDPD ≤ 2,5** | MD | 0 | 0% | 0 | 0% |
| **MDPD ≥ 2,5** | MDA | 0 | 0% | 0 | 0% |
| **Conformity Index PITV** | | | | | |
| **PITV > 2,5** | MAD | 0 | 0% | 0 | 0% |
| **2< PITV ≤ 2,5** | MD | 0 | 0% | 1 | 0,5% |
| **1 ≤ PITV ≤ 2** | PP | 102 | 45,8% | 94 | 50,8% |
| **0,9 ≤ PITV < 1** | MD | 46 | 20,6% | 31 | 16,8% |
| **PITV < 0,9** | MAD | 75 | 33,6% | 59 | 31,9% |

**Table 2** : RTOG classification of the 408 AVMs planned following SALT methodology

## Discussion and conclusion

The RTOG quality assurance guidelines are supposed to be used for all localisations in the head. We have restricted this study to only AVMs.
RTOG classification of our results shows that we are for the coverage index in the majority of cases classified 'major acceptable deviation' because we accept to underdose the lesion. For the homogeneity index, as our PI is always greater than 50%, we are 'per protocol'. Finally, for the conformity index, two third of the cases are between 0,9 and 2 (MD and PP).
SALT indices highlight that our strategy is to spare healthy tissues since in most of the cases OHTF is inferior to 0,3. It is important to notice that the geometric conformity index g is kept constant whatever the quality and the complexity of the treatment planning.
This study showed that in the SALT prescription methodology the adjacent healthy tissue protection is favoured relatively to the lesion coverage whereas in RTOG methodology the lesion coverage is prevailing over the adjacent healthy tissue overdosage.

Two point of view are discussed here. RTOG suggests to choose a prescription isodose close to the minimum isodose in the lesion. But this prescription isodose must be superior or equal to 50%. It is tolerated to irradiate up to 2 times the lesion volume.
SALT indices complete RTOG parameters in the sense that there is a volumetric description of the underdosed lesion and overdosed HT portions. Moreover the combination of these two factors (ULF and OHTF) defines a conformity factor g which seems to be more representative of the dose distribution conformity.
We think that it is interesting to complete RTOG indices by the sd of the lesion DDVH, OHTF, ULF and the geometric conformity index g. This would permit to consider a more complete set of evaluation tools.

## References

[1] Schlegel W., Pastyr O., Bortfeld T., Schad L., Gademann G., Lorenz WJ. 1992 Computer systems and mechanical tools for stereotactically guided conformation therapy with linear accelerators *Int J Radiat Oncol Biol Phys* **24** 781-7
[2] Shaw E., Kline R., Gillin M. et al 1993 RTOG:radiosurgery quality assurance guidelines *Int. J. Radiation Oncology Biol. Phys.* **27** 1231-39
[3 Betti O. and Derechinski V. 1983 Irradiation stéréotaxique multifaisceaux *Neurochirurgie* **29** 295-298
[4] Lefkopoulos D., Schlienger M., Mérienne L. et al 1994 The associated targets methodology and the multi-isocenters radiosurgery treatment planning system Artemis-3D *Bull. Cancer/Radiother.* **81** 111-125
[5] Grandjean P., Platoni K. and Lefkopoulos D. 1998 Use of a general inverse technique for the conformational stereotactic treatment of complex intracranial lesions *Int. J. Radiation Oncology Biol. Phys.* **41** 69-76

# BANG™ polymer gels applied to the verification of conformal heavy ion radiotherapy

**Ulla Ramm[1], Michael Bock[2], Ulrich Weber[3], Michael Krämer[3], Achim Bankamp[2], Marc Damrau[1], Heinz-Dietrich Böttcher[1], Lothar R. Schad[2], and Gerhard Kraft[3]**

[1]Universitätsklinikum, Strahlentherapie, Frankfurt/Main, [2]Deutsches Krebsforschungszentrum, Heidelberg, and [3]Gesellschaft für Schwerionenforschung, Darmstadt, Germany

## Introduction

Magnetic Resonance Imaging (MRI) can be used to measure the dose distribution produced by sparsely ionizing radiation absorbed in tissue-equivalent BANG™ polymer gels [1, 2]. In contrast to conventional dosimetry techniques using ionization chambers or thermoluminescence detectors (TLD) MR imaging of BANG™ gels allows the verification of complete three-dimensional dose distributions with one single measurement. It is not obvious, that this technique can immediately be extended to densely ionizing radiation like the $^{12}C^{6+}$ beam used in the radiotherapy project started at the Gesellschaft für Schwerionenforschung mbH (GSI), Darmstadt, Germany. For such high-LET radiation saturation effects can be expected, just like for any other condensed phase detector. Another difficulty arises from the fact that a $^{12}C$ beam in matter undergoes fragmentation and generates a mixed radiation field of various particles with different energies. Contributions of different particles with a spectrum of energies generate the signal in the detector and this is not necessarily identical to the physical dose $D(\vec{r})$. Hence, in analogy to the radiobiological efficiency or the response of other condensed phase detectors, such a TLDs, to high LET heavy ion radiation, systematic investigations on the dose response of BANG™ polymer gels relative to photon radiation were started. Our contribution reports on MR imaging of tissue-equivalent aqueous polymer gels irradiated with monoenergetic carbon beams. The extent of the saturation effects to be expected for this high-LET radiation has been explored and first efficiency values have been deduced.

## Material and methods

For calibration with sparsely ionizing radiation we have irradiated BANG™ polymer gel samples (BANG™-type 3, MGS Research Inc., Guilford, USA) with 6 MV photons generated at the electron linear accelerator (SL25, Elekta, Crawley, UK) at the department of radiotherapy of the University of Frankfurt/Main, Germany. Doses of up to 15 Gy were applied at a field size of 5 cm * 5 cm to determine the dose-response curve. Two opposing fields were used in order to ensure a homogeneous dose distribution within the irradiated volume. The MR images were measured at a 1.5 T whole body scanner (Magnetom, Siemens, Erlangen, FRG) using the standard quadrature head coil. The transverse MR relaxation rate $R_2 = 1/T_2$ of the water protons was taken as a measure of the radiation dose absorbed in the gel. A CP-CPMG phase cycling pulse sequence, that aquires 32 spin echos, was used for MR imaging. Repetition time $TR = 2000$ ms and echo times $TE = 20$ ms up to 640 ms (echo spacing $\Delta TE = 20$ ms) were chosen. The signal in a spin-echo MR image produced by a dose $D$ is given by:

$$S_i(TE) = S_0 \; e^{-R_2(D)TE_i} \tag{1}$$

where $S_i$ are the signal amplitudes at the echo times $TE_i$. Since the absolute value of transverse relaxation is not essential for dosimetry, the transverse MR relaxation rate $R_2$ is deduced from a fitting procedure on logarithmic signal amplitudes for the whole MR image series of variing $TE_i$. Figure 1 shows the results on transverse MR relaxation rate $R_2$ as a function of dose up to $D = 15$ Gy. The yield of polymerization increases linearly with the energy transferred to the gel. At higher doses the curve is known to show a saturation effect [2]. The linearity allows to generate a $R_2$ map at given acquisition parameters for converting the MR signal amplitudes to absolute dose. First heavy ion experiments were performed with the raster scan facility at the GSI in CAVE M [3]. BANG™ polymer gels were irradiated with a single beam of monoenergetic $^{12}C$ ions in the energy range of 90 MeV/u up to 430 MeV/u and projectile rates around $10^6$/s to $10^8$/s. The beam was scanned over an area of 3 cm * 3 cm to ensure homogeneous distribution of the ions. To avoid "trivial" deviations from the linearity of dose response, particle fluences were restricted to an expected maximum dose in the bragg peak of 10 Gy. The radiation dose is calculated from the measured particle fluence according to

$$\begin{aligned} D(r) = 1.602 \; & \times \; 10^{-10} \\ & \times \; \frac{1}{\rho}\left(\frac{dE}{dx}\right)_{gel} (\text{MeV cm}^2/\text{g}) \\ & \times \; \Phi(\text{particles/cm}^2) \end{aligned} \tag{2}$$

using the mean energy loss $\left(\frac{dE}{dx}\right)_{gel}$ in BANG™ polymer gel calculated from

$$\overline{dE/\rho dx}(\text{MeV cm}^2/\text{g}) = \frac{(E_i - E_f)(\text{MeV})}{\rho(\text{g/cm}^3) \times \Delta x(\text{cm})} \tag{3}$$

with the initial and final energies $E_i$ and $E_f$, respectively, and the gel density $\rho$. This algorithm is implemented into the treatment planning software TRiP [4], which is used for the patient treatment planning in the GSI therapy project. The MR images were aquired in the MR head coil from CP-CPMG sequences and the transverse MR relaxation rate $R_2$ were calculated as described above. Using the $R_2$ dose calibration derived from low LET irradiation (see Fig. 1) the transverse relaxation rate is converted into absolute dose.

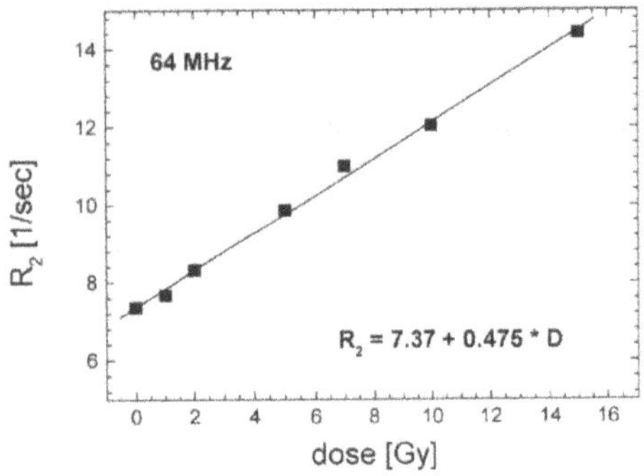


**Figure 1:** Dose response curve of BANG™ polymer gel on 6MV photon irradiation.

## Results and discussion

In Figure 2 depth dose profiles in BANG™ polymer gels after irradiation with monoenergetic carbon ion are graphed exemplarly. The results from MR image aquisition are compared with treatment planning calculations for $^{12}$C ions of 126, 154 and 166 MeV/u, respectively. The significant disagreement between the measured amplitude of the gel reponse and the planned physical dose profile in the region of the Bragg peak is a consequence of the strongly reduced efficiency of BANG™ polymers for high-LET $^{12}$C particles. Although the dose in the Bragg peak was chosen to be far below the saturation region for sparsely ionizing radiation such as photons or electrons, the experimental results exhibit a large saturation effect for heavy ions. These

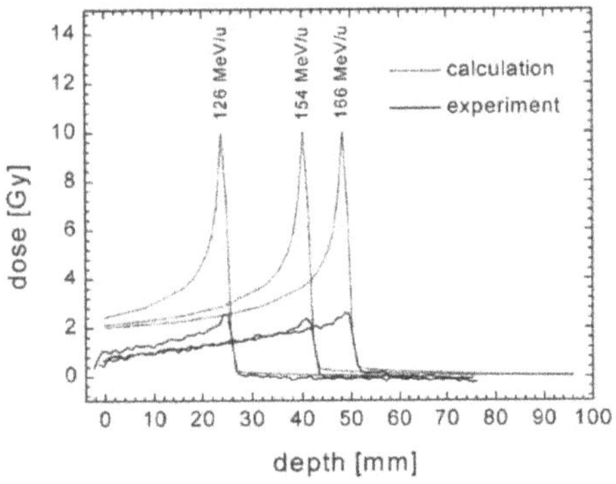


**Figure 2:** Depth dose curves for 126, 154 and 166 MeV/u $^{12}C^{6+}$ ions incident on BANG™ polymer gel. Dotted lines: calculated with TRiP, solid lines: measured with MR imaging.

results show the importance of the microscopic dose deposition pattern for high-LET radiation. Since the linear energy transfer (LET) of fast heavy ions increases with decreasing projectile energy, the local ionization density rises. High local ionization density in the center of the ion path causes saturation effects. As a consequence the efficiency is largely reduced at the end of the depth dose profile, where the energy of the heavy ions is low. In analogy to the radiobiological efficiency of high LET radiation or the dose response of other solid state detectors, such as TLDs, the efficiency $\epsilon$ of polymer gels is defined as the ratio of the transversal relaxation rate $R_2$ per dose $D$ for high LET heavy ions to transversal relaxation rate $R_2$ per dose $D$ for signal of low LET photon radiation:

$$\epsilon(E, Z) = \frac{[(R_2 - R_{2,0})/D]_{high}}{[(R_2 - R_{2,0})/D]_{low}} \tag{4}$$

Here, $R_{2,0}$ denotes the transverse relaxation rate without irradiation. The ratio is expected to depend on both, particle energy $E$ and charge $Z$. Although no dedicated measurements with monoenergetic particle beams have been carried out so far, first estimates for $\epsilon$ can be derived from the results shown in Figure 2. In the entrance region of the carbon beam nuclear fragmentation can be neglected and the ions can still be considered monoenergetic. Thus, it is possible to determine $\epsilon$ for $^{12}$C ions for the given energies. The results are shown in Figure 3. For high projectile energies, i.e. low LET values the efficiency is still close to a constant value, but for decreasing projectile energies (increasing LET) the efficiency decreases. A similar dose response was found by *Geiß* et al. [5] for TLDs exposed to high LET radiation.

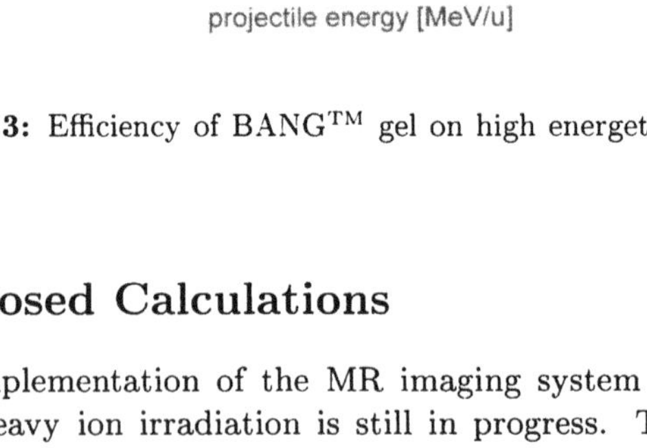


**Figure 3:** Efficiency of BANG™ gel on high energetic carbon ions.

## Proposed Calculations

The implementation of the MR imaging system for high LET heavy ion irradiation is still in progress. The fragmentation of the primary carbon beam along its path results in a mixed radiation field of ions from protons up to carbon, with energies from the initial beam energy down to the stopping region. Hence an efficiency table covering this range of ion species and energies needs to be established in order to allow a quantitative verification of 3D dose distributions with the BANG™ polymer gel method. Because not all ions and/or energies will be experimentally accessible, model calculations are necessary to complement the measurements. It is planned to use an adaption of a model developed at the GSI [6], which relies only on heavy ion track structure and the experimentally determined photon response. The model calculations are based on the assumption that knowledge of the radial dose $D(r)$ around the ion path and of the gel response to reference radiation $(R_2 - R_{2,0})_{ref}$ is sufficient to obtain the efficiency $\epsilon(E, Z)$. For the radial dose $D(r)$ at a distance $r$ from the particle track, results of track structure calculations [7] will be parametrized, leading to

$$D(r) = \begin{cases} k & : \ r \leq r_0 = 0.1\text{nm} \\ k(r_0/r)^2 & : \ r_0 < r < R_{el} \end{cases} \quad (5)$$

with the konstant $k$ normalized to the energy loss

$$2\pi \int_0^{R_{el}} D(r) r dr = \frac{1}{\rho} \left( \frac{dE}{dx} \right) \quad (6)$$

In the track structure calculations mentioned above the maximum range of the secondary electrons $R_{el}$ depends on the electron energy $E_e$ only, leading to $R_{el} \propto E_e^{3/2}$. The heavy ion energy loss $dE(E)/dx$ can be calculated using the code ATIMA [8]. Using Equation 5 and the dose response of BANG™ gels on sparsely ionizing radiation (see Fig. 1) it will be possible to calculate the dose deposition in a volume $\Delta V_i$. Summing up of all volumes $\Delta V_i$ in all layers $\Delta z_i$ yields the BANG™ gel signal after heavy ion irradiation. This procedure enables to calculate the efficiency $\epsilon(E, Z)$ for all ions and energies according to its definition given in Equation 4. This method was already successfully applied to describe the response of biological systems as well as thermoluminescence detector responses after heavy ion irradiation [5].

## Conclusion

The dependence of the BANG™ gel efficiency on energy and charge of heavy ions does not allow a direct dose measurement. However, once this dependence is determined by experimental data and extensive model calculations as suggested, MR imaging of tissue-equivalent aqueous polymer gel can be extended to the verification of three-dimensional dose distributions in high LET heavy ion radiotherapy.

## References

[1] Gore J C, Kang Y S, and Schulz R J 1984 Measurement of radiation dose distributions by nuclear magnetic resonance (NMR) imaging *Phys. Med. Biol.* **29** 1189–1197

[2] Maryanski M J et al. 1993 NMR relaxation enhancement in gels polymerized and cross-linked by ionizing radiation: A new approach to 3D dosimetry by MRI *Magn. Res. Imag.* **11** 253–258

[3] Haberer T et al. 1993 Magnetic scanning system for heavy ion therapy *Nucl. Instr. and Meth. in Phys. Res. A* **330** 296–305

[4] Jäckel O and Krämer M 1998 Treatment planning for heavy ion irradiation *Physica Medica* **14** Suppl. 1 53–62

[5] Geiß O et al. 1998 Efficiency of thermoluminescent detectors to heavy charged particles *Nucl. Instr. and Meth. in Phys. Res. B* **142** 592–598

[6] Scholz M and Kraft G 1994 Calculation of heavy ion inactivation probabilities based on track structure, X ray sensitivity and target size *Radiat. Prot. Dosim.* **52** 29–33

[7] Krämer M 1995 Calculations of heavy-ion track structure *Nucl. Instr. and Meth. in Phys. Res. B* **105** 14–20

[8] Schwab T 1991 Transport von Schwerionen durch Materie innerhalb ionenoptischer Systeme *GSI-Report* **91-10**

This work was presented in parts at DOSGEL99 - 1st International Workshop on Gel Dosimetry, Lexington, Kentucky, USA, July 1999

# Correlation between CT number and water-equivalent thickness for heavy charged particles

**Eike Rietzel, Oliver Geiß, Dieter Schardt, Bernd Voss, Michael Krämer and Gerhard Kraft**
Gesellschaft für Schwerionenforschung - Biophysik, Planckstraße 1, D-64291 Darmstadt, Germany

## Introduction

There are a number of advantages in using heavy charged particles like protons or carbon ions instead of photons for radiotherapy [1]. For example an improved conformity of the target volume and the irradiated volume can be achieved due to the small lateral scattering and the inverted depth dose profile.
For the treatment planning the precise knowledge of the particle ranges in different tissue types is one of the most important input parameters. The information about the tissue composition and densities of a volume to be irradiated usually is derived by Computer Tomography (CT). For the calibration of the CT numbers (measured in Hounsfield units) to tissue density several calibration curves exist [2, 4, 3, 5][1]. The relation between the water-equivalent path length and the CT number is stored in a so called Hounsfield look-up-table (HLUT) which allows fast interpolation.
The verification of the effective particle ranges by positron emission tomography (PET) [6] during the first patient treatments with carbon ions at GSI showed that the HLUT described in [3] needed further improvements.
Therefore the range of carbon ions in specific animal tissues like brain, muscle, fat and bone was measured. These measurements in combination with the corresponding CT data resulted in a new calibration curve. In addition a frozen pig head was irradiated with numerous pencil beams at different positions. The measured ranges are compared to modeled ranges which take into account the beam profile as well as the tissue quantities derived from CT and the HLUT. These comparisons are used to validate or even improve the new HLUT for the realistic but most complex situation of a compound of various different tissues in the target volume.

## Material and methods

For the measurement of the precise range of carbon ions in specific animal tissues each sample was irradiated separately without contributions from other tissues. The different tissues were packed into thin plastic bags each. These bags were then placed in a polysterene box (inner dimensions: 100x100x300 mm$^3$, wall thickness: 20 mm) applying slight pressure. In the computer tomograph Somatom Plus4 at 120 kV the filled box was scanned with a pixel size of 0.5 mm and a slice distance of 3 mm. The different tissue materials were irradiated with a 388 MeV/u carbon beam. Behind the box a water tank with variable thickness (telescope) as well as an ionization chamber were placed to measure the exact position of the resulting Bragg peak. The spatial resolution for measuring the Bragg peak was about 0.1 mm. In front of the box a second ionization chamber was used as reference. The different shifts of the measured Bragg peaks for the different tissues give their corresponding water-equvalent path lengths.
The frozen pig head was scanned in the Somatom Plus4 with a pixel size of 1.1mm and a slice distance of 1.0 mm. At 441 different positions the head was irradiated with a carbon ion pencil beam at 400 MeV/u (FWHM = 2.3 mm). The different Bragg peaks were measured in an ionization chamber (IC) stack [7] with a spatial resolution of about 1 mm.
In contrast to the experiment described above the irradiated tissue is not homogeneous within the spread of the beam. For a comparison of the measured and the expected ranges therefore the profile of the beam has to be considered.
The expected ranges are modeled by a combination of the CT data and the HLUT to calculate the water-equivalent thicknesses of the head at each voxel. To obtain the expected signals in the ICs in the stack the stack itself and the beam profile have to be considered. The beam profile requires the use of weighting factors for the different parts of the beam traversing the pig head through different voxels. These factors are calculated by an integration over the Gaussian beam profile in the range of the corresponding voxel. To compute the expected signals in the IC stack the beam is split into smaller sub-beams. The dimensions of these sub-beams are defined by the CT voxel size. The sum of all the weighted sub-beams yields the expected signals. The water-equivalent path length of the experimental set up was measured without the pig head in the beam line and taken into account as a fixed offset.

## Results and Discussion

From the carbon range measurements in the homogeneous tissues and bone materials a new calibration curve was obtained (figure 1). In figure 2 the region of soft tissues is shown enlarged. Here the deviations from the calibration curve described in [3] can be observed. The precise measurements presented here result in a sort of fine structure in the calibration curve.

For muscle tissue the difference of the computed ranges between the new HLUT and the one used before is shown in figure 3. The Bragg peak is shifted about 1.5 mm. The

[1] The calibration curves strongly depend on the CT scanner system.

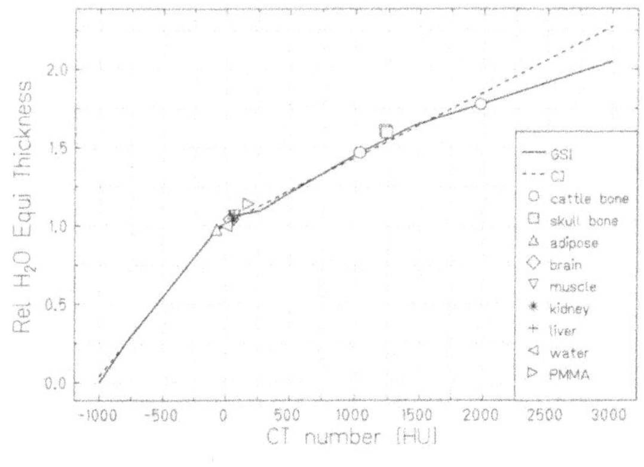


**Figure 1:** Correlation between CT number and water-equivalent thickness. The calibration used for tumor treatment is shown as full curve (GSI), experimental data are shown as symbols. The dashed curve shows the calibration used before (CJ, [3]).

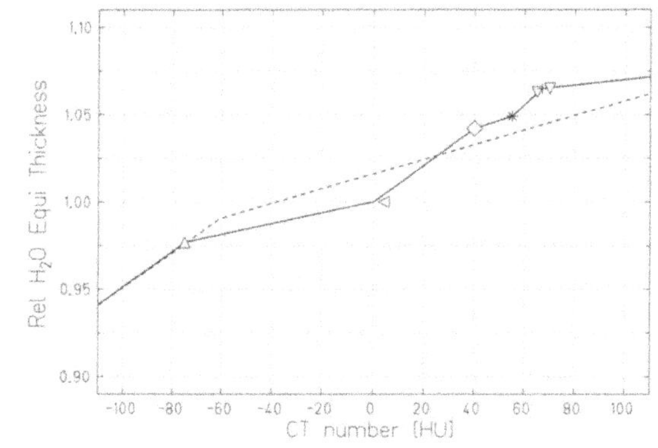


**Figure 2:** Correlation between CT number and water-equivalent thickness, enlarged region of soft tissues. See fig. 1 for details.

experimental data is in good agreement with the peak calculated using the new HLUT.

The water-equivalent thickness of the experimental set up for the pig head measurements was measured with a carbon beam (183 MeV/u) and no sample in the beam line. This measurement was also used to test the model to compute the signals in the IC stack depending on the beam energy and profile, the CT data and the HLUT. Since no sample was in the beam line the complete CT data was set to the CT number of air (-1000). Figure 4 shows measured (markers) compared to the modeled (new HLUT) signals (curve) in the IC stack. The agreement between the model and the experiment is sufficient for the inspection of the pig head experiment.

The measurements performed with the pig head were compared with the corresponding modeled signals. Figure 5 shows one of the measured as well as the corresponding modeled Bragg peaks. The peak modeled with the new HLUT is in good agreement with the measured data whereas the previous used HLUT results in an obvious difference.

At other positions the agreement between the measured

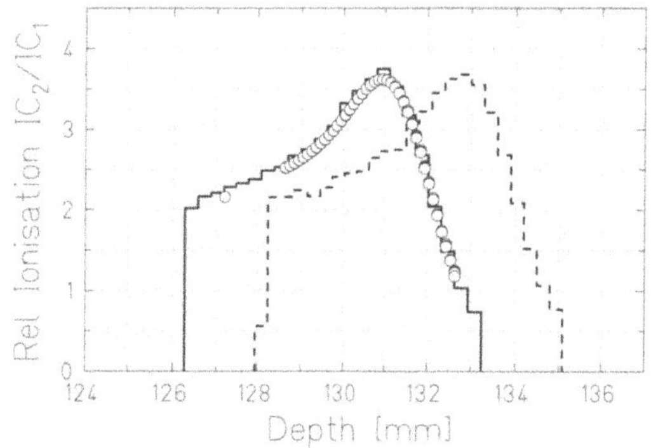


**Figure 3:** Comparison between measured (symbols) and calculated (curves) depth dose distributions after irradiation of muscle tissue with 388 Mev/u carbon ions. The bragg peak (full curve) computed with the new HLUT is in good agreement with the measured data whereas for the previous used calibration curve (dashed curve) a shift of about 1.5 mm can be observed.

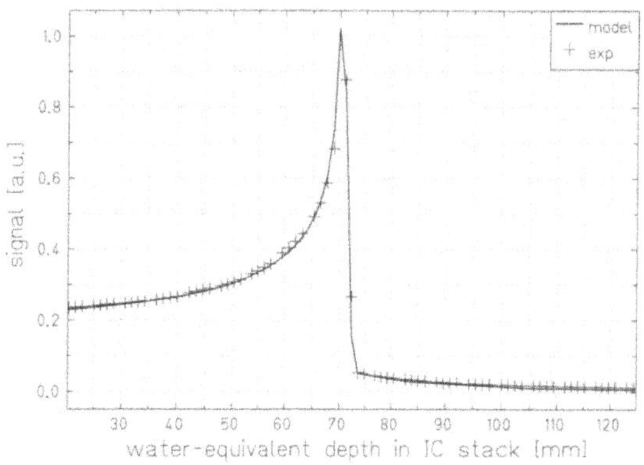


**Figure 4:** Test of the model to compute the signals in the stack of ionization chambers, 183 MeV/u carbon ions without the pig head in the beam line. The modeled peak is shown as curve, the measured signals as markers.

and the modeled peak is not as good as shown in figure 5. Assuming that the model yields correct results this means a further improvement of the Hounsfield look-up-table should be possible. At the moment this is limited by the measurements of the Bragg peaks as well as the CT data.

The resolution for the peak measurements is limited by the characteristics of the ionisation chamber stack and the accuracy in positioning the pig head. Therefore more precise results could be obtained by measuring the Bragg peaks with the telescope water tank.

The spatial resolution of the peak modeling depends on the voxel size of the CT data. This is especially the case for the splitting of the beam in sub-beams. The calculation of the weighting factors due to the beam profile does not depend on the CT voxels. Here accurate results can be obtained by the integration over the Gaussian beam distribution.

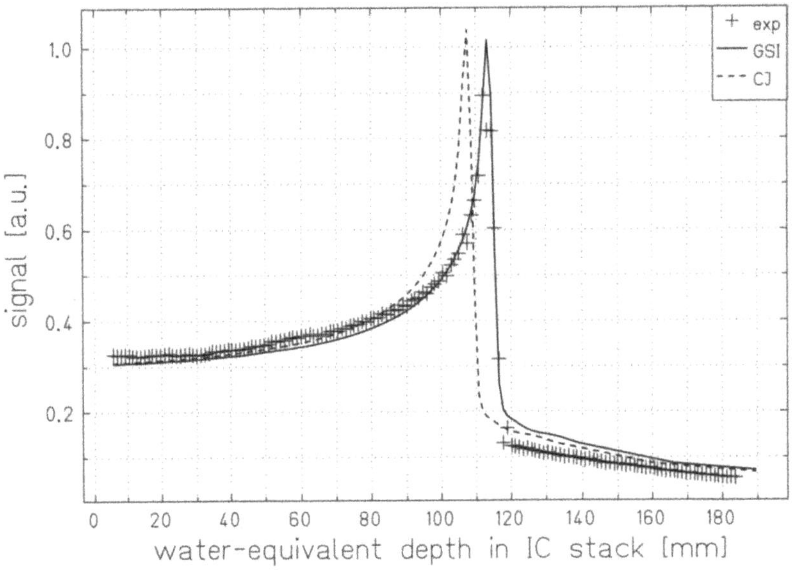


**Figure 5:** Irradiation of the frozen pig head, comparison of the measured and the modeled residual ranges. The full curve shows the modeled Bragg peak computed with the new HLUT (GSI), the dashed line the one computed with the HLUT described in [3] (CJ). The use of the new HLUT results in a better agreement between modeled and measured peak.

## Conclusion

The new Hounsfield look-up-table presented here results in a better agreement for the computed and the measured range of carbon ions in tissue. But the pig head experiment shows that further improvement of the HLUT should be possible. The presented model for the computation of the expected signals in the stack of ionization chambers yields precise results. In a next step we will therefore try to fit the modeled to the measured signals by varying the Hounsfield look-up-table.

## References

[1] Kraft G 1990 The radiobiological and physical basis for radiotherapy with protons and heavier ions. *Strahlentherapie und Onkologie* **166** 10–13.

[2] Minohara S, Kanai T, Endo M and Kawachi K 1993 Effects of object size on a function to convert X-ray CT numbers into water equivalent path length of charged particle beams. *Proc. 3rd workshop on physical and biological research with heavy ions* NIRS-M-99, HIMAC report No. 6.

[3] Jacob C 1997 Reichweite CT-Zahl Beziehung von Phantommaterialien und Messungen mit einer neuentwickelten multisegmentierten Ionisationskammer zur Dosisverifikation bei Schwerionenbestarhlung. *PhD thesis* University Heidelberg.

[4] Schneider U, Pedroni E and Lomax A 1996 The calibration of CT Hounsfield units for radiotherapy treatment planning. *Phys. Med. Biol.* **41** 111-124.

[5] Schaffner B and Pedroni E 1998 The precision of proton range calculations in proton radiotherapy treatment planning: experimental verification of the relation between CT-HU and proton stopping power. *Phys. Med. Biol.* **43** 1579–1592.

[6] Enghardt W, Fromm WD, Geissel H, Keller H, Kraft G, Magel A, ManfraßP, Münzenberg G, Nickel F, Pawelke J, Schardt D, Scheidenberger C and Sobiella M 1992 The spatial distribution of positron-emitting nuclei generated by relativistic light ion beams in organic matter. *Phys. Med. Biol.* **37** 2127.

[7] Brusasco C 1999 A detector system for the verification of three-dimensional dose distributions in the tumor therapy with heavy ions. *PhD thesis* University Kassel.

# Parameter adjustment of a proton pencil beam algorithm using experimental data from complex compensators

H. Szymanowski[1], S. Caneva[1], A. Mazal[1,2], C. Nauraye[2], R. Ferrand[2], M.-C. Murillo[1], G. Gaboriaud[1] and J.-C. Rosenwald[1]

[1]Institut Curie, 26 rue d'Ulm, 75005 Paris, France, and [2]Centre de Protonthérapie d'Orsay (C.P.O.), B.P.65, 91402 Orsay, France

## Introduction

We report on an experimental procedure for the adjustment of various parameters used in a proton pencil beam algorithm recently developed by our group. The procedure is aimed at determining the most adequate modeling of the influence from compensator and from the beam line elements in order to improve the dose computation accuracy.

## Material and methods

Our proton pencil beam algorithm is based on the principles described by Gottschalk *et al.* [1] for proton scattering within the medium. For clinical conditions, the algorithm features simple specific parameters accounting individually for the beam modulation, the contribution of scattering from compensator at depth in the patient, and the influence of the proton beam line as a whole. The adjustment procedure of these algorithm parameters relies on comparisons between computed and measured dose distributions. In order to enhance specifically the effects induced by the variation of each model parameter, different complex shaped compensators have been designed. Dose distribution measurements have been performed in water in presence of these compensators on the 200 MeV therapeutic proton beam line at C.P.O. with a diode detector. The same conditions have been reproduced for the dose calculation algorithm implemented in the commercial treatment planning system ISIS3D.

## Results and discussion

The outcome of a well defined methodology carried out for investigating the parameter values with the complex compensators is twofold. First the computation accuracy has been significantly improved by a simple and accurate modeling of the compensator influence on the pencil beam radial spread. Second the adjustment procedure has allowed to determine a quantification method of the beam line scattering by the means of additional measurements of the lateral penumbra in air. The proton pencil beam algorithm supplied with the adjusted parameter values provides predictions in excellent agreement with all the measurements. In particular the mean deviations over the dose distributions are about 1.0% in terms of dose, and 0.1mm in terms of position. The maximum deviations in dose and position do not exceed respectively 5.0% and 1.0mm for the most extreme geometric configurations.

## Conclusion

The optimal parameters entering our proton pencil beam algorithm have been determined by using experimental data from complex shaped compensators. Since the knowledge of the physical and geometrical characteristics of the beam line elements is not needed, the algorithm can be easily adapted to any therapeutic proton beam line, following the same adjustment procedure. Despite the complexity of the geometries involved, this adjustment procedure is not meant to replace a thorough validation procedure, which can be performed at a first level by comparison with measurements obtained under simple irradiation conditions. Beside their role for adjustment, the complex compensator geometries, which have no clinical relevance, belong to a second level of validation. This level of algorithm testing needs to be complemented with geometries closer to clinical cases. For a more practical evaluation of its performances, our proton dose algorithm is currently being assessed with real patient compensators.

## Reference

[1] Gottschalk B *et al.* 1993 Multiple Coulomb scattering of 160 MeV protons *Nucl. Instrum. Method* B **74** 467-90

# The "X-Sting": a new, PC-based, 3D stereotactic treatment planning system

**Kiki Theodorou, Eduard Schrebmann, George Nikiforidis and Constantin Kappas**

Medical Physics Department, Medical School, University of Patras, 26 500 Patras, Hellas

## Introduction

Stereotactic radiotherapy (SRT) aims to treat intracranial lesions considered to be inoperable or carrying excessive risk from conventional surgery as well as to irradiate small volumes where high precision and high dose gradient are required. Stereotactic radiotherapy is a multi-task radiotherapy treatment technique, which involves multi-modality imaging technologies as well as complex mechanical and computational procedures. Therefore, a dedicated stereotactic radiotherapy treatment planning system is necessary for the management of the above information, for the design and computation of the irradiation technique as well as for the evaluation and, if possible, the optimization of the treatment plan. The purpose of this study is to present a new 3D treatment planning system dedicated for stereotactic radiotherapy treatments, the *X-STING*. The treatment planning system has been based on personal computer (PC) taking into account the wide availability of those platforms as well as their increasing performance capabilities. Furthermore, we have incorporated into the system new features and algorithms for stereotactic radiotherapy purposes as well as it has been designed to be flexible for future developments.

## Material and methods

The whole treatment planning application has been developed and implemented to a Personal Computer (PC). The implementation of the application to a PC system, was decided to two reasons: (a) the wide availability of PCs and (b) the easy and fast hardware connection to other peripheral systems (scanner, printer, water-phantom etc.). The hardware characteristics are: PC Intel Pentium II at 420 MHz with 64 Mb RAM memory plus 400 Mb virtual memory and 4 Gb hard disk. The basic software specifications for the development of the treatment planning system were: Windows NT Server, Service Pack 4, Borland C++ Builder, The Visualization Toolkit Library (vtk), version 2.2 and a DICOM converter.

### Specifications

According to the requirements of a stereotactic radiotherapy treatment planning system, the specifications for the development of the *X-STING* are: **(i)** Modelization of the treatment machine and development of a treatment machine database. The treatment machine model includes the definition of all the mechanical and dosimetric characteristics of the treatment machine (linear accelerator) [1], **(ii)** Image acquisition from different imaging modalities. The *X-STING* is able to receive CT, MRI and Angiographic images and is DICOM 3.0 compatible, **(iii)** CT and Angiographic localization algorithm, **(iv)** Image correlation between CT and Angiographic images [2], **(v)** Delineation process. The delineation could be done in any slice orientation. **(vi)** Patient Model. The patient model is a 3D matrix which includes anatomical information derived from the images available, biological information as well as information concerning the dose distribution. **(vii)** Beam definition via the BEV module, **(viii)** 3D-dose calculation, **(ix)** Dose-Volume Histograms (DVHs), **(x)** Visualization tools.

### Design Characteristics

The design was based on the following principles: **(i)** Build a system, which is flexible enough for future changes, **(ii)** Construct algorithms independent of visualization libraries and **(iii)** Compatibility with the DICOM standard. Special attention has been paied to the design of the user interface which is not in the philosophy of the "pop-up windows" but a common graphical user interface is applied through out the application (Fig. 1).

### Visualization

For the visualization processes of the *X-STING*, the Visualization ToolKit (vtk) has been used, which is a software system for 3D computer graphics, image processing, and visualization. Vtk includes a C++ class library, and several interpreted interface layers including Tcl/Tk, Java, and Python. According to the opitions offered by the vtk libraries, the main visualization capabilities of the *X-STING* are: **(i)** Visualization of 2D images of any orientation, **(ii)** Automatic delineation, **(iii)** Beam's Eye View (BEV), **(iv)** Visualization of the dose distribution.

## Results and discussion

The structure of the application is based on 3 levels. At the bottom level, specific radiotherapy algorithms are implemented using pure C++ code. The result of these algorithms is passed to the Visualization ToolKit (vtk) libraries, which are used mainly for visualization and non-radiotherapy related purposes. On the highest level, the user interface (based on C++ Builder) displays the results obtained from the vtk libraries. The performance of the system has been assessed as far as the speed of the different calculations is concerned. The results are the following:

- The automatic contour extraction takes 1 sec for the whole volume (35 slices) while it is real-time for each slice.
- The slice reconstruction in any arbitrary orientation (sagital, coronal, and oblique) is performed real-time.
- The 3D reconstruction of the whole volume (35 slices) is around 10 sec.

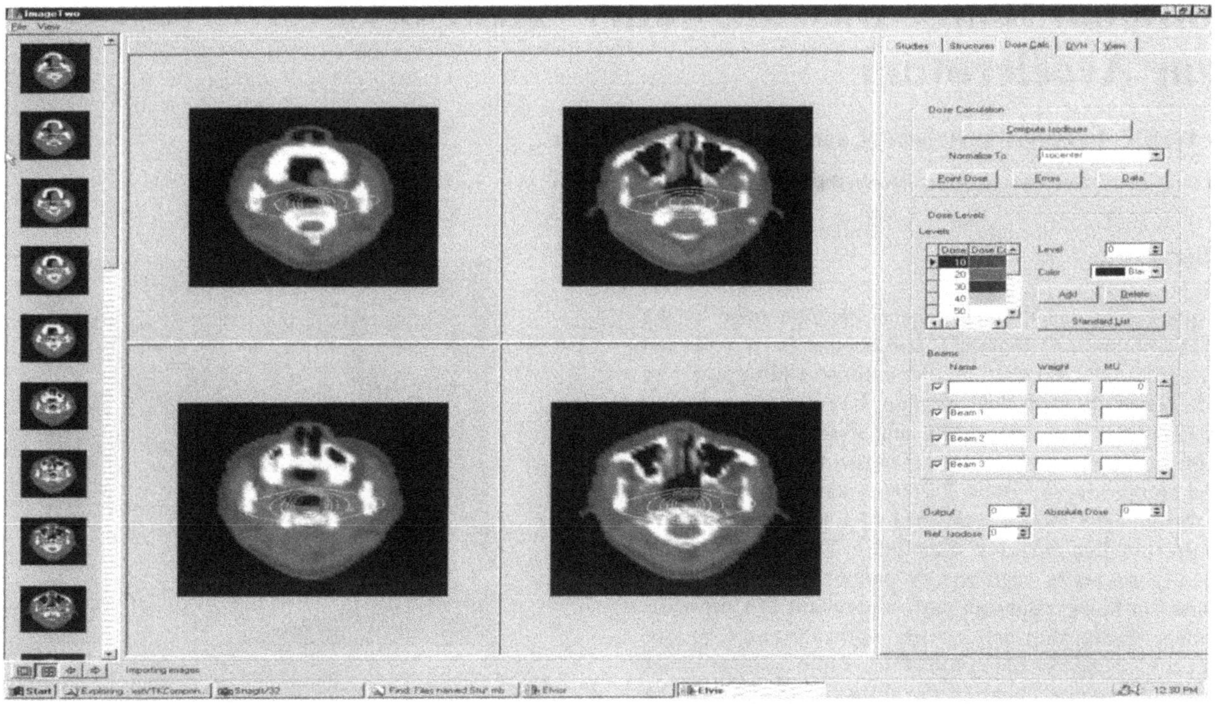


**Figure 1:** Example of the X-Sting interface. 2D visualization of the dose distribution superimposed on transverse CT images

- The dose calculation performed for the default dose matrix (50 x 50 x 50 points) takes around 30 sec for a complete irradiation scheme (6 arcs of 120° each).
- The isodose display is real-time both in 2D and 3D representation.
- The DVH calculation is real-time.

The above results are comparable with the computation times presented by the currently available commercial systems. Nevertheless, the performance of the system could be significantly improved by just increasing the RAM memory of the computer.

## Conclusion

The stereotactic radiotherapy treatment planning system *X-STING* has been designed and implemented in order to meet the current and as much as possible the future needs of the stereotactic techniques. It is in accordance with the intentional standards as far as communication protocols and conventions are concern. The *X-STING* is fully DICOM 3.0 standard compatible while the DICOM RT standard referring specifically to radiotherapy objects is integrated into the system. Furthermore, several innovative algorithms have been incorporated to the presented system in order to meet the current requirements of the stereotactic treatments. Nevertheless, the performance of the *X-STING* TPS cannot be fully exploited unless a high degree of accuracy and reliability is reached, which is only possible through exhaustive quality assurance effort. Several tests have been performed for the assessment of the accuracy of the dose calculation where the results of the treatment planning system have been compared with the actual dose measurements. The results are in accordance with the international recommendations. The whole system is currently under systematic testing for the quality control of its specifications.

## References

[1] Theodorou K, Kappas C, Rosenwald J C 1998 Modelization of the external radiotherapy machine into radiotherapy treatment planning system. *Physica Medica* **3** 111-118

[2] Theodorou K, Kappas C, Gaboriaud G, Mazal A D, Petrascu O, Rosenwald J C 1997 A simple method for 3D lesion reconstruction from two projected angiographic images: implementation. to a stereotactic RTPS. *Radiotherapy and Oncology* **43** 281-284

# Automated Image Based Quality Assurance for Medical Linear Accelerators

**Keith T. Welsh[1], Lawrence E. Reinstein[1] and Robert A. Wlodarczyk[1]**

[1] State University of New York at Stony Brook, Stony Brook, NY 11794-7028

## Introduction

Regular quality assurance measurements recommended by the AAPM TG-40 are an important component of a radiation oncology department's overall quality assurance program. The increased availability of dual photon beam multi-modality LINACs creates a time consuming and exacting task for the medical physicist who performs these measurements. We have developed an innovative system for computerized Image Based Quality Assurance (IBQA) composed of a software program and a corresponding imaging phantom. The IBQA system automatically measures regular QA parameters and monitor any changes in those values as part of standard QA regimen. The intimate relationship between the software and a unique phantom provides nearly full automation. From a single image and a total of 3 mouse clicks in the software, the TG-40 QA parameters are quickly and automatically calculated. The IBQA system includes many other features that aid in the process and evaluation of QA parameters.

## Material and methods

The plastic IBQA phantom (Fig. 1) contains a unique set of radio-opaque fiducial markers that are used to establish the coordinate system, x-y magnification factors and non-linearity of the image. Additional markers are embedded in 8 rotatable disks that are situated around the edge of the 20X20 $cm^2$ field

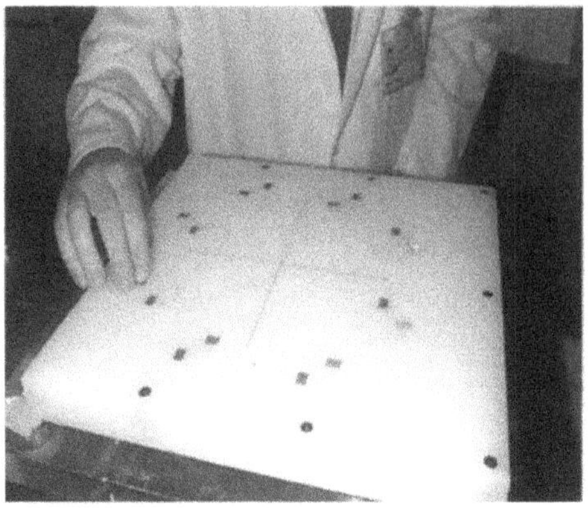

**Fig. 1** Picture of the IBQA phantom. Visible are the scribed lines to line up with the LINAC's cross hairs and the rotating disks used to mark the light field edges..

region and are used to localize the light field.
The IBQA software contains image processing and registration algorithms which analysis the recorded digital image. A screen shot of the program is shown in Fig. 2. The software automatically detects the fiducial markers, adjusts x-y magnifications and corrects for image warping and rotations. Curve fitting and smoothing techniques are used to improve the SNR. The associated database, stored in MS Access© format, stores baseline and tolerance values for each modality and

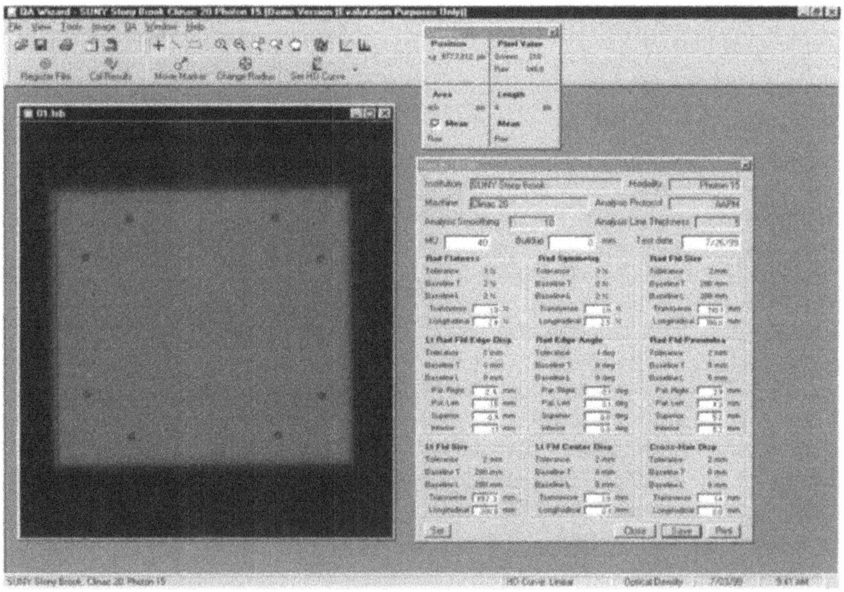

**Fig. 2** Screen shot of IBQA system program showing the results of the analysis of a film irradiated in the IBQA phantom. On the left, is shown the digital image of the film and the detected fiducial markers and radiation field edges, the calculated light field edges and the centers of the light field, radiation field and phantom. The results screen is on the right; note the parameters in red are out of tolerance. The entire process is fully automated and takes only 3 mouse presses!

energy of all associated radiation machines as established by the user during the setup of the "preference." After analysis of the image, the results can be saved to the database and printed in report form to be included as part of QA documentation. All calculated results are then available for easily retrieval and "data mining."

The accuracy of the IBQA system was tested by comparing its results to conventional point densitometer measurements, direct geometric measurements, or to measured pre-defined changes from a reference beam. Reproducibility and the effects of image digitization, in both spatial and gray scale resolution, were also tested.

## Results and discussion

The IBQA system measures *Radiation Field Flatness* and *Symmetry*, *Radiation Field Penumbra Widths*, *Radiation* and *Light Field Sizes*, *Field Edge Orthogonality* and *Light Field, Cross Hair and Radiation Field Center Centricity*. By designing the analysis algorithms around a unique IBQA phantom we were able to make the system automated, fast and easy to use. The entire accelerator QA process of the IBQA system involves only four routine steps. They are setting up the phantom in the therapy machine and irradiating, obtaining a digital file of the transmitted radiation field either from an EPID or by scanning a film through a digital scanner, analysis of the file by the IBQA software and generation of a printed Report from the IBQA software.

Table 1 show the reproducibility from a cumulative number of test films. Individual parameter results were averaged from all test films The results of less than 0.3 mm reproducibility for all spatial parameters is well within most protocol tolerences of 2 mm. Table 2 shows results from testing the systems ability to track changes in the reference beam parameters. Again the system was able to accurately track the changes within 0.3 mm for most changes.

The IBQA system improves on conventional methods for measuring parameters suggested by AAPM TG-40. It is fast, easy to use and is capable of measuring QA parameters with precision that is consistent with TG 40 recommended tolerances. Most of the IBQA system's results have standard deviations approximately 0.3 mm as shown in tables 1 and 2. In contrast manual measurement of the radiation field parameters, which were measured with a point densitometer with a 1 mm sensor aperture, have an uncertainty of ± 0.5 mm and ± 0.5 % for position and OD measurements, respectively. The manual measurements of the shifts values also have uncertainties of ± 0.5 mm.

The IBQA system is capable of correcting imaging artifacts, such as spatial distance variation across an image and background density variation across an image, that can be introduced by image scanners or developers. The spatial variation correction is only dependent on the phantom the density correction requires a blank file to be scanned as a template.

Although the IBQA system performs its analysis automatically, it also provides analysis preferences and tools, which give the user the ability to influence how the image is analysis and to study accelerator beam image in much greater detail. The use can specify smoothing mask size, line thickness averaging width and calculation protocols the routines use to analyze the film and return its results. The user can choose from several different protocols. After image registration the user can inspect and adjust the position of the detected markers before the image parameters are actually calculated. The program also includes an H&D mapping control that allows the user to define an H&D curve to convert the intensity image to a dose map image prior to QA analysis. Another tool is an interactive profiler that displays the pixels values of a user defined line along with the locations of detected markers and field edge-lines, and also has optional smoothing and line thickness averaging of pixels. Other tools and features include a histogram, color coded detection markers, and an image palette control. Also the preliminary data tables suggest that the IBQA Phantom may also be used with good accuracy in a film less mode through direct accelerator field digitization using an EPID. The feasibility of this method is still under study.

## Conclusion

We were successful in creating an automated, easy to use, fast and robust system for regular QA accelerator measurements. The IBQA system was able to track changes in all parameters with an acceptable degree of accuracy and precision. Its integrated database makes it possible to establish baseline and tolerance tables for all QA parameters for each accelerator modality and energy, record and retrieve QA parameter results for trend analysis and "data mining" for most AAPM TG-40 beam parameters and select specific protocols for defining the QA parameters. The unique coupling of the image analysis

| | Number of Images | Number of Measurements | Average | SD | Units |
|---|---|---|---|---|---|
| **Radiation Field Size** | 11 | 22 | 198.90 | 0.21 | mm |
| **Light Field Size** | 11 | 22 | 198.60 | 0.37 | mm |
| **Crosshair Shift** | 3 | 6 | 0.63 | 0.03 | mm |
| **Radiation/Light Field Edge Coincidence** | 3 | 6 | 1.07 | 0.11 | mm |
| **Light Field Shift** | 3 | 6 | 0.92 | 0.11 | mm |
| **Jaw Angle** | 11 | 44 | 0.00 | 0.00 | deg |
| **Flatness** | 11 | 22 | 3.15 | 0.36 | % |
| **Symmetry** | 11 | 22 | 1.65 | 0.32 | % |
| **Penumbra** | 11 | 44 | 4.39 | 0.17 | mm |

**Table 1** Shown is the reproducibility of the system. IBQA measured values, for each parameter values shown above, are average over all dimensions. The standard deviations (SD) are also reported.

| | Number of Images | Number of Measurements | Shift From Reference | Average Error | SD | Units |
|---|---|---|---|---|---|---|
| **Crosshair Shifts** | 8 | 12 | +3, -3, +6, -6 | -0.18 | 0.25 | mm |
| **Radiation/Light Field Edge Coincidence** | 4 | 6 | +3, -3, +6, -6 | -0.15 | 0.31 | mm |
| **Light Field Shift** | 4 | 6 | +3, -3, +6, -6 | -0.08 | 0.27 | mm |
| **Jaw Angle** | 1 | 4 | -5 | -0.13 | 0.10 | deg |
| **Radiation Field Size** | 2 | 4 | -10,+10 | -0.91 | 0.53 | mm |
| **Light Field Size** | 2 | 4 | -10,+10 | -0.20 | 1.00 | mm |

**Table 2** Shown is a list of the intended shifts in parameter values with respect to the reference setup, and the average error in detection and measurement of these shifts by the IBQA system.

software and the IBQA phantom provides nearly full automation of analysis and report generation.

## References

[1] AAPM Task Group No. 40, "Comprehensive QA for radiation Oncology", 1994, American Association of Physicist in Medicine

[2] Constantinou, C, Protocol and Procedures for Quality Assurance of Linear Accelerators, Library of Congress Cataloging-in-Publication, 1993

# A multi-purpose quality assurance tool for MLC-based IMRT

**Yan Chen, Lei Xing, Gary Luxton, Jonathan G. Li and Arthur L. Boyer**

Radiation Oncology Department, Stanford University School of Medicine, Stanford, CA 94305

## Introduction

Intensity modulated radiation therapy (IMRT) has emerged as a maturing clinical technology. More fields are often used in an IMRT treatment than in conventional conformal therapy. Complex intensity distributions in the fields are planned in order to spare critical structures adjacent to the planning target volume (PTV). The complexity of IMRT has led most facilities gaining experience with this new technology to adopt a conservative quality assurance (QA) process. This extensive QA has been a limiting factor to the wide spread use of IMRT. A QA program involves virtually every aspects of treatment planning and delivery, including verification of intensity maps for each field, absolute dose at given points, and the integrity of the hardware and software of the beam delivery systems. In order to verify the patient position, digitally reconstructed radiographs (DRR) in the beam's eye view (BEV) are computed as references for checking the setup accuracy and target localization during treatment using portal imaging. In our clinic, a QA protocol, which is similar to the prototype IMRT QA program described by Burman *et al*, has been implemented.[1] Such a QA process is a very labor-intensive undertaking. It demands not only many physicist hours, but also a large block of machine time on the linear accelerator, which obviously conflicts with treating patients, especially in a busy clinic. We have developed a software tool in an attempt to speed up the QA procedure. A network connection is established between a personal computer (PC) on which the in-house QA program resides, the CT virtual simulation system, the treatment planning system, and the record and verifying system. The QA program reads in the parameters of a treatment plan from various sources, and modifies and creates several files for beam delivery and verification. It also calculates the dose to isocenter as an independent check of the monitor units (MU) computed by the treatment planning system. It can accomplish all the QA tasks in one step, except verification of the intensity profiles, thus considerably reducing the time required for the QA process.

## Material and methods

As illustrated by the diagram in Fig. 1, the contours of each target and critical structure for IMRT treatment planning are outlined on axial CT slices using a virtual simulation workstation (AcQSim, Picker International, Cleveland, OH, USA). The CT study along with the structure information is transferred in DICOM format[2] to an inverse planning workstation (Corvus, NOMOS Corporation, Sewickley, PA, USA). The step-and-shoot technique is used for beam delivery. After the treatment plan has been approved by the physician, the leaf sequence information is transferred to a record-and-verify system (VARIS, Varian Medical Systems, Palo Alto, CA, USA) using a program called Varian RTP Exchange (Varian Medical Systems, Palo Alto). The RTP Exchange file contains the leaf sequences for all fields in ASCII format.

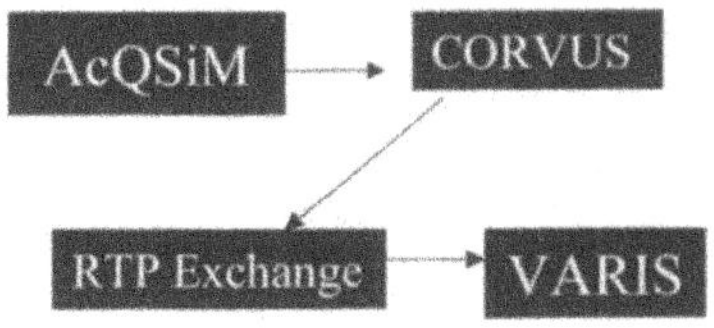


**Figure 1:** Flow-chart diagram for IMRT treatment planning

The QA tasks following the approval of a treatment plan can be described as the following:

1. verification of the two-dimensional intensity profiles of the fields using an electronic beam imaging system or film.
2. patient-specific dose measurement using a phantom for verifying the MU settings.
3. generating AP and lateral DRRs for isocenter verification using AcQSim.
4. generating the DRR for each field marked with the multileaf collimator (MLC) boundary for patient setup verification during treatment.
5. generating a file for an open MLC field for the boundary of each IMRT field to make a portal imaging film using a double exposure technique.
6. generating the graphics for the initial position of the MLC (the first segment in the leaf sequence) for each field for confirmation during treatment.

Items *1* and *2* are the QA tasks to confirm that the treatment plan actually produces a dose distribution as reported by the treatment planning system. The intensity distribution can be acquired using film or a Beam Imaging System (BIS, Wellhöfer Dosimetrie, Schwartzenbruck, Germany), and the images are compared with the intensity maps generated by the treatment planning system. The patient-specific dose measurement is performed using a phantom and the same MLC leaf sequences. A Corvus utility is used to perform a forward calculation for the dose distribution in the phantom. The absolute dose at one or more points is measured using an ion chamber. The dose distribution in the phantom can be verified using TLD or film.[3] Acquiring the intensity profile and measuring the dose are performed using the linear accelerator. It is good QA practice to "dry-run" the treatment plan at least once before actually treating the patient. However, setting up a phantom for dose measurement can be quite time consuming. Until a reliable three-dimensional dosimeter is available, absolute dose measurement and intensity map verification must be carried out separately. Each procedure requires 1 – 2 hours of accelerator time. We decided to use an independent dose calculation similar to the manual MU calculation for conventional treatment to replace absolute dose measurement for every case. In principle, if the dose calculation model is reasonably accurate, an independent calculation by computer can provide a similar degree of confidence as for treatment involving conventional fields. The leaf sequence and the source-to-surface distance (SSD) for each field are used as input for the dose calculation.

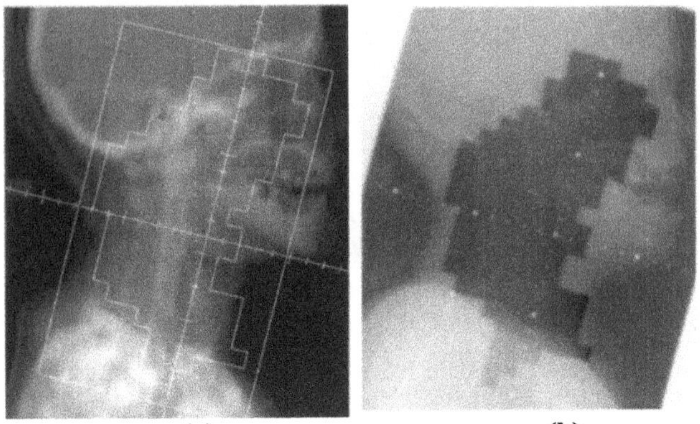

**(a)** **(b)**

**Figure 2: (a)** DRR in BEV with marked field boundary of an IMRT field, and **(b)** Portal image for the same field.

The QA tasks listed in Items *3*-5 are for setup and localization verification before and during the treatment. A pair of orthogonal DRRs is used to verify the patient position by comparison with simulation films from a conventional simulator. Portal images are used for detecting any significant variations during daily treatment. A portal image for a conventional treatment can be taken using the double exposure technique, one with the customized radiation port and the other with a larger rectangular open field, so that both the field boundary and some patient anatomy can be seen on the image. A "conventional" portal image for an IMRT field can be created as well, using the MLC boundary as the port of the radiation field. An example of such portal image is shown in Fig. 2(b). For portal image exposure, an MLC field to define the field boundary is needed. The DRR in the beam's eye view (BEV), as shown in Fig. 2(a), can be used as a reference for comparing with the portal image for target localization during the treatment. It is useful to mark the field boundary also on the DRR.

The graph of the first MLC segment of each field is used for the final confirmation before each treatment is started. This graph is compared with the initial MLC position shown on a computer screen of VARIS.

A convenient vehicle for transferring the leaf sequence information to VARIS is the RTP Exchange program from Varian. The machine parameters and MU settings are transferred at the same time, eliminating the need to manually enter the data. We use an in-house program to read in the leaf sequences and find the field boundary by concatenating all the segments for each field. Although generating an open MLC field for portal imaging is straightforward, it is time consuming to load these portal fields one by one into VARIS. A quick solution is to append these fields to the original RTP file for the treatment. This process is represented by the two one-sided arrows that connect the Corvus and the RTP Exchange through our in-house program in the diagram in Fig. 3. A current hardware limitation in the Varian system is that, for a field with intensity modulation, the field width has a maximum of 14.5 cm. The treatment planning system uses two or more abutted intensity-modulated fields for a wider field. For the purpose of verifying the target localization, it is unnecessary to take the portal image for two split fields separately. Therefore a "glued" portal MLC field is generated by our program for abutted fields with the same gantry angle.

To mark the boundary manually on the DRR in the field's BEV is extremely laborious. To automate this task, we create a treatment plan on AcQSim, which is called an RT plan in AcQSim terminology, in the *Virtual Simulation* mode using open beams with the same field orientations as planned by Corvus. This plan is modified by our program to define the actual field portals. The double-sided arrow in Fig. 3 connecting AcQSim and Corvus illustrates the fact that Corvus has imported the anatomy information from AcQSim for planning, and the beam geometry information is sent back to AcQSim for generating an RT plan. The RT plan is modified by the in-house program and sent back to AcQSim. The DRRs in BEV with field boundaries can be displayed and printed in the *Verification* mode on AcQSim.

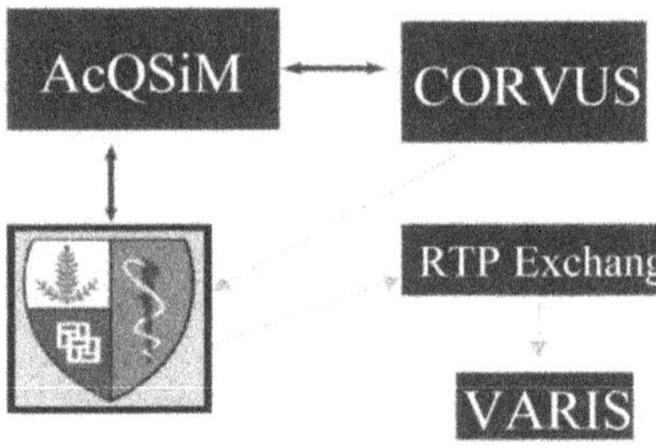


**Figure 3.** Schematic representation of data flow.

Our program reads in the field SSD, a parameter available for each field in the RT plan from AcQSim. Although it may not be difficult to extract the SSD information from Corvus, we decided to use the geometry of the original patient anatomy, so that the dose calculation is truly independent of Corvus.

The dose to isocenter by an intensity-modulated field is calculated from the leaf sequence and the SSD. A simple algorithm is used to sum the contribution from each segment to the dose at the isocenter. Following the idea of Clarkson summation, one can decompose the output factor, assumed to be the product of the collimator scatter factor and the phantom scatter factor, into a summation of the contributions from many finite-size beamlets. We further assume that the collimator scatter factor is dependent only on the jaw setting for a linear accelerator using an MLC. The phantom scatter contribution from each beamlet for an open field can then be decomposed by differentiating the tissue-to-maximum ratio (TMR) data with respect to field size. For a segment shaped by an MLC in a step-and-shoot IMRT field, each beamlet is either open or blocked by the MLC. Therefore, the phantom scatter factor can be approximated by the summation of each beamlet contribution weighted by a transmission factor. The transmission factor is 1 for an open beamlet or the leakage factor for a closed beamlet. For an intensity-modulated field, a resultant modulating factor for each beamlet can be calculated by summing the transmission factor for each segment, weighted by the fractional MU of the segment.

In summary, our QA program takes the leaf sequence file in the RTP Exchange format and the AcQSim RT file corresponding to an IMRT plan as input, and generates four files, namely, the report for calculated dose to isocenter, the RTP Exchange file appended with portal imaging MLC fields, a modified AcQSim RT file for DRRs marked with MLC field boundaries, and a PostScript graphic file for the initial MLC positions.

## Results and discussion

Our QA program has been implemented as a routine clinical process. Since its implementation, the manpower needed for IMRT QA has been reduced significantly. The program runs on a PC in a few seconds for tasks that formerly demanded several hours. Listed in Table 1 is the time it would take to carry out each of these tasks manually for a typical case.

| | time |
|---|---|
| Mark field boundaries on DRRs | 1.0 - 1.5 h |
| Transfer MLC fields to VARIS | 15 - 30 min |
| Copy initial MLC position from Shaper | 15 - 30 min |
| Measure the dose using an ion chamber | 1.0 - 1.5 h |
| Total | 2.5 – 4.0 h |

**Table 1:** Time consumed for various QA tasks.

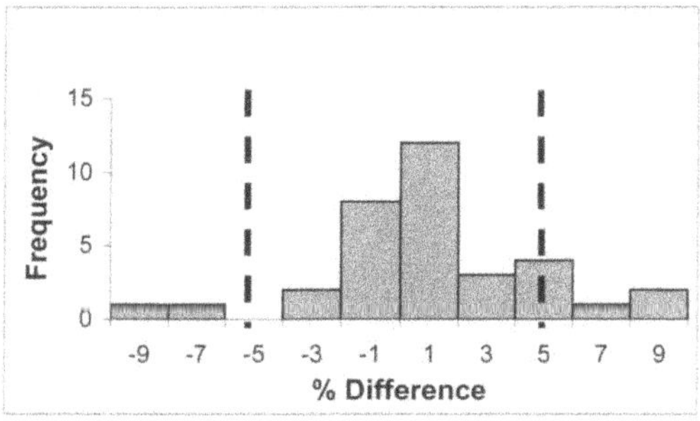


**Figure 4** Difference histogram of dose calculation.

Verification of the absolute dose to the isocenter is a major task carried out by our QA software. It gives us enough confidence to omit the ion chamber measurement in the QA process for IMRT. This has benefited us multilaterally in freeing the physicists from taking the measurements, saving machine time on the linear accelerator, and lowering operational cost. If the isocenter is inside the PTV, and no appreciable tissue heterogeneity in the paths of the beams, our calculated dose to the patient agrees with Corvus and chamber measurement within ±5%. Larger discrepancies as much as ±10% have been encountered, but in a predictable way. The fixed collimator scatter factor in our simple dose calculation algorithm is problematic in the case that a substantial amount of flattening filter scattered photons are blocked by the MLC. As a result, the scatter dose may be overestimated if the isocenter happens to be a location of low dose. In the case that a beam passes through a large air volume, the dose will be underestimated since no heterogeneity correction is considered in our calculation. In Fig. 4, we report the error distribution of the calculated isocenter dose compared to Corvus calculation for 34 clinical cases. The percentage difference in 29 cases is less than ±5%. The results of 10 phantom plans comparing Corvus calculation, measurement, and QA calculation are presented in Table 2. Our results are comparable with the *in vivo* measurement results of Tsai *et al.*[4]

| Calculation | Measurement | Corvus |
|---|---|---|
| 230.6 (-2.3) | 241.0 (+2.1)) | 236.0 |
| 171.2 (+5.7) | 162.9 (+0.6) | 162.0 |
| 192.9 (-1.6) | 197.7 (+0.9) | 196.0 |
| 211.6 (-0.7) | 218.8 (+2.7) | 213.0 |
| 218.6 (-3.7) | 218.7 (-3.7) | 227.0 |
| 248.1 (-2.3) | 249.7 (-1.7) | 254.0 |
| 226.7 (+1.2) | 231.3 (+3.3) | 224.0 |
| 207.7 (+0.8) | 217.7 (+5.4) | 206.0 |
| 216.4 (-1.6) | 227.0 (+3.2) | 220.0 |
| 176.2 (+0.1) | 176.2 (+0.1) | 176.0 |

**Table 2**: Comparisons of isocenter dose (in cGy) per treatment fraction from calculation, Corvus, and measurement. Percentage differences from Corvus are listed in parentheses.

## Conclusion

Clinical implementation of IMRT is a complex process involving several commercial systems that may be acquired from one or more vendors. A comprehensive QA program is needed to verify that a treatment plan is correctly delivered. We have developed a software program that performs dose calculations, automatic data transfer, and various graphic utilities simultaneously. The program substantially improves the efficiency of the QA process.

## References

[1] Burman C, Chui C S, Kutcher G, Leibel S, Zelefsky M, LoSasso T, Spirou S, Wu Q, Yang J, Stein J, Mohan R, Fuks Z, Ling C C 1997 Planning, delivery, and quality assurance of intensity-modulated radiotherapy using dynamic multileaf collimator: a strategy for large-scale implementation for the treatment of carcinoma of the prostate *Int J Radiat Oncol Biol Phys* **39** 863-73

[2] Xing L, Curran B, Hill R, Holmes T, Ma L, Forster K M, Boyer A L 1999 Dosimetric verification of a commercial inverse treatment planning system *Phys Med Biol* **44** 463-78.

[3] Low D A, Mutic S, Dempsey J F, Gerber R L, Bosch W R, Perez C A and Purdy J A 1998 Quantitative dosimetric verification of an IMRT planning and delivery system *Radiother Oncol* **49** 305-16

[4] Tsai J S, Wazer D E, Ling M N, Wu J K, Fagundes M, DiPetrillo T, Kramer B, Koistinen M, Engler M J 1998 Dosimetric verification of the dynamic intensity-modulated radiation therapy of 92 patients *Int J Radiat Oncol Biol Phys* **40** 1213-30

# Monitor Unit Calculation for Intensity Modulated Photon Field

**Lei Xing, Yan Chen, Gary Luxton, Jonathan G. Li, and Arthur L. Boyer**

Department of Radiation Oncology, Stanford University School of Medicine, Stanford, California 94305-5304, USA

## 1. Introduction

Intensity-modulated radiation therapy (IMRT) has recently been emerged as a new radiation therapy modality arising from the development of inverse planning and the computer-controlled delivery using multileaf collimators (MLC). While IMRT improves the dose distribution for many clinically complicated cases, it also entails new techniques for treatment verification because of the intensity modulation of the incident photon beams. Among various issues related to verifying the treatment, a pressing problem is how to verify efficiently the calculation of monitor units (MU) from a commercial inverse planning system. An independent MU check is required for a patient treatment based on primitive machine data, e.g., output factor, TMR, etc. For a conventional treatment plan this is typically done using an independent manual calculation. Because of the lack of an effective tool for the MU calculation, ion chamber measurement has been employed to verify the patient dose in a surrogate phantom in many institutions, which is time consuming and costly.

The most straightforward way to verify the MU or dose calculation of an IMRT treatment planning system is perhaps to sum the fractional MUs corresponding to the segmented fields. The MU calculation for a multileaf collimated static field has been described in the literature.[1] A few attempts have been made to develop more efficient techniques for the verification of dynamic delivery. Boyer and Xing *et al.* have investigated some theoretical aspects of the MU calculation for intensity modulated field.[2] Recently, Kung and Chen have developed an approach for the "forward" dose verification.[3] In their calculation, the MUs and leaf sequence files for a patient treatment were used as input to compute the dose at a given point in the patient. A modified Clarkson method was used to determine the dose for a given non-uniform fluence map. The purpose of this paper is to bridge the gap between the intuitive approach of Kung and Chen and the theoretical framework by Boyer and Xing *et al.*, and to provide a close formula for MU calculation in IMRT. The formula is general and suitable for any delivery method of intensity modulated beam. The method will be illustrated for MLC modulated IMRT using a Varian accelerator (Varian Oncology Systems, Palo Alto, CA). The data of a few clinical IMRT cases will be presented.

## 2. Material and methods

We will concentrate on IMRT based on fixed-gantry delivery. As will be seen below, the methodology is quite general and can be generalized for dynamic arc IMRT. For convenience, let us first consider the case of a single incident beam. Multiple beams can be dealt with similarly as long as their relative weights are known. Assume that a treatment field defined by the jaws can be partitioned into $M$ beamlets. Also, assume that there are $K$ segments in the dynamic treatment field. The field shapes of these segments are known from the given leaf sequence file. The dose at a given point in the patient is a summation of the contributions of all segments of treatment, i.e.,

$$D = \sum_{k}^{K} MU_k d_k = MU \sum_{k}^{K} f_k d_k \ , \qquad (1)$$

where $MU_k$ is the number of monitor units delivered by the $k^{th}$ segment, $MU$ is the total monitor unit delivered by the beam, $f_k = \mathrm{MU}_k / \mathrm{MU}$ is the fractional MU of the $k^{th}$ segment, and $d_k$ is the dose per unit MU from the $k^{th}$ segment. Let $d^0_m$ be the dose contribution from the $m^{th}$ beamlet when it is open, and $d^t_m$ be the leakage dose per unit MU from the $m^{th}$ beamlet when it is blocked by the MLC. If we denote the set of beamlets inside the open field area of the $k^{th}$ beam segment by $A_k$, the dose from the $k^{th}$ segment per unit MU is given by

$$d_k = \sum_{m \in A_k}^{M} d^0{}_m + \sum_{m \notin A_k}^{M} d^t_m \ . \qquad (2)$$

We introduce a notation

$$\delta_{m,A_k} = \begin{cases} 1 & \text{if} \quad m \in A_k \\ 0 & \text{if} \quad m \notin A_k \end{cases} , \qquad (3)$$

and further assume that the leakage dose can be related to the open beamlet dose by

$$d^t_m = \alpha\, d^0_m \ ,$$

where $\alpha$ is the transmission factor. Then, by exchanging the order of summations, we can recast equation (1) as

$$D = MU \sum_{m}^{M} C_m d^0_m \ , \qquad (4)$$

where

$$C_m = \sum_{k}^{K} \left[ \delta_{m,A_k} + \alpha \left( 1 - \delta_{m,A_k} \right) \right] f_k \ . \qquad (5)$$

Equation (4) relates the dose at a given point to the setting of the monitor units, *MU*, and is the main result of this paper. Equation (4) shows that, in order to obtain the dose of a multi-segment dynamic field, one only needs to perform the dose calculation of the contributing beamlets once. The increase in MUs required to deliver a modulated field is reflected by the $C_m$ factor defined by the summation in equation (5). The calculation is facilitated by separating the open and blocked sets of beamlets, assuming that any beamlet is either completely open or blocked. Except for the beamlet size, which can be dependent of step size in a specific leaf sequence algorithm, our approach is independent of leaf sequence algorithms and delivery machines. All one needs for the calculation is the dose/MU and the transmission factor for each beamlet. The beamlet dose, $d_m^0$, can be calculated using a variety of methods, as simple as a Clarkson type of approach or as complex as Monte Carlo simulation.

The remaining problems are computational. To obtain the absolute value of MU using equation (4), it is required to calculate the dose contributions from the beamlets. Given a collection of beamlets, there are many ways to calculate their dose contributions to a point. Instead of dividing the field into a series of annular rings[3], we proceed by using the beamlets as the elementary building blocks. This decomposition seems to be more natural since it utilizes the field boundaries defined by the MLC. In the following we describe a simple way to carry out the MU calculation based on a modified Clarkson method.[4]

The calculation point can be anywhere inside the field. As in the conventional treatment, it is convenient to choose the isocenter as the verification point because the source-to-skin distance (SSD) of the beam can be easily obtained and no off-axis ratio is involved. In this case, we consider the contribution from the central four beamlets as the "primary dose", denoted by $D_p$, and the contributions from the rest of the beamlets as "scatter". To be specific, let us assume that the beamlet size is 1cm×1cm. In reality each of the four beamlets in the central 2cm×2cm square can be either open or blocked. When all the four beamlets are open in the beam, the primary dose is given by

$$D_p(\text{cGy}) = MU \times C_f(\text{cGy/MU}) \times S_c(l_{eq}) \times S_p(l = 2\text{ cm}) \times TMR(d, l = 2\text{ cm}) , \tag{6}$$

where $C_f$ is the calibration factor of the linac, $S_c$ is the collimator scatter factor obtained by in-air measurement, $S_p$ is the phantom scatter factor defined as the ratio of the dose rate for a given field at reference depth to the dose rate at the same depth for the reference field size with the same collimator opening, $l_{eq}$ is the equivalent square of the field defined by the opening jaws, and $TMR(d, l)$ is the tissue-to-maximum ratio for a square field of side $l$ at the depth $d$.[4] The total scatter dose is calculated by summing up the contributions of all non-central beamlets. Each non-central beamlet acts as a scatter source and its contribution to the isocenter can be computed using the modified Clarkson method.[4] To the first order approximation, the scatter contribution from a beamlet centered at a distance $r_m$ from the isocenter is given by $D_m = D_m^u a^2$. Here $a$ is the beamlet size, and $D_m^u$ is the scatter dose from a unit area at the center of the $m^{\text{th}}$ beamlet. To obtain $D_m^u$, one may first compute the scatter dose from a circular ring with radius $r_m$ and then divide it by the area of the ring, $2\pi r_m \Delta r_m$. To improve the accuracy, a beamlet can be further divided into a number of sub-beamlets and the dose from these sub-beamlets can be dealt in a similar manner as described above. A sum of the contributions of the corresponding sub-beamlets gives the scatter dose of the beamlet. We found that a sub-beamlet size of 0.5cm×0.5cm can yield satisfactory results consistent with experimental measurements for all clinical cases we have tested and further reduction in the sub-beamlet size does not give notable improvement. Of course, equation (4) is quite general and allows one to use any other method for MU calculation based on the beamlet information.

The case of multiple incident beams can be dealt with similarly. One can proceed along two directions to verify the system calculation. One is to use the prescription information and fractional weighting of each beam to derive the monitor units for each beam. These MUs can then be compared with the system calculation. When the information of fractional weighting is not available, one can proceed to use $MU_j$ for each field provided by the treatment planning system to calculate the dose at a point using

$$D = \sum_{j=1}^{J} D_j = \sum_{j=1}^{J} MU_j \left( \sum_{m=1}^{M_j} C_{m,j} d_{m,j}^0 \right) , \tag{7}$$

where index $j$ has been added to label each individual incident beam, and $J$ is the total number of beams. The dose given by equation (7) is then compared with that given by the treatment planning system. One should note that this method only verifies the composite dose, not that of individual beam.

# 3. Results and Discussion

## 3.1 Simplified examples

Let us consider the delivery of a simple fluence profile shown in figure 1a. There are a few ways to generate the fluence map by segmented delivery; two are shown in figures 1b and 1c. In the first delivery scheme, the MLC leaf pair delivers the three fluence blocks in sequences. In this case, $f_1$=1/4, $f_2$=1/2, and $f_3$=1/4. Substituting the $f_k$'s into equation (4) and equation (5) we have

$$MU = \frac{4D}{(1+2\alpha)d_1 + 2d_2 + (1+\alpha)d_3} . \tag{8}$$

If we ignore the transmission dose, the above result indicates that in order to deliver a dose $D$ to a point using the segmented delivery shown in figure 1b, the delivery time is four times longer than that required by a delivery using a physical compensator. This agrees with an intuitive calculation based on the simple shape of the fluence map. For the delivery

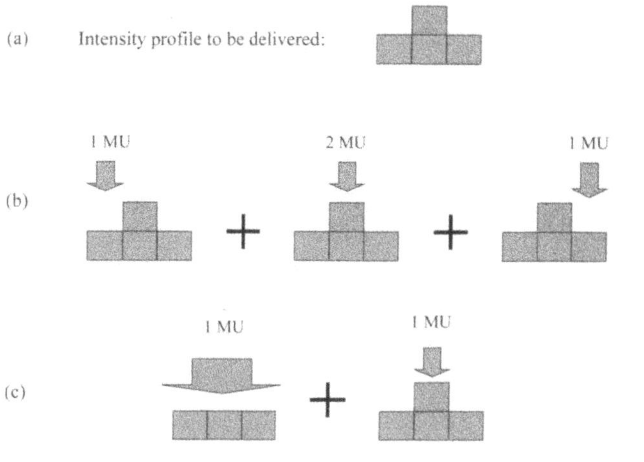


**Fig. 1** A simple example to illustrate the MU calculation. (a) is the intensity profile to be delivered. (b) and (c) represent two different delivery schemes.

scheme shown in figure 1c, it can be similarly shown that the delivery time is two times longer than that required by a physical compensator delivery if the leaf transmission is ignored. Note that the transmission doses in the two delivery schemes are different. The transmission is less if the delivery is more efficient.

### 3.2 Clinical examples

The above method has been applied to over fifty clinical IMRT cases, including head and neck, brain, and prostate patients, as well as in the surrogate phantoms for chamber measurement. The clinical IMRT plans were generated using the CORVUS inverse planning system.[5] The leaf sequence files were read into the software module. The fractional MU factors, $f_k$'s, and the primary and scatter doses are then computed. In table 1 we show the detailed calculation for a nine-field prostate phantom plan together with ion chamber measurement data. The measurement for each field in a cylindrical water phantom was used as a surrogate for measurements in the patient. For comparison, the primary and the scatter doses for each field are separately listed along with the total contribution of the field.

Table 1: Data for a 9-field prostate IMRT treatment using a 15 MV photon beam. The original patient plan was used to generate the dose distribution in a surrogate cylindrical water phantom (See Ref. 4 for detailed description about the phantom). At the isocenter, the Corvus dose is 253.6 cGy, the calculated dose using the current approach is 249.2 cGy, and an ion chamber measurement gives 249.6 cGy.

| Gantry angle (degree) | Corvus cal. (cGy) | Primary dose (cGy) | Scatter dose (cGy) | Beam dose (P.+S.) (cGy) | Measure-ment (cGy) |
|---|---|---|---|---|---|
| 30 | 45.4 | 41.9 | 3.0 | 45.0 | 43.8 |
| 65 | 22.8 | 20.5 | 1.9 | 22.5 | 24.1 |
| 95 | 30.0 | 27.8 | 1.8 | 29.6 | 28.8 |
| 135 | 29.4 | 26.2 | 2.0 | 28.2 | 29.0 |
| 225 | 33.7 | 30.4 | 2.1 | 32.5 | 33.3 |
| 265 | 25.3 | 23.4 | 1.9 | 25.3 | 24.5 |
| 295 | 20.7 | 18.3 | 1.8 | 20.1 | 20.8 |
| 330 | 46.3 | 43.0 | 2.9 | 46.0 | 45.1 |
| Total dose | 253.6 | 231.7 | 17.5 | 249.2 | 249.6 |

Table 2 summarizes the results of five clinical IMRT cases.

Table 2: Summary of dose verification for five IMRT patients.

| Disease site | Patient plan Corvus dose (cGy) | Patient plan Current cal. (cGy) | Phantom plan Corvus dose (cGy) | Phantom plan Current cal. (cGy) | Measure ment (cGy) |
|---|---|---|---|---|---|
| Prostate #1 (15 MV) | 222.6 | 232.5 | 224.0 | 226.7 | 231.3 |
| Prostate #2 (15 MV) | 208.4 | 209.1 | 220.0 | 216.4 | 227.0 |
| Brain (4MV) | 173.3 | 173.5 | 196.0 | 192.9 | 197.7 |
| Liver (6MV) | 234.3 | 251.4 | 237.0 | 238.3 | 231.1 |
| Abdomen (15MV) | 179.0 | 177.7 | 178.0 | 176.2 | 176.3 |

Both original patient plan and the corresponding surrogate phantom plan data are listed. An ion chamber measurement for each patient in a cylindrical water phantom is also presented in the table 2. In all cases, the calculated dose agreed with the CORVUS calculation within 4%, except for the 6MV liver case where the deviation is larger than 7%. According to the report of AAPM TG-40,[6] a disparity should be resolved before commencing or continuing a treatment if the independent calculation differs by more than 5% from the treatment plan. Our calculation did not take into account of the contour variation. In the liver case, we noticed that there was a significant variation of the skin contour within the treatment fields. The irregular skin surface lead to a large discrepancy in the final dose. An ion chamber measurement was used to resolve the discrepancy in this case.

## 4. Conclusion

We have provided a close formula for MU calculation from a prescribed dose and a given leaf sequence file for IMRT treatment. The MU is expressed as a function of the contributing beamlet doses and the dynamic modulation factors. The formula is quite general and can be implemented as an independent MU verification tool for any leaf sequence algorithm and delivery machine. It may also find an application in dose calculation from a known leaf sequence file and finite pencil beam kernels. The approach was illustrated in verification of the isocenter dose for CORVUS treatment plans and our results indicated that it is robust and efficient for clinical use.

We wish to thank J. Kung and B. Curran for useful discussions. This work was supported in part by Grants from the Whitaker Foundation and the NCI (No. CA43840).

## References

[1] Boyer A L , Xing L, Ma C, Curran B, Hill R, Kinia A, and Bleier A 1999. Theoretical considerations of monitor unit calculations for intensity modulated beam treatment planning. *Med. Phys.* 26, 187-195.

[2] Georg D and Dutreix A 1997. A formalism to calculate the output ratio in a mini-phantom for a GE multileaf collimator, *Phys. Med. Biol.* 42, 521-536.

[3] Kung J and Chen G 1999. A modified Clarkson integration for IMRT. *Med. Phys.* 26: 1135 (abstract).

[4] Khan F 1994. The physics of radiation therapy. Baltimore: Williams & Wilkins.

[5] Xing L, Curran B, Hill R, Holmes T, Ma L, Forster K, Boyer AL 1999, Dosimetric verification of a commercial inverse treatment planning system, *Phys. Med. Biol.* 44, 463-478.

[6] Kutcher G *et al* 1994. Comprehensive QA for radiation oncology: Report of AAPM Radiation Therapy Committee Task Group 40. *Med. Phys.* 21, 581-618.

# Image Correlation and *In Vivo* Dosimetry in IMRT

**Mark H. Phillips, Ph.D.[1], Homayoon Parsaei, M.Sc.[1,2], Paul S. Cho, Ph.D.[1], Görkem H. Kuterdem, M.Sc.[1,3], Hege Kippenes, DVM[4], and Pat Gavin, Ph.D., DVM[4]**
[1]University of Washington, Department of Radiation Oncology, Seattle, WA, USA
[2]University of British Columbia, Department of Physics, Vancouver, BC, Canada
[3]University of Washington, Department of Electrical Engineering, Seattle, WA, USA
[4]Washington State University, School of Veterinary Medicine, Pullman, WA, USA

## Introduction

Intensity modulated radiation therapy is pushing the frontiers of radiation therapy in several different areas simultaneously. Broadly speaking, these areas are (a) the dose calculation algorithms, (b) the use of inverse planning or plan optimization algorithms, (c) the complexity of the treatment plan in terms of the large increase in the number of variables that define the treatment, and (d) the enlarged scope of manufacturer-provided software needed to deliver the entire treatment. These advances are, of course, not independent. The optimization algorithms produce fluence distributions that result in a large number of time-dependent variables being required. In turn, this increase in the number of states of the delivery needing to be modelled (such as leaf edge penumbra at nearly every point within the field) has required a more sophisticated dose calculation algorithm, since relatively small errors per field become much more important with so many segments. And finally, the large number of variables results in the need for computer control of the treatment delivery since no person could manage the complexity.

All of these factors have resulted in increased uncertainty in the dose actually delivered to the patient. Questions arise including: (a) the degree to which the new dose calculation algorithms model the time dependent machine variables; (b) how well does the dose calculation algorithm deal with the irregular, small, and off-center fields that are part of the treatment; and (c) how accurately is the dose delivered by the linac/MLC? In addition to these issues which can be addressed to a large degree by the use of phantoms, a very important question is: "How accurately is the dose actually delivered given the fact that each beam's 2-dimensional fluence must interdigitate precisely with the fluence of every other beam in the treatment over the course of fractionation in the face of set-up errors, inhomogeneities, and irregular surfaces?"

Our approach to answering these questions has been to develop an *in vivo* dosimetry model that utilizes canine irradiation, TLD measurements and image correlation of serial CT image sets.

## Material and Methods

As described elsewhere in these proceedings [2], a collaboration between University of Washington Medical Center (UWMC) and Washington State University Veterinary Hospital (WSU) has been established in which canines are treated for head and neck tumors using IMRT. The patients were staged, imaged and treated at WSU; treatment plans calculations, IMRT QA, and dosimetry were performed at UWMC. Even though the two institutions are 500 km apart, the use of X Windows protocols and standard file transfer protocols removed all obstacles from the interchange of imaging, planning and treatment data between the two institutions.

Implementation of this model has proceeded in stages. Verification of the positioning accuracy of the immobilization devices has been measured on a series of dogs presenting with spontaneous tumors and prescribed a course of radiation therapy. Implementation of IMRT and the use of image correlation and diode dosimetry was commenced on a series of deceased dogs. The mature phase of the project, which is currently underway, includes 15 purpose-bred dogs; six were controls undergoing conventional therapy for a paraspinal tumor, and nine were treated with IMRT.

### Imaging

The dogs were fitted with biteblock and alpha cradle immobilization devices at WSU and were imaged using CT (PLAN-CT). The images were transferred to the UWMC planning computer, and the veterinary radiologists drew target and normal structure contours remotely using the treatment plan contouring tools. An intensity modulated plan was designed and tested at UWMC, and transferred electronically to the WSU linac, an Elekta SL15 fitted with MLC [1, 2].

Treatments were typically carried out over four weeks. Once a week, a catheter (7 French) was loaded with TLD's (50 TLD's, 2 mm long, 1 mm diameter) and inserted into the airway. For nasal tumors, the catheter was inserted directly into the target volume if possible. For paraspinal tumors, the catheter was located in the low dose invagination region. Several cases were done in cadavers, in which cases, catheters were placed longitudinally in the spinal cord (low dose) and laterally through the target volume (high dose and gradient regions). The animal was placed in the immobilization device and re-imaged with CT (TREAT-CT). It was then transferred to the linac couch where a port film was taken. If necessary, the port film was used to reposition the dog. The treatment was delivered, and the TLD's and the CT images were sent to UWMC.

### Image Correlation

Each TREAT-CT image set was correlated with the PLAN-CT image set using an image correlation software package provided by the Department of Radiation Oncology, University of North Carolina. The correlation was optimized manually by the operator using radiographically apparent anatomy. The location of each TLD within the CT images was determined with the aid of small radiographically opaque spacers located in the TLD catheter. After image correlation was complete, the anatomical locations of each TLD was determined within the PLAN-CT image set, and the planned treatment dose to each of those points within the anatomy was calculated.

Part of the biteblock immobilization device is a "stereotactic ring" that contains easily imaged fiducial markers. The dogs were set-up by table offsets from the stereotactic ring, although the final treatment may be modified by the port film information. This ring provided an easy means to assess the repositioning reproducibility of the animals. If the rings were aligned, the deviation in anatomical correlation between the TREAT-CT and PLAN-CT image sets was the measure of the accuracy of the patient set-up.

A simpler method of image correlation has also been used in this study–namely, the visual comparison of daily port films. Using bony landmarks, the daily setup errors were quantified. These errors were corrected before treatment commenced.

### TLD Dosimetry

The TLD's were cylindrical LiF diodes [1]; they were read using the Harshaw Model 3500 reader. Since the catheters must be shipped to UWMC for reading, all TLD's, including calibration TLD's, were decayed for at least 24 hr before reading. The manufacturer-recommended annealing schedule was followed. The standard deviation in readings in a calibration irradiation was $\pm$ 2%. For each irradiation, each TLD was identified as to its coordinates in the CT image set; individual calibration constants were applied to the readings of each TLD. The final comparison is made between the measured dose of each TLD and the corresponding anatomical point in the PLAN-CT.

## Results and Discussion

The aim of this work has been to develop a system in which all of the uncertainties in the IMRT process could be quantified by comparing the measured dose in the tissue to the planned dose. The means has been to use TLD dosimetry in deceased and living canines, and to use image correlation techniques to map the positions at which dose measurements have been made onto the planned dose distribution.

[1]Bicron/Harshaw, Solon, OH

Preliminary work focussed on using sequential port images to determine the accuracy of the patient immobilization system. It was found that for tumors in the head, setup accuracy was 1-2 mm. In the neck, the daily setup errors were found to be approximately 5 mm.

The most data has been obtained for the irradiation of deceased dogs. Figure 1 illustrates a transverse CT image in which the target volume is outlined, as are the positions of TLD-loaded catheters. One catheter is located in the esophagus, one in the spinal column, and one placed through the target volume and lying in the plane of the CT image. Figures 2 and 3 illustrate the dose to the TLD's in the spinal and coplanar catheters for a seven beam IMRT irradiation. The esophagus catheter was in place for only one beam. The planned target dose was 400 cGy. In the inverse planning program, the spine was constrained to receive no more than 200 cGy, and 200 cGy was the planned dose resulting from the optimization. These and the results of other cadaver experiments were used to refine the imaging, planning, correlation and dosimetry procedures.

In correlating the five images sets from a single dog's treatment, the amount of time and data involved was quite large, and we have not yet completely analyzed the data for the fifteen dogs that were treated for paraspinal tumors. In addition to the dosimetry, clinical examinations and pathology studies will be conducted. The biological and dosimetric results will be combined with the treatment planning to evaluate the accuracy of the IMRT process.

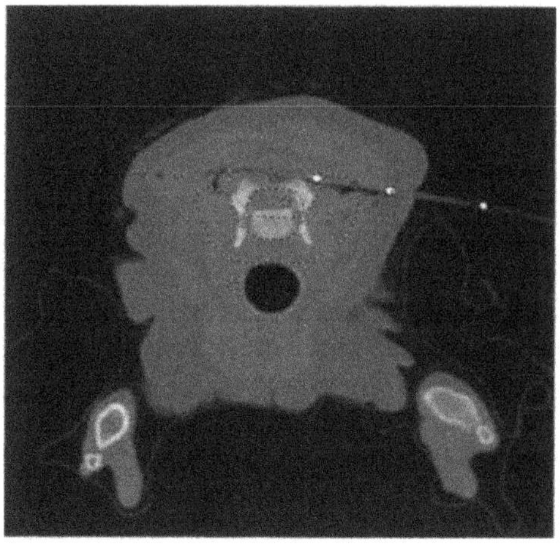

**Figure 1:** The immobilization bed with the bite-block in place used both for planning and treatment.

## Conclusion

A model has been proposed that will provide a means of correlating calculated doses for IMRT treatments with doses measured *in vivo* in a clinical setting. The purpose of these measurements is to determine the extent to which uncertainties in a number of complex algorithms and procedures

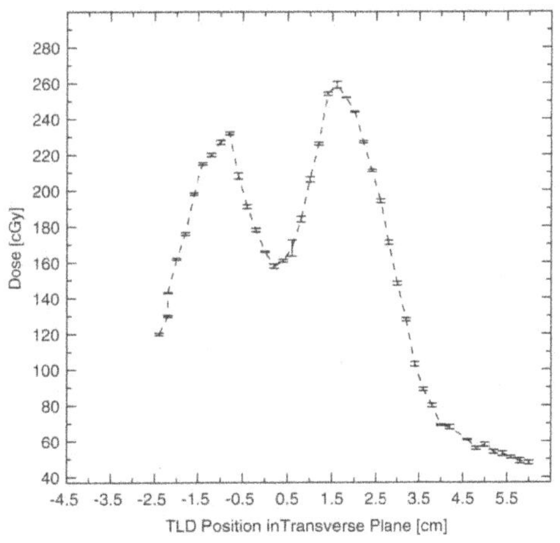


**Figure 2:** The immobilization bed with the bite-block in place used both for planning and treatment.

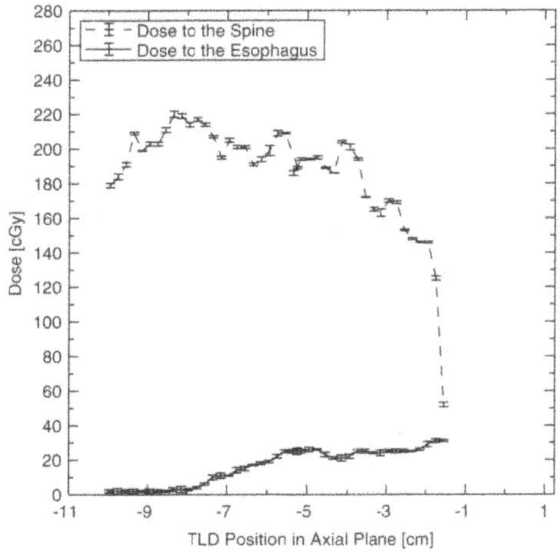


**Figure 3:** The immobilization bed with the bite-block in place used both for planning and treatment.

affects the clinical delivery of this type of radiation therapy. To date, we have worked to implement and optimize each stage in the process. This has included phantom measurements and measurements in deceased dogs. Currently, we are collecting and analyzing data in the treatment of fifteen dogs with paraspinal target volumes. The results of this study, the correlation of measured doses with anatomy and planned doses, will be combined with clinical and radiobiological endpoints to help establish both the limits and the potential of IMRT.

## Acknowledgements

This work was supported in part by grants from Elekta Oncology Systems and the Whitaker Foundation.

## References

[1] Cho P, Phillips M, Sutlief S, Gavin P, Kippenes H. In vivo measurements of intensity modulated radiation therapy, *Med Phys*, 25(7), Part 1: A201, 1998.

[2] Parsaei H, Phillips MH, Cho PS, Kuterdem G, Kippenes H, Gavin P. Delivery and *In-vivo* Dose Verification in IMRT, Proceedings of XIIIth ICCR, 2000.

# On the chemical stability of 3D monomer/polymer gel dosimetry

**Yves De Deene[1,2], Carlos De Wagter[1], Eric Achten[2] and Wilfried De Neve[1]**
[1]Department for Radiotherapy, Nuclear Medicine and Experimental Cancerology, University Hospital of Gent, Belgium and [2]Department for Magnetic Resonance, University Hospital of Gent, Belgium

## Introduction

In monomer/polymer gel dosimetry, the spin-spin relaxation rate, R2 = 1/T2 is related to radiation dose that has been delivered to the gel phantom. This makes the gel a suitable 3D dosimeter that can be applied for the verification of complex dose distributions as they occur in conformal radiotherapy [1, 2, 3, 4]. However, severe long-term instabilities of the gel have been reported recently [5].

The purpose of this study was to investigate the long-term stability of our BANG-type gel. We repeated the stability measurements of McJury *et al* for a more extended set of gel samples irradiated with different doses.

As a result, we were able to extract two different kinds of instabilities. The first kind affects the slope of the dose-R2 plot and saturates within one day while the second kind affects the intercept of the dose-R2 plot and continues for more than one month. It is demonstrated that the two instabilities originate from completely different chemical mechanisms.

The effect of the chemical instabilities on the applicability of monomer/polymer gels is discussed and possible strategies to overcome chemical instability related dose errors are suggested.

## Material and methods

A solution of acrylamide (3%(w/w)) and N,N'-methylene-bis-acrylamide (3%(w/w)) was heated to 45 °C in order to dissolve the crosslinking monomer. Another solution containing gelatin was also heated to 45 °C to obtain a sol. Subsequently, both solutions were cooled down to 30 °C before mixing to avoid 'spontaneous' polymerization. All processing steps were completed in one production set-up containing interconnected airtight reaction flasks that were bubbled by nitrogen to expel oxygen that would inhibit the radiation-induced polymerization reaction [6]. Finally, the gel was pumped over by use of a peristaltic pump into several test tubes placed in a perspex glove box that was flushed with nitrogen in order to keep the oxygen concentration lower than 0.01 mg.l$^{-1}$.

The dose-response of the gel-batch was determined by exposing the test tubes containing gel to different known doses. Each tube was irradiated separately in a cubic water tank with 6-MV photons at a depth of 5 cm and respecting a source-to-surface distance (SSD) of 95 cm.

The gels were scanned in a Siemens SP 1.5 T whole body scanner using the standard RF CP head coil with a multiple spin-echo sequence with phase-alternating-phase shift (PHAPS) and 32 equidistant echo times (TE/TR/FOV/MS = 20ms-640ms/3s/200mm/256) to obtain the R2 images. The sequence was modified in order to compensate for artifacts arising from eddy currents, stimulated echoes and temperature drift. The gel temperature was recorded during the image by use of a fluoroptic thermometry system.

The R2 images were computed applying a $\chi^2$-minimization algorithm. The first two base images were not used in the fitting as the first two echoes deviate from the mono-exponential relaxation course due to stimulated echoes [7].

## Results and discussion

An instability of the dose-R2 curve is observed although the change in R2 over a certain period is an order of magnitude smaller than the changes observed in previous work by McJury *et al* in an irradiated sample [5]. Restricting to the linear part of the dose-R2 plot, a variation can be observed in both the slope and the intercept of the dose-R2 curve (see Figure 1). However, it can be seen that while the variation in the slope saturates after a time period of about 12 hours, the variation in the intercept progresses over a much longer period and reaches a saturation level only after about one month.

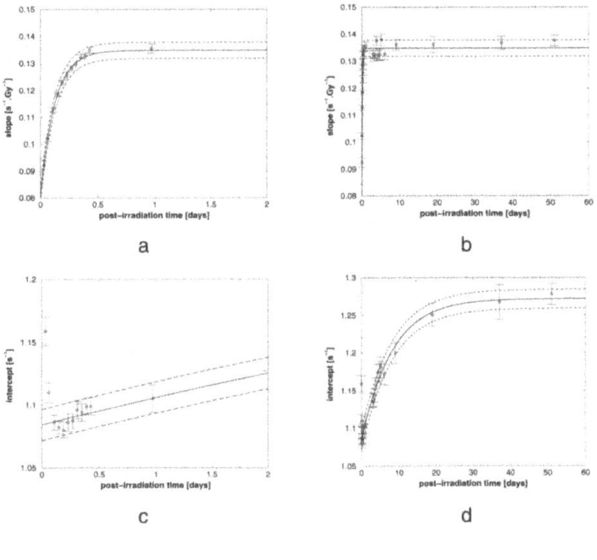


**Figure 1:** The slope (a-b) and intercept (c-d) from the dose-R2 plot as a function of post-irradiation time. Graphs (a) and (c) are for the first two days. Graphs (b) and (d) cover two months.

The variation in the slope of the linear part in the R2-versus-dose plot is due to post-irradiation polymerization. The same time constant for the post-irradiation polymerization was also found by Audet [8]. Other groups that investigated polymerization kinetics in highly cross-linked polyacrylamide gels by use of spectrophotometry have also observed poorer kinetics with increasing concentration of cross-linking agents [9]. The fact that the post-irradiation polymerization saturates after 12 hours post-irradiation implies that this kind of instability will not cause a systematic dose error when the dosimeter gels are stored during one night after irradiation and prior to scanning.

The variation in the intercept of the linear part in the R2-versus-dose plot originates from the continuation of the gelation process of the gelatin. Evidence for this is also provided from the observation of both an unirradiated BANG gel sample and from a gel sample containing only gelatin immediately after manufacture (see Figure 2: samples #5 (#6) and #3 respectively and Figure 4a). It can be noticed that there is no difference in aging behavior between a gelatin gel sample and an unirradiated BANG gel sample although the R2 of the unirradiated BANG gel sample is smaller than the R2 of the sample containing only gelatin. While the increase in R2 is highest during the first day post-manufacture, a smaller increase is still noticeable the second day.

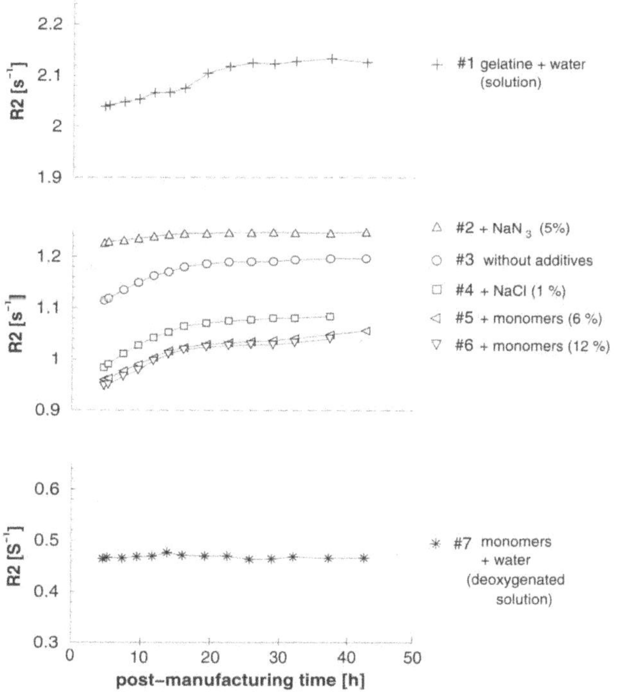


**Figure 2:** The R2 of several mixtures containing different chemicals recorded immediately after manufacture. Mixture #1 contains an unheated solution of gelatin powder. Mixture #2 to #6 are gelatin gels containing various chemicals and mixture #7 is a deoxygenated monomer solution.

The variation in the intercept deserves some attention as a systematic error of about 1.5% of the maximum dose is made if calibration and dose mapping occur at a time seperation of one day. This systematic error is proportional to the time delay between calibration and dose mapping for dosimeter gels that are scanned within the first 10 days after manufacture.

No change in R2 of a deoxygenated monomer solution was found. Adding sodium azide ($NaN_3$) alters the R2 aging curve significantly as almost no variation in R2 was still observable. It was also seen that the stabilizing effect of sodium azide is concentration dependent. A change in the viscosity of the gel was observed for various concentrations of sodium azide. Gels with sodium azide concentration higher than 10% did not gel but remained fluid.

The gelation of aqueous gelatin solutions is governed by the growth of a three-dimensional network of biopolymer chains (see Figure 3).

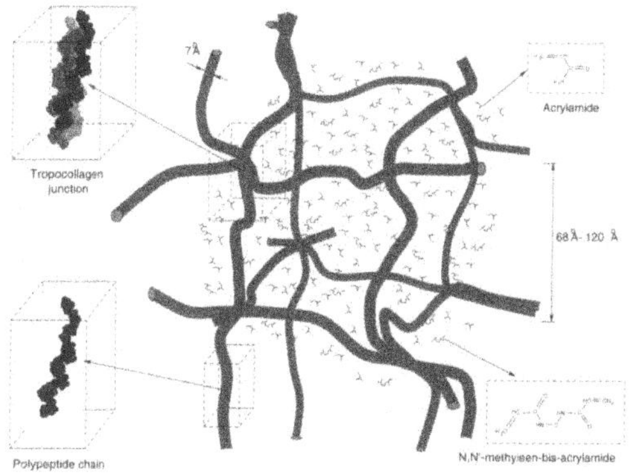


**Figure 3:** Simplified model of the microscopic structure of the monomer/polymer gel based on stoechiometric calculations. For reasons of clarity, water molecules are not shown.

The junctions of the network result from renaturing of collagen as the temperature is lowered below 35 °C. The collagen unit (tropocollagen) is a rod made of three polypeptide chains, each one being twisted into a left-handed helix and all three being wrapped into a super-right-handed helix [10].

The gelation process of aqueous gelatin solutions has been investigated by the observation of different physico-chemical properties such as by use of viscosimetry [11], atomic force microscopy [12], dye fluorescence [13], dielectric measurements [14], polarimetry and MR relaxometry [15]. The sol-gel transition can be described by use of the percolation dynamic approach [16]. All of these studies demonstrate that the gelation is extremely rapid during the first minutes after quenching the sol at temperatures below 35 °C but that although the evolution is much slower after the first hours, no equilibrium is found even after a week.

Different temperature treatments during the manufacture of the gelatin gels results in a significant change in R2 but does not change the magnitude of R2 variation due to aging (see Figure 4b-c).

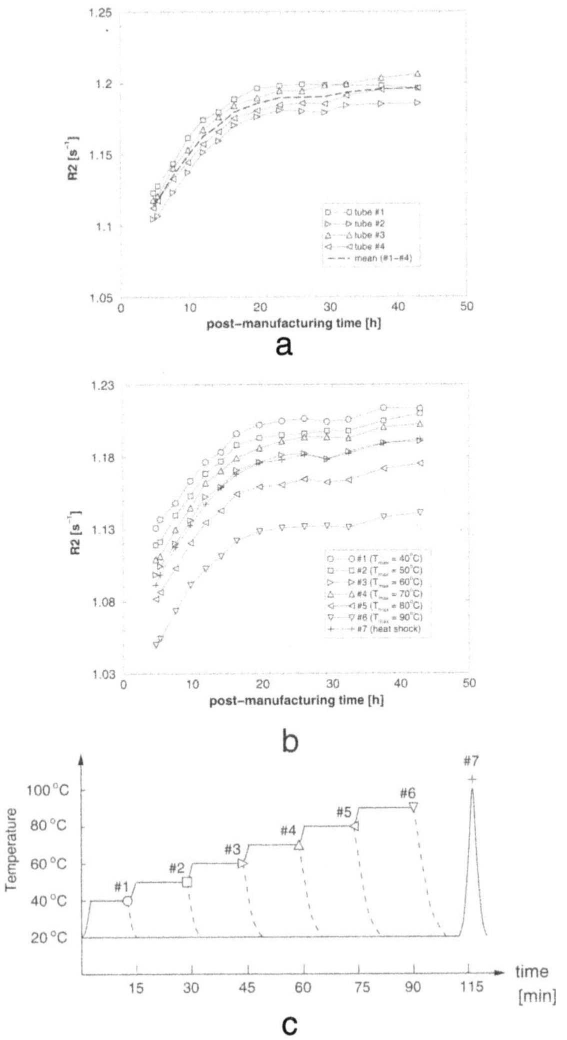


**Figure 4:** The R2 of a 6% (w/w) gelatin gel immediately after manufacture. (a) Four samples of the gelatin gel heated to 50 °C for 15 minutes showing the inter-batch reproducibility. (b) The R2 of the gelatin gel heated at different temperatures during manufacture. The corresponding temperature history of each gel is shown in graph (c).

From the gel sample given a temperature treatment in the form of a boost (sample #7) it is seen that not only the maximum temperature determines the change in R2 but also the time period a certain temperature treatment is given.

## Conclusion

Two kinds of chemical instability in monomer/polymer dosimeters have been observed. The first kind acts on the slope of the R2-versus-dose plot but is limited to the first 12 hours after irradiation and is related to post-irradiation polymerization of the monomer/polymer aggregates. The second kind of instability acts on the intercept of the R2-versus-dose plot and continues for more than a month. The mechanism responsible for this instability is the formation of macromolecular collagen structures that provokes a change in the local mobility of water molecules.

It was found that the addition of sodium azide to the gel has a significant influence on the stability of gelatin gels. It may be worth looking for other chemical additives or how the molecular composition of the peptide chains of gelatin can be modified in order to stabilize the gelation of gelatin gels.

## References

[1] Ibbott G S, Maryanski M J, Eastman P, Holcomb S D, Zhang Y, Avison R G, Sanders M and Gore J C 1997 *Int J Rad Oncol Biol Phys* **38** 1097–1103

[2] Oldham M, Baustert I, Lord C, Smith T A D, McJury M, Warrington A P, Leach M O and Webb S 1998 *Phys Med Biol* **43** 1113–1131

[3] De Deene Y, De Wagter C, Van Duyse B, Derycke S, De Neve W and Achten E 1998 *Radioth Oncol*, **48** 283–291.

[4] De Deene Y, De Wagter C, Van Duyse B, Derycke S, Mersseman B, De Gersem W, Voet T, Achten E and De Neve W 1999 *Magn Reson Med, In press* .

[5] McJury M, Oldham M, Leach M O and Webb S 1999 *Phys Med Biol* **44** 1863–1873

[6] Maryanski M J, Ibbott G S, Eastman P, Schulz R J and Gore J C 1996 *Med Phys* **23** 699–705

[7] Fransson A, Ericsson A, Jung B and Sperber G O 1993 *Magn Reson Imaging* **11** 771–784

[8] Audet C 1995 NMR-Dose Response Studies of the Gels Used for 3-D Radiation Dosimetry by Magnetic Resonance Imaging *PhDthesis* McGill University, Montréal

[9] Gelfi C and Righetti P G 1981 *Electrophoresis* **2** 213–228

[10] Ward A G 1977 *The science and technology of gelatin* (Academic Press, London)

[11] Huang H, Sorensen C M 1996 *Phys. Rev. E* **53** 5075–5078

[12] Mackie A R, Gunning A P, Ridout M J and Morris V J 1998 *Biopolymers* **46** 245–252

[13] Bozena R 1999 *J. Phys. B: At. Mol. Phys.* **32** 3463–3468

[14] Bohidar H B, Jena S S, Maity S and Saxena A 1998 *Colloid. Polym. Sci.* **276** 81–86

[15] Maquet J, Théveneau H, Djabourov M, Leblond J and Papon P 1986 *Polymer* **27** 1103–1110

[16] Daoud M 1987 *Kinetics of nonhomogeneous processes* (Ed. Freeman G R) (Alberta: John Wiley and Sons) 651–723

# An initial investigation of Optical CT and MR scanning of gel dosimeters

**Mark Oldham, Jeffrey H Siewerdsen and David A Jaffray**

Radiation Oncology, William Beaumont Hospital, 3601 W 13 Mile Road, Royal Oak MI USA

## Introduction

Radiation sensitive gels, including BANG and Fricke-gels, are at the forefront of research into improved dosimetry techniques. Despite being the only dosimeter that offers true 3D information about the dose-distribution, radiation sensitive gels have to-date made little impact in most clinics. This is due to the fact that the field is still new and rapidly developing, but also due to the high cost and high noise characteristics of the standard way of reading these gels – MR scanning. To circumvent these difficulties several groups are looking at an alternative low-cost approach to reading the gels, using laser based optical-CT scanning [1-4].

In this paper we report on an optical CT scanning system recently developed in our lab, and a preliminary study which compares, for the same gel samples, MR with optical scanning. The comparison has two parts: a) calibration methods and accuracy, and b) noise and resolution in dosimetric images. We also outline a novel optical calibration method with primary advantages in terms of speed and robustness. The important feature of the study is that each scanning method was applied to the same gel samples.

## Material and methods

Four identical cylindrical barex flasks, each 14cm long and 5.3cm diameter, were filled with BANG3 gel (MGS Research Inc., Guilford CT 06437 USA). The BANG3 formulation is particularly suitable for this study as the nature of polymerisation causes a strong signal-change in both optical and MR modalities, more-so than the original BANG formulation for example. Three of the flasks were used to investigate gel calibration issues, and the fourth flask was used as a dosimeter to study an intricate radiosurgical QA delivery.

### Calibration by optical and MR modalities

Three of the flasks were sequentially placed in a water-bath and irradiated with a single 6MV beam from an Elekta SL20 linac, with field-size 10x10cm. The beam was orientated such that a standard depth-dose was deposited along the long axis of the flask [5,6]. The flasks were irradiated to a dose of 0.5, 1.25 and 2.5Gy at dmax respectively. Each flask was then scanned by both optical and MR (1.5T Siemens Vision scanner) modalities. A novel technique was developed to determine the optical calibration of $\Delta\mu$ (i.e. the change in optical attenuation coefficient) versus dose. Conventionally $\Delta\mu$ is obtained from 2D optical CT reconstructions at multiple doses, here equivalent to various depths in the gel. In this prototype scanner the time for data collection for a single 2D reconstruction is about 25 minutes. Acquiring at 1mm steps along 3 gels, each 10cm long, would require >5days for data collection. However the equivalent data can be obtained in <5minutes by exploiting the fact that in the calibration depth-dose irradiation, all gel at the same depth in a flask receives the same dose (i.e. has the same optical attenuation). A simplified optical set-up is thus permissible *for calibration,* which measures the amount of laser-light transmitted through the diameter of each flask at 1mm depth increments along the flask (figure 1).

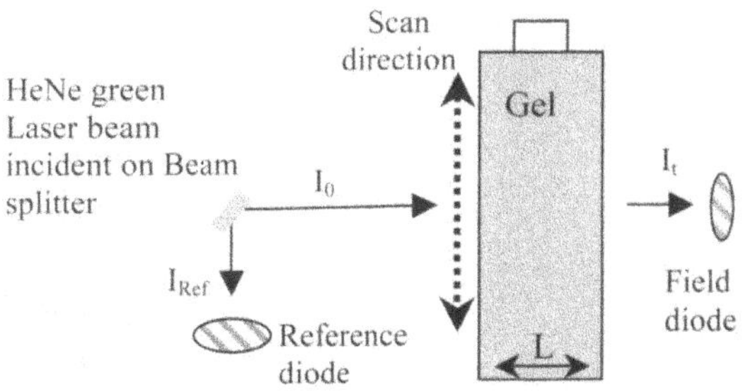


**Figure 1:** schematic of optical set-up for calibration.

The optical scanning acquisition was configured to return the ratio $R=I_{Ref}/I_t$. A calibration plot of $\Delta\mu$ versus dose was obtained by determining $\Delta\mu$ from two measured ratio values for the same trajectory in the gel, corresponding to before and after irradiation, $R^U$ and $R^I$ respectively.

$$\Delta\mu = \ln[R^I / R^U]/L \qquad \text{Equation 1}$$

In equation 1, $\Delta\mu$ is the change in optical attenuation coefficient, and L=diameter of flask. This simple relation holds because $I_0 \propto I_{ref}$ and taking the log of ratios allows common terms (e.g. effects of the flask wall) to subtract out. Each line scan gives $\Delta\mu$ values versus dose for the depth-dose delivery along the flask. Using this method $\Delta\mu$ values versus dose were obtained at 1mm steps along the entire gel flask in about 1 minute. Statistics can be improved by averaging any number of line profiles taken with the phantom at different degrees of rotation about its long axis. The proposed method assumes that light scattered and reflected back onto the field detector is small, and also independent of the amount of polymerisation.

The MR protocol followed was that recommended by the BANG gel manufacturer and produces R2 values in the gel, from two single echo images with TE=20 and 100ms respectively. The spatial resolution was set as 0.98x0.98x3mm$^3$. These values push the MR scanner toward the limit of its spatial resolution; indeed the 3mm slice thickness was the smallest available on this scanner.

### Experimental radiosurgery delivery

The remaining dosimetric flask (#4) was irradiated with a standard radiosurgery QA configuration consisting of 3 6MV equi-angularly spaced fields, each with field-size 7mm diameter at the isocentre. The purpose of the configuration is to verify accurate collimator alignment on the linac-head, which is confirmed by visualisation of concentric cross-firing of the three beams. The highly collimated 'sharp' beams of radiosurgery make this distribution an ideal test for studying the performance of optical and MR scanning in regards to noise and spatial resolution. The dosimetric flask was scanned ≈ 24 hours post irradiation by both MR and optical CT modalities. Optical CT scanning was performed using the apparatus of figure 2.

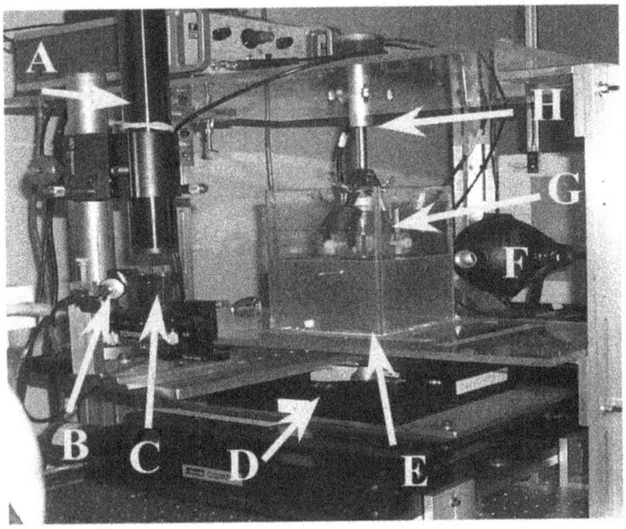


**Figure 2:** Optical CT scanning set-up. A=vertically mounted laser, B=reference detector, C= beam-splitter, D=translation stage, E=perspex water-bath containing anti-freeze, F=lab-sphere containing field detector, G=gel flask suspended vertically, H=gel flask suspension arm attached to rotational motor. The laser and lab-sphere (containing field detector) translate horizontally on a computer-controlled stage. The water bath remains stationary avoiding ripples [Jordan K, 4]. The gel phantom is suspended from above and rotates about the vertical.

Optical CT scanning was performed as follows. First optical matching between the anti-freeze in the water-bath and the gel was achieved by diluting the antifreeze until the deflection of the laser-beam under translation across the flask was minimised. Zero deflection can be achieved except at the edges of the flask where strong refraction occurs. Line scans were taken with the laser stepping in 1mm increments across the flask with an additional 1.5cm either side, allowing padding for the reconstruction. Between each line-scan, the flask was rotated by 1.8degrees, until data for 180 degrees of rotation had been acquired. The total time was about 45 minutes when scanning was only allowed from left-to-right (i.e. the scanner was 're-wound' after each line-scan). Reconstructions were performed using the MATLAB inverse-radon transform, and taking the difference image of optical CT scans before and after irradiation yielded the values for Δμ.

## Results and discussion

The calibration plots for MR and optical scanning are shown in figure 3A,B and C. The figures show the measurement of the active parameter (Δμ for optical and R2 for MR) versus dose at all depths down each of the three flasks. The noisiness of the single pixel profile (0.98mm) in the MR image is shown in figure 3A and is clearly poor.

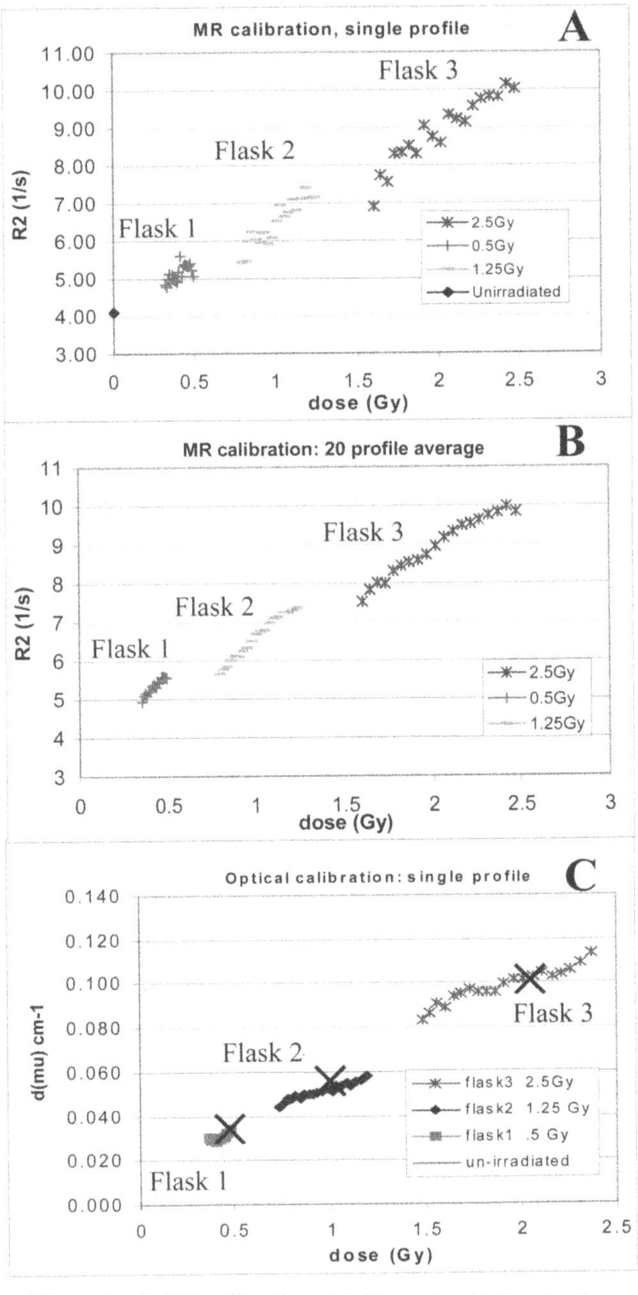


**Figure 3:** A) MR calibration plot illustrating high noise for a high spatial resolution of 0.98mm per pixel, B) averaging 20 profiles gives better statistics, C) optical calibration profiles. X's indicate values obtained by 2D reconstruction, small points were obtained by the novel profile method outlined in the text and equation 1.

Better statistics are achieved by averaging 20 profiles (B), although this corresponds to a spatial resolution of 2cm, not reasonable for dosimetric verification. The optical and MR axial images through the central plane of the 3field SRS distribution in the dosimetric phantom (#4) are shown in figures 4A and B respectively.

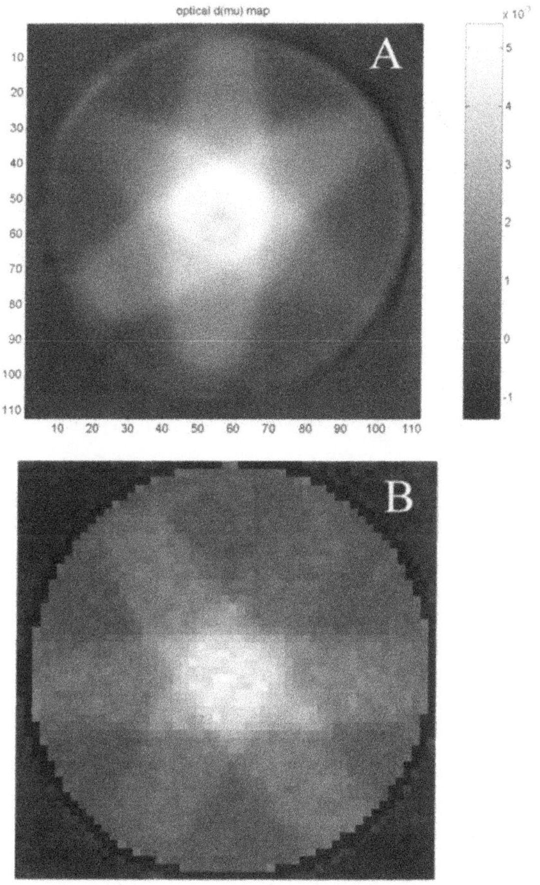


**Figure 4:** A) optical CT difference image post-pre irradiation, axis units are mm/2, B) MR R2 image of the same plane in the same gel. Note the two images are not rotationally aligned.

Comparing the optical CT image with the corresponding MR image, the superior quality of the optical approach is clearly demonstrated. The performance of the optical scanner is even more impressive considering that the slice width was a 1/3rd that of the MR (1mm as opposed to 3mm). The principle reason for the improvement in quality is the higher signal to noise observed in the optical measurements. Better MR images can be obtained, without loss of resolution, by further averaging. In the data presented here, TE=20 images were averaged 3 times and TE=100 images were averaged 5 times due to the intrinsic lower signal in the latter. The scanning time took 1hour, which is all that can be reasonably expected for this purpose.

## Conclusions

In this paper we present the following;

1) An optical CT scanning system developed in our lab based on previous designs [1,3]. The features of note include,
   a) Stationary water-tank to eliminate rippling effects
   b) Use of an optical lab-sphere, which averages the collected incident light at a specific solid angle, and renders the system insensitive to small deviations of the incident beam due to deflections.
   c) The use of green anti-freeze as a convenient optical matching solution, which dilutes readily at room temperature, unlike alternatives such as glycerine.

2) The outline of a novel and fast optical calibration method, where $\Delta\mu$ (=change in optical attenuation coefficient) values are obtained from line-scans as opposed to full 2D reconstructions. In the example presented equivalent data collection time was reduced from 5 days to <5 minutes.
   a) The method is particularly suitable for purely attenuating gels where the influence of scatter and re-reflection onto the field diode is negligible.
   b) For scattering gels (like the BANG3) the method still holds away from the edges of the flask as illustrated by the agreement with reconstructed values in figure 3C.

3) A comparison of the performance of opticalCT with MR imaging for the same plane through a radisosurgery delivery (figures 4B,C). High spatial resolution was required from both modalities, as necessitated by the intricate nature of the radiosurgery delivery. The superior quality of the optical modality is clearly demonstrated. The main reason for the increased quality of optical scanning is the higher signal to noise.

## References

[1] J. C. Gore, M. Ranade, M. J. Maryanski, and R. J. Schulz, I: Development of the Optical Scanner, Phys.Med. Biol. 41, pp.2695-704, 1996

[2] M.J.Maryanski, Y.Z.Zastavker, and J.C.Gore, II: Optical Properties of the BANG Polymer Gel, Phys. Med. Biol. 41, pp. 2705-2717, 1996

[3] Kelly BG, Jordan KJ, Battista JJ Optical CT reconstruction of 3D dose distributions using the (FBX) gel dosimeter ,Med Phys 1998 Sep;25(9):1741-50

[4] Jordan K, Developmental issues for opticalCT and gel dosimetry, Proc 1st Int Conf. on Rad. Ther. And Gel Dosimetry, available CDROM ISBN 0-9684873-2-7

[5] Oldham M, McJury M, Baustert IB, Webb S, Leach MO Improving calibration accuracy in gel dosimetry, Phys Med Biol 1998 Oct;43(10):2709-20

[6] McJury M, Tapper PD, Cosgrove VP, Murphy PS, Griffin S, Leach MO, Webb S, Oldham M, 3D dosimetry around a HDR 192Ir source using a PAG dosimeter, Phys Med Biol 1999 Oct;44(10):2431-44

# Analyzing dose distributions from a treatment planning system, Monte Carlo simulations and polymer gel measurements

**P A Love, D G Lewis and C W Smith**
Department of Medical Physics, Velindre Hospital, Cardiff, CF14 2TL, UK

## Introduction

As planning algorithms become increasingly accurate, quality assurance tests need to become more sophisticated to uncover discrepancies between reality and calculations which may only present themselves in complex geometrical situations (inhomogeneities etc.). Gel dosimetry and Monte Carlo simulations are capable of providing detailed dose information for comparison where more conventional dosimetry has limitations. In this work we aim to use both Monte Carlo calculations and polymer gel dosimetry to compare with results from a treatment planning system. A variety of gel phantoms were constructed to test the performance of calculations in different situation such as homogeneous and inhomogeneous phantoms.

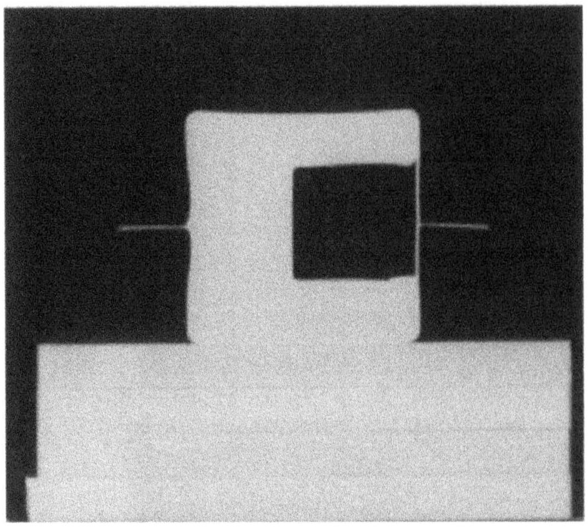

**Figure 1:** CT scan of the air cavity phantom showing the geometry used. The air cavity is 7 cm thick and the phantom is sitting on several layers of backscatter material to be irradiated from above.

## Material and methods

Three polymer gel (see below) phantoms of different geometry were constructed, 1) rectangular homogeneous phantom of dimension $14 \times 13 \times 13\,\mathrm{cm}^3$ 2) rectangular phantom containing a 7 cm deep air cavity located on one half of the phantom 3 cm below the surface (Figure 1) and 3) rectangular phantom containing a 2 cm thick aluminum slab located on one half of the phantom 3 cm below the surface (Figure 2. The homogeneous phantom was irradiated to 7 Gy at depth of maximum dose with a $5 \times 5\,\mathrm{cm}^2$ 6 MV photon beam with a focus-to-surface distance (FSD) of 100 cm. The two inhomogeneous phantoms were irradiated to 4 Gy to ensure the dose fell within the region where the gel dose response is linear (typically $< 8$ Gy). A field size of $10 \times 10\,\mathrm{cm}^2$ was used with the FSD = 100 cm.

The method of comparison is based on the $\gamma$-index analysis presented by Low *et al.* [1]. This method is used to compare two dose distributions and provides a quantitative representation of differences based on the combined dose-difference and DTA criteria. The criteria used here are dose-difference $\Delta D_M = 3\%$ and DTA $\Delta d_M = 3\,\mathrm{mm}$. Regions where the dose distribution fail to meet these criteria have values of $\gamma > 1$. Values of $\gamma$ below 1.0 show differences in the dose distributions which are within the specified criteria.

### Poly-acrylamide gel

Poly-acrylamide gels (PAG) are used for the measurement of 3D dose distributions. The PAG manufacturing procedure used by our group is similar to that published previously [2, 3] with a composition of 5% gelatin, 3% acrylamide and 3% N, N'-methylene-bis-acrylamide added to deionized water. Barex containers are used which allow the gel phantom to have thin walls (1 mm), various shapes and inhomogeneous inserts [4]. After irradiation the PAG is scanned using MRI on a 1.0 T Siemens Magnetom Impact. The pulse sequence used is a multiple spin-echo with a repetition time $T_{\mathrm{R}} = 4000$ ms and 16 echo times $T_{\mathrm{E}} = 50, 100, 150...800$ ms using 2 acquisitions giving a scan time of under 30 minutes. The field of view was 256 mm with $1 \times 1\,\mathrm{mm}^2$ pixels and a slice thickness of 5 mm. Single slices were used in the current work.

### Monte Carlo simulations

Monte Carlo simulations are performed using the BEAM code [5] from the National Research Council of Canada. A linear accelerator model was used to produce phase space data for various field sizes the used in the BEAM user-code called DOSXYZ [6] to simulate the radiation transport within a rectilinear array of voxels representing the gel phantom. CT scans were used to describe the geometry and material information used in the DOSXYZ simulation using so-called ramp functions to convert CT number into material and density. Individual ramp functions were used for each phantom with a single mass density assigned to

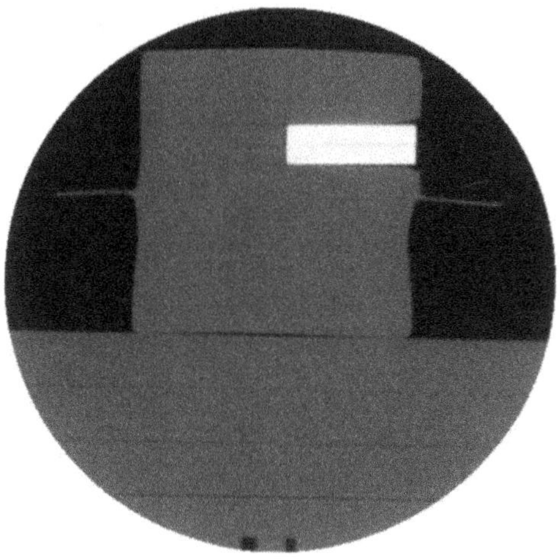

**Figure 2:** CT scan of the aluminum insert phantom showing the geometry used. The aluminum slab is 2 cm thick and the phantom is sitting on several layers of backscatter material to be irradiated from above.

materials to enable similar density description in the treatment planning system.

### Treatment planning system

The treatment planning system (TPS) used in this work is Helax-TMS version 5.0 (Helax AB, Sweden). This TPS incorporates both pencil beam and collapsed cone algorithms. The same CT data used for the Monte Carlo simulation is imported into the TPS to define the phantom geometry. Material definition can be achieved not only by conversion from CT numbers but also by defining volumes of interest and explicitly defining the material type using the dose plan basis module in the planning system.

## Results and discussion

The calculated (Monte Carlo and TPS) and measured (gel dosimetry) results for the homogeneous phantom had good agreement over the entire volume with $\gamma < 1.0$ when dose-difference and distance-to-agreement criteria are set to 3% and 3 mm respectively. Although there are no regions which fail these criteria, discrepancies are observed in the Monte Carlo data at shallow depths due to the accelerator model used. This has been confirmed with comparison with diode line dose measurements in a water tank and improvements to the model are currently being made.

Results from the air-cavity phantom are shown in Figures 3 and 4 where the black areas have $\gamma > 1$ and therefore fail the criteria. The failed region within the air cavity itself is expected because dose data is obviously not available from gel dosimetry and the TPS does not consider the dose in air. Other regions pass the criteria of $\Delta D_M = 3\%$ and $\Delta d_M = 3$ mm but smaller differences are present. For the Monte Carlo and TPS comparison these small discrepancies may be attributed to limitations in the Monte Carlo accelerator model used and TPS pencil beam algorithm not handling scatter changes from lateral inhomogeneities [7] (around the air cavity). The difference in the gel and TPS data outside the air cavity is thought to be resulting from the calibration procedure of the gel. It is widely thought that the gels are linear up to 8 Gy but correlations with diode data [8] suggest a second order polynomial describes the dose response more accurately even at lower doses (4 Gy).

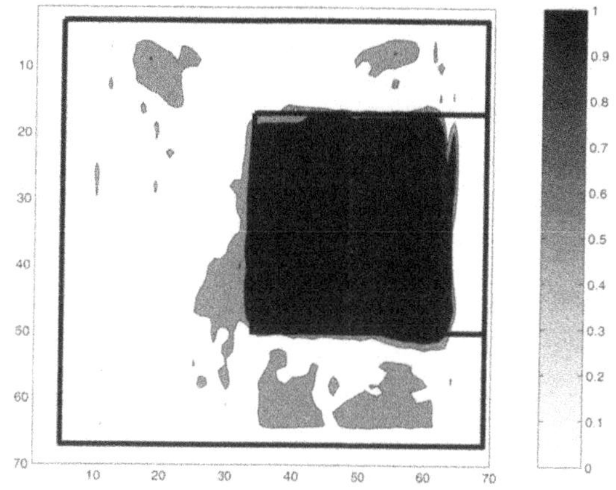

**Figure 3:** Gamma map for the air cavity phantom comparing Monte Carlo and TPS dose distributions. The black areas fail the criteria of dose difference < 3% and distance-to-agreement < 3 mm

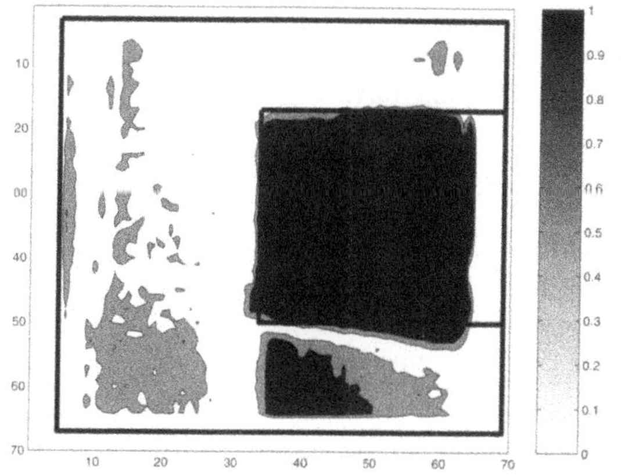

**Figure 4:** Gamma map for the air cavity phantom comparing polymer gel and TPS dose distributions. The black areas fail the criteria of dose difference < 3% and distance-to-agreement < 3 mm

Results from the aluminum insert phantom are shown in Figure 5. Using the same criteria as above, the failed region for this phantom is below the aluminum insert when comparing TPS results with Monte Carlo results. This is believed to be due to material specification differences between the Monte Carlo simulation and TPS which are currently being investigated.

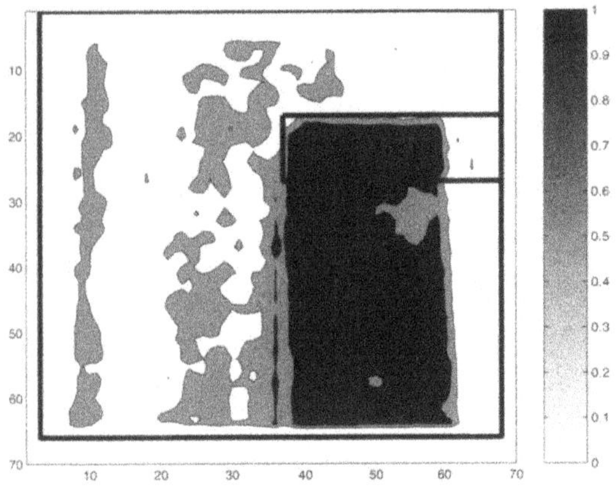

**Figure 5:** Gamma map for the aluminum slab phantom comparing Monte Carlo and TPS dose distributions. The black areas fail the criteria of dose difference < 3% and distance-to-agreement < 3 mm

## Conclusion

The three-way comparison of dose distributions produced by Monte Carlo simulations, treatment planning algorithms and polymer gel measurements has been examined for three different phantoms. Homogeneous phantoms have good agreement ($\Delta D_M < 3\%$, $\Delta d_M < 3\,\mathrm{mm}$) throughout the entire volume. The air cavity phantom also passes these criteria, however some small local differences were observed. The third phantom containing an aluminum slab has yielded differences between calculation and measurement which are currently undergoing further investigation.

## Acknowledgments

We would like to thank Dan Low from the Mallinckrodt Institute of Radiology for making the $\gamma$-code freely available. This project is funded by Cancer Research Wales (W E Fry) and Tregaron studentships.

## References

[1] Low D A, Harms W B, Mutic S and Purdy J A 1998 A technique for the quantitative evaluation of dose distributions *Medical Physics* **25** 656–661

[2] Maryanski M J, Schulz R J, Ibbott G S, Gatenby J C, Xie J, Horton D and Gore J C 1994 Magnetic resonance imaging of radiation dose distributions using a polymer-gel dosimeter *Phys. Med. Biol.* **39** 1437–1455

[3] Baldock C, Burford R P, Billingham N, Wagner G S, Patval S, Badawi R D and Keevil S F 1998 Experimental procedure for the manufacture and calibration of polyacrylamide gel (PAG) for magnetic resonance imaging (MRI) radiation dosimetry *Phys. Med. Biol.* **43** 695–702

[4] Love P A, Lewis D G and Smith C W 1999 Experiences of producing and MRI scanning large volume Barex gel phantoms *Proceedings of the 1st International Workshop on Radiation Therapy Gel Dosimetry* Schreiner L J *Editor* Canadian Organization of Medical Physicists **ISBN:0-9684873-1-9**

[5] Rogers D W O, Faddegon B A, Ding G X, Ma C M, Wei J and Mackie T R 1995 BEAM: A Monte Carlo code to simulate radiotherapy treatment units *Med. Phys.* **22** 503–524

[6] Ma C M, Reckwerdt P, Holmes M, Rogers D W O and Geiser B 1995 DOSXYZ Users Manual *National Research Council of Canada* **PIRS-0509B** (NRC, Ottawa)

[7] Knöös T, Ahnesjö A, Nilsson P, Weber L 1995 Limitations of pencil beam approach to photon dose calculations in lung tissue *Phys. Med. Biol.* **40** 1411–1420

[8] Oldham M, McJury M, Baustert I B, Webb S and Leach M O 1998 Improving calibration accuracy in gel dosimetry *Phys. Med. Biol.* **43** 2709–2720

# Automated verification of 3D-Conformal and IMRT treatment planning using polymer gels

Gary Gluckman[1], Terry Button[1], Allen Meek[1], Marek Maryanski[2] and Lawrence Reinstein[1]

[1]SUNY Stony Brook, New York, USA, and [2]MGS Research Guildford, Connecticut, USA

## Introduction

A major stumbling block to the growth of high-tech treatment modalities such as 3D-conformal radiotherapy and IMRT is the lack of an acceptable methodology to test the agreement between planned and delivered patient dose distributions (1-3). Conventional 1D or 2D radiation dosimetry systems that are used to verify treatment-planning calculations are not capable of efficiently providing the integrated dose information throughout a clinically relevant volume with adequate spatial resolution. Recently BANG©-gels (MGS Research Inc., Guilford, CT) in combination with MRI have been shown to record and accurately map 3D dose distributions with high spatial resolution and precision (4). In BANG-gels, radiation-induced polymerization of acrylic monomers dissolved in an aqueous gel produces a permanent, self-developing three-dimensional image of dose distributions that can be appreciated visually (see Figure 1) or measured quantitatively by MRI scanning (5). However, to utilize the full potential of BANG-gel technique, we have developed a software package (Stony Brook Gel Dosimetry Analysis, SBGDA), which provides completely automated verification. The SBGDA software is DICOM (6) compatible, enabling it to compare gel/MRI dosimetry to the 3D-RTP calculations. The dose distribution is calculated from R2 maps derived from spin-echo images and automatically registered. Several color-graphic tools (e.g., dose difference histograms with color-wash) are included to facilitate validation of the plan calculations.

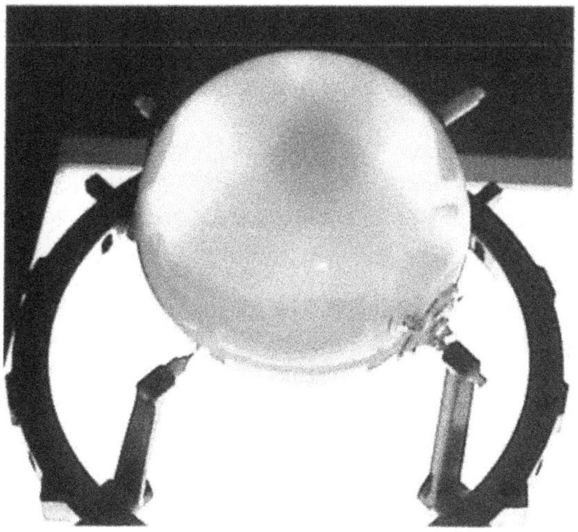

**Figure 1:** Spherical flask (15.3 cm inner diameter) containing BANG-gel. The flask is attached to a BRW head-frame.

## Material and methods

The BANG-gel formulations were prepared and poured into 16 cm diameter spherical Pyrex glass flasks (15.3 cm inner diameter) with an 11.5 cm long neck. As a preliminary study to stringently test spatial accuracy, each flask filled with BANG-gel was attached to a BRW head-frame (using a set of four suction cups) prior to CT imaging and irradiation. High-resolution CT scans with in-plane pixel resolutions ranging from 0.66 to 0.94 mm, 1 to 3 mm slice thickness' were used. After imaging, the flasks were placed in the treatment room and allowed to reach thermal equilibrium and the CT images transferred to our radiosurgery treatment planning (RTP) system for planning. The plans were devised so that the maximum dose to the BANG-gel was 25 Gy (the gels were prepared so that the dose response curve is linear up to this range). We irradiated a set of 8 vials for dose calibration. The flasks were irradiated in a 6 MV photon field using a floor-stand based radiosurgery system. After irradiation, the flasks were transported to the MRI room and left there overnight for thermal equilibration. Imaging employed a multi-slice train of Hahn spin-echo pulse sequence with TR of 6000 ms and TE's of 30 ms and 90 ms, as well as a modified thirty two echo Carr-Purcell-Meiboom-Gill (CPMG) spin-echo sequence. Modifications included a crusher gradient in the read direction after the thirty-second echo and spoiler gradients about each phase encode gradient. These modifications served to eliminate stimulated echo artifacts, which were initially present. A FOV of 25.6 cm, 128x128 matrix and 2 mm slice thickness resulted in a voxel of 2x2x2 mm3. The gel was scanned in interleave mode to reduce magnetization cross-talk between noise from adjacent slices.

The CT images, the exported RTP dose matrix and the MRI images were imported into the SBGDA software for analysis. The measured dose distributions were then calculated from R2 maps derived from spin-echo images and automatically registered with the RTP dose matrix for comparison. Various tools are available for comparing the two dose distributions, such as dose-difference maps, overlay of fused images, point-by-point and profile dose comparisons.

Several phantoms were irradiated in this initial study, and example of one such study is given below:

**6-fields, single isocenter (example study) :** A 6-field, single isocenter plan was employed and irradiated in a 6 MV photon field to a maximum dose of 25 Gy. A 30.0 mm collimator was used and the isocenter position was A-P = 20.0 mm, Lateral = 0.0 mm, Vertical = 10.0 mm (Figure 1). The plan was intentionally devised so that the two of the 6 fields clipped the BRW head-frame in order to test the sensitivity of BANG-gel to detect such errors typically unaccounted for in most RTP systems (if not all). This results in a lower isocenter dose and skewing of the isodose lines.

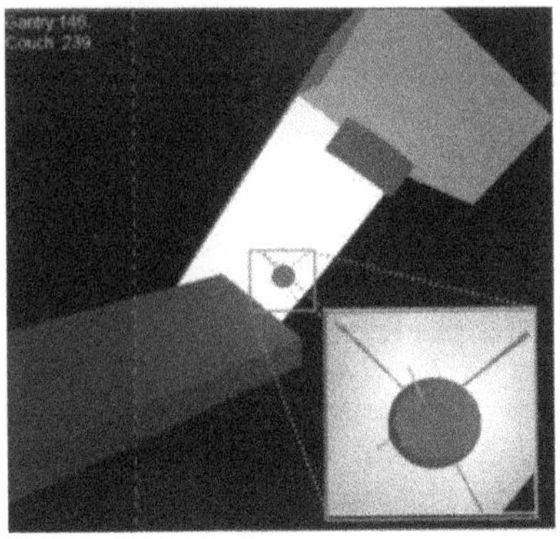


**Figure 2:** Perspective view of the 6-static field plan delivered to the BANG-gel phantom.

## Results and discussion

The calculated and measured isodose surfaces agreed to within 2 mm and in the low dose regions the percent differences were under 5%. The measured maximum dose was slightly lower than predicted, as expected since the treatment planning system uses a simple TMR/OAR algorithm (with slant-depth corrections) for calculating the dose distributions, and does not take into account any heterogeneities. The flask walls are approximately 3.5 mm thick, with a density of 2.2 g/cm3.

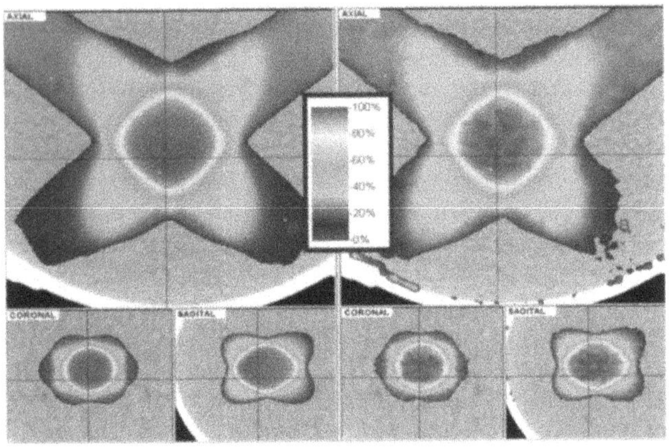


**Figure 3:** Dose color-wash comparison between the RTP dose distribution (left) and measured BANG-gel dose distribution (right). The dose distributions are overlayed on top of the CT data.

## Conclusion

We have developed an automated procedure for fusing the RTP and BANG-gel dose distributions providing a quantitative verification of the accuracy of 3D dose distributions. Effectiveness of our software is demonstrated using several BANG-gel phantoms irradiated to different multi-beam configurations. The dosimetric and spatial uncertainties (as well as its efficiency and ease of use) have been evaluated and found to conform to the recommended tolerances for RTP QA expressed by AAPM TG40 and TG53.

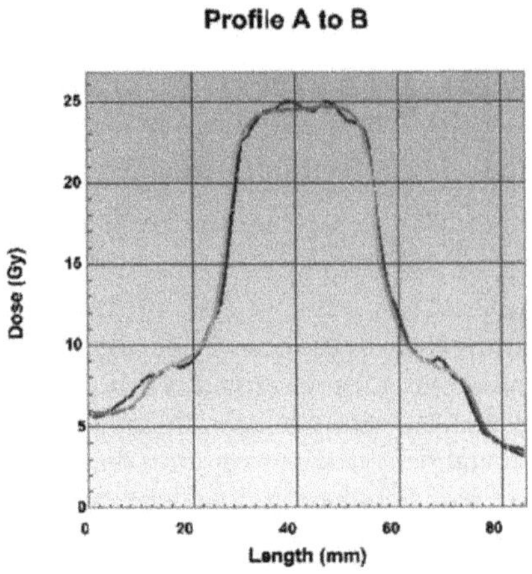


**Figure 4:** Comparison of the RTP predicted (color) and BANG-gel measured (black) dose profiles (see color-wash comparison).

## Acknowledgements

The research and development is supported in part by NIH-SBIR, CA82026 and the Stony Brook Radiation Oncology PC.

## References

[1] Suit H D 1986 Impact of Improved Local Control on Survival *IJROBP* **12** 453-458

[2] Purdy J, Klein E and Rowe D Quality Assurance and Safety of New Technologies *Seminars in Radiation Oncology* **5** 156-165

[3] TenHaken R K and Fraąss B 1996 Quality Assurance in 3-D Treatment Planning *Ed. by J.L. Meyer, J.A. Purdy, 3-D Conformal Radiotherapy, published Khager and Basil, Vol. 2* 104-114

[4] Meeks S L, Bova F J, Maryanski M J, Kendrick L A, Ranade M K, Buatti J M, Friedman W A 1999 Quantitative dosimetry evaluation through image correlation with BANG polymer gel dose maps *Int. J. Radiat. Oncol. Biol. Phys.* **43** 1135-1141

[5] Maryanski M J, Ibbott G S, Eastman P, Schulz R J and Gore J C 1996 Radiation Therapy Dosimetry using Magnetic Resonance Imaging of Polymer Gels *Med. Phys.* **23** 699-705

[6] ACR/NEMA: DICOM-RT Extension to DICOM Standard (1996).

# Future concepts for IMRT verification techniques derived from experiences gained in scanning heavy ion radiotherapy

**Christian P. Karger, Günther H. Hartmann, Oliver Jäkel and Peter Heeg**

Deutsches Krebsforschungszentrum, Abt. Medizinische Physik, INF 280, D-69120 Heidelberg

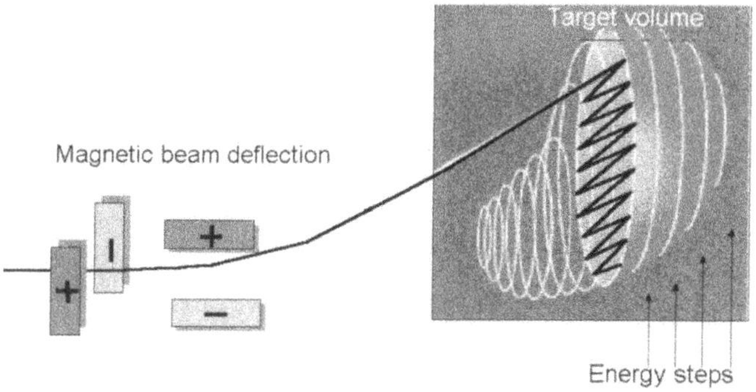


**Figure 1**. The principle of heavy ion therapy using a raster scanner.

## Introduction

There are far reaching similarities between intensity modulated radiotherapy (IMRT) using photons from a Linac and radiotherapy using a scanning ion beam. As a matter of fact scanning ion radiotherapy can also be regarded as an IMRT-technique. In both cases, a highly conformal dose distributions is achieved by decomposing the treatment field into multiple sub-fields. In IMRT with photons the sub-fields are created either statically (step and shoot technique) or dynamically (by moving leaves of an multi-leaf-collimator during irradiation). With heavy ions, the dose distribution is built up by a pencil beam which is scanned over the tumor cross section. The penetration depth of the ions is modulated actively by variation of the synchrotron energy (fig. 1). This new therapy modality using a horizontal scanning ion beam, is now brought into clinical routine at the Gesellschaft für Schwerionenforschung (GSI) [1,2].
All IMRT-applications demand thorough dosimetric verification of the beam delivery for each individual patient. This verification process differs in some characteristic features from that for simple static treatment fields:

1. Since each IMRT-field is composed of multiple sub-fields, the dose at one measurement point may comply with the calculated dose, while it may differ at another. Therefore the measurement at a single point is not sufficient to gain representative information about the actual dose distribution.
2. Each dose measurement requires the application of the complete treatment field. To gain representative information about the dose distribution in a reasonable amount of time, simultaneous measurements at multiple points are indispensable.
3. If the dose verification is to be performed routinely for each individual patient, an online procedure including an online-evaluation of the measurement should be preferred.

For the heavy ion facility, new and efficient verification techniques were developed. The experiences gained so far may also be of value for the development of future concepts for IMRT-verification.

## Material and methods

### Dosimetric verification

Dosimetric verification is performed in a water phantom for each individual patient prior to its irradiation [3]. The treatment field is recalculated to the geometry of the water phantom. Two multi-channel electrometers (Multidos, PTW, Germany) in combination with 24 small thimble ionization chambers (IC03, Wellhöfer, Germany) are used. The ionization chambers are densely packed into a PMMA-mounting, which is attached to the arm of the 3D-motor driven water phantom (MP3, PTW, Germany). The electrometers and the water phantom are controlled by a new developed software. After adjustment of the phantom, the calculated dose values at all measurement positions are available to the measurement system via an interface to the planning system [4]. The graphical display of the chamber positions within the dose distribution allows the selection of adequate measurement positions. The measurement is completely computer-controlled and a numerical as well as a graphical comparison of the measured and calculated dose is available immediately after the measurement is finished. The mean deviation and the standard deviation of all measured deviations are calculated to characterize the compliance between measurement and calculation. By printouts a complete documentation for the measurement is obtained and a quick decision can be made whether the dose distribution is acceptable.

### Geometrical verification

To check the shape and orientation of the actual treatment field with respect to the patient anatomy, a film is irradiated and is then compared with the target contour in beams eye view, calculated by the treatment planning system.

### Geometrical and dosimetric online-verification

Besides the dosimetric and geometric verification prior to the irradiation of the patient, an online-monitor of the particle number per scan position and the scan position was developed at GSI. The number of particles at each raster point is controlled by plane parallel transmission chambers and the actual scan position of the beam is acquired by multi-wire chambers. If the deviations in the beam position or in the particle number exceeds certain intervention thresholds, the control system generates an interlock and the irradiation process is interrupted. During the irradiation process, the actual beam position is displayed on a screen for each energy slice by the therapy online monitor.

Before the irradiation starts, the superposition of all scan positions of all energy slices is calculated for the beams eye view. By comparison with the irradiated film and the target contour, it can be assured that shape and orientation of the actual field are correct.

## Results and discussion

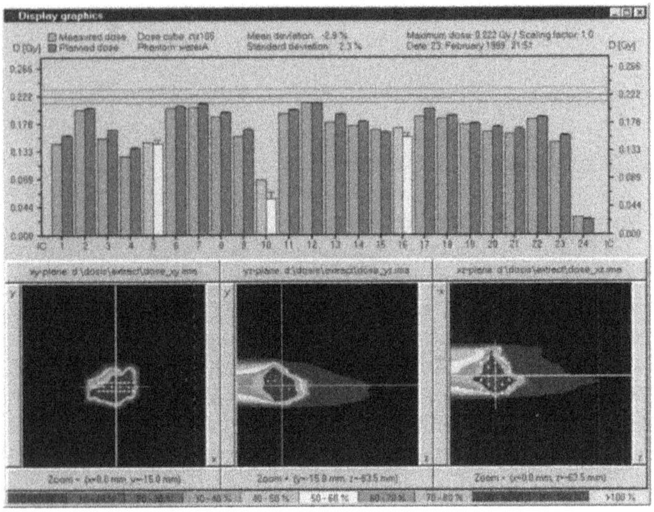

**Figure 2**. Example of an verification measurement

Up to now 48 patients have safely been treated with the scanning carbon beam at GSI. A total of 374 verification measurements have been carried out. Each treatment field of each patient was measured at least twice: once within the target volume and once at the distal edge of the target volume. Fig. 2 gives an example for a verification measurement within the target volume and fig. 3 summarizes the result of all measurements. Each data point corresponds to about 20 measurement positions.

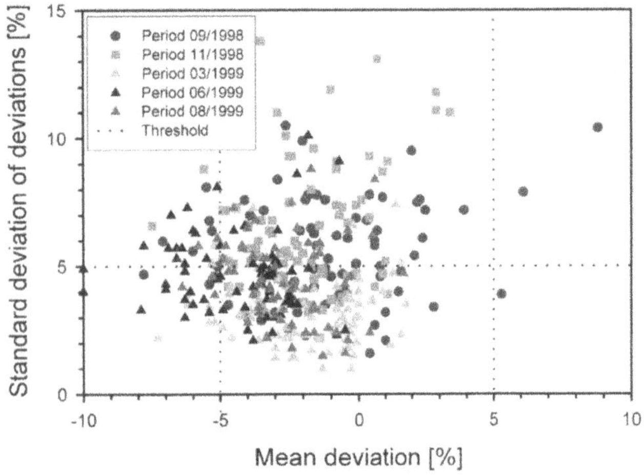


**Figure 3**. Summary of all verification measurements

It is important to note, that the deviations between measured and calculated dose depend on three error sources: (i) correctness of beam delivery, (ii) uncertainties in the beam model used for the dose calculation, (iii) uncertainties in the measurement system.

For each of the two displayed parameters intervention thresholds of 5% have been defined. If an intervention threshold is exceeded, the deviations are carefully analyzed in order to decide which of the error sources can be attributed to the observed deviation. If a malfunction of the beam delivery sytem can be excluded, the patient will be irradiated, however, only after consultation and permission of the responsible radio-oncologist.

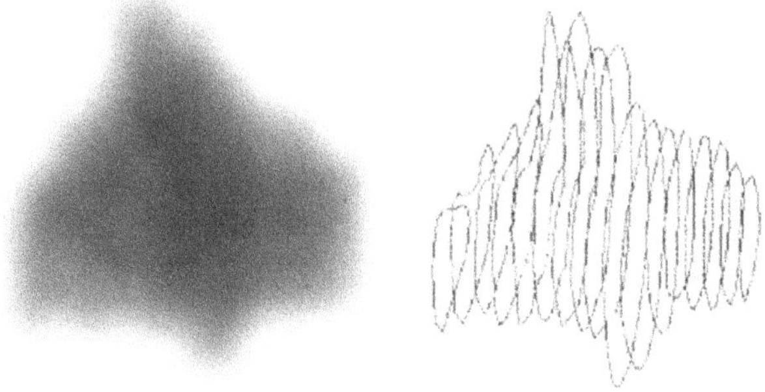

**Figure 4**. Target volume and irradiated Film in beams eye view

The comparison of the irradiated film with the target contour in beams eye view serves as a plausibility check in oderer to prevent an application of the wrong field or of the use of the wrong angle of the treatment table. This check is of great value for IMRT-fields, since they can not be vizualized by light-vizors like static fields produced by conventional collimators.

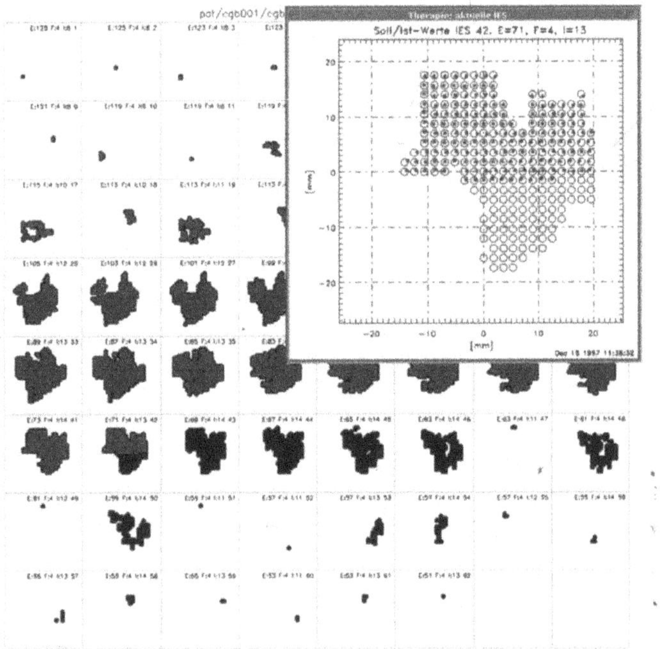

**Figure 5**. The therapy online monitor developed at GSI

The therapy online monitor reads out the information of the monitor chambers and the multi-wire chambers. In addition to the control of the particle number by the monitor chambers, which has ist counterpart in the monitor chambers in a

conventional Linac, the actual beam position is recorded and displayed. Both, monitor chambers and multi-wire chambers are part of the control system.
When IMRT-techniques are applied, the beam delivery should be checked by methods, which are independent and redundant to the methods used by the control system. Therefore the dose distribution of each individual field is verified, using the described verification system. Both, the therapy online monitor and an independent and efficient dose verification system, are prerequisites for a safe performance of heavy ion therapy.

## Conclusion

In heavy ion therapy as well as in IMRT with photons, the applied dose is controlled by monitor chambers during irradiation of the patient. The monitoring of the scan positions in heavy ion therapy can be regarded as counterpart to the control of the leaf positions of the multi-leaf-collimator, which define the sub-fields in IMRT with photons.
IMRT uses highly complex beam delivery techniques which offer more possibilities of malfunction compared with static field techniques. Therefore, great emphasis has to be put on verification of the delivered dose. The dose delivery should be verified prior to the irradiation of each patient using a system which is independent and redundant to that of the control system. On the other hand, the verification has to be performed within a reasonable amount of time. The latter is currently one of the limiting factors for wide clinical application of IMRT.
Regarding heavy ion therapy, the requirements with respect to verification of dose delivery are very similar. This is due to the fact that the main characteristics of IMRT also apply to this new modality. The following experiences gained in heavy ion therapy may be transferred to IMRT with photons:

1. The number of detectors must be high enough to cover a representative area of the dose distribution. The desired information should be attained by one or at most two measurements.
2. The use of detectors, should allow electronically readout (e.g. multiple ionization chambers or an array of them).
3. The comparison of measured and calculated dose should be performed online. The requires a computer interface to the planning system and the knowledge of the actual positions of the detectors with respect to the dose distribution.

In heavy ion therapy, these features are realized by the described verification system. There are however two features of the verification system which limit its use for IMRT with photons: (i) For photons the use of a water phantom may not be adequate, since it requires horizontally or vertically oriented beams. Gravity effect with respect to the leafs of a multi-leaf-collimator require verification under the gantry angle used for irradiation of the patient. (ii) On the other hand, it is not necessary for photons to determine the dose in different depths, since the dose at a single depth determines the dose at any depth when the depth dose distribution is known. This is one of the main differences to radiotherapy with a scanned ion beam, since in the latter multiple beams of different energy (and therefore different range in tissue) are superimposed. In each of these energy steps, the beam delivery may fail and the depth dose distribution would then be modified.
As a consequence of these specific features, on could think of a two-dimensional array of detectors, which is adapted to the accessory-holder of the gantry. By calculating the expected dose for this detector configuration, the correct application of dose could be verified for any gantry angle. A further developed system may also be operated during patient irradiation as an independent system to the control system, but with the possibility to generate an interlock, if significant deviations between measured and calculated doses occur. A first approach to develop such a system is currently undertaken in our institution.
Another frequently discussed approach uses a portal imaging device to verify the transmitted dose behind the patient. This technique has the disadvantage that the measured dose critically depends on the accuracy of patient positioning, which is completely independent and separable from the problem of a correct beam delivery.

## References

[1] Jäkel O, Hartmann G H, Heeg P, Jacob C, Karger C P, Krämer M, Kress J, Krießbach A, Lappe C and Debus J 1999, Erste Schwerionenbestrahlung von Patienten in Europa: Medizinphysikalische Aspekte. Zeitschrift für Medizinische Physik **9**, 88-95

[2] Kraft G 1998, Schwerionentherapie bei der GSI: Erste Patienten behandelt. Physikalische Blätter **54**, 104-105

[3] Karger C P, Jäkel O, Hartmann G H and Heeg P 1999, A system for three-dimensional dosimetric verification of treatment plans in intensity-modulated radiotherapy with heavy ions. *Medical Physics* **26** 2125-2132

[4] Jäkel O., Krämer M., Hartmann G H, Heeg P, Karger C P and Kraft G 1999, Treatment planning for the heavy-ion facility at GSI. *Strahlentherapie und Onkologie* **175** (Suppl. II), 15-17

# A software system for patient-specific quality control of intensity-modulated radiation treatments by Fricke-gel dosimetry

**Philippe Belanger[1], Yanic Bercier, William Parker and Dimitre Hristov**

[1]Medical Physics Unit, 1650 Cedar L5-112, Montreal, Canada, H3G 1A4

## Introduction

Current state of the art treatment techniques in radiation oncology include the use of intensity modulated radiation therapy (IMRT) to deliver highly conformal doses to precisely defined target volumes while maximising healthy tissue sparing. Intensity modulated beams (IMB) can be delivered with the use of multileaf collimators (MLC) either dynamically, or by using a segmented treatment delivery. Very complex IMBs require a dynamic dose delivery system, which provides the necessary dose resolution to deliver an accurate dose distribution. The use of dynamically delivered beams produced by MLCs pose unique problems for radiation dosimetry. Dynamic dose, delivery requires an integrating dosimeter, and the steep dose gradients that may be encountered in IMRT require a measuring instrument with high spatial resolution.

MRI-based dosimetry with ferrous sulphate (Fricke) gel phantoms is suited for dynamic beam delivery because it provides unprecedented advantages. Continuous, three dimensional dose information may be acquired in a single measurement. Also, the fact that the irradiated phantom is the actual radiation detector avoids any unnecessary perturbation that film or other dosimetric probes might introduce to the system. The high spatial resolution (sub-millimetre) attainable with this system is suited to measuring the steep dose gradients encountered in IMRT, and the integrating nature of the detector makes it effective in measuring dose distributions from dynamic dose delivery systems. Finally, the nature of the gel allows the dosimeter to be poured into arbitrary containers, and permits the easy insertion of inhomogeneities into the phantom. These properties of the gel dosimeter make it an attractive option for the complex quality assurance procedure of intensity-modulated radiation treatments.

## Description of the quality assurance procedure

A patient-specific acrylic mould is filled with Fricke-gel, irradiated, and MR imaged as part of the quality assurance procedure performed before any delivered treatment. The Fricke-gel solution constituents are given in Table 1.

| Component | Concentration |
|---|---|
| NaCl | 1 mM |
| Ferrous sulphate | 1 mM |
| Sulphuric acid | 0.5 M |
| Gelatin | 5% w/w |

**Table 1:** Fricke-gel constituents

The MR imaging is done on a General Electric *Signa 5X* 1.5 T MR imager (GE Medical System, Milwaukee, WI). The GE Quad Head coil is used. The different imaging parameters are in the Table 2. Those parameters have been set in order to get the best signal-to-noise ratio in a T1 weighted image.

| | |
|---|---|
| Excitation sequence | Spin echo |
| Echo time | 11 msec |
| Repetition time | 500 msec |
| Field of view | 24 cm |
| Matrix dimensions | 256 x 256 |
| Voxel dimensions | 0.9 x 0.9 x 3 $mm^3$ |

**Table 2:** MR imaging parameters

Dose-MR signal intensity calibration is performed by filling 6 lucite vials (radius 12 mm, length 43 mm, thickness 1 mm) with the Fricke-gel. Each of those vials is irradiated with a different dose (10 to 60 Gy) and the dose/MR-signal intensity data is fitted by an analytical calibration function reflecting the theoretically expected dose-MR signal relationship [1].

The 3D MR dataset of the irradiated patient mould is then mapped onto a 3D dose dataset with the calibration function. Assuming that the mould of the patient is accurate in shape, and that the phantom is irradiated exactly as the patient would be, the resulting MR-dose image can be registered (or fused) with a planning computed tomography (CT) scan of the patient. A quantitative analysis of the coverage of the target volume can be performed, and an objective evaluation of the treatment plan obtained. Below we describe the software system developed for this quality assurance and plan verification procedure.

## Software system

The system is developed with the AVS 5.4 software (Advanced Visual System Inc., Waltham, MA) running on a Pentium II class processor (Intel Corporation, Santa Clara, CA) 233 MHz., 256 megs of RAM, running on Red Hat Linux 6.0 OS (Red Hat Software Inc. North Carolina). Figure 1 shows the system structure.

### Calibration

At the calibration stage, the MR image of the irradiated calibration vials is registered (Figure 5) to the MR image of the unirradiated vials ("blank" image) and reformatted. After subtraction, the MR signal values in the difference image have been shown to correlate well with the absorbed dose [1]. The user selects regions of interest within the vials (Figure 3) and the average signal intensities are automatically used for the determination of the parameters in the calibration function.

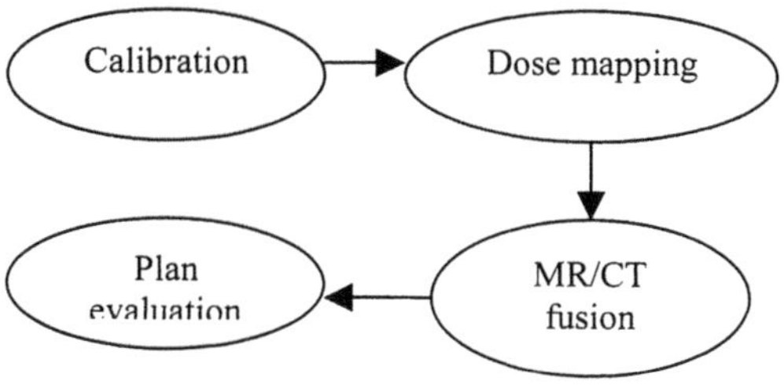


**Figure 1:** System structure

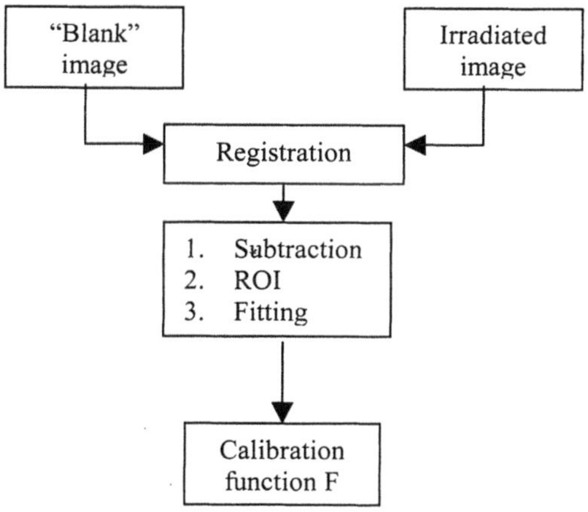


**Figure 2:** Calibration

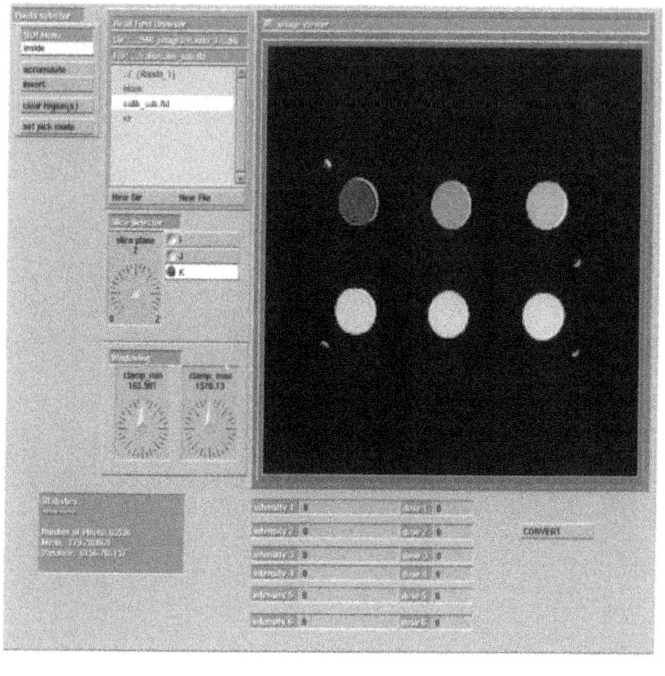

**Figure 3:** Calibration layout. The user selects an ROI within each vial in the difference image.

**Dose mapping**

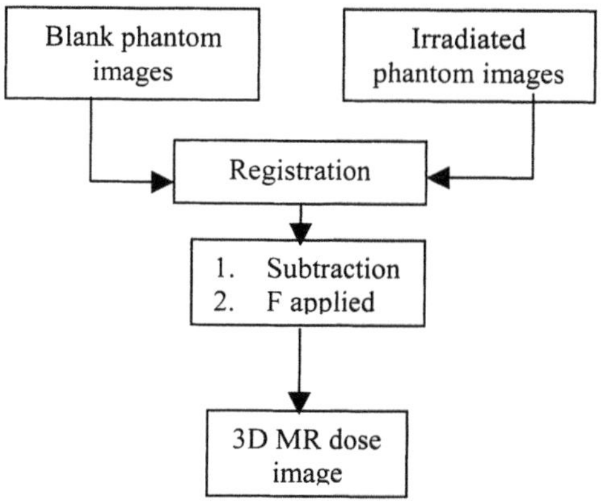


**Figure 4:** Dose mapping

After registration and reformatting, the MR dataset of the unirradiated patient mould is subtracted from the MR dataset of the irradiated mould. The calibration function is applied to the resulting dataset and 3D dose data is generated.

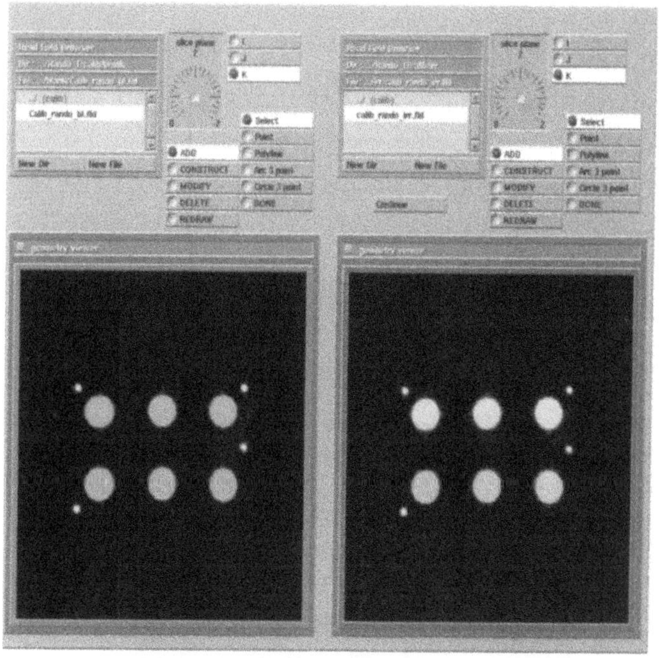

**Figure 5:** Registration. At left, the template image and at right, the image to register. User can select fiducial markers (small bright dots on both images) on any plane (axial, coronal or sagittal) for point-matching registration.

**MR/CT Fusion**

The point-matching method is used by selecting the fiducial markers on both images. A fine-tuning is done manually afterwards. After registration of the CT and the MR-dose datasets, the MR dataset is reformatted to match its CT counterpart.

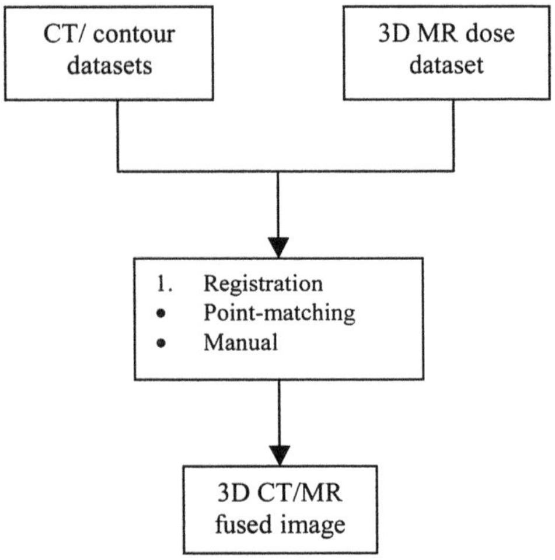


**Figure 6:** MR/CT fusion

**Plan evaluation**

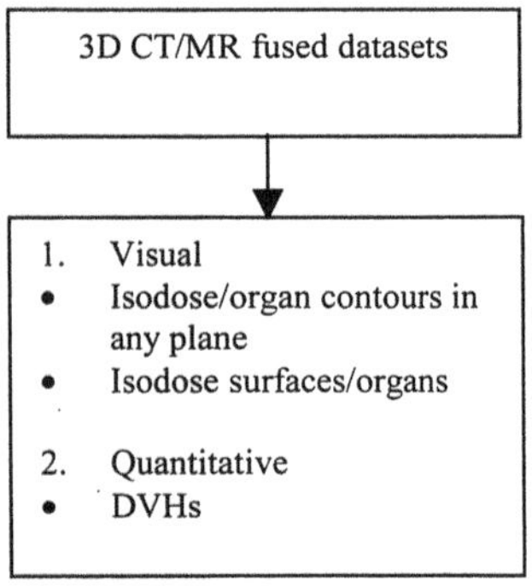


**Figure 7**: Plan evaluation

After the MR/CT fusion plan evaluation can be performed visually or quantitatively (Figure 7). An example of isodose surfaces/organ visualisation is shown in Figure 8. The DVH can be calculated and compared with the DVH calculated by the planning computer.

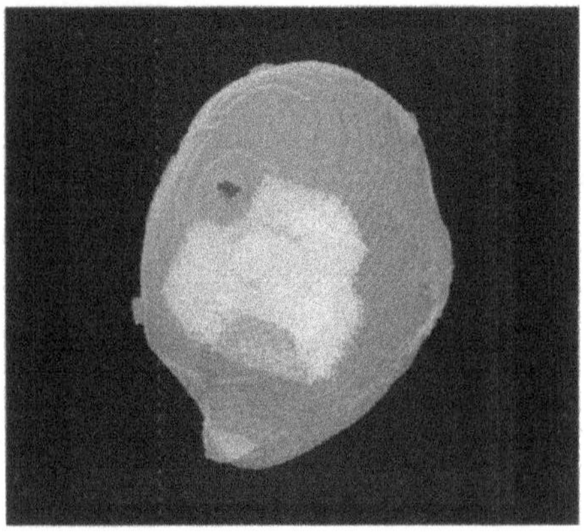

**Figure 8:** Anatomy/dose visualisation. The target is not completely covered by the 80% isodose surface.

## Conclusion

Ferrous sulphate gel dosimetry has shown potential in the evaluation of dose distributions from dynamically delivered beams. It can be further extended to provide patient-specific quality assurance of intensity modulated radiation treatments. We have presented a software system to analyse and quantify the results of the Fricke dosimetry in this quality assurance procedure.

## References

[1] Chu W C, Guo W Y, Wu M C, Chung W Y, Pan D H C, December 1998, The irradiation induced magnetic resonance image intensity change provides a more efficient three-dimensional dose measurement in MRI-Fricke-agarose gel dosimetry, *Medical Physics*, **25**(12), 2326-2332

# A simple and robust method for clinical implementation of midplane transit dosimetry using diodes and portal films

**Sara Broggi, Claudio Fiorino, Riccardo Calandrino**

Servizio di Fisica Sanitaria, H.S. Raffaele, Milano, Italy

## Introduction

This work investigates the possibilities of using a pair of diodes in correspondence with the beam axis in conjunction with a portal film at the exit to estimate in-vivo midline dose distributions, without any additional patient information. In particular, we wished to study the possibility of estimating midplane dose distributions without applying the inverse square correction factors, defined in previously published works [1,2].

These factors which take into account the different portal film-patient distances and the source-to-skin distances (SSD) in the entrance points, need an accurate knowledge *a priori* of the 3D shape of patient body contour.

## Material and methods

Our proposed method considers each patient with a curved profile equivalent to a parallelepiped phantom with a thickness z equal to the real patient's thickness on the field axis and with a variable electronic density ρ, depending on the water-equivalent thickness, crossed by the beam. ($\rho(z)*Z=T(y)$) (Figure 1)

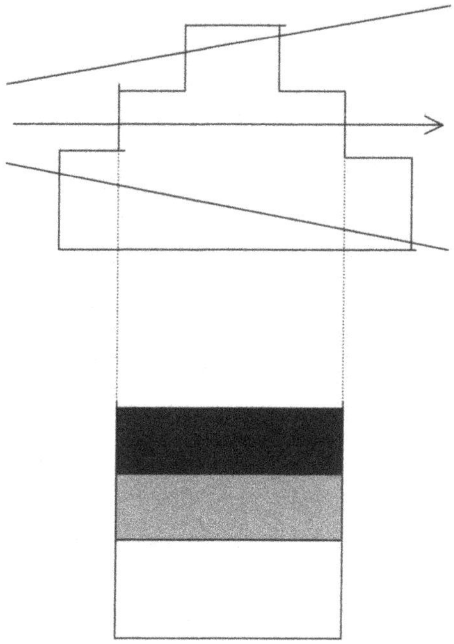

Figure 1: The proposed method: assumption for "curved" patient contours

Based on this assumption, the exit dose map is determined from the relative dose map measured at the portal detector level by the film (Kodak X-Omat in localization cassette) by geometrical backprojection to the corresponding exit points and normalised to the on-axis absolute exit dose value measured with the diode; in the same way the relative entrance dose map is derived by correcting the absolute dose value measured with the diode at the entrance surface by the (known) off-axis ratios, excluding penumbra region.

For each pair of $D_{in}$ and $D_{out}$, we calculated $D_{mid}$ by applying the Rizzotti and the Huyskens algorithms. [2,3]

For the on-axis entrance/exit dose measurements we used p-type silicon diodes (Scanditronix, EDP 10) connected to a multi-channel electrometer (DPD 510, Scanditronix) opportunely calibrated to convert the diode signal in absorbed dose.

The midline dose profiles were measured with a NE2571 cylindrical ionisation chamber or with a small volume PTW chamber (0.125 cc).

The method was tested for 6 MV beams in homogeneous cubic phantoms, homogeneous phantoms with varying thickness symmetrically (simulating head and neck regions) and asymmetrically (simulating abdomen/pelvis region) and a half-sphere phantom with simulating the breast.

For asymmetrical phantoms, the total midplane dose was estimated/measured for an irradiation with two opposing fields. A number of combinations of phantom thickness and field sizes were investigated. The minimum air gap between portal film and phantom was kept equal to 5 cm.

## Results and discussion

Results confirm that the proposed method can be used to estimate midplane dose maps within 2%-3% for most clinically suitable situations.(see for instance Fig 2,3)

For homogeneous symmetrical phantoms the agreement makes worse with the increase of the scattered radiation's weight: with the increase of the phantom-portal film distance, for larger field sizes and for phantoms with larger total thickness. This is congruent with the results of a number of investigations (see for instance [4,5])

For homogeneous asymmetrical phantoms the percentage deviation raises with the step thickness.

Discrepancies larger than 3% (up to 5-6%) are found for "stressed" irradiation geometries, not linked with any clinical condition.

## Conclusion

The obtained results not only show the accuracy of the proposed method but, due to its simplicity, suggest a rapid clinical implementation.
This method could allow to estimate midplane dose distributions in relevant clinical situations such as head-neck, breast and abdomen/pelvis irradiation.
We will clinically test in-vivo this method for these anatomic regions. Further investigations will be done in order to estimate the accuracy and the limits of the proposed method in inhomogeneous regions (i.e.: thorax).

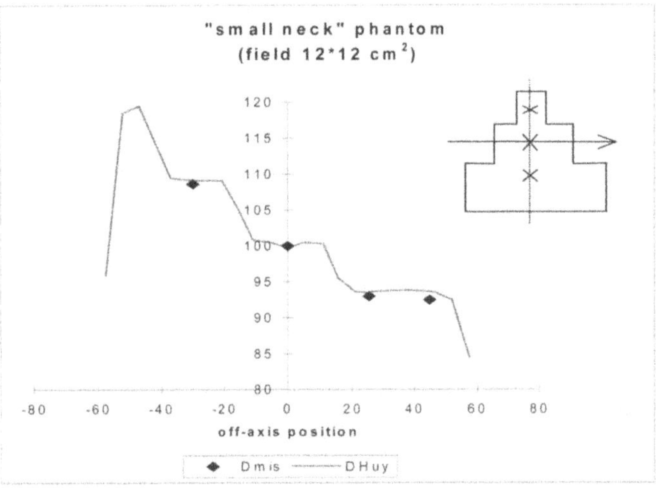


Figure 2: "small neck phantom": estimated vs measured midline doses

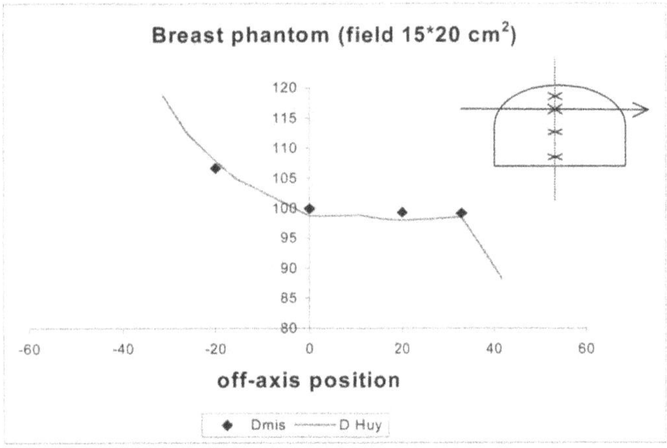


Figure 3: "breast phantom": estimated vs measured midline doses

## References

[1] Fiorino C, Del Vecchio A, Cattaneo G.M., Fusca M, Longobardi B, Signorotto P, Calandrino R 1993 Exit dose measurements by portal film dosimetry *Radiotherapy and Oncology* **29** 336-340

[2] Huyskens D, Van Dam J and Dutreix A 1994 Midplane dose determination using in vivo dose measurements in combination with portal imaging *Phys. Med. Biol.* **39** 1089-1101

[3] Rizzotti A, Compri C and Garusi G.F. 1985 Dose evaluation to patient irradiated by $^{60}$Co beams, by means of direct measurement on the incident and on the exit surfaces *Radiotherapy and Oncology* **3** 279-283

[4] Fiorino C, Uleri C, Cattaneo G.M., Calandrino R 1996 On-line exit dose profile measurements by a diode linear array *Phis.Med.Biol* **41** 1291-1304

[5] Essers M, Boellard M, van Herk M, Lanson J. H. and Mijnheer B.J. 1996 Transmission dosimetry with a liquid-filled electronic portal imaging device *Int. J. Radiat. Oncol. Biol. Phys.* **34** 931-941

# Comparison of MRI-Interrogated Fricke and BANG Gel Proton Dose Visualisation for a Therapy Cyclotron

John N H Brunt[1], Richard P Hagan[1,2] and Andrzej Kacperek[2]

[1]Physics Department, and [2]Douglas Cyclotron Unit, Clatterbridge Centre for Oncology, Bebington, near Liverpool, CH63 4JY, England

## Introduction

At the XI th ICCR, we reported on a methodology for using Magnetic Resonance Imaging (MRI) to interrogate irradiated Fricke gels in order to display and analyse the proton dose distributions[1] achievable with the Clatterbridge cyclotron[2], which provides a U.K. national facility for treatment of ocular melanomas.

Our discussion/conclusions section referred in particular to the low rate of fall of dose beyond the Bragg peak. We hypothesised that diffusion might be implicated; it would have relatively more significant effects for small-field, small penumbra proton irradiations than for other types of radiation therapy. We decided to investigate a greater variety of formulations of Fricke gels in which diffusion might be inhibited, in comparison with cross-linked polymer gels.

## Material and methods

Cuboid box phantoms for Fricke gels were constructed using Perspex and polycarbonate. To seek an optimal combination of dose-discrimination sensitivity and diffusion inhibition, various formulations involving agarose or gelatine gels with or without Xylenol orange[3] were used. Geometrically similar phantoms to our design were manufactured by MGS Research Inc and filled with BANG (max dose 25 Gy, max dose rate 6 Gy/min type).

The proton energy of the cyclotron is 62 MeV, and the effective energy at the irradiation port is 60 MeV. Dose rates of typically 15 Gy per minute for Fricke gels and 5 Gy per minute for BANG gels were used. Within the same phantom as the test fields, between 4 and 9 calibration fields were irradiated using a 20 mm collimated, fully modulated beam.

Investigations included:

- unmodulated Bragg peaks at a range of dose rates, using rectangular collimators with widths from 1 mm to 20 mm
- range-shifted fully modulated irradiations (as used for iris treatments)
- irradiations using wedging, blocking and abutted fields

MR imaging of gels was performed on a Philips Gyroscan T5-NT (0.5T) system using a quadrature head coil; quadrature neck and quadrature knee coils were also tested, but the head coil was found most suitable. A mixed IR (TR=2240 ms, TI=360 ms) and SE (TR=760 ms, TE = 50,100,150,200 ms) sequence was used. Signals were analysed using the scanner's software implementation of the ratios and least squares technique[4] to provide images consisting of pixel-by-pixel values of T1 and T2. A matrix of 256 x 256 pixels was used with voxel size usually 0.95 x 0.95 x 11.0 mm. For Fricke gels, the scan (which was commenced within 30 minutes of irradiation) had a duration of typically 12 minutes. Scans were repeated up to 5 times to obtain images over a period of approximately one hour, yielding data for diffusion rate calculations. Scans of similar duration were performed on BANG gels (24 hours or more after irradiation), for direct comparison, but were supplemented by scans of longer duration, enabled by the absence of diffusion in these gels.

The field of view (205 to 243 mm) encompassed the entire section through each phantom, and thus visualised several calibration irradiations and test fields simultaneously, together with a T1/T2 reference container and a spatial resolution phantom.

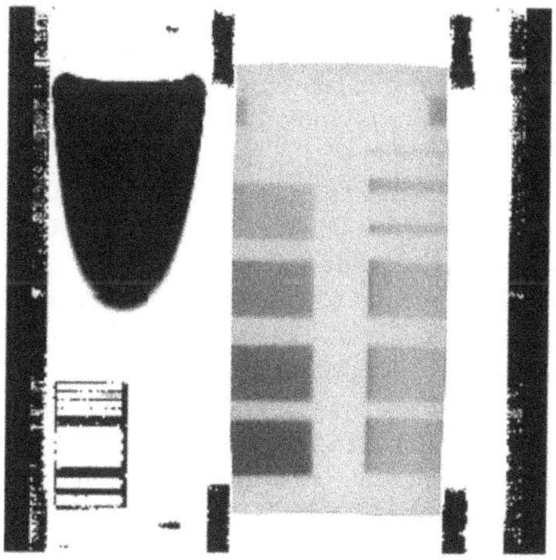

**Figure 1:** T1 image of proton-irradiated BANG-25 gel phantom, placed in a water trough, together with a T1/T2 reference container and a spatial resolution phantom. Left side, calibration irradiations; right side, Bragg peaks obtained with different dose rates and with different widths of slit collimators.

## Results and discussion

The Fricke formulation offering the optimal combination of dose discrimination sensitivity and modest diffusion rate had a near-linear R1 versus dose curve with gradient 0.023 $s^{-1}$ per Gy. The corresponding gradient for the BANG-25 gel was 0.0083 $s^{-1}$ per Gy. Because, however, the longer scan durations permitted by BANG gel enabled higher signal-to-noise ratios (SNR) to be achieved, its dose discrimination sensitivity exceeded that of our optimal Fricke formulation. While R2 images offer 5 times steeper response versus dose, the normalised SNR is 8 times lower, and we have therefore found no overall advantage in using R2 images of BANG gels.

In our previous Fricke work, the fall of dose from 90% to 10%, beyond a fully modulated field took place over a distance of nearly 6 mm, and our best subsequent efforts with Fricke gels could only reduce this by a factor of two. The equivalent distance in BANG gel is approximately 1.7 mm.

## Conclusion

Despite considerable effort, proof of the suitability of Fricke gels, for precise visualisation of dose distributions for ocular treatments by protons, remains elusive. Our results so far indicate, however, that BANG-25 gel offers adequate dose discrimination sensitivity, together with sufficient geometrical precision.

## References

[1] Brunt J N H, Eagle J A, Kacperek A, Lawrence G P, and Shaw JE 1994 Display and analysis of proton dose distributions from a therapy cyclotron using magnetic resonance imaging of fricke gels *Proceedings of XI ICCR.* pp 360-1.

[2] Bonnett D E et al, 1993 The 62 MeV proton beam for the treatment of ocular melanoma at Clatterbridge *British Journal of Radiology* **66** 907-914.

[3] Rae W I D, Willemse C A, Lotter M G, Engelbrecht J S and Swarts J C 1996 Chelator effect on ion diffusion in ferrous-sulfate-gelatin gel dosimeters as analyzed by MRI *Med Phys* **23** 15-23

[4] In den Kleef J J E and Cuppen J J M, 1987 RLSQ: T1, T2 and rho calculations, combining ratios and least squares *Magnetic Resonance in Medicine* **5** 513-524.

# Concave Dose Distributions in Dynamic Arc Radiosurgery

**Mathias Pfaender[1], Gerhard Grebe[2], Julia Ahlswede[1], Martin Roll[2], Lutz Lüdemann[1], Volker Budach[1], Reinhard Wurm[1]**

[1]Humboldt University Berlin, Charité-Mitte, Germany, [2]TFH Berlin, University of Applied Science, Medical Physics Department, Germany

## Introduction

Conformal stereotactic radiosurgery (SRS) and radiotherapy (SRT) using a linear accelerator and a micro-multileaf-collimator (mMLC) offer the possibility to irradiate irregulary shaped target volumes. The target volume is irradiated at several fixed gantry angels whereas the leaves of the mMLC replicate the shape of the volume in beams-eye-view. The conformity of the dose distribution with a concave target volumes is limited. With the dynamic arc radiosurgery it is possible to improve the conformity [1]. It is an arc treatment with moving leaves of the mMLC. This method combines the advantages of arc treatments with holed collimators and of mMLC treatments at fixed gantry angels. In this paper dose distributions with concave forms were verified by polymergel dosimetry [2].

## Material and methods

Dose distributions with concave structures in spherical BANG-2 phantoms from MGS Research, Inc. were calculated with the BrainSCAN stereotactic planning software, version 4.0, from BrainLAB. The dose distribution was calculated using a simple Clarkson algorithm. The therapy plans provided 5 arcs, taking care that the isocenter in the planning target volume were shielded by the leaves of the mMLC at no time during the movement of the gantry. The images for the planning process were taken with a CT PQ 2000 from Picker with a slice thickness of 2mm. The phantoms were irradiated using the computer controlled mMLC m3 from BrainLAB mounted to a Varian Clinac 2100C with 6 MV x-rays.

The radiation polymerises the gel in the phantoms. To measure the polymerisation MR images of the phantoms were taken with a Magnetom Vision VB 31 from Siemens. The phantoms were positioned in a head coil. Transversal slices were taken with a spin echo sequence with two variable echo times using the MR parameters TR = 1000 ms, TE1 = 70 ms, TE2 = 140 ms, FOV = 200 mm, matrix size 256x256, pixel size 0.78 mm x 0.78 mm, slice thickness 3mm and 8 acquisitions. With the image data the relaxation rate R2 and the dose were calculated pixel by pixel with MathCad Plus (MathSoft, Inc., Livingston, UK). The dose response of the gel was measured with phantoms of the same kind radiated with known doses and investigated simultaneously with the same MR parameters. The dose distribution in the phantoms was compared with the planned isodoses using image processing tools.

## Results and discussion

The dose-response of the BANG-2 gel was obtained from the R2 map of the calibration phantoms. An example is shown in fig.1. The data ware fitted very well with a linear function. The squared correlation coefficient is $r^2 = 0.998$. With this calibration function the dose map of the dynamic arc radiation was calculated and the 50% and 90% isodoses were contoured (fig 2). The planned 50% and 90% isodoses in the isocenter plane (fig. 3) fit within 1 mm, in small regions within 2 mm, with the corresponding calculated isodoses. The deviations are not systematic and caused first of all by the pixel size of the CT and the MRT, the grid of the dose calculation and the statistical noise of the signal intensities in the MR images. The deviation at the dorsal part of the dose distribution reported ealier [3] was not registered.

Due to the simple algorithm used for the calculation of the dose distribution it was nessecary to position the isocenter within the radiation field at any angle of the gantry. If the isocenter were shielded by one or more leaves the algorithm delivers too much monitor units for the whole arc in question and a false dose distribution.

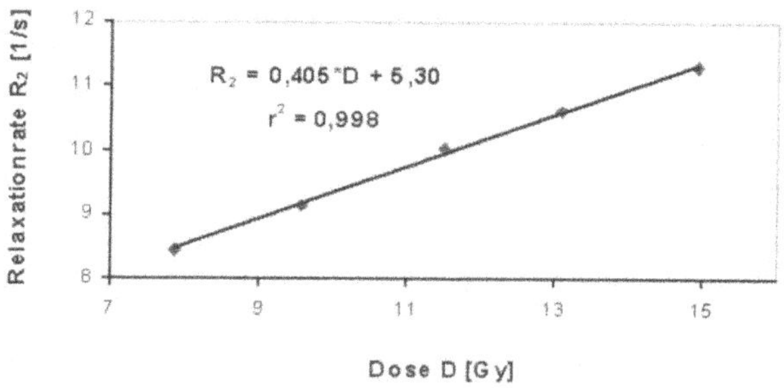


Fig.1 Relaxationrate depending on the dose

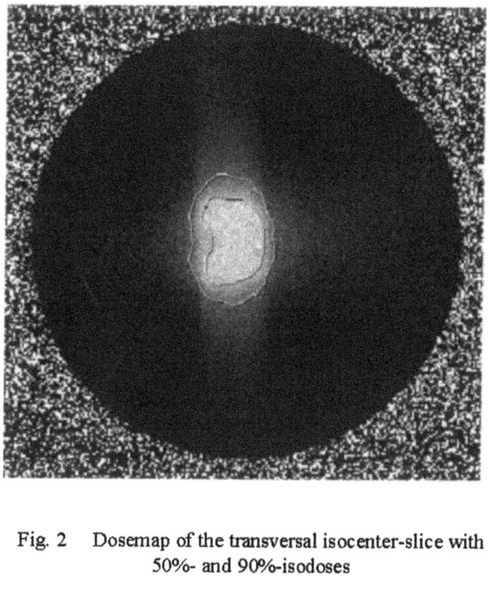

Fig. 2 Dosemap of the transversal isocenter-slice with 50%- and 90%-isodoses

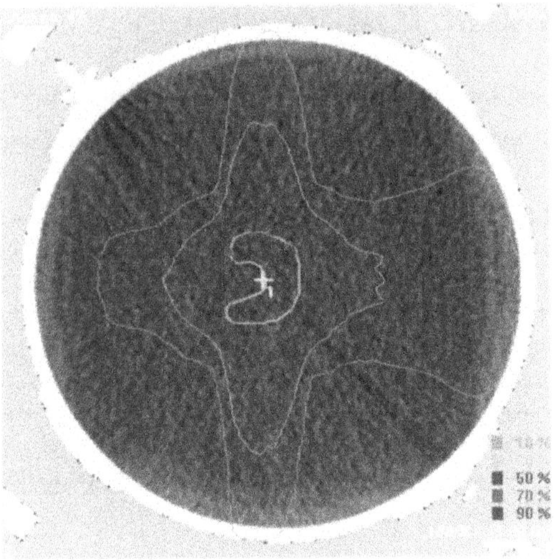


Fig. 3 Transversal CT-isocenter-slice with PTV and selected isodoses

## Conclusion

Calculated dose distributions with concave forms were verified with BANG phantoms within 1 mm, in small regions within 2 mm. The steep dose gradient near the 90% isodose was confirmed. These results are correct, if the isocenter is not blocked by the leaves. With this restriction the radiosurgery of concave target volumes is possible with optimized conformity using the dynamic arc method.

## References

[1] Leavitt D D 1998 Beam Shaping for SRT/SRS *Medical Dosimetry* **23** 229-236

[2] Maryanski M J, Ibbott G S, Eastman P, SchulzR J, Gore J C 1996 Radiation therapy dosimetry using magnetic resonance imaging of polymer gels *Med. Phys* **23** 699-705

[3] Pfaender M, Grebe G, Roll M, Jahn U, Budach V, Wurm R 1999 Dynamic Arc Radiochirurgie: Verifikation der räumlichen Dosisverteilung *Strahlenther Onkol* **175** *Sondernr 1* 170

# Is Monte Carlo noise removal feasible?

**Joseph O. Deasy, PhD**

Mallinckrodt Institute of Radiology, Washington University School of Medicine, Saint Louis, Missouri, USA; deasy@radonc.wustl.edu

## Introduction

The Monte Carlo (MC) method has long been viewed as the ultimate dose distribution computational technique, due to its capability of realistically accounting for underlying physical processes and anatomical information. The inherent stochastic fluctuations (i.e., noise) in the resulting dose distributions, however, have several important effects: noise will affect estimations of all the relevant dosimetric and radiobiological indices [1]; noise degrades the resulting visualizations, e.g. isodose plots, which are used to guide treatment planning; and the noise level dictates the computation time.

We ask the question here whether it is feasible to introduce a post-processing step which reduces statistical fluctuations in the MC dose distribution. We call this process 'denoising'. It may also be refered to as filtering or smoothing. In this abstract we only have space to present a few limited results for a homogeneous and a step-heterogeneity phantom. Complete results will be submitted for publication elsewhere.

Our initial investigations, however, support the hypothesis that denoising of MC dose distributions is, to some degree, feasible.

### Motivation

Consider a small region in a 3-D dose distribution where the path-length spectrum as a function of secondary electron energy is relatively unchanging. Let the number of Monte Carlo simulated particle tracks through a voxel be denoted $N$, and let the average dose per particle track be denoted $<d>$. As the number of particle events in a voxel becomes large ($N >> 10$), the probability distribution of $N$ becomes Gaussian, with a coefficient of variation propotional to $1/\sqrt{N}$. This implies that

$$d = <d> \times \mu, \quad (1)$$

where $d$ is the array of MC generated values, $<d>$ is the array of true values and $\mu$ is an array of random variables. If we take the logarithm of both sides we get:

$$\log(d) = \log(<d>) + \log(\mu). \quad (2)$$

### Monte Carlo post-processing as an image restoration problem

Equation (2) can be rewritten as

$$g = f + n. \quad (3)$$

From this point of view, we are dealing with an array set of data $g$ (equal to $\log(d)$), which is comprised of the 'true' values $f$ (equal to $\log(<d>)$), plus a random variable noise term $n$ (equal to $\log(\mu)$). We epect that $\mu$ (and $n$) will vary slowly across the dose distribution. This logarithmic transformation is known in statistical applications as a variance stabilizing transform[2].

Equation (3) arises in many different technical areas, especially statistics, digital filtering, and digital image processing. A vast number of techniques and algorithms have been applied to reduce noise or otherwise enhance data in this form. Image restoration in particular is distinguished from other types of digital image processing by the fact that some useful knowledge is available about the noise term $n$, as is the case here.

Just being able to write equation (3), however, does not guarantee that noise removal (or 'denoising') methods will be applicable. Concerning this, we further observe that the 'data term' $f$ is typically much smoother than the noise term $n$. Although there can be some noise correlation between neighboring voxels (depending on a number of factors such as particle type, beam direction, beam energy, etc.) we hypothesize that this observation about smoothness will hold, and this will generally make denoising/smoothing algorithms applicable. Similar to what is observed in image processing, however, there are regions where the dose distribution tends to vary sharply, thus containing high frequency components which smoothing will tend to blur out. This can happen, for example, near the edge of the dose distribution or in a dip due to an upstream heterogeneity.

## Material and methods

### The ITS MC computer code

We modified the ITS fortran MC computer code [3] to compile and run on the Win32 platform using the freely available and fast g77 (GNU-licensed) fortran compiler. The modifications were in the form of a source code update patch which is easily applied using the UPEML update processor (distributed with the ITS package). Batch processing scripts were written using the REXX language to automatically rerun routines using unique random number seeds based on the date and time. REXX scripts also were written to strip the resulting dose distributions from the ITS output file in a form which is suitable for direct input into another program (Matlab).

### Denoising method

In this initial report, we describe results using uniform data-smoothing methods (i.e. the numerical method is independent of the local image information). Quantitative indices of the extent of denoising will be reported elsewhere.

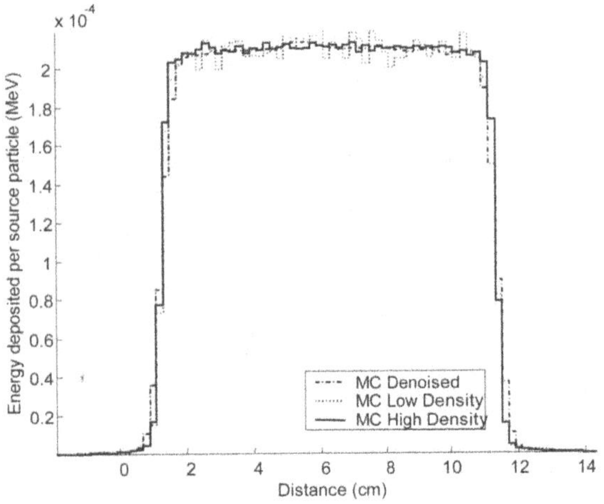


**Figure 1: Profile plot comparing MC results for 10-MeV electrons incident on a uniform phantom (depth of 1.0 cm).**

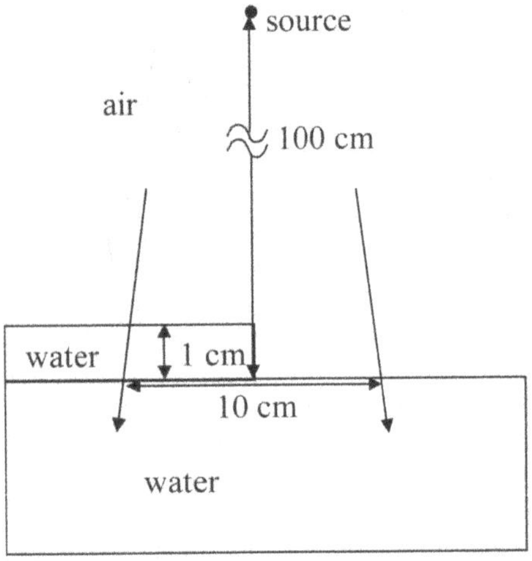


**Figure 2: Step-heterogeneity MC phantom for 10-MeV electrons.**

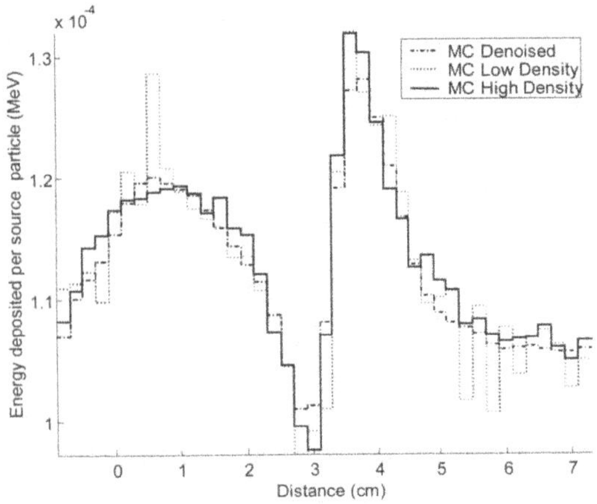


**Figure 3: Profile plot comparing MC results for step heterogeneity phantom.**

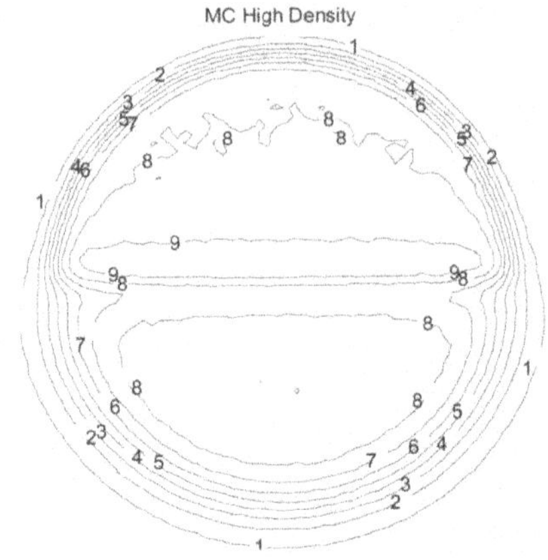


**Figure 4: Contour plot of high density MC result (80 million histories) for heterogeneity phantom. Dose values are rescaled to a maximum of 10.**

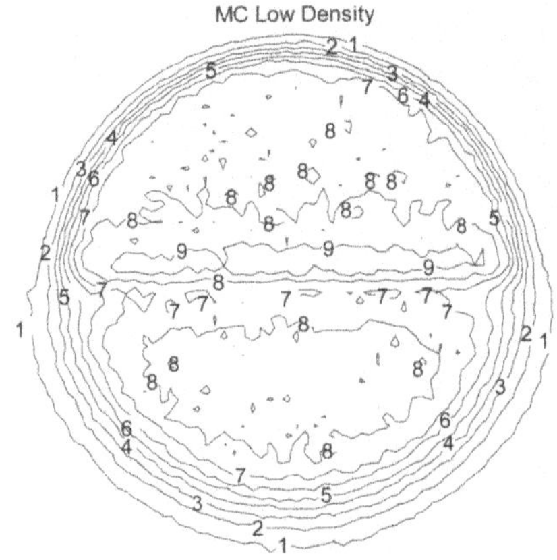


**Figure 5: Contour plot of low density MC result (4 million histories) for phantom 2.**

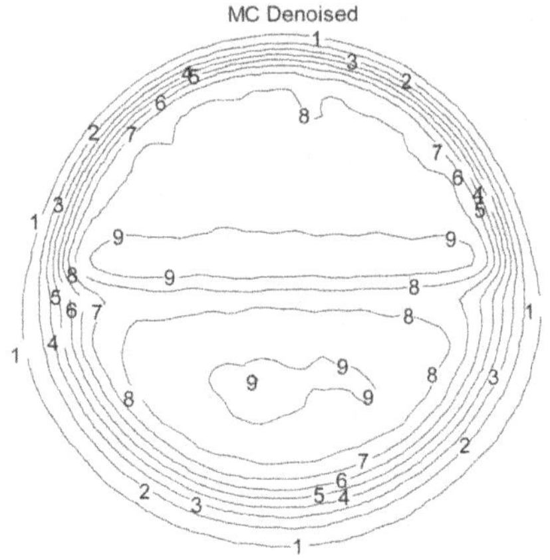


**Figure 6: Contour plot of denoised low density MC result (4 million histories) for phantom 2. A binomial filter was used.**

In the techniques tested thus far, we sample a plane of the dose distribution, thus creating a digital dose 'image'. It is this image which is filtered. All of the filtering techniques are applied to the variance stabilized (log-transformed) dose image $\log(d)$, which is thereafter transformed back to dose-space.

Denoising routines were written in Matlab (version 5.3). Several types of denoising filters have been applied, but we will report here on results from a single interesting linear filter. The data is convolved with a fourth-order 5x5 binomial smoothing filter described by Jahne[4]. Binomial filters are especially interesting because their Fourier transform transfer functions have no ripples and monotonically decrease to zero.

Figure 1 shows the result of applying the filter to a MC 10-MeV electron beam profile in water. Three curves are shown: a low density curve (4 million histories), a high density curve (80 million histories), and the 'denoised' curve resulting from applying the binary filter to the image of the low density dose distribution in the plane at 1 cm depth. Voxels are rectangular and of width 2 mm. In brief, the result shows that the denoised curve tends to estimate the high density curve significantly better than the low density curve. There is, however, a slight widening of the penumbral region. This penumbral widening is due to the sharpness of this dose profile, which implies a high frequency component. Other profiles at greater depth (not shown here) have less steep penumbraa and show even more succesful denoising.

Figures 2 shows the geometry for a heterogeneous phantom used for results shown in Figures 3-6. This geometry is designed to be a demanding test of the performance of the binomial filter. 10-MeV electrons are released with directions sampled uniformly over a cone restricted to have a projected width at the phantom surface of 10 cm. Figure 3 shows another profile comparison between low density (4 million particles), high density (80 million particles), and a denoised distribution based on filtering the low density simulation. Once again the denoised distribution shows that, over most of the profile, the denoised result is an improvement on the low density result. However, we can clearly see that there is some "rounding'' or blurring of the denoised dose near the valley of the trough. The scoring plane is at a depth of 2.55 cm.

Figures 4, 5, and 6 show contour plots of the dose distributions resulting from the heterogeneity phantom. The distributions have all been scaled to make the maximum dose equal to 10. The denoised distribution is clearly much cleaner visually than the low density MC simulation. The ability to visually inspect the dose distribution has been significantly improved using the denoising filter.

All uniform filtering approaches share a common weakness, however, which is the smoothing out of sharp features in the actual dose distributions, such as the cold-trough or the dose profile shoulders. We are currently investigating adaptive filtering methods, where the local filtering would be modified based on some local dose characteristics.

## Conclusion

The apparent appropriateness of applying some type of denoising/smoothing/filtering to MC dose distributions leads to the formulation of several hypotheses concerning the potential advantages of Monte Carlo noise removal. In particular, we hypothesize that appropriate denoising of Monte Carlo dose distributions will have three advantages:

1. Visually, the dose distribution images will be easier to inspect, and therefore more clinically appropriate.
2. Dosimetrically, the results will be more accurate for given computational effort/time. The minimum target dose, in particular, will be better estimated.
3. Computationally, the time required to reach a dosimetrically satisfactory answer will be reduced.

Of course, 2 and 3 imply each other.

Much work will be necessary to understand and fully exploit possibilities apparent in MC denoising. Many different questions can be asked about Monte Carlo denoising, both in terms of how applicable it will be (electrons and photons?), what denoising methods are appropriate (will adaptive methods be necessary?), and what quantitative tests should be done to evaluate denoising methods. We hope to further investigate some of these interesting questions.

This research was supported by NIH grant CA85181.

## References

[1] Buffa F, Nahum A, and Mubata, C 1999 Influence of Statistical Fluctuations in Monte-Carlo Dose Calculations and Radiobiological Modelling and Dose Volume Histograms *Med Phys* **26** 1120

[2] Madansky A, 1988 Prescriptions For Working Statisticians, Springer, Berlin, p. 156.

[3] Halbleib et. al 1994 Integrated TIGER Series of Coupled Electron/Photon Monte Carlo Transport Code System, version 3.0, RSICC Code Package CCC-467, distributed by the Radiation Shielding Information Center, Oak Ridge, TN, http://www-rsicc.ornl.gov/rsic.html.

[4] Jahne B, 1997 Digital Image Processing, Springer, Berlin, p. 297.

# Implementation of several variance reduction techniques into the XVMC Monte Carlo algorithm for photon beams

**Matthias Fippel[1], Iwan Kawrakow[2], Fridtjof Nüsslin[1] and David W. O. Rogers[2]**
[1] Abteilung für Medizinische Physik, Radiologische Universitätsklinik, Hoppe-Seyler-Str. 3, 72076 Tübingen, Germany,
[2] Institute for National Measurement Standards, National Research Council, Ottawa, Ontario K1A 0R6, Canada

## Introduction

The accuracy of dose calculation for patient treatment planning in cancer radiation therapy should be better than ±2% taking into account a maximum uncertainty of ±5% for the delivery of dose [1]. The Monte Carlo (MC) technique is potentially the most promising method to achieve this criterion if radiation sources and patients are modelled accurately and a large number of particle tracks are simulated. Because of the increasing speed of modern computer systems and the introduction of new variance reduction techniques, MC dose calculation time could be reduced dramatically during the last few years. This paper deals with the implementation of such variance reduction techniques into the recently developed XVMC [2, 3] code for photon beam dose calculation.

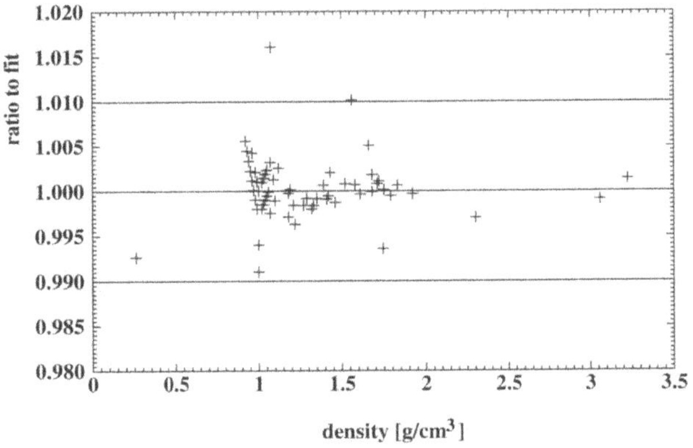


**Figure 1:** Ratio of electron densities from ICRU Report 46 [5] to the mapping function (2) used by XVMC.

## Material and methods

### XVMC

XVMC is the extension of the Voxel Monte Carlo (VMC) algorithm for electron beams [4] also allowing the simulation of photon radiation within the patient. This has been realized by including Compton interactions, pair production and photo electric absorption. Analysing the energy and density behaviour of the three different photon processes for human tissue leads to the conclusion that the cross sections $\mu_{c(p,a)}(E,\rho)$ can be calculated from the corresponding cross sections in water multiplied by a function giving the material dependence, i.e.

$$\mu_{c(p,a)}(E,\rho) = \mu^{w}_{c(p,a)}(E)\ f_{c(p,a)}(\rho). \tag{1}$$

For example, the density dependent part of the Compton cross section for a tissue material with mass density $\rho$ can be calculated by the ratio of tissue electron density to water electron density:

$$f_c(\rho) = \frac{n_e(\rho)}{n_e^w} \approx \begin{cases} \rho/\rho^w, & \rho \leq \rho^w \\ 0.85\rho/\rho^w + 0.15, & \rho \geq \rho^w. \end{cases} \tag{2}$$

The second part of equation (2) is the function implemented in XVMC to extract the electron density from CT information. Figure 1 shows the ratio of $n_e(\rho)/n_e^w$ taken from [5] to this function for all tissue types. Only Gallstone ($\rho$ = 1.075 $g/cm^3$) does not satisfy 1% accuracy. Similar procedures exist to calculate the cross sections for pair production and photo electric absorption as well as electron collision stopping power, radiation stopping power and scattering power. This strategy is more accurate than the common approach of selecting a representative material for a definite Hounsfield number range and interpolating linearly between these materials because in general the cross section density dependence is not linear as the Compton coefficient of equation (2). However, if the tissue type is known exact values can be used instead of fit functions.

Secondary particle parameters (energy, momentum) are sampled from differential cross sections. Photons are transported by ray tracing. Electrons are simulated by a class II condensed history scheme with continuous boundary crossing. Delta electrons and bremsstrahlung photons can be produced. However in most cases these photons are cancelled by Russian Roulette. Positrons are approximated by electrons. The accelerator head is modelled by a primary point source collimated to the given field size. The initial photon energy is sampled from a spectral distribution extracted from measurements in water. An additional head scatter contribution models the particle fluence outside the beam limits. The initial ray tracing technique described in [2] provides the optimum distribution of primary interaction sites but restricts beam modelling. For example, this disadvantage prevents the use of phase space files generated by the BEAM MC code [6]. To circumvent the restrictions, alternative variance reductions have been investigated.

### Variance reduction techniques

The total error of MC dose calculation (stochastic and systematic) is given mainly by the statistical fluctuations, because of the small influence of approximations in the energy and material range of interest. Therefore, the accuracy (specified by the standard deviation $s$) depends on the number of particle histories simulated. This however, requires a definite calculation time $T$ using a given computer system. Methods decreasing the product $s^2T$ (or increasing the efficiency $\epsilon = 1/(s^2T)$) for the same treatment geometry and the same computer are called variance reduction techniques. The following new techniques have been implemented into the XVMC photon transport routine.

*Photon splitting:* Instead of tracing only one single photon through the patient geometry, a specified number $n_{split}$ of identical photons with decreased weight $1/n_{split}$ will be tracked on one straight line. Additionally, the photon interaction sites are distributed optimally along this line and identical secondary particle parameters are selected if the interaction types (Compton, pair or photo effects) are identical.

*Electron history repetition:* Photon splitting into subphotons allows repetition of electron histories. For instance, if a Compton interaction is selected for the first sub-photon, one electron history in water is simulated and the parameters are stored. Then, this history is applied to the patient geometry by scaling the electron step lengths and multiple scattering angles. Because of the identical starting energies, the history can be reused for further Compton electrons of the split photon. The same method is used for photo electrons, pair electrons and positrons.

*Russian Roulette:* Photon splitting leads (depending on $n_{split}$) to a large number of Compton photons. However, their contribution to dose is much smaller than for the original photon. Wasting CPU time for Compton photon transport can be avoided by Russian Roulette, i.e. they are only simulated with the probability $1/n_{split}$. Therefore, their weight must be increased by $n_{split}$ leading to the original weight. The remaining photons are simulated again using the splitting and history repetition technique by calling the corresponding routine recursively. Russian Roulette is also used to cancel the majority of bremsstrahlung photons.

*Quasi-random numbers:* Generally, for MC simulations a sequence of uncorrelated random numbers is used. However, for specific problems quasi-random sequences could be more beneficial. These numbers, e.g. the Sobol' sequence [7], provide better uniform distributions than uncorrelated random numbers and have been implemented to determine starting position and free path length of the primary photons.

*Parameter settings:* The transport parameters $P_{cut}$ (photon energy cut-off), $K_{cut}$ (secondary photons are simulated using KERMA approximation if their energy is below $K_{cut}$), $E_{cut}$ (electron energy cut-off, electrons with energy below $E_{cut}$ are transported by continuous slowing approximation) and $E_{step}$ (maximum electron energy step size) are optimised in terms of calculation speed and systematical accuracy.

## Results and discussion

XVMC including the new variance reduction techniques have been benchmarked against EGSnrc [8, 9] calculations. An example is demonstrated in figure 2. The water phantom contains lung and bone inhomogeneities. The results have been normalised with respect to initial photon fluence leading to absolute dose distributions. Figure 2 shows the XVMC/EGSnrc ratio of central axis depth dose curves derived by this means. The combined standard deviation ($1\sigma$)

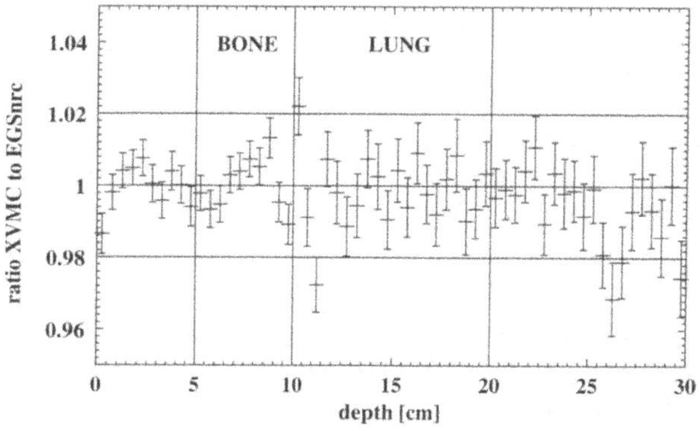


**Figure 2:** Ratio of depth dose distributions for a 6 MV photon beam with field size 10 × 10 $cm^2$ calculated with XVMC and EGSnrc. The phantom consists of water, lung ($\rho = 0.26\ g\ cm^{-3}$) and bone ($\rho = 1.85\ g\ cm^{-3}$). The voxel size is $(0.5\ cm)^3$.

of both calculations is represented by the error bars. Because the ratio of two MC calculated dose distributions is given by a Gaussian, the probability for differences larger than 2% is not zero. To separate statistical fluctuations from systematical errors a new method has been developed [3]. This method applied to the above situation implies agreement to be better than 1% between both MC algorithms. The results of XVMC and EGSnrc represented by depth or cross dose profiles would not show visible deviations. Therefore, such figures are not plotted here.

The new XVMC code has been cross checked also by comparisons to the early version with initial ray tracing. Significant differences have not been observed. Therefore, we conclude that agreement to the measurements of [10] continues. But the calculation time could be reduced by a factor of 5 to 10 because of the variance reduction techniques mentioned above. In table 1 typical CPU times to calculate dose distributions in water for different beam sizes and energies are presented. Here, the relative statistical uncertainty in each voxel is given by the ratio of standard deviation to dose maximum. The specified statistical error of 1.5% in table 1 has been derived by averaging the errors of all voxels with dose larger than 90% of the maximum dose.

An automatic procedure was developed to obtain a statistical accuracy $\sigma_n^2$ specified by the program user. First of all, the total number of particle histories $n$ is estimated depending on voxel size, field size, energy and $\sigma_n^2$, leading

| | beam size [$cm^2$] | | |
|---|---|---|---|
| | 5 × 5 | 10 × 10 | 20 × 20 |
| 6 MV | 65 | 242 | 928 |
| 18 MV | 78 | 318 | 1230 |

**Table 1:** CPU time for XVMC (in seconds) to calculate dose distributions in water for different photon energy spectra and collimator settings using a 450 MHz PentiumII PC. The phantom consists of $(0.5\ cm)^3$ voxels. The average statistical error in the region with at least 90% of the maximum dose is 1.5%.

to an estimated number of histories per batch. After each batch a "present" standard deviation $\sigma_i^2$ can be calculated. This value depends on the number of finished histories $i$. A new estimate for the total number of histories is then calculated by

$$n = i\ \frac{\sigma_i^2}{\sigma_n^2}. \tag{3}$$

The number of histories per batch varies using this approach. This leads to different weights for each batch and must be taken into account when calculating average dose and standard deviation.

## Conclusion

The implementation of several new variance reduction techniques into the XVMC algorithm has increased the speed for photon beam dose calculation by a factor of 5 to 10 compared to the previous version with initial ray tracing. Therefore, the computation time on a grid with $(0.5\ cm)^3$ spacial resolution could be reduced to a few minutes (1 to 20 minutes) using a single CPU personal computer.

Furthermore, the new program version permits complete decoupling of beam modelling and patient dose calculation. The interface is given by a source sampling sub-routine allowing the implementation of various accelerator head models, e.g. phase space files. For clinical purposes empirical models are preferred. The free parameters can be determined from measurements supported by a beam parameter generation utility.

Another utility program transfers patient density matrices and beam parameters from commercial planning systems into the VMC file format. Implementation of the code for routine treatment planning of clinical electron and photon beams is planned for the near future.

## Acknowledgements

Financial support for the work presented here was provided by the Deutsche Forschungsgemeinschaft under contract number FI 757.

## References

[1] Brahme A, Chavaudra J, Landberg T, McCullough E C, Nüsslin F, Rawlinson J A, Svensson G and Svensson H 1988 Accuracy requirements and quality assurance of external beam therapy with photons and electrons *Acta Oncologica* **27** Suppl. 1, 1-76

[2] Fippel M 1999 Fast Monte Carlo dose calculation for photon beams based on the VMC electron algorithm *Med. Phys.* **26** 1466–1475

[3] Kawrakow I and Fippel M 1999 Investigation of variance reduction techniques for Monte Carlo photon dose calculation using XVMC *submitted to Phys. Med. Biol.*

[4] Kawrakow I, Fippel M and Friedrich K 1996 3D electron dose calculation using a voxel based Monte Carlo algorithm (VMC) *Med. Phys.* **23** 445–457

[5] Photon, electron, proton and neutron interaction data for body tissues *ICRU-Report* **46** International Commission on Radiation Units and Measurements 1992

[6] Rogers D W O, Faddegon B A, Ding G X, Ma C M, Wie J and Mackie T R 1995 BEAM: A Monte Carlo code to simulate radiotherapy treatment units *Med. Phys.* **22** 503–524

[7] Press W H, Teukolsky S A, Vetterling W T and Flannery B P 1997 *Numerical Recipes in Fortran 77* (Cambridge: Cambridge University Press) pp 309

[8] Kawrakow I 1999 Accurate condensed history Monte Carlo simulation of electron transport, I. EGSnrc, the new EGS4 version *to be published in Med. Phys.*

[9] Kawrakow I 1999 Accurate condensed history Monte Carlo simulation of electron transport, II. Application to ion chamber response simulations *to be published in Med. Phys.*

[10] Fippel M, Laub W, Huber B and Nüsslin F 1999 Experimental investigation of a fast Monte Carlo photon beam dose calculation algorithm *Phys. Med. Biol.* **44** 3039–3054

# Parallel processing of radiotherapy Monte Carlo simulations on a remote Beowulf cluster

**Peter Love[1], Emiliano Spezi[1], Geraint Lewis[1], Cyril Smith[1] Edward Morton[2] and Dave Munro[2]**
[1]Department of Medical Physics, Velindre Hospital, Cardiff, CF14 2TL, UK;
[2]Department of Physics, University of Surrey, Guildford, GU2 5XH, UK

## Introduction

Radiotherapy and radiation protection Monte Carlo calculations have been carried out on a remote Beowulf cluster. Beowulf [1] clusters are now common in academic departments because of their high performance to cost ratios. The Department of Physics at the University of Surrey is in the process of building a 128 processor Beowulf cluster (called Remus) with 1.2 Gigabit/s network for real-time image processing of fluoroscopic x-ray image data. Surplus processor time has been available for Monte Carlo calculations.

## Material and methods

Preliminary performance tests were carried out on a small cluster (Romulus) of five computers consisting of 1 Master 350 MHz and 4 Slave 300 MHz Intel Pentium II processors. The Monte Carlo codes used for this study were MCNP [2] (Los Alamos National Laboratory) and BEAM [3] (National Research Council of Canada). These codes are currently used as part of our research into radiotherapy bunker design and treatment planning calculations. All computers were running the Linux operating system (version 2.2.5) with Parallel Virtual Machine (PVM) software [4] installed allowing the PVM version of MCNP to be used. Parallel jobs using BEAM were started with a modification of the pprocess script from the BEAM code which splits input files to be distribtued to computing nodes.

The MCNP test simulates the transport of 10 million particles through a radiotherapy linear accelerator maze [5]. Firstly PVM was configured with all available hosts then various jobs were started by specifying the number of tasks to spawn. The elapsed time was used when calculating the efficiency. The efficiency is relative to a single machine (300 MHz) transporting 10 million initial particles.

The BEAM test uses the DOSXYZ [6] usercode to simulate the transport of 10 million initial particles through a rectilinear water phantom designed to measure beam profiles. The script used to start the simulation simply splits the single 10 million particle job into $n$ jobs of each $10/n$ million particles. Each job is then started on a particluar machine specified in a file of hostnames. All $n$ jobs are accessing the same phase-space file located on the master NFS-exported disk. These tests were run in isolation with no other users present on the system. The time used for efficiency calculations was the elapsed time given by the difference between START times and END OF RUN times as recorded in the log file. The efficiency is relative to a single machine (300 MHz) transporting 10 million initial particles.

## Results and discussion

A summary of the efficiency for the MCNP simulation is in Table 1 and graphed in Figure 1. Results indicate that the efficiency (defined above) scales linearly with the number of processors used for calculations. This is expected when using only 5 machines but network and disk congestion will occur when the number of computers involved rises to 128, which will be studied in due course. Note that PVM starts $n$ tasks on slaves and 1 additional controlling task on the master therefore when $n = 5$ six processes are run on five computers which cause the performance decrease observed.

| Tasks $n$ | Total MHz | Efficiency |
|---|---|---|
| - | 300 | 1.00 |
| 2 | 600 | 1.98 |
| 3 | 900 | 2.94 |
| 4 | 1200 | 3.80 |
| 5 | 1550 | 3.34 |

**Table 1:** Efficiency of distributed MCNP calculation compared to a single machine when increasing the number of PVM tasks.

The same linear scaling was observed with the BEAM jobs as listed in Table 2 and shown in Figure 1. The master machine had a higher efficiency of 1.24 compared to the expected 1.17 (350 MHz/300 MHz) since the phase-space data was located on the local disk and not mounted over a (less efficient) network file system. This will not be an issue when beam models are used for input to BEAM simulations.

| Split# | Total MHz | Efficiency |
|---|---|---|
| 1 | 300 | 1.00 |
| 1 | 350 | 1.24 |
| 2 | 600 | 1.99 |
| 3 | 900 | 2.97 |
| 4 | 1200 | 4.00 |
| 5 | 1550 | 4.94 |

**Table 2:** Efficiency of distributed BEAM calculation compared to a single machine when increasing the number of CPUs involved.

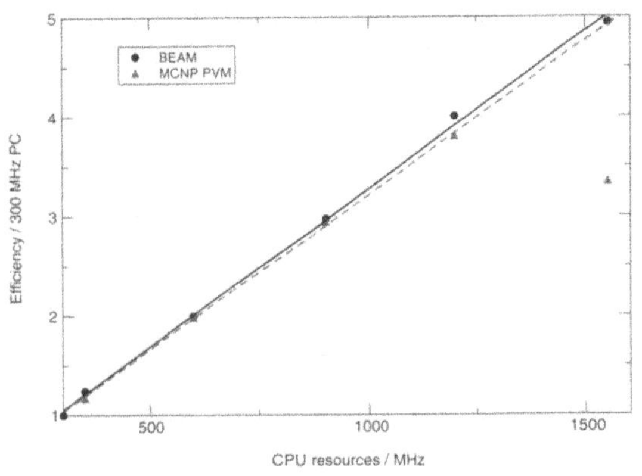


**Figure 1:** Efficiency of distributed MCNP and BEAM calculations compared to a single machine when increasing the CPU resources. The MCNP point at 1550 MHz is explained in the discussion.

## Conclusion

The efficiency of using a remote Beowulf cluster has been evaluated when performing radiotherapy Monte Carlo calculations. There is a linear relationship between calculation efficiency and number of processors used for both MCNP and BEAM simulations. It is expected that a centralized and remote Beowulf Cluster may supply enough computing power for calculation of full Monte Carlo treatment plans on the order of minutes. Having high speed computations may avoid the requirement to introduce the physics approximations which are present in most emerging Monte Carlo treatment planning codes. The resource may be shared and accessed by multiple radiotherapy departments who require fast but infrequent calculations with minimal effort to setup and configure.

## References

[1] www.beowulf.org

[2] Briesmeister J F editor 1997 *MCNP - A General Monte Carlo N-Particle Transport Code, Version 4B, LA-12625-M* (Los Alamos National Laboratory, Los Alamos, NM)

[3] Rogers D W O, Faddegon B A, Ding G X, Ma C M, Wei J and Mackie T R 1995 BEAM: A Monte Carlo code to simulate radiotherapy treatment units *Med. Phys.* **22** 503–524

[4] www.epm.ornl.gov/pvm/pvm_home.html

[5] Al-Affan I A M, Smith C W, Morgan H M and Lillicrap S C 1998 Dose rate and energy distributions of x-rays from a linear accelerator at the maze entrance of a radiotherapy room by measurement and Monte Carlo simulation *Radiation Protection Dosimetry* **78** 273–277

[6] Ma C M, Reckwerdt P, Holmes M, Rogers D W O and Geiser B 1995 DOSXYZ Users Manual *National Research Council of Canada* **PIRS-0509B** (NRC, Ottawa)

# A Scaling Method for Multiple Source Models (SMSM)

C. Cris[1], E. Born[1], D. Frey[1] R. Mini[1], H. Neuenschwander[2], W. Volken[1]

[1]Inselspital – University of Bern, Bern, Switzerland, and [2]Radio-Oncology, Lindenhofspital, Bern, Switzerland

## Introduction

Fast MC algorithms for electron beam dose calculation are a promising alternative to actual conventional dose calculation methods.
The potential of these methods can only be fully exploited by providing accurate input data for the electron beams involved. The Multiple Source Model (MSM) ([1]) provides a compact way to describe clinical electron beams. It relies on MC simulation of particle transport through accelerator heads and samples particle properties from fluence distributions corresponding to the accelerator head components which are looked upon as individual particle sources.
The scaling method for MSM (SMSM) allows to develop MSM representations starting from measured dose distributions in water and MSM beam characterization for a reference machine.

The new method has been developed and tested for VARIAN CLINAC 2300 C/D treatment units.

## Material and methods

The SMSM method relies on the beam description for a reference clinical linear accelerator.
MSM descriptions of the electron beams delivered by this machine are developed from the detailed beam data calculated using BEAM ([2]), a traditional MC code designed for simulations of particle transport through clinical accelerator heads. BEAM is part of the OMEGA project ([3]) conducted by the National Research Council of Canada (NRCC) and the University of Wisconsin.
The MSM characterization of the electron beams delivered by our reference machine contains six particle sources (Figure 1):

- -one point source of direct electrons;
- -one planar source for particles originating in the jaws;
- -three planar sources for particles originating from the three applicator scrapers;
- -one point source for the contaminating photons.

Fluence distributions for each of these sources are extracted from beam data using BEAMDP ([1]), a code which is also part of the OMEGA project. Energy and particle position distributions are not correlated. The extracted distributions are stored in an ASCII file, the so-called MSM parameter file, from now on just designated as parameter file. MSM also includes methods for sampling of individual particle properties from the calculated fluence distributions. Therefore parameter files can be directly used as input for MC dose calculations.
Our reference machine is a VARIAN CLINAC 2300 C/D of the Clinic of Radio-Oncology at Inselspital in Bern. Therefore the SMSM can only be applied to such treatment units. This restriction is due to the definition of *similar beams* which are those beams to which our method applies: They have the same parameters (nominal energy and beam size) and are delivered by treatment units showing differences among corresponding dose distributions only due to technical tolerances and beam adjustment.

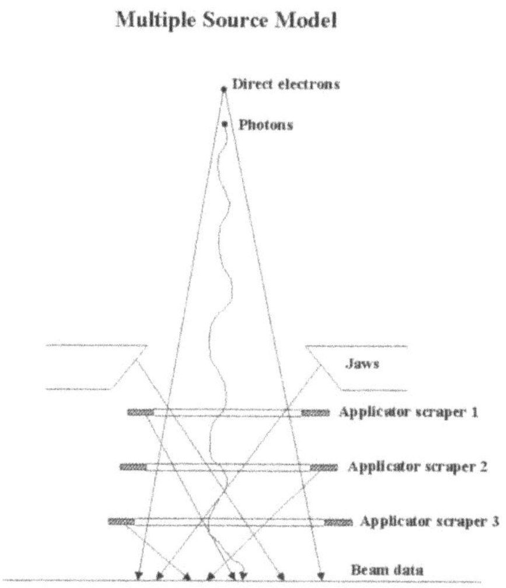


Figure 1

Following this definition SMSM requires only the knowledge of the parameter files of the reference machine and measured distributions of the dose released in water by the beam to be modelled.
The new method relies upon two assumptions:

1. Scaling the energy distribution of the direct electrons is sufficient to reproduce dose distributions correctly;
2. The energy spectrum of the direct electrons can be approximated by a Landau distribution.

The first assumption is confirmed by analyzing dose distributions computed using beam data calculated by BEAM which reveals that dose distributions are mainly determined by the direct electrons and the definition of *similar beams* which assumes both treatment units to have identical scattering foils and therefore to show very similar flight direction distributions of the direct electrons. The second assumption follows straightforward from the analysis of beam data determined by BEAM.
The Landau distribution $\Lambda_E(E)$ can be written as a function of the particle energy $E$ using $E_p$ (the most probable energy) and $\Gamma$ (FWHM of the energy distribution) as

$$\Lambda_E(E) = \frac{3.58}{\sqrt{2\pi}\Gamma} e^{-\frac{1}{2}\left[e^{\frac{3.58}{\Gamma}(E-E_p)} - \frac{3.58}{\Gamma}(E-E_p)\right]}.$$

$E_p$ and $\Gamma$ are connected to $R_p$ and $G$, two parameters of measured depth dose curves, by formulas given in ([4]).

SMSM computes the energy spectrum of the direct electrons $f'(E')$ of a *similar beam* starting from the corresponding spectrum $f(E)$ of the reference machine. The latter is approximated by $\Lambda_E(E)$ with parameters $E_p$ and $\Gamma$, and the former is approximated by $\Lambda'_E(E')$ with parameters $E'_p$ and $\Gamma'$. $E_p$ and $\Gamma$ are determined directly from $f(E)$ while $E'_p$ and $\Gamma'$ are calculated from the measured parameters $R_p$ and $G$. $E'$ is calculated as $E' = \frac{E'_p}{E_p} E$.

The scaling method consists in a mapping of the differences $f(E) - \Lambda_E(E)$ upon $f'(E') - \Lambda'_E(E')$. For this purpose the slopes A,B,C and D of the straight lines $g_1$, $g_2$, $g_3$ and $g_4$ (Figure 2) are used. The scaling is mathematically expressed by $\frac{A}{B} = \frac{C}{D}$. Writing down A,B,C and D and solving for $f'(E')$ leads to

$$f'(E') = f'_{max} - (f_{max} - f(E)) \frac{\Lambda'_{E'_{max}} - \Lambda'_E(E')}{\Lambda_{E_{max}} - \Lambda_E(E)}.$$

$f'_{max}$ is determined by requiering $f'(E')$ to be normalized.

SMSM has been implemented in a computer code which applies the scaling procedure to the parameter file of a reference machine beam. The result is a new parameter file which contains the scaled energy distribution for the direct electrons. The energy scale for all sources within the new parameter file is also scaled by $E' = \frac{E'_p}{E_p} E$.

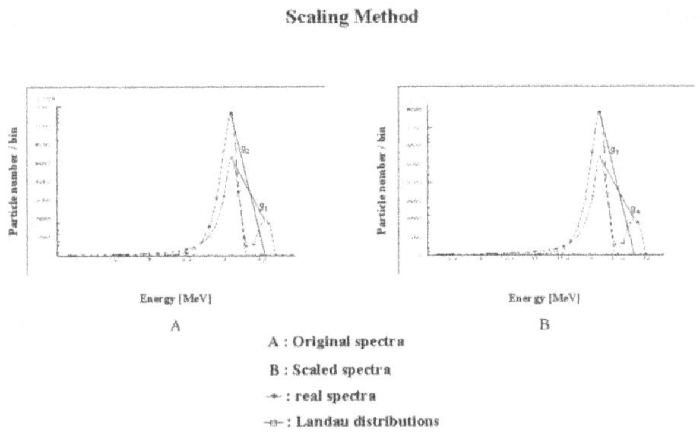


Figure 2

## Results and discussion

SMSM has been tested by scaling MSM parameter files of different beams delivered by our reference machine. Scaling such beams is even more difficult a task than scaling *similar beams*. Therefore the examples shown further down represent a severe test for our method.

The criterium to assess the performance of our scaling method has been the accuracy of dose distributions reproduced by scaled parameter files as compared to the corresponding measured dose distributions. Dose distributions are characterized by depth dose curves.

The dose distribution calculations were carried out using the EGS4 ([5]) code DOSXYZ. The transport parameters ([5]) were set as follows: AE=521keV; AP=10keV; ECUT=700keV; PCUT=10keV; ESTEPE=4%. The simulated water phantoms had a resolution of 0.25cm x 0.25cm x 0.2cm. 32Mio. primary electron histories have been simulated for every nominal beam energy.

Dose distribution measurements were effectuated with a Scanditronix RFA300 system using semiconductor diodes.

Depth dose curves are normalized at the depth of the dose maximum. The uncertainty of measurements amounts to ca. 0.5% of the dose maximum. The total statistical fluctuations of the calculated depth dose curves is $\pm 1.0\%$ to $\pm 1.5\%$ of the dose maximum.

The original and scaled energy distributions (scaling of 16 to 18MeV beam) of the direct electrons are compared in Figure 3. The ordinate values are computed as percent values represented by the electron numbers of the individual energy bins with respect to the total number of direct electrons.The spectra show good agreement.

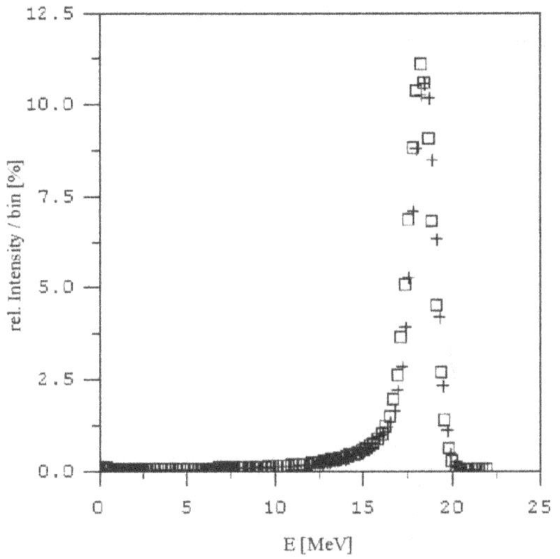


Comparison of the scaled 16MeV energy distribution to MSM energy distribution of the 18MeV beam

□ MSM; E=16MeV
+ SMSM 16 → 18MeV

Figure 3

The depth dose curves obtained from dose calculations using the original and the scaled parameter files for this example are shown in Figure 4. The electron range and the slope of the depth dose curves show very good agreement. The slight differences appearing in the build-up region and in the position of the depth dose maximum are explained by the statistical fluctuations and the approximations involved in the scaling method. Figure 5 shows the same comparison as Figure 3 for the scaling of the 18 to the 20MeV beam. As for Figure3 the spectra exhibit good agreement. Figure 6 shows the same depth dose curves as Figure 4 for the scaling of the 18 to the 20 MeV beam. As for Figure 4 the electron range and the slope of the depth dose curves show very good agreement. The slight differences in the build-up region have the same reasons as those observed in Figure 4.

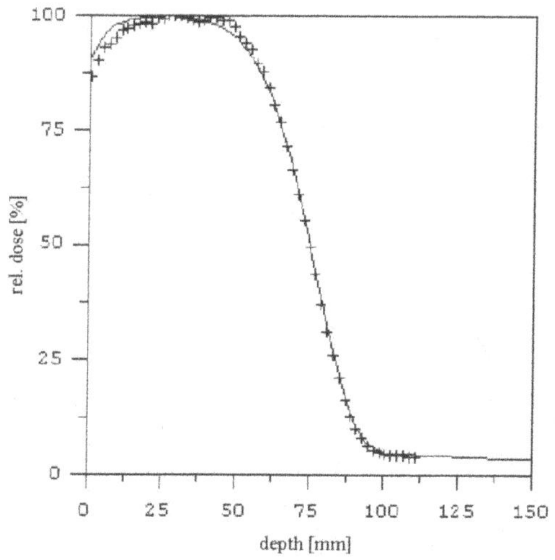


Nominal beam energy : 18MeV

Figure 4

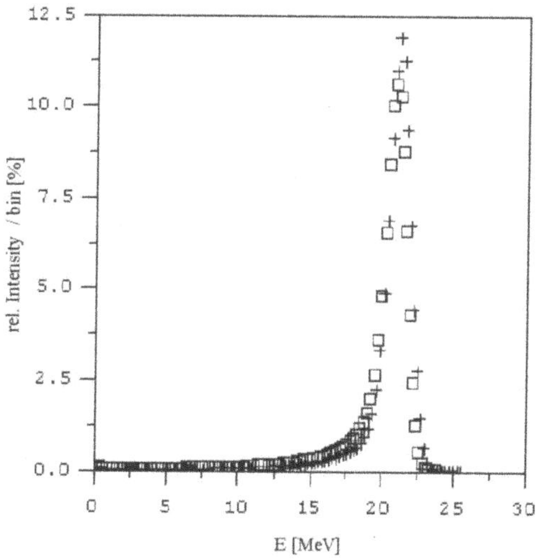


Nominal beam energy : 20 MeV

Figure 6

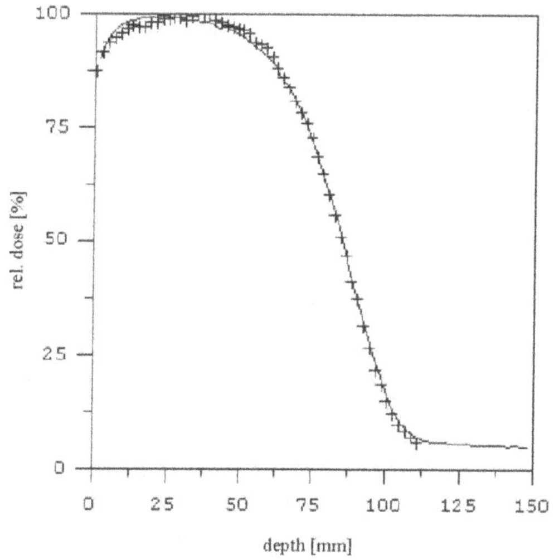


Comparison of the scaled 18MeV energy distribution to MSM energy distribution of the 20MeV beam

□ MSM; E=18MeV
+ SMSM 18→ 20MeV

Figure 5

## Conclusion

The presented method for scaling parameter files between *similar beams* shows good results for VARIAN CLINAC 2300 C/D accelerators. The presented examples are a severe test for our method. The differences which are still observed between scaled and measured dose distributions might be removed by improving the approximations used by the actual method. SMSM will be subjected to further validation involving measured dose distributions produced by clinical accelerators different from the reference machine.

## References

[1] Ma C M and Rogers D W O 1999 Beam Characterization: a Multiple-source Model *NRCC Report PIRS-0509(D)rev*

[2] Rogers D W O, Faddegon B A, Ding G X, Ma C M, Wie J, Mackie T R 1999 BEAM: A Monte Carlo code to simulate radiotherapy treatment units *Med. Phys.* **22** 503-24

[3] Mackie T R, Sohn W, Lindstrom M, Kubsad S S, Reckwerdt P J, Kinsella T J, Bielajew A F and Rogers D W O 1999 The Ottawa-Madison Electron Gamma Algorithm (OMEGA) project: Feasibility of two Monte Carlo techniques. *Proceedings of the X ICCR* (Lucknow, India) pp 250-53

[4] *ICRU Report 35* 1984

[5] Nelson W R, Hirayama H and Rogers D W O 1999 The EGS4 Code System (Stanford Linear Accelerator Center Report SLAC-265 (Stanford Calif))

# Effect of CT Streaking Artifacts in Monte Carlo Dose Distributions for Head and Neck Cancer

**Todd Pawlicki and C.-M. Ma**

Department of Radiation Oncology, Stanford University School of Medicine, Stanford, CA 94306, USA

## Introduction

Unlike any other anatomical site in the human body, CT streaking artifacts are routinely observed in the head of patient. This is due to dental work that consists of a localized high Z material. All model based dose calculation algorithms that use CT scan data should be influenced by regions of artifically increased CT numbers within a patient's scan to be used for treatment planning and dose calculation. The purpose of this work is to study the effects of streaking artifacts in CT scans on Monte Carlo calculated dose distributions for a treatment site in the head and neck.

Monte Carlo dose calculations use the data from a patient's CT scan set in a way that is somewhat different from other model based dose calculation algorithms. The physical density *and* type of material in each voxel are required for simulation. The usual approach to obtain these data is to develop a conversion table of CT number to physical density. Then, one selects a range of CT numbers to denote the various materials in a patient's body. Streaking artifacts in a patient CT scan can effect these relationships by introducing an artifical increase in the local CT number and subsequent determination of physical density. This problem is further compounded, in regard to Monte Carlo simulations, because the material in a voxel will change as well, usually going from soft tissue to cortical bone. The effects of these types of perturbations or a "typical" patient CT scan set are investigated for treatment of the RT parotid in the head and neck. The magnitude of errors in Monte Carlo calculated dose distributions due to CT streaking artifacts for this case are reported here.

## Material and methods

### Clinical case with CT artifacts

We obtained the CT scan set of a patient of the head & neck using the Picker AcQSim (Picker International, Cleveland, OH). For this patient, with dental work, there are streaking artifacts from the dental fillings. A narrow tumor in the region of the RT parotid gland was delineated for treatment. Actual size of the target was 2.25 x 2.25 x 1.0 cm$^3$. Due to the dental work of this patient, there are typical CT streaking artifacts in the region of the tumor. This CT scan, with the streaking artifacts, was then modified to remove the streaking artifacts from the CT slices in the scan set. One CT slice with, and one CT slice without the presence of streaking artifacts are shown in Figure 1 a and b. Two treatment strategies were then applied to both CT scan sets. The treatment types investigated are a single lateral 20 MeV electron beam and a single lateral 4

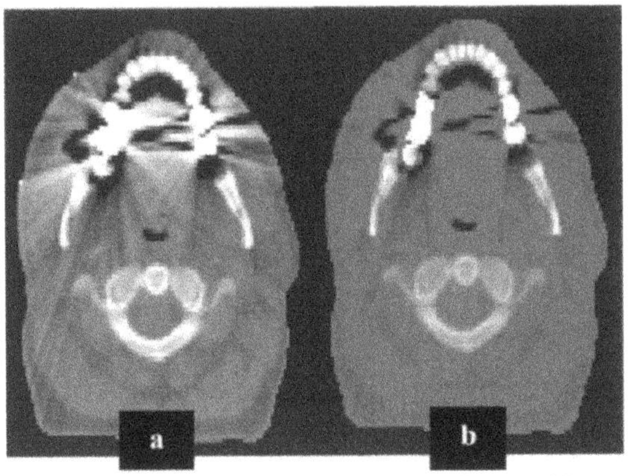


**Figure 1:** Example of a CT scan of the head with streaking artifacts (a) and with the streaking artifacts removed (b).

MV photon beam. The field size was about 1.5 cm x 3.5 cm for both beams. The beams were oriented enface at 100 cm source-to-surface distance. The effect of the CT artifact was evaluted in regard to the target coverage as well as the dose to the contralateral parotid gland and mandible.

### The Monte Carlo code

The Monte Carlo code system used in this study is an EGS4 [1] based user code called MCDOSE [2] which has been developed at Stanford. MCDOSE has been implemented as a general purpose clincal dose calculation system. Conventional electron and photon 3D dose calculation, IMRT dose calculation as well as additional investigative treatments like modulated electron beams can be performed with this code. A complete description of MCDOSE is given in reference [3].

## Results and discussion

The voxel sizes for the CT scan data set were 0.14 cm in the left-right direction, 0.18 cm in the anterior-posterior direction and 0.30 cm in the superior-inferior direction. Mass density in each voxel was obtained from the measured CT number and for the scan set with CT artifacts the range of mass densities for the RT parotid was 0.77-1.41 g/cm$^3$, LT parotid was 0.83-1.62 g/cm$^3$ and mandible was 0.96-1.60 g/cm3. The maximum mass density anywhere in the phantom was 2.96 g/cm$^3$ and this was located directly inside the filling of a cavity in one of the teeth.

**Photon beam plan**

The isodose distribution for the photon beam plan is shown in Figure 2. The isodose lines for the simulation with and without the streaking artifacts show similar coverage of the target (RT

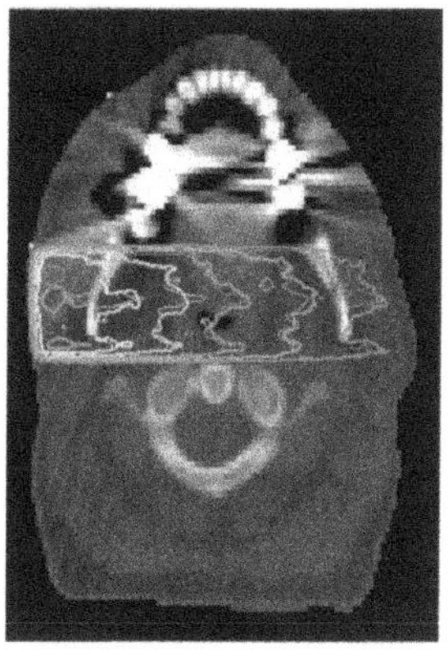

**Figure 2:** A single 4 MV photon beam to treat the RT parotid gland calculated by Monte Carlo. The isodose lines are normalized to the delivered dose at dmax. Isodose lines represent 100, 90, 80, 70, 60 & 50 percent of the prescription dose.

parotid). However, some greater differences are observed for the contralateral parotid as shown in Figure 3.

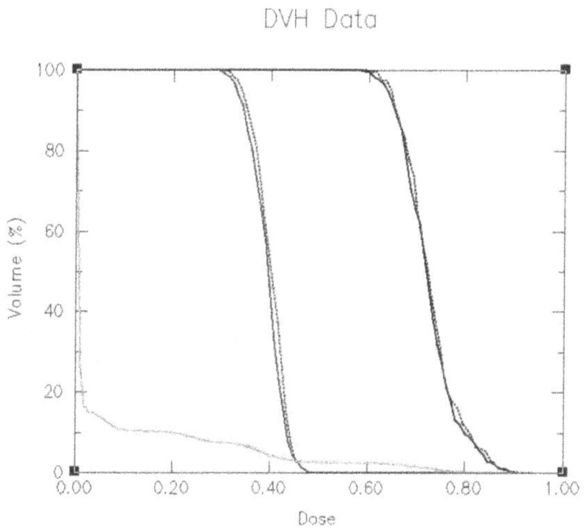


**Figure 3:** DVH for the single 4 MV photon beam. The solid line is a result of Monte Carlo calculation in the presence of CT artifacts. The dotted line is the same calculation with the CT artifacts removed.

**Electron beam plan**

The isodose distribution for the electron beam plan is shown in Figure 4. The isodose lines for the simulation with and without the streaking artifacts show a larger difference in the target than for the photon beam plan. But the the LT parotid and mandible DVHs are similar for each simulation as shown in Figure 5.

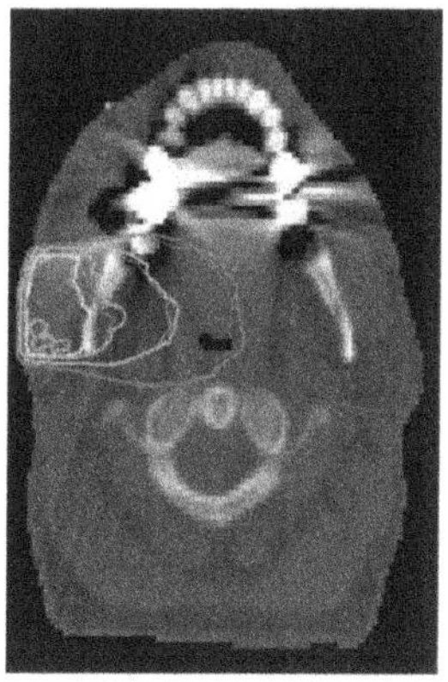

**Figure 4:** Asingle 20 MeV electron beam to treat the RT parotid gland calculated by Monte Carlo. The isodose lines are normalized to the delivered dose at dmax. Isodose lines represent 100, 90, 80, 50, 20 percent of the prescription dose.

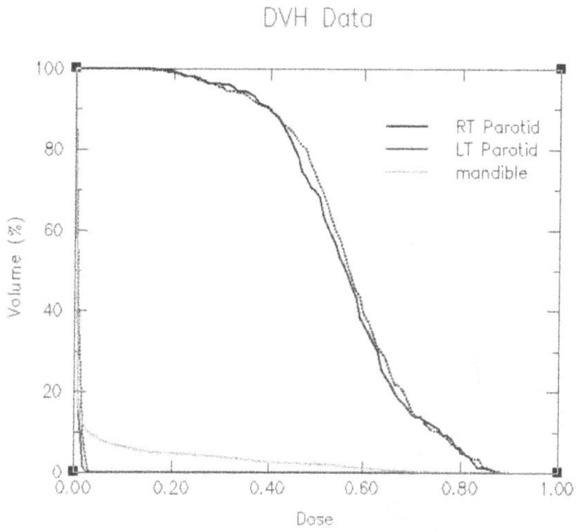


**Figure 5:** DVH for the single 20 MeV electron beam. The solid line is a result of Monte Carlo calculation in the presence of CT artifacts. The dotted line is the same calculation with the CT artifacts removed.

## Conclusion

We have investigated a clinical situation where CT steaking artifacts are routinely observed, namely, in the head and neck. These artifacts are typically due to the dental work associated with a patient. It is important to note that this study merely represents a "typical" case. There are clinical cases with more severe CT streaking artifacts. To illustrate this effect, we artificially increased the mass density of the CT streaks and then performed another simulation. The DVHs for these simulations are shown in Figure 6. In this case we find larger differences between the Monte Carlo dose distribution calculated with and without streaking artifacts. We expect similar results for cases where the target is located in the region of severe streaking artifacts.

Further study needs to be conducted on the maximum extent of the CT artifacts and their effect on Monte Carlo dose distributions. This is needed especially for rare clinical

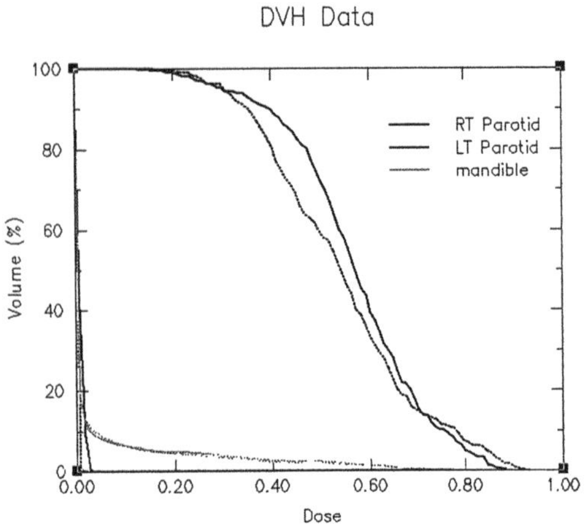


**Figure 6:** DVH for the single 20 MeV electron beam. The solid line is a result of Monte Carlo calculation in the presence of CT artifacts. The dotted line is the same calculation with the CT artifacts removed. In this comparison, the CT streaking artifacts were increased by a factor of 2 to demonstate the possible effect in serve cases.

situations like and CT streaks from hip replacements or other Titanium rods placed in a patient to support their spinal column following surgery of the vertebra. In addition to this, more routine clinical situations need to be studied, such as, surgical clips and fudicuial makers placed near or in the tumor at the time of surgery.

## References

[1] Nelson R, Hirayama H and Rogers DWO (1985). The EGS4 code system, Stanford Linear Accelerator Center Report SLAC-265 (SLAC, Stanford, CA)

[2] Ma C-M, Pawlicki T, Li JS, Jiang SB, Deng J, Kapur A., Mok E, Luxton G, Boyer AL (1999). MCDOSE – A dose calculation tool for radiotherapy treatment planning, Med. Phys. 26 1148 (Abstract)

[3] Ma C-M, Pawlicki T, Lee MC, Jiang SB, Li JS, Deng J, Yi B, Mok E and Boyer AL (1999) Energy- and intensity-modulated electron beam radiotherapy for breast cancer Phys. Med. Biol. (submitted)

# PEREGRINE: Bringing Monte Carlo based Treatment Planning Calculations to Today's Clinic

**Ralph Patterson, Tom Daly, Dewey Garrett, Christine Hartmann Siantar, Ron House and Sarita May**

Lawrence Livermore National Laboratory

## Introduction

Monte Carlo simulation of radiotherapy is now available for routine clinical use. It brings improved accuracy of dose calculations for treatments where important physics comes into play, and provides a robust, general tool for planning where empirical solutions have not been implemented. Through the use of Monte Carlo, new information, including the effects of the composition of materials in the patient, the effects of electron transport, and the details of the distribution of energy deposition, can be applied to the field.

PEREGRINE™ is a Monte Carlo dose calculation solution that was designed and built specifically for the purpose of providing a practical, affordable Monte Carlo capability to the clinic. The system solution (see Figure 1) was crafted to facilitate insertion of this powerful tool into day-to-day treatment planning, while being extensible to accommodate improvements in techniques, computers, and interfaces.

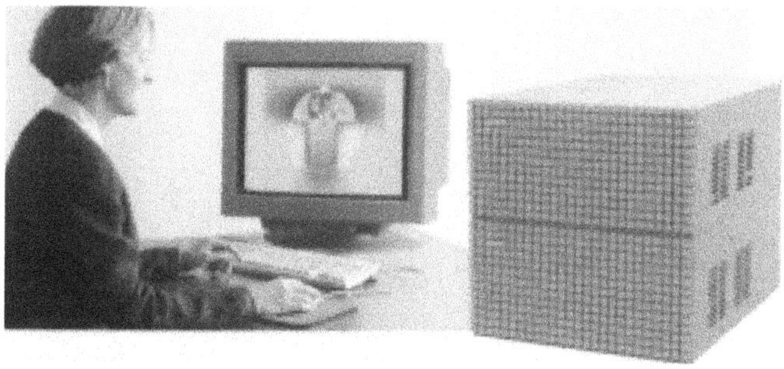

**Figure 1:** PEREGRINE dose calculation system.

## History

Although the idea of solving equations through stochastic simulation was known for some time by statisticians, its power for solving complex, real-world problems was first recognized by von Neumann and Ulam in 1949. The advantage of the Monte Carlo method is that it allows one to arrive at an exact solution for a wide variety of problems that are too complex to be solved analytically.

Monte Carlo radiation transport has served an important role at Lawrence Livermore Laboratory since its founding in 1952. In the 1950's, transport was based on von Neumann's work, constrained to neutrons, and limited by knowledge of physical cross sections. Computations were performed on the ENIAC computer. Throughout the intervening years, LLNL physicists using increasingly powerful IBM, CDC, and Cray computers improved the physics representations and broadened the included particles, developed efficient algorithms, and implemented a plethora of special and general-purpose codes. In addition, LLNL physicists developed all-particle (photon, neutron, electron, and other charged particle) databases, many of which serve as the world standard today. In the early 1990s, the neutron and proton cross sections were extended to 250 MeV, driven by a growing number of requests from the medical community.

Each decade, efforts were made to apply Monte Carlo calculations to radiation therapy. However, until the 1990's, computers were too slow and expensive to support day-to-day use of Monte Carlo calculations to predict dose delivered to patients.

Several Monte Carlo codes have been used in the medical physics community for years for research, verification of dose calculation algorithms, shielding calculations, and limited clinical treatment planning. The most prominent general purpose Monte Carlo implementations used include EGS[1] and MCNP[2] (and codes based on them). Other Monte Carlo based approaches (such as those that use Monte Carlo to precalculate kernels and voxel Monte Carlo) have also been used in order to gain speed by incorporating simplifying assumptions.

The PEREGRINE program was undertaken to provide a system solution that makes Monte Carlo transport practical for day-to-day treatment planning. In order to accomplish this, we utilized the knowledge base gained in over 45 years of Monte Carlo development to design a new, single-purpose code for use in treatment planning for radiotherapy. Our purpose was to make Monte Carlo fast, inexpensive, and, most importantly, simple enough to be used by medical physicists, dosimetrists, and physicians in a working clinical environment. By creating a new system, we were able to include all the relevant physics (but only the relevant physics), utilize only geometries relevant to the clinical setting, create simple interfaces to existing treatment planning systems, and implement an application which very efficiently utilizes modern multi-cpu computer architectures and commodity hardware.

## Physics and verification testing

PEREGRINE[3,4] simulates radiation therapy starting with a set of representative particles randomly sampled from distributions determined from offline simulations of the treatment-independent portion of the radiation source[4,5,6]. It tracks each photon, electron, and positron through the treatment-dependent beam delivery system and then through the patient using standard full-physics Monte Carlo transport methods. Treatment-specific beam modifiers such as collimators, apertures, blocks, multileaf collimators and wedges are modeled explicitly during each PEREGRINE calculation. The patient is described as a Cartesian map of material composition and density determined from the patient's CT scan.

PEREGRINE is designed to be accurate and fast. The accuracy derives from the high-fidelity cross-sections and proven transport methods used in modeling the particle transport and in the accuracy of the CT scan description of the patient. Speed is attained by numerous design techniques including:

- modeling the patient-independent radiation source offline
- the use of delta scattering in photon tracking
- the use of electron range rejection
- support for user specification of the resolution and extent of the dose reporting region

An extensive, measurement-based validation and verification process was undertaken to ensure the accuracy of PEREGRINE[7]. The simplest and most direct radiation source tests are open fields incident on water phantoms: depth dose for small to large fields, field flatness or horns for large fields, and relative output for small, large, and high aspect-ratio (rectangular) fields. In addition, depth dose comparisons for independent-jaw fields tests the adequacy of off-axis photon energy distributions.

Accurate photon particle-interaction data and transport algorithms are critical for determining relative attenuation and scatter in accelerator-head components, beam modifiers, and the patient. Their accuracy has been demonstrated by experimentally verifying the water-phantom dose distributions resulting from beam modifiers such as blocks, block trays, wedges, multileaf collimators, and compensators, in phantoms with step (discontinuous) and partial-cylinder (continuously changing) surface irregularities, and in phantoms with internal heterogeneities with high- and low-atomic number and high- and low-densities.

Accurate electron and positron transport is most important in regions of electron disequilibrium. These regions are located less than one electron range from a significant material boundary, such as the outer surface of the phantom or internal-heterogeneity surfaces. The dose predicted in the dose-buildup region near the initial patient or phantom surface depends on accurate electron transport for two reasons. First, dose is contributed directly by contaminant electrons produced in the beam delivery system and the air. Second, dose is contributed from electrons created by photon interactions in the patient or phantom (this is also an electronic disequilibrium area).

Finally, electron scatter into the monitor chamber may contribute to uncertainty in relative dose predictions. PEREGRINE™ uses published collimator jaw-dependent backscatter measurements[8] to estimate this correction to the absolute output per monitor unit. The accuracy of this approach is assessed in the beam delivery system tests.

## Software architecture and implementation

The PEREGRINE system software design process was based upon a traditional top-down, process-driven, structured design methodology intended to reduce software complexity, enhance software reliability, and promote efficient software maintenance.

The software is organized into three specialized library component packages (see Figure 2). The PEREGRINE Monte Carlo library provides the single simple interface which all dose calculation executives utilize to perform each phase of the dose calculation: setup, particle transport, and finalization. This central library is designed to take advantage of both shared memory and message-based distributed computing environments and depends upon two supporting libraries that each focus on input/output (I/O). The Teletherapy Source Library (TSL) provides the interface for I/O of patient-independent beam delivery characterization data. The Treatment Planning Interface (TPI) provides the interface for I/O of patient-specific treatment planning data.

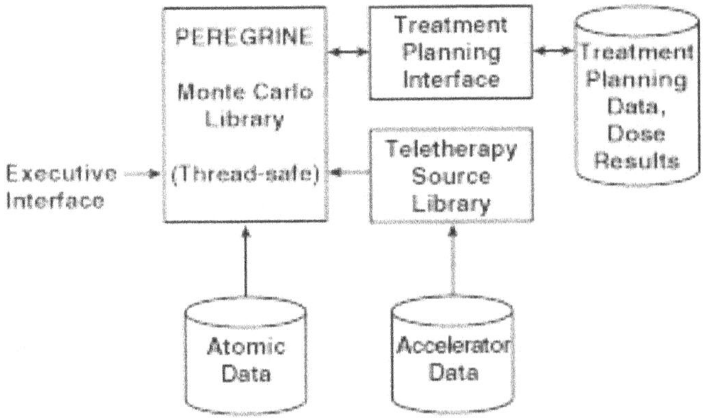


**Figure 2:** PEREGRINE software architecture.

In addition to the library interfaces, a common executive interface is defined to control access to critical shared resources which provides for increased flexibility during software development and testing. A simple single-threaded executive is utilized as a primary test-jacket to develop, debug, and test library code. The PEREGRINE product system is based upon a high-performance, two-tiered, distributed master/slave architecture designed to exploit computational resources in a scalable manner. The master focuses on the I/O bound phases of the dose calculation (setup and finish) and controls and coordinates multiple slaves. Master and slaves communicate using messages over standard networking protocols, including TCP/IP and UDP. Each slave focuses on the compute bound particle transport phase of processing and is designed to take performance advantage of multiple CPUs using shared memory and POSIX threads.

## Hardware realization (PEREGRINE engine)

PEREGRINE is implemented with a master-slave, distributed architecture that runs on commodity, multi-processor x86 mainboards interconnected on a private network.

Each board runs the Solaris (Sun TM) operating system — the master board boots from a local disk, slaves are booted diskless by the master. The hardware components are assembled in a chassis module that contains power supplies, a hard disk, up to 6 mainboards, a small 100MB ethernet hub, and floppy drives (used to boot slave boards). Each mainboard supplies controllers for all peripherals used for operation on the private network; a single network card is required to access a public network. Mainboards are currently available with 733MHz, dual Pentium III (Intel™) cpus; the chassis will accommodate future board designs with faster processors and additional cpus. A typical 24 processor configuration uses two modules interconnected by a single network cable; additional modules can be added by a connection through an ethernet switch.

A PEREGRINE engine is attached to a treatment planning system via a conventional office network; dose calculation jobs are scheduled through a networked file system and a runtime fifo (first-in-first-out) queue.

The master executive is a tcl (tool-command-language) interpreter extended with routines from the PEREGRINE libraries and additional routines for threading and network distribution. A slave executive is a custom interpreter that incorporates and threads the key Monte Carlo transport routine. In operation, a master script implements a state machine that processes jobs submitted on the job queue. The master sequences a case through the routines of the PEREGRINE api for input and setup, distributes the job to all slaves (including slaves running on the master main board), collects and aggregates computed dose, and writes out result files. While a case is in progress, real-time statistics and dose views are available through an rpc (remote procedure call) interface for view on the host treatment planning system.

The PEREGRINE engine design achieves the following goals:

- simple setup
- expandable number of processors
- low life-cycle costs
- adaptable to new technologies

## Conclusions

The PEREGRINE system has achieved the goal of providing practical Monte Carlo for use in clinical radiotherapy practice. A dose calculation engine has been designed, implemented, tested, and verified[3-7,9]. The technology has been licensed to NOMOS Corporation of Sewickly, PA, USA, and routine implementation in clinics is imminent. The challenges at hand include discovery of the specific uses which deliver the full potential of Monte Carlo, and furtherance of Monte Carlo in radiotherapy applications through improved measurement programs and the continued development of clinical solutions.



Work performed under the auspices of the U.S. Department of Energy by the Lawrence Livermore National Laboratory under Contract W-7405-ENG-48.

## References

[1] W. R. Nelson, H. H. Hirayama, D. W. O. Rogers, "The EGS4 Code System", SLAC-Report-265, (Stanford Linear Accelerator Center, Stanford, CA, 1985)

[2] J. F. Briesmeister, editor "MCNP™ - A General Monte Carlo N-particle Transport Code, Version 4a", LA-12625, (Los Alamos National Laboratory, Los Alamos, NM, 1988)

[3] C. L. Hartmann Siantar, P. M. Bergstrom, W. P. Chandler, L. Chase, L. J. Cox, T. P. Daly, D. Garrett, S. M. Hornstein, R. K. House, E. I. Moses, R. W. Patterson, J. A. Rathkopf, A. Schach von Wittenau, "Lawrence Livermore National Laboratory's PEREGRINE Project", 1997 XII th International Conference on the use of Computers in Radiation Therapy, D. D. Leavitt and G. Starkschall, ed. Medical Physics Publishing, p. 19.

[4] C. L. Hartmann Siantar, P. M. Bergstrom, L. J. Cox, T. P. Daly, D. H. Fujino, M. Descalle, D. Garrett, B. Guidry, R. K. House, D. Jong, D. K. Knapp, S. H. May, E. I. Moses, R. W. Patterson, C. Powell, D. M. Williams, A. E. Schach von Wittenenau, R. S. Walling, J. A. White, N. Albright, L. Verhey, D. Wieczorek and M. C. Schell, "Implementation of the PEREGRINE Monte Carlo Dose Calculation System for Photon Beam Therapy," submitted to Phys. Med. Biol.

[5] C. L. Hartmann Siantar and E. I. Moses, The PEREGRINE Programme: Using Physics and Computer Simulation to Improve Radiation Therapy for Cancer, European Journal of Physics, 19 513-521 (1998).

[6] A. E. Schach von Wittenau, L. J. Cox, P.M. Bergstrom, W. P. Chandler, C.L. Hartmann Siantar, and R. Mohan, "Correlated histogram representation of Monte Carlo derived medical accelerator photon-output phase space," Med. Phys. 26:7 1196-1211 (1999).

[7] E. Schach von Wittenau, L. J. Cox, P. M. Bergstrom, S. M. Hornstein, R. Mohan, et.al., p. 146-149, XII th International Conference on the use of Computers in Radiation Therapy, D. Medical Physics Publishing, Madison, Wisconsin,1997.

[8] A. Duzenli, B. McClean and C. Field, "Backscatter into the beam monitor chamber: Implications for dosimetry of asymmetric collimators," Med. Phys. 20:2, Pt. 1 363-367 (1993).

[8] C. L. Hartmann Siantar, P. M. Bergstrom, T. P. Daly, M.-A. Descalle, D. Garrett, R. K. House, D. K. Knapp, S. May, R. W. Patterson, R. S. Walling, N. Albright, L. Verhey, and D. Weiczorek, "Clinical Implementation of the PEREGRINE Monte Carlo Dose Calculations System for Photon Beam Therapy", Proceedings of the Eleventh International Congress of Radiation Research, Dublin, Ireland July 18-23, 1999, Lawrence Livermore National Laboratory, Livermore CA, and University of California San Francisco, San Francisco, CA 94143

# Modification of a Virtual Source Model for Monte Carlo Based IMRT Verification

**Randi Fogg[1], Indrin Chetty[1], John J. DeMarco[1,2], Nzhde Agazaryan[1] and Timothy D. Solberg[1,2]**

[1]Department of Radiation Oncology and [2]Jonsson Comprehensive Cancer Center, 200 UCLA Medical Plaza, suite B265, Los Angeles, CA 90095

## Introduction

The recent growth of advanced treatment modalities in radiation therapy, such as IMRT and 3D-conformal radiotherapy, brings an increased need for accurate treatment verification. These treatment methods are primarily indicated in heterogeneous regions and for target volumes that are irregularly shaped or near critical structures. A Monte Carlo based dosimetry algorithm provides the ability to accurately simulate dose distributions for clinical situations in radiation therapy. It has been well established that Monte Carlo simulation represents one of the most accurate methods for dose calculation within heterogeneous media. The purpose of this study is to describe the development and modifications of a Monte Carlo based phase space source model for IMRT dose verification. A phase space source model has been previously developed for simulation of arbitrary intensity distributions for conventional clinical treatment planning [1,2]. This work represents an extension of that model to incorporate the necessary features for simulation of intensity modulated radiotherapy fields.

## Material and methods

### The Monte Carlo Phase Space Source Model

The phase space source model was developed by first simulating the components of the linear accelerator treatment head using the code MCNP4B (Monte Carlo N-Particle version 4B) [3]. The calculated fluence distributions were reconstructed into a beam model consisting of a cartesian fluence grid with discrete photon fluence elements. Fluence weights may be adjusted to match the physical beam for an arbitrary field shape by assigning a value of 0.015 (relative to the central axis) to regions of the beam that are blocked by a leaf from the multi-leaf collimator. The small positive value represents a first order approximation that is used to account for leakage and transmission through the field shaping collimators. This method allows for the simulation of arbitrary intensity distributions without the inefficient step of calculating particle transport through the field defining collimators. The model also includes an electron contamination subsource developed using the code BEAM [4], as well as a correction to incorporate scattering effects from the extra-focal radiation component.

### Modifications of the Model

The virtual source model, which has been shown to accurately simulate arbitrarily shaped radiation beams for conventional treatments, has been modified to allow for verification of IMRT and Conformal Stereotactic Radiotherapy treatments on a Novalis 6MV linear accelerator (BrainLAB AG, Heimstetten, Germany). Novalis is equipped with a micro-multileaf collimator (mMLC) with a maximum field size of 10 x 10 $cm^2$. The collimator leaves vary in width from 3 mm in the center to 5.5 mm on the outside, projected at isocenter. The geometry of the specific accelerator was simulated to determine the photon fluence at a plane just above the mMLC, and the fluence values were transformed to a 200 x 200 square pixel matrix. The fluence map is used to sample the starting particle's position ($x$, $y$). In addition, the particle's energy and direction are also sampled within the virtual source model.

Once the linear accelerator (LINAC) source has been simulated, the fluence grid can be used for dosimetric calculations for any arbitrarily shaped beam or series of beams. For IMRT treatments, the leaf sequence is obtained from a translation algorithm. The algorithm, based on that of Bortfeld et al, uses a sliding window technique to minimize beam time and accounts for leaf leakage and transmission [5]. An additional parameter can be specified to minimize the tongue-and-groove effect. The sequencing algorithm produces the necessary leaf prescription in a format that can be read directly by the Novalis mMLC controller.

A second program has been written that reads the sequence file and constructs the corresponding intensity map for the Monte Carlo simulation. IMRT treatments can be delivered in either dynamic or step-and-shoot mode; dynamic treatments are approximated as a series of static beams for calculations. In both techniques, each set of leaf positions is associated with a beam weight, or index. This index represents the proportion of the total dose that has been delivered when the leaves reach that position. For each beam, any grid space that is open is given a value of the dose proportion given in that segment, and each grid element covered by a collimator leaf is assigned a value of 0.015 times the dose proportion, to account for leakage. The sum of all beams provides a treatment-specific intensity map, which is multiplied by the discrete phase space fluence map determined in the LINAC simulation, to produce the cumulative fluence grid for the leaf sequence.

## Results and discussion

The modified phase space source was benchmarked against standard depth dose and profile ion chamber measurements and compared with measurement in various theoretical and clinical examples. The low energy cutoffs for all calculations were 10 keV for photons and 500 keV for electrons. The field sizes used for benchmarking were 2.4x2.4 $cm^2$, 5.1x5.1 $cm^2$ and 8x8 $cm^2$. Depth dose and profile calculations were carried out in a 30x30x30 $cm^2$ simulated water phantom using a cylindrical tally cell with a grid spacing of 2 mm. Figure 1 shows a

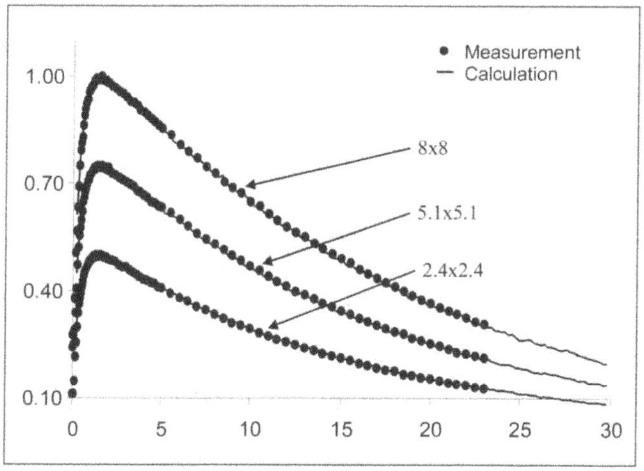


**Figure 1:** A comparison of Monte Carlo depth dose calculations and water phantom measurements for Novalis. The 8x8 $cm^2$, 5.1x5.1 $cm^2$ and 2.4x2.4 $cm^2$ field size data were normalized to $d_{max}$, and they have been scaled to 1, 0.75 and 0.5, respectively, for inclusion on the same graph.

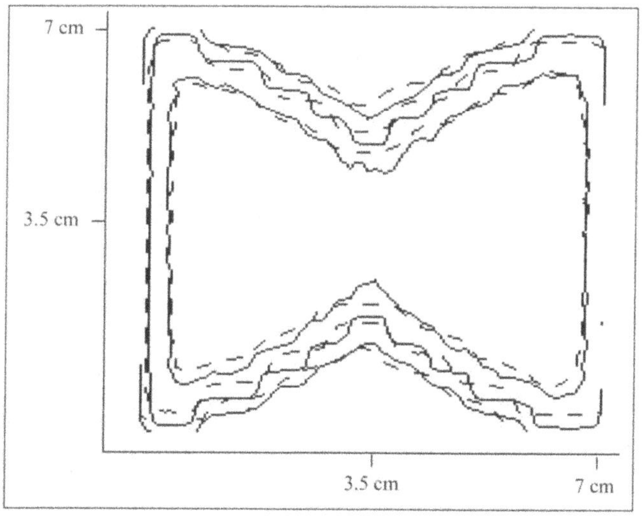


**Figure 2:** A comparison of Monte Carlo calculation (solid lines) and film measurement (dashed lines) for a single beam. Isodose lines shown are, from the center of the distribution outwards, 90%, 50%, 15%.

comparison of measured and calculated relative depth dose values for the three benchmark field sizes. Calculated depth dose curves were found to be within 2% of measurement in all regions of the curves.

Table 1 provides a quantitative comparison of the measured and calculated profiles of the benchmark fields. The Task Group 53 criteria for acceptable agreement in the inner (dose > 90%) and outer (dose < 10%) regions of the curve is 2% of the normalization dose, and the recommended distance to agreement in the penumbral region (10% < dose < 90%) is 2 mm. The agreement between the calculation and measurement is well within these criteria.

In addition to benchmarks, comparisons of Monte Carlo calculation to film measurement were made with various field shapes. We will present two comparisons here; the first is a single arbitrary field shape, and the second is an IMRT delivered distribution of an image. Film measurements were made using Kodak X-OMAT V film placed at 10 cm depth in a 30x30x20 $cm^3$ solid water phantom. Calculations were made in a simulated water phantom of the same size, also at a depth of 10 cm, with a tally voxel size of 0.2x0.2x1.0 $cm^3$. Figure 2 shows a comparison of measurement and calculation for an AP beam with an arbitrary field shape defined by the mMLC. There are small differences seen in regions with highly irregular leaf positions, but in general there is good agreement.

The final example is a step-and-shoot IMRT dose distribution of an arbitrary intensity pattern derived from a photograph of Dr. H. Rodney Withers, Chair of the UCLA Department of Radiation Oncology. The intensity pattern (photograph) was broken into 14 intensity levels which produced 152 leaf segments. The film measurement and Monte Carlo calculations of the distribution are shown in Figure 3. The qualitative agreement between these images indicates that the modified virtual source model is an accurate method for dosimetric verification of IMRT treatments with arbitrarily shaped fields.

## Conclusion

This study describes a modified photon virtual source model, which has been shown to provide accurate Monte Carlo based IMRT verification. A unique feature of the source model that makes the Monte Carlo calculation more efficient is the ability to simulate an arbitrary field shape without tracking photons

| Novalis | | Inner Beam Dose > 90% | | Penumbra 10% < Dose < 90% | | Outer Beam Dose < 10% | |
|---|---|---|---|---|---|---|---|
| | Field Size ($cm^2$) | Percent (%) difference | | Distance to agreement (mm) | | Percent (%) difference | |
| | | Ave. | Max. | Ave. | Max. | Ave. | Max. |
| 6 MV | 2.4 x 2.4 | 0.2 | 0.6 | 0.5 | 0.7 | 0.1 | 0.5 |
| | 5.1 x 5.1 | 0.3 | 1.5 | 0.6 | 0.9 | 0.5 | 0.9 |
| | 8.0 x 8.0 | 0.4 | 1.9 | 1.0 | 1.9 | 1.2 | 1.5 |

**Table 1:** A quantitative comparison of calculated and measured profile curves for benchmark fields. Agreement is well within Task Group 53 criteria.

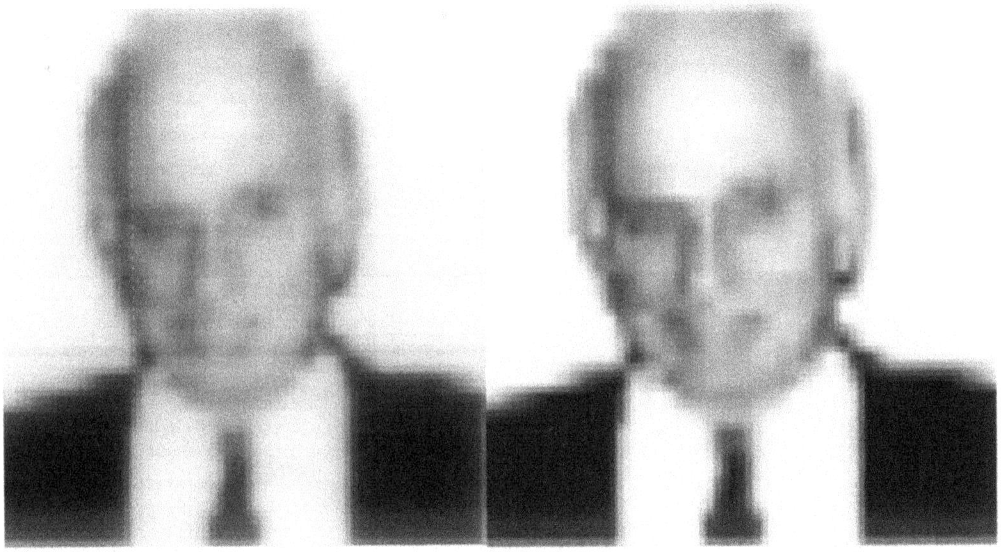

**Figure 3:** Left: film measurement of an IMRT fluence map delivered on Novalis. Right: beam's-eye-view of a Monte Carlo calculation of the distribution.

through the field defining collimators. The creation of a fluence matrix from a leaf-sequencing file allows verification of both single field conformal treatments and multi-segment IMRT treatments. Depth dose and square field profiles calculations demonstrate the accuracy of this model. In addition, irregular field and IMRT treatments are found to be in good agreement with measurement. The modifications and unique features of this model show it to be a valueable and accurate tool for IMRT dose verification.

## References

[1] Chetty I, DeMarco JJ and Solberg TD A virtual source model for Monte Carlo modeling of arbitrary intensity distributions. *Medical Physics* January, 2000

[2] DeMarco JJ, Chetty I and Solberg TD 1999 Incorporating conventional treatment planning parameters into a Monte Carlo based dosimetry algorithm. *Medical Physics* **26** 1752

[3] Briesmeister JF 1997 "MCNP™ - A general Monte Carlo N-Particle transport code" Los Alamos National Laboratory Report LA-12625-M

[4] Rogers DWO, Faddegon DA, Ding GX, Ma CM, We J and Mackie TR 1995 BEAM: A Monte Carlo code to simulate radiotherapy treatment units *Medical Physics* **22** 503-524

[5] Bortfeld TR, Kahler DL, Waldron TJ, Boyer AL 1994 X-ray field conpensation with multileaf collimators *International Journal of Radiation Oncology Biology and Physics* **28** 723-730

# IMRT with Monte Carlo dose computation: what is the benefit?

**W. Laub, M. Alber, M. Birkner and F. Nüsslin**
Department of Medical Physics, University of Tuebingen, Germany

## Introduction

Monte Carlo simulations arguably offer the most readily explorable route to computing radiation transport in complex geometries and inhomogeneous media. With IMRT, not only the dose computation in the patient poses problems, but also the predominantly small field sizes and the modulation devices in the accelerator head. However, IMRT also offers abundant degrees of freedom to compensate for the dose loss due to lateral electron transport at low density surfaces by adjustments to the primary fluence.

Instead of only providing MC dose verification where indicated, an inclusion of the MC dose calculation into the optimisation process would be desirable. This study shows how MC can be incorporated to full accuracy into an existing IM algorithm as a second stage of optimisation at a minute increase in overall MC computation time. The method is essentially independent of the first IM optimisation stage if the objective function is convex and a scatter is taken into account by the conventional algorithm which is used to compute the fluence updates. The viability of the method is shown in two cases of target volumes adjacent to low density surfaces: a lung tumour and a tumour close to the sinuses and nasal cavities.

## Material and methods

The idea behind this development is to construct a converging sequence of 'verification' dose distributions which form the basis of the fluence update computations. The MC dose computations can be run under full consideration of the accelerator head, which in turn bears on the subsequent optimisation.

We propose to start the algorithm with a fluence $\Phi^0$ obtained from an initial optimisation step with pencil beam dose computation. The PB algorithm will be employed also for the fluence updates. The MC/IM algorithm reads:

1. Compute TERMA operator $T_{PB}$ with a finite-size Pencil Beam algorithm and solve optimisation problem defined by minimising the objective function $f(D = T\Phi)$ as a function of dose $D$, to yield $\Phi^0$.
2. MC loop counter $k = 0$.
3. Compute $D^0 = T_{MC}\Phi^0$.
4. On the basis of the MC dose $D^k$, find fluence $\Phi^{k+1}$ by using $T_{PB}$.
5. Update MC Dose: $D^{k+1} = D^k + T_{MC}(\Phi^{k+1} - \Phi^k)$.
6. Converged? If no, k=k+1, goto 4.

The updated fluence elements in step 5 can also be negative, in which case the particle would be given negative statistical weight. Convergence can be checked by comparing the objective function value of the intermediate MC/PB dose and the corresponding MC dose. Typically, the IM/MC optimisation takes at most 20 per cent longer than MC verification alone. The MC code used in this study was EGS4, which is well established in Radiotherapy Physics [1,2]. In the patient geometry, the physical properties were attributed according to tissue type as defined by contouring and density. CT numbers (in Hounsfield units) were converted into electron densities. Thresholds of the CT numbers were set to distinguish a small number of different media or tissues. Voxel sizes were about $(3mm)^3$ for thorax cases, and about $(1.5mm)^3$ for head and neck cases. Full phase-space files of a scoring plane above the collimators were used to start MC events. These files resulted from BEAM simulations of an Elekta SL 20 Linac [3]. If intensity profiles are translated into compensators or MLC fields during the MC/IM process, the influence of intensity modifying equipment can be taken into account with MC methods during the IM/MC optimisation. In most cases, it would be sufficient to use a tuned down photon transport routine taylored to the particular geometry of the equipment.

## Results and discussion

A lung tumour was defined in an Alderson phantom and was planned with elective nodal irradiation to the mediastinum with five coplanar photon beams of 6MV. The resolution of the dose computation grid was $(3mm)^3$, the pencil beam resolution was $5mm^2$ at isocentre distance. The pencil beams were arranged on a hexagonal grid. The optimisation employed biological constraints of which only pneumonitis and myelitis as well as the maximum-dose constraint on the mediastium remained active, i.e. dose limiting. The total computation time was 13 h on a 533 MHz DEC Alpha with $1.2 \times 10^8$ particle histories.

The confounding factor in this settup which goes unnoticed with PB algorithm is the increased penumbra in lung, which leads to a dose loss along the edges of the PTV of some 5 Gy and an increased volume of the lung which receives low doses. The former can be picked up by lifting the fluence along the field edges which is known as penumbra sharpening, see figure 1. The PB optimisation yielded an isoeffective homogeneous dose to the GTV of 77.4 Gy, which was diminished to 73.1 Gy according to the EGS4 verification computation and restored to 75.4 Gy by the subsequent IM/MC optimisation. The full equivalent dose to the target volume could not be restored since active constraints were present which would have been violated by a further increase.

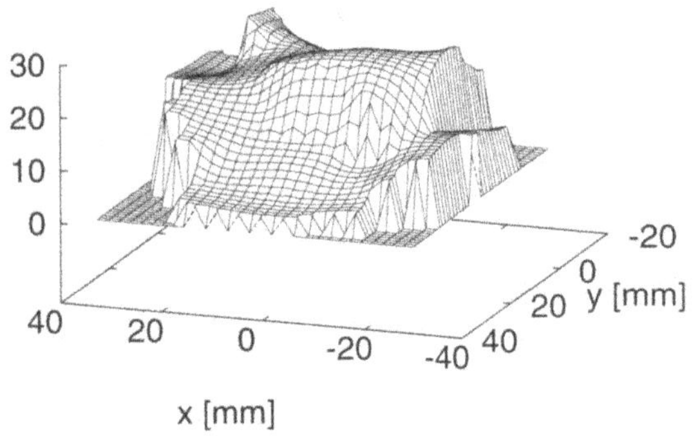


**Figure 1:** The bulk in the centre of the fluence profile corresponds to the boost (GTV) volume of a lung case. Along the left (caudal) and right outline of the volume, penumbra sharpening ridges can be seen, which are not present at the other outlines, because they would violate the maximum dose constraint on the PTV. Coordinates are given at a source distance of 500 mm.

The second case is a target volume adjacent to the sinuses which was planned with four non-coplanar photon beams of 6MV, of which three pass partially through air cavities. The resolution of the dose computation grid was $(1.75mm)^3$, the pencil beam resolution was $2mm^2$ at isocentre distance. Again, the pencil beams were arranged on a hexagonal grid. The biological constraints included both eyes, the contralateral optical nerve, the chiasm and the brain. The total computation time was 6 h with $5.5 \times 10^7$ particles.

The confounding factor of this treatment is the second dose buildup region of the frontal fields behind the cavities. With the small field sizes, this region can spread up to 1 cm into the GTV, which affects up to one third of the total volume. The IM/MC optimisation has to adjust the fluence elements which are tangental to these regions. The PB optimisation yielded an isoeffective homogeneous dose to the PTV of 70.9 Gy, which was diminished to a mere 63.8 Gy according to the EGS4 verification computation. At the same time, the constraint to the chiasma was violated due to increased scatter contributions. To meet the demand for higher primary fluence in some areas, the fluence had to be redistributed. The subsequent IM/MC optimisation improved the result to 68.1 Gy. Again, active constraints prevented a total restoration of the PB dose.

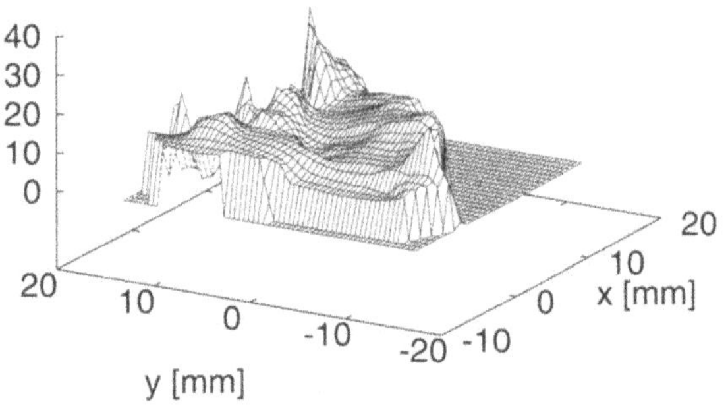


**Figure 2:** The pronounced peak at the rear of the fluence profile compensates for the dose re-buildup behind the nose and the frontal sinuses in the stereotactic case.

## Conclusion

The IM/MC optimisation proves to be a viable method to compensate for dose inhomogeneities near low-density surfaces, which in some cases result in significant underdosage of the target volume. Together with the advantage of the inclusion of detailed head scatter into the optimisation, which has yet to be fully explored, IM/MC optimisation offers substantial potential of increasing the accuracy of IMRT planning. The computation times did not appear to be prohibitively long. Since computation times scale with the speed of the MC code, total computation times of about an hour can be reached with highly efficient MC codes such as XVMC [4].

## References


[1] Nelson W R Hirayama H Rogers D W O 1985 The EGS 4 Code System *SLAC Report-265*

[2] Nahum A E 1995 Three-D dose calculation (III); application of Monte Carlo-methods *Workshop 95, DKFZ Heidelberg* 89–97

[3] Rogers D W O Faddegon B A et al 1995 A Monte Carlo code to simulate radiotherapy treatment units *Med. Phys.* **22** 503-524

[4] Fippel M 1999 Fast Monte Carlo dose calculation for photon beams based on the VMC electron algorithm *Med. Phys.* **26** 1466–1475

# The impact of Monte Carlo dose calculations on treatment outcomes

**Paul Keall, Jeffrey Siebers and Radhe Mohan**

Department of Radiation Oncology, MCV Hospitals, Virginia Commonwealth University, Richmond, VA, USA

## Introduction

Accurate calculation of dose distributions for radiation therapy has long been a goal of medical physicists. The more advanced current dose calculation algorithms, such as the superposition/convolution method,[1-4] can accurately compute dose in most instances. However, the accuracy of currently available dose computation models for planning of radiation treatments is limited,[5-10] and in extreme cases, even these advanced methods can result in dose errors of several percent. Discrepancies compared to dose distributions may be clinically significant for some cases. Monte Carlo-based dose calculations can potentially compute dose with an accuracy that surpasses that of conventional algorithms.[10] Monte Carlo dose calculation is theoretically limited only by the daily change in patient anatomy (due to patient positioning, motion, or physiological changes), by the uncertainty with which patient materials can be estimated, and by the accuracy of the measured data used to commission the Monte Carlo dose calculation algorithm.

The aim of this research was to compare Monte Carlo calculated treatment plans with superposition calculated plans for a set of clinical cases, and to firstly quantify and dose distribution differences, and secondly to determine if any resulting differences are clinically significant.

## Material and methods

The Monte Carlo calculations used EGS4[11]/BEAM[12] for the phase space creation and MCVRTP* for the patient dose calculation, coupled to the ADAC† Pinnacle³ TPS, via the MCV system.[13] The calculated dose-to-material was converted to dose-to-water using the method of Siebers *et al.*[14] The plans were calculated to a statistical proecision of ~1% at $D_{max}$, which has been shown by Keall *et al.*[15] not to significantly affect isodose lines, dose volume histograms or biological indices.

The commissioning of MCV involved comparisons between MCV calculations and measurements. From the commissioning process[16] it was determined that the dose output calculated with the MCV code is accurate to within ±2 mm or ±2% of $D_{max}$. This accuracy means that horizontal error bars on the MC dose volume histograms are ±2% of $D_{max}$, for EUD calculations are ±2%, and for TCP calculations are $\pm<2\gamma_{50}$.

The superposition calculations were performed using Pinnacle³'s Collapsed Cone Convolution[17] (CCC) algorithm.

Clinical cases chosen were treatments of the lung, prostate, head and neck, and breast. The MCV calculations were performed on the same field set up as those planned for the patient treatment using Pinnacle. The same monitor units were used for both MCV and CCC calculations, and therefore absolute doses can be compared. The dose distribution differences were analysed visually from isodose plans, by determining the dose range within various contours, dose volume histograms (DVHs) and biological indices.

The biological indices were calculated from the DVHs. The TCP was calculated using

$$TCP = 0.5^{\exp\left[\frac{2\cdot\gamma_{50}}{\ln 2}\left(1-\frac{EUD}{D_{50}}\right)\right]}.$$

The dose yielding 50% TCP ($D_{50}$) was calculated from the information given in Munzenrider *et al*[18] and used their tabulated $\gamma_{50}$ values. The equivalent uniform dose[19] (*EUD*) was calculated from

$$EUD = 2\cdot\frac{\ln\left[\frac{1}{V}\sum_i v_i SF_2^{\frac{D_i}{2}}\right]}{\ln SF_2}.$$

$V$ is the volume composed of elements $v_i$, and $SF_2$, the surviving fraction of cells after irradiation of 2 Gy, was set to 0.5.

## Results and discussion

**Figure 1** shows sample MCV calculations and measured depth dose and lateral profile results for a 6 MV beam from our Varian‡ Cl2100C accelerator. These plots give examples of the accuracy of the MCV code.

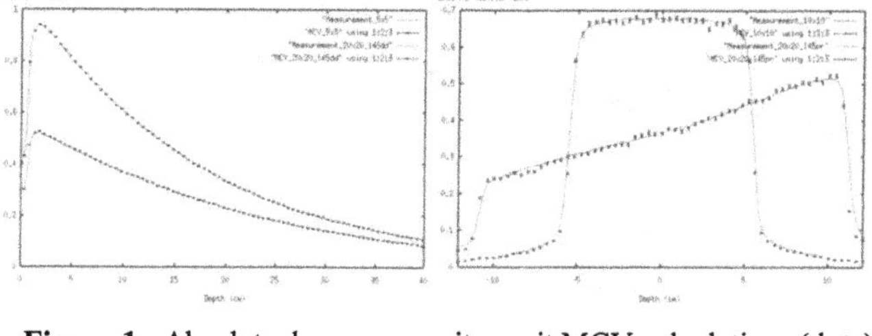

**Figure 1.** Absolute dose per monitor unit MCV calculations (dots) and experimental measurements (lines) for depth dose and profiles curves, in open and wedged fields.

* MCVRTP is a C++ Monte Carlo code provided by ADAC Laboratories that uses many of the published algorithms of EGS4.
† ADAC Laboratories, Milpitas, CA 95035.

‡ Varian Oncology Systems, Palo Alto, CA 94304.

The MCV and CCC calculations for the 4 clinical cases are presented in **Figure 2.** The isodose lines appear similar, however, closerr inspection reveals differences. The dose differences can be better observed from DVHs.

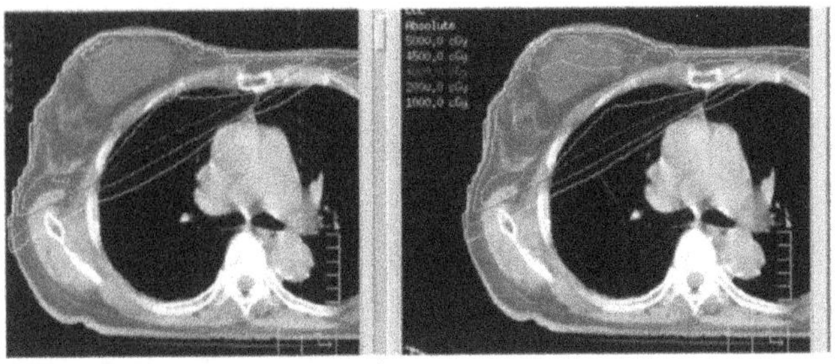

a) Breast treatment

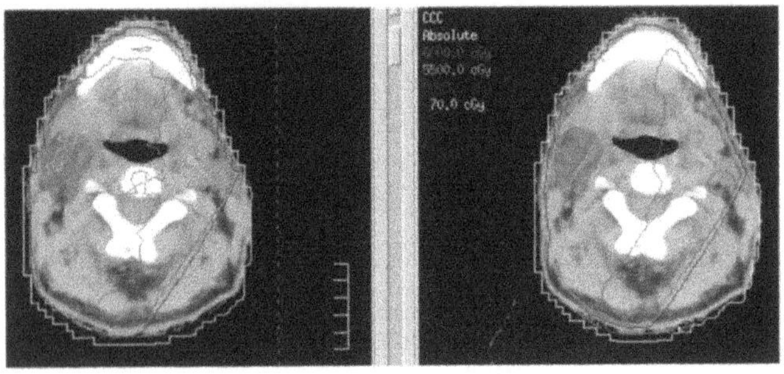

b) Head/Neck treatment

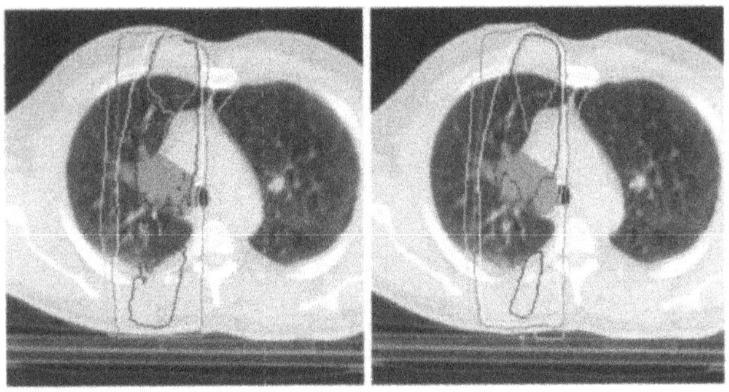

c) Lung treatment

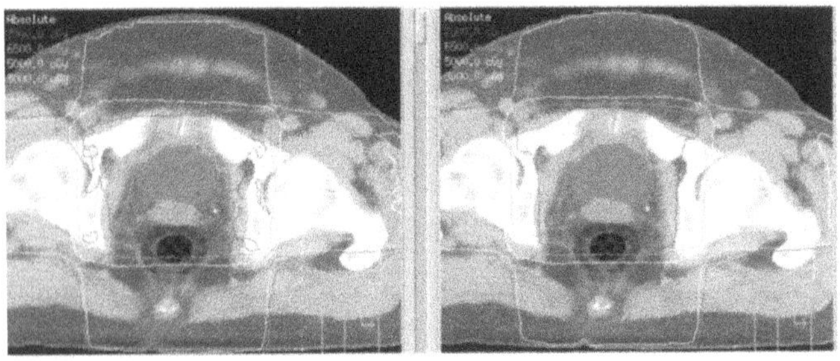

d) Prostate treatment

**Figure 2.** Isodose plots for the four clinical sites studied. MCV results are on the left, CCC results on the right.

DVHs for the head and neck, and prostate case are shown in **Figure 3**.

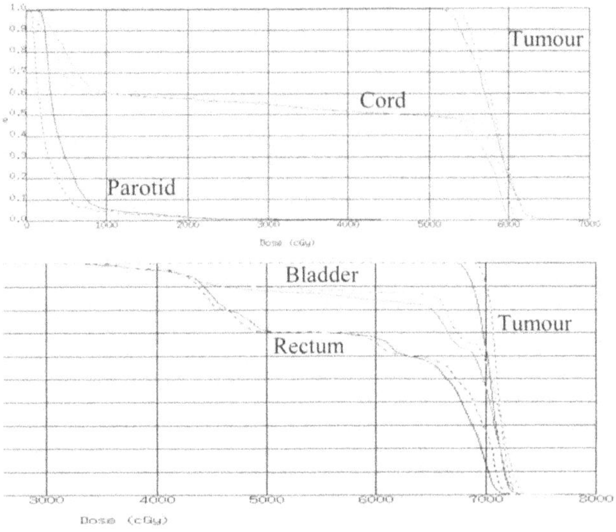


**Figure 3.** Dose volume histograms for the head and neck case (top) and prostate case (bottom). MCV results are solid lines, CCC results are dashed.

The significance of the difference seen in the DVHs can be quantified using biological indice calculations, as displayed in Table 1.

**Table 1.** TCP and NTCP values as determined from Monte Carlo and convolution calculations for several treatment sites.

| Treatment Site | MCV EUD | CCC EUD | MCV TCP | CCC TCP | MCV NTCP | CCC NTCP |
|---|---|---|---|---|---|---|
| Breast | 48 Gy | 28 Gy* | 96% | 24%* | 0% (lung) | 0% (lung) |
| Head/Neck | 16 Gy | 16 Gy | 0% | 0% | 21% (cord) | 24% (cord) |
| Lung | 70 Gy | 71 Gy | 64% | 65% | 10% (lung) | 7% (lung) |
| Prostate | 65 Gy | 66 Gy | 80% | 81% | 6% (bladder)<br>10% (rectum) | 7% (bladder)<br>11% (rectum) |

*Note that a small element of the breast CCC target volume had a low dose, thus significantly reducing the TCP and EUD.

Apart from the discrepancy in the breast plan, the CCC calculated EUD and TCP values were within calculation error of those calculated by MCV. CCC overpredicted the cord NTCP for the head/neck treatment, and underpredicted the lung NTCP by 3% as compared to MCV predictions.

## Conclusion

The dose differences between plans calculated by a commissioned Monte Carlo system, and a commercial superposition algorithm were assessed via isodose plots overlaid on the CT scan, DVHs and biological indices (TCP, NTCP and EUD).

Differences in isodose plots were observed which were also seen in the DVHs. Though the target DVHs differ, the EUDs and TCPs were similar for the Monte Carlo and superposition calculations (except for the breast case as discussed earlier) and are within the Monte Carlo calculation uncertainty. The critical structure DVHs also differ, and this difference was noted by the different NTCP values, especially for the lung which may be due to the known interface limitation of superposition,[5-9] and the cord, which is embedded inside a bone matrix.

There are arguments both to diminish and highlight the importance of these differences. When other uncertainties in treatment are taken into account, such as target outlining, organ motion, set-up errors, machine output variations etc, the importance of these differences is diminished.

However, highlighting the importance of these differences is that the biological data for the $\gamma_{50}$ and NTCP parameter values came from inaccurate data, blurring the curves which are in reality sharper, leading to a higher biological response of individual patients to dose.

Have we shown that superposition-based models are inaccurate? No. Is Monte Carlo more accurate than superposition? Yes. Is this increased accuracy clinically significant? Maybe. Though the results of this study are inconclusive as to the need for Monte Carlo, it cannot be proven in general that for all cases superposition-based models are sufficiently accurate.

## References

[1]A.L. Boyer and E.C. Mok, "A photon dose distribution model employing convolution calculations," *Med. Phys.* **12**, 169-177 (1985).

[2]T.R. Mackie, J.W. Scrimger, and J.J. Battista, "A Convolution Method of Calculating Dose for 15-MV X-rays," *Med. Phys.* **12**, 188-196 (1985).

[3]A. Ahnesjö, P. Andreo, and A. Brahme, "Calculation and Application of Point Spread Functions for Treatment Planning With High Energy Photon Beams," *Acta Oncol.* **26**, 49-56 (1987).

[4]R. Mohan, C. Chui, and L. Lidofsky, "Differential Pencil Beam Dose Computation Model for Photons," *Med. Phys.* **13**, 64-73 (1986).

[5]M.K. Woo and J.R. Cunningham, "The validity of the density scaling method in primary electron transport for electron and photon beams," *Med. Phys.* **17** (2), 187-194 (1990).

[6]P.E. Metcalfe, T.P.Y. Wong, and P.W. Hoban, "Radiotherapy x-ray beam inhomogeneity corrections: the problem of lateral electronic disequilibrium in lung," *Aust. Phys. Eng. Sci. Med.* **16** (4), 155-167 (1993).

[7]C. X. Yu, T. R. Mackie, and J. W. Wong, "Photon dose calculation incorporating explicit electron transport," *Med. Phys.* **22** (7), 1157-1165 (1995).

[8]P.J. Keall and P.W. Hoban, "Accounting for primary electron scatter in x-ray beam convolution calculations," *Med. Phys.* **22** (9), 1413-1418 (1995).

[9]P.J. Keall and P.W. Hoban, "Superposition dose calculation incorporating Monte Carlo generated electron track kernels," *Med. Phys.* **23** (4), 479-485 (1996).

[10]R. Mohan, "Why Monte Carlo?," presented at the XII International Conference on the Use of Computers in Radiotherapy, Salt Lake City, Utah, 1997.

[11]W.R. Nelson, H. Hirayama, and D.W.O. Rogers, *The EGS4 Code System*, Stanford Linear Accelerator Center, Report No. SLAC-265, 1985.

[12]D.W.O. Rogers, B.A. Faddegon, G.X. Ding *et al.*, "BEAM: a Monte Carlo code to simulate radiotherapy units," *Med. Phys.* **22** (5), 503-524 (1995).

[13]J.V. Siebers, P.J. Keall, B. Libby *et al.*, "A Monte Carlo System for Radiotherapy Dose Calculations: Integration Issues," *Med. Phys.* Submitted, October (1999).

[14]J.V. Siebers, P.J. Keall, A.E. Nahum *et al.*, "Converting absorbed dose to medium to absorbed dose to water for Monte Carlo-based photon beam dose calculations," *Phys. Med. Biol.* Accepted for publication Dec (1999).

[15]P.J. Keall, J.V. Siebers, R. Jeraj *et al.*, "The effect of dose calculation uncertainty on the evaluation of radiotherapy plans," *Med. Phys.* Accepted for publication (1999).

[16]P.J. Keall, J.V. Siebers, and R Mohan, *Acceptance testing and commissioning tests for a Monte Carlo-based photon dose calculation algorithm*, Medical College of Virginia Internal Report, 1999.

[17]Ahnesjö, "Collapsed cone convolution of radiant energy for photon dose calculation
in heterogeneous media," *Med. Phys.* **16** (4), 577-592 (1989).

[18]J.E. Munzenrider, A.P. Brown, J.C.H. Chu *et al.*, "Numerical Scoring of Treatment Plans," *International Journal of Radiation Oncology, Biology and Physics* **21** (May), 147-163 (1991).

[19]A. Niemierko, "Treatment Evaluation," in *Teletherapy: Present and Future*, edited by T.R. Mackie and J.R. Palta (Advanced Medical Publishing, Madison, WI, 1996).

# On the evaluation and implementation of efficient sampling algorithms for Monte Carlo based dose calculation

**Indrin J Chetty[1], John J DeMarco[1], Timothy D Solberg[1]**

[1]UCLA Department of Radiation Oncology, 200 UCLA Medical Plaza, Suite B-265, Los Angeles, CA, 90095

## Introduction

Despite its unparalleled accuracy for dose calculation in heterogeneous media, the Monte Carlo method is typically regarded as a "pie in the sky" approach for radiotherapy dosimetry studies. This opinion is fueled by the fact that a Monte Carlo treatment planning calculation may take up to several days to produce a statistically meaningful result. The availability of faster processor speeds and parallel processing, however, may soon make feasible the widespread implementation of Monte Carlo methods for clinical treatment planning. Several groups are currently actively pursuing the use of Monte Carlo methods for a wide variety of dosimetry studies. These include: the OMEGA/BEAM group at the NRCC, Stanford University Department of Radiation Oncology, Lawrence Livermore Peregrine Project, Memorial Sloan Kettering Department of Radiation Oncology and, the UCLA Department of Radiation Oncology. At the UCLA Department of Radiation Oncology, clinical treatment planning for research purposes is presently being conducted using an MCNP4B-based photon phase space source model that has been integrated with a commercially available treatment planning system [1,2]. Treatment plans are carried out using a networked configuration of 10 to 14 Windows NT (300 Mhz) machines setup to run the calculations in parallel, resulting in a processing time of between 8 and 10 hours for a treatment simulation with average sized ports (10x10 cm$^2$). This study focuses on the evaluation and implementation of effective sampling algorithms to improve the efficiency of the Monte Carlo calculation. Several areas were investigated including discrete probability distribution sampling, photon transport techniques, such as delta-scattering, and efficient random number generation.

### Material and methods

### Discrete probability sampling

The phase space source model that is used for Monte Carlo treatment planning calculations samples a discrete cumulative distribution function (CDF) for photon fluence because varying beam intensities, as encountered with intensity modulated beams cannot be accurately represented with continuous, parametric functions. The photon fluence grid consists of discrete fluence bins that may be adjusted to simulate a physical radiation distribution. Random sampling of discrete distributions may be accomplished using the inverse transform method. The inverse transform method for sampling a discrete distribution involves a sequential search through the CDF to find the smallest value of $i$ such that: $\sum_{i=1}^{n} P(i) \geq \xi$ where $\sum_{i=1}^{n} P(i)$ is the CDF, $\xi$ a uniform random deviate on the interval [0,1], and $i$ the bin index. If the number of bins is large, then the overhead associated with sequentially searching for a value that satisfies the above inequality becomes excessive, thereby reducing the efficiency of the inverse transform solution.

Chen et al [3] proposed an algorithm that increases the efficiency of the sequential search by use of an index table to search a subset of the given distribution. The algorithm first calculates $m$ integer values (cut-points) based on the values in the CDF. The range of the integers therefore extends between 1 and $n$, where $n$ represents the total number of bins in the discrete CDF. For each sample, the algorithm randomly selects an integer value (cut-point) and begins the sequential search at that point in the CDF, reducing the number of comparisons for generating the random sample.

### Photon transport schemes

The probability distribution function for photons interacting in a homogeneous medium is given by: $P(R) = \mu e^{-\mu R}$, where $\mu$ is the mass attenuation coefficient of the medium and $R$ the distance between successive collisions. Conventional Monte Carlo algorithms transport photons by first calculating the distance to next collision, $R$, using the inverse transform solution of the above equation: $R = -\frac{Ln\xi}{\mu}$, where $\xi$ represents a uniform random number on the interval [0, 1]. The photon's distance to nearest boundary crossing, $B$, is calculated based on the particle's position and direction cosines. A comparison is made between $B$ and the distance to next collision, $R$. If $R$ is less than $B$, there is a collision within the current cell and the appropriate sub-routines are called for interaction type and secondary particle production. If $R$ is greater than $B$, the particle's position is updated to the nearest boundary crossing and a new $R$ is calculated. The major drawback of this method is that as the lattice voxel size is decreased, the algorithm spends more time tracking the position of photons as opposed to producing and tracking secondary electrons and photons. This is an expected result given that a typical 6 MV photon travels an average distance of approximately 20 cm before interacting in a water phantom. The efficiency of conventional photon tracking is also reduced for smaller voxel sizes due to the increased number of boundary crossings.

Woodcock et al [4] describe an algorithm that significantly increases photon tracking efficiency by eliminating voxel boundary checking. The algorithm is used to transport neutral particles through a heterogeneous phantom composed of optically thin geometry regions. A majorant cross-section, $\mu_{max}$, representing the largest cross-section of all materials in the geometry, is selected. $\mu_{max}$ is defined to be the sum of real and imaginary cross-sections : $\mu_{max} = \mu + \mu_i$, where $\mu$ represents the cross-section for a physical (real) interaction, while $\mu_i$ denotes the cross-section for an imaginary interaction. An imaginary interaction is one in which the photon's energy and direction remain unchanged. The photon's distance to next collision is calculated using the relation : $x_{n+1} = x_n + \left(\frac{-Ln\xi}{\mu_{max}}\right)\omega_x$ ,where $x_n$ is the starting location, $x_{n+1}$ the new location, $\omega_x$ the direction cosine assuming travel in the *x*-direction, and $\xi$ a uniform random deviate $\in$ [0, 1]. A rejection game is played where a location is accepted as a real collision site if $\xi \le \frac{\mu_{n+1}}{\mu_{max}}$. If $\xi > \frac{\mu_{n+1}}{\mu_{max}}$ then the collision is imaginary and the particle's position is updated to the $(n+1)^{th}$ location with no change in energy or direction. The probability for a real collision is therefore $\frac{\mu_{n+1}}{\mu_{max}}$, while that for an imaginary collision is $1-\frac{\mu_{n+1}}{\mu_{max}}$.

## Results and discussion

### Discrete probability sampling

The inverse transform and cutpoint methods were compared as independent subroutines as well as in the context of the complete Monte Carlo simulation. Three probability distributions with 40, 400, and 6400 discrete bins were used for sampling purposes. The time to generate 1 x $10^7$ random samples from each distribution was determined for each algorithm. This data is reflected in Table 1. The cut point method ranged from being 3 times more efficient for the 40 bin distribution to 350 times more efficient for the 6400 bin distribution.

A timing benchmark was made to compare the performance of the cut point method with the inverse transform method in the complete Monte Carlo simulation. The source sampling distribution consisted of 102,400 (320x320) discrete probability bins representing the integrated photon fluence from the Philips SL-25, 6 MV, linear accelerator treatment head. The simulation geometry consisted of a cylindrical water phantom, with 1 cm diameter, 2 mm thick tally cells, setup to score central axis depth dose. Based on 1x$10^6$ histories, the simulation time required for the inverse transform method was 64.4 minutes while that for the cut point method was 17.2 minutes. The Monte Carlo simulation efficiency is therefore increased by a factor of four using the cut point method.

| Number of bins in probability distribution | Sampling Algorithm | Time (minutes) per 1x$10^7$ random samples |
|---|---|---|
| 40 | Inverse Transform | 0.73 |
| | Cut-point method (20 cut-points) | 0.25 |
| 400 | Inverse Transform | 5.45 |
| | Cut-point method (200 cut-points) | 0.25 |
| 6400 | Inverse Transform | 92.17 |
| | Cut-point method (5000 cut-points) | 0.28 |

**Table 1:** Timing comparison for the *cut-point*, *inverse transform* and methods for generating 1x$10^7$ random samples from discrete probability distributions with variable bin sizes..

### Photon Transport Schemes

The delta-scattering and conventional algorithms were compared as independent sub-routines and also in the context of the complete Monte Carlo simulation. A standard C-code was written to track primary particles only and the history was terminated after the first collision. The geometry consisted of a spherical phantom of radius 100 cm, segmented into 200 annuli, each with 5 mm thickness composed of five different materials ranging from lung to cortical bone. A 2 MeV, monoenergetic, isotropically directed photon source was located at the center of the phantom. The total number of photons crossing each annulus was scored to compare the accuracy of the delta-scattering transport versus conventional tracking. Table 2 shows the times required by the delta-scattering and conventional algorithms to track 1x$10^6$ photons.

| Photon Tracking Algorithm | Time (Seconds) Heterogeneous Geometry |
|---|---|
| Conventional | 93 |
| Delta-Scattering | 16 |

**Table 2:** Timing comparison of the conventional and delta-scattering transport schemes for transporting 1 x $10^6$ histories through a series of overlapping spheres, defined in a standard C routine.

It is noted that the delta-scattering method is approximately 6 times faster than the conventional method for the heterogeneous geometry. Figure1 illustrates the comparison of the delta-scattering simulation versus conventional calculation for attenuation through the heterogeneous geometry.

The results illustrate that the *delta-scattering* photon tracking scheme is equivalent to analytical exponential attenuation. By simulating a real or imaginary collision at every evaluation point, the delta-scattering method bypasses individual voxel boundary checking, thereby creating a very efficient transport scheme.

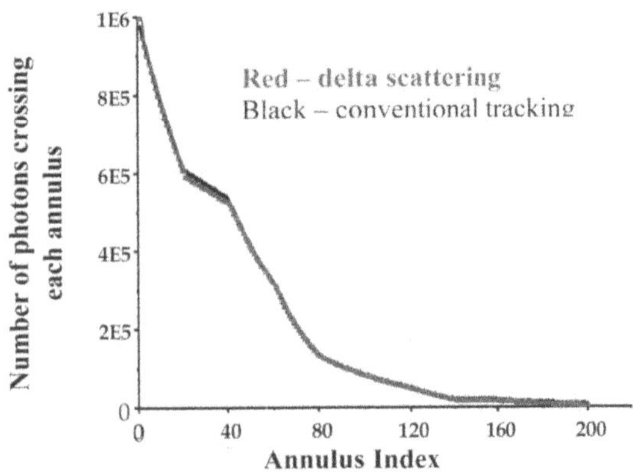


**Figure 1.** Accuracy comparison of the delta-scattering versus conventional tracking schemes for a C-code simulation consisting of primary beam attenuation in the heterogeneous geometry. The total number of particles crossing a given annulus is plotted as a function of the annulus index

A code modification was incorporated into the MCNP code to to evaluate the differences between the delta scattering and conventional tracking scheme in the complete Monte Carlo simulation. A 30x30x30 $cm^3$ water phantom was setup with a tracking plane consisting of 128x128x1 elements. The phase space source model, located at a distance of 100 cm from the phantom isocenter, was used for the simulation source description. Figure 2 represents a plot of the timing ratio of the conventional transport versus the delta-scattering method to track 1 x $10^5$ photon histories as a function of lattice cell size.

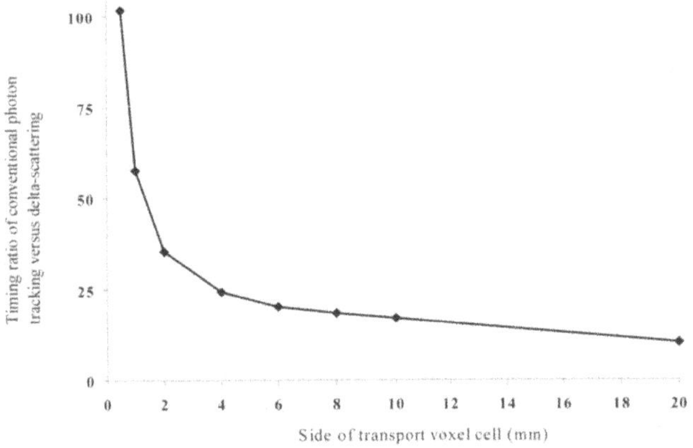


**Figure 2.**. Speedup of the delta-scattering photon tracking scheme relative to conventional transport as a function of the transport voxel cell size. For a typical tracking voxel size of 0.2x0.2x0.2 $cm^3$, the delta-scattering scheme is roughly 35 times more efficient than the conventional transport method.

It is worthy to note that the while the tracking time for the conventional method increased exponentially as the voxel size is reduced, the tracking time for the delta-scattering method remained constant as a function of voxel size. This is attributed to the increased overhead associated with boundary checking for conventional transport as the voxel size is reduced, which is contrary to delta-scattering where there is no boundary checking. The efficiency of delta-scattering transport relative to conventional transport, therefore, increases exponentially as the voxel cell size is reduced.

**Psuedo-random number generation**

We are also presently evaluating several psuedo-random number generators with respect to efficiency and accuracy [5]. These include a standard multiplicative congruential algorithm, and a generator based upon a subtractive method. Preliminary results show that the subtractive algorithm is roughly 15% more efficient than the random number generator used in the MCNP Monte Carlo code. Given that the random number generator is the most frequently called function in the Monte Carlo simulation, it is envisaged that further research in this area may produce notable increases in the calculation efficiency.

## Conclusion

Several efficient Monte Carlo algorithms were compared and tested as specific routines and in the context of a complete Monte Carlo simulation. In particular, algorithms were evaluated for: the generalized sampling of a discrete distribution, photon tracking, and psuedo-random number generation. Integration of the efficient algorithms with the MCNP transport code provided valuable insights with regard to areas where the code has the largest overhead. It is seen, for example, that relative to source sampling, the code spends an insignificant amount of time generating a single random sample. Photon tracking, on the other hand, requires significantly more time than source sampling. It can be concluded that efficient sampling algorithms may be used to increase the efficiency of the Monte Carlo simulation by at least an order of magnitude over conventional sampling methods.

## References

[1] DeMarco JJ, Solberg TD, and Smathers JB 1998. A CT-based Monte Carlo dosimetry tool for radiotherapy treatment planning and analysis. *Medical Physics* **25**:1-11.

[2] Chetty I, DeMarco JJ, Solberg TD 2000. A virtual source model for Monte Carlo modeling of arbitrary intensity distributions. (in press) *Medical Physics*, January.

[3] Chen HC, Asau Y. On generating random variates from an empirical distribution 1974. *AIIE Transactions* **6**:163-166.

[4] Woodcock ER, Murphy T, Hemmings PJ, Longworth SC 1965. Techniques used in the GEM code for Monte Carlo neutronics calculations. *Proc. on the Conf. Applications of Computing methods to Reactor problems*. ANL-7050 Report, Argonne National Laboratory, 557.

[5] DeMarco JJ, Solberg TD, Chetty I, Smathers JB 1998. Efficient sampling algorithms for Monte Carlo based treatment planning. *Radiation Physics and Chemistry* **53**:229-234.

# Electron Beam Commissioning for Monte Carlo Dose Calculation

**Jun Deng, Steve B. Jiang, Todd Pawlicki, Jinsheng Li and C.-M. Ma**

Department of Radiation Oncology, Stanford University School of Medicine, Stanford,CA 94305, USA

## Introduction

The pencil beam algorithm has been used in most of the current commericial treatment planning systems for electron beam dose calculations [1]. However, due to the inappropriate treatment of electron transport in inhomogeneous phantoms, large discrepancies (10% or more) have been observed between the pencil beam algorithm and the measurements in air cavities and bone [2, 3]. Recently, due to the development of computer technology and the variance reduction techniques, the Monte Carlo method has gained popularity as the most accurate approach for electron as well as photon dose calculations [4, 5, 6, 7]. In particular, the Monte Carlo method can handle electron multiple scattering in the presence of inhomogeneities much more accurately than any existing analytical dose models.

Although Monte Carlo method has unsurpassed accurancy over other models, there are some limitations to its application in the clinic. First, Monte Carlo experience is generally required in order to perform correct Monte Carlo simulations and dose calculations. Secondly, to perform dose calculations using the Monte Carlo method, large phase space files are needed, which contain the detailed information of particles, such as the energy, charge, position, and directions. It is time consuming to generate these phase space files, which puts a great burden on the computer resources in a regular medical institute. Thirdly, it requires large disk space to store the phase space data once they are generated, usually tens of Gigabytes.

To overcome these disadvantages, Ma et al. [8] have developed multiple sources to model the phase space data obtained from the Monte Carlo simulation of clinical linear accerelators. Based on these multiple sources, one can accurately represent and reconstruct each phase space file while keeping the storage requirement low. However, these multiple sources are generated by analyzing the corresponding phase space files, which if not totally impossible, is not practical in the clinic. Therefore, to fully make use of the advantages of the Monte Carlo method for accurate and fast dose calculations in the clinic, an automated beam commissioning procedure is required which depends entirely on the standard measured data of a clinical linear accelerator.

Several studies have been carried out on electron beam modeling and commissioning. Janssen et al. [9] have tried to extract phase space information from limited sets of measured data such as central axis depth dose curves and dose profiles at different surface source distances (SSD). Jiang et al. [10] employed a hrbrid approach to model and commission the clinical electron beams generated from a Varian Clinac 2100C. They utilized the combined information from measurement as well as original full phase space data to generate a four-source model such that they can use one reference accelerator to commission the beams from other linear accelerators of the same type.

In this work, we further develop an automated commissioning procedure for electron beams of arbitrary incident energies generated from different types of linear accelerators currently available for radiotherapy. The procedure is based entirely on the standard measured data to derive the source model parameters.

## Material and methods

Based on our previous Monte Carlo study, we have observed that, for the clinical electron beams, the primary dose contribution comes from the direct electrons which include those not interacting with the beam defining system and those scattered from the primary collimator, jaws and shielding rings. These direct electrons can be approxiamted by a virtual electron point source. The location of the point source can be determined using the pin-hole method.

An electron point source with a proper energy spectrum can give a reasonably accurate depth dose curve. By adding another photon point source, the bremsstrahlung tail in the measured depth dose curve can be reproduced accurately. However, it is found that the penumbra at the phantom surface generated with this two point source model is sharper compared to that generated with the full phase space data due to the lack of scattered electrons from the beam defining components in the linear accelerator. Therefore, scatter sources representing the applicator scrapers are needed in order to account for this effect.

Provided with the central axis percent depth dose (PDD) curve, dose profile at surface and dose profiles at $d_{max}$ for 100 cm SSD and 110 cm SSD for a certain field size and a nominal beam energy, we can commission the electron beam to generate a source parameter file which contains the relative intensity, position, energy distribution and fluence distribution of each source in the model.

The energy spectrum of direct electrons can be determined by fitting the relative weights for central axis PDDs of 100 mono-energetic beams in order to match the measured central axis PDD excluding photon tail. We employ a random creep method together with a smoothening technique to find the best solution, which makes the fitted energy spectrum more realistic as shown in Figure 1 in comparison to the electron energy spectrum obtained from Monte Carlo simulation.

The electron fluence is obtained by fitting the measured surface dose profile to an empirical dose response function. By doing this, we can recover the dose profiles along the major axes as well as along the diagonal field. Figure 2 shows a reconstructed dose profile from the measured dose profile at surface. When transporting onto the phantom surface at 100 cm SSD, the measured dose profiles along major axes and along diagonal are recovered accurately.

While the direct electron energy distribution determines the major part of the central axis PDD, the tail part is mainly due to the bremsstrahlung photons. By discreting the pure electron contribution from the tail in the central axis PDD provided, we can determine the relative photon intensity in our source parameter file.

Once the source parameter file has been created, we run MCDOSE to calculate dose distributions in water phantom and compare with the measurements.

## Results and discussion

Figure 1 shows the energy spectrum comparison for a 6 MeV clinical electron beam. The symbols are obtained using the random creep method while the solid lines are from the Monte Carlo simulations of the electron beams generated from a Varian Clinac 2100C accelerator at Stanford Medical Center. As shown, the fitted spectrum is very close in shape to the Monte Carlo spectrum. The fitted energy spectrum is shifted from the Monte Carlo spectra due to the different $R_{50}$.

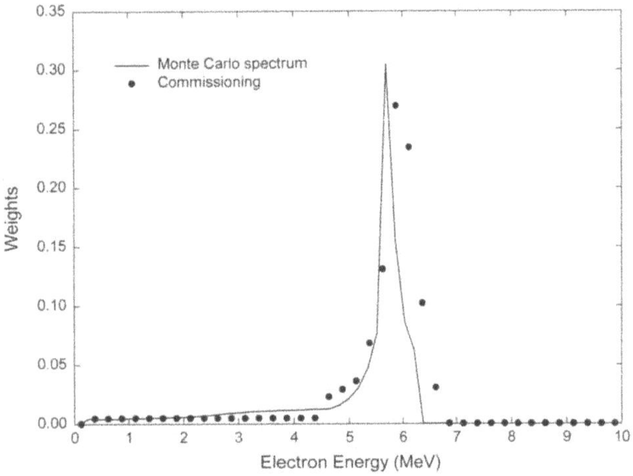


Fig. 1 Energy distribution of the direct electrons of a 6 MeV electron beam. The Monte Carlo simulated energy spectrum serves as a reference.

Figure 2 shows the reconstructed fluence profile for the 6 MeV electron beam with an applicator size of 20 x 20 $cm^2$ defined at 100 cm SSD. Due to the backprojection from the phantom surface to the phase space reconstrcution plane at 94 cm SSD, the fluence profile field size is a little narrower.

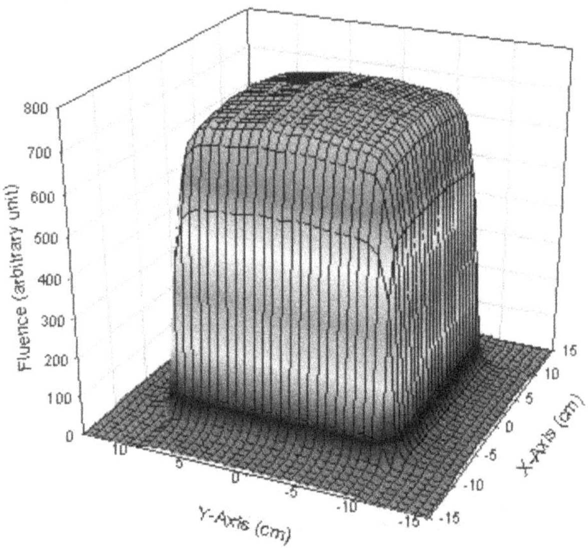


Fig. 2 The reconstructed fluence profile that can recover the measured profile at phantom surface.

The dose distribution compariosn for a 6 MeV electron beam with applicator size 20 x 20 $cm^2$ is shown in Fig. 3. The calculated central axis percent depth dose curve from the commissioning data agrees very well with the measured central axis percent depth dose curve. The dose profiles at different depths of 0.1 cm, 1.3 cm and 2.5 cm show good agreement between the measured and the commissioned data, even in the penumbra region, indicating that our commissioning procedure is suitable for accurate dose calculations clinically.

Similar comparisons have been performed on other electron beam energies with various applicator sizes in order to validate our commissioning procedure. Shown in Fig. 4 is the electron spectrum and dose distributions for a 20 MeV electron beam with applicator size of 10 x 10 $cm^2$. The spectra agreed well between the Monte Carlo simulated phase space and the commissioning data and central axis PDDs agreed very well between the measurements and commissioning results.

## Conclusion

An electron beam commissioning procedure has been proposed and tested using 6 MeV and 20 MeV electron beams for applicator sizes of 20 x 20 and 10 x 10 $cm^2$, respectively. The results have shown that good agreement has been achieved between measurements and the beam commissioning results in central axis PDDs and dose profiles at different depths. The proposed electron beam commissioning procedure is suitable for Monte Carlo electron beam dose calculations in clininal treatment planning systems.

This work is partially supported by NCI Grant No. CA 78331, DOD Grant No. BC971292, RSNA seed grant for radiological research and a consortium agreement with NumeriX, LLC. We would like to thank other members of our Monte Carlo group at Stanford University, Dr. Arthur Boyer, Dr. Gary Luxton and

Dr. Sam Brain for valuable discussions and comments on this work.

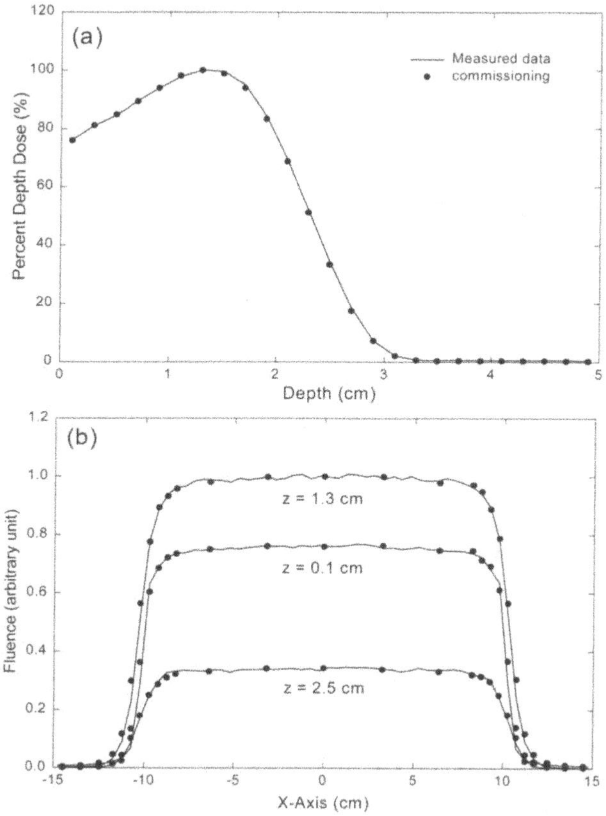


Fig. 3 Dose distribution comparison for a 6 MeV electron beam with applicator size 20 x 20 $cm^2$ between the commissioning results and measurements. The solid lines are the measured data while the symbols are the Monte Carlo calculations with the commissioning data.

## References

[1] Hogstrom K R, Mills M D and Almond P R 1981 Electron beam dose calculations *Phys. Med. Biol.* **26** 445-459.

[2] Cygler J, Battista J J, Scrimger J W, Mah E, and Antolak J 1987 Electron dose distributions in experimental phantoms: a comparison with 2D pencil beam calculations *Phys. Med. Biol.* **32** 1073-1086.

[3] Mah E, Antolak J, Scrimger J W, and Battista J J 1989 Experimental evaluation of a 2D and a 3D electron pencil beam algorithm *Phys. Med. Biol.* **34** 1179-1194.

[4] Jenkins T M, Nelson W R, Rindi A, Nahum A E and Rogers D W O *Monte Carlo transport of electrons and photons*, Plenum Press, New York, 1988.

[5] Mackie T R Applications of the Monte Carlo method in radiotherapy. In Kase K, Bjarngard B and Attix F H, editors, *Vol III of Dosimetry of Ionizing Radiation*, 541-620, Academic Press, New York, 1990.

[6] Rogers D W O and Bielajew A F Monte Carlo techniques of electron and photon transport for radiation dosimetry. In Kase K, Bjarngard B and Attix F H, editors, *Vol III of Dosimetry of Ionizing Radiation*, 427-539, Academic Press, New York, 1990.

[7] Andreo P 1991 Monte Carlo techniques in medical radiation physics *Phys. Med. Biol.* **36** 861-920.

[8] Ma C-M, Faddegon B A, Rogers D W O, and Mackie T R 1997 Accurate characterization of Monte Carlo calculated electron beams for radiotherapy *Med. Phys.* **24** 401-416.

[9] Janssen J J, Korevaar E W, van Battum L J, Storchi P R M, and Huizenga H 1997 Clinical Electron Beam Dose Calculations with the Phase Space Evolution Model *Procedings of The 12$^{th}$ International Conference on The Use of Computers in Radiation Therapy* Salt Lake City, Utah, USA 195-196.

[10] Jiang S B, Kapur A and Ma C-M 2000 Electron Beam Modeling and Commissioning for Monte Carlo Treatment Planning *Med. Phys.* **27**, 1111-22.

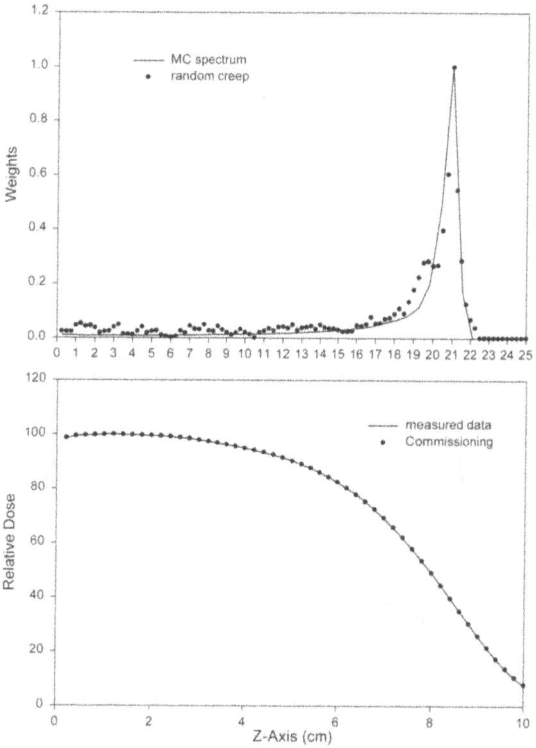


Fig. 4 Spectrum and dose distribution comparison for a 20 MeV electron beam with applicator size 10 x 10 $cm^2$ between the commissioning results and measurements. The solid lines are the measured data while the symbols are the Monte Carlo calculations with the commissioning data.

# Modeling and Commissioning of Clinical Photon Beams for Monte Carlo Treatment Planning

**Steve B. Jiang, Jun Deng, Jisheng Li, Todd Pawlicki, Arthur L. Boyer and C.-M. Ma**
Department of Radiation Oncology, Stanford University School of Medicine, Stanford, CA 94305-5304, USA

## Introduction

Monte Carlo treatment planning requires accurate beam information as input to generate accurate dose distributions. The phase space data of a clinical photon beam can be obtained by simulating the accelerator treatment head using a Monte Carlo code, such as BEAM [1-2]. The simulated phase space data (or the subsequently derived multiple source model) can be used for Monte Carlo treatment planning dose calculation [3]. However, it is not practical to simulate every individual clinical photon beam in a routine clinic [4-5].

In this work, we develop an efficient procedure to model and commission clinical photon beams for Monte Carlo treatment planning. A three-source model is used to represent clinical photon beams. Parameters in the model are extracted from standard measured data. The proposed procedure has been applied to, and tested for, 6 and 15 MV beams from a Varian Clinac 2300CD machine.

## Material and methods

### Clinical photon beam representation

A clinical photon beam mainly consists of three types of particles, *i.e.*, primary photons (those coming directly from the target to the patient), scattered photons, and contaminant electrons. Accordingly, the beam can be represented with a three-source model including a point source for primary photons, an extrafocal source for scattered photons, and an extended source for contaminant electrons.

The point source for primary photons is assumed to be located at the target. The off-axis softening effect and horn effect are taken into account for primary photons. For primary photons, both the energy spectrum and planar fluence are a function of radial distance from the central axis.

The scattered photons are mainly from the flattening filter and primary collimator. We model all scattered photons using a planar source which is located at the bottom of the flattening filter and referred to as the extrafocal source [6]. An important assumption is that the extrafocal source plane emits photons isotropically. The source intensity distribution at the extrafocal plane is assumed to be peaked at the central axis and monotonically decreasing with the off-axis distance. Therefore, it can be approximated by a series of Gaussian functions. The number of Gaussians can vary for different machines and beam energies. One energy spectrum is assumed for all scattered photons.

The monitor chamber backscatter is also accounted for in the model. We assume that the backscattered radiation to the monitor chamber has a linear relationship with the irradiated area of the jaw's upper surface.

We assume a planar source with uniform intensity distribution for contaminant electrons. All contaminant electrons are assumed to have same energy spectrum.

### Clinical photon beam reconstruction

During Monte Carlo dose calculation for treatment planning, we need to reconstruct the beam phase space using the model. At the sampling plane, we determine each particle's position, direction, energy, and weight from the model.

First, we determine the source from which source the particle has originated. This is done by sampling from the relative weights of sources. Then, we sample the particle's phase space using that source just determined.

If a photon originates from the point source, the procedure to determine its phase space on the sampling plane is as follows:

1. Determine the photon's position on the sampling plane.
2. Draw a rayline from the point source to photon's position on the sampling plane, which gives the photon's direction.
3. Determine the photon's energy based on its position on the sampling plane.
4. Find the relative planar fluence at the photon's position on the sampling plane and use it as the photon's weight.

If a photon is from the extrafocal source, the sampling procedure is as follows:

1. Determine from which Gaussian the photon is from.
2. Determine emitting position on the extrafocal plane.
3. Determine the position on the sampling plane.
4. Draw a line from the emitting position on the extrafocal plane to the position on the sampling plane, which gives the photon's direction.
5. Sample the energy from the energy spectrum and determine the weight.

For contaminant electrons, their transport in air from the source plane to the sampling plane can be handled with the Fermi-Eyges theory. The sampling procedure for a contaminant electron is as follows:

1. Determine the electron's initial position and direction on the sampling plane by projecting from the source plane directly.
2. Sample the electron's energy from the energy spectrum.
3. Perturb the electron's position and direction on the sampling plane around the initial position and direction using the Fermi-Eyges theory [7].

The beam model is used with an in-house developed EGS4

user code called MCDOSE [8]. For each particle, a weight is given according to the monitor unit, calibration factor, and monitor chamber backscatter factor. Therefore, the absolute dose value (in cGy) is given by a MCDOSE simulation.

### Clinical photon beam commissioning

To commission a clinical photon beam using our source model, we need to determine unknown parameters in the model for the beam. These parameters include the energy spectra for primary photons, scattered photons, and contaminant electrons, the relative planar fluence distribution for primary photons, the relative source intensity distribution for scattered photons, and the relative weight and position of the electron source.

We obtain the photon beam energy spectrum by fitting the measured percent depth dose (PDD) curve in water using the pre-calculated PDD curves for monoenergetic beams. It is important to note that the PDD is not sensitive to the energy spectrum at the phantom surface. Thus, fitted energy spectrum may be physically unrealistic (*i.e.*, negative fluence, more than one peak, *etc.*) even though it gives a good match to the measured PDD. To avoid these problems, we use the log-normal function to represent a photon beam energy spectrum. Using the least $\chi^2$ fitting method, the unknown parameters in the energy spectrum are determined by matching the calculated PDD with the measured PDD. We also add a constraint to peak energy position to make sure it is reasonable. The fitting is performed using the grid search method.

The measured central axis PDD for the 10×10 cm$^2$ field size and 100 cm SSD is used to determine the central axis spectrum for primary photons. The off-axis PDDs (obtained from the measured dose profiles for the maximum field size at several depths) are used to fit the off-axis energy spectra of primary photons. The off-axis energy spectra are fitted up to 10 cm off-axis distance. For off-axis distance larger than 10 cm, the energy spectra are obtained through the extrapolation of the fitted parameters. The energy spectra for the scattered photons and contaminant electrons are approximated with the central axis spectrum for primary photons.

The relative planar fluence distribution for primary photons at the phantom surface is extracted from the measured dose profile at $d_{max}$ in water. This is done by considering the variations of the energy spectrum and the mass energy absorption coefficient with the off-axis distance.

Using the model for extrafocal source and monitor chamber backscatter, the relative in-air output factor, $S_c$, can be calculated analytically [6]. The parameters in the model are then determined by fitting the calculated $S_c$values with the measured ones for three sets of field sizes, which are square fields from 4×4 cm$^2$ to 40×40 cm$^2$, and rectangular fields with one pair of jaws at fixed opening of 10 cm and the other pair moving from 4 cm to 40 cm.

The electron surface dose, defined at the central axis and depth of 5 mm, is calculated by subtracting the calculated photon surface dose from the measured surface dose for several field sizes from 4×4 cm$^2$ to 40×40 cm$^2$. The position of the electron source plane is determined by fitting the electron fluence at the sampling plane, which is calculated using the Fermi-Eyges theory, to the electron surface dose for selected field sizes [7]. The relative weight of the electron source is obtained by comparing the calculated with the extracted electron surface dose for the same MU.

## Results and discussion

The proposed procedure has been applied to 6 MV and 15 MV beams from a Varian Clinac 2300C/D accelerator. Figure 1 shows the central axis energy spectra for primary photons for both beams and the comparison with the responding Monte Carlo simulations. The Monte Carlo simulations were performed using the EGS4/BEAM code for the entire accelerator treatment head. To check the off-axis spectra, we also compared the mean energy as a function of off-axis distance with the Monte Carlo data, as shown in figure 2. We can see that, using the current approach, central axis and off-axis spectra can be extracted accurately from the standard measured data.

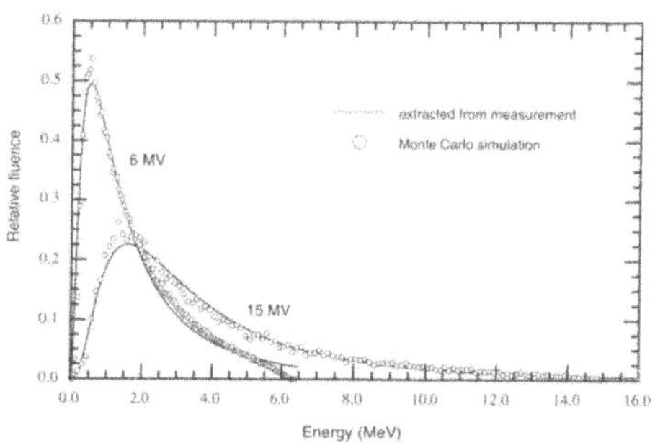


**Figure 1:** Central axis energy spectra for primary photons for 6 and 15 MV beams. Solid lines are spectra extracted from measured PDD using the proposed approach. Open circles are the Monte Carlo simulations using BEAM.

For each beam, the model is calibrated once the measurement using the dose values at 10 cm depth for the 10×10 cm$^2$ field. Table 1 gives the dose for both 6 and 15 MV beams at 10 cm depth for field sizes from 5×5 cm$^2$ to 40×40 cm$^2$ and the comparison with measured data. It can be seen that the current approach will predict the beam output within 1%.

The calculated dose distributions in water are also compared with the measurement and good agreement (within 1% or 1 mm) has been observed. Figure 3 shows the calculated and measured 15 MV depth dose curves in water for a few field sizes and at 100 cm SSD.

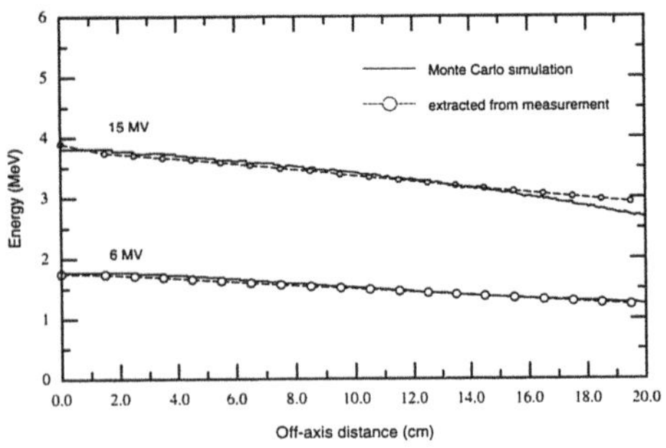


**Figure 2:** Primary photon mean energy as a function of off-axis distance for 6 and 15 MV beams. Solid lines with open circles are extracted from the measured central axis and off-axis PDDs. Histograms are the Monte Carlo simulations using BEAM

| field size ($cm^2$) | beam 6 MV | 15 MV |
|---|---|---|
| 5×5 | 0.604(0.3%) | 0.723(0.9%) |
| 10×10 | 0.674(0.1%) | 0.774(0.1%) |
| 20×20 | 0.743(0.4%) | 0.818(0.5%) |
| 30×30 | 0.782(0.8%) | 0.844(0.3%) |
| 40×40 | 0.799(0.4%) | 0.859(0.3%) |

**Table 1:** The calculated dose values (cGy/MU) at 10 cm depth in water for both 6 and 15 MV beams. The difference from the measurement is given in parenthesis.

## Conclusion

A practical procedure has been developed to model and commission clinical photon beams for Monte Carlo treatment planning. A clinical photon beam is represented with a three-source model including a primary photon point source, a scattered photon extrafocal source, and an electron extended source. All the source parameters can be determined using the standard measured data. The methods to represent a clinical photon beam using the proposed beam model, to determine the model parameters, and to sample the beam phase space from the model during Monte Carlo treatment planning, have been discussed. The accuracy of the model for the calculation of absolute and relative dose distributions in water has been demonstrated to be within 1% or 1mm. The proposed procedure has been implemented for Monte Carlo treatment planning using a newly-developed Monte Carlo code (MCDOSE).

### Acknowledgements

The work was supported in part by the US Army breast cancer research program (BC971292), the NCI grant CA78331, and a consortium agreement with the NumeriX, LLC.

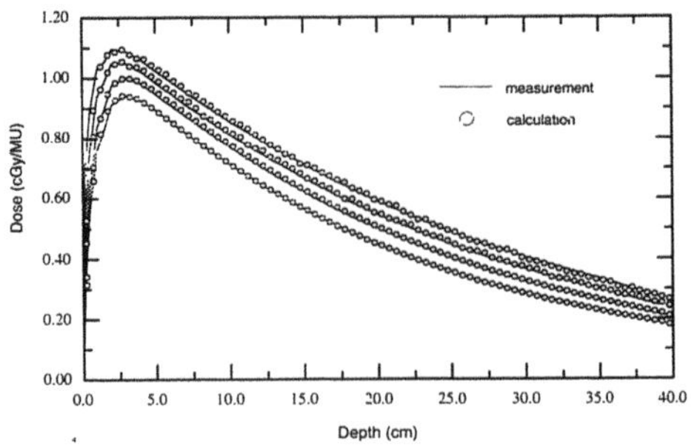


**Figure 3:** Depth dose curves in water for the 15 MV beam. Solid lines are measured data and open circles are calculated using the current beam model with the MCDOSE code.

## References

[1] Rogers D W O, Faddengon B A, Ding G X, Ma C M, We J and Mackie T R 1995 BEAM: A Monte Carlo code to simulate radiotherapy treatment units *Med. Phys.* **22** 503–524

[2] Ma C M and Jiang S B 1999 Monte Carlo modeling of electron beams from medical accelerators *Phys. Med. Bio.* **44** R156–R188

[3] Ma C M, Faddegon B A, Rogers D W O and Mackie T R 1997 Accurate characterization of Monte Carlo calculated electron beams for radiotherapy *Med. Phys.* **24** 401–416

[4] Jiang S B, Kapur A and Ma C M 2000 Electron beam modeling and commissioning for Monte Carlo treatment planning *Med. Phys.* **27** (in press)

[5] Deng J, Jiang S B, Kapur A, Li J S, Pawlicki T and Ma C M 2000 Photon beam characterization and modeling for Monte Carlo treatment planning *Phys. Med. Bio.* **45** (in press)

[6] Jiang S B, Boyer A L and Ma C M 2000 Modeling the extrafocal radiation and monitor chamber backscatter for photon beam dose calculation *Med. Phys.* **27** (accepted)

[7] Jiang S B, Luo Z M and Ayyangar K M 1998 Incorporation of the electron energy-loss straggling into the Fermi-Eyges equation *Rad. Phys. Chem.* **53** 477–482

[8] Ma C M, Pawlicki T, Li J S, Jiang S B, Deng J, Kapur A, Mok E, Luxton G and Boyer A L 1999 MCDOSE - A dose calculation tool for radiotherapy treatment planning *Med. Phys.* **26** 1148 (abstract)

# Simulation of Beam Modifiers for Monte Carlo Treatment Planing

J. S. Li, T. Pawlicki, J. Deng, S. B. Jiang and C.-M. Ma

Radiation Oncology Department, Stanford University School of Medicine, Stanford, CA 94305, USA

## Introduction

Beam modifiers, such as jaws, wedges, blocks, compensator, multi-leaf collimator (MLC), electron cutout and bolus need to be considered when the Monte Carlo method is applied to dose calculation in radiation therapy treatment planning. The most accurate method is to simulate particle transport in each beam modifier using the Monte Carlo method. The EGS4 [1] user code BEAM [2] was designed to perform treatment head simulations. Once the phase space data is obtained at the distal face of a beam modifier, another dose calculation tool, like DOSXYZ [3], is needed to perform the dose calculation in a phantom or a patient built from CT data. This two-step method works well but is not convenient. It requires additional time to perform the two-step simulation and large storage space for the temporary phase space data produced after the first step simulation. This is not suitable for routine clinical dose calculations. In this work we have implemented beam modifiers in an EGS4 user code called MCDOSE [4,5].

## Material and methods

MCDOSE is specially designed for clinical dose calculations for radiotherapy treatment planning. It has some special features, such as beam phase space reconstruction using source models, inclusion of beam modifiers in patient-specific simulations, implementation of several variance reduction techniques and forward dose calculation for intensity modulated radiation therapy (IMRT).

For photon beams, our multiple source models [6] cover all the fixed components above the jaws in the accelerator head. The beam modifiers considered in the MCDOSE code are those typically found in clinical use, namely, -jaws, wedges, blocks, compensators, MLCs and boluses. For electron beams, the multiple source models [7] cover all the components down to the applicator. Only the last scrapers, electron cutouts and boluses need to be considered. The source model parameters were derived from the phase space data simulated using the EGS4/BEAM system and verified using the measured beam data [8].

The jaws are modeled as two pairs of bars in X and Y dimension. The inner edges of bars focus to the target. The input parameters for jaws are only X1, X2, Y1, Y2 for the inner opening and the jaw material. The dimensions correspond to the jaw opening projected at the isocenter (at 100cm source-to-surface distance (SSD)).

Wedges are accurately simulated by MCDOSE using information input by the user. The required parameters are the wedge orientation, location, material and the two dimensional point coordinates to specify its shape. This approach is similar to wedge definition for conventional dose calculation algorithms, except that for one important point. For the Monte Carlo approach, the user enters the exact wedge specifications without any modifications or adjustments in the parameters so that the final dose calculation matches the measured dose profiles of the wedge under consideration. Thus, in our Monte Carlo approach, the physical transport of particles in the beam modifiers and the reproduction of the phase space must be accurate to obtain good agreement with measured results.

Both the treatment block and tray are simulated by MCDOSE. The location, thickness and material of the block and tray are required. The location was defined using the distance between target and the distal surface of the block tray. The user also needs to specify the opening by giving the coordinates of the vertices of the blocked portion of the beam at 100 cm SSD. The planes defining the inner surfaces of the block opening were divergent with a point source as is the case for the actual block at the linac. Compared with BEAM, the advantage of MCDOSE is that we do not need to divide the opening into subregions. The user inputs the points continuously around the perimeter of the opening. To speed up the simulation, the range rejection technique was applied in the code. The effects on the dose results are less than 1% when compared to a full BEAM simulation.

The compensator and tray are simulated by MCDOSE. The location, material and the thickness of the compensator and tray are required. The compensator was divided into different bins in X and Y directions. The X-Y coordinate and thickness for each bin are required.

Electron cutouts are handled similarly to the blocks. But it does not have the tray and the inner planes to define the opening are straight and parallel to the beam axis. However, we have also included the option to have a diverging electron block for those clinics using that approach. The location, material and coordinates of every vertex to specify the opening are required.

The bolus is simulated by adding extra layer of material to the patient's geometry (outside the patient external contour) according to the bolus's material and thickness.

## Results

### Wedge

The dose distribution of a 45° wedge (10 cm x 10 cm jaw setting and 100 cm SSD) in a water phantom was calculated by MCDOSE. The material of the wedge was lead. A 15 MV photon beam with a 20cm × 20cm field above the jaws from a Varian Clinac 2300C/D machine was used as source input. A comparison calculation was performed using BEAM plus DOSXYZ under the same conditions. Figure 1 shows the isodose distribution in the X-Z plane through the central axis. The agreement between the results of MCDOSE and BEAM plus DOSXYZ is within 1%. The CPU time required for this wedged beam simulation was only about 35% of that required for a 10cm × 10cm open beam.

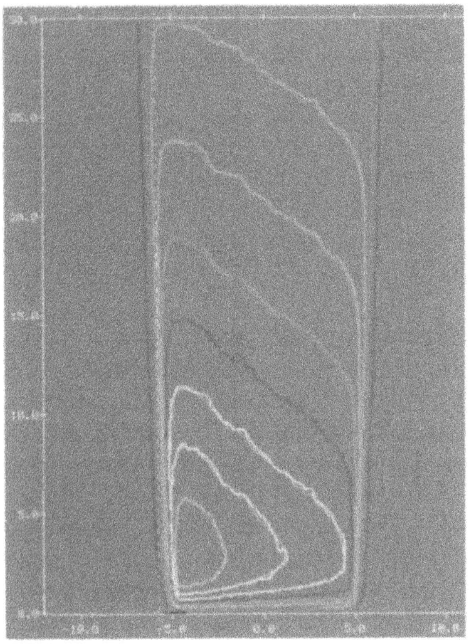

**Figure 1:** Comparisons of the isodose distribution in the X-Z plane through the central axis in a water phantom between MCDOSE (thin lines) and EGS4/BEAM plus DOSXYZ (thick lines). A 45° wedge were simulated for a 15MV photon beam, the field size was 10cm × 10cm defined at 100SSD.

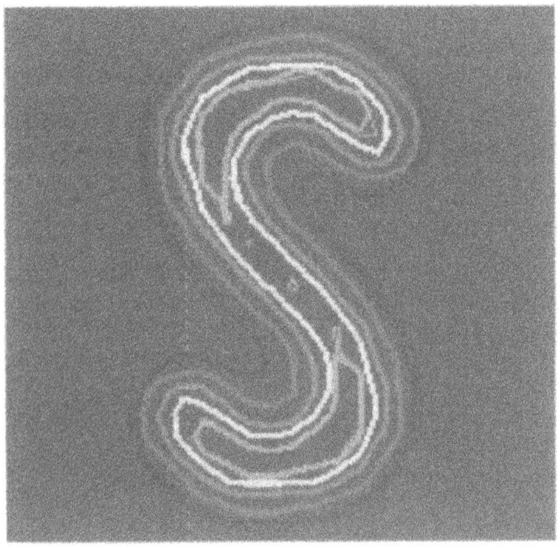

**Figure 2:** The isodose distributions at the depth of the maximum dose in a water phantom for a blocked 15MV photon beam. The field size is 10cm × 10cm defined at 100cm SSD. The block had an S-shaped opening. The simulation results of BEAM (thick lines) and MCDOSE (thin lines) are shown.

## Block

A block with a hypothetical S-shaped opening was simulated by MCDOSE and BEAM respectively. The material of the block was Cerrobend and that of the tray was PMMA. The isodose distributions at $D_{max}$ in a water phantom for a blocked 10cm x 10cm 15MV photon beam are shown in figure 2. A good agreement between them can be observed. The CPU time required for this blocked beam simulation was about 70% of that required for a 10cm × 10cm open beam.

## Compensator

The m-shaped isodose distributions in a water phantom were calculated by MCDOSE and BEAM plus DOSXYZ respectively. In the BEAM simulation, the component modules MLC and SLABS were used to simulate the compensator and the tray. The material of the compensator was copper and the tray material was PMMA. The thickness of the compensator was 2.0 cm except the area denoted by the m-shape where the thickness is 0.5 cm. The results are shown in Figure 3 and excellent agreement can be observed. Comparing to the dose calculation for a 10cm × 10cm open field, 60% extra CPU time was required to do dose calculation with this compensator by MCDOSE.

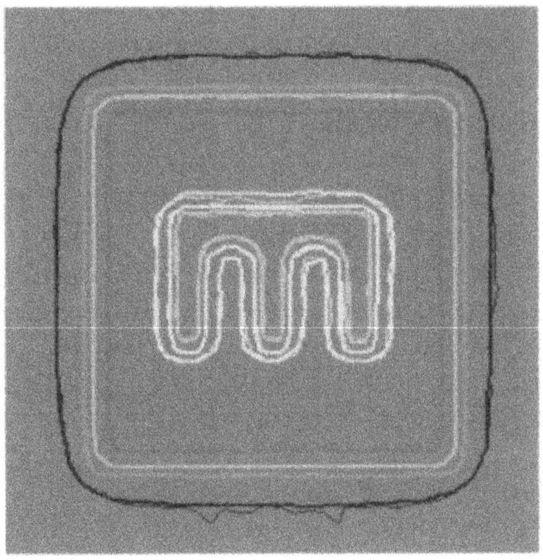

**Figure 3:** The isodose distributions at the depth of the maximum dose in a water phantom for a 10cm × 10cm 15MV photon beam. The beam was modified with a specially designed compensator. The simulation results of BEAM (thick line) and MCDOSE (thin line) are shown.

## Electron Cutout

The dose distributions in a water phantom were calculated using BEAM plus DOSXYZ and MCDOSE for a 12 MeV electron beam with a butterfly-shaped cutout. The material of the cutout was Cerrobend. A phase space of a 10cm x 10cm electron beam above the last scraper from a Varian Clinac 2100C machine was used as source input. Good agreement (within 1%) was achieved between the results of MCDOSE and BEAM. Comparing to the dose calculation for a 10cm x 10cm open field, MCDOSE required a 35% additional CPU time for the dose calculation with this complex butterfly-shaped cutout.

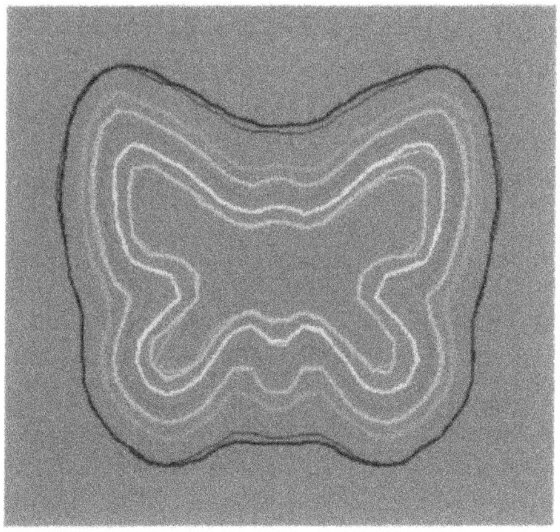

**Figure 4:** The isodose distributions at the depth of the maximum dose in a water phantom for a 10cm × 10cm 12 MeV electron beam. The beam was modified with an electron cutout that had a butterfly-shaped opening. The simulation results of BEAM plus DOSXYZ (thick line) and MCDOSE (thin line) are shown.

**Bolus**

For the same patient phantom, bolus material was added outside the external contour of the patient and dose calculations were performed using DOSXYZ and MCDOSE respectively. The difference found between their results was within the statistical uncertainty of 0.5% of the maximum dose.

## Conclusion

The code for beam modifier simulation in a Monte Carlo dose calculation tool, MCDOSE, was implemented and validated. The simulation results with beam modifiers by MCDOSE were compared with those of EGS4/BEAM plus DOSXYZ. Excellent agreement has been achieved. The CPU time needed by the simulation depends on the type and shape of the beam modifier. Our results demonstrate that MCDOSE simulates beam modifiers accurately and efficiently, and is suitable for clinical dose calculations.

This work is partially supported by NCI Grant No. CA 78331, DOD Grant No. BC971292, RSNA seed grant for radiological research and a consortium agreement with NumeriX, LLC. We would like to thank other members of our Monte Carlo group at Stanford University, Dr. Arthur Boyer, Dr. Gary Luxton and Dr. Sam Brain for valuable discussions and comments on this work. We also like to thank Todd Koumrian and Michael Luxton for their invaluable computer hardware and software support.

## References

[1] Nelson R, Hirayama H and Rogers DWO (1985). The EGS4 code system, Stanford Linear Accelerator Center Report SLAC-265 (SLAC, Stanford, CA)

[2] Rogers DWO, Faddegon BA, Ding GX, Ma C-M, Wei JS, Mackie TR (1995). BEAM: A Monte Carlo code to simulate radiotherapy treatment units. Med. Phys. 22: 503-25.

[3] Ma C-M, Reckwerdt P, Holmes M, Rogers D W O, Geiser B, and Walters B, (1995) *DOSXYZ Users Manual*, NRCC Report No. PIRS-0509B

[4] J. S. Li, T. Pawlicki, J Deng, S.B. Jiang, A. Kapur, E. Mok, C-M Ma (1999). Clinical validation of a Monte Carlo dose calculation tool for radiotherapy treatment planning, Med. Phys. 26 1083 (Abstract)

[5] C-M Ma, T. Pawlicki, J. S. Li, S. B. Jiang, J Deng, S.B. A. Kapur, E. Mok, G. Luxton, A. Boyer (1999). MCDOSE – A dose calculation tool for radiotherapy treatment planning, Med. Phys. 26 1148 (Abstract)

[6] Deng J, Jiang S B, Kapur A, Li J S, Pawlicki T, Ma C-M (2000) Photon beam characterization and modeling for Monte Carlo treatment planning, Phys. Med. Biol. 45 in press

[7] Jiang S B, Kapur A and Ma C-M (2000) Electron beam modeling and commissioning for Monte Carlo treatment planning, Med. Phys. 27 (Jan) in press

[8] Ma C-M, Mok E, Kapur A, Pawlicki T A, Findley D, Brain S, Forster K and Boyer AL (1999) Clinical implementation of a Monte Carlo treatment planning system for radiotherapy, Med. Phys. 26: 2133-43

# Speeding up Monte Carlo simulation of electron cut-outs in treatment planning

**Dr Cephas D Mubata, Dr Frank Verhaegen and Dr Alan E Nahum**

The Royal Marsden NHS Trust, Fulham Road, London, UK

## Introduction

Treatment planning using Monte Carlo technique is becoming increasingly popular. This is especially the case for electron beams, since electrons are directly ionising, so a fewer number of histories are required to attain a given statistical uncertainty compared to photons. On most linear accelerators, there are a finite number of energies and applicators. The only patient dependent beam shaping device then is the electron cut-out at the end of the applicator or on the skin. It is possible to simulate and collect the beam characteristics in terms of phase space data or beam models at the top of the cerrobend or lead cut-outs, (see Figure 1). Simulation of

these cut-outs can be time consuming if variance reduction techniques are not used. These can take the form of sampling from particles inside the block and discarding the ones in the block material, raising the cut-off energies, and range reduction techniques.

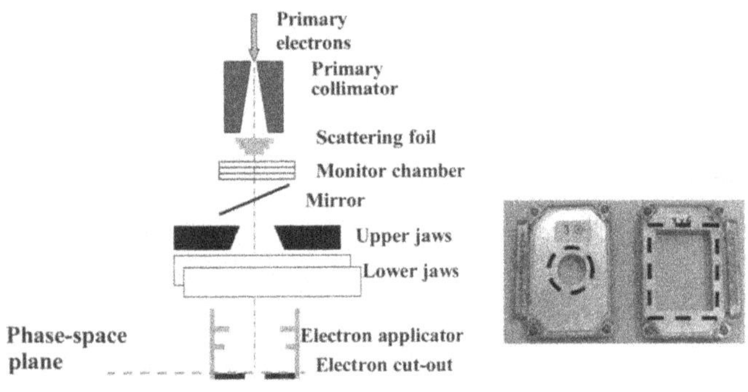


**Figure 1:** Schematic diagram of an electron linac showing the different beam shaping components. Photographs of typical electron cutouts are also shown.

### Aim

The aim of this investigation was to explore the possibility of speeding up MC of electron beams by minimization of time spent simulating beam shaping devices. All the particles with no significant contribution to the end result are discarded. The effect of the different variance reduction techniques on the dose distributions and the output factors was studied.

## Materials and Methods

The calculations were carried out for a Varian 2100C using the BEAM/DOSXYZ Monte Carlo codes, for beam energies between 6 and 20 MeV. Phase space data was calculated to the top of the cut-out for the different electron applicators. Transport of the particles through the cut-out was carried out by introducing a margin or 'skin' region around the block aperture in which the random trajectories where followed. The cut-outs in Fig.1 show the regions (dashed lines) around a circular and a rectangular aperture, in which the particle tracks are followed. Outside these regions the particles were discarded. Dose distributions were calculated using DOSXYZ with the Phase Space data from the block simulations. Relative output factors were calculated for cut-outs with and without particles from the cut-outs.

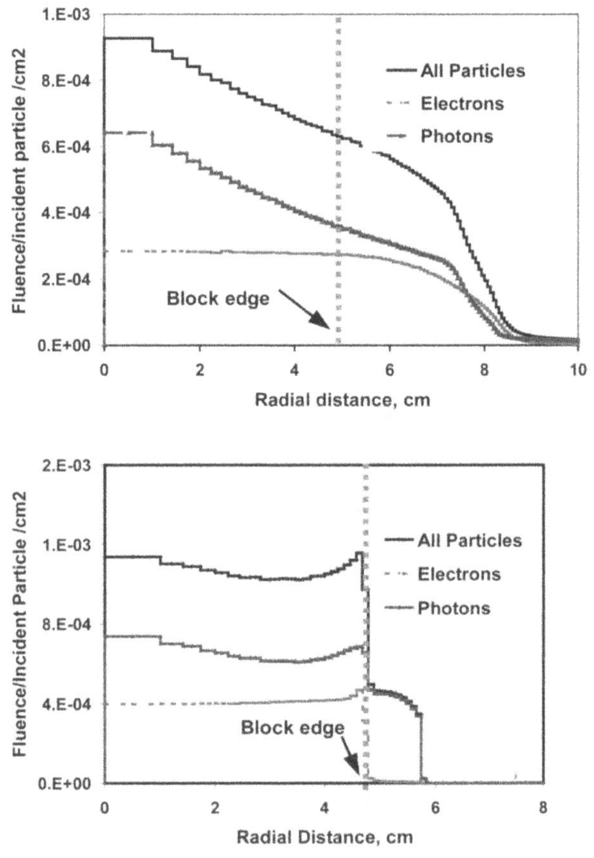


**Figure 2:** The radial distributions of the particles collected in the phase space file just above (top) and below (bottom) the cut-out

## Results and discusion

At low energies (≤ 9 MeV) the effect of the scatter from the block is marginal. However at higher energies, the scatter from the block walls has a significant effect on both the profiles, and on the central axis depth dose. At 16- and 20-MeV the scattered electrons increase the dose on the central axis by up

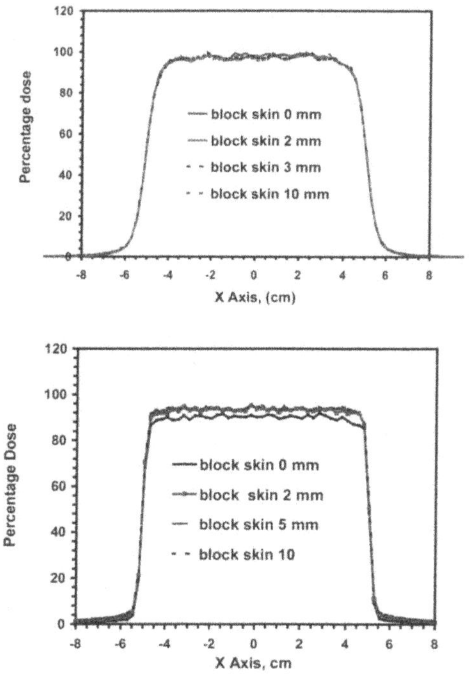


**Figure 3:** Effect of block thickness: 10x10cm$^2$ in 15x15 cm applicator, profile depth=0.5cm for (a) 6MeV and (b) 16MeV. ECUT=0.7MeV, PCUT=0.01MeV.

to 5% in the buildup region, especially for small field sizes (see for example Fig.4 for a 5x5cm2 at 16-MeV). Fig.3 (a) and (b) show the profiles at 0.5cm depth for a 10x10cm2 field. Although the profiles for the different skin thicknesses are inseparable at 6MeV, there are noticable differences at 16MeV.

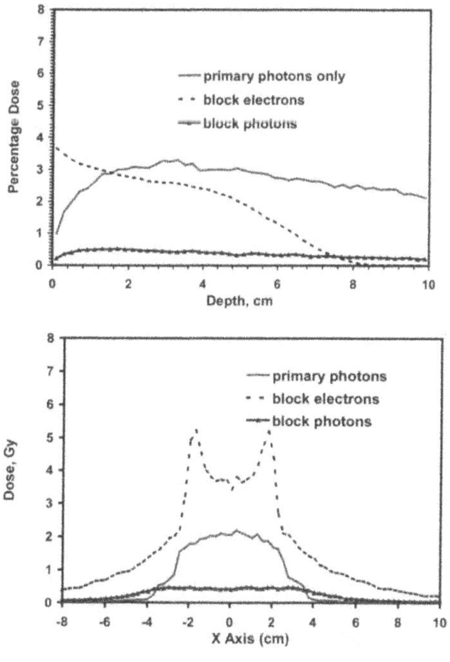


**Figure 4:** Relative contributions from particle from the block to the depth doses and profiles for a 5x5cm$^2$ field, 16MeV. The profiles were taken at $d_{max}$.

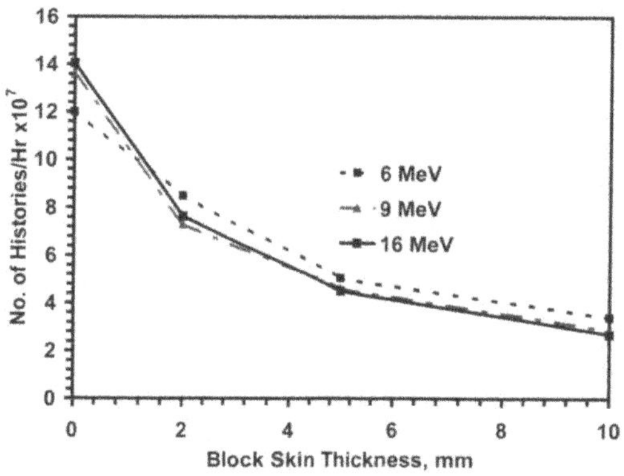


**Figure 5:** Effect of the simulated block 'skin' thickness on calculational speed to simulate the electron cutout. (6MeV on Pentium III 450 MHz, 9- and 16- MeV on PII 400MHz.)

However, using a 2mm margin round the aperture yields profiles which are in close agreement to a 10mm margin for the 16MeV beam.

The radial distributions of the particles collected in the phase space file just above and below the cut-out is shown in Fig.2a. The dotted line shows the position of the block edge. A sizable amount of time
can be saved by discarding the particles outside the simulation region during both the simulation and phase space sampling stage.
Block photons contribute less than 0.5% of the total dose over the whole field.
There is an increase of speed by a factor of up to 2.0 for no block simulation (skin 0 mm) compared to skin thickness of 2.0 mm. The speed increased by a factor 2.0 for 2.0mm compared to a 10.0mm block skin thickness.
In BEAM range rejection is used as one of the variance techniques. In cut-out simulation if the range of the electron is such that it will not escape from the block to reach the phantom then it can be discarded. This however ignores possible bremsstrahlung interactions. The choice of the maximum energy at which range rejection can be performed has to be chosen with care. The use of cut-off energy (ESAVE = 3.0 MeV), below which range rejection can be carried out, was found to increase the computational speed by a factor 2.0 compared to ESAVE=0.7MeV (see Fig.6) without affecting the dose distributions.

## Output

We have used BEAM to calculate output factors for electron cut-outs and there is excellent agreement with measurements. The results from the work has been presented elsewhere, (Verhaegen 1999). In the present study, output factors were also calculated with reduced block material, using a 2mm block skin. The output factors calculated were found to be within 2% of the those calculated using full simulations, as demonstrated in Fig.6, for 9MeV small fields. Output factors can therefore be calculated considerably faster for a given statistical accuracy. It might be possible to further speed up the process by leaving out the block particles completely or at least the photons produced in the blocks, in the calculation of these relative factors.

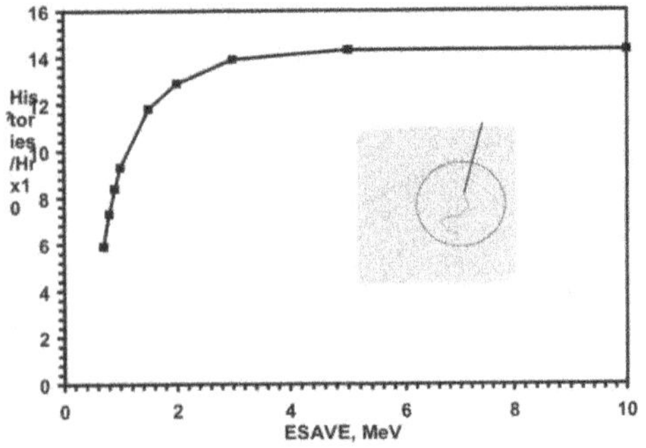


**Figure 6:** Gain in CPU speed with increase in the cutoff energy, ESAVE below which range rejection is switched on. 16MeV, for a 10.0 mm block skin.

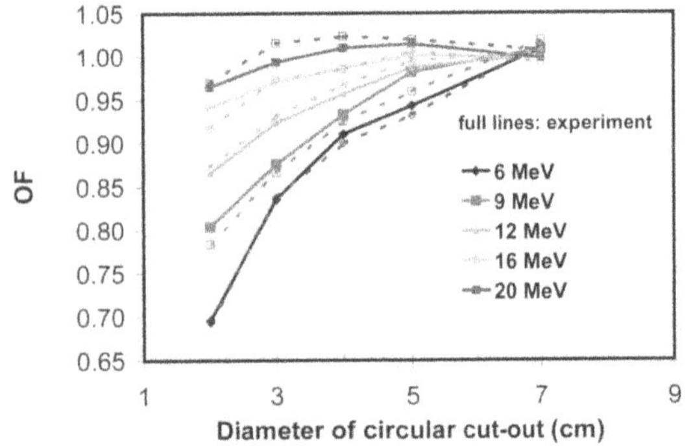


**Figure 7**: Output factors for circular electron cutouts for different energy beams, Monte Carlo (solid) and measurements with PTW Markus chamber (dotted).

| Cutout size | With 2mm block thickness | % difference with full MLC |
|---|---|---|
| 4 x 4 | 0.897 | - 2.1 |
| 5 x 5 | 0.94 | - 0.1 |
| 6 x 5 | 0.95 | - 0.3 |
| 8 x 6 | 0.991 | - 0.6 |
| 8 x 8 | 0.958 | + 0.5 |

**Table 1:** Output factors calculated using a 2mm block skin compared to full simulation for a 9 MeV beam

## Conclusions

Simulation of cutout can be speeded up by tracking particles in optimized block skin thicknesses. The use of a 2mm minimum block margin or skin has been found to be adequate to account for fluence from the cutout although this thickness may be increased for high energies A CPU time saving by a factor of 2.0 when using this margin has been observed compared to full simulation. Performing range rejection for electrons with kinetic energy of 3.0MeV has been found to have a CPU time saving by a factor of 2.0 compared to 0.7MeV. This high range rejection cut-off energy has been found to have no effect on dose distributions. Preliminary calculations have hinted at the possibility of omitting all block particles in relative output factor calculations.

## References

[1].Verhaegen F., Mubata C, Pettingel J, and Nahum A, 'Calculation of output factors for an electron accelerator (6-20 MeV) by Monte Carlo modelling', Med.Phys, **26(8)**, 1744,1999

# Influence of tissue composition on the results of Monte Carlo simulations for patient dose calculations

**Wilfried Schneider, Thomas Bortfeld and Wolfgang Schlegel**
Deutsches Krebsforschungszentrum, Dept. of Medical Physics, Im Neuenheimer Feld 280, 69120 Heidelberg, Germany

## Introduction

As input for Monte Carlo programs such as EGS4 [1] one needs the mass density and the elemental weights of all media which occur within the geometry. In the case of patient dose calculations, the geometry is given by the CT-data. A correlation between the CT-number and the mass density can be obtained following the procedure of a stoichiometric calibration presented by Schneider et al (1996) [2]. The conversion of CT-numbers to elemental weights was investigated by Schneider et al (1999) [3]. In their results, two points are outstanding. First, most of the soft tissues with a mass density greater than 1 (g $cm^{-3}$) cannot be clearly resolved by means of the CT-number. Due to the higly different contents of water, adipose and protein in these tissues, the elemental weights can only be determined with great uncertainties. On the other hand, the various skeletal tissues with mass densities from 1.1 to 1.9 (g $cm^{-3}$) are composed of only two components namely bone marrow and osseous tissue in different proportions. As consequence, skeletal tissues with different compositions can be distinguished by means of the CT-number. Nevertheless, in most of the applications of Monte Carlo simulations for patient dose calculations, the range of skeletal tissues is presented by only one bone composition. In this paper, we have investigated the effect of tissue composition on Monte Carlo dose calculations separately for the range of soft tissues as well as for skeletal tissues.

## Material and methods

### Monte Carlo simulations of dose distributions in soft tissues

Our data base of tissue parameters is taken from Woodard and White (1986) [4]. We have determined the mean composition of 35 soft tissues, whose mass densities are in the range from 1.02 to 1.12 (g $cm^{-3}$). Urine and skin are those tissues, whose elemental weights have the greatest deviations to the mean composition. In table 1 are listed the corresponding elemental weights. For the Monte Carlo simulations, which are carried out with EGS4, we have generated cross-sectional data files for urine, skin and the mean composition. The simulation geometry is such that a 2 x 2 $cm^2$ electron beam with 100 cm SSD is perpendiculary impinging a homogeneous cubic phantom with 20 cm side length. The beam energy is 6 or 21 MeV respectively. The maximum value of the dose distribution obtained using the mean composition as phantom media is set to 100 percent. To make a direct comparison with the corresponding distributions in urine and skin possible, the dose values obtained in these two cases are normalized as well to the maximum dos value in the mean composition.

### Monte Carlo simulations of dose distributions in skeletal tissues

The procedure is the same as described in the section about soft tissues. For our comparison, we have selected 3 different compositions. Sternum ($\rho = 1.25\,\mathrm{g\ cm^{-3}}$) and cortical bone ($\rho = 1.92\,\mathrm{g\ cm^{-3}}$) are taken from White et al (1987) [5], bone is a composition given in Johns-Cunningham (1983) [6]. The corresponding elemental weights are listed in table 2.

## Results and discussion

### Dose distributions in soft tissues

The calculated dose distributions are presented in figure 1 (a–d). Each plot shows a comparison of the depth dose profile in mean composition with that in urine or skin respectively. The mass density assigned to mean composition is always the same as the mass density of the tissue in comparison. The maximum difference of corresponding dose values occur in the comparison of mean composition with urine in case of the 6 MeV electron beam and takes a value of 1.6 % of the dose maximum. As can be seen from table 1, the main difference in the composition of soft tissues is given by the individual weights of carbon (Z=6) and oxygen (Z=8). Since the atomic numbers of both elements differ only slightly, the influence on the physical cross-sections determining the dose distributions is quite small. Considering photon beams, the most relevant quantity is the electron density, which depends, beside the mass density, only on the ratio of atomic number and atomic mass. This ratio is approximately 0.5 for carbon as well as for oxygen and therefore the individual weights of these elements are not critical.

### Dose distributions in skeletal tissues

Depth dose profiles in bone are compared with the corresponding profiles in sternum and cortical bone (s. figure 1 e–h). The mass density assigned to bone is always the same as the mass density of the tissue in comparison. The differences between corresponding dose distributions are clearly greater than in case of the soft tissues. In the comparison of the 21 MeV profiles in bone and cortical bone, the

| | H | C | N | O | Na | P | S | Cl | K |
|---|---|---|---|---|---|---|---|---|---|
| Urine | 11.0 | 0.5 | 1.0 | 86.2 | 0.4 | 0.1 | | 0.6 | 0.2 |
| Skin | 10.0 | 25.0 | 4.6 | 59.4 | 0.2 | 0.1 | 0.3 | 0.3 | 0.1 |
| Mean composition | 10.3 | 13.4 | 3.0 | 72.3 | 0.2 | 0.2 | 0.2 | 0.2 | 0.2 |

**Table 1:** Elemental weights of urine, skin and the mean compostion of 35 soft tissues. The values are given in percentage points on mass.

| | H | C | N | O | Na | Mg | P | S | Cl | K | Ca | Fe |
|---|---|---|---|---|---|---|---|---|---|---|---|---|
| Sternum | 7.8 | 31.6 | 3.7 | 43.8 | | 0.1 | 4.0 | 0.2 | 0.1 | 0.1 | 8.5 | 0.1 |
| Cortical bone | 3.4 | 15.5 | 4.2 | 43.5 | 0.1 | 0.2 | 10.3 | 0.3 | | | 22.5 | |
| Bone | 6.4 | 27.8 | 2.7 | 41.0 | | 0.2 | 7.0 | 0.2 | | | 14.7 | |

**Table 2:** Elemental weights of sternum, cortical bone and bone. The values are given in percentage points on mass.

maximum deviation is 5.7 % of the dose maximum. The origin for the higher differences is given by the content on high atomic number elements in skeletal tissues. From table 2 we can see that the weights of phosphorus (Z=15) and calcium (Z=20) differ significantly between the 3 compositions. Using bone as mean composition for all skeletal tissues, the real weight of calcium in the individual skeletal tissue can differ up to 7.8 percentage points from the mean value. Considering photon beam dose calculations, the different weights of hydrogen can cause deviations on dose distributions. This is because hydrogen is the only element within tissues, for which the ratio of atomic to mass number is 1 instead of 0.5.

## Conclusion

The effect of tissue composition on Monte Carlo dose calculations is quite different for soft and skeletal tissues. In case of soft tissues, the use of a mean composition seems to be sufficient for patient dose calculations. However, skeletal tissues should be distinguished by means of the CT-number. Because of the different content on the high atomic number elements phosphorus and calcium, significant deviations on the dose distributions can appear when using only one composition for the whole range of skeletal tissues.

## References

[1] Nelson W. R., Hirayama H. and Rogers D. W. O. 1985 The EGS4 code system *SLAC-Report 265, Stanford Linear Accelerator Center*

[2] Schneider U., Pedroni E. and Lomax A. 1996 The calibration of CT Hounsfield units for radiotherapy treatment planning *Phys. Med. Biol.* **41** 111–24

[3] Schneider W., Bortfeld T. and Schlegel W. 1999 Correlation between CT-numbers and tissue parameters needed for Monte Carlo simulations of clinical dose distributions *Radiotherapy & Oncology Suppl. 1* **51** S56

[4] Woodard H. Q. and White D. R. 1986 The composition of body tissues *Br. J. Radiol.* **59** 1209–19

[5] White D. R., Woodard H. Q. and Hammond S. M. 1987 Average soft-tissue and bone models for use in radiation dosimetry *Br. J. Radiol.* **60** 907–13

[6] Johns H. E. and Cunningham J. R. 1983 The physics of radiology *Thomas, Springfield, Illinois*

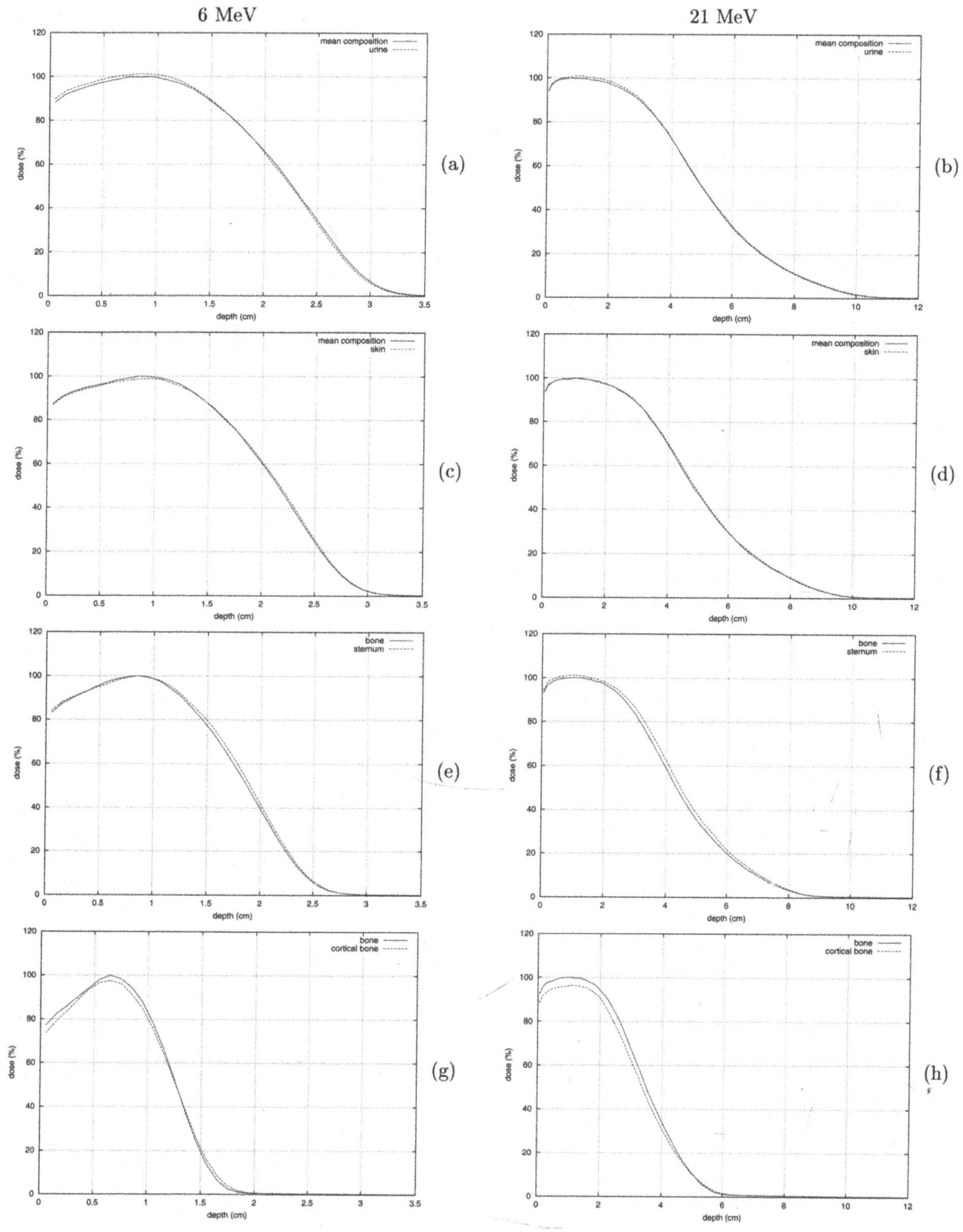


**Figure 1:** Comparison of calculated dose profiles of electron beams in a homogeneous phantom with the following compositions: (a) 6 MeV mean composition – urine ($\rho = 1.02$ g cm$^{-3}$), (b) 21 MeV mean composition – urine ($\rho = 1.02$ g cm$^{-3}$), (c) 6 MeV mean composition – skin ($\rho = 1.09$ g cm$^{-3}$), (d) 21 MeV mean composition – skin ($\rho = 1.09$ g cm$^{-3}$) (e) 6 MeV bone – sternum ($\rho = 1.25$ g cm$^{-3}$), (f) 21 MeV bone – sternum ($\rho = 1.25$ g cm$^{-3}$), (g) 6 MeV bone – cortical bone ($\rho = 1.92$ g cm$^{-3}$), (h) 21 MeV bone – cortical bone ($\rho = 1.92$ g cm$^{-3}$).

# A Virtual Linear Accelerator for Verification of Treatment planning systems

**Elinore Wieslander**[1] **and Tommy Knöös**[1]

[1] Radiation Physics, Lund University Hospital, SE-221 85 Lund, Sweden

## Introduction

An accurate determination of the absorbed dose in treatment planning is of highest importance. ICRU 42 states that computer-produced dose distributions can be considered accurate enough if they differ from relative dose measurements by less than 2 %, or 0.2 cm in position of isodose curves in very steep dose gradients. [1]

The accuracy of Treatment planning systems (TPS) can be determined by performing phantom measurements. The selection of detector and method, determined by the purpose of the study, limits the number of dose points, shape and composition of the phantoms.[2-5] The requirements on the accelerators, i.e. stability of output, energy, flatness and symmetry, are of the same order as those put on the TPS. Thus if characterisation and verification measurements for a TPS are separated in time deviations may occur. Recently the Monte Carlo BEAM code has been used to reconstruct accelerators in clinical use for the verification procedure of TPS.[6]

The aim of this work is to study whether measurements for the verification procedure of a pencil beam based TPS can be replaced with Monte Carlo simulations. This new approach, based on a virtual, Monte Carlo simulated generic treatment unit, eliminates the fluctuation in accelerator output. This could facilitate the commissioning process of a new TPS, and also simplify the determination of the limits of the TPS. An inhomogeneous geometry in which it usually is rather complicated to perform measurements is used to illustrate the advantage with this approach.

## Material and methods

The treatment planning system used in this study, HELAX-TMS 4.1A, is based on fluence modelling and a pencil-beam convolution concept introduced by Ahnesjö *et al* 1992.[7] The emphasis in this work lies on the accuracy of the dose modelling, thus a method is chosen where head-scatter fluence is absent.

The data needed to characterise a treatment unit in the TPS consist of depth doses for the pencil beam compilation, star profiles for the primary fluence matrix, output factors (OF) in air for head scatter modelling, absolute dose for monitor unit calculations and profiles in water for penumbra and filter determination. These data are listed in Table I. To be able to implement a treatment unit into the TPS, the machine geometry together with a measured characterising data set for each beam quality has to be supplied to the vendor. Earlier versions of this TPS has been extensively described and verified in several papers.[4, 5, 8-13]

| | SPD [cm] | Field size [cm] | Depth [cm] |
|---|---|---|---|
| Central depth dose | 90 | 5, 10, 15 & 20 | ---- |
| Profiles | 90 | 5, 10, 15 & 20 | 1.5,5,10 & 20 |
| Star shaped profiles | 90 | 40 | 10 |
| Output factors air | 100 | 5, 10, 15 & 20 | ---- |
| Output factors water | 90 | 5, 10, 15 & 20 | 10 |

**Table 1:** The characterisation data used to implement a treatment unit into the treatment planning system.

The Monte Carlo calculations are performed with the EGS4 module XYZP with PRESTA implemented.[14, 15] The possibility to use a photon spectrum and a divergent beam has been added.

For the purpose of this study, any spectra could be used. However, to get clinically relevant beam qualities, depth dose equivalent spectra extracted from the TPS are used. The parameters for the EGS4 transport are: AP = Pcut = 10 keV, AE = 521 keV and Ecut = 600/700 keV. The simulations are performed in ten batches and the statistical uncertainty, estimated as standard deviation, is kept below 0.8 % inside the primary radiation field. The TPS calculates absorbed dose to water, which is a consequence of the point-spread functions being generated in water. Therefore water, with density according to the actual medium in the TPS, is used in EGS4.

The virtual accelerator is set up to produce two photon energies, 6 and 18 MV, covering most conventional beam qualities. The beam characterisation data needed to implement an accelerator in the TPS is generated using a modified version of XYZP in a water phantom ($54\times54\times44$ $cm^2$) with source phantom distance 90 cm (characterisation geometry). An air layer is added in front of the phantom to account for electrons generated in the air column between the target and the phantom. All photons are selected from a distribution describing the spectrum and emitted from a point source into the rectangle describing the beam opening, consequently no collimator jaws are needed. The emission probability is kept constant over the whole beam leading to symmetry in the A-B and G-T directions.

To reduce the CPU time the Monte Carlo runs are divided in specific depth dose, profile and star simulations. In this way, the voxel geometry can be optimised for each simulation. Ecut equal to 600 keV is used for depth doses and 700 keV for profiles and star. Voxel size and number of histories are summarised in Table 2. Output factors in water, $OF_{water}$ and absolute dose calibration are obtained from the depth dose and star profiles since the EGS4 dose is normalised to the incoming fluence. The virtual accelerator has no treatment head, thus no variation in head scatter with field size results in output factors in air, $OF_{air}$, equal to unity. The data is then sent to the TPS vendor for implementation according to the same procedure as used for "real" accelerators.

| | Voxel size X direction [cm] | Voxel size Y direction [cm] | Voxel size Z direction [cm] | Histories [millions] |
|---|---|---|---|---|
| Depth doses | 0.75/4/5/6$^A$ | 0.75/4/5/6$^A$ | 0.25/0.50$^B$ | 35-150 |
| Profiles | 0.5 | 0.50/4/5/6$^A$ | 0.50 | 200-250 |
| Star | 1.0 | 1.0 | 2.0 | 400-440 |

**Table 2:** The voxel size and number of histories used for the characterisation data simulations for 6 and 18 MV.

The implementation of data into the TPS for this virtual linear accelerator is evaluated by comparing depth doses, profiles and OF for square fields with field sizes from 5 to 40 cm from the virtual Monte Carlo based accelerator, with the results from the TPS for exactly the same characterisation geometry. All data is normalised to a reference situation (isocentric set up with 10 cm depth for a 10×10 $cm^2$ field). With this approach both relative distribution and absolute level can be evaluated using the same data set.

The virtual accelerator and its corresponding unit in TPS is used to study the dose distribution in a mediastinum like geometry with water and lung (water with relative density 0.3).[9, 16-18] A 10×10 $cm^2$ open photon field with a SPD of 100 cm is used for both energies. The dose is scored along the x-axis in a cartesian grid with $\Delta x = 0.25$, $\Delta y = 4.00$ and $\Delta z = 0.25$ cm. The number of histories is 600×$10^6$ and Ecut is equal to 600 keV for both energies.

## Results and discussion

The implementation process of the virtual accelerator, made by the TPS vendor, turns out successfully. The virtual accelerator is extreme in the sense that it has a infinitely small target and headscatter is absent. Two small disagreements associated with target size and headscatter are found and minimised by minor adjustments in the TPS data base.

Output factor normalised depth doses and profiles calculated by the TPS are in good agreement with the simulations for both 6 and 18 MV in the characterisation geometry. Deviations are, however, seen in the build-up region. Depth doses and profiles for the 10×10 $cm^2$ 6 MV field are seen in figure 1. The difference between TPS calculated and Monte Carlo simulated depth doses is included. The deviations for the depth doses and the profiles, for both energies, are less than 2 % and for many points <1 %, except in the build-up region where the deviations are larger. This is of the same order as previously reported results based on measurements.[8] The larger deviations in the build-up region is due to insufficiencies in the TPS modelling of charged particle contamination. Consequently, in the characterisation geometry, the TPS fulfils the ICRU 42 requirements on computer-produced dose distribution, i.e. within 2 % or 2 mm. For the $OF_{water}$ deviations up to 2 % were found for both energies.

The results for the mediastinum case illustrate the well known fact that the pencil beam concept does not handle charged particle disequilibrium in other media than water.[9] A penumbra widening and decrease of absorbed dose in the lung is observed in the Monte Carlo simulations due to a prolonged range of the electrons in low-density regions, which causes gradual loss of lateral electron equilibrium. This effect is not modelled by the TPS. The difference between TPS and Monte Carlo simulations in the lung region increases with energy and is about 9.5 % for 18 MV compared to 3.5% for 6 MV.

The developed approach makes it possible to study the absorbed dose to the whole volume of interest in contrast to conventional measurements where the number of dose points is limited.[4, 19, 20]

The EGS4 code used does not account for scatter from irradiated parts of the treatment head, consequently the virtual accelerator can be used for studies of phenomena associated with the irradiated media, e.g. phantom scatter, inhomogenities etc. The method used is suited for isolated studies of the dose modelling of treatment planning systems.

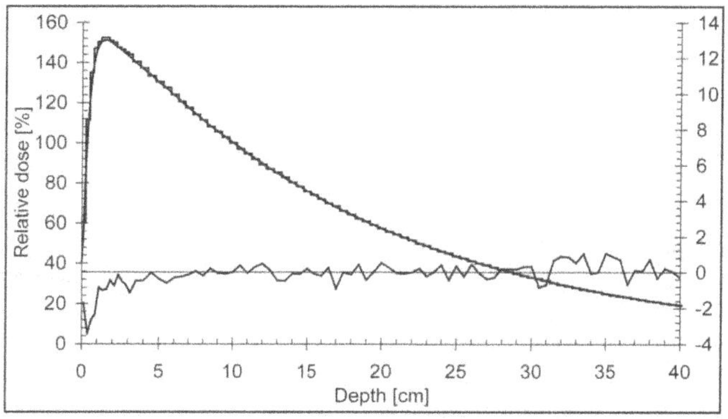


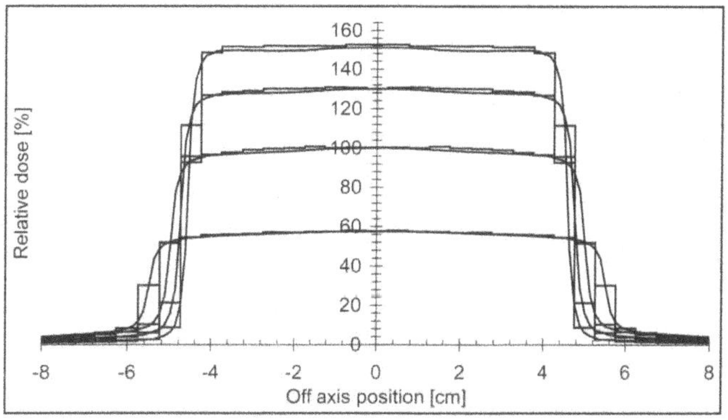


**Figure 1:** Depth doses and profiles for the characterisation geometry, equivalent field side 10 cm. Step shaped curve represents Monte Carlo simulations and dashed lines TPS calculation (left scale). The deviations between depth doses are shown in the lower part (right scale)

## Conclusion

The presented results show that it is possible to create a data set for characterisation of a treatment planning system with a Monte Carlo simulated linear accelerator and to use it for verification. In contradiction to conventional measurements there are no problems with fluctuating accelerator output, and additional verification geometries can easily be added. The lack of head scatter in the virtual accelerator makes it possible to study the dose modelling separately. One can more easily identify and isolate deficiencies in the dose model used by the

TPS. Further on, advanced and complicated geometries in which conventional measurements are complicated or even impossible can be studied as well.

In the future data sets for several energies and for various TPS can be made available for both users and vendors for verification of treatment planning systems.

## References

[1] International Commission on Radiation Units and Measurements (ICRU) 1987 Use of Computers in External Beam Radiotherapy Procedures with High-Energy Photons and Electrons *ICRU Report 42*

[2] Knöös T, Ahlgren L and Nilsson M 1986 Comparison of measured and calculated absorbed doses from tangential irradiation of the breast *Radiother. Oncol.* **7** 81-88

[3] van Bree N A M, Idezs M H M, Huizenga H and Mijnheer B J 1994 Film dosimetry for radiotherapy treatment planning verification of a 6 MV tangential breast irradiation *Radiother. Oncol.* **31** 251-55

[4] Hurkmans C, Knöös T, Nilsson P, Svahn-Tapper G and Danielsson H 1995 Limitation of a pencil beam approach to photon dose calculations in the head and neck region *Radiother. Oncol.* **37** 74-80

[5] Hurkmans C, Knöös T and Nilsson P 1996 Dosimetric verification of open asymmetric photon fields calculated with a treatment planning system based on dose-to-energy-fluence concepts *Phys. Med. Biol.* **41** 1277-90

[6] van der Zee W and Welleweerd J 1999 Calculationg photon beam characteristics with Monte Carlo techniques *Med. Phys.* **26** 1883-92

[7] Ahnesjö A, Saxner M and Trepp A 1992 A pencil beam model for photon dose calculation. *Med. Phys.* **19** 263-73

[8] Knöös T, Ceberg C, Weber L and Nilsson P 1994 The dosimetric verification of a pencil beam based treatment planning system *Phys. Med. Biol.* **39** 1609-28

[9] Knöös T, Ahnesjö A, Nilsson P and Weber L 1995 Limitations of a pencil beam approach to photon dose calculations in lung tissue *Phys. Med. Biol.* **40** 1411-20

[10] Weber L, Ahnesjö A, Nilsson P, Saxner M and Knöös T 1996 Verification and implementation of dynamic wedge calculations in a treatment planning system based on dose-to-energy-fluence formalism *Med. Phys.* **23** 307-16

[11] van't Veld A A 1997 Analysis of accuracy in dose and position in calculations of a treatment planning system for blocked photon fields *Radiother. Oncol.* **45** 245-51

[12] Basran P S, Ansbacher W, Field G C and Murray B R 1998 Evaluation of optimized compensators on a 3D planning system *Med. Phys.* **25** 1837-44

[13] Hansson H, Björk P, Knöös T and Nilsson P 1999 Verification of a pencil beam based treatment planning system: output factors for open photon beams shaped with MLC or blocks *Phys. Med. Biol.* **44** N201-07

[14] Nelson W R, Hirayama H and Rogers D W O 1985 The EGS4 code system Report SLAC-265 Stanford Linear Accelerator Center, Stanford CA

[15] Bielajew A F and Rogers D W O 1987 PRESTA: The parameter reduced electron-step transport algorithm for electron Monte Carlo transport *Nucl. Instrum, Meth. Phys. Res.* B **18** 165-81

[16] Rice R K, Mijnheer B J and Chin L M 1988 Benchmark measurements for lung dose corrections for x-ray beams *Int. J. Radiat. Oncol. Biol. Phys.* **15** 399-409

[17] Ahnesjö A 1989 Collapsed cone convolution of radiant energy for photon dose calculation in heterogeneous media *Med. Phys.* **16** 577-92

[18] Blomquist M and Karlsson M 1998 Measured lung dose correction factors for 50 MV photons *Phys. Med. Biol.* **43** 3225-34

[19] Mackie T R, El-Khatib E, Battista J and Scrimger J 1985 Lung dose corrections for 6- and 15-MV x rays *Med. Phys.* **12** 327-32

[20] Kosunen A, Järvinen H, Vatnitskij S, Ermakov I, Chervjakov A, Kulmala J, Pitkänen M, Väyrynen T and Väänänen A 1993 *Radiother. Oncol.* **29** 327-35

# A Monte Carlo method for commissioning electron beams

**John A. Antolak, Michael S. Bieda and Kenneth R. Hogstrom**

Department of Radiation Physics, The University of Texas M. D. Anderson Cancer Center, 1515 Holcombe Blvd.-94, Houston, TX 77030, USA

## Introduction

The dosimetric properties of electron beams produced by linear accelerators (linacs) exhibit small but significant variability between different manufacturers, mostly due to differences in the treatment head design [1, 2]. Even linacs produced by the same manufacturer can have different beam characteristics if a particular radiation oncology clinic requires electron beams that meet atypical specifications. For these reasons, institutions rely on linac-specific beam data that has been measured by a qualified medical physicist for treatment planning and beam-monitor unit calculations.

In this study, the feasibility of using a Monte Carlo approach for commissioning electron beams was investigated. The advantages of calculating electron dosimetry data include (1) significant decrease in the time from the arrival of the machine to it's initial use, (2) decreased time to accumulate machine data, and (3) the ability to produce a more extensive data set. The BEAM user code [3] provides a general framework for the simulation of the complex geometry found in linear accelerator treatment heads. BEAM uses the EGS4 code system [4] with the PRESTA algorithm [5] for electron transport. The BEAM user code is capable of recording a phase space, which can be used as input for other simulations.

Other investigators have shown, for selected conditions, that BEAM is capable of generating dosimetry data that are accurate to within 3% of $D_{max}$ when compared to measured results [3, 6-8]. They have shown that the Monte Carlo method can be used to predict machine-specific electron dosimetry data accurately for a limited set of clinical treatment parameters, i.e., limited combinations of energy, applicator, field size, and SSD. The purpose of this work was to investigate whether the Monte Carlo technique can be used to generate all beam commissioning dosimetry data with sufficient accuracy, and therefore be considered an acceptable substitute for measurement during the beam commissioning process.

The hypothesis of this research is that Monte Carlo-based dose calculations can generate electron beam commissioning data that are accurate within a specified criteria compared to measured data. The criteria for the calculated percent depth-dose and cross-beam profiles is that results must be within 2% of $D_{max}$ or 0.1 cm of measured data for the entire range of clinical treatment parameters. The criteria for output factors and air gap factors is that results must be within 2% of $D_{max}$ for the field size and SSD of interest for the entire range of clinical treatment parameters.

## Materials and methods

The measured data set utilized in this study was obtained during the commissioning of a Varian Clinac 2100C (Varian Oncology Systems, Palo Alto, CA) at The University of Texas M. D. Anderson Cancer Center (serial #492). It is a standing wave accelerator with a dual scattering-foil system that supports five customized electron energies. Klein *et al* [9] offer an extensive description of the scattering foils and applicators used in the Varian Clinac 2100C. The range of measured data and measurement techniques followed the recommendations of the AAPM TG-25 Report [10], and included the following for each of the five electron beam energies:

1. Central axis percentage depth dose (%DD) at 100 cm SSD for a range of square field sizes (2x2 to 25x25 $cm^2$), selected rectangular fields (3x12 and 6x12 $cm^2$), and selected square fields (6x6 and 15x15 $cm^2$) at 110 cm SSD.
2. Cross-beam profiles at 100 cm and 110 cm SSD at several depths for a range of field sizes (2x2 to 25x25 $cm^2$).
3. Output factors versus field size (2x2 $cm^2$ to open applicator) at 100 cm SSD for all applicator sizes.
4. Air gap correction factors at 105, 110, 115, and120 cm SSD for a range of field sizes.

A complete list of measured data and measurement techniques is described elsewhere [11].

The physical description (geometry and composition) of the Varian 2100C treatment head was supplied by the manufacturer. Some of the treatment head geometry (that was accessible and perhaps not supplied) was measured directly. Figure 1 shows a schematic of the treatment head model in this study.

To avoid redundant calculations, the treatment head simulation was divided into multiple, linked simulations. In the first simulation, the beam was transported from the accelerator exit window to the bottom of the light field mirror (ABOVE_JAWS in Figure 1). These simulations produced phase space files (one for each energy) that were used as the sources for the next set of simulations, which transported the beams from the top of the photon jaws to the bottom of the second scraper bar (BELOW_JAWS in Figure 1). The output of these calculations were phase space files (one for each energy and applicator) that were used as sources for the final simulations, which transported the beam through the cerrobend insert and a cylindrical water phantom (APPLICAT_PHAN in Figure 1). To calculate cross-beam profiles, a phase space file was collected below the cerrobend insert and used as input for a water phantom calculation using the DOSXYZ user code [12]. The electron source (incident on the accelerator exit window) was assumed to be mono-energetic and mono-directional, down the central axis of the treatment head. The spatial distribution of the source was Gaussian with a full-width at half-maximum of 1.5 mm [13], and a new BEAM source was added to simulate this spatial distribution. The initial energy of the beam was adjusted until the practical range of a calculated 10x10-$cm^2$

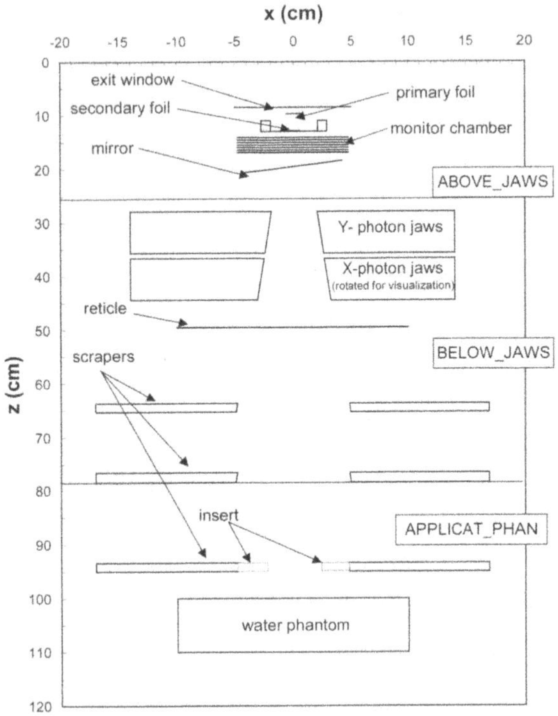


**Figure 1:** Schematic of the Varian Clinac 2100C treatment head used for BEAM simulation.

percentage depth dose agreed with measurement to within 0.5 mm. For the BEAM simulations, the secondary electron production threshold (AE) was set to 0.521 MeV (total energy) and the transport cutoff (ECUT) was set to 0.700 MeV. The DOSXYZ calculations used AE = 0.700 MeV. For all simulations, the PRESTA-default electron step-size was used. A more detailed description of the model and its approximations can be found elsewhere [11].

All of the data normally measured during commissioning (see above) was computed for energies of 6 MeV and 12 MeV. The 20-MeV data set was limited to the 10x10 $cm^2$ and 25x25 $cm^2$ applicators at 100-cm SSD because of time constraints. The calculated data was compared to the measured data and evaluated with respect to the criteria stated in the hypothesis above.

| | Applicator size ($cm^2$) | | | |
|---|---|---|---|---|
| Energy (MeV) | 10x10 | 15x15 | 20x20 | 25x25 |
| 6 | ok | ok | 2.7% (8.0 cm) | 4.0% (11.0 cm) |
| 12 | 2.7% (4.4 cm) | 3.4% (5.5 cm) | 3.3% (9.8 cm) | ok |
| 20 | --- | --- | --- | ok |

**Table 1:** Summary of cross-beam profile discrepancies for the open applicator fields. Those fields that met the 2%, 0.1 cm criteria are marked "ok". For those fields that didn't meet the criteria, the maximum difference in relative dose and the distance from central-axis is given.

## Results and discussion

Using the BEAM Monte Carlo code and the procedures presented above, a comparison of calculated with measured data for the Varian Clinac 2100C showed the following:

1. %DD curves and cone insert ratios can be predicted within our specified accuracy (2%) for energies from 6- to 20-MeV for the 10x10 $cm^2$ to 25x25 $cm^2$ applicators, and for field sizes ranging from 2x2 $cm^2$ to the open field size of the applicator.
2. Air gap factors can be predicted within an accuracy of 2.2% for energies of 6- and 12-MeV for field sizes ranging from 2x2 $cm^2$ to 25x25 $cm^2$, and for SSD ranging from 100 to 120 cm SSD. Considering that the calculated data had some uncertainty (~ 0.7%), a maximum difference of 2.2 % is not statistically different from the 2% criteria. Three air gap factors for the 6-MeV beam (2.8% for 2x2 $cm^2$, 120 cm SSD; 3.3% for 3x3 $cm^2$, 115 cm SSD; 3.8% for 3x3 $cm^2$, 120 cm SSD) fell outside this range. The air gap factors for these field size/SSD combinations were much less than unity, therefore the percentage difference was increased compared to other air gap factors. The standard errors for these air gap factors are greater than 1.0%, which means the large discrepancies are in part due to poor statistics.
3. Open cone ratios for energies 6-, 12-, and 20-MeV and for the 15x15 $cm^2$ to 25x25 $cm^2$ applicators differ from measurement by as much as 4.3%, The average of 9 comparisons was 2.1%, and 4 of the values exceeded the 2% criteria.
4. Cross-beam profiles for the small fields formed by Cerrobend inserts (3x3 $cm^2$ and 6x6 $cm^2$ for the 6- and 12-MeV beams) were within the 2% (0.1 cm) criteria. Cross-beam profiles for open applicator fields (10x10 $cm^2$ to 25x25 $cm^2$ at 6-, 12-, and 20-MeV frequently failed the 2% (0.1 cm) criteria. Table 1 summarizes the maximum discrepancies between measured and calculated cross-beam profiles for open fields.
5. To calculate a complete electron beam commissioning data set for the Varian Clinac 2100C (5 energies, 4 applicators) requires approximately 156 days of CPU-time, or 26 days on six DEC AlphaStation 255/300s. This workstation is approximately equivalent to a 200 MHz Pentium Pro PC.

Prior to this study, the most extensive comparison between measured and calculated (BEAM) data for the Varian 2100C was published by Kapur *et al* [7]. However, their comparison was restricted to field sizes smaller than 20x20 $cm^2$, and a single SSD (100 cm). The data in this study is very similar to data presented in that paper, as might be expected. However, during the course of this study, we discovered that the manufacturer's specification for the geometry of the scattering foils was incorrect [14]. The effect was largest at higher energies and large field sizes. For a field size of 25x25 $cm^2$, the difference between calculated and measured cross-beam profiles was approximately 10% at 11-cm off-axis distance. Kapur *et al* [7] did not show cross-beam profiles for field sizes larger than 15x15 $cm^2$, so they may not have seen this problem. Another apparent difference in the two studies is that while we

| Energy (MeV) | Applicator Size ($cm^2$) | Calc. OCR | Standard Error (%) | Meas. OCR | Difference (%) |
|---|---|---|---|---|---|
| 6 | 15x15 | 0.995 | 0.8 | 0.997 | -0.2 |
| | 20x20 | 1.022 | 0.8 | 1.003 | 1.9 |
| | 25x25 | 1.038 | 0.7 | 0.995 | 4.3 |
| 12 | 15x15 | 1.017 | 0.5 | 0.987 | 3.0 |
| | 20x20 | 1.000 | 0.5 | 0.969 | 3.2 |
| | 25x25 | 0.963 | 0.5 | 0.946 | 1.8 |
| 20 | 15x15 | 1.006 | 0.5 | 0.975 | 3.2 |
| | 20x20 | 0.964 | 0.5 | 0.953 | 1.1 |
| | 25x25 | 0.923 | 0.5 | 0.917 | 0.6 |

**Table 2:** Open Cone Ratios for the 6-, 12-, and 20-MeV beams. The percentage difference [((calculated – measured)/measured)x100%] is tabulated in the final column. The standard error of the calculated OCR is given as a percentage of the calculated OCR.

found that open cone ratios could not be computed reliably, they found agreement to within 2%. However, the normalization field sizes are different, and if we renormalize our open cone ratios to the 15x15-$cm^2$ field size, our results are in agreement with theirs.

## Conclusion

First, the results do not support the hypothesis that Monte Carlo calculations can generate electron commissioning data that is accurate within 2% of $D_{max}$ or 0.1 cm for the entire range of clinical treatment parameters. If the criteria were relaxed to 4% of $D_{max}$ or 0.3 cm for cross-beam profiles and %DD and 4% of $D_{max}$ for the other data, the hypothesis would be supported; however, this is not clinically acceptable.

Second, the BEAM Monte Carlo code can be used for the determination of relative central-axis quantities such as percent depth dose, cone insert ratios, and air gap factors for all energies and applicators. However, ratios of dose output for open cones should be measured.

Third, a full comparison over the entire range of clinical treatment parameters is necessary to adequately assess the accuracy of the Monte Carlo method for electron-beam calculations.

**Acknowledgements**
This work was supported by SRA97-015 from Varian Oncology Systems.

## References

[1] Hogstrom K R 1991 Clinical electron beam dosimetry: basic dosimetry data *Advances in Radiation Oncology Physics - 1990 Proceedings of the Summer School of the AAPM* ed. J Purdy (New York: American Institute of Physics) pp 390-429

[2] American Association of Physicists in Medicine Task Group 21 1983 A protocol for the determination of absorbed dose from high-energy photon and electron beams *Med Phys* **10** 741-771

[3] Rogers D W, Faddegon B A, Ding G X *et al* 1995 BEAM: a Monte Carlo code to simulate radiotherapy treatment units *Med Phys* **22** 503-24

[4] Nelson W R, Hirayama H and Rogers D W O 1985 The EGS4 code system: Stanford Linear Accelerator Center.

[5] Bielajew A F and Rogers D W O 1987 PRESTA–The parameter reduced electron-step transport algorithm for electron Monte Carlo transport *Nucl Instrum Meth B* **18** 165-181

[6] Ding G X and Rogers D W O 1995 Energy Spectra, angular spread, and dose distributions of electron beams from various accelerators used in radiotherapy. Ottawa: National Research Council of Canada.

[7] Kapur A, Ma C M, Mok E C *et al* 1998 Monte Carlo calculations of electron beam output factors for a medical linear accelerator *Physics in Medicine & Biology* **43** 3479-94

[8] Zhang G G, Rogers D W, Cygler J E *et al* 1999 Monte Carlo investigation of electron beam output factors versus size of square cutout *Med Phys* **26** 743-50

[9] Klein E E, Low D A and Purdy J A 1995 Changes in electron beam dosimetry with a new scattering foil-applicator system on a CL2100C [published erratum appears in Int J Radiat Oncol Biol Phys 1995 Sep 30;33(2):545] *Int J Radiat Oncol, Biol, Phys* **32** 483-90

[10] Khan F M, Doppke K P, Hogstrom K R *et al* 1991 Clinical electron-beam dosimetry: report of AAPM Radiation Therapy Committee Task Group No. 25 *Med Phys* **18** 73-109

[11] Bieda M S 1999 A Monte Carlo method for commissioning electron beams, M.S. thesis, University of Texas Graduate School of Biomedical Sciences

[12] Ma C-M, Reckwerdt P, Holmes M *et al* 1995 DOSXYZ Users Manual. Ottawa: National Research Council of Canada.

[13] Jaffray D A, Battista J J, Fenster A *et al* 1993 X-ray sources of medical linear accelerators: focal and extra-focal radiation *Med Phys* **20** 1417-27

[14] Bieda M S, Hogstrom K R and Antolak J A 1999 Modification of input data for electron beam Monte Carlo calculations *Med Phys* **26** 1122-1123

# Add a Dynamic Swing to Monte Carlo simulation —— Modeling Dynamic Jaw Motion Using Three Sampling Techniques

**H. Helen Liu, Ph.D.**, [1], **Frank Verhaegen, Ph.D.**[2]
[1]Radiation Physics, UT MD Anderson Cancer Center, Houston, U.S.A., and [2]Physics Department, Royal Marsden Hospital (Institute of Cancer Research), London, UK

## Introduction

In radiation dosimetry, Monte Carlo simulation offers unique and superb opportunities in studying the generation of radiation and its path through patients. This technique is gaining a wider recognition in radiotherapy treatment planning because of improved computer performance and availability of more user-friendly Monte Carlo programs, such as the BEAM Monte Carlo code [1]. Monte Carlo simulation improves the accuracy of dose calculation in treatment planning, especially for inhomogeneous regions such as head and neck, and lungs. However, the Monte Carlo technique is still time consuming in nature and requires significant computational power in order to simulate transport of large number of particles.

Recently, advanced treatment techniques such as intensity modulated radiotherapy (IMRT), relies on more sophisticated beam delivery systems, including dynamic jaws and multi-leaf collimators (MLCs). These dynamic treatments pose additional challenges to Monte Carlo simulation because a fourth dimension, time, is being introduced to the dose distributions. To compute the accumulative dose, a straight-forward approach is to treat the dynamic field to be composed of individual component fields, as in a step-shoot fashion [2]. However, this approach requires simulation for each component field, and its accuracy may be limited by the spatial resolution between the stepping fields. The purpose of this research is to extend the application of the Monte Carlo technique to dynamic fields. We developed a more efficient and automated approach based on random sampling of the jaw positions in simulating the dynamic jaw motion. The accuracy of this approach was verified and compared to two different component sampling techniques. The principle behind this work can be extended to the IMRT fields using dynamic MLCs.

## Materials and Methods

On Varian linear accelerators, a dynamic wedge creates wedge-shaped dose profiles by moving one of the upper jaws (Y1 or Y2) across the field. The dose output for the dynamic wedge is controlled by a segmented treatment table (STT), which specifies the monitor units (MUs) as a function of the jaw position. In this work, a Varian 2100C linear accelerator equipped with the dynamic wedge was simulated using the BEAM Monte Carlo code [1]. The simulation of the accelerator was performed in two stages. The static components in the accelerator, including the electron target, primary collimator, and flattening filter were simulated in the first stage. The phase space particles were collected at the front surface of the monitor chamber. These phase space particles were used as the input for the second stage of the simulation, which included the monitor chamber and the jaws. The final phase space particles were collected at the isocenter plane of 100 cm SAD.

To simulate the dynamic jaw motion using the Monte Carlo technique, three methods were studied in this work. For the first two methods, the STT was divided into small bins with a finite spatial resolution. The corresponding component fields were simulated, from which the individual phase space data were combined for the dynamic wedge. The first approach ("NH") was to simulate the number of histories that is proportional to the MUs of each component field which was given by the STT. The second approach ("WT") was to simulate the same number of histories for each component field, but weight the particles from a component field by its MUs.

A third and more efficient approach ("RS") in simulating the dynamic wedge was to treat the jaw as a true moving component. To achieve this, for each starting particle history, the position of the jaw was re-sampled from a probability distribution function, which was computed from the STT of the dynamic wedge. An example of the probability distribution function of a 10 cm wide 60 degree wedge is shown in Fig. 1. In the BEAM code, a jaw position sampling routine was added to the component module of "JAWS". The position of the front surface of the moving jaw piece (facing the electron target) was sampled from the distribution function. The position of the back surface of the moving jaw was also recomputed during the simulation based on the divergence of the beam. This reflects closely the design of the jaws moved in an arc fashion to define the beam edge on Varian machines.

In simulating the dynamic wedge shown in Fig. 1., 10 million 6 MeV electrons were used for the first stage of the simulation, which resulted in approximately 17 million phase space particles used for the subsequent simulations. In using the component field technique, the STT was divided with 1 cm spatial bin. Using the first simulation method ("NH"), the number of histories simulated for each component field ranged from 6.25 million for the largest 10 cm wide field to 14.76 million for the smallest 1 cm wide field. For the second simulation method ("WT"), 10 million histories were used for each of the 10 component fields. A weighting factor ranging from 0.625 for the 10 cm wide field to 1.476 for the 1 cm wide field were applied to the resulting phase space particles. For the third simulation method ("RS"), a total of 100 million histories were used in one single run of the simulation. The jaw position was sampled discretely with 1 cm spatial resolution in order to compare the results to those of the component sampling techniques. To compute realistic dose distributions, the position was sampled from the continuous probability distribution function (Fig. 1), which represents the true dynamic motion of the jaw.

## Results and Discussion

Fig. 2 shows comparisons of the fluence and energy fluence distributions of the 60 degree dynamic wedge using the two component techniques ("NH" and "WT"). The agreement between the results of the two methods indicates that there is no significant difference between using the number of histories versus weighting the particles in simulating the component fields. This also validates the basic assumption used in the random sampling method ("RS") that the fluence or energy fluence output is proportional to the number of simulated histories, provided that there is significant number of particles being simulated to represent the beam with statistical confidence.

Fig. 3 shows comparisons of the fluence and energy fluence distributions of the same wedge using the first component technique ("NH") and the random sampling technique ("RS"). There is an excellent agreement between the results from the two methods. This verifies the accuracy of the random sampling technique for simulating the dynamic jaw motion. A stepping effect is shown by the fluence and energy fluence distributions because each component field moves by 1 cm increments. The advantage of using the random sampling technique is the flexibility of either simulating the dynamic motion via a step-shoot fashion, as used for the component sampling techniques, or sampling the the jaw position continuously to simulate the true dynamic motion on the Varian machines. The CPU times for the simulations were comparable between the random sampling technique and the component sampling technique ("NH") because the same number of histories were simulated. Yet the random sampling technique is much more efficient to use and requires less data storage space, because only one simulation needs to be performed with one single phase space file output.

In reality, the machine output during the dynamic wedge beam delivery is controlled by the collected charge from the monitor chamber in the machine head. The monitor chamber reading can be affected by the backscattered radiation from the jaws. This effect has been studied in full detail in separate works [3, 4], from which the backscatter correction can be applied to compute realistic dose distributions using Monte Carlo simulation. The computed dose distributions will be verified by those from the measurements. The simulation of the dynamic wedge is a step forward towards applying Monte Carlo simulation for IMRT beam delivery.

## Conclusions

In this work, three sampling techniques were investigated in Monte Carlo simulation of dynamic jaw motion for the Varian dynamic wedges. Using the first two methods, the dynamic wedge was approximated by individual static component fields. The number of histories or the weighting of the particles used in the simulation was proportional to the MUs of the component field. In a third approach, the jaw motion was sampled from a probability distribution derived from the STT of the wedge. Results of the Monte Carlo simulation showed excellent agreement among all three methods. This indicates that the primary output of the machine (excluding the effect of the jaw backscatter) is proportional to the number of simulation histories. Thus for the component sampling techniques, it is equivalent to use either the number of the histories or weight the particles by the MUs of the component fields. The random sampling technique can be used for both the step-shoot and true dynamic beam delivery. This approach is more efficient and accurate in simulating the dynamic jaw motion, and can be generalized towards simulation of dynamic MLCs for IMRT.

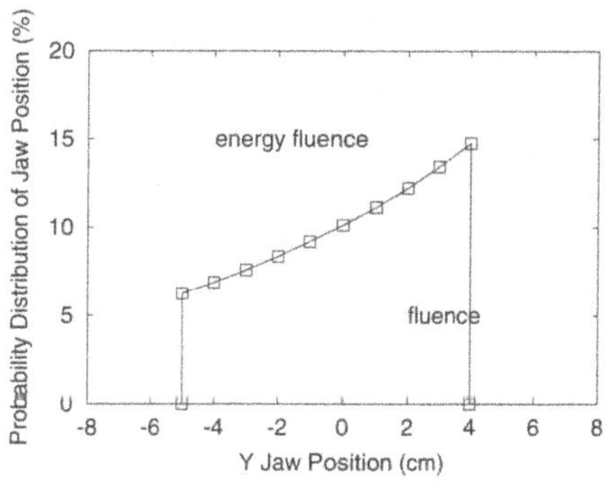


**Figure 1:** Probability distribution function of jaw position based on STT of the Varian 60 degree dynamic wedge.

## Acknowledgments

This research is in part funded by a Marie Curie Research Training Grant from the European communities. The authors would like to thank Dr. Dave Rogers and his physics group for making the BEAM Monte Carlo available for this work.

## References

1. Rogers D W O, Faddegon B A, Ding G X, Ma C M, We J, Mackie T R, BEAM: A Monte Carlo code to simulate

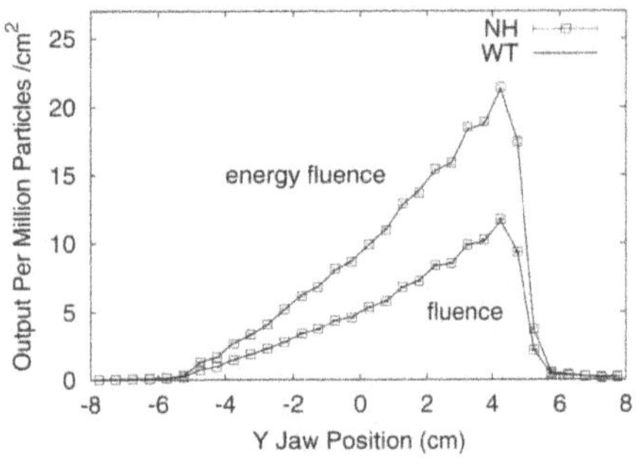


**Figure 2:** Fluence and energy fluence distributions across the wedge gradient direction of the 60 degree dynamic wedge from the two component sampling techniques: "NH" uses different number of histories and "WT" uses different particle weighting for individual component fields. The standard errors of the Monte Carlo data are approximately 1% of the values inside the field.

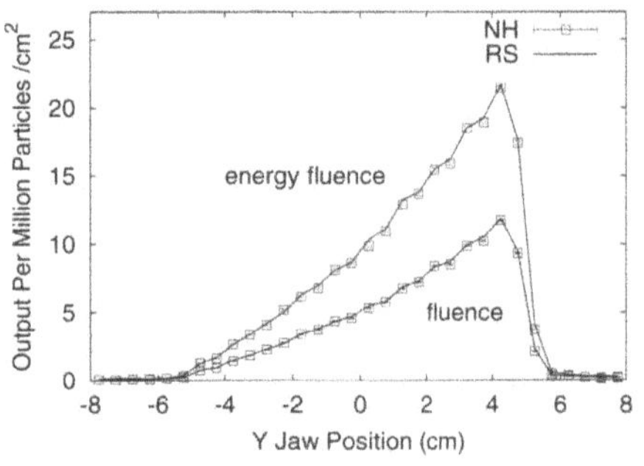


**Figure 3:** Fluence and energy fluence distributions across the wedge gradient direction of the 60 degree dynamic wedge from the component sampling technique "NH" and from the random sampling technique "RS". The standard errors of the Monte Carlo data are approximately 1% of the values inside the field.

radiotherapy treatment units, *Med. Phy.* **22** 503 – 524, 1995;

2. Verhaegen F and Das I J, Monte Carlo modeling of a virtual wedge, *Phys. Med. Biol.* **44** N251 – 259, 1999;

3. Liu H H, Mackie T R, McCullough E C, Modeling photon output caused by backscattered radiation into the monitor chamber from collimator jaws using a Monte Carlo technique, *submitted to Med. Phy.*;

4. Verhaegen F, Symonds-Tayler R, Mubata C, Bidmead M, Nahum A, and Liu HH, A Monte Carlo study of backscatter in the monitor ino chamber for clinical photon and electron beams, *submitted to the XIII International Conference on the use of computers in radiation therapy, Heidelberg, Germany, 2000.*

# Dynamic-MLC Modeling for Monte Carlo dose calculations

**Jeffrey V. Siebers, Paul J. Keall, Mark Arnfield, Jong Oh Kim and Radhe Mohan**

Department of Radiation Oncology, MCV Hospitals, Virginia Commonwealth University, Richmond, VA, USA

## Introduction

In the near future, the Monte Carlo method will be used for simulating intensity-modulated treatments delivered with dynamic multi-leaf collimators (DMLCs). Monte Carlo (MC) dose calculation algorithms are being recognized as the most accurate way of predicting patient dose.[1] However, for IMRT delivered with DMLCs, accurate dose calculation is non-trivial, even with Monte Carlo.

For treatment fields treated with static (non-moving) multileaf collimators, radiation transmitted through and scattered from the MLC leaves is ~2% of the open-field dose.[2] This radiation is called the MLC leakage radiation. For IMRT delivered with DMLCs, the minimum intensity deliverable to a location within the fixed accelerator jaws is the static field leakage rate divided by the "efficiency" of the IMRT field delivery, where efficiency is defined as the number of monitor units required to deliver the prescribed maximum dose with an open field divided by the number of monitor units required to deliver the IMRT treatment. For delivery of complex IMRT intensity distributions, efficiency can be less than 0.2, resulting in MLC leakage dose contributions (minimum deliverable intensities) of greater than 10% of the maximum in-field dose. Note, at some points in the treatment field, all of the local dose may be due to leakage. Thus, accurate accounting of leakage dose in the patient dose calculation must exist.

Many approaches are possible for modeling MLCs for MC dose calculations. Exact simulation of DMLCs using MC requires a "time-dependent" MC geometry. Even without time-dependent geometry, the complex geometry of the MLC (i.e. the tongue-and-groove features) makes accurate simulation computationally time consuming. DMLC modeling can be simplified by discretizing the field into $N$ static fields, which are then computed in a sequential manner, however, unless $N$ is large (sufficient to account for the moving rounded leaf tips and the in-field intensity variations) this method will not accurately model the dose delivery. Without using variance reduction schemes, exact MC DMLC models require an increase in the number of source particles sampled to obtain the same statistical dose uncertainty in the patient. Compared to static field delivery, the number of source particles must increase by approximately the inverse of the efficiency of beam delivery. This increases the dose computation time.

The purpose of this paper is to show the components of radiation transmitted through and scattered from a multileaf collimator to the dose deposited beneath a MLC. A simplified model of the MLC for use with Monte Carlo dose calculations is developed and tested, and the range of validity of the model is discussed. Although this model is applicable to dynamic field delivery, in this work, only static, blocked MLC field results are presented.

## Material and methods

An 80-leaf multileaf collimator for a Varian* 2100c accelerator was modeled for this study. This multileaf collimator has the tongue-and-groove design to reduce inter-leaf radiation leakage. The 6 MV mode of the accelerator was used for all calculations presented here.

**Figure 1:** Cross-section of MLC leaves modeled for the MCNP4b2 simulations. The tongue-and-groove of the leaves were fully modeled.

### Determination of MLC leakage components

MCNP4b2[3] was used to model a fully closed MLC to determine the components of radiation exiting the MLC as a function of the field size incident upon the MLC. A cross-section of the MLC leaf model is shown in Figure 1. The rounded leaf tips were ignored and the leaf lengths were set to be larger than the irradiated field area for this study. Particles from a pre-generated phase space file[4] were transported through the treatment head to the MLC entrance surface. The jaw settings were set to 5×5, 10×10, and 15×15 $cm^2$ during these simulations. Each particle incident upon the MLC (configured to fully block the field) was re-used twenty times for transport through the MLC. Following the MLC, the particles were sorted according to their point of origin, either the target, the MLC, or other treatment head components, corresponding to primary, MLC-scatter, and head-scatter beam components. Particles exiting the MLC were transported through a 30×30×30 $cm^3$ water phantom whose entrance surface was located at 95 cm SSD. Lateral dose profiles were scored in 0.1×4.0×2.0 $cm^3$ voxels, 0.1 cm normal to the long axis of the leaves, 4 cm along the leaves and 2 cm along the depth axis, centered at a depth of 5 cm. The total dose from the three components was normalized to the dose for an open field

* Varian Oncology Systems, Palo Alto, California, USA

of the same field size. Dose components for the target, head-scatter, and MLC-scatter components were thus determined.

**Analytic MLC Model**

A simplified model of the MLC was developed for MC simulations for use with the MCV Monte Carlo code.[5] Photons incident upon the MLC have their beam weights modified by the attenuation through the MLC leaf, including the effect of the rounded leaf tip,

$$w_f = w_i / T_{total} \times \left( T_{open} + T_{closed} e^{-\mu(E)l} + S_{tip} \right)$$

with

$$S_{tip} = T_{in} \int_0^{T_{in}} e^{-\mu(E)l(T)} dT + T_{out} \int_0^{T_{out}} e^{-\mu(E)l(T)} dT .$$

Initial and final beam weights are designated $w_i$ and $w_f$. The total time, $T_{total}$, consists of the time the MLC is open and closed, $T_{open}$ and $T_{closed}$, (neglecting the time that the leaf tips are at the point), and the time the incoming and outgoing leaves are passing by the point, $T_{in}$ and $T_{out}$. $\mu(E)$ is the linear attenuation coefficient of the MLC material (tungsten) for the particle with energy $E$, and $l$ is the pathlength of the particle through the MLC.

In this model of the MLC, electron transport through the MLC leaves and scattered photons and electrons produced in the MLC are ignored. Electrons incident on the MLC have their weight reduced by the fraction of time that the MLC is open. Furthermore, photons are assumed to travel only within a single leaf. Transport of photons from one leaf to the next (or from a leaf to an open area) is neglected.

Comparisons between the analytic MLC model and full MLC simulations were performed as follows. The MCV code was used to transport particles from an EGS4 created phase space distribution file, through jaws defining a 10×10 $cm^2$ field size, to the entrance of the MLC. This phase space file was operated on by the analytic MLC model, with resulting phase-space particles transported through a 40×40×40 $cm^3$ water phantom whose surface was located at 100 cm SSD. Dose was scored in 0.2×1.0×0.2 $cm^3$ voxels. The same EGS4 phase space file of particles incident upon the MLC was also used as an input file for an MCNP simulation of a closed MLC, with particles incident upon the MLC being re-used twenty times. Particles exiting the MCNP simulation were transported using MCV through the same water phantom as the analytic MLC model. Resulting dose distributions for the two models were compared.

## Results and Discussion

**Determination of MLC leakage components**

Figure 2 graphically shows the components of the MLC leakage for the 10×10 $cm^2$ field at 5 cm depth in a water phantom computed using MCNP4b2. The primary beam results clearly show the differential transmission through the full leaf thickness and the leaf-overlap regions. The MLC scatter contribution, however, can be approximated by a broad Gaussian distribution.

Table 1 shows the components of the radiation exiting the MLC averaged from -1.5 cm to 1.5 cm on the lateral profiles. The total leakage increases with field size due to increased scatter from the multileaf collimator. For the 10×10 $cm^2$ field, the MLC scatter contributes ~11% of the dose from radiation exiting the MLC at a depth of 5 cm. Given that the total leakage for a blocked MLC field is ~1.7% of the open field dose for static delivery, the MLC scatter component is insignificant (less than 1% of the maximum dose in the field) for dynamic fields with efficiencies greater than ~0.18. Similarly, for a 5×5 $cm^2$, efficiencies greater than ~0.06 yield insignificant dose from MLC scatter, while for a 15×15 $cm^2$ field, the efficiency should be greater than ~0.3.

**Figure 2:** Components of radiation exiting the MLC for irradiation with a 10×10 field.

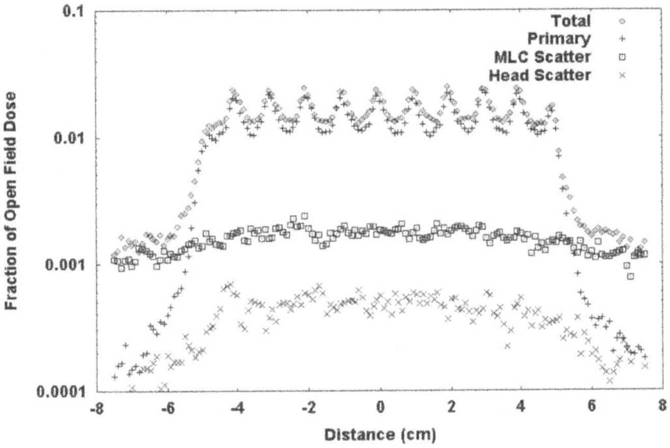


| | 5×5 | 10×10 | 15×15 |
|---|---|---|---|
| Total | 1.61% | 1.65% | 1.84% |
| Primary | 1.51% | 1.42% | 1.46% |
| Head Scatter | 0.04% | 0.05% | 0.07% |
| MLC Scatter | 0.06% | 0.18% | 0.31% |

**Table 1:** Components of radiation exiting the field fully blocked by a multileaf collimator. Values are given as percentage of dose for an open field.

**Figure 3:** Comparison of full MCNP MLC model and the analytic MLC model at a depth of 5 cm for closed MLC leaves covering a 10×10 $cm^2$field.

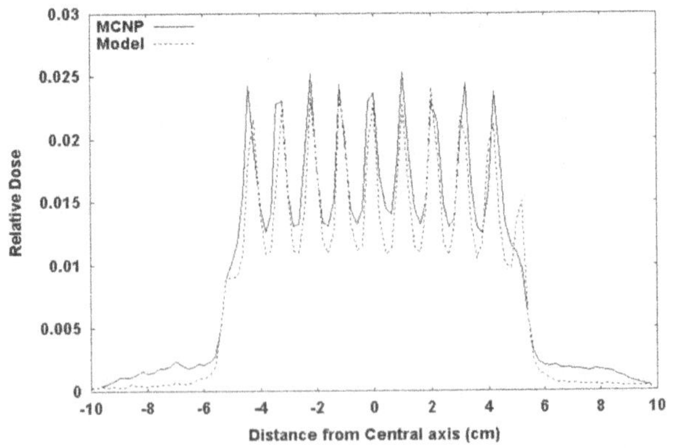

**Analytic MLC Model**

Figure 3 compares Monte Carlo dose calculations done with the analytic MLC model and with the full MC MLC simulation at a depth of 5 cm in the water phantom. The jaws were set to produce a 10×10 cm$^2$ for these simulations and the MLC configured to fully block the field. The in-field agreement is good, with the analytic model underestimating the full MC simulation by the MLC scatter contribution (as determined by integrating the profile). Outside the 10×10 cm$^2$ field, the MCNP MLC simulation predicts more dose due to the fact that this area was open during the simulation (no leaves existed to attenuate the jaw leakage in this region). The average output (determined by integrating between -4 cm and +4 cm on the profiles) as a function of depth in the water phantom was determined for both MLC simulations. The ratio between the full MC simulation and the analytic model is shown in Figure 4. Neglecting the MLC-scatter contribution has the greatest effect at the surface, with reducing significance at depth. However, even at 30 cm depth, neglecting the MLC-scatter results in a ~10% under-prediction of MLC leakage.

**Figure 4:** Ratio of the output for the analytic MLC simulation to the full MCNP MLC simulation as a function of depth in the phantom.

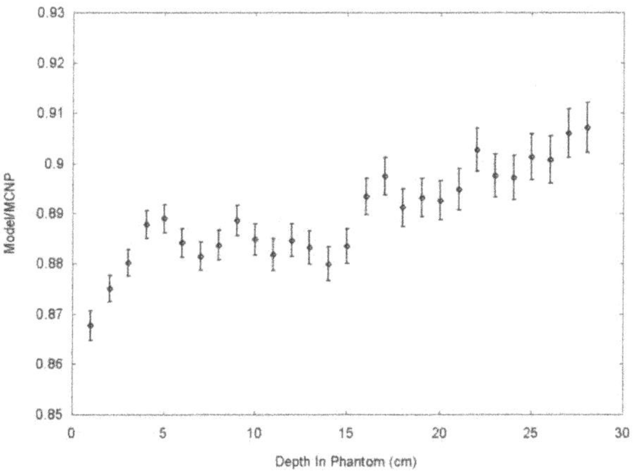


# Conclusions

The MLC scatter contribution to dose in-field for MLC blocked fields is a function of the area of the MLC leaves exposed to the radiation beam. Since the dose contribution for MLC leakage is small, this contribution can be ignored for static field delivery. For dynamic field delivery (IMRT delivered with a DMLC), however, the leakage contribution increases as the efficiency of beam delivery decreases. The MLC scatter contribution may become important for large field sizes and low efficiency fields.

A simple analytical model of the MLC has been developed that is appropriate for application to dynamic IMRT dose calculations. This model modifies the beam weight of particles incident upon the MLC by the probability that they will be attenuated by the MLC. The model ignores the MLC scatter contribution; however, such a contribution could be added to the model. One advantage of this MLC model is that particles are conserved, obviating the need to run additional beam-line phase space particles for dynamic IMRT Monte Carlo simulations. The analytic model agrees with predictions based upon a full MLC simulation, under-predicting the true MLC leakage by the MLC scatter component. The model will be sufficiently accurate for small fields and fields with high delivery efficiencies, however, the model will underestimate the MLC leakage, particularly for large fields and inefficient fields.

These results are also useful for modeling leaf characteristics for non-Monte Carlo IMRT implementations.

# Acknowledgements

The authors acknowledge the financial support of NIH Grant CA 74158-02

# References

[1]R. Mohan, "Why Monte Carlo?," presented at the XII International Conference on the Use of Computers in Radiotherapy, Salt Lake City, Utah, 1997.

[2]T. LoSasso, C.-S. Chui, and C. C. Ling, "Physical and dosimetric aspects of a multileaf collimation system used in the dynamic mode for implementing intensity modulated radiotherapy," Medical Physics **25**, 1919-1917 (1998).

[3]J. F. Briesmeister, "MCNP- A General Monte Carlo N-Particle Transport Code, Version 4B," Report No. LA-13181, Los Alamos National Laboratory, 1997.

[4]J. V. Siebers, P. J. Keall, B. Libby, and R. Mohan, "Comparison of EGS4 and MCNP4b Monte Carlo Codes for generation of photon phase space distributions for a Varian 2100C," Phys. Med. Bio. **44** (5) (1999).

[5]J. V. Siebers, P. J. Keall, B. Libby, and R. Mohan, "A Monte Carlo System for Radiotherapy Dose Calculations: Integration Issues," Med. Phys. **Submitted, October 1999** (1999).

# Considerations for modelling MLCs with Monte Carlo techniques

**Hugo Palmans[1], PhD, Frank Verhaegen[2], PhD, Francesca M. Buffa[2], Cephas Mubata[2], PhD**

[1]Biomedical Physics Dept, University of Gent (Belgium), and [2]Physics Dept, Royal Marsden Hospital, London (UK)

## Introduction

In order to avoid systematic errors when sometimes a large number of small radiation fields are superimposed in intensity modulated photon radiation therapy (IMRT), accurate knowledge of the influence of the beam defining multileaf collimator (MLC) leaves on the radiation field is essential. Measuring the two-dimensional dose distributions of all radiation fields that might contribute to an IMRT treatment is impractical. An alternative is Monte Carlo (MC) simulations of the individual field arrangements. This requires an exact model of the MLC leaves. The current BEAM distribution provides two modules; one with a flat leaf end surface and one that models the curved shape of a cylindrical leaf end. The former is the standard MLC module in BEAM, the latter, MLCQ, is an extension of the module MLCP, developed by us and described in [1]. In this work, lateral dose profiles for two different accelerators equipped with MLCs are calculated. The differences in the penumbral regions are shown in a homogeneous phantom and in patient geometry.

## Material and methods

Using the Monte Carlo code EGS4/BEAM [2], models for two accelerators were built; an Elekta SL25 and a Varian 2100C, both equipped with MLCs. In the SL25 the MLC is situated between flattening filter and jaws whereas for the 2100C it is the final beam-collimating device, located after the jaws. Manufacturer's information was used to model the machines. The model for the SL25 is similar to the one presented by us earlier [1], except for some minor differences in the construction details of the accelerator head. In the same publication [1], a new BEAM CM for an MLC with rounded leave ends, was presented. This model, called MLCQ, takes the rounded MLC leave end shape of Elekta and Varian accelerators correctly into account.

Lateral dose distributions obtained with the new model, MLCQ, were compared to those obtained with the standard BEAM model for MLCs (CM MLC) and to measurements. For the SL25, besides a 10x10 $cm^2$ reference field centred at central axis, rectangular fields with field sizes of 10x1 $cm^2$ and 10x2 $cm^2$ were used which were centred at the central axis and at off-axis positions of 5.0 cm and 10.0 cm.

To demonstrate the importance of a correct MLC model for Monte Carlo treatment planning, a clinical case was studied. An 8-field plan with identical equi-angular square fields (6.4x6.4 $cm^2$) for a prostate tumour was planned on the Dosigray Monte Carlo treatment planning system with the two different models for the MLC. For this case, the bladder is exposed to eight overlapping penumbral regions. The resolution of the calculation grid was 5 mm in the lateral directions and 2 mm in the sup-inf direction, which was also the MLC leave direction.

## Results and discussion

### Comparison of lateral dose profiles

For field sizes of 10x10 $cm^2$ and 10x4 $cm^2$ for the 6 MV photon beam from the SL25 the differences obtained with both models were not significant. Figures 1 and 2 show lateral profiles at 10 cm depth for field sizes of 10x2 $cm^2$ and 10x1 $cm^2$. Figure 1 gives data for fields centred at the central axis, while in figure 2 off-axis fields are given. Compared are profiles calculated using CM MLC and CM MLCQ. The differences as a percentage of the maximum dose are also shown.

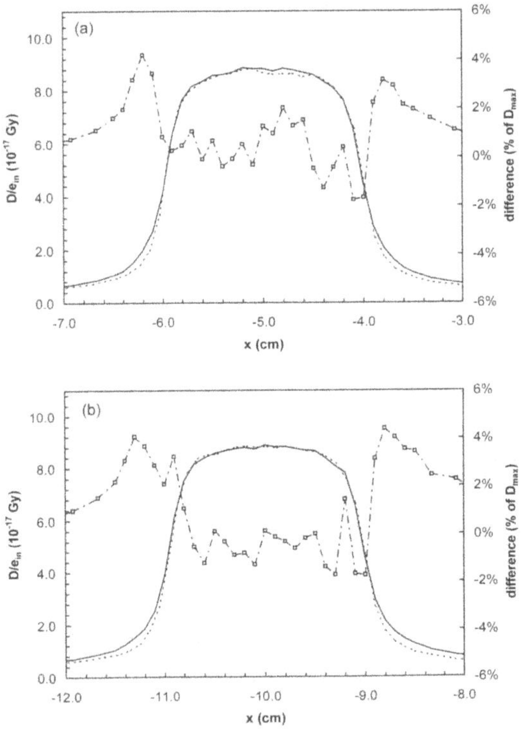


**Figure 1.** Calculated lateral dose profiles at 10 cm depth with CM MLCQ (full line) and CM MLC (dashed line) and differences as a percentage of the maximum dose (symbols and right vertical axis) for a 6 MV beam from a SL25 linac for centred fields with field sizes of (a) 10x2 $cm^2$ and (b) 10x1 $cm^2$. Fields are such that the 50% dose levels are equal.

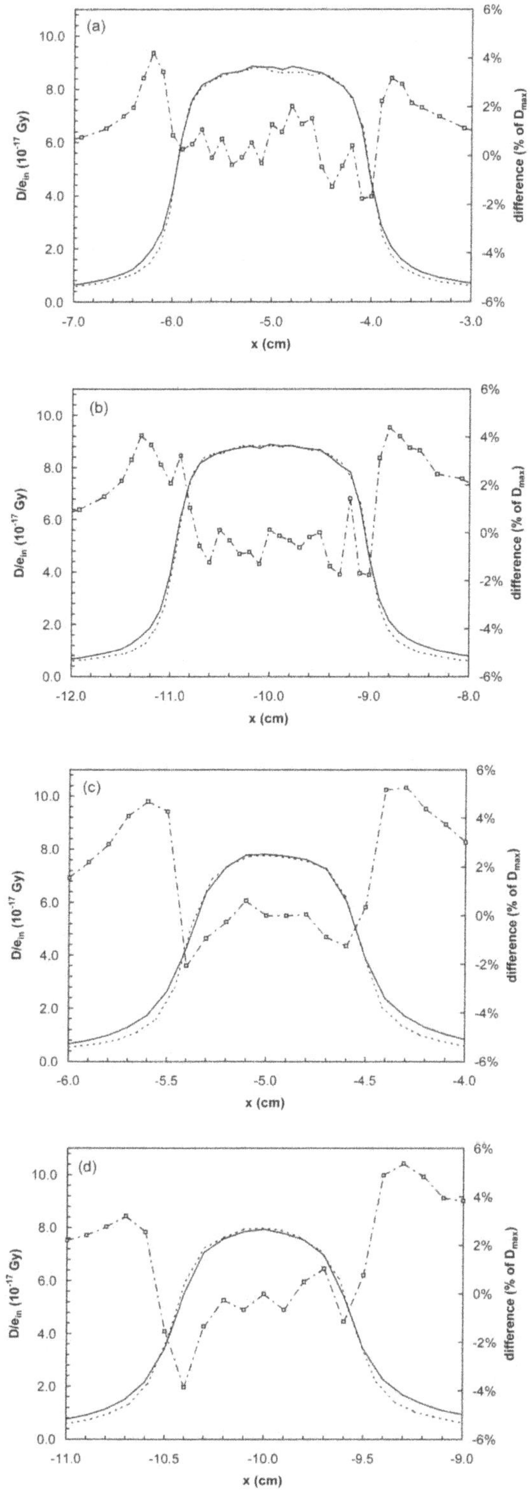


**Figure 2.** Same as figure 1 for field sizes of (a) 10x2 cm$^2$ at 5 cm off-axis, (b) 10x2 cm$^2$ at 10 cm off-axis, (c) 10x1 cm$^2$ at 5 cm off-axis and (d) 10x1 cm$^2$ at 10 cm off-axis.

The settings of the leaves in both models were such that the 50% dose levels coincide, so that only the differences in the MC models will show up and not the differences due to different field widths for the same light field setting. Differences up to 5% of the maximum dose near the edge of the field can be observed for the smallest field sizes.

In earlier work by our group, it was shown that calculations with CM MLCQ, which takes the roundness of the leaves into account, give a good agreement with measurements [1]. Comparing the data in this reference with the results from figures 1 and 2 it is clear that the results obtained with CM MLC deviate more from the measurements than the results obtained with CM MLCQ.

When using the same light field calibration for determining the opening between opposite leaves, results with CM MLC indicate a smaller field (judged by the 50% dose level) and a smaller penumbra. Thus, when these MLC models are used for Monte Carlo treatment planning in the clinical situation, the differences between the two models will be even larger. This is demonstrated for a 10 MV beam from the Varian 2100C linac. In figures 3 and 4, lateral dose distributions at 10 cm depth for centred and off-axis fields of 4x4 cm$^2$ and 2x2 cm$^2$ are compared for the two CMs MLC and MLCQ. Differences up to 15% or 1 mm can be seen for the centred fields. For the off-axis fields, which are of importance for IMRT treatments, the differences are even larger.

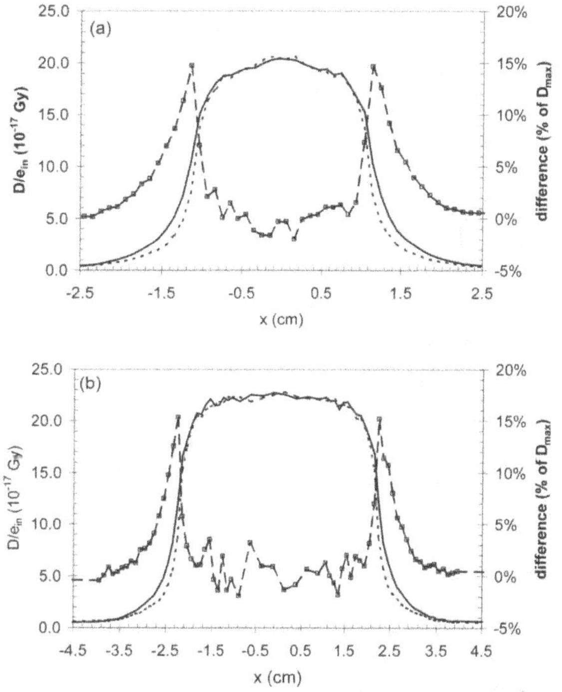


**Figure 3**. Calculated lateral dose profiles at 10 cm depth with CM MLCQ (full line) and CM MLC (dashed line) and differences as a percentage of the maximum dose (symbols and right vertical axis) for a 10 MV beam from a 2100C linac for centred fields with field sizes of (a) 2x2 cm$^2$ and (b) 4x4 cm$^2$. Fields are such that the light field settings are identical.

Simulations with an even more precise MC model for the 2100C MLC leaves, which takes into account that only the central 50% is curved while the outer segments are tangential to the curved segment (labelled MLCRF) resulted in lateral fluences that were not significantly different from the MLCQ model, even for the fields with the largest offset (14 cm). This is shown in figure 5 for a 2x2 $cm^2$ field.

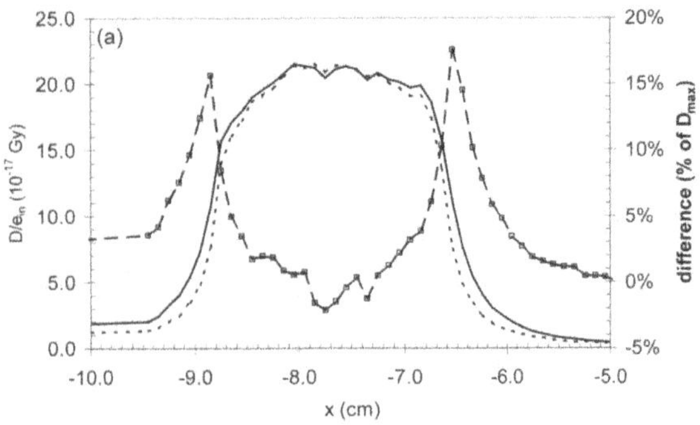


**Figure 4.** Same as figure 3 for an off-axis position of 7 cm for a 2x2 $cm^2$ field.

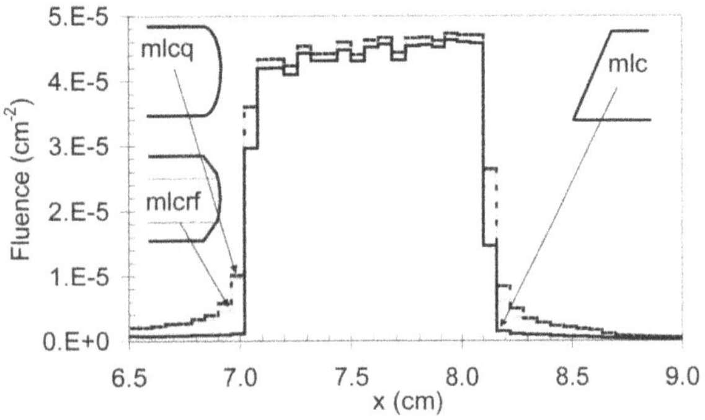


**Figure 5.** Lateral fluence at the level immediately after the Varian 2100C MLC for the three MLC models MLC, MLCQ and MLCRF for a 2x2 $cm^2$ field for a 10 MV photon beam.

**A clinical example**

Figure 6 shows the dose volume histogram for the clinical case studied. A prostate patient was planned with 8 equi-angular lateral beams of 10 MV photon beams with a target dose of 60 Gy. The bladder was considered. Although the lateral dose distribution extends a bit more in the bladder for the MLCQ module compared to the MLC module, the dose volume histogram for the bladder does not indicate significant differences. This is probably due to the tissue heterogeneities, which tend to obliterate the small dose differences in the penumbra. More clinical cases are being studied in this project.

## Conclusion

In this work lateral dose profiles from 6 MV and 10 MV photon beams, shaped with MLCs with rounded leaf ends, were studied for two different clinical accelerators.

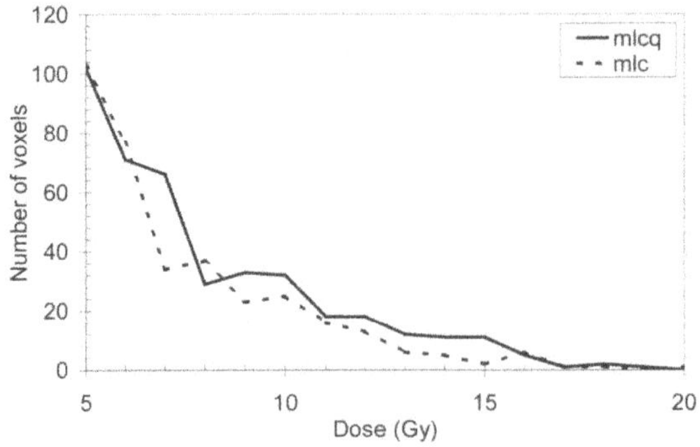


**Figure 6**. Dose volume histogram for the clinical case studied.

Monte Carlo simulations with two different models for the MLC leaves were compared. By comparing to measured dose profiles in an earlier work [1], it was found that an accurate model of the MLC leaves, taking into account the curvature of the leaves, is required for the simulations. Using the default EGS4/BEAM model of an MLC with focused leaves in stead of a model with rounded leaves can in the penumbral regions lead to differences of up to 15% in dose or 1mm in position of $d_{50}$ for a single field.

Superimposing several of these fields with an inaccurate model for the MLC leaves can lead to errors in penumbral regions. However, a preliminary study of a clinical case for an eight-field prostate plan, calculated with a Monte Carlo treatment planning system, indicates that the differences in the penumbral regions will be very small.

## Acknowledgements

John Pettingell and Shakilah Patval from the Royal Marsden Hospital, London, are thanked for their assistance in this work. F.V. is sponsored by a Marie Curie Research Training Grant from the European Communities.

## References

[1] De Vlamynck K, Palmans H, Verhaegen F, De Wagter C, De Neve W and Thierens H 1999 Dose measurements compared with Monte Carlo simulations of narrow 6 MV multi-leaf collimator shaped photon beams. *Med. Phys.* **26**, 1874-1882

[2] Rogers D, Faddegon B, Ding G, Ma C-M, We J and Mackie T 1995 BEAM: a Monte Carlo code to simulate radiotherapy treatment units. *Med. Phys.* **22**, 503-524

# Monte Carlo simulation of wax compensating filters for radiotherapy of the head and neck.

**E. Spezi[1], D.G.Lewis, K. Gray and C.W.Smith**

Department of Medical Physics, Velindre Hospital Cardiff CF14 2TL, UK. [1]Email: emiliano.spezi@physics.org

## Introduction

The use of individualised compensating filters has long been established in radiotherapy to modify dose distributions to allow for contour and tissue variations [1]. Compensators are designed to replace the missing tissue required to produce a uniform patient surface but are retracted away from the skin in order to preserve the skin-sparing effect in megavoltage photon beams. Compensators, made from tissue-equivalent or from higher density materials, are commonly used for radiotherapy of the head and neck. The dose to the patient can be calculated by modelling measured data for the reduction in dose due to loss of scattered radiation from the missing tissue [2] [3]. However the anatomical complexity of the treatment region and the tissue inhomogeneities present requires an accurate calculation of the effects of scattered radiation and electron contamination produced when modelling the thickness of compensator material required [4] [5]. Moreover there is a clinical need to etablish more firmly 3D dose distribution in patient arising by using wax compensators [6], for a better evaluation of Intensity Modulated Radiation Therapy benefits.
Monte Carlo dose calculation engines nowadays represent the most advanced and suitable technique for elaborate radiotherapy treatment plans involving tissue inhomogeneities [7]. The Monte Carlo Code System BEAM/EGS4 [8,11] has been used among others in our centre for efficient simulation of megavoltage photon beams [9]. This study investigates the capabilities of BEAM in simulating photon beams modulated with wax compensators. A comparison with experimental data for different wax slab thicknesses is reported. Charged particle contamination effects have also been analysed.

## Material and methods

Simulating "non-standard" materials (i.e. those not included in ICRU tables [10]) using the BEAM code requires building such material data from composition information provided by the manufacturer. Wax compensator data have been generated for this study using the EGS4 data preprocessor code PEGS4 [10]. Initial BEAM simulations for the wax material were performed. Consequently the material characterisation parameters, such as density, were tested and adjusted to produce a good match between calculated and experimental depth dose data for a $(10\times10)cm^2$ 6MV photon field. This test and the following BEAM simulations were carried out using a pre stored BEAM 'phase space' data file. The file contained $25.0\cdot10^6$ particles (99.98% of which are photons) and was generated using $400.0\cdot10^6$ e- incident on the target. The phase space data were recorded in a plane at the exit window of a Varian Clinac 2100CD. These data were were checked for quality assurance purposes against measured reference data sets.
To test calculation accuracy for a wax compensation system using the Monte Carlo technique, we compared both depth doses and profiles, and central axis retraction factors, for wax slab compensators of different thicknesses (2cm, 4cm, 7cm, 10cm). As shown in Figure 1 the retraction factor f at P' is defined as

$$f=(\text{dose at } P')/(\text{dose at } P) \qquad (eq.\ 1)$$

In this configuration the distance from the lower compensator surface and the phantom surface was 25cm for each slab thickness.
Doses from a $(10\times10)cm^2$ 6MV photon beam were measured for open and compensated fields incident on a water phantom using a fixed number of Monitor Units (400). The compensator data were normalised to the dose value for the open field at 5cm deep.
BEAM phase space files were generated for the different slab thickness by using the $25.0\cdot10^6$ particles stored in the 'open field' phase space file as a source incident on the upper compensator surface. These phase space files, representing the radiation output from the compensator, were then used as input to the DOSXYZ code [12] simulating the water phantom irradiation. In this case a common recycling factor of 8 was applied in reusing phase space particles. It has been verified that this approach does not produce artefacts nor underestimate the error in the final dose calculation [13].

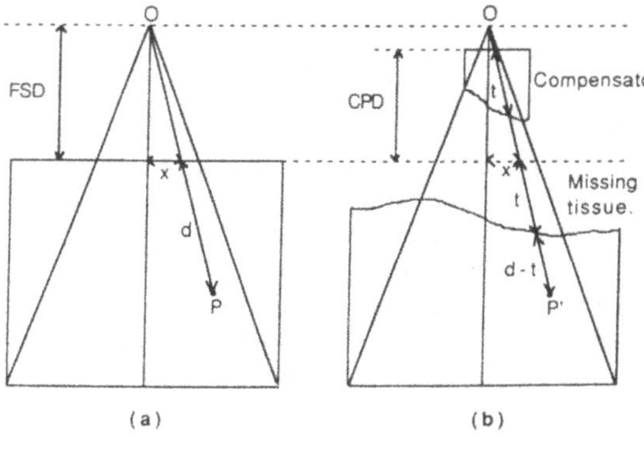


**Figure1:** Definition of retraction factor. P and P' are corresponding points in (a) the full phantom and (b) the compensated phantom (FSD = Focus to Surface Distance, CPD = Compensator to Phantom Distance).

Two different phantom configurations and different electron and photon cut-off energies (ECUT and PCUT respectively) were used, depending on the subject of the study.

(1) *Depth doses and central axis retraction factors*: a phantom (25x25x40)$cm^3$ with a fine grid of (2.5x2.5x0.2)$cm^3$ voxels along the first 2cm in depth, and a coarser grid of (2.5x2.5x1.0)$cm^3$ for depths > 2cm, was used for a achieving better particle transport control and resolution around depth of dose maximum (dmax), (ECUT= 0.621keV, PCUT= 10KeV, 521ICRU PEGS data set and PRESTA [14] switched on);

(2) *Transverse profiles*: a phantom (25x25x40)$cm^3$ with a (0.5x0.5x1.0)$cm^3$ grid was used; (ECUT= 0.700keV, PCUT= 10keV, 521ICRU pegs data set and PRESTA switched on).

Doses were normalised to the dose value for the open field at 5cm deep obtained with phantom (1). It was verified that there was good agreement between that depth dose value and the dose obtained in phantom (2) at the 5cm reference depth in the same geometrical volume.
The contaminant dose arising from charged particles generated in the compensator has been evaluated with separate DOSXYZ runs using phantom (1). The Monte Carlo simulations were carried out by restarting only charged particles from the compensator output phase space files and using the same recycling factor as above. Results are presented in next section.

## Results and discussion

Figure 2 shows the comparison between calculated and measured depth doses for different wax slab compensator thickness. The Z-axis represents the depth of point of measurement in the phantom plus the thickness of missing tissue (equivalent to d+t in Figure1). The Monte Carlo calculated percentage depth dose produced by contaminant particles is also shown. The statistical uncertainty associated with the calculated depth doses is 1%. Uncertainties for contaminant depth doses range from 3% to 5% because of the relatively small number of particles simulated (~$55 \cdot 10^3$ for 2cm slab wax - ~ $47.5 \cdot 10^3$ for 10cm slab wax). As it is impossible to present a comparison of measured and calculated transverse profiles for all the compensator thickness and all the depths, one slab thickness (7 cm) has been selected and shown in Figure 3. In this case the uncertainty associated with the calculations is displayed and ranges from 1% to 3%.
The agreement between calculations and experiments is very good. Moreover, the Monte Carlo calculations predict very well the variation of depth dose with wax thickness considering that both sets of data were normalized independently at the same point. The agreement in the penumbra region could be improved by using a finer dose calculation grid, but otherwise the profiles almost exactly match the experimental data.

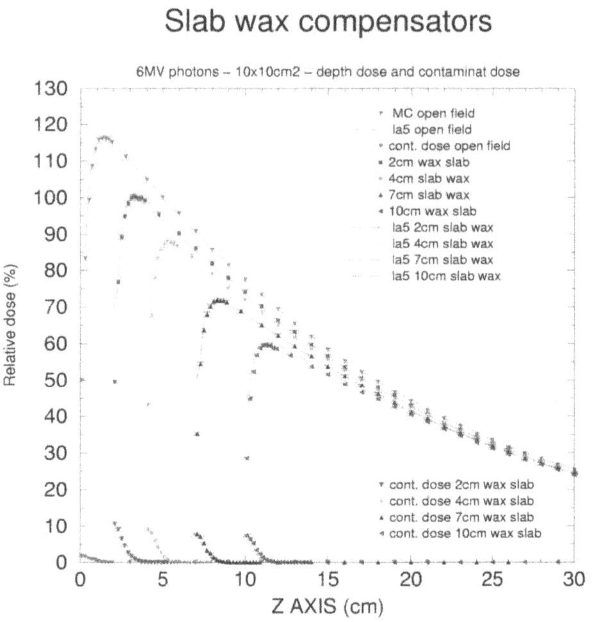


**Figure 2:** Monte Carlo and measured depth doses for different uniform wax compensator thickness. Calculated contaminant dose is shown.

The charged particle contamination study emphasises a fairly constant value of the ratio (contaminant dose)/(total dose) with increasing compensator thickness (Figure 2). This value ranges between 8% (2cm slab wax) and 11% (10cm slab wax) in the first half-cm. Nevertheless this appears significant if compared with 1% contaminant dose obtained from the open field data.

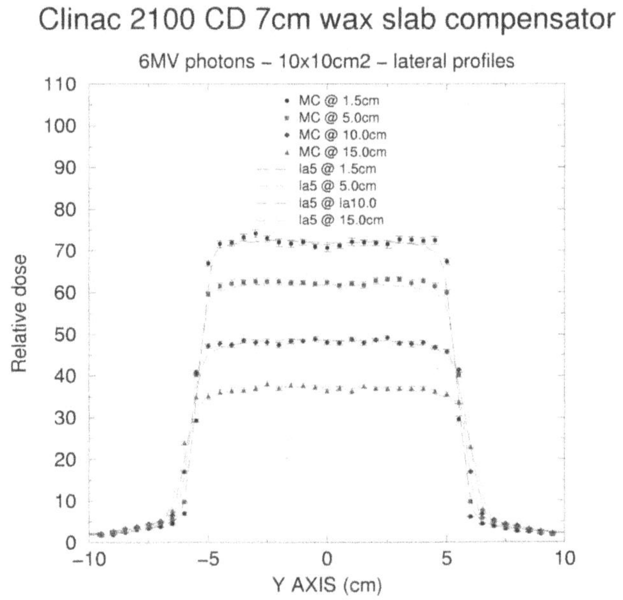


**Figure 3:** Monte Carlo and measured profiles for wax compensator thickness =7cm. Normalisation point is 5cm deep for both sets of data.

The comparison between computed and measured central axis retraction factors for all the compensator thickness is shown in Figure 4. Both the data sets were independently normalised at 5cm deep. The agreement is in the order of a few percent.

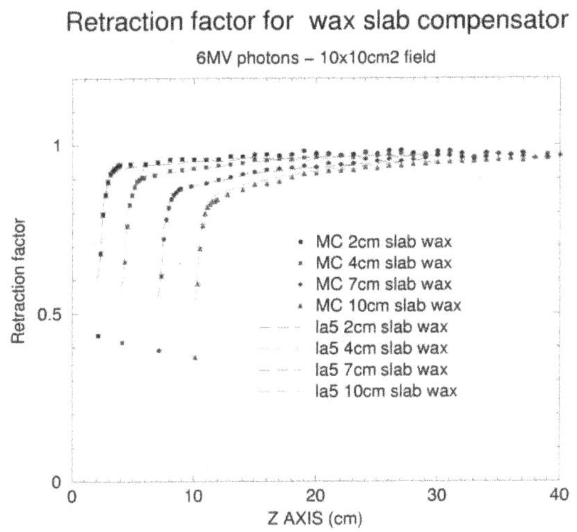


**Figure 4:** Retraction factor for different slab wax thickness (see eq. 1).

## Conclusion

Wax compensators routinely used in radiotherapy of the head and neck have been successfully simulated using the BEAM code based on an accurate accelerator model for a Varian Clinac 2100CD and a reliable implementation of material data. Charged particle contamination has been studied. The simulations indicate that contaminant dose arising from the compensator can reach significant levels (up to 10%) when compared with total dose at the patient surface. Moreover the prediction of the contaminant dose spatial distribution when using more complex shaped compensating filters is likely to benefit from further Monte Carlo calculations. This study has generated results which require further dosimetric and analytical investigations. This work forms part of a current project whose objective is a comparison of the effectiveness of intensity modulation technique with compensating filters for radiotherapy of head and neck. MLC implementation in the present Clinac model is in progress and static field IMRT simulation will also be considered, together with full 3-D shape modelling and characterisation of wax compensators.

## Acknowledgments

This work is supported by a Cancer Research Wales (WE Fry)/Tregaron studentship to ES.

## References

[1]Hall E J and Oliver R 1961, The use of standard isodose distributions with high energy radiation beams - the accuracy of a compensator technique in correcting for body contours, *Br. J. Radiol.* **34** 43-52.

[2]Jackson W 1970, Wax retraction as a technique for compensating effect of surface irregularities in high-energy radiotherapy, *Br. J. Radiol.* **43** 859-867.

[3]Gray K and Smith C W 1994, Accuracy of dose calculation methods for retracted tissue compensators, *Phys. Med. Biol.* **39** 2355-2365.

[4]Wilks R and Casebow M P 1969, Tissue compensation with lead for 60Co teletherapy, *Br. J. Radiol.* **42** 452-458.

[5]Boyer A L 1982, Compensating filters for high energy x-rays, *Med. Phys.* **9** 429-433.

[6]Basran P S, Ansbacher W, Field G C and Muray B R 1998, Evaluation of optimized compensators on a 3D planning system, Med. Phys. 25, 1837-1844.

[7]Ma C M, Mok E, Kapur A, Pawlicki T, Findley D, Brain S, Foster K and Boyer A L 1999, Clinical implementation of a Monte Carlo treatment planning system, *Med. Phys.* **26** 2133-2143.

[8]Rogers D W O, Faddegon B A 1995, Ding G X, Ma C M, We J and Mackie T R, BEAM: A Monte Carlo code to simulate radiotherapy treatment units, *Med. Phys.* **22** 503-524

[9]Love P A, Lewis D G, Al-Affan I A M and Smith C W 1998, Comparison of EGS4 and MCNP Monte Carlo codes when calculating radiotherapy depth doses, *Phys. Med. Biol.* **43** 1351-1357.

[10]ICRU Report 37, Stopping Power for Electrons and Positrons, 1984.

[11]Nelson W R, Hirayama H and Rogers D W O., The EGS4 Code System, SLAC-Report-256, Stanford 1985.

[12]Ma C M, Reckwerdt P, Holmes M,. Rogers D W O, Geiser B and Walters B, DOSXYZ User's Manual, NRCC Report PIRS 509B, NRC Ottawa 1997.

[13]Van der Zee W and Welleweerd J 1999, Calculating photon beam characteristics with Monte Carlo techniques, *Med. Phys.* **26** 1883-1892.

[14]Bielajew A F and Rogers D W O 1987, PRESTA: The parameter reduced electron-step transport algorithm for electron Monte Carlo transport, *Phys. Med. Biol.* **35** 163-181.

# OMEGA Monte Carlo verification of dosimetric data for Gamma Knife®

**Komanduri Ayyangar, Rob Mooij[1] and Paul Nizin[2]**

Medical College of Ohio, Toledo, OH, ıColumbia Presbyterian Medical Center, New York, NY, □Baylor College of Medicine, Houston, TX

## Introduction

In the dosimetry of narrow Cobalt-60 beams from Gamma Knife®, there are 3 elements of importance viz. the central axis depth-dose data , beam profiles and collimator output factors. These present a challenge to the current data acquisition and verification methods. Using the OMEGA Monte Carlo Codes, we have simulated one of the 201 source positions and thereby analyzed single beam data. Simulation geometry and source dimensions are consistent with data provided by the Gamma Knife manufacturer.

## Materials and methods

The BEAM routine from OMEGA beam[1] (version beam98 distribution)is used to model the Gamma Knife geometry in three steps. The simulation geometry is depicted in Fig.1. In the first step the source geometry and the primary collimators are modeled and a phase space file is obtained. In the second step, one of the four helmet collimators ie. 4mm, 8mm , 14mm and 18mm is modeled arriving at four different phase space files. In the final step DOSXYZ program is used to calculate doses in water phantom and generate a 3D beam. The voxel size was 1mm x1mm x 2mm. The simulations were carried out using BEAM98 code on an SGI workstation. Nearly 1 billion histories were used in the first step and 12 million histories in the second step. The standard deviation for central axis depth dose was nearly 0.7%.

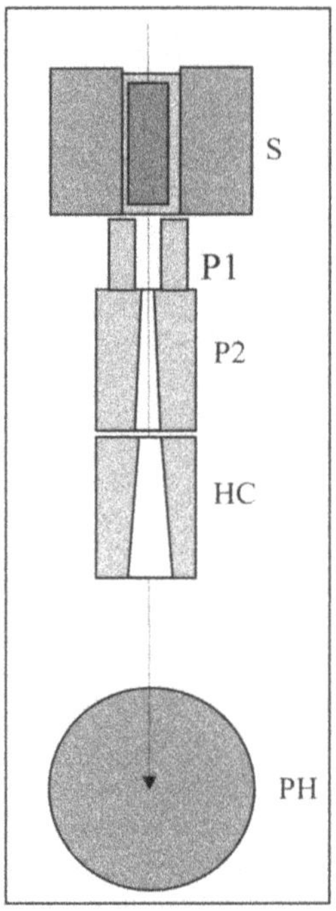


**Figure1:** Schematic of simulation geometry. S –source Capsule housing; P1 -Primary Collimator 1; P2 -Primary Collimator 2; HC – Helmet Collimator; PH –Spherical Phantom.

## Results and discussion

### DEPTH DOSE DATA:

For comparison of Monte Carlo simulated depth dose data, no reference percent depth dose data are available. However, TAR values for narrow Co-60 beams are available from Nizin and Mooij[2] that are consistent with tabulated broad beam tars of BJR25[3] . Using the Monte Carlo calculated depth dose data, TAR values were calculated and compared with those derived analytically. The average percent deviation of the OMEGA derived TAR values are 1.5%, 1.8%, 2.7% and 3.2% respectively for the 18mm, 14mm, 8mm and 4mm diameter collimators at isocenter. The comparison of TAR values with those of Nizin and Mooij[2] for the 18mm and 4mm collimators are shown in Fig.2 and 3 respectively. Similar results were obtained for the 14mm and 8mm collimators.

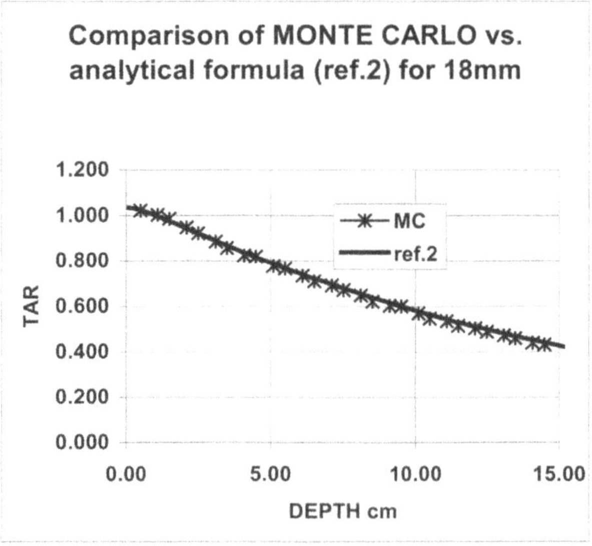


**Figure 2:** Comparison of MONTE CARLO vs. analytical formula (ref.2) for 18mm collimator

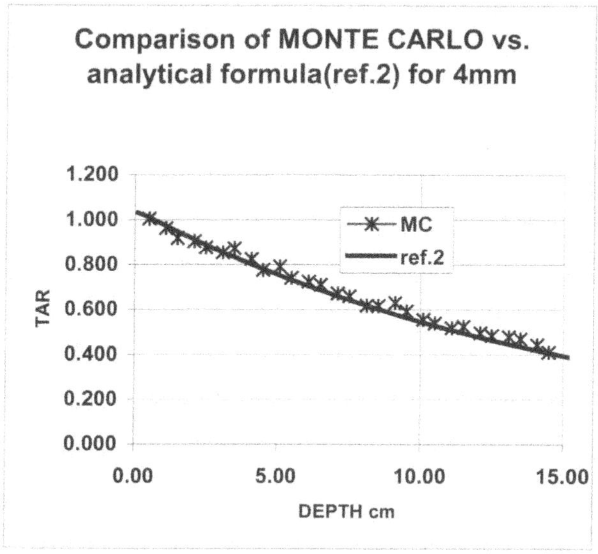


**Figure3:** Comparison of MONTE CARLO vs. analytical formula (ref.2) for 4mm collimator

**BEAM PROFILES:**

Beam profiles were compared with Gamma Plan data from the manufacturer and good agreement was observed as shown in Fig.4. However, there seem to be a larger penumbra for the OMEGA calculation which was not observed in a previous EGS4 calculation[5]. While the central axis standard deviation is nearly 0.7%, the standard deviation for profiles typically is 20% at beam edge (50% of central axis value). In view of this a variance reduction technique based on circular symmetry is being developed to get better accuracy for the profiles.

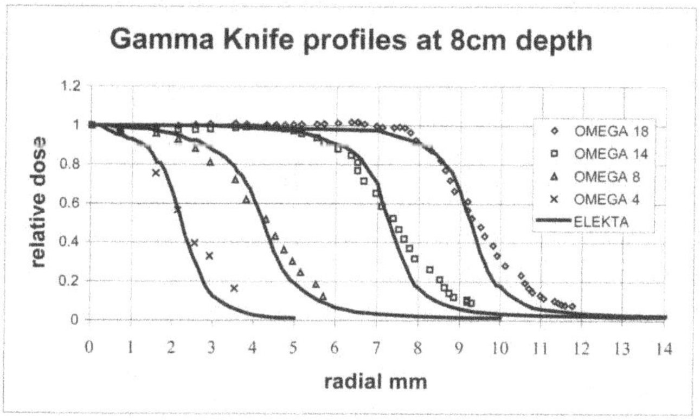


**Figure 4:** Comparison of ELEKTA supplied and OMEGA calculated beam profiles for the 4mm, 8mm, 14mm and 18mm collimators.

**OUTPUT FACTORS:**

The output factors, relative to the 18mm collimator, at 8cm depth are tabulated below.

| | OMEGA | ELEKTA | % Diff. | Ref.4 |
|---|---|---|---|---|
| 4mm | $0.914 \pm 0.008$ | 0.870 | 5 | 0.871 |
| 8mm | $0.979 \pm 0.007$ | 0.956 | 2.4 | 0.943 |
| 14mm | $1.004 \pm 0.008$ | 0.984 | 2 | 0.979 |
| 18mm | 1.000 | 1.000 | 1.000 | 1.000 |

**Table 1:** Gamma Knife output factors at 8cm depth in water

## Conclusion

In conclusion, experimental and analytical data pertinent to the Gamma Knife dosimetry are independently verified using similar data generated via OMEGA Monte Carlo Codes. The agreement between these two sets of data is found to be very good.

## References

[1] Rogers D W O, Faddengon B A, Ding G X, Ma C M, We J and Mackie T R 1995 BEAM: A Monte Carlo code to simulate radiotherapy treatment units, *Med. Phys.*, **22** 503-524

[2] Nizin P, Mooij R, 1998 Tissue-air ratios for narrow Co-60 gamma-ray beams Med.Phys. **25** 1458-1463

[3] Central Axis Depth Dose data for use in Radiotherapy 1996 *British Journal of Radiology* Suppl.**25** 52-53

[4] Nizin P 1998 On absorbed dose in narrow Co-60 gamma-ray beams and dosimetry of the Gamma Knife *Med.Phys.*, **25** 2347-2351

[5] Cheung J Y C, Yu K N,Yu C P and Ho T K Monte Carlo calculation of single-beam dose profiles used in a gamma knife treatment planning system *Med. Phys.* **25** 1673-1675

# A Monte Carlo study of backscatter in the monitor ion chamber for clinical photon and electron beams

**Frank Verhaegen[1], PhD, Richard Symonds-Tayler[1], Cephas Mubata[1], PhD, Margaret Bidmead[1], Alan Nahum[1], PhD and H. Helen Liu[2], PhD**

[1]Physics Dept, Royal Marsden Hospital, London and Sutton (UK) and [2]Dept of Radiation Physics, Univ. of Texas M. D. Anderson Cancer Center, Houston, Texas, USA.

## Introduction

For monitor unit calculations based on dose-to-fluence formalisms [1] the contribution of backscattered radiation from the jaws into the monitor ion chamber of a linear accelerator has to be known. In principle, Monte Carlo (MC) simulations of the complete accelerator geometry for Monte Carlo treatment planning can take the backscatter to the monitor chamber into account, provided an accurate model for the energy deposited in it is available. Output factors for different fields are influenced by forward scatter towards the measuring point and by backscatter towards the monitor chamber. When MC simulations are used to calculate output factors, only the first effect is automatically taken into account. In order to be able to compare MC calculated output factors to measured ones, the backscatter contribution should be used as a correction to the MC output factors. The effect is also of importance when modelling a dynamic wedge.

In this work, using a Monte Carlo model, the contribution of backscattered radiation from accelerator jaws to the energy deposited in the monitor ion chamber was studied for photon and electron beams as a function of jaw position. The results were compared to measurements and literature data. The spectra of the backscattered particles were obtained from the MC simulations.

## Material and methods

### The Monte Carlo model for the accelerator

A Monte Carlo model for a Varian 2100C accelerator was built for electron beams (6, 9, 12, 16, 20 MeV) and photon beams (6 and 10 MV), using the MC code EGS4/BEAM [2]. The energy of the primary electron beam (assumed mono-energetic) was tuned to match measured depth dose profiles in water Calculated depth dose, using DOSXYZ [3], was found to be usually well within 1% (for some point close to the surface a 2% difference was obtained) at all depths for photon and electron beams of all energies. Good agreement was also obtained when calculated and measured lateral dose profiles were compared. These results have been already partly described elsewhere [4].

### Modelling the monitor ion chamber

The monitor ion chamber of the Varian 2100C accelerator consists of a number of thin copper-coated kapton windows. A detailed model of the monitor ion chamber according to the manufacturer's information was built. The monitor ion chamber was described earlier by Duzenli et al [5]. The dose deposited in the top ion chamber by the primary beam was calculated by modelling the accelerator up to the monitor chamber. A phase-space file, containing information on the particles in the primary beam was constructed at a level after the monitor chamber. In a second step in the simulation, particles were sampled from this phase-space file and transported further in the complete geometry of the accelerator. This step includes the modelling of backscatter towards the monitor chamber from the shielding ring and the upper and lower jaws. A second phase-space file, containing information on the backscattered particles, is obtained at the level right after the monitor chamber. Since the geometry of the shielding ring never varies, the contribution to the backscatter from it is counted as part of the primary beam. This contribution is always very small. Particles that scatter from the jaws and then go through the shielding ring are counted as backscatter from the jaws. The backscatter in the monitor as a function of jaw setting was studied for photon beams of 6 MV and 10 MV and for electron energies between 6 and 20 MeV.

### Measuring backscatter in the monitor ion chamber for photon beams

There is more backscatter to the monitor chamber when the jaws are closed so for a given monitor unit (MU) setting the beam is switched off sooner when the field size is decreased. The upper jaws have the largest effect due to their proximity to the chamber. As in reference [6] we assume that the primary radiation coming from the X-ray target is proportional to the total beam energy impinging on it. In this work, the target charge was measured using one channel of a 6-channel pulse electrometer system which was made at the ICR for use with the ion chamber described in [7]. The electrometer records the target charge following each linac synchronisation pulse.

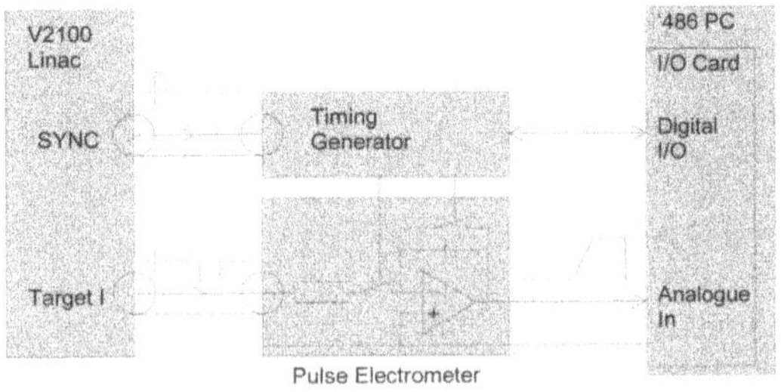


**Figure 1**: Schematic of the target current measurement hardware. The electrometer is based upon Burr-Brown IVC102 devices. The pulse electrometer system is controlled by a program on the PC.

The linac does not 'fire' at every SYNC pulse so some of the recorded values are at offset level. An advantage of the pulse electrometer is that the offset is known and well controlled because the charge integrator is reset at every SYNC pulse. The target charge readings in each run are summed to get the total beam charge.

About 8000 pulses were collected during 200 MU. Measurements were done for 6 and 10 MV photon beams. A number of positions for upper and lower jaws forming field sizes ranging from 0.5 cm to 40 cm (projected at 100 cm SSD) were used. For each field, target charge was collected 10 times. After subtraction of the constant noise level, the total collected charge was obtained, as a measure of the total delivered beam energy.

## Results and discussion

### Monitor ion chamber backscatter for photon beams

Figures 2 and 3 show that the measured collected target charge decreases with decreasing field size for 6 MV and 10 MV photon beams, respectively. Although the pulse shape of the 6 MV photon beam exhibited more noise and distortion than the pulse shape for the 10 MV beam, the statistical uncertainty on the target charge for a fixed number of MU was less.

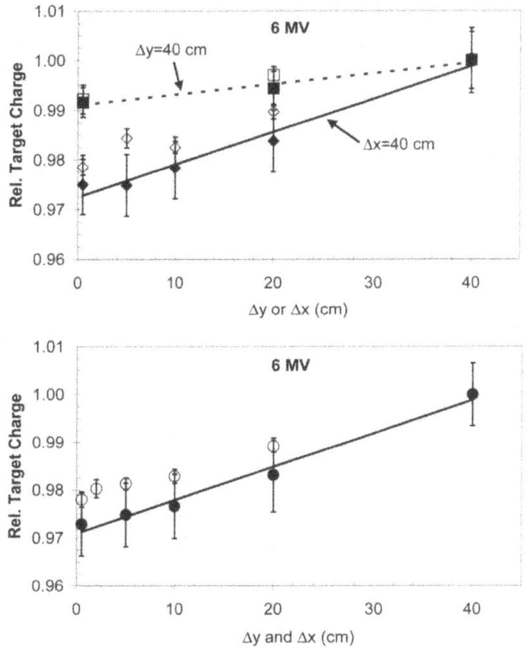


**Figure 2:** Decrease in the collected target charge with decreasing field for a 6 MV photon beam. Results are shown for rectangular fields (top panel) with either the lower jaws retracted and variable position of the upper jaws (diamonds) or vice versa (squares) and for square fields (bottom panel). Full symbols represent measurements, open symbols are derived from Monte Carlo simulations. The lines are linear fits through the measurements (full: Δx=40 cm, dashed: Δy=40 cm).

Also shown in the graphs are the results derived from MC simulations, where the calculated backscatter contribution is defined as $D_{jaws}/(D_{jaws}+D_{shielding}+D_{primary})$. This quantity is related to the reciprocal of the quantity that is given in fig. 2. Within the uncertainties, a good agreement between simulations and measurements was obtained. Results from the simulations tend to predict a slightly smaller decrease with decreasing field size for 6 MV photons and the opposite for 10 MV photons. The difference in backscatter between the smallest and largest fields, used in this study, amounts to about 2-3%. This has to be taken into account when comparing MC calculated or experimentally derived output factors. This effect should also be taken into account when modelling a dynamic wedge for the 2100C accelerator [8,9].

The results obtained for 6 MV photons are in good agreement with published results [6,10]. For 10 MV photons, no published data is available. Our results indicate that monitor backscatter in 6 MV and 10 MV beams is of comparable magnitude. It has to be remarked that the target-charge-pulse counting technique that was used by Yu et al [10] did not produce sensible results in our case, indicating that the number of target pulses is not a good measure of total charge collected by the monitor ion chamber for our accelerator. This can be the case when the shape or amplitude of the pulses varies slightly with jaw setting.

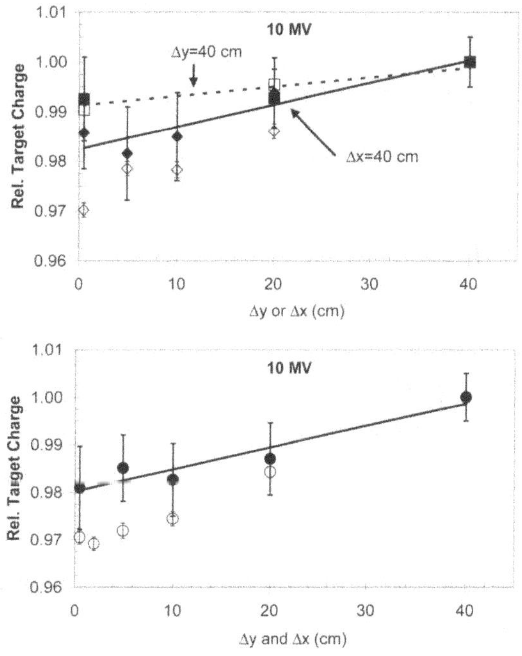


**Figure 3:** Same as fig 1 but for 10 MV photons.

Monte Carlo simulations also allow determination of spectral information for the backscattered particles. Figure 4 compares photon and electron spectra for the direct beam and the backscattered radiation for a 6 MV photon beam and a 0.5x0.5 $cm^2$ field.

In the spectrum of backscattered particles fluorescent photons from the jaws are present at low energies. The mean energy of the backscattered photons and electrons is 0.3 MeV and 0.7 MeV, respectively, whereas for the primary beam it is 1.3 MeV and 1.2 MeV, respectively. The majority of the backscattered dose deposited originates from electrons that were created in the jaws.

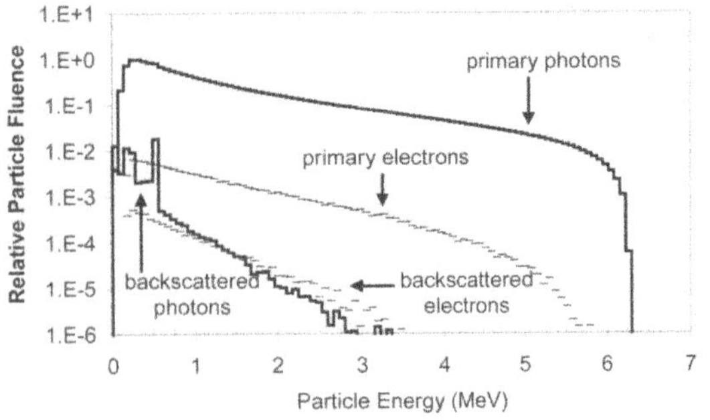


**Figure 4:** Primary and backscattered photon and electron spectra for a 6 MV photon beam and a 0.5x0.5 $cm^2$ field. The maximum of the fluence for the primary photons has been normalised to unity.

#### Monitor ion chamber backscatter for electron beams

Backscatter from the jaws to the monitor chamber is expected to be a smaller problem in electron beams because normally electron beams are mostly defined by the applicators and cut-outs whereas the jaws are set to relatively large fields. To verify this, MC simulations were done for electron beams with energies ranging from 6-20 MeV for a number of field sizes. Figure 5 gives the backscatter from the jaws to the monitor for electron beams (6, 9, 12, 20 MeV) as a function of jaw setting. The lower jaws (X) are separated symmetrically by 20 cm (projected at 100 cm SSD) and the upper jaws (Y) change position symmetrically. The dashed lines in the graphs are for the contribution of the upper jaws only.

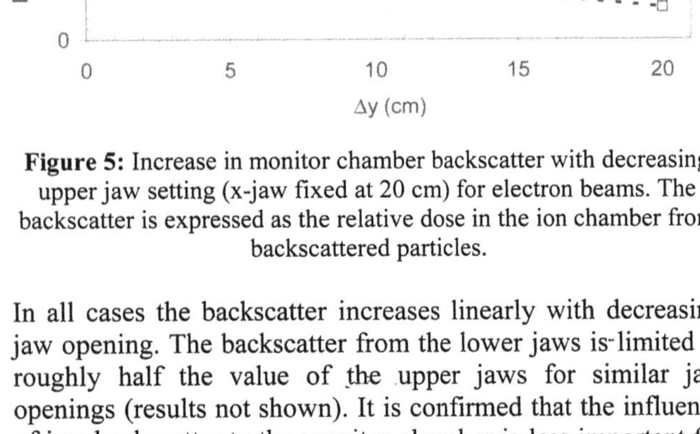


**Figure 5:** Increase in monitor chamber backscatter with decreasing upper jaw setting (x-jaw fixed at 20 cm) for electron beams. The backscatter is expressed as the relative dose in the ion chamber from backscattered particles.

In all cases the backscatter increases linearly with decreasing jaw opening. The backscatter from the lower jaws is limited to roughly half the value of the upper jaws for similar jaw openings (results not shown). It is confirmed that the influence of jaw backscatter to the monitor chamber is less important for electron beams than for photon beams. Even for the lowest electron energy, the relative difference in backscatter between the largest and smallest fields used in clinical practice, is less than 1%. Therefore, no corrections to MC derived output factors, caused by this effect, are required in practice.

## Conclusion

In this work a Monte Carlo model was built for photon and electron beams from a Varian 2100C accelerator. An accurate model of the monitor ion chamber was included. Using the Monte Carlo model, the backscatter from the jaws to the monitor chamber was studied. For photon beams, the results were compared to measurements based on target charge collection. Good agreement between the two techniques was obtained. From the results in this work, correction factors for Monte Carlo derived output factors can be derived.

## Acknowledgements

Steve Butler is thanked for his assistance in the measurements. F.V. is sponsored by a Marie Curie Research Training Grant from the European Communities. R. S-T. is supported by a Programme grant from The Cancer Research Campaign [CRC] under grant reference SP2312/0201.

## References

[1] Ahnesjö A and Aspradakis M M 1999 Dose calculations for external photon beams in radiotherapy *Phys. Med. Biol* **44** R99-R155

[2] Rogers D, Faddegon B, Ding G, Ma C-M, We J and Mackie T 1995 BEAM: a Monte Carlo code to simulate radiotherapy treatment units. *Med. Phys.* **22**, 503-524

[3] Ma C-M, Reckwerdt P, Holmes M, Rogers D W O, Geiser B and Walters B 1996 DOSXYZ users manual *NRCC Report* PIRS-0509B (Ottawa: NRC)

[4] Verhaegen F, Mubata C, Pettingell J and Nahum A 1999 Calculation of output factors for an electron accelerator (6-20 MeV) by Monte Carlo modelling. Abstract for the 41st annual meeting of the AAPM, Nashville, July 25-29, 1999, *Med. Phys.* **26/8** p1744

[5] Duzenli C, McClean B and Field C 1993 Backscatter into the beam monitor chamber: implications for dosimetry of asymmetric collimators. *Med. Phys.* **20**, 363-367

[6] Lam K L, Muthuswamy M S and Ten Haken R K 1998 Measurement of backscatter to the monitor chamber of medical accelerators using target charge. *Med. Phys.* **25**, 334-338

[7] Partridge M, Symonds-Tayler JRN and Evans PM 1999 A large-area ionisation chamber for portal image calibration. Phys. Med. Biol. **44,** 271-279

[8] Verhaegen F and Das I 1999 Monte Carlo modelling of a virtual wedge. *Phys. Med. Biol* **44** N251-N259

[9] Liu H H and Verhaegen F Add a dynamic swing to Monte Carlo simulation – Modelling dynamic jaw motion using three sampling techniques, submitted to the XIII International Conference on the use of Computers in Radiotherapy, heidelberg, Germany, 2000.

[10] Yu M K, Sloboda R S and Mansour F 1996 Measurement of photon beam backscatter from collimators to the beam monitor chamber using target-current-pulse-counting and telescopic techniques. *Phys. Med. Biol* **41** 1107-1117

# Monte Carlo simulation of the effective point of measurement of the Markus chamber for electrons, the upright PinPoint chamber for photons, and other chambers

**Ulf F. Rosenow[1], Christian Thieke[1] and Marc Lauterbach[2]**

[1]Georg-August-University Göttingen, Department Clinical Radiation Biology and Clinical Radiation Physics, Göttingen, Germany, and [2]Massey Cancer Center, Medical College of Virginia, Richmond, VA, USA

## Introduction

Recently it was demonstrated in careful experiments by Roos et al.[1] that for the Markus chamber a downstream shift of 0.5 mm of the effective point of measurement, $P_{eff}$, should be assumed nearly independently of electron energy and in-phantom depth. This effect may be attributed to an ineffective guard-ring which allows scatter from the side wall to reach the sensitive volume, thus providing some similarity of this chamber to a cylindrical one. Rosenow et al. [2] have shown that, at the very low end of clinically applied electron energies, a plate separation of 2 mm will necessarily lead to a steep rise of the perturbation correction factor, $p_u$, above unity with decreasing electron energy. There is reason to assume that a shift of $P_{eff}$ may also be involved since the effect is due to reduced back scatter. In the dosimetry of small field stereotactic photon beams the highest spatial resolution achievable with ionization chambers is with a PinPoint chamber [3] in an upright orientation, i. e. with the tip of the chamber pointing upstream, since the chambers inner diameter is only 2 mm. In this situation the position of $P_{eff}$ is not only unknown but may vary with photon or electron energy and position in the beam. Monte Carlo simulation is a preferable method to determine $P_{eff}$ in these and other circumstances. It enables an in-depth analysis of the factors influencing $P_{eff}$ and a clear distinction from other corrections such as the perturbation correction factor. We present results of our investigations in $P_{eff}$ in the PTW-Markus, the PTW-PinPoint, an improved Markus-type and other plane-parallel chambers.

## Material and Methods

The Monte Carlo simulations are performed with the EGS4/PRESTA/BEAM codes.[4,5] These had previously been intensively tested and there suitability for structures as small as the chambers used confirmed.[6,7] The sub-code DOSRZ was used for the dose calculations which handles cylindrical structures. The chambers were modeled in all details such as wall materials, entrance windows, guard-rings or central electrodes, respectively, including even the inner graphite coating, excluding however the chamber cables and connecting filaments. The PinPoint chamber was only modeled in the upright orientation. All data input for the simulations was by means of the graphical user interface XInput developed in this group.[8]

The following ionization chambers were included in this investigation: The Markus chamber (PTW 23343), a newly developed small electron chamber with 1 mm plate separation and 2 mm guard-ring (which we will denote P1S2), the Roos chamber (PTW 34001), the NACP chamber and the PinPoint chamber (PTW 31006). The radiation modalities employed were monoenergetic electrons of 2, 4, 6, 10 and 15 MeV, cobalt-60 gammas and linear accelerator photons of 6 MV. The beams were assumed as to be parallel rays vertically impinging on a semi-infinite PMMA phantom in which the chambers were embedded at various depths. Circular beams of 3.5 cm radius were generally assumed. In some simulations monoenergetic radiation was replaced by BEAM-generated "real" phase-space spectra in order to verify that this would not affect the general validity of the results. The simulations were run on a dual processor 200 Mhz Pentium Pro PC under LINUX and on a parallel array of LINUX systems in the computing center common to this University and the Max-Planck-Society of Göttingen.

$P_{eff}$ was determined as follows: Depth-dose curves were first derived in PMMA by defining dose score regions of 5 mm diameter and 0.1 mm thickness positioned in the central axis of the beams in steps of 0.5, 1 or 2 mm depending on energy and sufficient depth resolution. Simulations were then done for the chambers positioned at corresponding depths in the PMMA phantom. The sensitive chamber volumes were defined as score regions and their dose determined from ICRU stopping power ratios water-to-air.[9] The chamber-derived depth-dose curves were scaled in order to achieve the same dose maximum as in the "pure" PMMA curves and then shifted in depth to make the fall-off regions optically coincide. The shift then represents the position of $P_{eff}$.

## Results and Discussion

Since our initial interest was in $P_{eff}$ of the Markus chamber we will show results of that chamber here as an example. In Figure 1 the simulated depth-dose curves as simulated in pure PMMA and for the Markus chamber in PMMA are shown for monoenergetic 6 MeV electrons. The scale factor necessary to equalize the maximum of the chamber curve to the PMMA curve was 1.01 which corresponds to a perturbation correction factor of 0.99. This is the factor determined experimentally with Fricke dosimetry [10] or from the corresponding fitting curve of Wittkämper et al.[11] Figure 2 shows the Markus chamber curve scaled and shifted to fit the PMMA curve optimally by eye judgment. The resulting shift is 0.7 mm at about the $R_{50}$ depth. This corresponds exactly to the experimental result of Roos et al. [1] since a 0.2 mm air gap added constructively in front of the entrance window to prevent damage of the thin entrance window needs to be accounted for. Roos et al. stated a negligible dependence of $P_{eff}$ on energy or depth which can also be taken from Figure 2 since the curves coincide even in the build-up region. For the other energies investigated the same $P_{eff}$ was found.

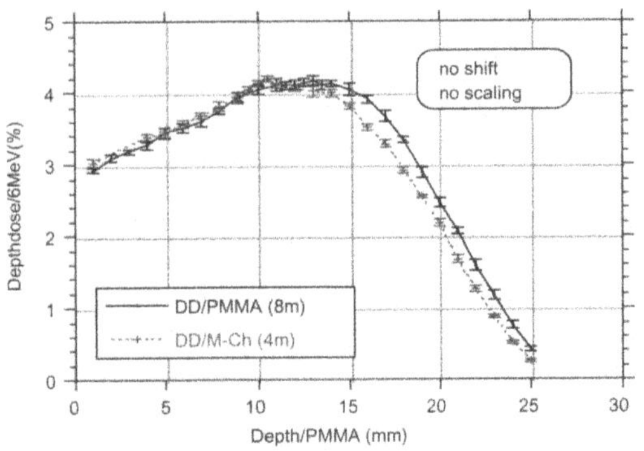


**Figure 1:** Monochromatic 6 MeV depth-dose curves simulated for PMMA with 8 million histories and the Markus chamber in PMMA with 4 million histories. Error bars represent ±1 SD

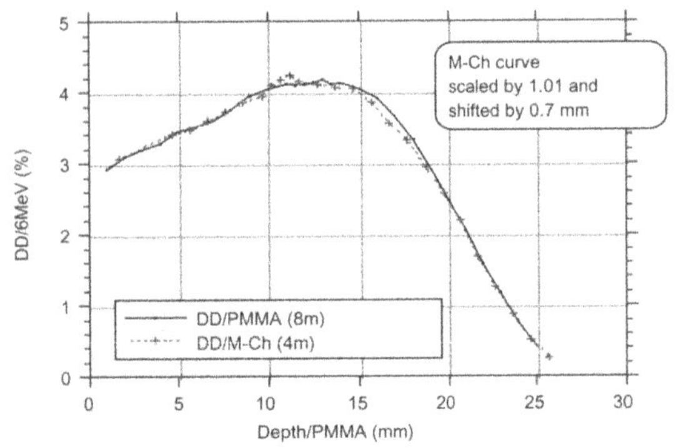


**Figure 2:** As in Fig. 1 with the Markus chamber curve scaled and shifted to coincide with the PMMA curve.

As expected, $P_{eff}$ of the P1S2 chamber does not show any shift since optimization of this chamber in order to eliminate the perturbation correction involves also avoidance of a shift in $P_{eff}$. The common assumption of $P_{eff}$ at the center of the inner entrance window surface holds. However, the scaling factor necessary to align the curve maxima of the chamber and PMMA depth-dose curves was 1.026 where one would have expected unity. This finding will be further investigated. According to our preliminary studies, plane-parallel chambers with 2 mm plate separation tend to show a slight shift of $P_{eff}$ at energies around and below 2 MeV. Although this needs further confirmation one would have expected such a result from our detailed simulations of the perturbation effect of such chambers [2]. The PinPoint chamber exhibits some energy (and depth) dependence of the position of $P_{eff}$ in electron and photon beams which only needs to be accounted for in measurements of high intended accuracy. Further details will be shown.

## Conclusions

Monte Carlo simulations provide an ideal tool for the study of $P_{eff}$ shifts in some electron chambers such as the Markus chamber at all energies or chambers of 2 mm plate separation at very low electron energies. Furthermore it enables the definition of $P_{eff}$ for the PinPoint chamber in the upright orientation in photon and electron beams.

## References


[1] Roos M, Derikum A and Kraus A 1998 On the effective point of measurement of plane parallel chambers in electron beams *Radioth Oncol* **51** Suppl. 1 Abstract 44

[2] Rosenow U F, Lauterbach M and Lehmann J 1999 A small-volume electron chamber with flat energy response at all phantom depths: Result of an analysis by Monte-Carlo simulation and experiment *Med. Phys.* **26**, 1118 Abstract TH-C1-02

[3] Rosenow U F, Kasten G, Lehmann J and Lauterbach M Dosimetric characteristics of the small cylindrical chamber, or "PinPoint Chamber", in electron and photon beams 1997 *Med. Phys.* **24**, 1006 Abstract TH-DU-09

[4] Nelson W R, Hirayama H and Rogers D W O 1985 The EGS4 Code System Stanford Linear Accelerator Center Report SLAC-265 Stanford University

[5] Bielajew A F, Rogers D W O 1987 PRESTA: The parameter reduced electron-step transport algorithm for electron Monte Carlo transport *Nucl Instr Meth in Phys Res B* **18**, 165-181

[6] Lauterbach M, Lehmann J and Rosenow U F 1999 Energy deposition of electrons in low-, medium- and high-Z material. Comparison of the Monte Carlo transport code EGS4 with experiment *Nuc Inst. and Meth in Phys Res B* **152**, 212-220

[7] Lauterbach M, Lehmann J and Rosenow U F 1999 Exploration of the Monte Carlo code system EGS4 for the simulation of plane-parallel electron chambers *Zeitschr Med Phys* **9**, 38-46

[8] Lauterbach M, Lehmann J, Rosenow U F 1999 XInput: A program to edit "DOSRZ" input files *Med Phys* **26**, 760-762

[9] International Commission on Radiation Units and Measurements 1984 ICRU Report 37 *Stopping Powers for Electrons and Positrons* Bethesda.MD

[10] Rosenow U F 1993 Comments on the experimental determination of the replacement correction factor for parallel-plate ionization chambers in high energy electron beams *Med Phys* **20**:739-741

[11] Wittkämper F W Q, Thierens H, Van der Plaetsen A, de Wagter C and Mijnheer B J 1991 Perturbation correction factors for some ionization chambers commonly applied in electron beams *Phys Med Biol* **36**, 1639-1652

# A Fast Dose Calculation Algorithm for Deformable Liquid-Filled Brachytherapy Applicators with Low Energy Photon Emitting Radionuclides

**James F. Dempsey and Jeffery F. Williamson**

Radiation Oncology Center, Mallinckrodt Institute of Radiology, Washington University School of Medicine, St. Louis, MO USA.

## Introduction

Determining the dosimetric characteristics of novel sealed brachytherapy sources has developed into a well defined practice standard (1-2). Experimentally validated Monte Carlo photon transport (MCPT) simulations or measured data are used to produce treatment planning data for commerically available source designs. These data are then applied in brachytherapy treatment planning by interpolation or point source modeling of the characterized source. As most all

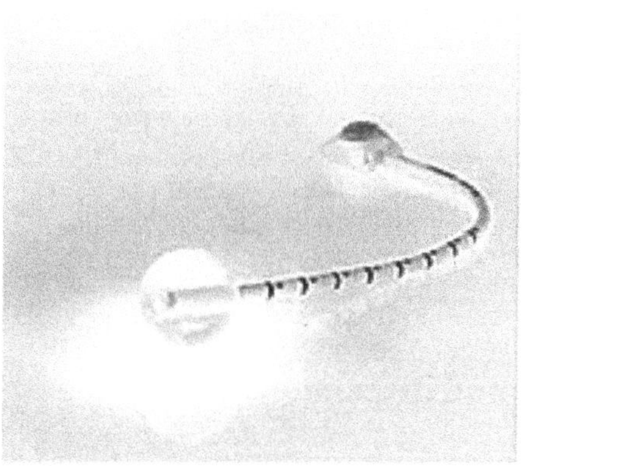

**Figure 1:** A novel $^{125}$I liquid-filled brachytherapy balloon applicator (the GliaSite RTS Proxima Therapeutics, Inc, Alpharetta, GA USA) designed for the treatment of malignant brain-tumor resection-cavity margins

brachytherapy sources are constructed of rigid materials and the planning data is normalized to a quantity of doismetric output, e.g. air kerma strength (3), this program produces fairly accurate clinical dosimetry (inter-source attenuation and tissue heterogeneities are often ignored).

However, this approach is not applicable to a novel class of liquid filled balloon brachytherapy applicators. Dempsey et al.(4) has described the dosimetric characteristics of a novel $^{125}$I liquid-filled brachytherapy balloon applicator see figure 1.(4) . The applicator consists of a double-walled silicone balloon resevoir attached to a subcutaneous infusion port by a multi-lumen Ba-loaded silicone catheter. While the balloon resevoir is expected to maintain a fairly uniform shape, there is no mechanism to prevent deformation of the revevoir geometry. This makes the use of tabulated MCPT simulation data or experimental measurement impractical. Treatment planning for the applicator requires an imaging technique that allows evaluation of the source geometry and a dose calcualtion that can accurately account for the influence of the geometry on the delivered dose. While MCPT simulation could be employed for each individual case, the time required for accurate dosimetry would be prohibitive.

A simple point dose kernel, valid only in a homogeneous water medium, was originally employed to parametrically study the dosimetric characteristics of this applicator. In this model the dose rate, $\dot{D}(\vec{\mathbf{r}})$, at the location $\vec{\mathbf{r}}$ outside of the applicator is given by,

$$\dot{D}(\vec{\mathbf{r}}) = \Gamma_k \left(\overline{\mu_{en/\rho}}\right)_{air}^{water} \int_V d^3\vec{\mathbf{r}}'\rho(\vec{\mathbf{r}}') \frac{T(|\vec{\mathbf{r}} - \vec{\mathbf{r}}'|)}{|\vec{\mathbf{r}} - \vec{\mathbf{r}}'|^2} \quad [1]$$

where $\rho(\vec{\mathbf{r}}')$ is the activity density, $T(r)$ is the attenuation and build-up factor as a function of distance r from the source, $\left(\overline{\mu_{en/\rho}}\right)_{air}^{water}$ is the ratio of mass energy absorption coefficients in water to that of air averaged over the photon energy spectrum, $\Gamma_k$ is the air kerma-rate constant and $T(|\vec{\mathbf{r}} - \vec{\mathbf{r}}'|)/|\vec{\mathbf{r}} - \vec{\mathbf{r}}'|^2$ accounts for contributions of all infinitesimal components of the source at positions $\vec{\mathbf{r}}'$ contained in the source volume V to the dose rate at the positions $\vec{\mathbf{r}}$. Unfortunately, this model produces unacceptably large errors (up to 25%) for when compared to MCPT simulation results, severely limiting its clinical use. In this study we develop a modified point dose kernel model more appropriate for treatment planning purposes. This model is based on equation [1] and has analytically derived correction factors for $\Gamma_k$ and for heterogeneities introduced by the applicator.

## Material and methods

### MCPT Simulations

A MCPT code, PTRAN, was used to calculate: the dose rate distribution at points along the cather and transverse axis of 1 cm radius balloon applicator at the center of a 30 cm diameter liquid water sphere. PTRAN simulates incoherent scattering, coherent scattering, and emission of K-, L-, or M-edge characteristic x-rays following photoelectric interaction. Vacancy probabilities, transition probabilities and fluorescent yields were taken from Plechaty [5]. Photon cross sections came from the DLC-99 library, distributed by the Radiation Shielding Information Center[6] Energy fluence was converted to kerma using the mass energy absorption coefficients of the

target media. The I-125 primary photon spectrum published by NCRP report 58 [7] was used for the source photon spectrum. Since PTRAN transports only photons, energy transferred to secondary electron energy by photon collisions is assumed to be deposited locally. For the low-energy photons emitted by $^{125}$I this assumption is quite valid and kerma will closely approximate absorbed dose (Valicenti *et al* 1995). The Once More Collided Flux (OMCF) [9] was used to evaluate kerma with separate runs of two million histories each, with standard deviations of less than 1 %.
The geometric modeling of PTRAN can ray trace through geometrically complex arrangements cuboidal, ellipsoidal, cylindrical and cone-shaped volumes: combined using set-theoretic operations into regions[10]. Complex shapes can be constructed, and queried for point classification and ray tracing. A detailed model of the applicator balloon resevoir was constructed including the geometry and properties of the Ba-loaded silicone multi-lumen catheter, a Ti positioning wire in the catheter, the $^{125}$I radiotherapy solution, and the silicone balloon.

### .The Modified Model

The modified model was used to calculate: the same dose rate distributions as the MPCT simulationsm; at points along the cather and transverse axis of a 1 cm radius balloon applicator at the center of a 30 cm diameter liquid water sphere. The modified model solves the following equation

$$\dot{D}(\vec{\mathbf{r}}) = \overline{(\mu_{en/\rho})}^{water}_{air} \int_V d^3\vec{\mathbf{r}}' \Gamma^{Atten}{}_k(|\vec{\mathbf{r}}-\vec{\mathbf{r}}'|)\rho(\vec{\mathbf{r}}')\frac{T(|\vec{\mathbf{r}}-\vec{\mathbf{r}}'|)}{|\vec{\mathbf{r}}-\vec{\mathbf{r}}'|^2}\frac{D^{Het}}{D^{Hom}} \quad [2]$$

where three new quantities are introduced; a position dependent air kerma strength, $\Gamma^{Atten}{}_k(|\vec{\mathbf{r}}-\vec{\mathbf{r}}'|)$, and a modified heterogeneous and homogeneous dose rate, $D^{Het}$ and $D^{Hom}$, respectively. The source strength of each source in active volume $\Gamma^{Atten}{}_k(|\vec{\mathbf{r}}-\vec{\mathbf{r}}'|)$, replaces the single value $\Gamma_k$ and is given by

$$\Gamma^{Atten}{}_k(|\vec{\mathbf{r}}-\vec{\mathbf{r}}'|) = \sum_i n_i \varepsilon_i (\mu_{en}/\rho)^{air}{}_i \exp(-\sum_k \mu_k \lambda_k) \quad [3]$$

where $n_i$ is the probability of emission for the ith photon, $\varepsilon_i$ is energy of the ith photon, $(\mu_{en/\rho})^{air}_i$ is the mass energy absorption coefffficent in air for the ith photon, and $\exp(-\sum_k \mu_k \lambda_k)$ is an applicator attenuation factor, accounting for non-water attenuation over path lengths $\lambda_k$ with linear attenuation coefficents $\mu_k$ for the kth non-water material traversed by $|\vec{\mathbf{r}}-\vec{\mathbf{r}}'|$. The $\lambda_k$'s are determined using the geometric modeling and ray tracing of the PTRAN simulation code. The a modified heterogeneous and homogeneous dose rates, $D^{Het}$ and $D^{Hom}$, are calculated following a simple derivation of the scattter to primary ratio (SPR) for a point source in a homogeneous medium given by Evans[11]. Assuming a linear relationship between the mean free path of a photon and the SPR Evans showed that for a point source in a homogeneous medium

$$SPR \cong \frac{\sigma_s}{(\mu_{en}/\rho)}(\mu r) \quad [4]$$

where $\sigma_s$ is the Klein Nishina linear scattering coefficent, $(\mu_{en/\rho})$ is the mass energy absorption coeffficent of the medium, $\mu$ is the linear attenuation of the medium, and $r$ is the distance fron the point source. Equation [4] was adapted for a heterogeneous medium such that

$$SPR = \frac{\sigma^i{}_s}{(\mu_{en}/\rho)^{wat}_i}\left(\sum_k \mu_k \lambda_k\right)$$

where $\sigma_s^{\ i}$ is the Klein Nishina linear scattering coefficent for the ith photon in water, and $\lambda_k$ and $\mu_k$ are as defined above
Total dose is evaluated by calculating primary dose and multiplying by (1+SPR). Equation [2] was evaluated using simple Monte Carlo Integration(12,13), evaluating $(T(|\vec{\mathbf{r}}-\vec{\mathbf{r}}'|)/|\vec{\mathbf{r}}-\vec{\mathbf{r}}'|^2)$, $\Gamma^{Atten}{}_k(|\vec{\mathbf{r}}-\vec{\mathbf{r}}'|)$, $D^{Het}$ and $D^{Hom}$ for each sampled point using the geometric modeling and ray tracing of the PTRAN simulation code.

## Results and discussion

Figure two shows the ratio of dose calculated by the modified model to that calculated by MCPT simulation as a function of distance from the 1 cm radius balloon surface. Excellent agreement is seen given the heuristic nature of the modified point dose kernel model. Between distances of 5 and 90 mm the agreement of the calculations is better than $\pm$3%. In clinical use, prescription depths will typically lie between 5 and 30 mm where the algorithm is quite accurate. A large discrepancy (up to 17%) exists at a few milimeters distance from the polar axis is observed. This is expected as the model has a limited ability to deal with situations of severe attenuation of primary photons. Although the software implimentation of this model has not been optimized for speed, its naive implimentation is approximately 50 times faster than the MCPT simulation using the same plateform and compiler settings.

## Conclusion

The simple model presented here is in excellent agreement with MCPT simulation. These results are very promising however, a parametric study of the agreement of algorithm with MCPT as a function of balloon geometry and deformation must be performed to validate its clinical use. A study has recently been completed to validate MCPT dose calculations

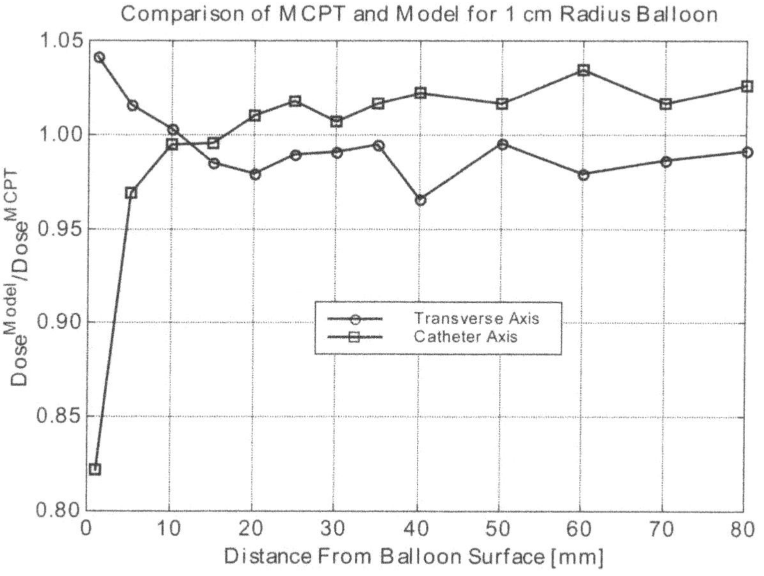


**Figure 2:** Ratios of dose calculated by the modified model to MCPT dose are a funtion of distance from the balloon surface along the transverse (circles ) and catheter (squares) axes of the balloon resevor

for this device and the combined works will provide a complete dosimetric characterization for this device.

This work supported by a grant from the National Institues of Health, grant number R01 CA46640.

## References

[1] Nath R, Anderson LL, Luxton G, Weaver KA, Williamson JF, Meigooni AS 1999 Dosimetry of interstitial brachytherapy sources: recommendations of the AAPM Radiation Therapy Committee Task Group No. 43. American Association of Physicists in Medicine. *Med Phys* **22** 209-34

[2] Williamson JF, Coursey BM, DeWerd LA, HansonWF, Nath R 1998 Dosimetric prerequisites for routine clinical use of new low energy photon interstitial brachytherapy sources *Med Phys* **25** 2269-2270

[3] Williamson JF, Coursey BM, DeWerd LA, HansonWF, Nath R, Rivard MJ, Ibbott G 1999 On the use of apparent activity (Aapp) for treatment planning of 125I and 103Pd interstitial brachytherapy sources: Recommendations of the American Association of Physicists in Medicine Radiation Therapy Committee Subcommittee on Low-Energy Brachytherapy Source Dosimetry *Med Phys* **26** 2529-2530

[4] Dempsey JF, Williams JA, Stubbs JB, Patrick TJ, Williamson JF 1999 Dosimetric properties of a novel brachytherapy balloon applicator for the treatment of malignant brain-tumor resection-cavity margins. *Int J Radiat Oncol Biol Phys* **42** 421-9

[5]Plechaty E F, Cullen D E and Howerton R J 1978 Tables and graphs of photon-interaction cross sections from 0.1 keV to 100 MeV derived from the LLL evaluated-nuclear-data-library (Lawrence Livermore Laboratory) *Report No. UCRL-50400 Vol 6 Rev. 2*

[6]Roussin W, Knight J R, Hubbell J H and Howerton R J 1983 Report No. ORNL/RSIC-46 *RSIC Data Library Collection*

[7]NCRP 1983 A handbook of radioactivity measurements *NCRP Report No. 58*

[8]Valicenti R K, Kirov A S, Meigooni A S, Mishra V, Das R K and Williamson J F 1995 Experimental validation of Monte Carlo dose-calculations about a high-intensity $^{192}$Ir source for pulsed dose-rate brachytherapy *Med. Phys.* **22** 821-830

[9] Li Z, Williamson JF, Perera H 1999 Monte Carlo calculation of kerma to a point in the vicinity of media interfaces. *Phys Med Biol* **38** 1825-40

[10] Li Z, Williamson JF 1999 Volume-based geometric modeling for radiation transport calculations. *Med Phys* **19** 667-77

[11] Evans RD *The Atomic Nucleus* (Cambridge University Press) 738-740.

[12]Press W, Flannery B, Teukolsky S and Vetterling W 1988 *Numerical Recipe in C* (Cambridge University Press) 523-527

[13]Baltas D, Giannouli S, Garbi A, Diakonos F, Geramani K, Ioannidis GT, Tsalpatouros A, Uzunoglu N, Kolotas C and Zamboglou N 1998 Application of the Monte Carlo integration (MCI) method for calculation of the anisotropy of $^{192}$Ir brachytherapy sources . *Phys. Med. Biol.* **43** 1783-1801

[14]Monroe JI, Dempsey, Dorton JA, Mutic S, Stubbs JB, Williamson JF 1999 Experimental Validation of Dose Calculation Algorithms for the GliaSite™ RTS, a Novel $^{125}$I Liquid-Filled Balloon Brachytherapy Applicator *Med Phys.* in submission

# Accounting for heterogeneities and shields in brachytherapy dose calculation by use of collapsed cone superposition

**Åsa K Carlsson[1] and Anders Ahnesjö[2]**

[1]Department of Medical Radiation Physics, Stockholm University and Karolinska Institute, Box 260, S-171 76 Stockholm, SWEDEN and [2]MDS Nordion Therapy Systems, Box 1704, Klostergatan 12, S-751 47 Uppsala, SWEDEN.

## Introduction

Dose calculation algorithms used in clinical brachytherapy treatment planning assume that patient dose distributions are identical to those in extended water phantoms. Effective attenuation corrections are sometimes performed to account for shields made of tungsten or lead[1], however, essentially a 1D method it is correct only for the primary dose. Approximate treatments of the scatter dose yields largest errors for photon energies with high scatter-to-primary ratios and for geometries where scattering conditions are very different from those in large water phantoms. Implants close to patient surfaces and sources shielded with high atomic-number materials are examples of such situations. Kernel superposition algorithms account for how the absorbed dose is influenced by the 3D spatial distribution of heterogeneities in the irradiated volume. The collapsed cone algorithm is a method for fast integration of point kernels to yield dose[2], which is considerably faster than straightforward superposition. It has recently been adapted for calculations of scatter-doses in brachytherapy[3]. In this work we investigate its use for scatter-dose calculations around a 350 keV point source in two heterogeneous geometries.

## Materials and methods

The collapsed cone algorithm with successive-scattering superposition[3] is used to derive distributions of scatter-doses around a 350 keV monoenergetic point source, for the geometries shown in Figure 1. The primary dose is approximated with the collision kerma and determined analytically. Results are compared to full Monte Carlo simulations using the code from Williamson[4] for the shielded source and EGS4 for the other cases.

### Scatter dose calculation using the collapsed cone algorithm with successive-scattering superposition

For calculations with the collapsed cone algorithm, point kernels are binned into a set of discrete cone axes and fitted to exponential functions. Speed is achieved by collapsing the transport of energy onto the axes of the cones and arranging a suitable lattice of lines[5] covering all voxels of the calculation matrix. When the algorithm was adapted for use in brachytherapy[3] it was shown that best results were achieved by a successive-scattering approach[6]. Successive-scattering is considerably less sensitive to the steep fluence gradients typical for brachytherapy than conventional, single-kernel superposition. Successive-scattering superposition divides scatter-dose calculations into calculations of once- and multiply-scattered photons as: *i*) calculation of first-scatter dose using the distribution of energy released by primary photons and a point kernel for once-scattered photons *ii*) use the first-scatter dose to derive the distribution of energy transferred to twice-scattered photons *iii*) calculation of the multiple-scatter dose using the distribution of energy transferred to twice-scattered photons and a multiple-scatter kernel for the dose distribution around the interaction sites of once-scattered photons.

### Monte Carlo simulations

A version of EGS4 including extensions[7,8] for improved transport of low energy photons was used in simulating the source localised close to the phantom surface. The source shielded with lead was simulated using the Monte Carlo code from Williamson[4]. This code approximates dose with collision kerma and allows more rapid estimates of dose in asymmetric geometries by supporting several non-analogue estimators. In the current simulation absorbed dose were derived in a selected number of points using a bounded next flight estimator[9].

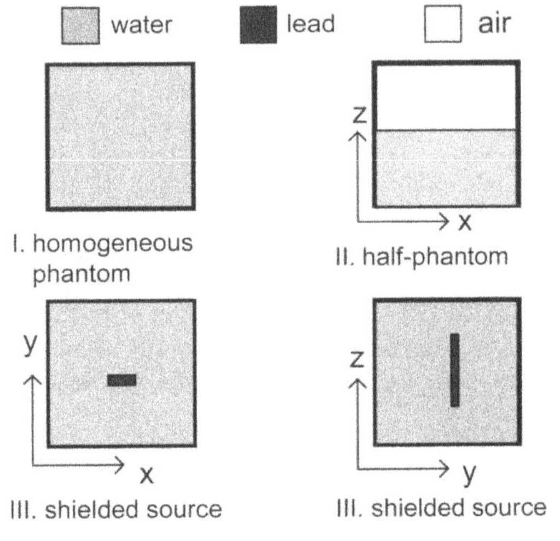


**Figure 1:** The outer dimension of all three geometries is a 20·20·20 cm$^3$ box with the source in the centre. The half-phantom is filled with water up to 0.5 cm above the source. The lead block for the shielded source has dimensions (Δx, Δy, Δz)=(2.5 cm, 1.0 cm, 10 cm) and are shown in two planes. The lead shield is centred in the phantom in the x and z directions and translated 0.5 cm from the centre along y.

## Results and discussion

Total absorbed dose distributions in the homogeneous water phantom and in the half-phantom are shown in Figure 2. The same isodose levels are shown in both phantoms and the effect of reducing the scattering medium by almost one-half can thereby be seen. Except for overestimating the dose slightly close to the phantom surfaces, due to the point kernel being generated in a large water phantom, collapsed cone results agree well with the Monte Carlo results. Note that currently used dose calculation algorithms would predict identical dose distributions in both these phantoms.

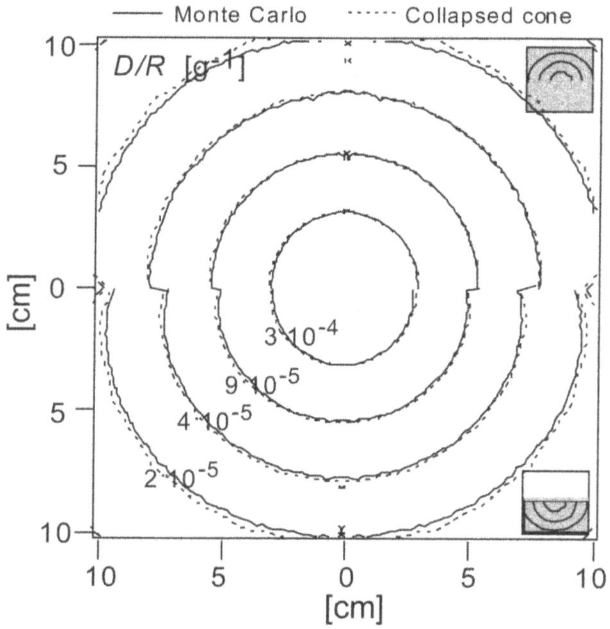


**Figure 2.** Absorbed dose distributions in the homogeneous water phantom (top) and the half-phantom (bottom).

The distribution of absorbed dose in the XY-plane of the shielded source calculated with collapsed cone superposition is shown in Figure 3.

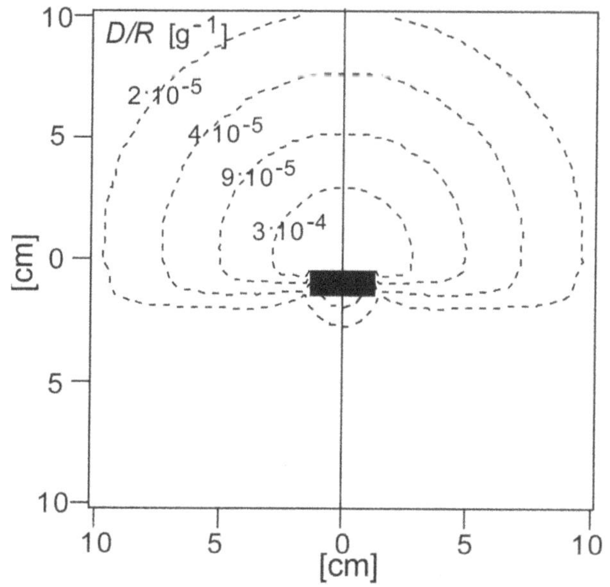


**Figure 3:** Dose distribution in the XY-plane around the shielded source derived by collapsed cone superposition. The full lines indicate the directions along which doses for comparisons were determined with Monte Carlo simulations.

In the Monte Carlo simulations of the shielded geometry, the dose was determined along the directions indicated in Figure 3, in front of and behind the lead shield. The comparison with Monte Carlo simulations along these lines is shown in Figure 4. Results from calculations in the homogeneous water phantom are also inserted in Figure 4. A small decrease in dose on the unshielded side of the shielded phantom as compared to the homogeneous phantom can be seen at some distance from the source.

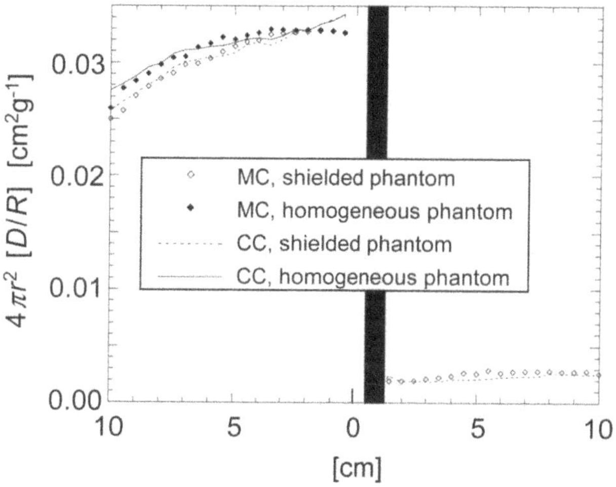


**Figure 4:** Comparison between collapsed cone superposition and Monte Carlo in front of and behind the lead shield. Results of calculations in the homogeneous water phantom are inserted on the unshielded side.

## Conclusion

The collapsed cone algorithm can be used to account for heterogeneities in brachytherapy. Results for a 350 keV point source located close to a phantom surface and shielded with lead are in good agreement with full Monte Carlo simulations.

## References

[1]Meertens H and van der Laarse R 1985 Screens in ovoids of a Selectron cervix applicator *Radiother. Oncol.* **3** 69-80

[2]Ahnesjö A 1989 Collapsed cone convolution of radiant energy for photon dose calculation in heterogeneous media *Med. Phys.* **16** 577-592

[3]Carlsson Å K and Ahnesjö A 2000 The collapsed cone superposition algorithm applied to scatter dose calculations in brachytherapy *Med. Phys.* Submitted

[4]Williamson J F 1988 Monte Carlo simulation of photon transport phenomena. In: *Morin RL (ed) Monte Carlo simulation in the radiological sciences* CRC Press, Boca Raton, Fl, p 53-102

[5]Ahnesjö A 1997 Cone discretization for the collapsed cone algorithm *International conference on the use of computers*

*in radiation therapy* XII *ICCR*, Salt Lake City, Utah, USA 114-166

[6]Carlsson Å K and Ahnesjö A 2000 Point kernels and superposition methods for scatter dose calculations in brachytherapy *Phys. Med. Biol.* Accepted for publication

[7]Namito Y, Ban S and Hirayama H 1995 LSCAT: Low-energy photon-scattering expansion for the EGS4 code *KEK Internal Report 95-10* (Tsukuba, Japan: National Laboratory for High Energy Physics)

[8]Leliveld C J, Maas J G, Bom V R and van Eijk C W E 1995 Monte Carlo modelling of coherent scatter: influence on interference *IEEE Nuclear Science Symp. and Medicaql Imaging Conf.* ed. P A Moonier (San Fransisco: IEEE) 1543-1547

[9]Williamson J F Monte Carlo evaluation of kerma at a point for photon transport problems *Med. Phys.* **14** 567-576

# Planning of Cardiovascular Brachytherapy

**Ulrich Quast[1], Dirk Flühs[1], Markus Bambynek[1], Clemens von Birgelen[2] and Dietrich Baumgart[2]**

[1]Clin. Radiation Physics, Dept. of Radiotherapy, and [2]Dept. of Cardiology, Essen Univ. Hospital, Essen, Germany

## Introduction

Cardiovascular diseases are the main cause of death in the western world primarily due to stenosis and finally occlusion of coronary arteries, leading to infarction. For the treatment of stenosis, percutaneous transluminal coronary artery angioplasty (PTCA), stenting (to overcome acute recoil effects), or atherectomy are commonly applied. But, they all lead to a high rate of restenosis resulting from acute recoil, neointimal hyperplasia (developing within a few weeks), and late unfavorable remodeling (shrinkage of the vessel after several months of wall thickening). After 20 years of cardiovascular research the great surprise came with the evidence that vascular radiotherapy applied immediately after intervention significantly reduced the high risk of recurrent stenosis from 30-60 % in 3 month after intervention to less than 10 % [2-4,10,11]. Radiation induced complications are reported.

However, many questions remain unanswered: Where is the target volume: intima, media, and/or adventitia? How to localize the target under treatment conditions? Which dose and dose distribution, which timing schedule, which sources and techniques are optimal for intracoronary radiotherapy? Which are the requirements for dosimetry and planning?

As a solution for some of these problems, the task group 60 of the American Association of Physicists in Medicine, AAPM TG 60, has prepared recommendations for the most relevant physical aspects of cardiovascular brachytherapy [3]. It was the goal of their report to review the physical, radiobiological and clinical rationales, irradiation techniques, diagnostic imaging procedures, and dosimetry methods used for treatment planning and evaluation, and especially to recommend procedures for dose specification, calibration, dosimetry, and quality assurance. The main problem, however, remains unsolved, how to determine these data for treatment planning and reporting with sufficient precision and within an acceptable time frame.

Treatment planning of intracoronary brachytherapy means a great challenge for medical physicists. For dosimetry, several basic and special requirements need to be fulfilled. The physical situation to be measured must not be disturbed by the measurement procedure itself. The extreme steep dose distribution - for ß-radiation a drop of 4 to 5 orders of magnitude of dose within a few millimeters - demands very high spatial resolution and precision. For the calibration of intravascular sources standard calibration conditions have to be chosen as close as possible to the clinical situation to measure the absolute absorbed dose to water. Then, any special physical situation can be described relative to these standard calibration conditions from measurements under systematic variation of the physical parameters.

The calculation of dose distributions can only be an additional method as the exact knowledge is required of all physical parameters of source, radiation, phantom material and interactions. Thus, in treatment planning dose calculations are insufficient without the corresponding measurements.

## IVUS and dosimetry based planning

*Intravascular ultrasound (IVUS)* provides excellent morphological and functional information of coronary arteries, needed to localize and define the target structures and to guide intracoronary brachytherapy planning, treatment, and follow-up [9], s. **Fig. 1**. Target volume is the whole vessel wall - including plaque/intima, media and adventitia - in the full extent of the injured section of the artery [8]. A mismatch of treatment volume and target volume can lead to edge-restenosis. Thus, sufficient safety margines are needed.

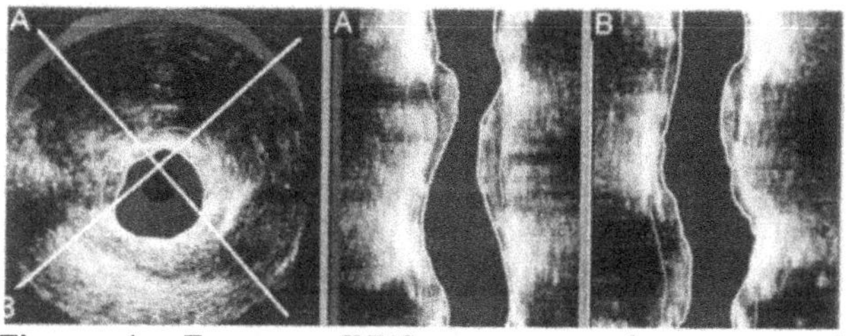

**Figure 1:** Transvers IVUS-tomogram and reconstructed longitudinal ultrasonic views of a coronary artery [7].

*Plastic scintillator dosimetry* [1,5-7] fulfills the special requirements for calibration, basic dosimetry, dosimetric treatment planning, and quality assurance of intracoronary brachytherapy: The absorbed dose to water can be determined:

- with high precision (about ±2% relative reproducibility and ±10% absolute accuracy for ß-radiation);
- at a high spatial resolution and positioning precision (about 0.1 mm);
- with a wide dynamic range (5-6 orders of magnitude of dose) with a linearity of ±2%; and
- fast (to provide for on-line results within a few minutes).

The high sensitivity allows to use very tiny plastic scintillator detector sizes (e.g. 0.3 mm x 1 mm ∅) providing the high spatial resolution. The detector response is independent of dose rate, accumulated dose, direction of incidence of radiation, temperature, or pressure.

The scintillation light proportional to the absorbed dose in the scintillator is guided by plastic fibers, converted by a high precision and long term stable photomultiplier into an electrical current, integrated by a PC within fractions of a second, and displayed as absorbed dose distribution. Thus, within a few minutes a complete depth dose distribution - e.g. from the surface of a high dose rate (HDR) vascular brachytherapy source down to the background of bremsstrahlung in the case of a ß-source - can be measured within 2 % reproducibility, s. **Fig. 2**. A two-dimensional distribution of dose requires some ten minutes, only.

Calibrated at NIST (National Institute of Standards and Technology, Gaithersburg, MD) together with a precision $^{90}$Sr-check source, the plastic scintillator dosemeter enables to measure directly the absolute absorbed dose to water.

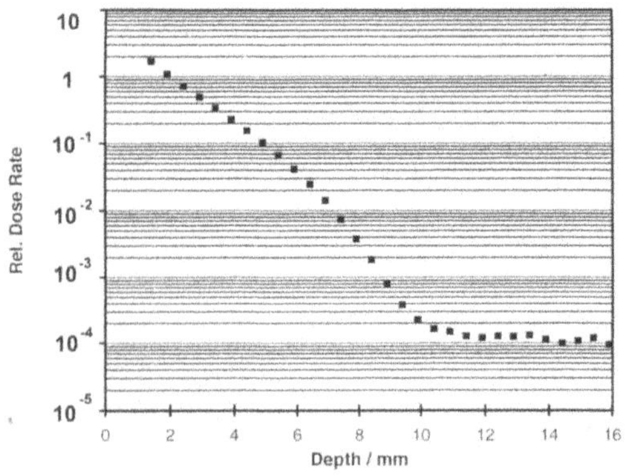


**Figure 2:** Radial depth dose distribution of an $^{90}Y$ line source measured in water with plastic scintillator dosimetry within 5 minutes [7], and normalized to the AAPM TG 60 calibration depth of 2 mm from the center of the source.

*IVUS and dosimetry based treatment planning* should be required for all experimental and clinical trials as well as for clinical routine treatment to be reported [7]. As the vessel wall thickness of diseased coronary arteries is extremely nonuniform, s. **Fig. 1**, it is impossible to center up a catheter with respect to all vessel layers inside a spatially curved artery. Thus, large distance variations lead to even larger dose variations and dose uncertainties in the layers of the vessel wall. Intravascular ultrasound, IVUS, shows the individual vessel wall architecture immediately prior to brachytherapy, and under treatment conditions, as seen from the assumed position of the source.

IVUS based dosimetric planning also enables the determination of all relevant treatment parameters: the irradiation time and the irradiation length, or the dwell times and number of source steps and positions, as well as the dose statistics (dose-volume-histogram) of the spatial distribution of dose delivered delivered to partial target structures and the whole target volume.

## Results

All dose data requested by the AAPM TG 60 for source calibration, basic dosimetry, treatment planning and quality assurance can be determined by plastic scintillator dosimetry and IVUS based dosimetric treatment planning.

For source calibration and specification, the plastic scintillator dosemeter allows to measure the absolute absorbed dose to water at a given reference distance with high precision and resolution. For ß-radiation, the absolute dose traced to NIST, can be determined with a precision of about 7.5 % (1 $\sigma$). For photon-radiation the dosemeter is traced to the PTB (Physikalisch-Technische Bundesanstalt at Braunschweig, Germany).

For source characterization, basic dosimetry and quality assurance, the plastic scintillator dosemeter allows to measure these dose data for all endovascular brachytherapy ß- or $\gamma$-sources used. The measurement has the great advantage to directly take into account all influences on the dose distribution, e.g. the non-uniformity or unsymmetry caused by an unequal activity distribution in a source or by the geometry of the source, by self-absorption in the material of the source (e.g. stent or balloon filled with radioactivity), or by differences in attenuation by a guide wire or by a contrast agent (liquid or gaseous). The AAPM TG 60 recommends to determine the radial dose function, geometry function, and anisotropy function for each specific source design of a commercial catheter-based system. These data can now be measured directly. Further influences on the dose inhomogeneity, e.g. due to differences in attenuation by a stent or by different tissue compositions can be taken into account.

Several clinical parameters influence the spatial distribution of dose and its variation, too, the extent of atherosclerosis, the thickness, density and atomic composition of the plaque, and the vessel bending. In addition, dynamic influences such as heart beating and breathing have to be considered. The dominant influences, however, are the strong distance dependence of dose (e.g. for ß-radiation at least 200 % per mm of water in the region of the reference depth at 2 mm), s. **Fig. 2** and the large distance variations in the vessel wall, s. **Fig. 1**.

For dose prescription and specification the variation of dose in the target volume must be reported in addition to the prescribed dose, specified to the AAPM TG 60 reference points. Primarily, however, the target volume must be defined. IVUS based dosimetric treatment planning provides then all requested information. Three-dimensional IVUS localization in addition allows to determine the dose-volume-histograms (DVH) for relevant target structures, e.g. media and adventitia, s. **Fig. 3**.

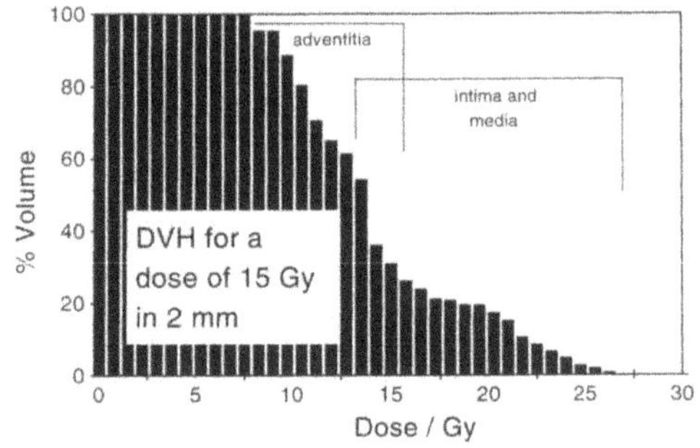


**Figure 3:** Dose-volume-histogram for the intracoronary brachytherapy with an $^{90}Y$-line source [7]

## Discussion and conclusion

Based on these experiences some conclusions can be drawn for dosimetry, planning and quality assurance of intracoronary brachytherapy.

*For source calibration* the general requirements and concepts for dosimetry have to be considered. In conclusion it can be proposed to calibrate also all photon sources used in vascular brachytherapy the same way as recommended by the AAPM TG 60 for therapeutic beta-sources, namely in terms of absorbed dose (rate) to water through precise direct dose measurement under physical conditions close to those in the clinical situation, and at the AAPM TG 60 reference distances. Although the activity can be determined easily, the conversion of activity to dose is unprecise. It requires to know the physical situation in advance.

For the calibration of therapeutic beta-sources applied in the USA, the American National Institute of Standards and Technology, NIST, uses a precision extrapolation chamber for absolute absorbed dose calibration, GafChromic™ film dosimetry for uniformity checks, Monte Carlo simulation for theoretical confirmation, a well type ionization chamber for activity calibration, and the Essen type plastic scintillator dosemeter for 3D-absorbed dose measurements.

*The biologically relevant parameters* can be defined, determined, recorded, and reported for each vascular brachytherapy treatment [3-6]:

- The position and length of the injured section of the coronary artery;
- the target volume including safety margins;
- the spatial distribution of absorbed dose to water (for radioactive stents accumulated over the biologically relevant time period of 48 hours): the absolute dose at the AAPM TG 60 reference point (and additionally the target related dose at 1.0 mm mean tissue depth), the mean dose, and the dose variation, or the dose-volume-histogram in plaque/intima, media and adventitia; and
- the temporal distribution of dose: namely the dose rate at the reference point and the irradiation time (for radioactive stents a suitable measure, e.g. three half-lifes of the source).

*Intracoronary brachytherapy* is a new, successful and – so far – complication-free application of radiotherapy to non-malignant, but severe coronary-artery diseases – if applied correctly. Precise three-dimensional treatment planning based on IVUS localization and plastic scintillator dosimetry, a work in progress, will be suitable for optimal irradiation treatment planning and complete reporting. These are essential prerequisites for later evaluation, comparison and hopefully understanding of the clinical results.

## References

[1] Flühs D, Heintz M, Indenkämpen F, et al. 1996 Direct reading measurement of absorbed dose with plastic scintillators. *Med Phys* **23** 427-434

[2] Jani S K, Teirstein P S, Massullo V, editors 1999 *Radiotherapy to Reduce Restenosis III.* La Jolla (CA): Scripps Clinic

[3] Nath R (chair), Amols H, Coffey C, et al. editors 1999 Intravascular brachytherapy physics: Report of the AAPM Radiation Therapy Committee Task Group No. 60. *Med Phys* **26** 119-152

[4] Quast U 1999 Definition and determination of the relevant parameters of vascular brachytherapy. In: P Levendag, editor: *Vascular Brachytherapy - New Perspectives* London (UK): Remedica Publishing, London pp 51-74

[5] Quast U, Flühs D, Bambynek M 1998 Endovascular brachytherapy treatment planning and radiation protection. *Herz* **23** 337-346

[6] Quast U, Flühs D, Bambynek M, et al. 1997 Fast 3D dosimetric treatment planning. The solution for precise cardiovascular ß-radiotherapy. In: Waksman R, Leon MB, editors. *Advances in Cardiovascular Radiation Therapy.* Washington (DC): Washington Hospital Center pp 8

[7] Quast U, Flühs D, Bambynek M, Baumgart D, von Birgelen, C 1999 3-D Endovascular brachytherapy *Frontiers of Radiation Therapy and Oncology: 3-D Radiation Treatment.* Basel: Karger, in press.

[8] Rubin P, Williams J P, Riggs P, et al. 1998 Cellular and molecular mechanisms of radiation inhibition of restenosis. Part I: Role of the macrophage and plattelet-derived growth factor. *Int J Radiat Oncol Biol Phys* **40** 929-941

[9] von Birgelen C, Erbel R, Di Mario C, et al. 1995 Three-dimensional reconstruction of coronary arteries with intravascular ultrasound. *Herz* **20** 277-289

[10] Waksman R, editor 1999 *Vascular Brachytherapy.* 2nd ed. Armonk (NY) Futura Publishing

[11] Waksman R, editor 1999 *Cardiovascular Radiation Therapy III.* Washington (DC): Washington Hospital Center

## Acknowledgment

Supported in part by a grant Qu 39/16-1 of the German Research Foundation DFG. The authors wish to thank their colleagues R. Erbel and H. Sack.

# An Iterative Mixed-integer Programming Approach to Brachytherapy Treatment Plan Optimization for Prostate Cancer

**Warren D'Souza**[1], **Robert Meyer**[2] **and Bruce Thomadsen**[1]
[1]Department Of Medical Physics, University of Wisconsin, Madison, 53706 USA, and [2]Department of Computer Sciences, University of Wisconsin, Madison, 53706 USA

## Introduction

Ultrasound-guided transperineal radioactive implantation of the prostate is one of the fastest growing medical procedures in the country. The number of yearly implant treatments is projected to increase to over 100,000 by 2005. Conventional treatment planning for interstitial brachytherapy is generally a trial and error process in which improved treatment plans are generated by iteratively changing via expert judgement the configuration of approximately 100 sources within the target volume in order to achieve a satisfactory dose distribution while minimizing damage to normal tissues. Automated stochastic algorithms such as simulated annealing (Pouliot *et al.*) and genetic algorithms (Yu *et al.*, Yang *et al.*) have been proposed. The limitation of stochastic algorithms is their tendency to get trapped in local optima rather than producing global optima. Gallagher *et al.* have utilized mixed integer programming (MIP) and the branch-and-bound method to generate treatment plans. However, their method uses a sampling approach that provides a coarse approximation (which may be inadequate) to the full set of points within the target volume. The rapidity of falloff in dose from an interstitial radioactive source requires a fine sample of the space in which the dose is calculated. We have implemented an iterative sequential approach using mixed integer programming and branch-and-bound to generate treatment plans. Our technique iteratively optimizes pseudo- independent 2-D slices to achieve a full-scale 3-D optimization.

## Material and methods

Mixed integer programming utilizes real continuous and integer variables. The MIP model for prostate seed implants involves the use of binary variables i.e., $y_P = 0,1$ corresponding to the placement or non-placement of seeds in a potential grid locations pre-determined by the ultrasound template. If $y_P$ is the binary (0/1) variable indicating the presence or absence of a seed at a potential seed grid location P, then the total dose $D_{ijk}$ delivered by all seeds to a point (i,j,k) in the dose calculation grid is obtained by summing the doses from all of the seeds:

$$D_{ijk} = \sum_{P=1}^{N} y_P D_{ijk}^P \qquad (1)$$

where $D_{ijk}^P$ is the dose contribution from seed P, and N is the number of possible seed positions. The total dose delivered to a point (i,j,k) therefore, is the weighted sum of the contribution from each possible seed position.

The primary goal in prostate seed implant brachytherapy is to deliver a prescribed dose to the prostate gland while maintaining the dose to organs at risk such as the urethra and rectum below harmful levels. We have implemented this by placing "soft" constraints for the dose over the target and sensitive structure region, and a combination of "soft" and "hard" constraints on the doses to the urethra and the rectum. The soft constraint over the target regions is described as:

$$D_{target} + z_{target} \geq T_d$$

where $T_d$ is the prescribed dose (145 Gy) to the prostate, $z_{target}$ is a non-negative variable that measures the deviation below the precribed dose level. For the urethra and the rectum, constraints can be stated as:

$$D_{urethra} - w_{urethra} \leq U_d$$
$$D_{rectum} - x_{rectum} \leq R_d$$

where $U_d$ (217.5 Gy for I-125 implants) and $R_d$ (101.5 Gy for I-125 implants) are critical doses to the urethra and the rectum respectively, and $w_{urethra}$ and $x_{rectum}$ are penalty variables that assume positive values if the dose to any voxel is above the critical dose level. Hard constraints are also placed on the doses to the urethra ($U_u$) and the rectum ($R_u$). This mandates that no voxel in the sensitive structures receives a dose above this level. The upper limits on the doses to the urethra and rectum are set at 275 Gy and 145 Gy respectively. The objective criterion that is minimized is comprised of a weighted sum of terms representing underdoses and overdoses (as described above), seeds, and needles.

The optimization is executed through an iterative process wherein three dimensional treatment plans are generated by sequentially optimizing the positions of sources in each of 10-15 two-dimensional slices (the number of slices is determined by the size of the prostate). The dose contribution of neigboring slices on the slice is calculated and the orientation of sources in this slice is then optimized. The iterative process begins with an *apriori* estimate of dose to each 2-D slice during the first iteration. During the second iteration, the dose contribution from the most recent source locations are considered from slices upto 4cm away. In this manner multiple iterations are carried out to generate the resulting treatment plan.

The optimization is carried out using the General Algebraic Modelling System (GAMS) and the Cplex mixed integer programming solver. The target and critical structures are contoured in the planning system. This data is pre-processed and transferred to GAMS, where constraints are set up and the objective/scoring function is described. The MIP model is passed to the branch-and-bound solver CPLEX, which returns an optimal solution. Branch-and-bound is a deterministic technique used to solve integer programs and guarantees a global optimum solution. This approach uses linear programming as its initial relaxation and then employs either-or restrictions derived from integrality constraints.

**Dose-Volume (DV) Constraints**

In some instances, it may not be possible to prevent overdosing a substantial volume of the urethra within the framework of the MIP model described above. Hence, it may become necessary to stipulate that no more than a certain volume be exposed to a dose above the critical dose. We implemented DV constraints through the use of more binary variables which can lead to longer solution times. For this reason, DV constraints were only imposed over the urethra. These constraints are stated as:

$$Dose_{urethra} \leq M * hd_{urethra} + U_d$$

where M $\gg$ 1, and $hd_{urethra}$ is a binary variable that determines if a voxel in the urethra exceeds the critical dose or not.

Since our approach involves sequentially optimizing each 2-D slice, DV constraints are enforced in a two-tier manner. One set of DV constraints is placed on the location of the urethra in plane for the slice being optimized and another set of constraints is imposed on the projection of the urehtra on the 2-D slice. This accounts for the curvature of the urethra in the inferior-superior direction.

## Results and discussion

We determined that 3 iterations (passes through the complete set of 2-D slices) were sufficient in terms of quality of solutions obtained. The dose-volume histograms (DVH's) obtained for the target, urethra and rectum display an oscillatory phenomena after successive iterations as can be seen from Figures 1 and 2 respectively. The DVH for the rectum showed marginal changes between successive iterations and therefore is not shown. The amount of change in the location of the DVH decreases after every iteration.

In all of the patients we have considered, when no DV constraints are enforced, target coverage (volume of target receiving at least the prescribed dose) is greater than or equal to 97.0%, (i.e. 97% of all points in the target. This approach therefore consistently yields this level of target coverage in contrast to manual plans (see Table 1). Imposition of DV constraints tends to lower the target coverage marginally but still yields acceptable coverage.

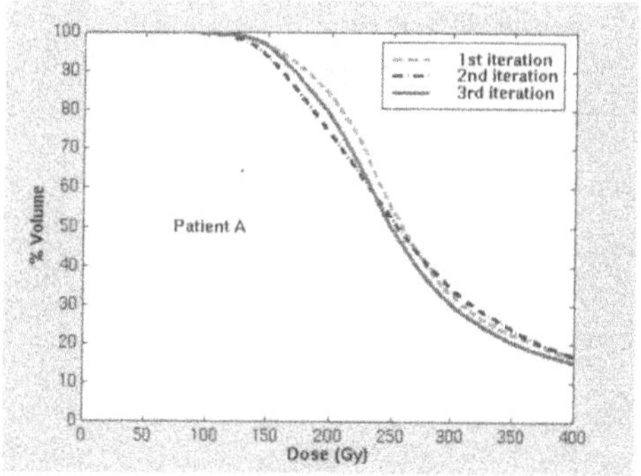


**Figure 1:** Target DVH resulting from 3 iterations of the mixed-integer programmi ng approach.

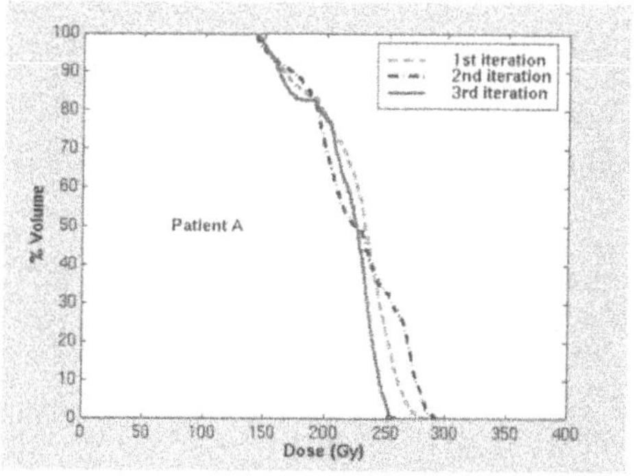


**Figure 2:** Urethra DVH resulting from 3 iterations of the mixed-integer programming approach.

| | Pre-DV | Post-DV | Manual |
|---|---|---|---|
| Patient A | 97.4% | 97.1% | 98.3% |
| Patient B | 97.6% | 97.5% | 94.9% |
| Patient C | 97.0% | 94.6% | 94.2% |
| Patient D | 97.9% | 95.5% | 96.4% |

**Table 1:** Volume of target receiving prescription dose before and after DV constraints and a comparison with the manual (clinical) plan.

Evaluation of the urethra DVH's shows that an appreciable volume of the urethra may receive greater than 150% (217.5 Gy for I-125 implants) of the target prescription dose. It may however, be misleading to evaluate DVH's based solely on this criteria because they tend to be very steep in the region of the dose being discussed. Thus, a slight shift in the DVH can result in significantly higher radiation estimates. There may also be some cross-over of the DVH's resulting from the automated plans and the clinical plan. The volume of the urethra receiving greater than 150% of the target prescription dose is reduced with the

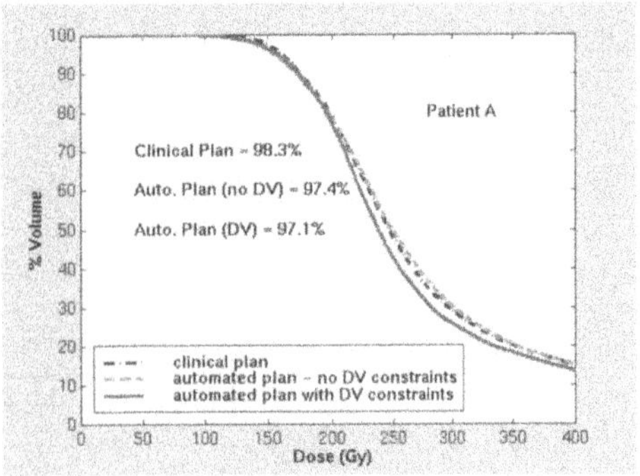


**Figure 3:** A comparison of the target DVH between the automated plans (pre-DV con straints and post-DV constraints) and the manual/clinical plan.

introduction of DVH constraints as can be seen in Table 2. No rectal DVH's are shown because they were comparable for the automated and manual plans.

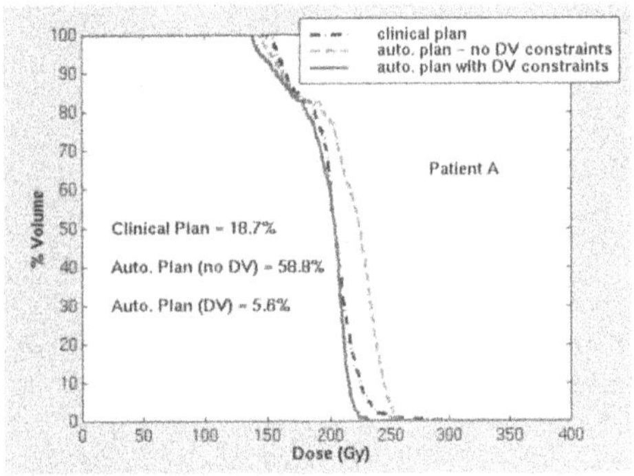


**Figure 4:** A comparison of the urethra DVH between the automated plans and the manual/clinical plan.

| | Pre-DV | Post-DV | Manual |
|---|---|---|---|
| Patient A | 58.8% | 5.6% | 18.7% |
| Patient B | 54.5% | 7.7% | 45.2% |
| Patient C | 48.9% | 15.1% | 0.0% |
| Patient D | 8.0% | 4.7% | 2.5% |

**Table 2:** Volume of urethra receiving receiving 150% of prescription dose (217.5 Gy) or higher before and after DV constraints and a comparison with the manual plan.

The number of needles used in the automated and clinical plans are both comparable. However, more seeds are utilized in the automated plan when no DV constraints are imposed. This can be justified by the superior target coverage of the automated plans. With DV constraints, the number of seeds is reduced but is still greater than or equal to the clinical plans.

| | Pre-DV | Post-DV | Manual |
|---|---|---|---|
| Patient A | 108 (25) | 104 (24) | 104 (26) |
| Patient B | 117 (24) | 112 (24) | 104 (23) |
| Patient C | 113 (22) | 108 (21) | 99 (20) |
| Patient D | 116 (20) | 100 (22) | 100 (22) |

**Table 3:** A comparison of the numbers of seeds (needles) for the automated plan (pre and post-DV constraints) and the manual plan.

## Conclusion

Treatment plans using mixed integer programming and the branch-and-bound solution method can be generated in 20-45 minutes on a Sun Ultra2, 200 MHz machine. We estimate that the planning time can be significantly reduced on a faster processor. The iterative approach involving the optimization of 2-D pseudo-independent slices yielded very good results. The volume of the target receiving at least the prescription dose (target coverage) is greater than 97% in all cases when DVH constraints are not used. The maximum dose to the urethra is maintained below harmful levels to avoid strictures. There are instances in which a certain volume of the urethra is exposed to an undesirable dose which may be a cause for concern regarding urethritis. In such cases, we have employed DVH constraints. The target coverage is marginally lower when these constraints are added, but is still greater than 94.6%, and the urethra overdosage is reduced to acceptable levels. In summary, the automated approach efficiently generates treatment plans comparable or superior to manually-generated treatment plans. These results also domonstrate the ease with which the mathematical models generated via this approach may be adapted as needed to generate solutions that achieve a variety of clinical goals.

## References

[1] Pouliot J, Tremblay D, Roy J and Filice S 1996 Optimization of permanent $^{125}$I prostate implants using fast simulated annealing *Int. J. Rad. Oncol. Biol.* **36** 711–720.

[2] Yu Y and Schell M 1996 A genetic algorithm for the optimization of prostate implants *Med. Phys.* **23** 2085–2091.

[3] Gallagher R, Lee E, Silvern D, Wuu C-S and Zaider M 1999 Treatment planning for brachytherapy: an integer programming model, two computational approaches and experiments with permanent prostate implant planning *Phys. Med. Biol.* **44** 145–165.

# Database infrastructure for multi-institutional clinical trials in 3D conformal radiotherapy and prostate brachytherapy

**Walter R. Bosch, William B. Harms, Sr., John W. Matthews, and James A. Purdy**

3D Quality Assurance Center, Mallinckrodt Institute of Radiology, Washington University School of Medicine, St. Louis, MO, 63110, USA

## Introduction

The practice of three-dimensional conformal radiation therapy (3DCRT) is heavily dependent on the use of image, geometric, and dosimetric data for treatment planning and verification. Several Radiation Therapy Oncology Group (RTOG) multi-institutional clinical protocols involving relationships of radiation dose and response in 3DCRT have been designed to acquire and collect both these treatment planning and verification (TPV) data as well as clinical endpoints. These TPV data have been evaluated by the 3DQA Center at Washington University in an effort (a) to evaluate the consistency of data and (b) to establish a database which can be linked to clinical outcomes for evaluating response statistics and developing dose-response models. To address these aims, two databases have been developed in the 3DQA Center. The first is a quality-assurance process-tracking database, the second a repository for evaluated TPV data for protocol cases.

## Material and methods

### QA Process Database

TPV data for three ongoing RTOG 3DCRT clinical trials are submitted to the 3DQA Center via internet FTP transfers or tape cartridges[1]. When these data are received, they are examined using a 3D radiotherapy treatment planning and review system (RTPRS) and its associated software tools. Submitted data are evaluated for completeness and consistency with protocol requirements. This QA process involves evaluation and scoring of CT scan coverage, target and organ contours, radiation field shape and placement, dose prescription, and dose uniformity.

### Treatment Planning and Verification Database

Once TPV data submitted by participating institutions have been evaluated and scored in the 3DQA Center, they are loaded into a second database which serves as a repository for this data and a means for correlation of treatment planning information with clinical outcomes. Information obtained in the QA evaluation process and stored in the QA Process database are used to facilitate the loading of TPV data into the data repository. Besides tracking the progress of evaluation and indicating readiness of data for loading, the QA Process database identifies initial, boost, and composite treatment plans in the RTPRS with data to be loaded.

### Data Model

The database schemas for the QA Process and TPV databases were developed using an entity-relationship model[2]. The data model used for the QA Process database consists of two main sets of entities. The first and most important set of entities are identified by a particular patient data set or "protocol case" and describe some feature of the data or QA evaluation for that case. Entities in this set include those describing

- the timeliness and completeness of data submitted to the QA center,
- QA scores for organ/target volume definition, field shaping and placement,
- dosimetric analysis for normal structures (total volume; prescription, maximum, and mean doses; and percent of volume receiving $\geq$ TD5/5 dose),
- dosimetric analysis for target volumes (total volume; prescription, ICRU reference, maximum, minimum, and mean doses; percentage of volume receiving $\geq$ prescription dose; and target coverage score),
- dose heterogeneity and conformity indices for target volumes,
- dates on which each fraction group was treated,
- a record of dates on which various portions of the case review were completed and the individuals responsible for each portion,
- a log of problems identified in the format or content of submitted data and their resolutions, and
- identification of tape volumes containing backup copies of submitted data.

A second set of entities are identified by institutions submitting data to the QA center. Entities in this set describe

- the credential status of institutions and date on which this status last changed and
- contact information for individuals in participating institutions.

The entities described above correspond directly to tables in the relational database implementation. Several additional tables are used as dictionaries for lookup of protocol-specific information including prescription dose levels, stratification groups, target volumes, organs at risk, and QA scoring definitions. Other tables are used to identify compatible versions of user interface programs and generate unique identifiers ("surrogate keys") for database tables.

The database schemas for QA Process and TPV databases were designed from the outset to support multiple protocols. Small changes in these schemas have been made as the QA process itself has matured, but no major, protocol-specific alteration has been required for new 3DCRT external beam studies. However, development of support for prostate brachytherapy protocols is prompting an update of TPV data submission methods (RTOG Data Exchange Format) and of the TPV database to include brachytherapy source specifications and new imaging modalities (MR and US).

The data model for the TPV database was originally conceived as including both patient imaging and treatment planning data as well as clinical outcomes contained on protocol forms. It has since become clear that maintaining both TPV and primary clinical data in a single database is not a practical goal because the quality assurance processes for TPV and clinical data are best carried out separately by the respective physics and statistical centers. Thus, effort has shifted to maintaining the TPV and clinical data subsets in separate databases maintained by the organizations responsible for assuring the quality of the data.

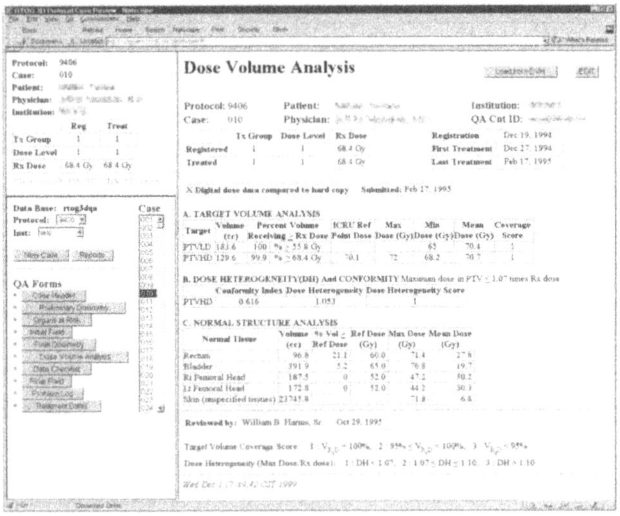


**Figure 1:** WWW-based user interface for QA Process database

The correlation of dose information (TPV data subset) with response (clinical data subset) requires access to both of these components. With these components stored in two separate (and geographically remote) database systems, both are needed to satisfy queries related to dose and response. Thus, some method must be used to link them. This linkage can be accomplished either by replication of data from one database to the other, or by accessing both databases to satisfy user queries.

Replication of data between database systems allows users to pose queries related to either or both TPV and clinical components within a single database system. This approach has been implemented in the 3DQA Center for data obtained in one protocol study. Queries are based on a single data model incorporating both TPV data and a replicated portion of clinical data supplied by the RTOG statistical support center. Data are copied between systems and updated through the exchange of text files.

Accessing two separate databases requires users to structure queries as two separate sub-queries, one restricted to TPV data, the other to clinical data. Fortunately, many questions related to dose and response are naturally structured as a partitioning of protocol cases based on one subset of the data (e.g., dose) and an evaluation of some parameter in the other subset (e.g., occurrence of some complication) for each group in this partition. While the widespread implementation of the open database connectivity (ODBC) interface makes such implementations possible, this approach requires knowledge of two different database schemas and access permission for two distinct systems maintained by two separate quality assurance entities.

**Internal Access to Database**

A web-browser interface has been developed to provide access to the QA process database for review and editing of protocol case QA scores and status information within the 3DQA Center. This interface has been realized using HTML frames as seen in the example screen shown in Figure 1. The user selects a protocol study and a case number within the study in the lower left hand frame. Ten buttons in this frame are used to display various QA forms for the selected case in the large, right hand frame. The small frame in the upper left hand corner displays basic information about the selected case including the patient name, physician name, submitting institution, as well as the dose level, stratification group, and prescription dose for the case. Along the bottom of this frame are codes which indicate which QA review forms are yet to be completed. When a QA form is selected, the relevant information for that case currently resident in the QA process database is displayed. This "browse" mode display can be printed using the print command of the web browser. An "edit" button in the top right-hand corner of this frame causes the "browse" display to be replaced by an "edit" display with editable fields containing the current information. The user can make changes to existing values or enter new values in these fields. A "Save" button on the edit page commits changes to the database, a "cancel" button returns to the "browse" page without updating the database, and a "reset" button resets editable fields to reflect the current contents of the database.

**External Access to Database**

Protocol participants can obtain feedback regarding the status and QA scores of cases they have submitted by accessing this information via the 3DQA Center web server (http://rtog3dqa.wustl.edu). This interface allows users with assigned passwords to view several QA forms, logs of unresolved problems, and a checklist of submitted data for protocol cases they have submitted to the 3D QA Center.

Participants can also submit protocol T2 (Digital Patient Submission Information) Forms for their protocol cases or dry run submissions online using an HTML-forms-based web interface. Online T2 forms are printed in the 3D QA Center and delivered via email to QA center personnel.

As the number of supported study protocols expands, the need to involve physicians at remote sites in the QA process grows, as does the importance of tools for remote review of submitted TPV data. By eliminating the need to distribute and configure software applications at remote sites, the ubiquitous web-browser interface greatly simplifies the deployment of remote review tools. Image-based tools are being developed to evaluate target-volume and critical-structure definitions as well as portal shape and placement. A web-based CT image review tool displays organ and target-volume contours on selected CT image slices. Treatment verification images can be reviewed using the Web View-Box tool, which displays pairs of pre-aligned simulation (or DRR) and portal images.

**Web Server Database Connectivity**

The architecture used implementing web-based access tools is shown schematically in figure 2. These tools have been realized using PERL-language CGI scripts performing database query and update functions as well as the formatting of retrieved information. Image formatting utilities are invoked by the CGI script to generate GIF and/or JPEG images for inclusion in HTML documents. Using such a utility, data retrieved from the database can be used to annotate images, e.g., for drawing organ contours or isodose curves on CT images or portal apertures on treatment verification images.

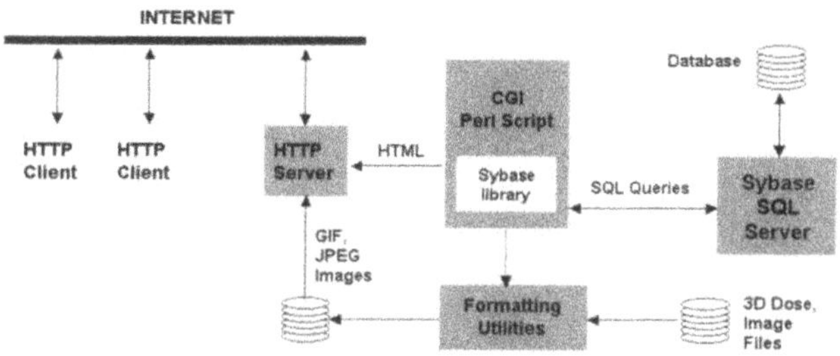


**Figure 2:** WWW-server architecture

## Results and discussion

The process of preparing data for loading into the TPV database has exposed several issues including the preservation of patient anonymity and the standardization of target-volume and organ identifiers.

**Anonymization and Confidentiality**

While it is possible (and helpful) to retain the identity of patients, physicians, and submitting institutions in the QA process database, such information must be withheld when providing access to TPV data. In contrast to the QA process database, the TPV database contains no explicit patient identification. Thus, guarding confidentiality is largely a matter of preventing inappropriate access to the QA process database. An important exception is the annotation written on digital films. Names of patients, physicians and institutions on these images must be made illegible before they can be loaded into the database. A web-based interface is currently used to "anonymize" submitted films in the 3D QA Center. The user identifies regions of the image which contain confidential identification by clicking on vertices of polygonal boundaries around these areas. Once identified, these regions are "pixelated" by replacing pixels in 8x8-pixel squares by the average value of the pixels they contain.

**Dual-use Data**

Three considerations make it attractive to use the same image/dose data files for both database and 3D RTPRS access. First, these data are large and dominate storage requirements for TPV data. Second, once the QA review has been completed, these data do not change. Third, while these image data may be retrieved for later study, there is at present no meaningful way to construct queries based on their content. Consequently, image and dose distributions have been stored in data files outside the database.

**Standardization of Structure Identifiers**

In order to compare dosimetric data for organ and target volumes in multiple cases of a protocol, the comparable volumes must be identified in the same way for each case in the database. While the RTOG 3DCRT protocols specify which organs and target volumes must be defined, there is considerable variability in the names used by protocol participants to identify the same volumes. Before being loaded into the TPV database, user-supplied organ and target-volume names in submitted data sets must be mapped to standard identifiers using software developed in the 3D QA Center.

## Conclusion

The development of a database infrastructure to support quality assurance in multi-institutional 3DCRT trials has been described. Segregation of data into a QA process database (dynamic) and TPV database (archival) simplifies the protection of confidential information. Patient confidentiality and data standardization issues must be addressed as part of the QA process. Web-based database tools are an essential part of the 3DQA center information infrastructure. Web-based access to provide feedback of QA information to participants has proven useful. Web-based QA review tools have the potential to allow physician review remote from the 3DQA Center.

This work has been supported in part by NIH grant 1 U22 CA81647 and DOD Medical Research Grant DAMD 17-98-1-8573.

## References

[1] Harms, W B, Bosch, W R, and Purdy J A 1997 An interim digital data exchange standard for multi-institutional 3D conformal radiation therapy trials *XII International Conference on the Use of Computers in Radiation Therapy*, D D Leavitt and G Starkschall eds. 465-468

[2] Bosch W R, Lakanen T L, Kahn M G, Harms W B, and Purdy J A 1997 An image/clinical database for multi-institutional clinical trials in 3D conformal radiation therapy *XII International Conference on the Use of Computers in Radiation Therapy*, D D Leavitt and G Starkschall eds. 455-457

# Evaluation of the Treatment Planning of Interstitial Hyperthermia of Glioblastomas

**B.W. Raaymakers[1], J.J.W. Lagendijk[1], J. Crezee[1], C.J.G. Bakker[1] and M.C.C.M. Hulshof[2]**
[1]University Medical Centre Utrecht, The Netherlands, and [2]Academic Medical Centre Amsterdam, The Netherlands

## Introduction

Currently a phase I study Interstitial hyperthermia combined with radiotherapy in patients with cerebral glioblastoma' is going on as a collaboration of the University Medical Centre Utrecht and the Academic Medical Centre Amsterdam. Within this study both the clinical feasibility of the treatment with the Multi Electrode Current Source Interstitial Hyperthermia heating system (MECS-IHT) [7] and the feasibility of the hyperthermia treatment planning system are being evaluated. This note reports on the treatment planning of the first four glioblastoma patients being treated.

## Heating technique

The target volume is implanted with plastic catheters which are loaded with capacitively coupled 27 MHz rf applicators [2]. The MECS-IHT system allows the simultaneous use of 64 individually controlled electrodes. Typically, in brain implants 12 catheters are being used with a total of about 20 electrodes (figure 1). Massive on-line temperature control (typically 84 individual sensors) is provided from seven-point thermocouple probes (sensor spacing 7-10 mm) integrated with each heating applicator.

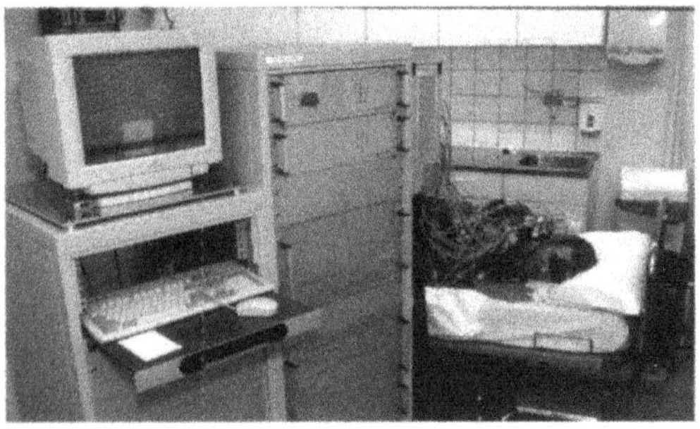

**Figure 1:** MECS-IHT system during treatment of a glioblastoma patient.

## Treatment planning system

Hyperthermia treatment planning consists of two processes: first the absorbed power distribution has to be calculated followed by the calculation of the resulting temperature distribution. In the hyperthermia treatment planning system the 3D absorbed power distribution is calculated with a quasi-static model [2]. An essential feature of the thermal model is its capability to describe the complex heat transfer related to discrete vasculature. The discrete vasculature (DIVA) thermal model [5] not only describes the heat transfer related to the discrete vasculature but also the distributed perfusion related heatsink coupled to the real arterial temperatures and the effective thermal conductivity. This model has been successfully tested theoretically [10] and in bovine tongues [8]. An extensive set of visualization and evaluation tools completes the treatment planning system. The treatment planning system runs on a Linux Intel platform.

## Data acquisition

The treatment planning system must be loaded with both the anatomy (mm resolution) and information about perfusion and discrete vasculature. To obtain the dielectric anatomy 3D MRI techniques are used. We studied the sensitivity of the absorbed power distribution for errors in the dielectric properties and showed that the use of literature based values [4] in combination with segmented images suffice for treatment planning purposes [9]. Phase contrast MRA with or without using Gd-DTPA contrast is clinically tested for determination of stenosis and quantification of flow. We showed that 3D phase contrast MRA is capable of supplying detailed geometrical vascular network information. We compared both MRA of the vasculature of bovine tongues with their vascular casts and MRI of the brains of healthy volunteers with anatomy hand book information and concluded that vessels with a diameter larger than 0.6 mm are visible. This resolution is currently available for sites accessible for surface coils. Within the glioblastoma study we use high resolution surface coil 3D phase contrast MRA for visualization of the anatomy and the delineation of the discrete vasculature. An example is given in figure 2. The implant defines the target volume, the MRA shows almost no large vessels in this post-operative tumour volume.

We image perfusion quantitatively with a dynamic segmented EPI dual gradient echo sequence. This two-dimensional, first passage gadolinium technique uses two surface coils; one on the neck for arterial input function determination and the other around the implant of catheters for depicting the volume of interest [1, 11]. Figure 3 shows the Cerebral Blood Flow map through the tumour site. Central tumour perfusions seems lower than the perfusion in the tumour periphery. Absolute figures are hard to obtain, the average tumour perfusion in figure 3 is 65 ml/100gr/min, slightly higher than that of the normal brain in the contra lateral site.

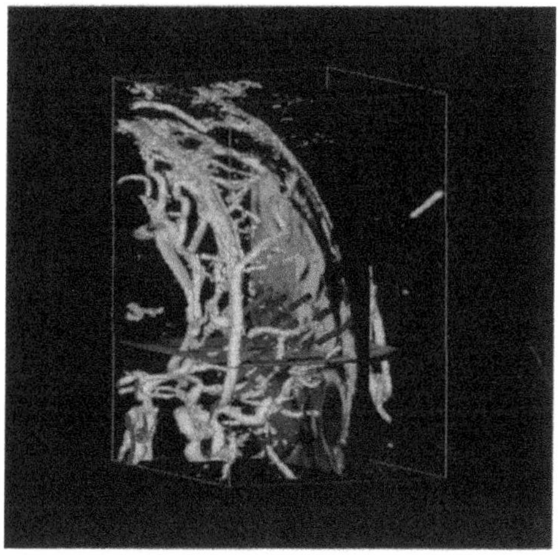

Figure 2: 3D phase contrast anatomy and vasculature in the target volume

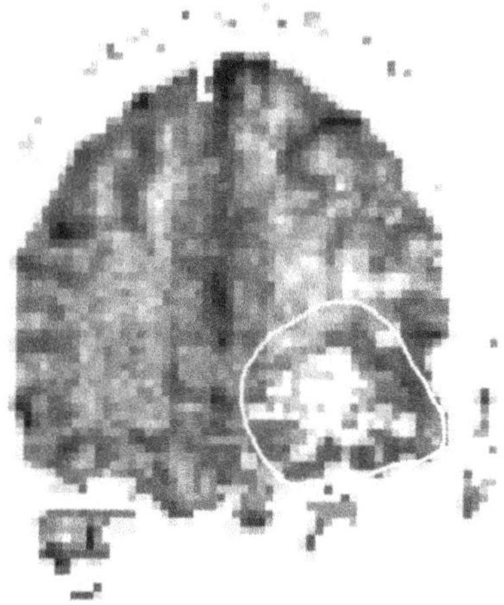

Figure 3: Cerebral blood flow image of the target volume (scale: white-black/20-70 ml/100gr/min)

## Treatment planning

The thermometry inside the heating catheters provides a detailed 3D map of the temperature distribution and the local perfusion for each thermocouple can be estimated from temperature decays at the end of treatment [6], also yielding a 3D perfusion map. The DIVA thermal model is used to approximate the 3D temperature distribution of the treatment. The heads are segmented manually in bone, liquor and brain. The electrodes are placed at the correct position and the power to each electrode is adjusted in such a way that the control temperature of that particular electrode during treatment is established. For the four patient studies blood flow was taken into account in the model by a heatsink. Discrete vessels where taken into account as much as possible. The four patient case studies yield good correspondence between the measured and simulated temperature distributions and temperature decays. Unfortunately, the first two patients showed that, the efficiency of the MECS-IHT system when operating with loss-less catheters proved to be insufficient to obtain the goal temperature of 42 °C in this high perfusion area at a catheter spacing of 15 mm. The use of low-loss catheters with 13 mm spacing was evaluated in the last two patients. In these patients a real 3D power control could be obtained resulting in nearly homogeneous temperature distributions at the electrodes. Due to the integration of the thermometry sensors in the applicators, maximum tissue temperatures are being measured. By switching off the power of individual electrodes for longer periods (several minutes) the corresponding thermometry sensors provide, together with the planning system, a good estimate of the minimum tissue temperatures. The perfusion map derived from the treatment data showed qualitative agreement with the MR findings. The estimation of the perfusion is obtained by simulating the treatment volume with various perfusion levels and compare those decays with the actual decays from the treatment. In spite of the large uncertainties in both methods and the fact that the MR perfusion values are before treatment and the transient values during treatment, the preliminary results are in reasonable quantitative agreement.

The detailed 3D temperature distributions from the last two patients clearly show the relative cold spots in between the catheters and high temperatures at the electrodes. From that it could be concluded that for glioblastomas the optimal spacing of the catheters is approximately 12–13 mm, with electrode lengths of 10–15 mm, in order to obtain clinically acceptable temperature homogeneity.

## New template technique

To minimize implant related risks we developed a hyperthermia angiography template technique (HATT) which uses a needle eye view through the anatomy to prevent accidental bleeding. This template technology may replace the stereotactic frame technology presently in use [3](figure 5).

## Conclusions

A complete 3D hyperthermia treatment planning system is available for the evaluation of interstitial hyperthermia. This system is now being tested in the interstitial hyperthermia treatment of glioblastomas. The full 3D temperature distribution can be analysed. The 13 mm catheter spacing treatment with low loss catheters provides good temperature homogeneity. We will continue this feasibility study.

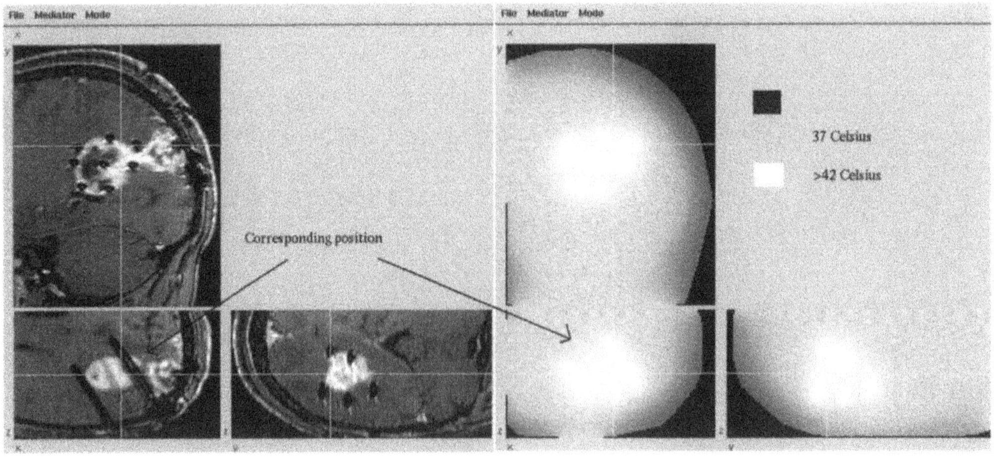


**Figure 4:** Anatomy and corresponding temperature distribution in the target volume

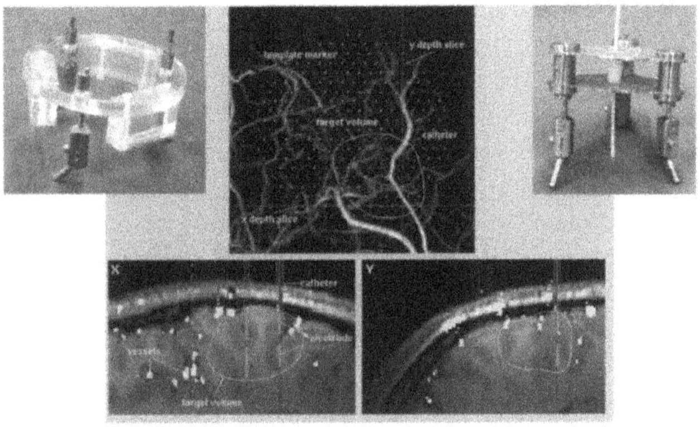

**Figure 5:** HATT imaging- (a) and drill template (b) and implant planning system (c)

## References

[1] Bakker CJG, Hoogeveen RM, Viergever MA, 1999 Construction of a protocol for measuring blood flow by two-dimensional phase-contrast MRA. *J Magn Reson Imaging* **9(1)** 119–27

[2] De Bree J, van der Koijk JF, Lagendijk JJW, 1996 A 3-D SAR model for current source interstitial hyperthermia. *IEEE Trans Biomed Eng* **43** 1038–45

[3] De Bree J, Lagendijk JJW, Raaymakers BW, Bakker CJG, Hulshof MCCM, Koot RW, Hanlo PW, Struikmans H, Ramos LM, Battermann JJ, 1998 Treatment planning of brain implants using vascular information and a new template technique. *IEEE Trans Med Imaging* **17** 729–36

[4] Gabriel C, Gabriel S, Corthout E, 1996 The dielectric properties of biological tissues: I. Literature survey. *Phys Med Biol* **41** 2231–49

[5] Kotte ANTJ, Van Leeuwen GMJ, Lagendijk JJW, 1999 Modelling the thermal impact of a discrete vessel tree *Phys. Med. Biol* **44** 57–74

[6] Lagendijk JJW, Hofman P, Schipper J, 1988 Perfusion analyses in advanced breast carcinoma during hyperthermia. *Int J Hyperthermia* **4(5)** 479–95

[7] Lagendijk JJW, Visser AG, Kaatee RS, Crezee J, van der Koijk JF, de Bree J, Kotte ANTJ, Kanis AP, Kroeze H, Levendag PC, Battermann JJ, 1995 Interstitial hyperthermia & treatment planning: the 27 MHz multi-electrode current source method *Activity, Special report* **6** 83–90

[8] Raaymakers BW, Crezee J, Lagendijk JJW, Comparison of temperature distributions in interstitial hyperthermia: experiments in bovine tongues versus generic simulations. 1998 *Phys Med Biol* **43(5)** 1199–214

[9] Van de Kamer JB, Van Wieringen N, De Leeuw AAC, Lagendijk JJW. Dependence of the SAR distribution on the dielectric parameters 1998 *Proc 17th ESHO Nancy* **47**

[10] Van Leeuwen GMJ, Kotte ANTJ, De Bree J, Van der Koijk JF, Crezee J, Lagendijk JJW, 1997 Accuracy of geometrical modelling of heat transfer from tissue to blood vessels *Phys Med Biol* **42** 1451–60

[11] Vonken EPA, Beekman FJ, Bakker CJG, Viergever MA. Maximum likelihood estimation of cerebral flow in dynamic susceptibility contrast MRI, 1999 *Magn Res Med* **41** 343–250

# Monte Carlo dosimetry for intravascular brachytherapy

**X.Allen Li, Ruqing Wang, Cedric Yu, Lance Weems and Mohan Suntharalingam**

Department of Radiation Oncology, University of Maryland, 22 South Greene Street, Baltimore, MD 21201-1595, USA

## Introduction

Intravascular Brachytherapy (IVBT) has been rapidly recognized as a potential treatment modality for reducing coronary restenosis after angioplasty [1]. There are many clinical trials currently underway to determine the efficacy of IVBT. At this stage, the optimum dose and the treatment target are largely unknown. Accurate dosimetry is crucial in analyzing data from these trails in order to both determine the most effective dose window and to improve our understanding of treatment failure. The region of interest for IVBT is very small (in the sub-mm to a-few-mm range). The dosimetric uncertainty on patient is generally high at the current time due to: (1) steep dose gradients in the immediate vicinity of the radioactive sources; (2) significant contributions from low energy secondary radiations; (3) complicated effects of specific source, applicator and radioactive stent design; (4) complicated patient geometry (such as heterogeneities due to calcified plaque, stent, vessel curvatures and source non-centering). Another contribution to dosimetric uncertainty is the fact that measurements are difficult (due to the extremely high dose gradient and other technical considerations). Also, analytical and empirical dose calculations are inaccurate (due to the perturbations caused by delivery devices, heterogeneities, and scatter and self-absorption of low energy secondary radiation). The AAPM TG-60 protocol for IVBT physics states that "ideally a three-dimensional dose distribution over the entire irradiated volume should be generated for each specific patient" [1]. Unfortunately, there is no easy way to accomplish this recommendation with the available brachytherapy treatment planning systems.

The purpose of this work is to develop a highly versatile, efficient, and accurate Monte Carlo dosimetry system to calculate 3-D dose distributions in patients for IVBT using intravascular ultrasound images and angiography. Because Monte Carlo uses particle-by-particle methods, it has the following advantages in IVBT dose calculations: (1) high accuracy and high resolution (only limited by computing time); (2) not subject to any geometrical constraints; (3) accurate and intrinsic calculation for inhomogeneity corrections; (4) all particle (electrons and photons) calculations. Monte Carlo calculation times can be prohibitively long for general routine clinical use. There has been considerable progress in the last few years in improving the speed and accuracy by choosing proper simulation parameters (such as electron step size) and by using more standard techniques of variance reduction. In addition, the computer hardware has also advanced rapidly. Moreover, for IVBT, the computing time will be further reduced because (1) the region of interest is small (i.e, the time required to trace each particle is short); and (2) the energies of photons and electrons are relatively low (i.e, electron ranges are short).

## Material and methods

The EGS4 Monte Carlo system [2] is used in this project. Comparing with other Monte Carlo codes, EGS4 has more flexibility in handling geometries and it can be more easily modified. Based on the standard EGS4 codes with PRESTA-II algorithm, a dedicate EGS4 user code, called MCIVBT, is being developed, according to the requirement of IVBT in geometry, accuracy and resolution. The intravascular ultrasound and angiography images is used to localize source positions and patient subjects (vessel wall, curvature, heterogeneties, et al). In addition to the standard particle transport algorithms, the following processes are incorporated into the MCIVBT, to further improve the modeling of low-energy transport: (1) electron binding correction for Compton scattering; (2) electron impact ionization; and (3) the production of L-edge characteristic X-rays.

A variety of tools are being developed to simulate different type of radioactive devices. A radioactive source is pre-modeled using its realistic structure and the result is stored in a source database. The data for each individual particle crossing the detailed source geometry is stored in a phase-space data file, which contains the information of the particle's history, energy, charge, position and direction. This phase-space data file is then used as input in the subsequent 3-D dose calculation.

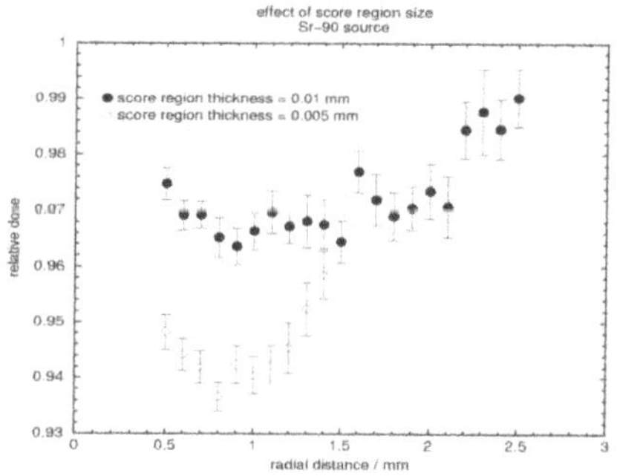


Fig. 1. Dose relative to 0.1-mm score region

## Results and discussion

This is a work-in-progress project. Some preliminary results are presented.

### 1. Accuracy of EGS4 for IVBT

The small source size and the small volume of interest in IVBT require very fine spatial resolution, which may violate the theoretical boundary conditions of the electron transport algorithms in EGS4. When step sizes are too small to allow at least 2.7138 collisions, as may be necessitated by the fine geometry, the algorithm may switch off multiple scattering (MS), producing dosimetric artifacts. Furthermore, the appropriateness of the algorithm in PRESTA to handle boundary crossing in very small regions also needs to evaluated. Our study for a $Sr^{90}$ β source showed that switching off multiple scattering could produce a dose deviation up to 6 % when the half thickness (d/2) of the dose scoring region is comparable with the Moliere minimum step size ($t_{min}$). The effect of switching off MS is negligible if d/2 >> $t_{min}$. Fig.1 presents the radial dose calculated with the score-region thickness of 0.01 or 0.005 mm relative to that calculated with 0.1-mm-thick score region. It is found that the calculation with 0.05-mm-thick score regions differs by 1% from that with 0.1-mm-thick score regions. The study shows that, if the electron step sizes are chosen to allow 5 to 40 collisions, with increasing step size, the doses surrounding the source increase and the error decreases. On the other hand, when larger step sizes are chosen, the dose calculation voxel size must also be increased in order for the calculations to converge. A good compromise between accuracy and applicability for IVBT simulation can be made, if the thickness of the scoring-region is greater than 0.05 mm and the electron step sizes are in the range allowing 10 to 30 collisions. The effects of other transport parameters were also evaluated. From these evaluations, we have found that the EGS4/PRESTA system is accurate for calculating the dose distribution fir IVBT provided the simulation parameters are chosen correctly.

The EGS4 calculation was validated by a variety of measurements and by an independent Monte Carlo system, MCNP (Fig.2). The agreement was within 5% (within 3% in the radial distance range of 0.7 – 4.0 mm).

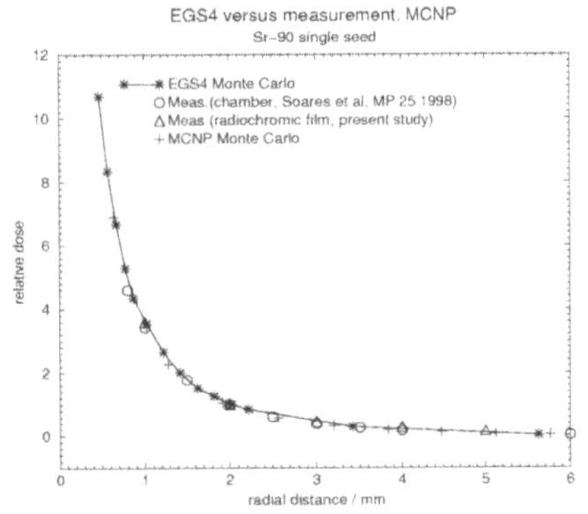


Fig.2. Comparison of relative radial dose, normalized at r = 2mm.

## 2. Evaluation of computing speed

Table.1 shows the CPU time required using EGS4 to calculate a 3-D dose distribution with a resolution of 0.2 mm for radial distance less than 3 mm and a resolution of 0.5 mm for r > 3 mm. The standard variance reduction techniques were used, and no care was taken to optimize the transport parameters for computing efficiency. It was found that the CPU times required for MCNP were generally double of those for the EGS4 codes.

| sources | $^{192}Ir$ | $^{125}I$ | $^{90}Sr$ |
|---|---|---|---|
| SUN Ultra 10 | 16 | 27 | 32 |
| Pentium II 450MHz | 18 | 25 | 38 |

**Table 1.** CPU time (min.) of using EGS4 codes to produce a statistical uncertainty of ± 1% at radial distance of 2 mm.

## 3. Various applications

To demonstrate the usefulness of the newly developed Monte Carlo system, preliminary calculations have been performed for various dosimetric situations encountered in IVBT.

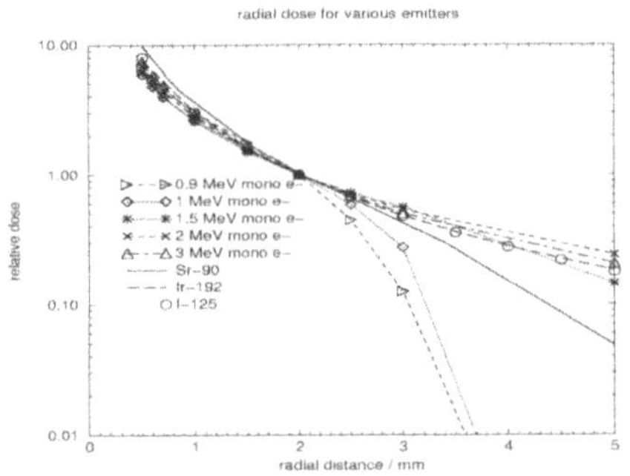


Fig.3. Comparison of relative radial dose for various sources.

3.1. Radial dose distribution: β versus γ. Fig. 3 compares the radial dose distributions for various sources. It is clear that a β emitter with energy around 1.5 MeV can produce a similar radial dose as those from the γ emitters.

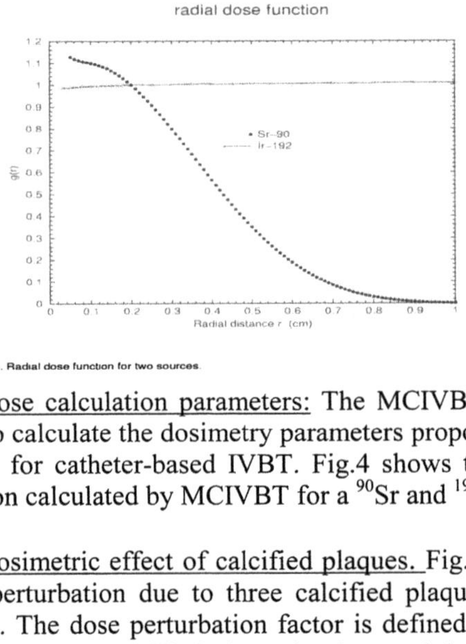


Fig.4. Radial dose function for two sources.

3.2. Dose calculation parameters: The MCIVBT code can be used to calculate the dosimetry parameters proposed by AAPM TG-60 for catheter-based IVBT. Fig.4 shows the radial dose function calculated by MCIVBT for a $^{90}Sr$ and $^{192}Ir$ sources.

3.3. Dosimetric effect of calcified plaques. Fig. 5 presents the dose perturbation due to three calcified plaques for the $^{90}Sr$ source. The dose perturbation factor is defined as the ratio of the dose with a calcified plaque in place and the dose in water. The plaques have a cylindrical shell shape with density of 1.45 g/cm$^3$. The data indicate that, for the $^{90}Sr$ source, up to 25% dose reduction behind the plaques is observed. Similar calculation for the $^{192}Ir$ source shows that a 6% dose increase within the plaques and no dose perturbation is found behind the plaques.

3.4. Dosimetric effect of of metallic stents. Fig.6 presents the dose pertubation as a function of the axial distance for the $^{90}Sr$ source in the presence of a stent. The inner radius of the stent is 1.45 mm. The positions of the stainless-steel wire along axial direction are indicated. It can be seen that, due to the perturbation from the stent, the doses at points 0.05 mm outside the stent varied by 25%. Calculation showed the dose in a region outside of stent (target region) can be reduced by up to 20% for the the $^{90}Sr$ source.

3.5. Dosimetric effect of contrast media. A contrast media may be injected during a catheter-based IVBT procedure. Fig. 7 presents the dose perturbation of a 1-mm thick contrast media.

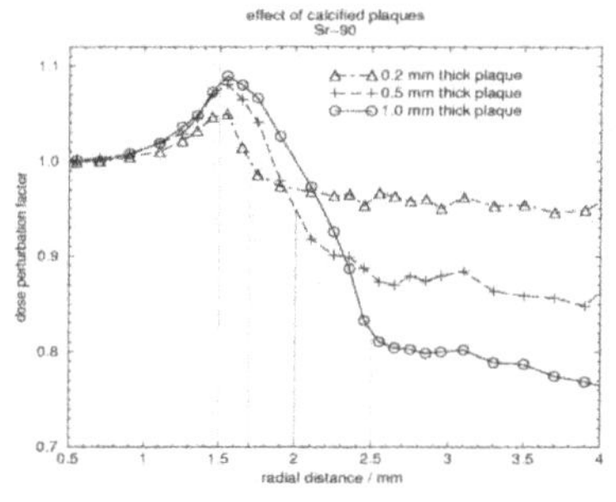


Fig.5. Dose perturbation for three cylindrical-shaped plaques.

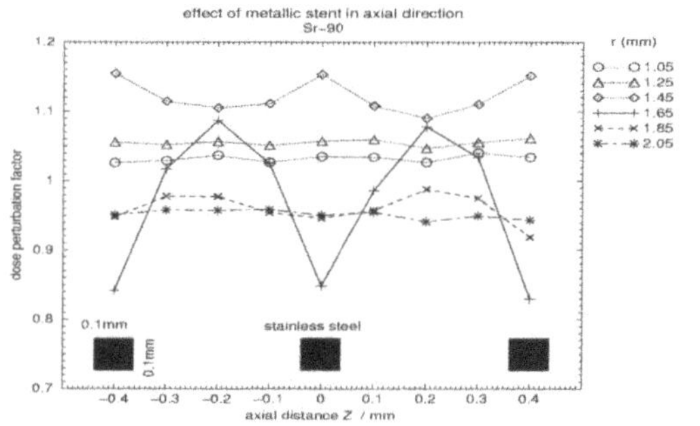


Fig.6. Dose perturbation of a metallic stent at various radial distances (r).

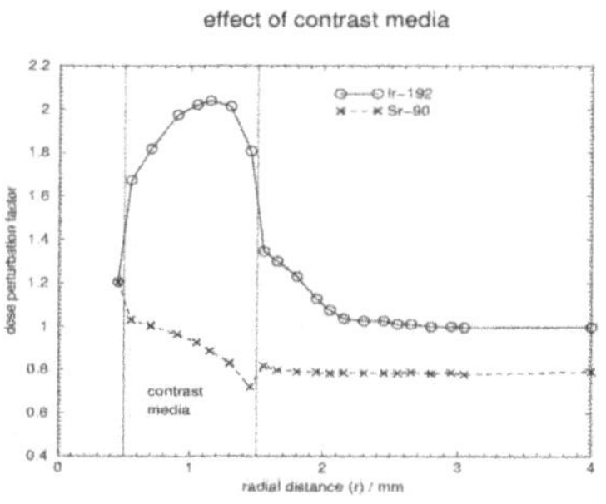


Fig.7. Dose perturbation of 1-mm thick Visipaque contrast media.

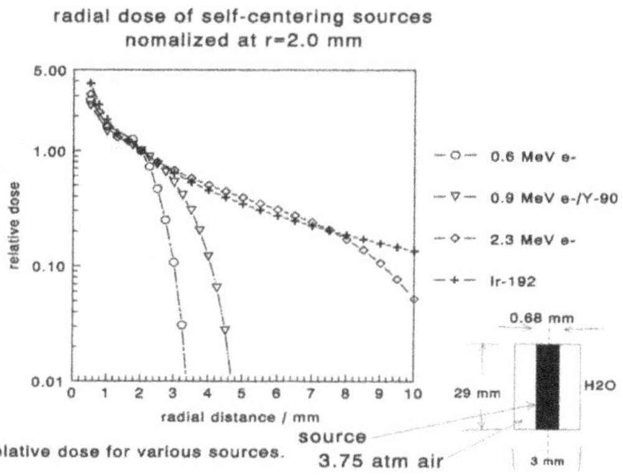


Fig.8. Relative dose for various sources.

3.6. Dose distribution of a self-centering radioactive wire. Figure 8 presents the radial dose distribution for a self-centering radioactive wire. Radioactive materials are uniformly distributed on a titanium wire of 29 mm long and 0.34 mm in radius. The radioisotope $^{192}$Ir and three hypothetical beta sources, emitting monoenergetic electrons of 0.6, 0.9 and 2.3 MeV respectively, are considered. A sketch of the calculation geometry is given in the lower-right corner.

3.7. Dose distribution for a radioactive stent. The radial dose distributions for two radioactive stents emitting 0.694 and 1.0 MeV electrons are shown in Fig. 9. It was assumed that the radioactive materials were uniformly distributed on the stainless-steel surface of the stent. The outer and inner diameters of the stent are 3.5 and 2.5 mm respectively, and the length is 20 mm. A sketch of the geometry is included in the lower-right corner.

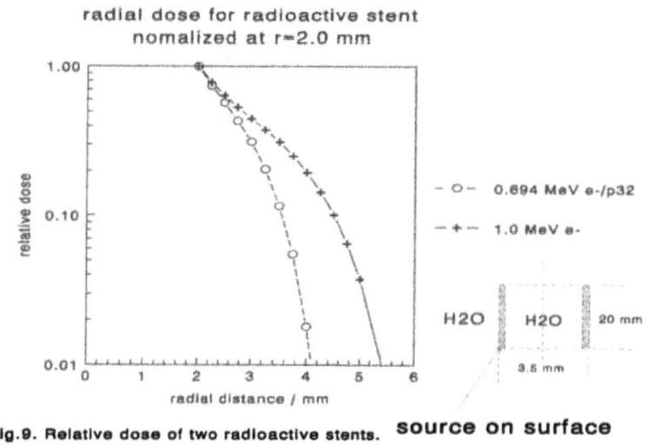


Fig.9. Relative dose of two radioactive stents.

## Conclusion

An accurate dosimetry system is required for intravascular brachytherapy. The EGS4 system are accurate and efficient for IVBT. Our newly-developed Monte Carlo package is powerful in resolving various IVBT dosimetric issues. The data obtained with this package are clinically important.

## References

[1] Nath R, Amols H, Coffey C, et al. 1999 Intravascular brachytherapy physics: Report of AAPM Radiation Therapy Committee Task Group No.60, Med. Phys. **26** 119-151

[2] Nelson W R, Hirayama H., Rogers D W O 1985 The EGS4 code system," SLAC-265 (Stanford Linear Accelerator Center, Stanford, CA)

# Monte Carlo Investigation of Typical and Potential Sources for Endovascular Brachytherapy

**Jörg Lehmann**[1], **Kenneth M. Forster**[2], **and Chang-Ming Ma**[1]
[1]Department of Radiation Oncology, Stanford University School of Medicine, Stanford CA 94305-5304, USA
[2]MD Anderson Cancer Center, University of Texas, Houston, TX 77030, USA

## Introduction

Coronary disease is the leading cause of death in developed countries. The cost of care for coronary patients is increasing while our ability to preserve life incrementally improves.

The use of balloon angioplastie to open arteries that have a stenosis (more than 50% reduction in lumen diameter of the artery) is an example of a modern, less invasive method of addressing this disease. In the United States alone over 500,000 angioplasties are performed every year, with nearly half of these patients experiencing re-stenosis. As a result, many patients receive an arterial stent directly following the balloon angioplastie. Even with the advent of arterial stents, the re-stenosis rate remains at 30 – 40% [1, 2]. A study at Emory University found that surgery is required for 25% of these patients within 5 years of their first angioplastie [3].

A leading hypothesis for the cause of re-stenosis is a hyperproliferation of smooth muscle cells via migration through micro-cracks in the arterial wall which result from the intervention itself. This process leaves deposits of neointima lining the arterial wall and eventually slowing the blood flow.

Early clinical trials at the Scripps Clinic [4] and at Emory University [5] have demonstrated a reduction in re-stenosis rates when radiation is administered directly following the arterial intervention. In the Scripps trial, patients with in-stent re-stenosis were randomized to receive radiation (at least 8 $Gy$ to the lumen wall, but not more than 30 $Gy$) or placebo following angioplastie. In this study there was a dramatic reduction in stenosis rate from 53.6 % for the control group to 16.7 % in the radiation group, approximately one third the re-stenosis rate [4].

In animal studies researchers have found that delivering an inadequate dose enhances the probability of a re-stenosis, and in the event of a re-stenosis the extent of the amount of neointima is increased with this under-dosing [6].

Some evidence of this effect in humans has been seen in subsequent analysis of the data from the Scripps trail. The choice of source and quality of the dosimetry is important for the success of any endovascular brachytherapy-trial.

In this work we have simulated the dose distributions for a variety of sources currently in clinical use, and we have also examined models of some theoretical sources that may be of interest in the future for this therapy.

## Material and methods

### Monte Carlo Simulations

The Monte Carlo Code EGS4 [7, 8] was used to simulate the dose distributions. The user code DOSRZ has been adapted for these simulations. To handle the complex input geometries the graphical user interface XInput [9] was employed.

Material input files were generated for the materials involved using PEGS4. To ensure high accuracy the energy range for these files started at 0.001 $MeV$ and ended just above the maximal energy of the source. Based on the results of preliminary simulations, PCUT and ECUT were set to 0.001 $MeV$ and 0.521 $MeV$, respectively. Simulations have been performed with PRESTA [10] and an improved electron transport algorithm (PRESTA II) [11].

The dose distribution for each source was calculated in water. The dose in tissue can be assumed less than 1 % higher than the dose to water [12].

The treated coronary arteries are located in the anterior or left lateral part of the heart. In the anterior direction the thickness of tissue can be approximated with 5 $cm$. Posteriorly often more than 15 $cm$ tissue have to be accounted for. To investigate the effect of this fact on the backscatter conditions, simulations with a 30 $cm$ diameter and a 5 $cm$ diameter phantom have been performed with the highest energy photon source used here. Differences were found to be in the order of 0.1 $mm$ for the 60, 80 and 100 % isodose lines. A phantom diameter of 20 $cm$ was then used for all simulations. 10 cm water were simulated on either side of the source in z-direction.

To evaluate the accuracy of the method, comparisons with measurements and Monte Carlo simulations by other investigators have been performed. Figure 1 shows the radial dose distribution for a $^{32}P$ source as simulated, compared to film measurements [13] with reasonable agreement in the typical therapeutic range.

### Isodose display - Xiso

To calculate the isodose lines, a utility program with a graphical interface was written in Tcl/Tk and called Xiso. The philosophy behind the program is to process output data from EGS4 user code DOSRZ after the simulation as oppose to changing the output routine of the code. The program, Xiso, reads the plotdat files that are produced by DOSRZ. It corrects for the fact that the radial dose distributions in the plotdat file specify the dose over the mean

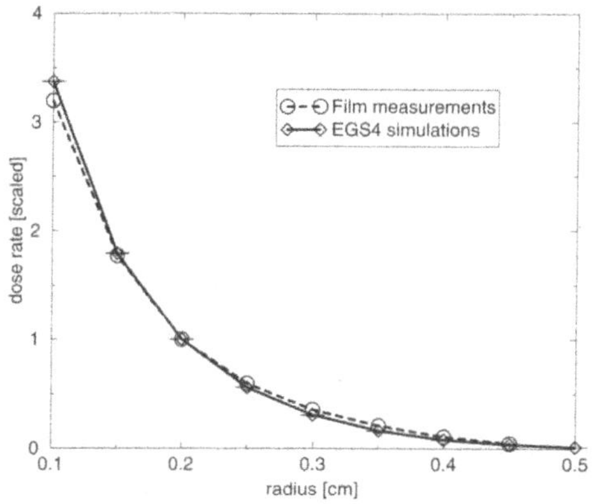


**Figure 1:** Comparison of the radial dose distribution as determined for a $^{32}P$ source with film measurements [13]. The error bars for the dose rate represent on standard deviation in each direction in this and the following figure.

of the inner and outer radius of a particular scoring region whereas the radius $r_{eff}$ that divides the volume (and mass) of the scoring region in half is located at

$$r_{eff} = \sqrt{\frac{r_{inner}^2 + r_{outer}^2}{2}}, \qquad (1)$$

$r_{inner}$ and $r_{outer}$ being the inner and outer radial boundary of the region. Interpolations between scoring regions use a linear approach. This introduces a slight bias in the radial direction, but the dose regions were set small enough so that this effect could be essentially eliminated.

Xiso creates isodose lines for user chosen levels and can write them to xmgrace files. It is possible to load additional simulation results with the same geometry but a different source configuration. This feature can be used to display the result of combined treatments.

Xiso can generate dose profiles radial or parallel to the source wire. Treatment time tables based on prescription information can be calculated.

### Sources

The sources investigated include the $^{32}P$ source by Guidant as used in the INHIBIT trail [14], a ribbon of $^{192}Ir$ sources [15], modified $^{125}I$ seeds and potential sources with $^{106}Rh$ and $^{169}Yb$.

The model 6711 $^{125}I$ seeds [15] have been modified for the needs of endovascular brachytherapy. The titanium housing material is replaced by aluminum (less dense). Furthermore, an implantation of the $^{125}I$ into the silver rod has been assumed to achieve adequate dose rates.

For the $^{169}Yb$ seeds a geometry analog to the modified $^{125}I$ seeds has been assumed. However, silver rod of the $^{125}I$ seeds is here replaced with aluminum. The originally empty inner cylinder of the source is filled with $^{169}Yb$ powder.

The $^{106}Rh$ source was modeled analog to the $^{32}P$ source. Several variation of the source design have been looked at.

A focus of this investigation was on the effect of the thickness of the actual source material which displays a high self absorption.

The spectra of the sources have been obtained from the literature [16, 17, 18, 19] . Adopting them for the EGS4 spectrum input format a line width of 2 $eV$ was assumed for line spectra.

The effects of arterial stents on the dose distribution have also been investigated.

## Results and discussion

Radial dose distributions for different sources are compared in figure 2. Each of them is normalized to the dose at a radial distance of 2 $mm$.

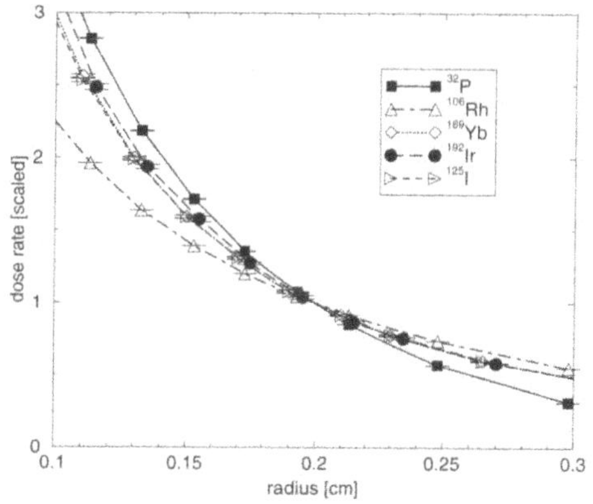


**Figure 2:** Simulated radial dose distributions at the longitudinal center of a $^{32}P$ source, a $^{106}Rh$ source, an $^{192}Ir$ seed, an $^{169}Yb$ seed, and an $^{125}I$ seed.

Figure 3 shows the influence of a simple intraluminal stent made of stainless steel on the isodose distribution around the center part of a $^{32}P$ source. The stent has an inner diameter of 2.6 $mm$, its wires are 0.2 $mm$ thick (radial direction) and 0.6 $mm$ wide. Between two wires is a gap of 1.8 $mm$. The dose is normalized at a radius of 2 $mm$ at the center of the source.

To investigate the difference between isotopes, for the following simulation only the input spectrum (and charge) has been modified to $^{192}Ir$ leaving the geometry unchanged. Results are displayed in figure 4. As expected, the distortion is significantly less pronounced in the case of the photons.

## Conclusion

A practical method for calculating detailed dose distribution for endovascular (and other) brachytherapy sources was presented.

This technique may now be used to assess the clinical viability of new sources as they are suggested.

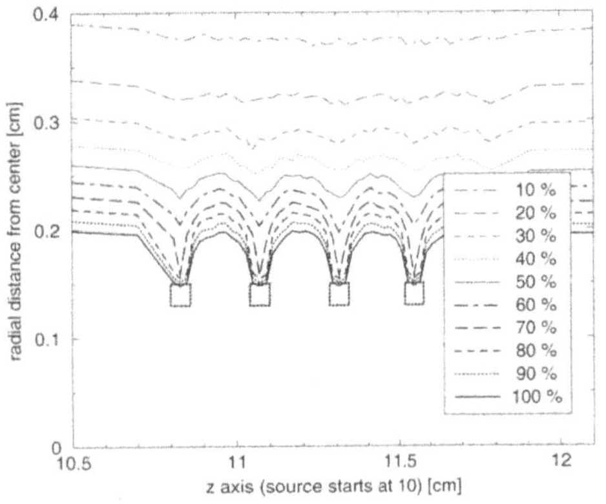


**Figure 3:** Simulated dose distribution around the center part of a $^{32}P$ source wire with an intraluminal stainless steel stent in place. The stent wires are symbolized by the boxes.

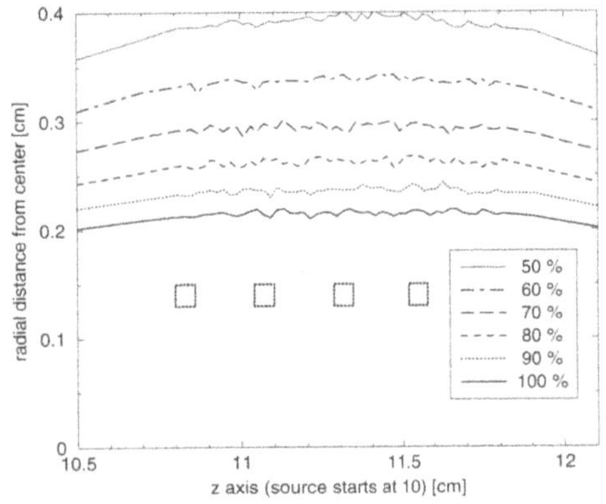


**Figure 4:** Simulated dose distribution around the center part of the source wire from figure 3 using $^{192}Ir$ instead of $^{32}P$. The stent wires are symbolized by the boxes.

## References


[1] Serruys P W, de Jaegere P, Kiemeneij F, et al 1994 A comparison of balloon expandable stent implantation with balloon angioplastie in patients with coronary artery disease *N Engl J Med* **331** 489–495

[2] Fischman D L, Leon M B, Baim D, et al 1994 A randomized comparison of coronary-stent placement and balloon angioplasty in the treatment of coronary artery disease *N Engl J Med* **331** 496–501

[3] Weintraub W S, Ghazzal ZM, Douglas JS Jr, et al 1993 Long-term clinical follow-up in patients with angiographic restudy after successful angioplasty *Circulation* **87** 831–840

[4] Tierstein P, et al 1997 Catheter based radiotherapy to inhibit the restenosis after coronary stenting *N Engl J Med* **336** 1697–1703

[5] King S, et al 1996 Coronary endovascular beta radiation for restenosis using a novel catheter system *Circulation* **46** 619

[6] Weinberger J, Amols H, Ennis RD, et al 1996 Intracoronary irradiation: dose response for the prevention of restenosis in swine *Int J Radiat Oncol Biol Phys* **36** 767–775

[7] Nelson W R, Hirayama H, and Rogers D W O 1985 The EGS4 Code System, *Report SLAC-265*, Stanford Linear Accelerator Center, Stanford, California

[8] Rogers D W O and Bielajew A F 1990 Monte Carlo techniques of electron and photon transport for radiation dosimetry *The Dosimetry of Ionizing Radiation, Vol III* edited by Kase K, Bjärngard B, and Attix F, pages 427–539, Academic Press

[9] Lauterbach M, Lehmann J, and Rosenow U F 1999 XINPUT: A program to edit "DOSRZ" input files *Med Phys* **26** 760–762

[10] Bielajew A F and Rogers D W O 1987 PRESTA: The parameter reduced electron-step transport algorithm for electron Monte Carlo transport *Nucl Inst and Meth* **B 18** 165–181

[11] Kawrakow I 1998 personal communication

[12] Sloboda R S and Wang R 1998 Influence of catheter materials and tissue composition on low dose rate iridium-192 seed implant dosimetry *Int J Radiat Oncol Biol Phys* **40** 249–255

[13] data from Guidant Inc.

[14] Lott S 1998 *Guidant Inc.* personal communication

[15] Weaver K A, Anderson L L, and Meli J A 1990 Source characteristics *Interstitial Brachytherapy by the Interstitial Collaborative Working Group* Raven Press, Ltd., New York

[16] Grove Engineering, Inc. 1987 "RADDECAY.EXE," 15215 Shady Grove Rd., Suite 202, Rockville, MD 20850

[17] Kocher D C 1981 Radioactive decay data tables *Report DOE/TIC-11026* Technical Information Center, U.S. Department of Energy, Washington, D.C.

[18] Borg J and Rogers D W O 1999 Monte Carlo Calculations of Photon Spectra in Air from $^{192}Ir$ sources *PIRS-629r* IRS NRCC

[19] Leighton R B 1959 *Principles of modern physics* McGraw-Hill Book Company

# Derivation of dosimetry data for brachytherapy sources using Monte Carlo for primary and scatter dose separation

**Kellie R. Russell[1], Anders Ahnesjö[1] and Åsa K. Carlsson[2]**

[1]MDS Nordion Therapy Systems, Uppsala, Sweden and [2]Dept. of Medical Radiation Physics, Karolinska Institute and Stockholm University, Stockholm Sweden

## Introduction

The scatter dose around brachytherapy sources is dependent on the characteristics and geometry of the scattering volume, while the primary dose depends only on the material along the source to calculation point path. Hence, algorithms based on primary and scatter dose separation will facilitate scatter dose integration and heterogeneity corrections. Source characterisation by means of Monte Carlo simulation of dose deposition per source emitted radiant energy allows dose separation into primary and scatter dose contributions [1]. The effects on the source geometry, self-absorption and attenuation in the source, encapsulation and wall material of the source channel are thus included in the calculated dose and kerma deposition. Radial dose distributions for the primary and total scatter dose were parameterised by exponential functions based on simple one-dimensional transport theory. Appropriate scaling and/or convolution techniques may be applied to each dose contribution separately to account for effects from scatter volume size, source placement and density variations [2]. The kerma in air at the reference point, per radiant energy emitted from the source, was also calculated by Monte Carlo simulation for each source and channel combination and used, together with the measured air kerma rate, to determine absolute dose rate to an arbitrary calculation point. Dosimetry data, inherent in the dose separation formalism, were extracted and compared with functions and parameter values recommended in the literature.

## Theory

Monte Carlo calculations can keep track of absolute dose by scoring energy deposition normalised to the radiant energy emitted from the source per atomic decay. The dose per radiant energy to point *pos* in a large water phantom is denoted as $[D/R]_c^{w,pos}$. The calculated total dose per radiant energy is the sum of the primary and scatter dose contributions. The dose contributions were parameterized to exponential functions based on simple 1D transport theory. The primary dose contribution has the form

$$\left[\frac{D}{R}\right]_{c,prim}^{w,pos} = \frac{1}{4\pi r^2 \rho}\left[a_1\, e^{-(a_2 - a_3 r) r}\right]$$

where the angular variations of $a_1$ depict the anisotropy, $a_2$ is a measure of the effective attenuation coefficient and $a_3$ corrects for the decrease of the attenuation coefficient due to primary spectrum hardening. The total scatter dose contribution is expressed by a convolution of a forward, one-dimensional, exponential scatter kernel with the SCERMA (difference in the total and kinetic energy released per mass). The result of the convolution integral motivates the double exponential function

$$\left[\frac{D}{R}\right]_{c,scat}^{w,pos} = \frac{1}{4\pi r^2 \rho}\left\{b_1\left[\left(1+b_2\right)-e^{-b_3 r}\right]\right\} e^{-b_4 r}$$

where $b_1$ insures energy balance, $b_2$ allows for backscatter at r=0, $b_3$ reflects the effective attenuation coefficient and $b_4$ accounts for the anisotropy of the primary spectrum. The $a$ and $b$ parameters are functions of the angle to the source axis to include angular variance in the distribution. The kerma in air was simulated for each source and channel combination. The parameter $[K/R]_c^{a,ref}$ is the calculated air kerma per radiant energy in air at the reference point, *ref*, 1 m from the source and was determined by

$$\left[\frac{K}{R}\right]_c^{a,ref} = \frac{1}{R}\left[\sum_i \frac{l_i}{V} E_i \frac{\mu_{tr}(E_i)}{\rho}\right]_c^{a,ref}$$

where $\mu_{tr}(E_i)/\rho$ is the mass energy transfer coefficient for photon $i$ of energy $E_i$ and $l_i$ is the tracklength in the scoring volume $V$. The calculated dose rate to position *pos* in a large water phantom is then

$$\dot{D}_c^{w,pos} = \dot{K}_m^{a,ref} \frac{\left[\frac{D}{R}\right]_c^{w,pos}}{\left[\frac{K}{R}\right]_c^{a,ref}} e^{-\lambda T}$$

where $\dot{K}_m^{a,ref}$ is the measured kerma rate in air at the same reference point, $T$ is the source decay time and $\lambda$ is the radioactive decay constant. The dose calculation formalism is thus directly comparable to the AAPM Task Group 43 (TG43) protocol formalism [3].

## Methods

Monte Carlo simulations were made in water and air for $^{192}$Ir sources used in the MicroSelectron HDR/PDR and GammaMed 12i HDR afterloading units and four interstitial sources; $^{192}$Ir (3 mm stainless steel-clad), $^{125}$I (Amersham models 6702 and 6711) and $^{103}$Pd (Theragenics model 200). Sources were positioned freely in unbounded water and air phantoms for the dose and kerma deposition simulations. The HDR/PDR sources were also positioned in combination with air-filled nylon and stainless steel source channels with inner/outer diameters of 5/6 mm and 1.5/2.0 mm, respectively. The EGS4/PRESTA [4] computer code was used together with a large cylindrical scoring geometry. The EGS4 code has been updated to improve low energy photon transport. Binding effects of atomic electrons, molecular interference on coherent cross-section in water and simulation of K- and L-shell fluorescent X-rays have been added [5]. The decay spectra were taken from MIRD [6] for the $^{192}$IR and $^{103}$Pd sources and Weaver [7] for the $^{125}$I sources. The $^{192}$Ir sources were described as specified by the manufactures including the source encapsulation and steel wire for the HDR/PDR sources. The $^{125}$I and $^{103}$Pd sources were described as 3 mm long vacuum filled cylinders with a diameter of 0.5 mm. The intrinsic radiation emission patterns suggested by Weaver [7] were used as input to the Monte Carlo simulations for the $^{103}$Pd and $^{125}$I sources to account for the anisotropy of the fluence distributions.

## Results and Discussion

Monte Carlo results for primary and scatter dose were parameterized to exponential functions of the radial distance from the source and stored in a table as functions of the angle $\theta$, where $0 \leq \theta \leq 180$. The Monte Carlo result for the GammaMed 12i HDR source is shown in figure 1 with the parameterized functions for primary and scatter dose.

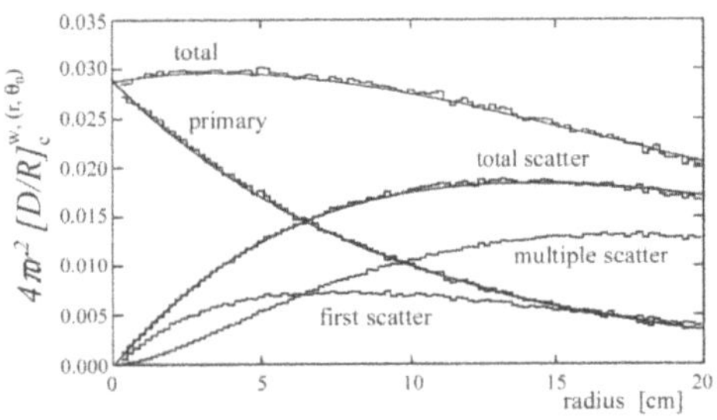


**Figure 1:** Monte Carlo simulation and parameterized primary and scatter dose functions for a GammaMed 12i HDR source in water.

Dosimetry data including radial dose profiles, anisotropy functions and dose rate constants, inherent in the dose separation formalism, were extracted and compared with functions and values recommended by the TG43 protocol and other published data. Radial dose functions *g(r)* for the interstitial sources and the GammaMed 12i HDR source, positioned freely in water, are shown in figure 2. The discrepancies at larger radial distances for the $^{192}$Ir sources are due to the differences in water phantom geometries used in the different studies, i.e. bound or unbound phantoms. The finite dimensions of a bound phantom reduce the scatter dose contribution, which dominates at radial distances larger than 6 cm. Specific dose rate constants, $\Lambda_0$, were calculated for $^{192}$Ir source and channel combinations and listed in table 1. $\Lambda_0$ values for the $^{192}$Ir sources agree to within ±1% of the value recommended by TG43. For the higher energy sources, $\Lambda_0$ is relatively insensitive to the material of the source channel. The Monte Carlo determination of kerma deposition for low energy sources, such as $^{103}$Pd and $^{125}$I, is sensitive to the geometric description of the source, the choice of decay spectrum and photon cross section libraries and to the handling of low energy photon transport [11,12]. These factors cause uncertainties in Monte Carlo determined values of $\Lambda_0$. Therefore, it is recommend that $\Lambda_0$ values based on measurements be used for low energy sources [11, 14] until better confidence in low energy simulation is gained.

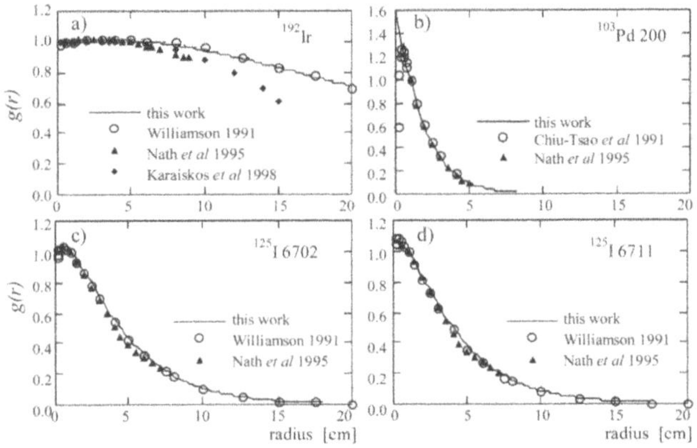


**Figure 2:** Radial dose functions, *g(r)*, for a) GammaMed 12i HDR, b) $^{103}$Pd (model 200) c) $^{125}$I (model 6711) and d) $^{125}$I (model 6702).

| Source | reference | inner/outer channel wall | $\Lambda_0$ (μGym²h⁻¹U⁻¹) |
|---|---|---|---|
| MicroSelectron | this work | water/water | 1.115±0.8% |
| HDR Classic | this work | air/nylon | 1.119±0.8% |
| | this work | air/steel | 1.112±0.8% |
| | ref. [8] | | 1.116±0.05% |
| | ref. [9] | | 1.115±0.5% |
| MicroSelectron | this work | water/water | 1.123±0.8% |
| HDR New | this work | air/nylon | 1.121±0.8% |
| | this work | air/steel | 1.117±0.8% |
| | ref. [10] | | 1.108±0.13% |
| GammaMed | this work | water/water | 1.113±0.8% |
| 12i HDR | this work | air/nylon | 1.114±0.8% |
| | this work | air/steel | 1.111±0.8% |
| MicroSelectron | this work | water/water | 1.131±0.8% |
| PDR | this work | air/nylon | 1.125±0.8% |
| | this work | air/steel | 1.130±0.8% |
| | ref. [9] | | 1.128±0.5% |
| $^{192}$Ir seed | this work | | 1.125±0.8% |
| | this work | | 1.120±0.8% |
| | ref. [11] | | 1.110±0.2% |
| | ref. [12] | | 1.105±0.008 |

**Table 1:** Specific dose rate constants, $\Lambda_0$, for $^{192}$Ir sources.

Anisotropy functions, *F(r,θ)*, at a radial distance of 3 cm and $0 \leq \theta \leq 180°$ were derived for sources positioned freely in water. Functions for $^{192}$Ir are shown in figure 3 and agree within ±3% with published Monte Carlo calculated functions and ±5% with measured values at angles between $10 \leq \theta \leq 170°$ to the axis. The calculated anisotropy is lower than measured values near 0 and 180° due most likely to measurement detector size limitations near the source axis. The anisotropy functions were reduced by 15% for steel channels compared with nylon channels at angles close to the source axis. Anisotropy functions for $^{125}$I and $^{103}$Pd are shown in figure 4. The dose deposition and thus the calculated anisotropy function for low energy sources is dependent on an accurate description of the source geometry and configuration. For this reason, we have followed the recommendations of Weaver [7] and base Monte Carlo simulation of dose on measured radiation emission patterns.

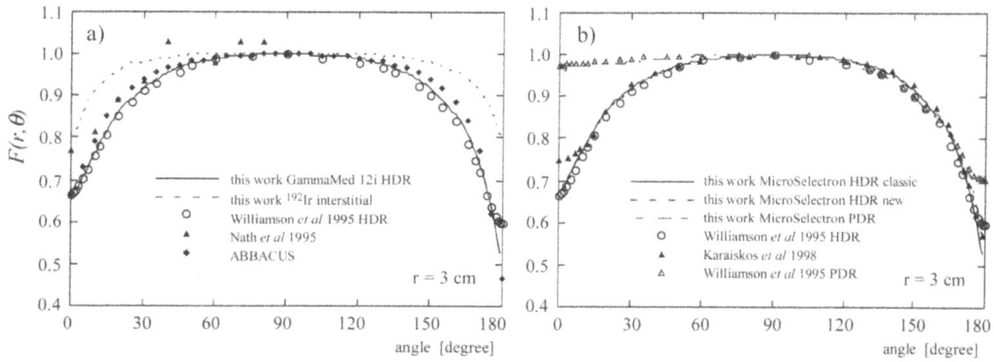


**Figure 3:** Anisotropy functions $F(r,\theta)$ for a) interstitial and GammaMed 12i HDR $^{192}$Ir sources and b) MicroSelectron HDR/PDR sources.

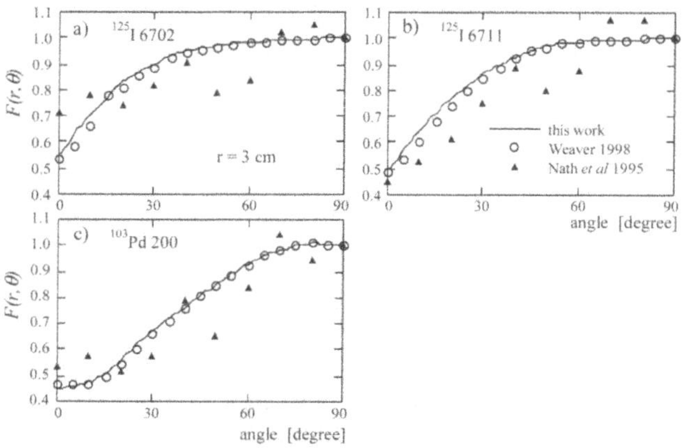


**Figure 4:** Anisotropy functions $F(r,\theta)$ for $^{125}$I and $^{103}$Pd sources.

## Conclusion

The use of Monte Carlo for simulation of source and channel combinations accounts for the dimensions of the source, self-absorption and attenuation in the encapsulation and channel wall. Separation of primary and scatter dose in a physical manner allows each contribution to be treated individually to account for changes in density of the scatter medium, use of internal shields and superficially positioned sources and geometry of the patient volume.

We have also Monte Carlo simulated other high energy sources such as $^{192}$Ir seeds, wires and hairpins, $^{137}$Cs tubes and spherical sources. The resulting distributions have been parameterized for brachytherapy applications. Anisotropy functions and specific dose rate constants inherent in the dose separation formalism agree well with functions and parameter values recommended in the literature for these sources.

The dose separation technique was designed absolute dose calculation from high energy brachytherapy sources and has been extended to describe dose deposition in the lower energy range. Monte Carlo simulations of dose deposition, i.e. radial dose and anisotropy functions, from low energy sources agree well with published data.

## References

[1]Russell K R and Ahnesjö A 1996 Dose calculation in brachytherapy for a $^{192}$Ir source using a primary and scatter dose separation technique *Phys. Med. Biol.* **41** 1007-1024

[2]Carlsson Å K and Ahnesjö A 2000 Point kernels and superposition methods for scatter dose calculations in brachytherapy *Phys. Med. Biol.* (Accepted for publication)

[3]Nath R, Anderson L L, Luxton G, Weaver K A, Williamson J F and Meigooni A S Dosimetry of interstitial brachytherapy sources: Reommendations of the AAPM Radiation Therapy Committee Task Group No. 43 *Med. Phys.* **22** 209-234

[4]Nelson W R, Hirayama H and Rogers D W O 1995 The EGS4 code system *Stanford Linear Accelerator Report* SLAC-265

[5]Hirayama H, Namito Y and Ban S 1996 Implementation of an L-shell photoelectron and an L x-ray for elements into the EGS4 code *KEK Internal Report* 96-10 (National Laboratory for High Energy Physics)

[6]Shirley V S 1991 Nucl. Data Sheets **64** 205

[7]Weaver K 1998 Anisotropy functions for $^{125}$I and $^{103}$Pd sources *Med. Phys.* **25** 2271-2278

[8]Karaiskos P, Angelopoulos A, Sakelliou L, Sandilos P, Antypas C, Vlachos L and Koutsouveli E 1998 Monte Carlo and TLD dosimetry of an $^{192}$Ir high dose-rate brachytherapy source *Med. Phys.* **25** 1975-1984

[9]Williamson J and Li Z 1995 Monte Carlo aided dosimetry of the microSelectron pulsed and high dose-rate $^{192}$Ir sources *Med. Phys.* **22** 809-819

[10]Daskalov G M, Löffler E and Williamson J F 1998 Monte Carlo-aided dosimetry of a new high dose-rate brachytherapy source *Med. Phys.* **25** 2200-2208

[11]Williamson J 1991 Comparison of measured and calculated dose rates in water near I-125 and Ir-192 seeds *Med. Phys.* **18** 776-786

[12]Mainegra E, Capote R and López E 1998 Dose rate constants for $^{125}$I, $^{103}$Pd, $^{192}$Ir and $^{169}$Yb brachytherapy sources: and EGS4 Monte Carlo study *Phys. Med. Biol.* **43** 1557-1566

[13]Chiu-Tsao S-T and Anderson L L 1991 Thermoluminescent dosimetry for $^{103}$Pd seeds (model 200) in solid water phantom *Med. Phys.* **18** 449-452

[14]Kubo H D, Coursey B M Hanson W F, Kline R W, Seltzer, S M, Shuping R E and Williamson J F 1998 Report of the ad hoc committee of the AAPM Radiation Therapy Committee on $^{125}$I sealed source dosimetry *Int. J. Radiation Oncology Biol. Phys.* 40 697-702

# Dose –Area Analysis for Endovascular Brachytherapy

**Martin Ebert[1], Nina Boeing[2] and Sean Geoghegan[3]**

[1]Department of Radiation Oncology, Sir Charles Gairdner Hospital, Nedlands, Western Australia 6009; [2]Department of Physics, University of Western Australia, Western Australia 6907; and [3]Department of Medical Physics, Royal Perth Hospital, Western Australia 6000.

## Introduction

The optimal choice of isotope and form (i.e., wire, liquid etc) for endovascular brachytherapy depends on many factors including dose uniformity across arterial structures, the influence of source centering, cost/availability, half-life and consideration of radiation protection. The centering issue was considered by calculating dose distributions due to several sources, and examining the dose-area relationship for artery wall as sources are moved off-centre.

## Material and methods

### Sources Considered and Dose Calculation

Several sources currently being used in clinical trials were considered - $^{32}P$ [1], $^{192}Ir$ [2] and $^{188}Re$ [3] – with characteristics as detailed in Table1. EGS4 Monte Carlo was used with a cylindrical user-code in calculation of dose distributions around the various sources (assuming in a water-equivalent medium), and to obtain dose fall-off curves with distance from the centre of each source.

| Isotope | Emissions | $T_{1/2}$ | Form |
|---|---|---|---|
| $^{32}P$ | β ($E_{mean}$=0.69 MeV; $E_{max}$=1.71 MeV) | 14.26d | Wire encapsulated by nitinol |
| $^{192}Ir$ | γ (0.317 MeV; 0.468 MeV; 0.308 MeV, 0.296 MeV) | 74.2d | Wire encapsulated by stainless steel |
| $^{188}Re$ | 85% β ($E_{mean}$=0.77 MeV; $E_{max}$=2.12 MeV)<br>15% γ (0.155 MeV) | 17h | Saline solution in angioplasty balloon with nitinol guide-wire |

**Table 1:** Isotopes and characteristics as modelled.

### Dose-Area Calculation

A medium-sized coronary artery was considered (radius 3mm, wall thickness 1mm). The artery wall was broken up into multiple sectors, and dose to these sectors due to an off-centre wire calculated using the Monte Carlo-derived dose distributions. Dose-Area information was then derived from the resulting arterial dose distributions (only 2D information was considered). This calculation was repeated for several off-axis positions of the two wire-based sources (see Table 1) to yield a series of dose-area hisotgrams (DAHs). For the solution-based source ($^{188}Re$), only a single DAH was obtained since the balloon used for irradiation with $^{188}Re$ is self-centering.

## Results and discussion

Dose fall-off plots running perpendicular to the sources are shown in Figure 1.

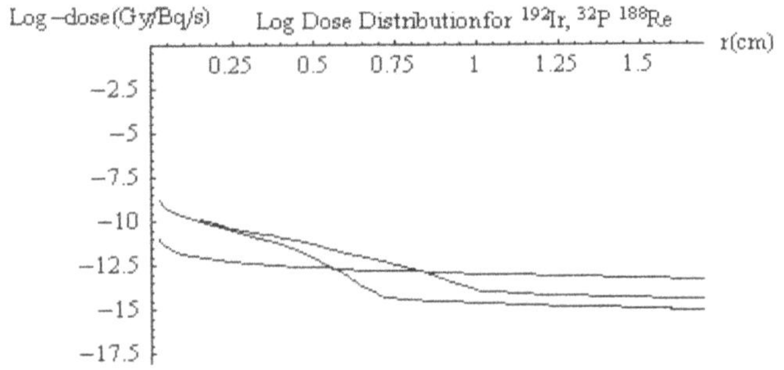


**Figure 1:** Logarithmic dose fall-off plots for three isotopes considered. Dose units are per unit source activity.

Figures 2 to 4 display DAHs for the $^{32}P$, $^{192}Ir$ and $^{188}Re$ sources respectively. These histograms have been normalised so that a minimum dose of 10 Gy is received by the artery wall in each case. DAHs at a number of off-centre distances are shown except for the $^{188}Re$ sourse which is always centred within the artery. Note the benefits for uniformity of using a γ-emitting source, at the cost of increased dose to distal normal tissue. The γ-emitting source has a slower dose fall-off with resulting higher distal-doses. The β-emitters have a more rapid dose fall-off with a small bremsstrahlung tail past the maximum electron range. This more rapid dose fall-off leads to a potentially broader range of doses to the artery wall when sources are not centred .This should be considered in light of the general inaccuracy associated with dose-prescription in endovascular brachytherapy.

The effect of dose-gradient on artery-doses as sources are moved off-centre is displayed in Figure 5. This figure plots the ratio of maximum artery-wall dose to minimum artery wall dose as the wire sources are moved off-centre.

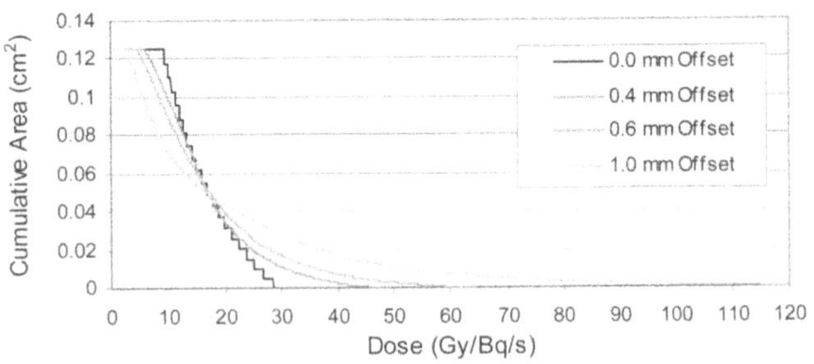


**Figure 2:** Arterial DAHs for $^{32}P$-wire source as the wire is moved off centre.

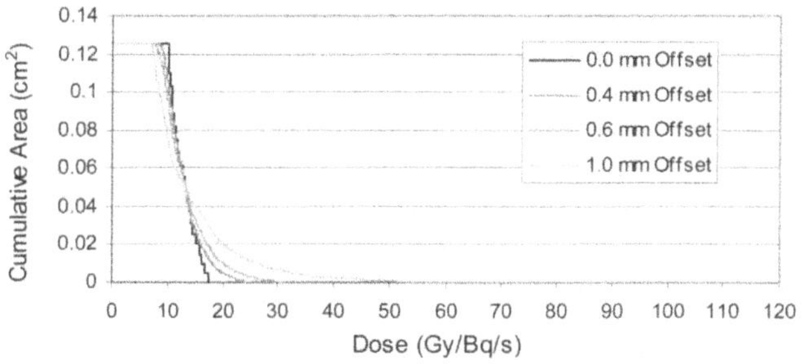


**Figure 3:** Arterial DAHs for $^{192}$Ir-wire source as the wire is moved off centre.

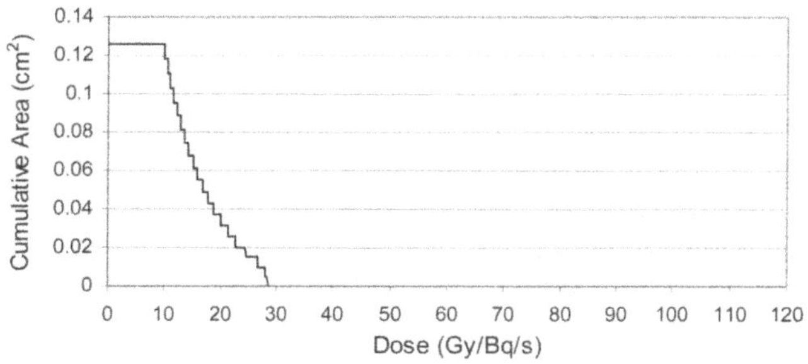


**Figure 4:** Arterial DAH for $^{188}$Re-liquid source.

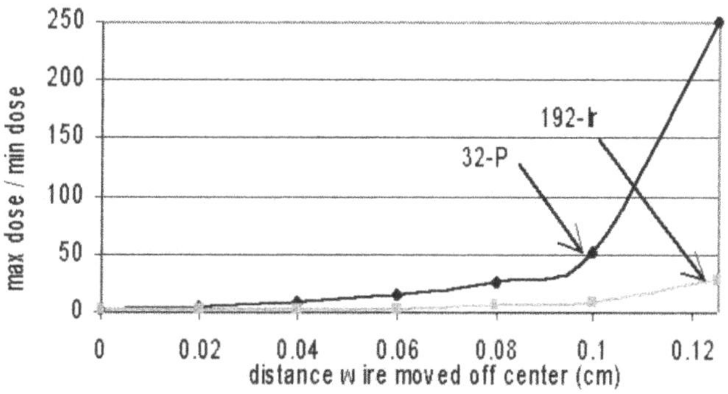


**Figure 5:** Ratio of maximum artery-wall dose to minimum artery-wall dose for the $^{32}$P and $^{192}$Ir sources as the wires are moved off-centre in the artery.

## Conclusion

This investigation confirms the benefits of using $\gamma$-emitters in terms of dose uniformity. This benefit should be weighed up against the benefits/detriments of using alternative isotopes (e.g., cost, radiation-protection, distal late-effects, non-uniform arteries, supply), as well as the technicalities of irradiation with various isotopes and their various forms.

## References

[1] Zhigang, X., Reinstein, L.E., Guozhen Yang, Pai, S. and Gluckman, G. (1997) The investigation of $^{32}$P wire for catheter-based endovascular irradiation *Med. Phys.* **24** 1788-1792

[2] Condado *et al.* 1997 Long term angiographic and clinical outcome after percutaneous transluminal coronary angioplasty and intracoronary radiation therapy in humans *Circulation* **96** 727-732

[3] Weinberger, J. 1998 Intracoronary radiation using radioisotope solution-filled balloons *Herz* **23** 366-372

# The application of GEANT4 simulation code to the verification of a brachytherapy calibration procedure

**Franca Foppiano[1], Stefania Garelli[1], Paola Moresco[1], Gabriella Paoli[1], Stefano Agostinelli[2]**

[1]Istituto Nazionale per la Ricerca sul Cancro di Genova, Largo Rosanna Benzi 10 16132 Genova, and [2]INFM and Università di Genova, Dipartimento di Fisica, Via Dodecaneso 33, 16100 Genova

## Introduction

The MicroSelectron High Dose Rate (HDR) system, installed at the National Institute for Cancer Research of Genova, uses a high activity Iridium-192 source which can be programmed to stay in specific positions for defined periods of time. The source consists of a cylinder of 0.6 mm of diameter and 3.5 mm length which is packed into a stainless steel tube of 1.1. mm of diameter and 5.0 mm length.
Calibration of the radionuclide source strenght is an essential part of any brachytherapy quality assurance programme.
The MicroSelectron sources are supplied by Mallinckrodt Medical B. V. - Holland with a calibration certificate that specifies the Air Kerma Rate measure at a distance of 1 m with an uncertainty of ± 5 %.
For every new $^{192}$Ir source we perform the measure of the Air Kerma Rate at a distance of 1 m following the Protocol for the Basic Dosimetry in Radiotherapy with Brachytherapy Sources of the Italian Association of Biomedical Physics (AIFB) [1] using a 0.6 cc Capintec chamber with a Capintec 192 Electrometer calibrated at the SIT Italian Calibration Service.
To verify the procedure used to calibrate each new MicroSelectron HDR brachytherapy source we are testing an in-house developed GEANT4 class to obtain simulated source Air Kerma Rate at distance of 1 m and simulated isodose distribution for the calculation of anisotropy coefficients for unshielded and shielded vaginal treatments.

## Material and methods

At every source change we perform the measure of the Air Kerma Rate at a distance of 1 m from the source comparing it with the certificated value.

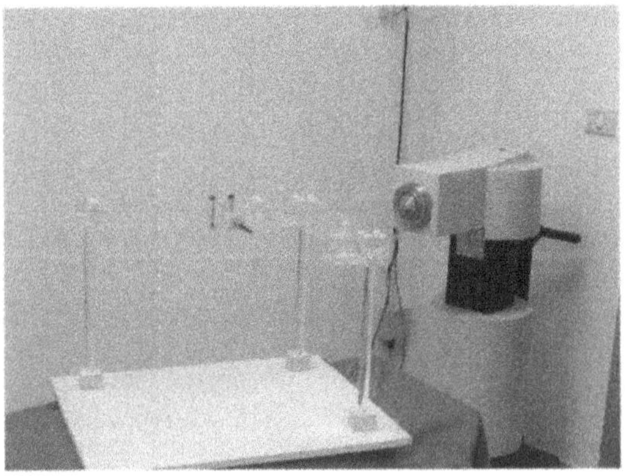

**Figure 1:** The custom calibration jig used for in air calibration.

Fig. 1 shows our custom calibration plexiglas jig, used for in air measurements. The source holder is a standard endobronchial treatment catheter, the chamber is a 0.6 cc Capintec chamber connected to a Capintec 192 electrometer.
We follow the direction of Basic Dosimetry on Radiotherapy with Brachytherapy Source of the Italian Association of Biomedical Physics (AIFB).
First of all we must obtain the chamber calibration factor $N_K^{sorg}$ for $^{192}$Ir. Our chamber is calibrated , by the SIT Italian Calibration Service, at the energy of $^{60}$Co and at a reference orthovoltage radiation with mean energy of 139 keV. A linear interpolation is used to find $N_k^{sorg}$ for $^{192}$Ir.
The reference dosimeter signal $M'(d_r)$ placed at a distance $d_r$ from the source must be multiplied for some correction factor to obtain the correct signal value $M_p(d_r)$ for the determination of Air Kerma Rate. The relation for $M_p(d_r)$ is:

$$M_p(d_r) = [(M'(d_r) \times K_{T,P} \times K_{sat} \times K_{dec}) - M_s(d_r)] \times P_{geom}(d_r) \times P_{air}(d_r)$$

$K_{T,P}$ is the correction factor which takes in account the air density difference during measurement and calibration,
$K_{sat}$ considers ricombination ion loss,
$K_{dec}$ is the correction factor for source decay,
$M_s(d_r)$ is the contribution due to photons scattered from air and room walls,
$P_{geom}(d_r)$ is the factor due to finite chamber dimensions,
$P_{air}(d_r)$ is the correction factor which takes in account the photon attenuation by air.
All these factors are obtained in our situation following the above cited Protocol.

The MicroSelectron HDR treatment planning system (PLATO), in order to account for the internal absorption and source encapsulation, uses a list of anisotropy correction factors $F_i(\varphi)$ where $\varphi$ refers to the longitudinal axial angle. Nucletron provides a standard anisotropy correction factors set which should be verified with on-site measurements.

To verify the calibration procedure and to obtain simulated anisotropy correction factors we are testing an in-house developed GEANT4 class. GEANT4 is a new-generation toolkit for full and fast Monte Carlo simulations available for the most common computer platforms. It is based on Object Oriented technology and has been developed using the C++ computer language. In GEANT4 [2] a set of models for the interactions of photons and electrons with matter is available with the following lower energy limits:

- photoelectric effect: 10 keV,
- Compton effect: 10 keV,
- Rayleight effect for optical photons,
- bremsstrahlung: 1 keV;
- ionisation: 1 keV,
- multiple scattering: 1 keV.

We are also evaluating a new set of models, the so called GEANT4 Low Energy, developed and validated [3] to extend the previous interactions to the energy range 250 eV-100 GeV for elements with atomic number between 1 and 100, in order to improve the verification process.

## Conclusions

For every new $^{192}$Ir source we perform the measure of the Air Kerma Rate at a distance of 1 m following the Protocol for the Basic Dosimetry in Radiotherapy with Brachytherapy Sources of the Italian AIFB. The usage of GEANT4 simulation code and of the GEANT4 Low Energy extensions for electrons and photons allows us to verify the calibration procedure followed in our Institute.

## References

[1] Protocollo per la dosimetria di base nella radioterapia con sorgenti brachiterapiche Aprile 1997. *Associazione Italiana di Fisica Biomedica.*
[2] http://wwwinfo.cern.ch/asd/geant4/geant4.html
[3] J. Apostolakis, S. Giani, M. Maire, P.Nieminen et al. GEANT4 Low Energy Electromagnetic Models for electrons and photons. Istituto Nazionale di Fisica Nucleare

# Autoreconstruction of Catheters in CT Based Brachytherapy Treatment Planning

**Natasa B. Milickovic[1,2], Dimos Baltas[1,3], Stavroula Giannouli[1,2], Michalis Lahanas[1], Nikolaos Uzunoglu[2,3] and Nikolaos Zamboglu[1,3]**

[1]Dept. of Med. Physics & Eng., Strahlenklinik, Städtische Kliniken Offenbach, 63069 Offenbach, Germany, [2]Dept. of Electrical & Comp. Eng. and [3]Institute of Communication & Comp. Systems, National Technical University of Athens, 15773 Zografou, Athens, Greece

## Introduction

The aim of this study was to develop an automatic reconstruction of brachytherapy catheters using CT data. Previously no such automatic facility has existed in any treatment planning software. To achieve this aim we have developed for the automatic reconstruction (which we term autoreconstruction) of plastic and metallic catheters. Our algorithms overcome a number of difficulties which arrise when a large number of catheters are present. These include situations with intersecting catheters and with loop techniques.
Modern brachytherapy treatment planning is image based[1-4] and frequently used imaging modality is CT scanning. CT based reconstruction accuracy depends on the CT imaging parameters such as the slice thickness, interslice distance and image resolution. In addition, accuracy also depends on observational ability of the user.
Image based treatment planning methods can significantly reduce the time required for the treatment planning process, to the use of projectional reconstruction methods using radiographs. Even so, a significant part of the treatment planning time is still spent in the reconstruction of catheters. From the analysis we made on 30 clinical implants the manual catheter reconstruction procedure took an average of 43.4% of the total treatment planning time: range of 22.6% to 71%. These times does not include those for image processing and contouring. The reconstruction time per catheter was an average of 151.2 s: range of 42.9 s to 312 s.

## Material and methods

### Introduction

The autoreconstruction process is based on post-implantation acquired CT images with the catheters *in situ* in their final positions. This includes the relevant patient anatomy, target volume(s), organs at risk, and the catheters. Catheter searching is made on a sequence of CT slices and is based on the Hounsfield number (HU) of the catheter material, catheter outer diameter, interslice distance, slice thickness and geometry of the catheter shape on the CT slices.
The slice thickness and interslice thickness must be adequately selected in order to take into account the curvatures of the catheters because these are not regular small diameter cylindres. We must therefore avoid loss of catheter area contrast in the reconstruction process during the CT slice acquisition. In general 3mm slice thickness and a 3mm interslice distance are satisfactory especiallly in cases when catheters *pass through* CT slices almost parallel to them, or when they lie on only a single CT slice and the neighboring region has very similar or significantly different (more than 2000HU) HU properties to that of catheters.

### Definitions

The area on a CT image which represents a cross-section through the catheter volume within the slice is termed the *catheter area.* The terms *catheter poin/pixel* are used to describe any point/pixel which is automatically recognized by the algorithm or manually identified by user, and belongs to a given *catheter area.* From a catheter area one central point is considered to represent the *catheter describing point*[1] on the CT slice. Each catheter is considered to be a geometrical entity that can be described by a set of arbitrary points laying on the CT slices, the *catheter describing points*[1].

### Hounsfield properties of the catheters

We analysed profiles of few different types of catheters which derived the default HU ranges for the plastic catheters to be (-600÷-200) and for the metallic catheters (2800÷3071).

### User defined parameters

Before the process of catheter autoreconstruction starts, the user must define some of the parameters that will be used in the search algorithm. These are: (a) catheter type: *plastic* or *metallic*, (b) serch region: *on-plane* (whole catheter lies in a single plane) or *in-volume*, (c) catheter tip position: *forward, backward* of the current slice (+ and – z direction in the DICOM definition) and (d) catheter loop option.

### Description of algorithms

*1.In-volume case*

As input data, we have a single catheter point **P**(x,y,z), that the user defines through GUI on any CT slice for each catheter where catheter can be easily identified and does not intersect with another catheter. Firstly, the pixel region around that given point is searched until the last two connected pixels of the group are found with HU values within the selected catheter HU range. While there is any unsearched pixel in the tree-like process, this routine is repeated. Finally a list of all *catheter recognized pixels* on the CT-slice is built. The central point $\mathbf{P}_C$(x,y,z) of the *catheter recognized area* is given by the equations below.

$$P_C = \frac{1}{n}\cdot\sum_{i=1}^{n} C_i.x,\ P_C = \frac{1}{n}\cdot\sum_{i=1}^{n} C_i.x,\ P_C = Z_{CT}$$

n is the total number of *catheter recognized pixels* and $C_i$.x and $C_i$.y are their x and y coordinates. $Z_{CT}$ is the z coordinate of the current CT slice where the recognition process was made. This central point is accepted as the first *catheter describing point.*

We now find the two most distant pixels in the *catheter recognized area.* They will be assigned as $P_1$ and $P_2$. From the Fig. 1 we can establish following relationship:

$$\cos(\varphi) = {r_1}/{r_2} \quad \textit{and} \quad \varphi = \arccos\left({r_1}/{r_2}\right)$$

where $r_1$ is the catheter outer diameter which depends on the type of catheter used, and $r_2$ is the distance between the centers of pixels $P_1$ and $P_2$.

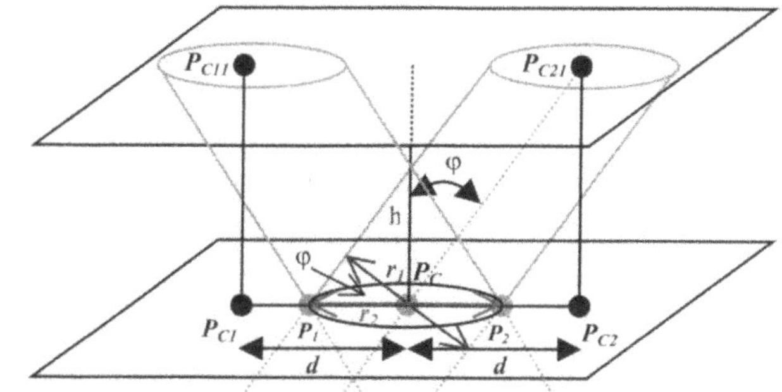


**Figure 1:** Catheter geometry and possible catheter positions on the next slice. It is analogous for the previous slice.

From Fig. 1 we see that catheter can have two possible directions. Distance d is given by, Fig. 1:

$$d = dist(P_C, P_{C1}) = dist(P_C, P_{C2}) = h \cdot \tan(\varphi)$$

where h is the distance between the two successive slices.

We now search for the next two *catheter describing points*, on the previous and on the next slice, based on the calculated distance d, the angle φ and direction of line $l(P_C,P_{C1})$, and $l(P_C,P_{C2})$ in the second case. We first find coordinates of two points $P_{C1}$ and $P_{C2}$. The possible catheter centers on the previous and on the next slices will be points $P_{C11}$ and $P_{C22}$ in the first case, or $P_{C21}$ and $P_{C12}$ in the second case, Fig. 1. Points $P_{C11}$ and $P_{C12}$ have the same x and y coordinates as the point $P_{C1}$, and their coordinate z is the coordinate z of the next and previous slice respectively. It is analogous for points $P_{C21}$ and $P_{C12}$. As we now have all possible catheter central points we need next to find which of these two point pairs ($P_{C11}$,$P_{C22}$) and ($P_{C12}$,$P_{C21}$) will determine the true catheter direction.

We first check if the HU number of the pixel to which point $P_{11}$ belongs, lies in the selected HU range of catheter. If it does, then we set a distance $d_{11}$ to 0mm, which means that this pixel belongs to catheter area. Otherwise, we search for the pixel $P'_{11}$ with satisfying HU number in the four *rings* area around the pixel $P_{11}$. If there is no pixel found $d_{11}$ is set to 100mm. Otherwise, $d_{11}$ is set to the distance between the $P_{C11}$ and $P'_{C11}$. In the same way we calculate distances $d_{12}$, $d_{21}$ and $d_{22}$, that are distances from the points $P_{C12}$, $P_{C21}$ and $P_{C22}$ respectively to the nearest pixel that belong to catheter area. Then we calculate:

$$d_1=d_{11}+d_{22} \text{ and } d_2=d_{21}+d_{12}.$$

If $d_1<d_2$, we accept the point pair ($P'_{C11}$,$P'_{C22}$) as recognized catheter points, othervise we accept ($P'_{C12}$,$P'_{C21}$). For example, if the pair ($P'_{C11}$,$P'_{C22}$) is accepted, and $d_{11}$=100mm, this means that we will search for the *catheter describing points* only in backward direction, as no catheter recognized point $P'_{C11}$ was found on the next slice. If $d_{11}=d_{22}$=200mm the algorithm stop searching because no new catheter point can automatically be found. In that case, the algorithm requires manual intervention for the determination of the next searching direction.

The algorithm consists of searching backward and forward from the giving catheter point P in the –z and +z direction according to the DICOM definition. The backward searching algorithm is given below.

*<u>Input data:</u>*
*$P_C$ - center of the catheter recognized area;*
*$P'_{C12}$($P'_{C22}$) – recognized catheter point on the previous slice;*
*Current_slice=$P_C$ slice – 1;*
*<u>Processing</u>*
*put $P_C$ in catheter describing point list;*
*error_flag=false;*
*Previous_point=$P_C$;*
*while(Current_slice• First_slice && error_flag==FALSE)*
*{Find catheter area A around the $P'_{C12}$ ($P'_{C21}$);*
*$CP_C$=central point of the catheter area A on a Current_slice;*
*put $CP_C$ in catheter describing point list;*

*search_direction_line=extrapolated from points (Previous_point, $CP_C$);*
*New=the nearest catheter point to the intersection of the search_direction_line and the previous CT slice (Current_sliice-1). A search is made in a four rings around the proposed pixel.*
*If New is empty: error_flag=TRUE;*
*else{*
*Previous_point=$CP_C$;*
*$P'_{C12}$ ($P'_{C21}$)=New;*
*Current_slice=Current_slice-1;*
*}*
*}*

After this the whole set of catheter describing points is available.

In the case of metallic catheters, artifacts can occur because of theirs significantly higher HU characteristic then this of other tissues. This is overcomed by checking the reconstructed catheter points, and *fix* the possible errors by *intential* over-jumping of the error-segment[3,4].

*2.Loops in the volume*

If catheter makes loops in the volume, we search it in the same way as previously described, except of the last step that need to be applied here. When the last point in the *forward* and *backward* direction is found, we analyse the shape of the catheter area on the CT slices of both the last found points in order to derive the next search direction from these, Fig. 2. After that we continue the process in exactly the same way.

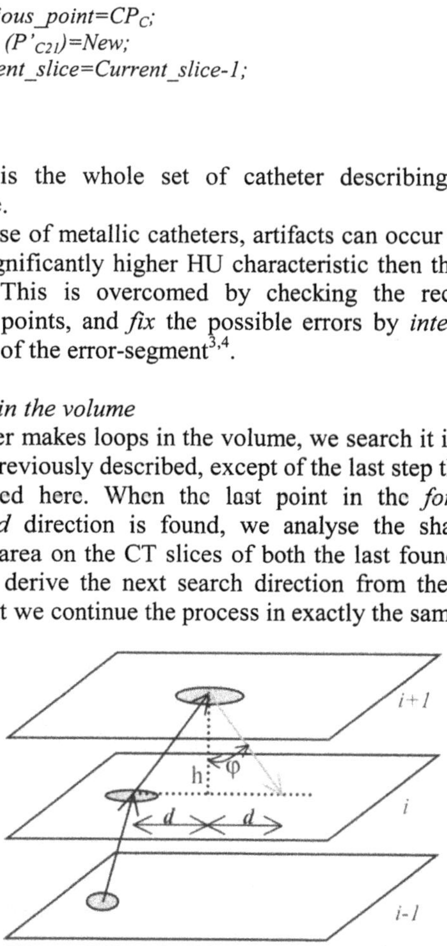


**Figure 2:** Search of the next catheter point in the case when catheter makes a loop in-volume.

*3. On-plane case*
If the entire catheter lies in a single plane, CT slice or calculated oblique cut, the search is made only in two dimensions.
*(a) On-CT-slice*
From the user given point, the algorithm automatically finds the entire group of *recognized catheter points* in that plane. From this group, the *catheter describing points* are extracted in a simple way as catheter skeleton points[3,4].
*(b) On-Oblique plane*
The same method for deriving the catheter skeleton on a single CT slice from the group of *cateheter recognized points* is used in this case. Since the *catheter describing points* per definition belong to CT slices we distinguish between the following cases: (a) If the oblique cut lies on the CT plane the *catheter describing points* are obtained in the same way as for the on-CT-slice case. (b) If the oblique plane is perpendicular to the z-axis and lies between two CT slices, the *catheter describing points* are obtained in the same way as for the on-CT-slice case where they are assumed to belong to the neaier slice. (c) In the general case, the oblique plane cuts the CT volume and has six degrees of freedom. Then, the catheter describing points are defined as the intersections of the sequential segments of the catheter skeleton with the CT slices.
*(c) Loops on-plane*
In this case, we make use of the property of the constant catheter outer diameter and use the logic of one stepping algorithm to extract *catheter describing points* from the entire group of recognized points[3,4].

**Materials**
Our algorithms have been tested in routine clinical practice. The implants were selected to include a representative spectrum of anatomical sites as well as implant geometry and different catheter types and materials. The sccuracy and time analysis have been done for 30 different clinical implants: prostate, breast, cervix, brain, chest, scapula, skin, neck and glioblastoma implants, and one phantom implant with three looped plastic catheters. Representative CT image and 3D view are shown in Fig. 3 for the case cervix tumor.
A comparison of the accuracy and the time required was made for the classical manual catheter reconstruction from the CT slices, as implemented in Plato* BPS (Vs. 13.5) and for our autoreconstruction method.

## Results and discussion

The accuracy and time analysis have been done for implants described in *Materials*.
The *catheter describing point* difference analysis shows mean geometrical differences varying from (0.36±0.25)mm to (1.12±0.35)mm with a mean value over all 31 implants of (0.67±0.36)mm, whereas source dwell position based analysis (dwell positions produced at each 2.5mm starting from a given catheter tip) gave mean geometrical difference varying from (0.38±0.22)mm to (1.41±0.44)mm with a mean value of (0.87±0.36)mm.
The reconstruction time analysis presented next shows that our algorithm is extremely time-efficient. In 27 of 30 clinical cases (90%) no manual intervention by user was needed duting the autoreconstruction based process. With our algorithm reconstruction was 25.7 times faster than the manual reconstruction (21.4 s compared to 547.2 s for the manual procedure). For the cases where the manual intervention was needed, reconstruction based on our algorithm s 8.2 times faster than the manual one (81.7 s compared to 739.8 s for the manual procedure).

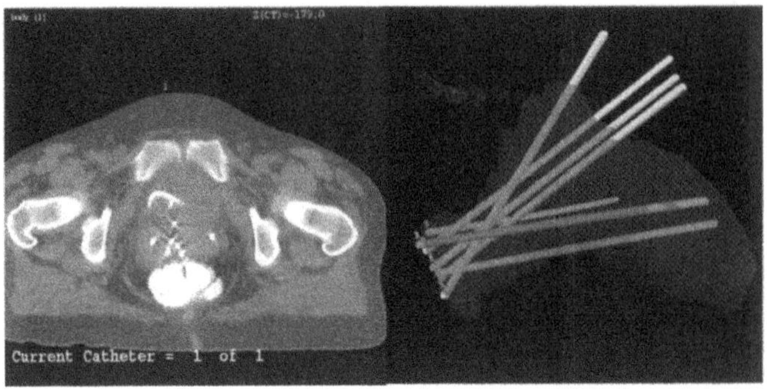


(a) (b)
**Figure 3:** (a) CT presentation and (b) 3D view of 8 plastic catheters in the case of cervix tumor.

## Conclusion

Our autorecostruction algorithm significantly improves, simplifies and accelerates the imaging based brachytherapy treatment planning procedure. Therefore the time needed for catheter reconstruction decreases to only the time that the user spends defining the input parameters through the GUI. The entire process is fully controled by user, who can accept or reject the reconstructed catheters. The success rate of our method in the cases tested was found to be as high as 90%. This improves the safety and reliability of the catheter reconstruction process. This innovative algorithm can revolutionize brachytherapy treatment planning in the $21^{st}$ century.

## References

[1]Tsalpaturos A, Baltas D, Kolotas C, van der Larse R, Koutsouris D, Uzunoglu N and Zamboglou N 1997 "CT-based software for 3-D localization and reconstruction in stepping source brachytherapy", *IEEE Trans. Inf. Techn. in Biomed.* **1** 229-242
[2]Zamboglou N 1997 "Interstitial Brachytherapy Possibilities" *New Developments in Interstitial Remote Controlled Brachytherapy* edited by Zamboglou N 174-180
[3]Milickovic N 1999 "Three Dimensional 3D Based Reconstruction Techniques in Modern Brachytherapy Treatment Planning" *Ph.D. Thesis 6th Chapter* NTUA-Dept. of Elec. & Comp. Eng.
[4]Milickovic N, Giannouli S, Baltas D, Lahanas M, Uzunoglu N, Kolotas C and Zamboglou N 1999 "Catheter autoreconstruction in CT based brachytherapy treatment planning" *Med. Phys.* submitted August 1999.

* Nucletron B.V., Veenendaal, The Netherlands

# EGS4 Energy Deposition Kernels at Low Photon Energy including the Molecular Coherent Scattering Form Factor

**Joseph M. Modrick, Thomas R. Mackie and Bruce R. Thomadsen**
Department of Medical Physics, University of Wisconsin, Madsion, WI 53706-1532, USA

## Introduction

At photon energies below 100 keV, coherent (Rayleigh) scattering can account for as much as 10 % of the total photon interaction cross section (see Figure 1). Rayleigh scatter at these low photon energies is primarily of interest to diagnostic physics, however it is also of paramount importance to the dosimetry of low energy brachytherapy sources such as I-125 and Pd-103. While it accurately can be argued that Rayleigh scatter does not contribute to the deposition of energy, coherent scattering does affect the distribution of energy deposited for low enrgy photons. The effects of coherent scatter on the distribution of deposited energy will be particularly crucial in the calculation of an energy deposition kernel where photons are forced to interact at a point and Monte Carlo is used to simulation the transport of secondary particles and deposition of energy away from the initial interaction point.

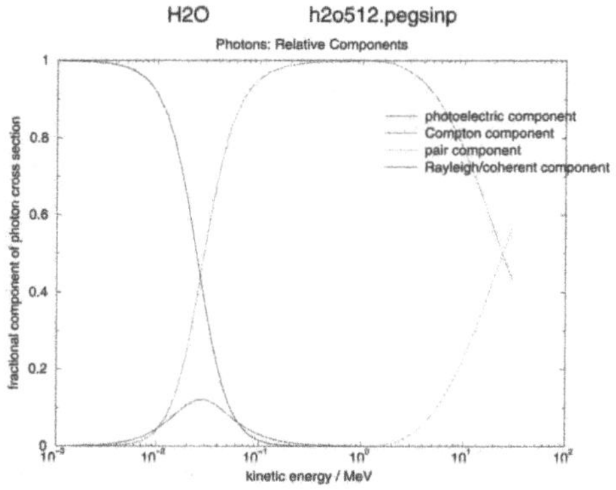


**Figure 1:** Fractional relative photon cross section components for water as a function of energy from the input file `h2o521.pegsinp`. Approximately 10 % of the total cross section is due to coherent scattering around 30 keV. The input file was generated using the EGS4 preprocessor PEGS4.

The EGS4 Monte Carlo system can simulate the coupled transport of photons and electrons including the effects of coherent scatter. However, it is well documented [1] that the atomic coherent scattering cross section data utilized in the default version of EGS4 system [2] are not in agreement with experimental results for material substances [3]. The atomic cross section data neglect interference effects, evident in measured form factors, and predict that the cross section is peaked at zero scattering angle. The recently measured coherent scattering form factor for water [5] clearly demonstrates the distinction between atomic and molecular form factors and shows the cross section is peaked at a non-zero scattering angle (see Figure 2).

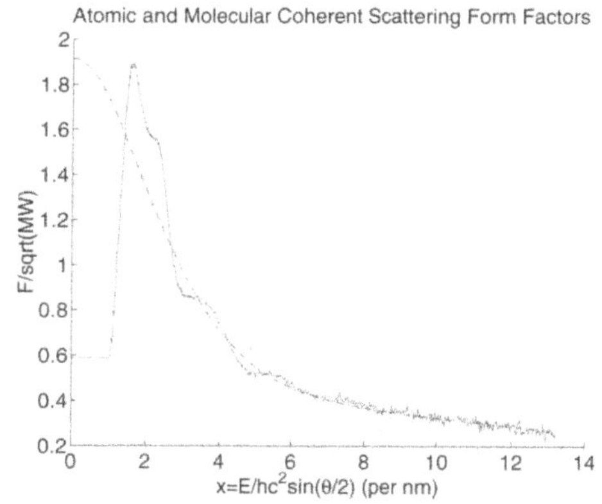


**Figure 2:** Comparison of atomic (dashed) and molecular (solid) coherent scattering form factors for water. Interference effects are evident in the measured molecular form factor [5].

## Material and methods

We have implemented the Low-Energy Photon-Scattering (LSCAT) expansion for the EGS4 code system [4], and applied these changes to the EGS4 "scatter sphere" code `scasph.mortran` [6] to compute energy deposition kernels at photon energies below 100 keV using the molecular coherent scattering form factor for water from recent measurements [5] to replace the default values in the EGS4 system. The 'scatter sphere" code computes the energy deposition in a 60 cm radius water sphere from mono-energetic unidirectional photons forced to interact at the center of the sphere. The energy deposition kernel results are expressed in terms of energy deposited per unit energy fluence. The LSCAT expansion extends the EGS4 Monte Carlo system to account for the effects of bound Compton cross sections, doppler broadening, and linear photon polarization. The `pegs4nb.mortran` file included in the LSCAT package has been modified by Taibi *et. al.* [7]. This modification is based upon the Leliveld contribution to the EGS4 system [8] which allows the EGS4 preprocessor PEGS4 to read new data files (form factors and cross sections) that take into account the effects of molecular interference in coherent scattering. The inclusion of the recently measured molecular form factor for water was accomplished by following the example of Taibi *et. al.* [7]. The Monte Carlo simulations were run on a 667 MHz Alpha processor and the energy deposition kernel plots were generated using PV-WAVE.

## Results and discussion

The effect of coherent scattering on energy deposition kernels was investigated by computing kernels with and without Rayleigh scatter included at photon energies below 100 keV. Representative kernels results are shown below for 30 keV energy deposition kernels. Each of these kernels were generated with EGS4 parameter values of 10 keV for the photon and electron (521 keV) transport cut-offs and an ESTEPE value of 2 % using $10^6$ photon histories. Energy deposition kernels at 30 keV were chosen because coherent scattering effects are maximal for these kernels since the fractional relative cross section of Rayleigh scatter is at its maximum value of approximately 10 % for 30 keV photons in water (see Figure 1). Each kernel plot displays isovalues of energy deposition (per unit mass) in units of cGy/photon-MeV on a polar plot with a radius of 10 cm. The initial uni-directional photons originate near the origin in the negative vertical direction and are forced to interact.

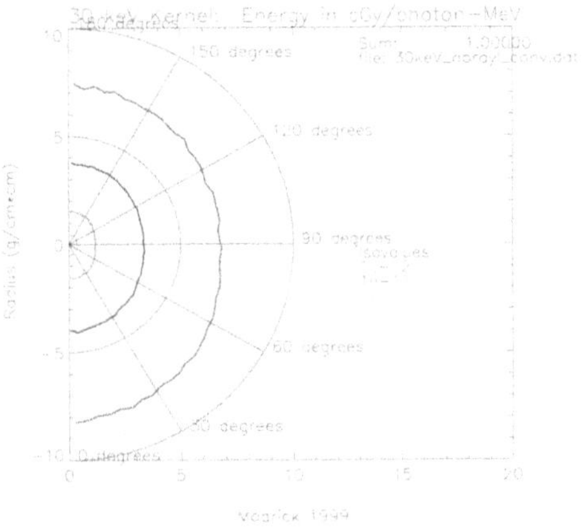


**Figure 3:** Isovalue kernel plot for a 30 keV kernel using default EGS4 with no Rayleigh scatter included. This kernel appears almost spherically symmetric. The isovalues in all these plots are $10^{-12}, 10^{-11}, 10^{-10}$, and $10^{-9}$ cGy/photon-MeV.

The first kernel plot (see Figure 3) shows a 30 keV energy deposition kernel computed using the default version of EGS4 with the Rayleigh scatter option switched off. This kernel plot is almost spherically symmetric about the center point of the initial photon forced interaction. This kernel result appears to be consistent with the neglect of Rayleigh scatter and the relatively isotropic distribution of Compton scatter at low photon energies.

The next kernel plot (see Figure 4) shows a 30 keV energy deposition kernel computed using the default version of EGS4 with Rayleigh scatter included using the default EGS4 atomic coherent scattering form factor. This kernel is slightly forward peaked in the distribution of energy deposition with the peak energy deposition occurring in the forward direction. This kernel result is consistent with the atomic form factor showing the coherent scatter cross section peaked in the forward direction.

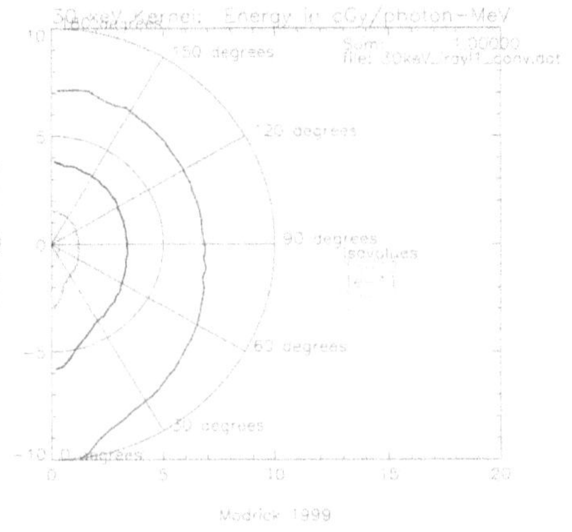


**Figure 4:** Isovalue kernel plot for a 30 keV kernel using default EGS4 with Rayleigh scatter included using the default EGS4 atomic form factor. This kernel appears slightly peaked in the forward direction.

The 30 keV kernel produced using the modified version of EGS4 with Rayleigh scatter included using the molecular coherent scattering form factor is shown below (see Figure 5). This kernel plot is slightly forward peaked in the distribution of energy deposition with the peak energy deposition occurring at a slight angle away from the forward direction. This kernel result appears to be consistent with the molecular coherent scattering form factor showing the coherent scatter cross section peaked at a slight angle away from the forward direction. This kernel result also exhibits distinct differences from the kernel result obtained with the atomic coherent scattering form factor. These differences appear consistent with the differences between the molecular and atomic coherent scattering form factors. The values in the backward directions (> 90°) are nearly identical, which is also consistent with the form factor curves.

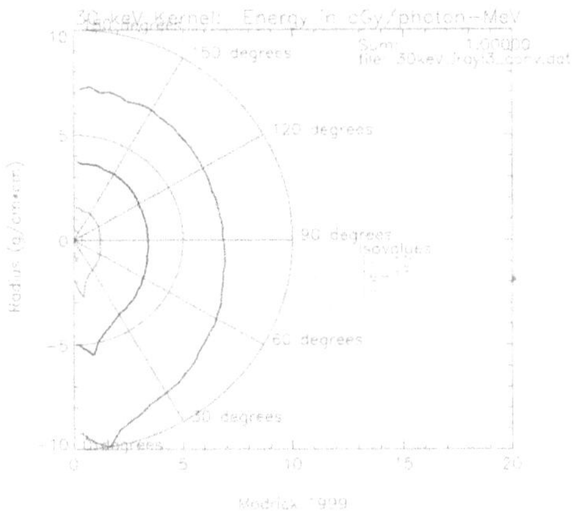


**Figure 5:** Isovalue kernel plot for a 30 keV kernel using the modified EGS4 with Rayleigh scatter included using the molecular form factor. This kernel appears slightly peaked in the forward direction with the peak energy deposition at a slight angle to the forward direction.

## Conclusion

The effects of coherent scattering on energy deposition kernels has been demonstrated. The inclusion of Rayleigh scatter in the computation of an energy deposition kernel has a distinct effect upon the distribution of energy deposition. With Rayleigh scatter neglected, the energy deposition kernel is spherically symmetric. This is consistent with the isotropic distribution of Compton scatter at low photon enrgies.

When Rayleigh scatter is included, the energy deposition kernel becomes forward peaked. This increase in the deposition of energy in the forward direction can be attributed to Rayleigh scattered photons being scattered primarily in the forward direction, rather than isotropically in the case of Compton scatter, and then subsequently undergoing a photoelectric interaction and depositing their energy locally.

When Rayleigh scatter is modeled using the atomic coherent form factor, the peak energy deposition is in the forward direction. This is consistent with the atomic coherent cross section also being peaked in the forward direction. This increased energy deposition in the forward direction can be atributed to the Rayleigh scattered photons being transported primarily with zero scattering angle in the Monte Carlo simulation.

When Rayleigh scatter is modeled using the molecular coherent form factor, the peak energy distribution is at an angle slightly away from the forward direction. This is consistent with the molecular coherent cross section also being peaked at an angle slightly away from the forward direction. This increased energy deposition at a small angle away from the forward direction can be attributed to the Rayleigh scattered photons being transported primarily with a small non-zero scattering angle in the Monte Carlo simulation. Since the molecular coherent form factor more accurately describes the scattering of low energy photons in material substances, the energy deposition kernels generated with the molecular form factor should be utilized for dose calculations at low photon energies.

These energy deposition kernels are being developed for use in a collasped-cone convolution/superposition code generalized to 3-dimensional brachytherapy geometries. To be applicable to the low photon energies of brachytherapy source such as I-125 and Pd-103, the energy deposition kernels must be developed with cross section data that realisticly describe the behavior of low energy photons in mater. The next low photon energy correction that should be applied to these deposition kernels is to account for the electron-binding effect of Doppler broading of Compton-scattered photons.

## References


[1] Nelson W R, Hirayama H and Rogers D W O 1985 The EGS4 Code System *SLAC-265* Stanford Linear Accelerator Center 93–95

[2] Hubbell J H and Øverbø I 1979 Relativistic atomic form factors and photon cross sections *J. Phys. Chem. Ref. Data* **8** 69–105

[3] Johns P C and Yaffe M J 1983 Coherent scatter in diagnostic radiology *Med. Phys.* **10** 40–50

[4] Namito Y, Ban S and Hirayama H 1995 LSCAT:Low-Energy Photon-Scattering expansion for the EGS4 code *KEK Internal* **95-10** High Energy Accelerator Research Organization

[5] Peplow D E and Kuruvilla V 1998 Measured molecular coherent scattering form factors of animal tissues, plastics and human breast tissue *Phys. Med. Biol.* **43** 2431–2452

[6] Mackie T R, Bielajew A F, Rogers D W O and Battista J J 1988 Generation of photon energy deposition kernels using the EGS Monte Carlo code *Phys. Med. Biol.* **33**, 1–20

[7] Taibi A, Royce G J and Speller R D 1999 A Monte Carlo study to investigate the potential of diffraction enhanced breast imaging *presented at the 6th international conference on Application of Nuclear Techniques, Crete, Greece, June 20-26*

[8] Leliveld C J, Mass J G, Bom V R, and van Eijk C W E 1996 Monte Carlo modeling of coherent scattering: influence of interference *IEEE Trans. Nucl. Science* **43** 3315–3321

# Advances in Patient Immobilisation and Positioning Techniques

**Wolfgang Schlegel[1], Otto Pastyr[1], Klaus Herfarth[2], Gernot Kuhr[1], Christian Lappe[1], Gernot Echner[1] and Marc Schneberger[1]**

[1]DKFZ, Department of Medical Physics , Im Neuenheimer Feld 280, D69120 Heidelberg, Germany
[2]DKFZ, Clinical Cooperation Unit Radiation Oncology , Im Neuenheimer Feld 280, D69120 Heidelberg, Germany

## Introduction

Radiation therapy is in the process of a continuos change. This movement has mainly been driven by the rapid and exciting achievements in computer technology, which led to the development of three dimensional radiation treatment planning and to completely new treatment delivery systems. As a result, real 3D conformal therapy is now becoming reality in clinical practice. Being able to plan and deliver conformal dose distributions with steep dose gradients, we have now especially to worry about the errors and uncertainties which arise when transferring treatment plans to the real patient. The involved task of patient immobilisation and positioning is still a weak link in the chain of radiotherapy and needs further improvement in order to meet the high requirements of 3D conformal radiotherapy. In this contribution, developments and experiences in patient immobilisation and positioning at the DKFZ will be reported.

## Material and methods

The field of patient immobilisation and positioning profited especially from stereotactic and navigational techniques as applied in modern neurosurgery. In our institute, where we are only treating patients in the frame of clinical studies, all conformal irradiations are performed under stereotactic conditions. Two different strategies exist for stereotactically guided radiotherapy procedures: Those for single dose irradiation ("radiosurgery", [1]) and those for fractionated treatments ("precision radiotherapy", [2,3]). Depending on the indication, the degree of precision which has to be reached and on the localisation of the target volume, invasive or non-invasive immobilisation techniques are used (Table 1).

| Invasive immobilization | | Non –invasive immobilization | |
|---|---|---|---|
| Head and Neck | Whole Body | Head and Neck | Whole body |
| Stereotactic ceramics frame | Extracranial stereotactic system with clamps (not used at DKFZ) | relocatable scotch cast system | relocatable scotch cast system or vacuum cushion |

**Table 1:** Immobilization techniques developed at DKFZ

### Fixation systems for single dose irradiation

For single dose irradiation (the main indications of which are AVMs and metastases), a stereotactic ceramic frame, designed for the use in CT, MRI, PET and DSA is applied. Using ceramics as immobilisation material allows to obtain MR-images which are completely free of artefacts. With this system stereotactic image registration can be performed at utmost precision [4].

### Fixation systems for fractionated treatments

For fractionated treatments of lesions in the brain and head and neck, special mask systems have been developed. The one used in our department is made from scotch cast bandages. This relocatable mask system results with a standard deviation of 1-2 mm in fixation and repositioning accuracy in the head and neck area ([2,3,5]).
For conformal stereotactic treatments in the body, a relocatable stereotactic extracranial fixation system has been introduced. The system which was developed in cooperation with the University of Tucson can be used in connection with a vacuum cushion, a scotch cast torso or with a rigid fixation to the spinal column (figures 1 and 2).

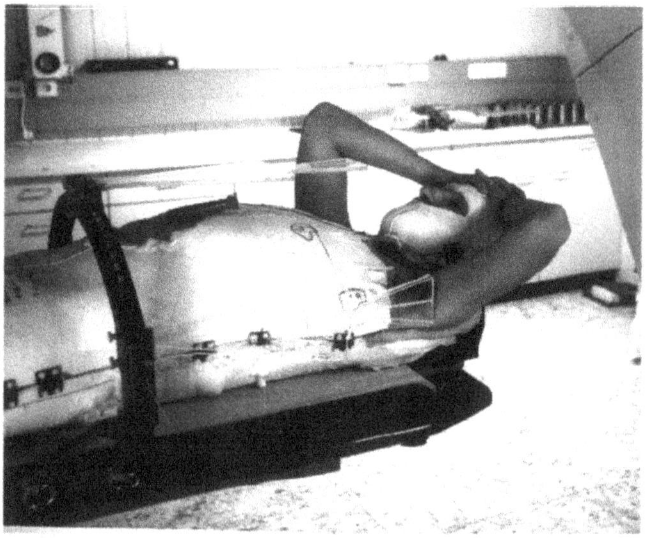

**Figure 1:** Extracranial stereotactic fixation of a patient undergoing conformal treatment of a parasinal tumour. For such indications, the scotch cast torso in combination with a mask gives best results in terms of repsoisitiong and immobilisation

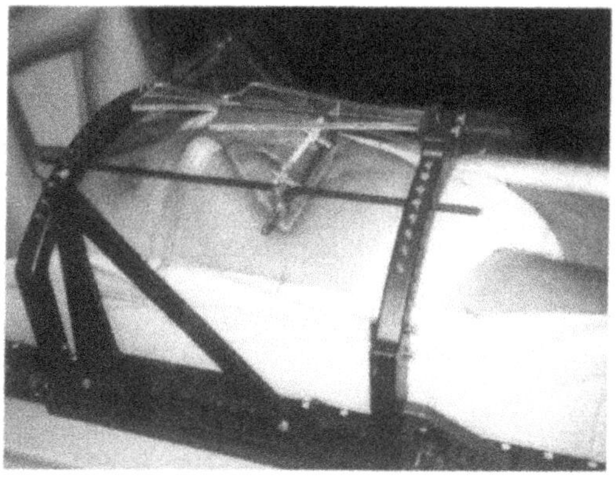

**Figure 2:** Extracranial stereotactic system in use for a patient with a liver lesion. For single dose irradiations of liver metastases a vacuum cushion is used as immobilization device. Recognize the compression plate which is used to reduce liver movement.

**Target localisation**

We use the localisation procedure as described for Linac-Radiosurgery by Pastyr [6]. The same target-localiser consisting of 4 Plexiglas-squares with imbedded V-shaped fiducial wires is used for single dose and fractionated treatments. After the same principle, a system was developed by our group to enable stereotactic target localisation for lesions in the body.

**Stereotactic Patient Positioning**

Again, the same stereotactic positioning principles are used for Radiosurgery and precision radiotherapy, both for brain and head and neck patients as well as for treatments with the whole body fixation system (Fig. 3). The stereotactic co-ordinates of the target point, calculated during 3D treatment planning, are transferred to the x-, y- and z- callipers of the stereotactic target positioner. The patients couch is then adjusted in x-, y- and z-direction, until the laser crosses match to the fiducials on the callipers.

**Tracking systems for automated patient set-up, and movement detection and correction**

To improve and facilitate the patient set-up during positioning at the linear accelerator, tracking devices quite similar to those used in neuro-navigation are under development. The device which was developed at the DKFZ allows an automated patient positioning for head and neck patients with an accuracy below 1 mm. The system is also able to detect target movement by measuring the patient position up to 25 time per second. With a computer controlled table top, significant position deviations which occur due to patient movements can be automatically and instantly corrected [5,7]).

The prototype of the so called "patient positioning sensor unit" (PPSU) is now being extended to extracranial applications. We intend to intoduce arbitrary marker arrangement on the patients′ surface, and to include detection of internal markers by an ultrasound probe and by electronic portal imaging.

Work was also focused to use the system not only for relative repositioning, but also for position measurements in absolute co-ordinates. A video camera calibration and image distortion correction procedure has been developed for this purpose, which is just now being implemented into the system.

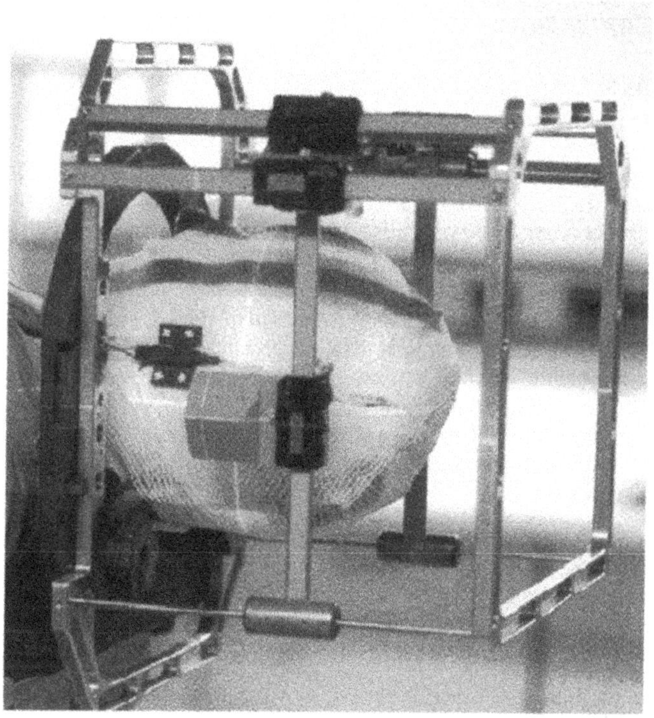

**Figure 3:** Stereotactic target positiong system for precision radiotherapy of patient with a brain lesion.

## Results and discussion

Stereotactic patient immobilisation and positioning techniques are the standard in our institute for all radiosurgical treatments and conformal irradiations. Having started with stereotactic irradiation of brain tumour patients in the early eighties, we found that and accuracy below 1 mm can be reached with rigid fixation and positioning systems, while the errors of the relocatable mask system were in the range of 1-2 mm.

In the last few years, we have started to transfer the stereotactic immobilisation and positioning principles to extracranial targets. Of course, the circumstances in extracranial stereotaxy are much more critical: First, due to the small gantry opening of MR units, it is not possible to perform stereotactic target delineation in MR images. Second, fixation and immobilisation of extracranial anatomical structures is more difficult, and last not least movement of internal organs and of the PTV introduces a much higher degree of uncertainty than in the head and neck area.

Nevertheless, some practical mechanical solutions have been introduced, which in the meanwhile allow stereotactic irradiation of paraspinal and prostate tumours (by using the extracranial localising and positioning system together with a scotch cast torso), of lung metastases (in combination with jet ventilation of the lungs which reduces the PTV movement to 2-3 mm) or of liver metastases (under application of a compression plate). Measurement of the repositioning of the target volume with radiographic and CT data showed, that the reproducibility of the PTV position was within 2-3 mm also in these extracranial cases.

## Conclusion

Stereotactic methods have been very effective to improve patient immobilisation and positioning in radiotherapy. The accuracy which can be reached for the brain and head and neck lesions are already within satisfying limits. Using the stereotactic approach, good results can also be reached for some extracranial targets, however the technical and time effort to be made is much higher.

Further improvement in patient immobilisation and positioning is urgently required to advance the field of high dose conformal radiotherapy for the most extracranial indications. The only way which seems to lead to a significant progress are navigational methods guided by ultrasound, radiographical methods or electronic portal imaging. Especially the problem of irradiating moving targets with IMRT has to be discussed in this context.

## References

[1] Hartmann G H, Schlegel W , Sturm V, Kober B, Pastyr O, Lorenz W J 1985 Cerebral radiation surgery using moving field irradiation at a linear accelerator facility *Int J Rad Oncol Biol Phys* **11** 1185-1192

[2] Schlegel W, Pastyr O, Bortfeld T, Becker G, Schad L, Gademann G, Lorenz W J 1992 Computer systems and mechanical tools for stereotactically guided conformation therapy with linear accelerators *Int J Rad Oncol Biol Phys* **24** 781-787

[3] Schlegel W, Pastyr O, Bortfeld T, Gademann G, Menke M, Maier-Borst W 1993 Stereotactically guided fractionated radiotherapy: technical aspects *Rad Oncol* **29** 197-204

[4] Schad L R, Boesecke R, Schlegel W, Hartmann G, Sturm V, Strauss L G, Lorenz W J 1987 Three dimensional image correlation of CT, MR, and PET studies in radiotherapy treatment planning of brain tumors *Journal of Computer Assisted Tomography* **11** 948-954

[5] Menke M, Hirschfeld F, Mack T, Pastyr O, Sturm V, Schlegel W 1994 Photogrammetric Accuracy Measurements of Head Holder Systems Used for Fractionated *Radiotherapy Int J Rad Oncol Biol Phys* **29** 1147-1155

[6] Pastyr O, Hartmann G H, Schlegel W, Schabbert S, Treuer H, Lorenz W J, Sturm V 1989 Stereotactically guided convergent beam irradiation with a linear accelerator: Localisation-technique *Acta Neurochirurgica* **99** 61-64

[7] Lappe C, Helfert S, Braun M, Pastyr O, Sturm V, Schlegel W 1997 A Videogrammetric System for Computer-Controlled Non-Invasive Patient Positioning in Leavitt, D (ed): Proc of the XIIth International Conference on the Use of Computers in Radiation Therapy Madison, Medical Physics Publishing 168-171

# Interventional strategies to counter the effects of inter-fraction treatment variation

**John W. Wong, Di Yan, David A. Jaffray, Greg Edmundson, and Alvaro A. Martinez**

Department of Radiation Oncology, William Beaumont Hospital, Royal Oak, Michigan, USA.

## Introduction

Great strides have been made in recent years in the development of important techniques for treatment planning and delivery. There is optimism that the new conformal treatment methods, such as intensity modulation (IMRT) will ultimately lead to improved local control and/or reduced toxicity. However, our expectations must be guarded. The higher degree of conformation means that the risk of treatment failure will also be higher. It is imperative to ensure that the treatments are not only optimally planned, but also accurately implemented. Failure to minimize treatment error will not only undermine the treatment outcome, but also lead to the erroneous and dire conclusion that the advanced treatment methods are ineffectively.

In order to satisfy the more stringent requirement of treatment accuracy, the characteristics of treatment error need to be re-examined such that their ill effects can be meaningfully minimized. One main cause of treatment inaccuracy is the variation in treatment geometry during the course of treatment. Geometric treatment inaccuracy in theory can be quantified and thus be systematically reduced. There are two types of geometric treatment variations. *Inter-fraction* variations pertain to the changes in patient positioning, organ shapes and positions between fractions. Field placement errors and changes in rectal filling during the course of prostate cancer treatment are prime examples. *Intra-fraction* variations pertain to the changes in the organ shapes and positions during a single treatment fraction. These include the motion of tumors and organs due to breathing and are particularly problematic in the thoracic and abdominal regions. This article addresses strategies to counter the effects of inter-fraction variations.

## Global vs. Patient-Specific Margins : A Need for Interventional Strategies

The conventional approach to alleviate the detrimental effects of setup variation is to "accommodate" them by prescribing a geometric margin around the target volume. Report 50 of the International Commission on Radiation Units and Measurements (ICRU) [1] recommends that such margin be prescribed according to the concept of planning target volume (PTV). The PTV depicts the volume that circumscribes the clinical target volume (CTV) to allow for field placement error, and for the inter-fraction and intra-fraction variation of the CTV.

At present, the prescription of the PTV is mostly based on the generic data on treatment variation observed in many patients. Strictly speaking, the population-based margin is specific to the institution and can be optimized for the disease site and the treatment technique [2]. Still, the approach would only provide an acceptable solution for the patient population, but which is not necessarily optimal for the individual patients. An appreciable portion of the population-based margin is spent accounting for the differences in the systematic variation between individual patients. It would be unnecessarily large for many patients, and yet inadequate for a few patients. For setup variation, systematic differences between prescription and treatment positions predominate [3, 4]. It follows that PTV margin can be greatly reduced by correcting the systematic setup error.

Implementing such an approach would require new *interventional strategies* that deviate from our conventional approach of setup correction using port films. Treatment variation is specific to the individual patient and not fully known prior to treatment. The foundation of intervention is to obtain as much information about the patient as reasonably possible such that an on-going treatment may be modified to attain an achievable and desirable treatment goal for the patient. Depending on the nature of the treatment variation, different strategies can be used to compensate, or minimize..

### Decision Rule for Setup Correction

For inter-fraction setup variation, a simple and highly effective means to correct for systematic error has been successfully implemented in Europe [5, 6]. By establishing an expected distribution of the systematic setup errors among the patients for the institution, a pre-defined threshold can be used to see if corrective action is warranted for a patient according to portal images on the first 1 or few treatment days. For prostate treatment, the approach has led to significant reduction in the margin for setup error for several institutions in the Netherlands [5,6].

### The Adaptive Radiation Therapy Strategy

The Adaptive Radiation Therapy (ART) strategy is a closed-loop feedback process where the PTV for the individual patient is systematically optimized based on the information measured during the course of treatment. [7-11]. It is particularly effective when the treatment variations are well behaved such that they can be characterized from a few initial treatment fractions. The information is then used to adjust subsequent treatments.

For setup error correction, ART differs somewhat from the Decision Rule approach by attempting to eliminate systematic error of the individual patient. For several disease sites, electronic portal images acquired for the first 5 days are typically adequate for deriving meaningful correction. Because the ART strategy relies on reproducible patient setup, setup correction is facilitated by moving the multileaf collimator (MLC) instead of the patient. For prostate treatment, retrospective and prospective studies have shown that after MLC adjustment, the systematic errors of the patients can be maintained to within $\pm$ 1 mm.

It is also possible to apply the ART strategy to compensate for inter-fraction organ motion. With the conformal 4-field box technique, a modified "convex hull" of the prostate segmented in CT scans acquired for initial treatment planning and the first 4 treatment fractions can be used to form an effective PTV for inter-fraction organ motion. This patient-specific PTV can be larger or smaller than the initial PTV based on conventional margin, such as that recommended by the RTOG. Most importantly, the approach brings to light on whether a patient is suitable for aggressive dose escalation.

**Image Guided Radiation Therapy (IGRT)**

While the ART strategy is a promising approach to compensate for treatment variation, its effectiveness diminishes for those treatments where variations have a large random component, or when the treatment involves only a few fractions. For example, our experience using ART for prostate treatment suggests that about 30% of the patients would not be suitable for significant dose escalation. A more direct interventional approach using on-line image guidance becomes necessary.

Image-Guided Brachytherapy for Prostate Boost Treatment
A good example of on-line IGRT is brachytherapy of prostate cancer that utilize ultrasound imaging [12-16], CT [17] or MRI [18]. Both inter- and intra- fraction variation of prostate motions are overcome. Highly accurate, user-independent high dose rate treatment can be delivered.

Image-Guided External Beam Conformal Therapy.
The simplest form of on-line IGRT in external beam is to employ optical [19] and radiographic MV or kV localization images to facilitate on-line correction of patient setup [20-24]. Such optical or ıadiographic guidance can be beneficial for those treatment sites where the approximation of the patient as a rigid body model is reasonable. However, if the treatment variation involves non-rigid organ displacement or deformation, then the use of 3D anatomic information would become necessary.
One approach to address the problem of internal organ motion is by implanting radio-opaque markers for radiographic guidance [25], or to use non-invasive ultra-sound imaging to identify shifts in the center of mass of the target [26]. Both methods can be effective in tracking the target, but with a cautionary note that a residual margin must be maintained since both approaches employ rigid body correction model that does not account for organ deformation. For the ultra-sound technique, the residual margin must also allow for possible organ rotation.
A comprehensive approach of image guidance is to use volumetric CT scans acquired prior to treatment. The scans can be acquired off-line with the complementary use of a body-frame for patient repositioning [27]. A more integrated approach is to acquire the tomographic images on-line. Uematsu et al had utilized a CT scanner opposite to, and co-axial with, a gantry-based linear accelerator to achieve on-line guidance [28]. Investigators at the University of Wisconsin have proposed to develop a tomotherapy machine which will have helical, MV or kV, CT scanning capability to guide and verify the delivery of slice-based IMRT [29]. At William Beaumont Hospital, on-board kV cone-beam CT capability has been installed on a medical accelerator (SL20 series, Elekta Oncology Systems) to facilitate IGRT [30]. Cone-beam reconstruction [31] employs 2D kV images acquired during one gantry rotation to generate full volumetric CT slices without the need for patient movement. With the use of an amorphous silicon flat panel imaging array as the 2D detector, exceptional image quality, comparable to that of a conventional helical scanner using equivalent exposure parameters [32,33]. While tomographic guidance is very powerful in principle, the degree of geometric margin reduction that is possible remains to be determined.

## Discussion

Advances in computer technology and the increase in imaging information have clearly improved many areas of radiation therapy. Yet, at present, the treatment process remains virtually unchanged. Most firmly entrenched is the use of population-averaged parameters in the optimization of patient treatment, despite the increasing availability of information specific to the individual patient.
The new wealth of imaging information can be used to improve radiation therapy of the individual patient. In this paper, several interventional strategies to minimize the effects of inter-fraction treatment variation are discussed. The results are promising. Commitment to adapt interventional treatment require re-thinking and re-structuring of the entire radiation therapy process. Several issues must also be addressed. These include the refinement of software and hardware tools, determination of sites which would most benefit, redefinition of the roles for the clinical personnel and possible alteration of fractionation schedule. Care must be taken be ensure that the cost of implementation be manageable, if not lessen. Finally, it needs to emphasized that PTV repesents only 1/3 of the radiation therapy problem (and perhaps the easiest 1/3). Efforts must now be directed to address the problem of accurately defining GTV and CTV.

## *Acknowledgments*

This work is supported in part by the NCI(US) grants R01-CA66074, R29-CA71785, R01-CA76182 and US Army Prostate Cancer Research Program (DAMD17-98-1-8497). The authors also wish to thank the support of Elekta Oncology Systems and ADAC Laboratories.

## References

1. ICRU (1993). Report No. 50: Prescribing, Recording and Reporting Photon Beam Therapy. Washington, D.C.: International Commission of Radiation Units and Measurements.
2. Mageras GS, Kutcher GJ, Leibel SA, Zelefsky MJ, Melian E, Mohan R, Fuks Z (1996). A method of incorporating organ motion uncertainties into Three-Dimensional conformal treatment plans. Int J Rad Oncol Biol Phys, 35:333-342,.
3. Rabinowitz I., Broomberg J., Goitein M., McCarthy K., Leong J. (1985). Accuracy of radiation field alignment in clinical practice. Int J Radiat Oncol Biol Phys, 11: 1857-1867.
4. Huizenga H., Levndag P.C., De Porre P.M.Z.R., Visser A.G. (1988). Accuracy in radiation field alignment in head and neck cancer: a prospective study. Radio Oncol, 11: 181-187.
5. Bel A., Vos P.H., Rodrigus P.T.R., Creutzberg C.L., Visser A.G., Stroom J.C., Lebesque J.V. (1996). High precision prostate cancer irradiation by a clinical application of an offline patient setup verification procedure using portal imaging. Int J Radiat Oncol Biol Phys, 35: 321-332.
6. Lebesque J.V., Remeijer P., Van Riel V., et al. (1998). Clinical evaluation of setup verification and correction protocols: results of multicentre studies of the Dutch Cooperative EPID Group, Proceedings of the 5th International Workshop on Electronic Portal Imaging. Pheonix, Arizona.
7. Yan D., Wong J.W., Gustafson G.S., Martinez A. A (1995). A new model for "accept or reject" strategies in off-line and on-

line megavoltage treatment evaluation. Int J Radiat Oncol Biol Phys, 31: 943-952.

8. Yan D., Vicini F., Wong J. Martinez A. (1997). Adaptive radiation therapy. Phys Med Biol, 42: 123-132.

9. Yan D., Wong J., Vicini F., Michalski J., Pan C., Frazier A., Martinez A. (1997). Adaptive modification of treatment planning to minimize the deleterious effect of treatment setup error. Int J Radiat Oncol Biol Phys, 38: 197-206.

10. Yan D., Ziaja E., Jaffray D., Wong J., Brabbins D., Vicini F., Martinez A. (1998). The use of adaptive radiation therapy to reduce setup error: a prospective clinical study. Int J Radiat Oncol Biol Phys, 41: 715-720.

11. Yan D., Lockman D., Brabbins D. (1998). A prediction model for defining a proactive planning target volume in external beam treatment of prostate cancer. Int J Radiat Oncol Biol Phys, 42:216 (Abstract).

12. Blasko J., Radge H., Schumacher D. (1987). Transperineal percutaneous iodine-125 implantation for prostate carcinoma using transrectal ultrasound and template guidance. Endocuriether Hyperther Oncol, 3: 131-139.

13. Edmundson G.K., Rizzo N.R., Teahan M., Brabbins D., Vicini F., Martinez A.A. (1993). Concurrent treatment planning for outpatient high dose rate prostate template implants. Int J Radiat Oncol Biol Phys, 27: 1215-1223.

14. Edmundson G.K., Yan D., Martinez A.A. (1995). Intraoperative optimization of needle placement and dwell times for conformal prostate brachytherapy. Int J Radiat Oncol Biol Phys, 33: 1257- 1263.

15. Martinez A., Gonzalez J., Stromberg J., Edmundson G., Plunkett M., Gustafson G., Brown D., Vicini F., Brabbins D. (1995). Conformal prostate brachytherapy: Initial experience of a Phase I/II dose escalating trial. Int J Radiat Oncol Biol Phys, 33: 1019- 1027.

16. Stromberg J., Martinez A., Gonzalez J., Edmundson G., Ohanian N., Vicini F., Hollander J., Gustafson G., Spencer W., Yan D., Brabbins D. (1995). Ultrasound guided high dose rate conformal brachytherapy boost in prostate cancer: Treatment description and preliminary results of a dose escalating clinical trial. Int J Radiat Oncol Biol Phys, 33: 161-171.

17. Zamboglou N., Kolotas C., Baltas D., Martin T., Rogge B., Strassman G., Tsalpatouros A., Vogt H.G. (1999). Clinical evaluation of CT based software in treatment planning for interstitial HDR brachytherapy. In Speiser B.L., Mould R.F., eds., Brachytherapy for the 21st Century, Nucletron B.V., The Netherlands. pp 312-326.

18. D'Amico A.V., Cormack R., Tempany C.M., Kumar S., Topulos G., Kooy H.M., Coleman C.N. (1998). Real-time magnetic resonance image-guided intersitial brachytherapy in the treatment of selected patients with clinically localized prostate cancer. Int J Radiat Oncol Biol Phys, 42: 507-515.

19. Johnson LS, Milliken BD, Hadley SW, Pelizzari CA, Haraf DJ, Chen GT (1999). Initial clinical experience with a video-based patient positioning system. Int J Radiat Oncol Biol Phys 45:205-213

20. Ezz A., Porter A., Munro P., Battista J., Jaffray D., Fenster A., Osborne S. (1991). Daily monitoring and correction of radiation field placement errors using a video-based portal imaging system: A pilot study. Int J Radiat Oncol Biol Phys, 22: 159-165.

21. De Neve W., Van den Heuvel F., De Beukeleer M., Coghe M., Thon L., De Roover P., Van Lancker M., Storme G. (1992) Routine clinical on-line portal imaging followed by immediate field adjustment using a tele-controlled patient couch. Radio Oncol, 24: 45-54.

22. Murphy M.J. (1997). An automatic six-degree-of-freedom image registration algorithm for image-guided frameless stereotaxic radiosurgery. Med Phys, 24: 857-886.

23. Van de Steene J., Van den Heuvel F., Bel A., et.al. (1998). Electronic portal imaging with on-line correction of setup error in thoracic irradiation: clinical evaluation. Int J Radiat Oncol Biol Phys, 40: 967-976.

24. Pisani L.J., Lockman D., Jaffray D., Yan D., Martinez A., Wong J. (1999) Factor limiting the accuracy of on-line setup correction using electronic localization radiographs. Int J Radiat Oncol Biol Phys, *submitted for publication.*

25. Balter J.M., McShan D.L., Lam K., et.al. (1997). Incorporation of patient setup measurement and adjustment within a computer controlled radiotherapy system. Proceedings of the 12th International Conference on the Use of Computers in Radiation Therapy. Eds. Leavitt D. and Starkschall G.: pp 182-184.

26. Lattanzi J., McNeeley S., Pinover W., et.al. (1998) A comparison of daily CT localization to a daily ultrasound-based system in prostate cancer. Int J Radiat Oncol Biol Phys, 43: 719-725.

27. Blomgren H., Lax I., Naslund I., et.al. (1995). Stereotactic high dose fraction radiation therapy of extracranial tumors using an accelerator. Acta Oncol, 34: 861-870.

28. Uematsu M., Fukui T., Shioda A., et.al. (1996). A dual computed tomography linear accelerator unit for stereotactic radiation therapy: a new approach without cranially fixated stereotactic frames. Int J Radiat Oncol Biol Phys, 35: 587-592.

29. Mackie T.R., Holmes T., Swerdloff S., Reckwerdt P., Deasy J.O., Yang J., Paliwal B., Kinsella T. (1993). Tomotherapy: a new concept for the delivery of dynamic conformal therapy. Med Phys, 20: 1709-1719.

30. Jaffray D.A., Drake D.G., Moreau M., et.al. (1999). Radiographic and tomographic localization of bone and soft-tissue targets on a clinical accelerator. Int J Radiat Oncol Biol Phys, 45:773-789.

31. Feldkamp L.A., Davis L.C., Kress J.W. (1984). Practical cone-beam algorithm. J Opt Soc Am. A1: 612-619.

32. Jaffray D.A., Drake D.G., Pisani L., et.al. (1999). Conebeam tomographic guidance of radiation field placement in radiation therapy of the prostate. Int J Radiat Oncol Biol Phys, *accepted for publication.*

33. Jaffray D.A., Siewerdsen J. H., Drake D. G. (1999). Performance of a volumetric CT scanner based upon a flat-panel imager. SPIE Physics of Medical Imaging Vol. 3659, *in press.*

# Interventional strategies for reducing respiratory-induced motion in external beam therapy

**Gig S. Mageras**

Department of Medical Physics, Memorial Sloan-Kettering Cancer Center, New York, NY 10021, USA

## Introduction

This presentation reviews recent developments in the measurement and control of respiratory motion-induced uncertainty in radiation treatments. These developments have been motivated by advances in high-precision radiotherapy in recent years, together with the recognition that physiological processes, among them respiration, play an important role in limiting the accuracy of dose delivery. In addition, advances in technology have spawned new types of detectors for measuring and reducing respiratory-induced motion.

Two different strategies have evolved to reduce the effect of respiratory motion in radiation treatments: controlled patient breathing, and respiration gating of the accelerator while the patient breathes normally.

## Controlled breathing techniques

In these techniques, breathing is altered either voluntarily by instructing the patient, or actively by means of an occlusion valve. A common feature is the use of breath-hold to immobilize the tumor, which is technologically relatively simple to implement and does not require any special capabilities of the treatment simulator, CT scanner, or treatment accelerator.

The University of Michigan has proposed a simple procedure for improving the accuracy of CT-based treatment planning and reducing margins for abdominal targets [1]. By acquiring CT data during breath-hold at normal end expiration, motion-induced artifacts are reduced. Furthermore, the CT images show the target at the exhalation extreme of its respiratory excursion, thus allowing reduced margins (consistent with the reproducibility of exhale position) superior to the target.

William Beaumont Hospital has developed a system of active breathing control (ABC), in which the patient breathes through a spirometer, and air flow is temporarily halted at a preset point in the respiratory cycle by means of an occlusion valve [2]. Functional reserve capacity (i.e., lung volume at end expiration) is used as the reference for determining the subsequent point in the respiration cycle for active breath-hold to occur. An initial study of 12 patients found the procedure to be well tolerated, with breath-holds of 15s up to 45s, depending on patient condition and degree of inspiration. Treatment plan studies have assessed the potential benefit of target margin reduction that would be possible by using ABC. A comparison of treatment plans of hepatic tumors in five patients showed a reduction in planning target volumes of 18-41% with ABC compared to free breathing [3]. Plan comparisons for Hodgkin's Disease at deep inspiration found reduced amounts of lung tissue irradiated, and reduced heart irradiation in splenic/para-aortic treatments, due to the combination of reduced margins and deep inspiration [4].

The Memorial Sloan-Kettering Cancer Center has developed a deep inspiration breath-hold (DIBH) technique for treatment of lung tumors [5,6,7]. The potential advantages of the technique are twofold: the breath-hold immobilizes the tumor, and deep inspiration reduces the normal lung density relative to the tumor, thus reducing the amount of normal lung receiving high dose. Using spirometry as a monitor of lung volume, the patient is coached through a modified slow vital capacity maneuver to achieve a reproducible inspiration level, followed by breath-hold. By using a high accelerator dose rate (500 monitor units/min), a treatment field is delivered during a breath-hold of about 12 seconds or less. Conformal treatments of non-small call lung cancer with the DIBH technique began in early 1998, and over 300 treatments to 12 patients have been administered to date. Fluoroscopy studies show diaphragm position to be reproducible to typically 1-3mm during and between breath-holds, while spirometry measurements acquired during treatment confirm this degree of reproducibility in lung inflation. Treatment plan comparisons of five patients suggest that the DIBH technique can reduce the volume of lung receiving more than 25Gy by 30% on average compared to free-breathing plans, due to the combined effect of reduced planning target margins and larger lung inflation [5]. Current clinical application uses the same planning target volume margins as for free breathing plans. Even so, dose to healthy lung is less in DIBH plans for all patients studied, due to the larger lung inflation [8]. As a result, patients treated with the DIBH technique have received higher prescription doses than would have otherwise been possible [6].

## Respiration gated radiotherapy

In this approach, a device monitors patient breathing and allows delivery of radiation during time intervals synchronized with the patient's respiratory cycle.

Respiration gated radiotherapy has been applied clinically already for several years in Japan. The Tsukuba Proton Medical Facility uses a strain gauge taped on the patient's abdomen or back (for prone treatments) to gate a proton beam [9]. The National Institute of Radiological Sciences uses a position sensor, consisting of a light emitting diode placed on the patient and camera, to gate a heavy ion beam [10]. An initial study of 36 patients (21 liver, 13 lung, 2 mediastinal) found that target volumes in gated treatments could be reduced 28% to 84% compared to those required for free-breathing treatments. Both centers have administered gated treatments on a routine basis, with over 200 patients treated.

More recently, a number of gating systems have been developed, using various means of monitoring respiration, among them spirometry [11], comparison of video images of the patient's chest with volume-rendered CT data [12], and fluoroscopic tracking of implanted gold markers [13].

The University of California at Davis and Varian Medical Systems have collaborated to develop a respiration-gated radiotherapy system [14]. The breathing monitor is based on infrared charge-coupled-device (CCD) video technology, together with passive reflective markers placed on the patient's chest or abdomen. On a treatment simulator, the system allows recording and playback of fluoroscopy synchronized with the external breathing motion signal. The planner specifies a treatment point (gate) in the breathing cycle by adjusting threshold levels with respect to the breathing motion signal, and examines anatomic motion in the fluoroscopy playback to evaluate and optimize the choice of gating thresholds. Currently under development is a means of triggering CT acquisition using the respiration gate signal.

Initial tests of the system's applicability to gated free-breathing treatments are currently underway, through the acquisition of breathing motion data, fluoroscopy and gated portal films with patients. Figure 1 compares the external marker position vs time with the observed diaphragm position of a patient during fluoroscopy [15], demonstrating the high degree of correlation between the two.

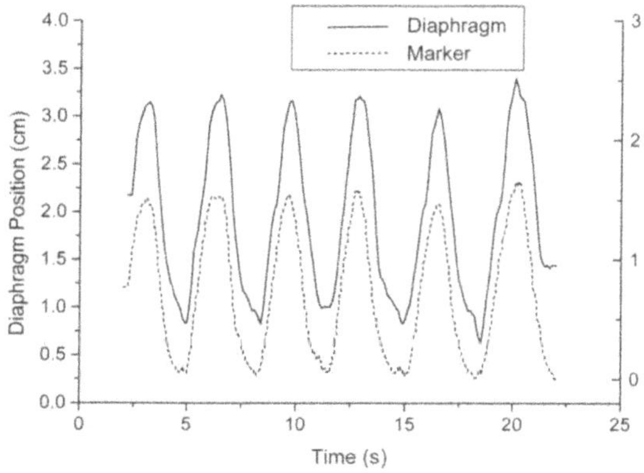


**Figure 1:** Example of external (marker placed on abdomen) and internal (diaphragm) breathing motion of a patient.

Preliminary results (including the examples shown here) also suggest that verbal breathing instruction (i.e., when to inhale and exhale), when matched to a patient's breathing period, helps to improve reproducibility in breathing. Figure 2 compares ungated and expiration gated diaphragm excursions in four patients. A factor 2 to 4 reduction in diaphragm excursion is achievable with gate widths corresponding to 30-50% beam duty cycle (ratio of beam-on time to total treatment time). Reduced diaphragm excursion is further confirmed through comparison of diaphragm position in gated simulation and portal films (Fig. 2).

Gated operation of intensity modulated radiotherapy (IMRT) by means of dynamic multileaf collimation is also possible. In

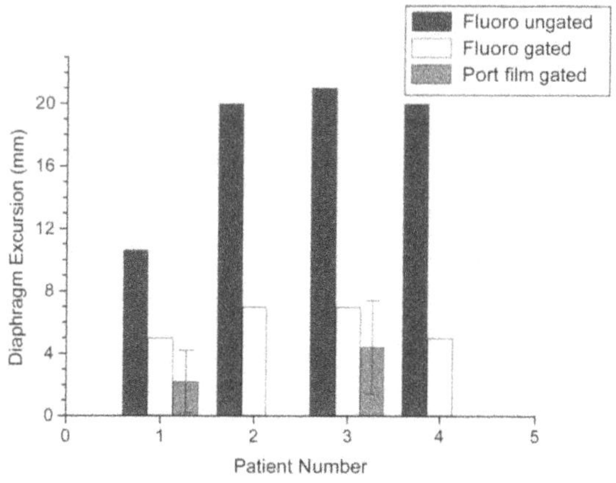


**Figure 2:** Range of variation in diaphragm position during fluoroscopy (ungated and gated). Grey bars denote mean deviation of diaphragm between gated port and simulation films, error bars denote range of deviations.

this mode of operation, both irradiation and leaf motion are suspended during intervals outside of the gate. Initial measurements with film indicate that gated operation has little effect on intensity modulated beam profiles. (Figure 3).

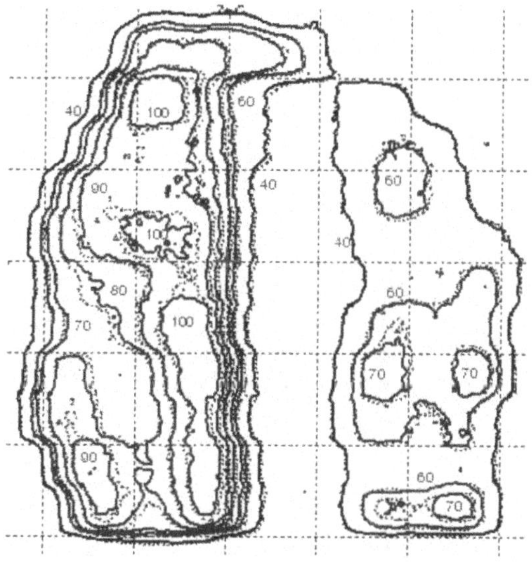


**Figure 3:** Isodose plots of a clinical intensity modulated field, with gated (dashed lines) and ungated (solid lines) operation.

## Discussion

The choice of controlled breathing vs gated techniques will depend on various factors such as disease site, patient cooperation, and staff time and effort. Hodgkin's Disease or tumors in the lung may benefit from treatment at deep inspiration, for which a breath-hold technique is more practical. However, nearly half of the patients initially instructed in the DIBH technique could not perform it satisfactorily; moreover, average time for simulation and treatment sessions in the first 8 patients was nearly double that for free-breathing treatments. By comparison, initial experience with gated treatment indicates that it is less demanding on patients, and requires little (1-2 min) additional treatment time. Gating at normal inspiration rather than at expiration for lung treatments may reduce lung toxicity due to the larger lung inflation, although the benefit is not as pronounced as at deep inspiration [8]. Dynamically delivered IMRT raises additional considerations, since intra-fractional organ motion can result in hot and cold spots in the dose distribution actually received by the target. [16,17]. IMRT using breath-hold techniques without accelerator gating may not be practical, due to the longer beam on times (factor of 2-3) that are required compared to static treatment fields. Accelerator gating can be integrated with IMRT, allowing treatment delivery either during normal breathing, or using short (3-5s) breath-holds to improve the beam duty cycle [14].

## Conclusions

A number of interventional techniques for controlling respiratory-induced motion have been developed in recent years, and clinical studies are underway at various centers. A common goal is to immobilize the tumor, and for some disease sites, treatment with increased lung inflation may be of additional benefit in sparing organs at risk. Although reduction in organ motion may indeed be achievable with these techniques, a word of caution is in order with regard to reducing treatment margins. Careful consideration must be given to other factors that can contribute to target underdose, including uncertainty in defining the extent of the clinical target volume, residual organ motion, patient setup deviations, and changes in beam penumbra and dose buildup in lung tissue.

## Acknowledgements

I thank Drs. Ken Rosenzweig, Ellen Yorke, and Mr. Eric Keatley for their assistance in obtaining some of the gated radiotherapy results presented here. This work was supported in part by U.S. National Institutes of Health grant #5 PO1 CA59017, and by Varian Medical Systems.

## References

[1] Balter J, Lam K, McGinn C et al 1998 Improvement of CT-based treatment-planning models of abdominal targets using static exchale imaging *Int J Radiat Oncol Biol Phys* **41** 939-943

[2] Wong J, Sharpe M, Jaffray D et al 1999 The use of active breathing control (ABC) to reduce margin for breathing motion *Int J Radiat Oncol Biol Phys* **44** 911-919

[3] Kini V, Sharpe M, Jaffray D et al 1998 Potential for dose escalation in the radiotherapy of hepatic tumors using active breathing control (ABC): a planning study *Int J Radiat Oncol Biol Phys* **42 (Suppl 1)** 141

[4] Stromberg J, Sharpe M, Kini V et al 1998 Active breathing control (ABC) for Hodgkin's Disease: reduction in normal tissue irradiation with deep inspiration and implications for treatment *Int J Radiat Oncol Biol Phys* **42 (Suppl 1)** 140

[5] Hanley J, Debois M, Mah D et al 1999 Deep inspiration breath-hold technique for lung tumors: the potential value of target immobilization and reduced lung density in dose escalation *Int J Radiat Oncol Biol Phys* **45** 603-611

[6] Rosenzweig K, Hanley J, Mah D et al 2000 The implementation of the deep inspiration breath hold technique in the treatment of inoperable non-small cell lung cancer *Int J Radiat Oncol Biol Phys* **(In press)**

[7] Mah D, Hanley J, Rosenzweig K et al 1999 The deep inspiration breath hold technique for the treatment of lung cancer: the first 200 treatments *Int J Radiat Oncol Biol Phys* **45 (Suppl 1)** 205

[8] Paoli J, Rosenzweig K, Yorke E et al 1999 Comparison of different phases of respiration in the treatment of lung cancer: implications for gated treatment. *Int J Radiat Oncol Biol Phys* **45 (Suppl 1)** 386-387

[9] Okumara T, Tsuji H, Hayakawa Y et al 1994 Respiration-gated irradiation system for proton radiotherapy. *In: Proceedings of the 11th International Conference on the Use of Computers in Radiation Therapy* 358-359

[10] Osaka Y, Kamada T, Matsuoka S et al 1997 Clinical Experience of heavy ion irradiation synchronous with respiration. *In: XIIth International Conference on the Use of Computers in Radiation Therapy* 176-177

[11] Sontag M, Merchant T, Burnham B et al 1998 Clinical experience with a system for pediatric respiratory gated radiotherapy *Int J Radiat Oncol Biol Phys* **42 (Suppl 1)** 140

[12] Johnson S, Hadley S and Pelizzari C 1998 A video-based technique to gate radiotherapy treatments for respiration *Int J Radiat Oncol Biol Phys* **42 (Suppl 1)** 139

[13] Shirato H, Shimizu S, Shimizu t et al 1999 Fluoroscopic real-time tumor tracking radiotherapy *Int J Radiat Oncol Biol Phys* **45 (Suppl 1)** 205

[14] Kubo H, Len P, Wang L et al 1999 Clinical experience of breathing synchronized radiotherapy procedure at the University of California Davis Cancer Center *Int J Radiat Oncol Biol Phys* **45 (Suppl 1)** 204

[15] Keatley E and Mageras G 2000 Computer automated quantification of respiratory motion in a fluoroscopic movie *In: XIII International Conference on the Use of Computers in Radiation Therapy* (these Proceedings)

[16] Yu C, Jaffray D and Wong J 1998 The effects of intra-fraction organ motion on the delivery of dynamic intensity modulation *Phys Med Biol* **43** 91-104

[17] Chui C 1999 The effects of intra-fraction organ motion on the delivery of intensity-modulated fields with a multileaf collimator *Med Phys* **26** 1087

# Ultrasound for Patient Positioning in Radiation Therapy

**Twyla Willoughby, MS, Patrick Kupelian, MD, Martin Weinhous, Ph.D.**

Cleveland Clinic Foundation 9500 Euclid Avenue, Tesk T28, Cleveland, OH 44195.

## Introduction

Ultrasound has been used in many applications in radiotherapy to determine anatomy. Even before the advent of CT, ultrasound was used to map organs and to illustrate isodose lines on treatment plans.[1,2] It is well documented that the prostate and bladder can be seen in the transabdominal ultrasound images. The ability to relate this information to the linear accelerator coordinate system and to obtain reliable position information for the prostate would allow the use of ultrasound as a positioning device. This could also be applied to other cases such as bladder, pancrease, kidney and liver.

## Material and methods

One device that has been commersially available for ultrasound alingments is the BAT™ system from NOMOS. This has been reported on in the literature.[3,4] This device consists of an ultrasound probe that is attached to a position-sension arm. The entire system is movable and is possitioned near the treatment table and is registered to the linear accelerator. After registration, images in two planes can be taken and the reconstructed contours from the patient treatment planning CT are overlaid on the ultrasound image. The patient is moved such that the position of the target in the ultrasound image corresponds to the target location in the treatment plan. An example of an axial and saggital image of a prostate, along with the corresponding CT contours is illustrated in Figure 1. This device has been used for prostate patient treatments at many centers. Other areas of application for such a device include liver, pancrease, chest wall, bladder, and kidney.

## Results and discussion

Studies have been performed on this device in order to determine the accuracy of this system and to determine its clinical useablilty. Studies at Fox Chase have compared the ultrasound device with daily CT scans. These studies have shown that the location of the prostate in the ultrasound relative to the location in the CT scan was AP 3.0 mm, LAT 2.4 mm, and S/I 4.6 mm [3]. Similar results have been seen at the Cleveland Clinic where comparisons were made between the possitining that is performed with the ultrasoudn device and the possition of the prostate as calculated based on implanted marker seeds in the prostate. In this study of 10 patients the mean difference were AP 4.2 mm, Lat 2.9 mm, S/I 4.7mm.

## Conclusion

These results indicate that ultrasound can be used in the localization of prostate. There are many areas that research can be done on this same type of device to determine the usability for other areas such as liver, kidney, and pancreas.

## References

[1] D. J. Brascho, 1975 "Radiation therapy planning with ultrasound," *Radiol Clin North Am* **13** (3), 505-21.

[2] R. O. Lowy, 1973 "The application of ultrasound tomography in radiation therapy," *J Can Assoc Radiol* **24** (4), 301-8.

[3] J.Lattanzi, S. McNeeley, W. Pinover, et al 1999 "A comparison of daily CT localization to a daily ultrasound-based system in prostate cancer. *Int J Radiat Oncol Biol Phys.* **43**(4): 719-25.

[4] D Mohan, MD, P Kupelina MD, T Willoughby M.S., 2000 "Short-Course Intensity Modulated Radiotherapy for Localized Prostate Cance with Daily Transabdominal Ultrasound Localization of the Prostate Gland." *Int J Radiat Oncol Biol Phys.* **46**(3) [accepted for publication]

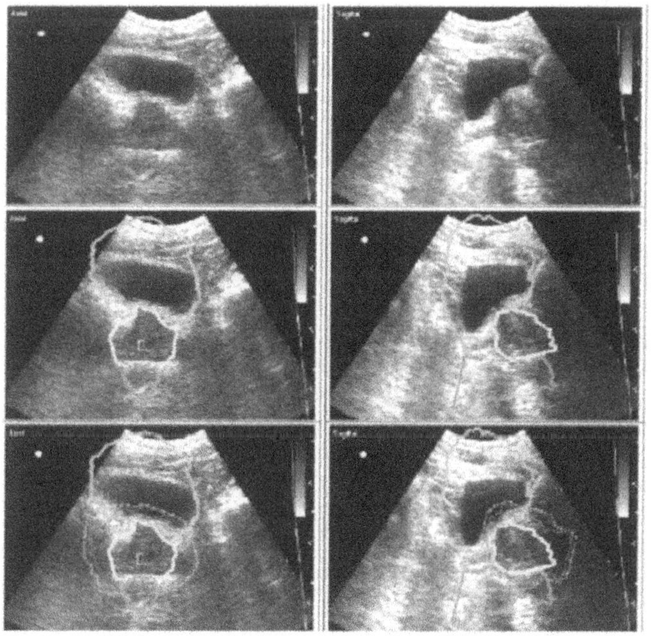

**Figure 1:** Ultrasound images with reconstructed contours and with sample isodose lines.

# Treatment Strategy For Daily Image Feedback Adaptive Radiotherapy

**Di Yan, PhD**

Radiation Oncology, William Beaumont Hospital, Royal Oak, Michigan, USA. This work was supported in part by NCI grant #CA71785

## Introduction

One of the major impediments to radiation treatment optimization is the inherent variability of patient and organ geometry during the course of radiation dose delivery. To overcome this obstacle, advanced technologies to facilitate image guidance and intensity modulated beam delivery are being rapidly developed. With these technologies, patient geometric variations can be repeatedly detected, and radiation dose can be better conformed to the target. However, accompanying the improving technology is a new challenge to the radiotherapy community, namely, how to utilize the information in daily patient images to maximize the treatment outcome.
In this study, a new treatment strategy is proposed by assuming daily volumetric image feedback in adaptive radiotherapy process. Utilizing daily image feedback and IMRT delivery, biological effective dose of the individual is optimized by means of selecting fraction dose in daily basis and total number of fractions.

## Material and methods

Figure 1 shows a flow chart of the daily image feedback treatment process. In this process, we assume that a volumetric image at each treatment day (i.e. the *k-th* fraction of treatment) is obtained for patient at treatment setup position before dose delivery. This technology has being developed by mounting kV x-ray source on the drum of an Elekta SL-20 medical linear accelerator [1] and designed in the prototype of Tomotherapy machine [2]. Target and normal volumes of interest (VOIs) for treatment planning are then defined, and imported to the organ deformation model [3] for the calculation of displacement mapping of VOIs by considering all rigid and non-rigid organ motion. An IMRT treatment plan is designed using the volumetric image by inverse planning to achieve a maximum separation (see Figure 2) between target prescription dose and the dose at a pre-defined critical volume for each of the VOIs. With also the displacement mappings of VOIs from the previous *k-1* volumetric images, the actual dose distribution in each of VOIs can be constructed [3]. The actual dosimetric differences, $g_1, \dots, g_k$, between the cumulative target dose at the prescription point (100%), and the minimum dose in the critical volume for each of $k$ treatments are then determined. Finally, the dosimetric differences, $g_1, \dots, g_k$, and the first *k-1* days of treatment dose, $d_1, \dots, d_{k-1}$, are input to an optimal **Controller** to decide the optimal daily prescription dose, $\hat{d}_k$, at the *k-th* treatment and estimate the total number of fractions, $\hat{N}_k$. The daily fraction dose and total number of fractions are optimized by maximizing the tumor biological effective dose (BED) [4] with respect to the constraints of equal BED for critical normal structures. The optimal controller is described as following.

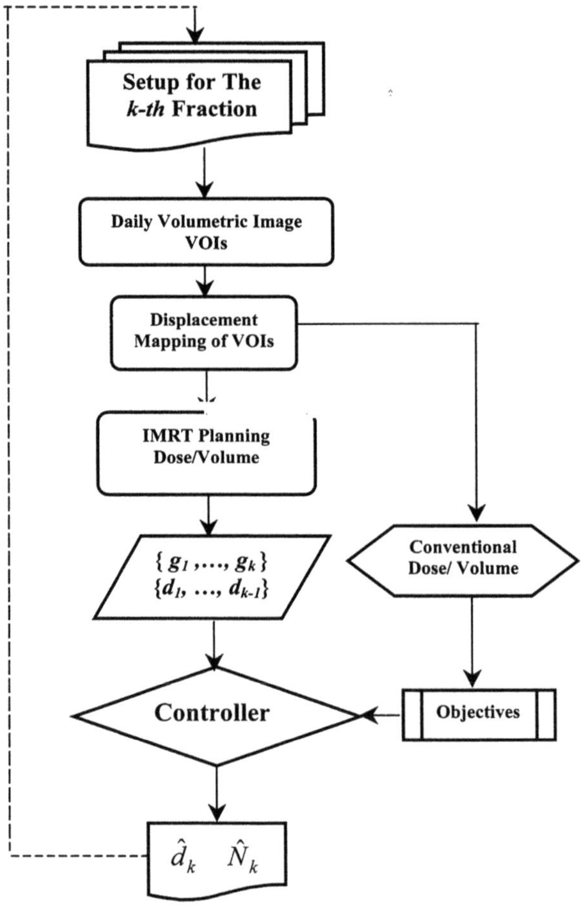


**Figure 1:** Flow chart of daily image feedback and optimal control process.

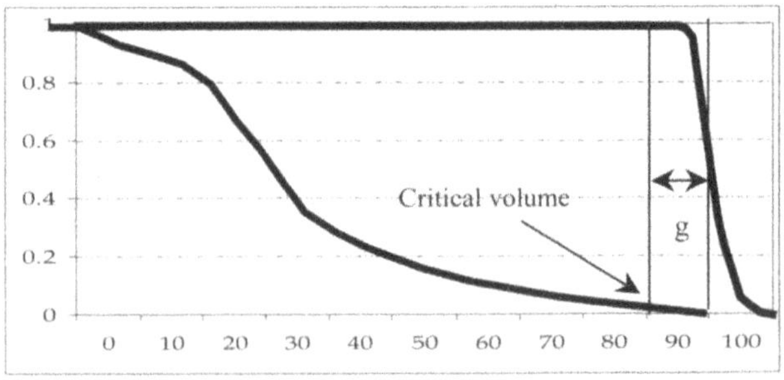


**Figure 2:** DVHs of target and small bowel for colo-rectal cancer treatment in the daily image feedback IMRT process. The critical volume of small bowel has size 1cc.

Considering the dynamic treatment process is ready for its *k*-th treatment after the first *k-1* fractions (*k* starts from 1). It is assumed that the *k-1* fractionation doses, $d_1, \dots, d_{k-1}$, and the one, $\hat{d}_k$, for the *k* treatment represent uniformly all possible daily doses for entire treatment ($\hat{N}_k$ fractions). Then, the tumor BED related to the daily prescription doses will be,

$$BED_t(d_1, \dots, d_{k-1}, \hat{d}_k, \hat{N}_k) =$$

$$\sum_{i=1}^{k-1} \frac{\hat{N}_k}{k} \cdot d_i \left(1+\frac{d_i}{\alpha_t/\beta_t}\right) + \frac{\hat{N}_k}{k} \cdot \hat{d}_k \left(1+\frac{\hat{d}_k}{\alpha_t/\beta_t}\right) - \frac{\ln 2(\hat{T}_k - t)}{\alpha_t\, T_{pot}}$$

where $T_{pot}$ is the average doubling time of the tumorigenic cells [5] or the effective cell doubling time in tumor. *t* is the time when tumor proliferation begins after the first treatment. $\hat{T}_k$ is the estimated total treatment time related to $\hat{N}_k$ and the time between the two adjacent fractions.

On the other hand, the BED related to the daily doses of critical volume for each VOI will be,

$$BED_n(g_1 d_1, \dots, g_{k-1} d_{k-1}, g_k \hat{d}_k, \hat{N}_k) =$$

$$\sum_{i=1}^{k-1} \frac{\hat{N}_k}{k} \cdot g_i d_i \left(1+\frac{g_i d_i}{\alpha_n/\beta_n}\right) + \frac{\hat{N}_k}{k} \cdot g_k \hat{d}_k \left(1+\frac{g_k \hat{d}_k}{\alpha_n/\beta_n}\right)$$

Here, we assume that the VOI injury after radiation is completely repaired i.e. the time between two fractions is more than 12 hours.

Now, a optimal **Controller (a)** will be designed by solving the following optimization problem, and determining the optimal daily dose for the *k-th* treatment, and the total number of fractions,

$$\underset{\{\hat{d}_k \;\; \hat{N}_k\}}{Max} \quad BED_t(d_1, \dots, d_{k-1}, \hat{d}_k, \hat{N}_k)$$

*w. r. t.* $BED_n = BED_{nc}(d, N)$.

Where $BED_{nc}(d, N)$ is the biological effective dose of VOI for the conventional treatment with respect to the dose fractionation *d* (i.e. 2Gy/per-fraction) and total number of *N* fractions.

This optimization problem has a continuous variable $\hat{d}_k$ (the *k-th* fraction dose) and a discrete variable $\hat{N}_k$ (the number of fractions). To determine the optimal solution, one can solve the Lagrange problem

$$\frac{\partial}{d_k} BED_t + \lambda \frac{\partial}{d_k} \{ BED_n - \underline{BED_{nc}} \} = 0, \text{ and}$$

$$BED_n - BED_{nc} = 0$$

by pre-selecting candidate of $\hat{N}_k$, and then find out the final solution among the candidates. This process will repeat at next *k+1*-th treatment to determine $\{\hat{d}_{k+1}; \hat{N}_{k+1}\}$ unless the actual number of treatments *k* is equal to the estimate $\hat{N}_{k+1}$.

The optimal solution from above optimal control model may not be always clinical practical, especially for tumor with long proliferation time ($T_{pot} > 7$ days) such as prostate adenocarcinoma. In this case, the tumor BED will be maximized by small dose per fraction and many fractions (i.e. LDR treatment). This is, of course, not clinically practical for the external beam treatment. With the daily image feedback process, one may also look for improving treatment outcome to an expected level, while keeping the total treatment time as short as possible. This problem can be modeled as following. For a desired tumor $BED_{tc}$, i.e. 15% dose escalation from the conventional tumor BED, we can determine the maximum fraction doses and the minimum total number of fractions, $\{\hat{d}_k; \hat{N}_k\}$, with which the desire can be achieved with respect to the equivalent $BED_{nc}$ for each of the VOIs. Therefore, we have,

$$BED_t(d_1, \dots, d_{k-1}, \hat{d}_k, \hat{N}_k) = BED_{tc} \quad \text{and}$$

$$BED_n(g_1 d_1, \dots, g_{k-1} d_{k-1}, g_k \hat{d}_k, \hat{N}_k) = BED_{nc}.$$

A **Controller (b)** for determining $\{\hat{d}_k; \hat{N}_k\}$ based on above consideration can be designed by solving the following equations,

$$\hat{d}_k \cdot \left\{ \frac{BED_{nc}}{BED_{tc}} - g_k + \left[ \frac{BED_{nc}/BED_{tc}}{\alpha_t/\beta_t} - \frac{g_k^2}{\alpha_n/\beta_n} \right] \cdot \hat{d}_k \right\} = \frac{\ln 2(\hat{T}_k - t)}{\alpha_t\, T_{pot}}$$

$$+ \sum_{i=1}^{k-1} \left[ \left( g_i - \frac{BED_{nc}}{BED_{tc}} \right) \cdot d_i + \left( \frac{g_i^2}{\alpha_n/\beta_n} - \frac{BED_{nc}/BED_{tc}}{\alpha_t/\beta_t} \right) \cdot d_i^2 \right]$$

$$\hat{N}_k = BED_{tc} \Big/ \left\{ \sum_{i=1}^{k-1} \left(1+\frac{d_i}{\alpha_t/\beta_t}\right) \frac{d_i}{k} + \left(1+\frac{\hat{d}_k}{\alpha_t/\beta_t}\right) \frac{\hat{d}_k}{k} \right\}$$

This controller outputs the $\{\hat{d}_k; \hat{N}_k\}$, starting at $k = 1$, before each treatment, and repeating until *k* equals $\hat{N}_k$.

## Discussion

Both of the Controller (a) and Controller (b) are designed by considering the daily volumetric image feedback and IMRT dose delivery, and can be applied to control the fractionation dose and total treatment time in the adaptive treatment process. The advantage of the Controller (a) is that it obtains a sequence of dose-per-fraction and total number of fractions, $\{(\hat{d}_k; \hat{N}_k)$:

$k = 1, 2, ...\}$, which maximize the biological effective dose of target. However, it also strongly depends on the knowledge of tumor proliferation during the treatment course, and the optimal solution may not be clinically practical. On the other hand, the Controller (b) is designed to find a sequence of feasible dose-per-fraction such that the total number of fractions or treatment time will be minimized with respect to a given desire for the tumor BED. It should be understand that an achievable clinical desire is dependent on the geometric and dosimetric separations between the treatment volume and critical normal structures. This separation is strongly dependent on the technology of imaging and IMRT delivery. Therefore, pre-study is required for a tumor site to decide what can be the reasonable and realizable clinical desire. Both controllers intend to remain the equivalent normal tissue toxicity at a clinically manageable level. It is assumed that this equivalence can be achieved if same biological effective dose is applied to a pre-defined critical volume for each of VOI.

The Controller (a) and (b) can also be designed by extending the BED model to include the entire dose distribution or dose/volume relation in the target and normal structures. In this case, the concept of the equivalent uniform dose (EDU) [6], the dose volume inhomogeneity corrected BED (DVIC-BED) [7], or the tumor control probability (TCP), after recasting them to include the dose-per-fraction and tumor proliferation effects, can also be adopted as the objective function for the controller design. In this case, the *k-th* treatment fraction dose should be determined by assuming the previous treatment doses and the one to be calculated, $\{d_1, ..., d_{k-1}, \hat{d}_k\}$, to be the samples of estimation that would be delivered with uniform distribution for total number of fractions, $\hat{N}_k$. The dose distribution in the target may also need to be evaluated by incorporating the displacement mappings of the target measured from the previous *k-1* images and the current *k-th* image for the actual dose distribution construction. Meanwhile, the effective dose, effective volume, which have been derived by the inclusion of the power law of the partial volume effect [8], or the normal tissue complication probability (NTCP) can be used for normal tissue constraints after recasting them to also include the dose-per-fraction effect. They, of course, have to be evaluated by incorporating the displacement mappings of VOIs. Furthermore, imcomplete repair of a normal structure should also be considered if the time between two adjacent fractions is short.

## References


[1] Jaffray D A, et al 1999 Radiographic and tomographic imaging system integrated into a medical linear accelerator for location of bone and soft-tissue target *International Journal of radiation Oncology, Biology Physics* 45 773-789

[2] Mackie R T, et al 1993 Tomotherapy: a new concept for the delivery of dynamic conformal radiotherapy *Medical Physics* 20 1709-1719

[3] Yan Di, et al 1999 A model to accumulate the fractionated dose in a deforming organ *International Journal of radiation Oncology, Biology Physics* 44 665-675

[4] Barensden G W 1982 Dose fractionation, dose rate and iso-effect relationships for normal tissue response *International Journal of radiation Oncology, Biology Physics* 8 1981-1997

[5] Fowler J F 1989 The linear quadratic formula and progress in fractionated radiotherapy-a review *Br J Radiol* 62 679-694

[6] Niemierko A 1997 Reporting and analysis dose distribution: a concept of equivalent uniform dose *Medical Physics* 24 103-110

[7] Bo Lennernas, Sten Nilsson 1999 Calculated effects of displacement errors in external beam radiotherapy of prostatic adenocarcinoma *Acta Oncologica* 38 203-208

[8] Kutcher G J, Burman C 1989 Calculation of complication probability factors for non-uniform normal tissue irradiation: the effective volume method *Int J Radiation Oncology Biol Phys* 16 0360-3016

# A Generalization of Adaptive Radiotherapy and the Registration of Deformable Dose Distributions

Weiguo Lu[1] T. Rockwell Mackie[1 2], Harald Keller[1], Kenneth J. Ruchala[2], and Gustavo H. Olivera[1 2]

[1]University of Wisconsin , Madison WI 53706, USA, and [2]Tomotherapy Incorporation, Middleton WI 53562, USA

## Introduction

Internal organ deformation throughout the course of radiation therapy is problematic to accurate determination of the dose delivered. Due to the internal motion and shape changes, the actual dose delivered to an organ volume could be significantly different from that of treatment planning. To incorporate internal organ variation into treatment optimization and evaluation, the difficult problems of determining the shape change, estimating the dose delivered and registering the cumulative dose mapping to one representation of the deformable organ must be solved. The development of tomotherapy makes such approaches possible.

We and others [1, 2, 3, 4] have shown that the detected megavoltage projection sinograms can be "tomographically reconstructed" to yield megavoltage (MV) CT images at the time of the treatment session. Objects with a 1 to 2% contrast can be resolved which is only slightly worse than the 0.5% to 1.0% contrast detectability of a conventional kilovoltage (kV) CT scanner (see Fig. 1). The high contrast resolution of low atomic number objects (e.g., between air and soft tissue) of MV CT is equivalent to that of kV CT scanners. CT images acquired during or after treatment would not improve the current treatment fraction but it could be used in conjunction with dose reconstruction to determine the dose received by the patient and used adaptively for future fractions.

"Dose reconstruction" may be the most important process introduced by the advent of tomotherapy. Dose reconstruction infers the dose distribution inside the patient based on the energy fluence measured during treatment and the CT scan generated at the time of delivery [5, 6, 7]. Accurate dose reconstruction requires a CT representation at the time of treatment. The isodose lines actually delivered that day can be superimposed on the CT representation that day and compared to the planning isodoses superimposed on planning CT's.

The critical step for cumulative dose mapping in a deformable organ is to track the displacement of each volume element in the organ between moments of dose delivery. By utilizing daily CT scanning, the organ shape can be accurately tracked. In this presentation, we use the "active contour" method [8, 9, 10, 11], which is usually used in computer vision and mechanical engineering, to track the organ shape in each delivery.

The term adaptive therapy[12, 13] was coined by Dr. Di Yan to describe the process of using portal images to guide alterations to subsequent delivery fractions to make up for geometric errors. In this presentation we propose a generalization of the meaning of adaptive radiotherapy to include all processes performed previously to improve the delivery of subsequent fractions of radiotherapy.

**Figure 1:** Low contrast phantom containing vials of varying contrast solutions. The vial diameters are 2.5 cm. The percentage contrast in terms of relative electron density with respect to water is indicated in the legend. Contrasts of 1% or higher are visable.

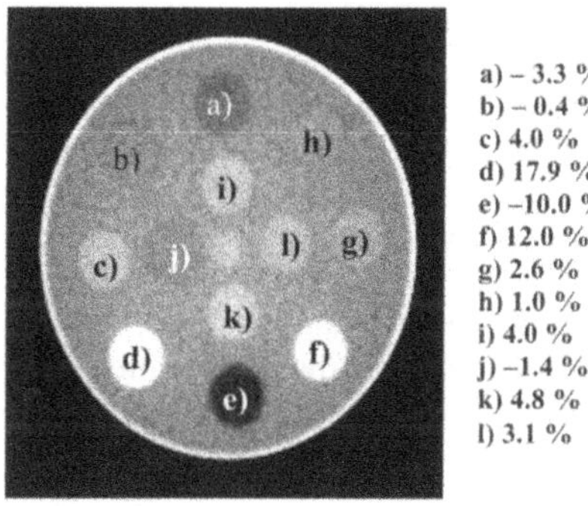


## Material and methods

### 1. Adaptive Radiotherapy

Adaptive radiotherapy reacts on subsequent fractions for verification results provided in previous fractions. MV CT and dose reconstruction is particularly well suited to this generalization of adaptive radiotherapy. This is because tomography can reveal geometrical deviations of soft tissues (portal images have limited ability to resolve soft tissue structures) and dose reconstruction can determine dosimetry information. We believe that the utility of dose reconstruction can be enhanced by being able to deformably register each of the reconstructed dose distributions together so that a composite dose distribution can be obtained.

**Figure 2:** Adaptive radiotherapy allows subsequent fractions to be modified on the basis of information gathered on previous fractions.

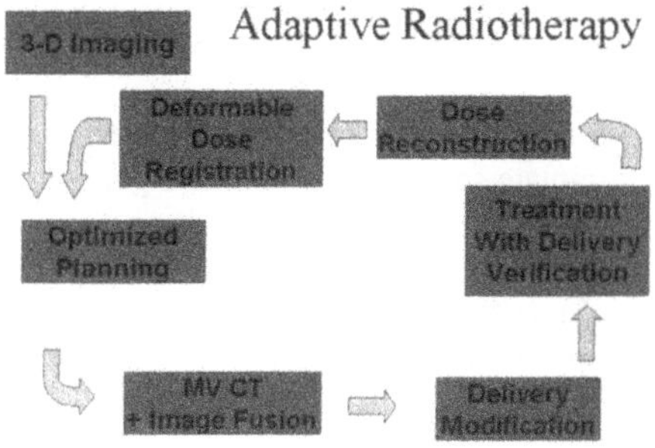

**2. Deformable Registration of Dose Distributions**

2.1 Active tracking of organ shape

The objects, such as organs, tumors, or other biological structures, are expected to have a tendency towards some average shape with a continuum of probabilities near that average shape. This tendency can be taken advantage of by its expression in an appropriately designed shape model. In this presentation, the boundary of the organ (contour) is represented as parametric B-spline curve. Parametric B-splines are attractive because they are capable of efficient represention of sets of contours in an image with smoothness controllable at each point.

Usually, images are "noisy" and therefore "regularization" is used to improve image quality by imposing prior constraints on the likely appearance of valid images. To actively track the organ shape in each fraction, we need to combine the "prediction" (template or prior information) and "observation" information. Prediction can be the physician contouring in the planning CT image or the prediction according to previous contouring. While the observation is the image feature measured from the daily CT image. The "observation" is done by locating the image features (edges, valleys or ridges) along the normal direction of the "predication" curve. To fit an image feature curve, the "shape-space" is used to reduce the shape variability and results in a smoother contour. The fitted curve is the solution of :

$$\min_{X}\{(X-\overline{X})^{T}\overline{S}(X-\overline{X})+\left\|WX+Q_{0}-Q_{f}\right\|^{2}\} \qquad (1)$$

The first term is the regularization term, which tends to pull any fitted curve towards the mean $\overline{X}$. It may be desirable for $\overline{X}$ to influence the shape of the fitted curve but not its position or orientation. Such a goal is achieved by adjusting the regularization matrix $\overline{S}$ to constrain the projection operator excluding an invariant subspace (we use Euclidean invariance shape space in this presentation.)

2.2 Deformable registration

The dose distribution can now be deformed using the deformed contour as the template constraining and providing a magnitude of the deformation. For deformable registration, volume elements (voxels) within an organ are generated using a volume mesh in both template and daily CT images. The dose mapping should be done voxel by voxel. Several standard methods for deformable registration are published, such as the methods based on elasticity between finite elements[14].

But since we know exactly the point to point mapping of organ contour between template and daily CT image, we can mapping the inner elements by a specific meshing technique. In this technique, meshing is done by shrinking the contour of organ step by step. In each step, the region between two contours are diveded into volume elements. By this method, we can map each volume element of daily CT image to the corresponding volume element in the template image. The mesh is especially constructed to approximately equalize the volume for all elements.

## Results and discussion

We presented some preliminary results about deformable organ shape tracking. For the results of other processes used in adaptive radiotherpy, we refer to [4, 7, 15]. Figure 3 is a simulation result of organ shape tracking by the active contour method. Panel A1 is the physician-contoured template of an organ of interest. Panel A2 is the B-spline curve constructed from the template image with the lateral marks indicating the direction of search for image features. Panel A3 is the " daily CT image" during delivery. Panel B1 is the measured contour of the organ of interest resulting from the search direction given in panel A2. Panel B2 is the fitted contour by the active contouring algorithm. Panel B3 is the resulting deformed contour of the organ of interest. As we can see from this figure, our tracking algorithm is quite accurate.

The distinction between delivering the radiation as precisely as possible and adaptive radiotherapy is time. Precision delivery is what is done today to make today's treatment more precise. Adaptive radiotherapy is what is done today to enable corrections in delivery to be done tomorrow. If computers algorithms for adaptive radiotherapy processes can be made faster, then the corrections can be made today instead of tomorrow.

## Conclusion

In this presentation we propose a generalization meaning of adaptive radiotherapy to include all processes performed in tomotherapy to improve the delivery of subsequent fractions. Adaptive radiotherapy hypothesize that it is possible to modify subsequent treatments on the basis of the verification information obtained from previous treatments. We argue that tomotherapy is suitable for adaptive radiotherapy since it provide greatly improved verification for each intensity modulated treatment. Dose reconstruction[15] and deformable dose registration are the key ideas for adaptive radiotherapy. These techniques use the CT data acquired at the time of treatment as well as information obtained during delivery verification. With dose reconstruction, the dose is associated with the daily CT representation. The deformable registration maps the daily dose received by each individual area of the tumor or organ back onto the original CT image so that the total dose can be more accurately determined. The difficulty of deformable registration is to track the shape of organ of interested. We present an active contour method to automatically tracking the deformable shape. Some preliminary results for deformable registration are presented. We will research and test the whole process associated with adaptive radiotherapy using the unique tomotherapy research benchtop (University of Wisconsin – Madison) and the world's first clinical tomotherapy unit.

**Figure 3.** Simulation results of avtive contour tracking of a deformable organ

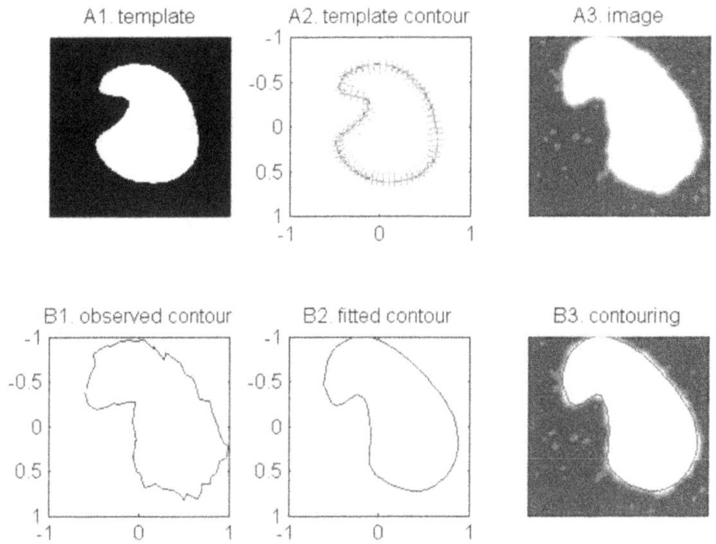


## References


[1] Swindell W 1983. A 4-MV CT Scanner for Radiation Therapy: Spectral Properties of the Therapy Beam. *Med. Phys.* **10**(3): 347-351.

[2] Swindell, W, Simpson R G, et al. 1983. Computed Tomography with a Linear Accelerator with Radiotherapy Applications. *Med. Phys.* **10**(4): 416-420

[3] Brahme A B Lind et al. 1987. Radiotherapeutic Computed Tomography with Scanned Photon Beams. *Int. J. of Radiat. Oncol., Biol., Phys.* **13**: 95-101

[4] Ruchala K, 1998. Megavoltage computed tomography for tomotherapy verification. *Ph.D thesis*, Dept. of Medical Physics. Madison, University of Wisconsin

[5] McNutt T R, Mackie T R, et al. 1997. Analysis and convergence of the iterative convolution/ superposition dose reconstruction technique for multiple beams and tomotherapy. *Med. Phys.* **24**: 1465-1476

[6] McNutt T R, Mackie T R, et al. 1996. Modeling dose distributions from portal dose images using the convolution/superposition method. *Med. Phys.* **23**(8): 1381-1392

[7] Olivera G H, Shepard D M, et al. 1999. Tomotherapy: *Modern Technology of Radiation Oncology* (in press). J. Van Dyk. Madison, Medical Physics Publishing.

[8] Blake A, Isard M, and Reynard D [1994] Learning to track curves in motion. *Proc. IEEE Int. Conf. Decision Theory and Control*, 3788—3793

[9] Blak A, Isard M, and Reynard D (1995), Learning to track the visual motion of contours *Artificial Intelligence*, **78**, 101--134, (1995).

[10] Blake A, Bascle B, Isard M and MacCormick J (1998), Statistical models of visual shape and motion *Proc. Roy. Soc. Lond. A*, **356**, 1283--1302, (1998).

[11] Blak A, Isard M, 1998, Active Contours, *Springer-Verlag Berlin Heidelberg*

[12] Yan D, Ziaja E, Jaffray D, Wong J, Brabbins D, Vicini F, Martinez A 1998 The use of adaptive radiation therapy to reduce setup error: a prospective clinical study. *Int J Radiat Oncol Biol Phys.* **41**(3):715-20.

[13] Yan D, Wong J, Vicini F, Michalski J, Pan C, Frazier A, Horwitz E, Martinez A 1997 Adaptive modification of treatment planning to minimize the deleterious effects of treatment setup errors. *Int J Radiat Oncol Biol Phys.***38**(1):197-206.

[14] Yan D, Jeffray D, Wong J, 1999, A model to accumulate fractionated dose in a deforming organ. *Int. J. Radiation Onclology Biol. Phys.* , **44**(3) 665-675

[15] Kapatoes J M, 1999, Radiation delivery verification and dose reconstruction in tomotherapy, *Ph.D thesis research prospectus*, University of Wisconsin-Madison

# Statistical control applications for dynamic refinement

**Randall K. Ten Haken, James M. Balter and Kwok L. Lam**

University of Michigan, Deparment of Radiation Oncology, 1500 E. Medical Center Drive, Ann Arbor, MI 48109-0010 USA

## Introduction

Electronic portal imaging devices, EPIDs, have the potential of providing daily information about the patient under treatment. Thus, daily imaging could provide about 40 measurements of patient position/configuration during the course of treatment, as opposed to less than 10 measurements from weekly port films. One class of correction strategies using this information involves rule based setup correction [1]. In this strategy, a correction is applied when statistical analysis indicates a systematic setup error above a predetermined threshold at a specified confidence level. These methods can effectively discover systematic setup errors. However, the corrections are discrete in time (in the sense that there is no correction before the rule is met), and they are based only on geometry (as opposed to their impact on the dose distribution). Thus, no advantage for improving patient setup results until after a given number of treatments have been delivered. Other geometrical approaches involve Adaptive Radiation Therapy (ART) schemes [2]. Patient-specific systematic and random errors are both determined statistically through daily imaging and offline analysis. The treatment field, originally planned according to population statistics, can be re-shaped in response to these errors. Thus, the method can provide patient specific treatment. However, the methods are still based on rules that are geometrical in nature; the estimated systematic and random errors are based on measured values when the threshold for correction is exceeded, or determined from population statistics when the threshold is not met. Therefore, the method does not fully integrate information from both the population statistics and individual patient measurements.

Another strategy [3] avoids the sudden change in treatment resulting from adaptive control methods. This algorithm uses stochastic control methods to design intensity profiles that are robust to uncorrectable parameters such as organ motion, and uses dynamic control methods to make frequent adaptive adjustments that correct for systematic and random setup errors. The dynamic control method is not inherently based on individual patient statistics. Although it can be modified to optimize the cost function based on the population distribution functions, the cost function does not make use of the patient specific errors to customize the treatment. It would be advantageous to have a treatment delivery scheme that combines the information from population statistics and measured data, including inter-fraction organ motion specific to the patient as elucidated during the course of treatment. The combined information could be used to dynamically refine the treatment by optimizing a cost function based on dose distributions and other clinical data.

## Material and methods

We have been investigating the application of optimal statistical decision theory [4] to dynamic refinement. One area that we have investigated is determination of patient setup error. During treatment planning, the best guess of the setup error distribution for a patient is the population distribution. During the course of treatment, we sample the setup error of the specific patient. We can then improve our estimation of the setup error distribution by combining our knowledge of the population distribution and the sampled data to obtain the *a posteriori* distribution using the conditional probability distribution.

We assume that the setup error of each patient is distributed according to a normal distribution characterized by a mean and a variance, or systematic error and random error, respectively. We also assume that the systematic and random setup errors of different patients are different and distribute according to a joint distribution represented by a normal-gamma probability density function, which describes the population of patients as a whole. The expected values of the systematic error and random error can be deduced from the normal-gamma distribution. As data on patient displacement are obtained during treatment, we can revise the joint probability distribution of systematic error and random error under the condition that the measured displacements have occurred. That is, in light of the findings that 1) the measured displacements have occurred and 2) the patient is part of the whole population, we can deduce the chances that the setup error of the patient has a particular systematic error and random error. This is the conditional probability distribution of the systematic error and random error posterior to the measurement of displacements. We can determine the revised expected values of the systematic error and random error after each measurement from the posterior distribution. It can be proven that the posterior distribution after N measurements of displacement is still a normal-gamma distribution function, but the parameters specifying distribution, and thus the expected values, are different from the a priori distribution function. The posterior joint distribution function and expected values of the systematic error and random error can be updated after each measurement of displacement.

## Results and discussion

Let us consider the case of one dimensional setup error (Figure 1).

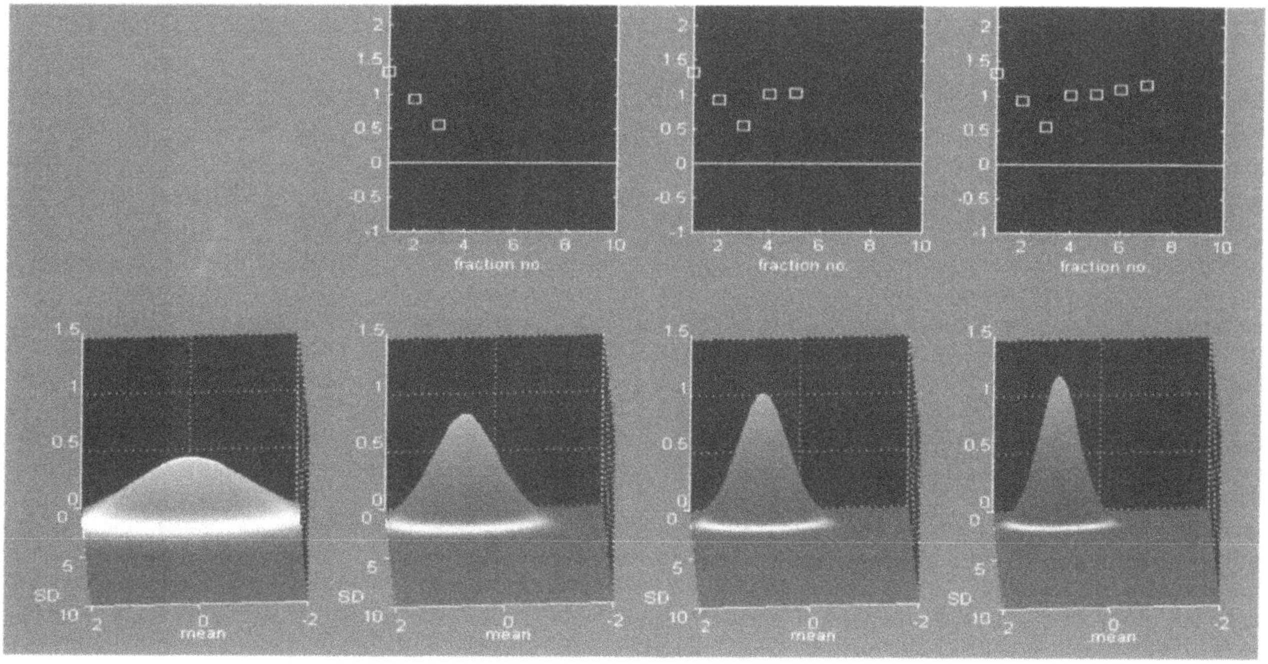


**Figure 1: 1D Simulation of posterior joint distribution function for setup.**

The top row (Fig. 1) shows the simulated 1D setup errors after 3, 5, and 7 fractions. The bottom row shows the corresponding probability density distribution of mean and standard deviation (SD) of setup error. The leftmost distribution is for overall the population. After three measurements, the base of the distribution already shifts significantly towards the 1 cm mean developing for the individual patient. The distribution narrows further as the number of measurements increases, indicating reduction of the confidence interval.

The results have been extended to multidimensional cases. The only different is that the normal-gamma distribution is replaced by the normal-Wishart distribution.

## Conclusion

Prior to patient treatment, little information is known about an individual patient, therefore population-based distributions must be used for dose modeling and optimization of the initial plan. It should be possible to use daily measurements to evaluate the *a posteriori* conditional probability of the systematic errors to give an estimate of "individual" variations based on the population models. As additional knowledge is gained about the setup uncertainties and organ motion of individual patients, the treatment plan and plan for further treatment can incorporate these individualized data, providing further assurance that predicted outcomes will be realized. This should result in clinical target volume coverage, together with more confident descriptions of normal tissue doses. Dynamic refinement of treatment techniques to customize treatment for individual patients should result in optimal safe treatments at a given prescription dose, or for further dose escalation at specified levels of risk

## References

[1] Bel A, Vos PH, Rodrigus PTR, Creutzberg CL, Visser AG, Stroom JC and Lebesque JV 1997. High-precision prostate cancer irradiation by clinical application of an offline patient setup verification procedure, using portal imaging. *Int J Radiat Oncol Biol Phys* **35** 321-332.

[2] Yan D, Wong J, Vicini F, Michalski J, Pan C, Frazier A, Horwitz E and Martinez A 1997. Adaptive modification of treatment planning to minimize the deleterious effects of treatment setup errors. *Int J Radiat Oncol Biol Phys* **38:** 197-206.

[3] Lof J, Lind BK and Brahme A 1998. An adaptive control algorithm for optimization of intensity modulated radiotherapy considering uncertainties in beam profiles, patient set-up and internal organ motion. *Phys Med Biol* **43**: 1605-1628.

[4] DeGroot MH 1970. Optimal Statistical Decisions. New York, McGraw-Hill.

# Clinical applications of combining IMRT with electron beams

**Jonathan G. Li, Arthur L. Boyer and Lei Xing**

Department of Radiation Oncology, Stanford University School of Medicine, Stanford, California 94305-5304, USA

## Introduction

The goal of radiation therapy is to achieve local tumor control while sparing as much as possible normal structures. An important step in producing an optimal treatment plan is the selection of beam modalities in order to utilize the different characteristics of different modalities [1]. Treatment plans involving a combination of electron and photon beams are routinely used in most cancer centers. However, direct abutting of electron and photon beams usually creates hot and/or cold spots in the abutting region [2,3]. To reduce dose inhomogeneity in the abutting region, several methods have been proposed, most of which utilize specially designed beam spoilers to broaden the penumbrae of the abutting beams [4]. Recent technological advancements in MLC and inverse planning provide a viable alternative for using dynamic MLC as a photon penumbra generator [5]. In this work, we describe a technique for optimizing combined electron and IMRT treatment plans using dynamic MLC. It generates patient-specific 3D treatment plans and is able to match the electron and photon beams at a pre-specified depth or in the target volume. The magnitudes of the hot and cold spots in the abutting regions are significantly reduced. The approach is not limited to abutting an electron field with one or two opposed photon beams. The optimization algorithm is quite general and can generate optimal plans for an arbitrary number of electron and photon fields and beam configurations. Both theoretical calculations and film measurements were carried out to characterize the dose distributions in the junction regions and to study the sensitivity of dose homogeneity to setup errors. Two clinical cases were presented to illustrate the application of the technique.

## Material and methods

Dose distributions in the abutting region of a 6-MV photon beam and a 9-MeV electron beam in a cubic phantom were generated using a clinical treatment planning system (PLUNC). Both beams were $10\times10\,cm^2$ with SSDs of 100 cm. Two photon beam setups were considered: a symmetric field (full beam setup), and an asymmetric field with a half-beam block on the electron beam side (half beam setup). Dose from the two beams was normalized to 100% at a reference depth of 2cm. An iterative algorithm was developed to optimized composite plans of electron fields with intensity modulated (IM) photon fields [6]. For a given patient, the algorithm can generate optimal weights of electron fields and beam profiles of IM photon fields. For the phantom study, the IM beam setup was the same as the half beam setup, with a margin of 2cm added on the abutting side. The goal of the optimization was to obtain a uniform dose at a 2-cm depth. To simulate setup errors, the electron beam was shifted from $-4$ mm (4mm gap) to $+4$ mm (4mm overlap) in steps of 2mm, where zero gap was defined as having the 50% isodose lines of the two beams match at the reference depth.

Film studies were conducted in a solid water phantom using a Varian Clinac 2300 C/D. Experiments were setup according to the parameters used in the computer simulations. A leaf sequence file was generated from the optimized intensity profile with a leaf step size of 2mm. Intensity modulation was restricted to a region within $\pm 2$ cm of the abutting line.

For more complex clinical cases, the IM photon profiles were optimized to achieve a compromise for the dose in the whole target volume. This was demonstrated by two clinical cases: a boost treatment of a head and neck cancer and a case involving chest wall irradiation in which an electron field was abutted with two opposed IM fields. Both the dose distributions and DVHs were used to evaluate the treatment plans.

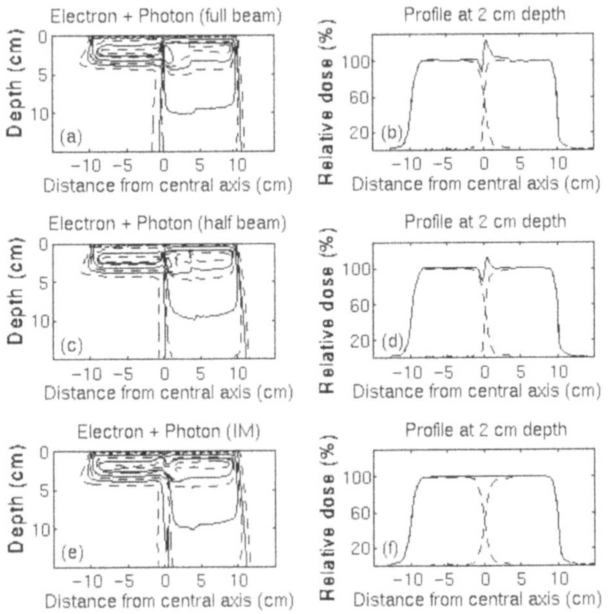


**Figure 1:** Computer calculations of the Isodose distributions and dose profiles at 2 cm depth for three different methods of matching a 6 MV photon beam with a 9 MeV electron. Isodose curves were drawn at 110%, 100%, 95%, 90%, 70%, 50%, 30%, and 10% levels, alternating with solid and dashed lines. Note there is no 110% isodose line in (e). The summed profiles were shown (solid lines) as well as the profiles of the respective electron and photon beams (dashed lines).

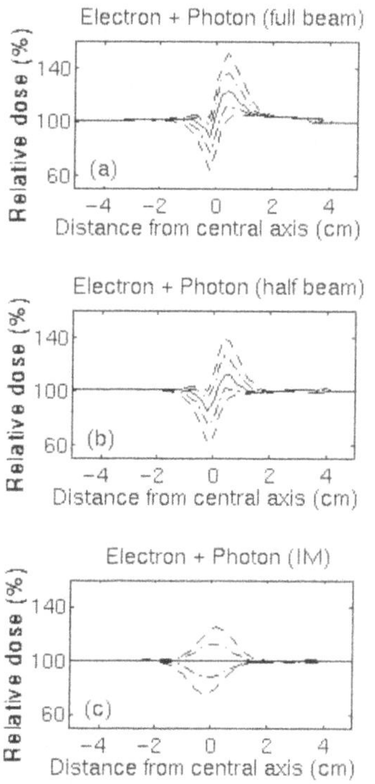


**Figure 2:** Comparison of the dose profiles of electron and photon beam matched fields at 2 cm depth for the three different photon beam setups as described in Figure 1 when patient setup errors were introduced. The five dose profiles in each subplot are, from the bottom curve up, for setup errors of –4, -2, 0, 2, and 4 mm, respectively.

## Results and discussion

Figure 1 compares the dose distributions of the electron beam combined with an unmodulated full beam photon beam, an unmodulated half beam photon beam, and an intensity modulated photon beam when there is zero gap between the two beams, and the corresponding dose profiles at the reference depth. Since the electron penumbra is wider than the unmodulated photon penumbra at 2-cm depth and beyond, when their 50% isodose curves are matched, a cold spot occurs on the electron beam side, and a hot spot occurs on the photon beam side. The non-divergent photon beam (half beam) is slightly advantageous over the divergent photon beam (full beam) in terms of dose homogeneity in the junction region, with magnitudes of over/under dosage of 13%/14% at the reference depth, compared with 23%/12% for the full beam setup. An exact match was achieved between the electron beam and IM photon beam at the reference depth. This is expected based on the geometry of the target. In fact, an exact match can be created at any depth where the electron penumbra is wider than the unmodulated photon penumbra. The intensity modulation effectively broadens the photon penumbra, making it complementary to the electron penumbra at the specified depth

Because of the broadened photon penumbra, the dose homogeneity in the junction region becomes less sensitive to patient setup errors. Figure 2 compares the dose profiles at the

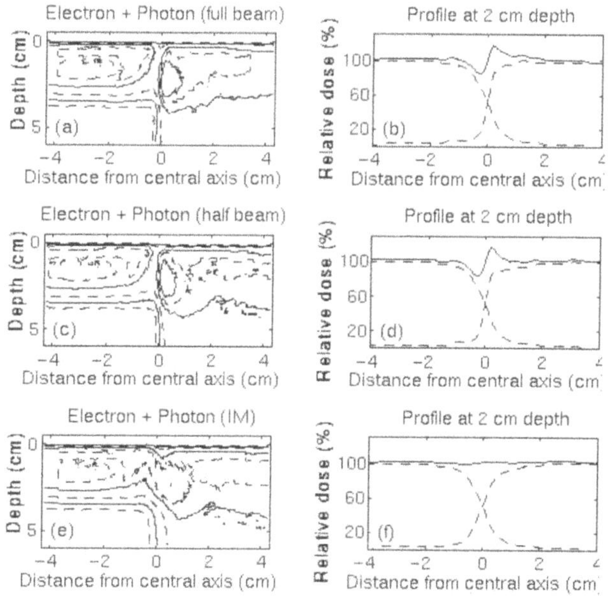


**Figure 3:** Measured Isodose distributions and dose profiles at 2 cm depth for three different methods of matching a 6 MV photon beam with a 9 MeV electron. Isodose curves were drawn at 110%, 100%, 90%, 70%, 50%, and 30% levels, alternating with solid and dashed lines. The experimental setups were the same as those used in the computer calculations of Figure 1.

reference depth when small patient setup errors were introduced. The magnitudes of the hot/cold spots when setup errors of $+4/-4$ mm were introduced were +50% and -36%, respectively, for the full beam setup (a). These were reduced to +25% and -23%, respectively, when IM photon beam was used (c).

The measured dose distributions of the matched fields and their corresponding dose profiles are shown in Fig. 3 for the three beam setups as in Fig. 1. The measured dose distributions compare well with the computer simulation, with hot and cold spots well matched in dimension and location.

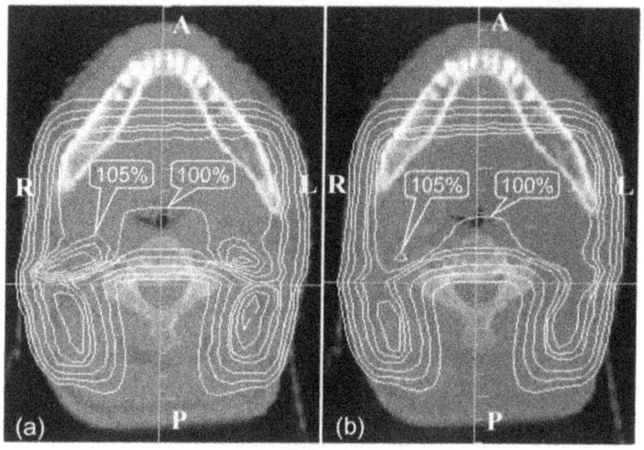


**Figure 4:** Comparison of the isodose distributions of the treatment plans in a transverse section of a head and neck cancer patient when the electron and photon beams were matched directly (a) and when dynamic intensity modulation was used for the photon beam.

The lateral distance between the 80% and 20% isodose levels at the reference depth was measured to be 3.6 mm for the full beam photon beam, compared with a distance of 9.3mm for the electron beam. The IM photon penumbra complemented the electron penumbra quite well, resulting in a uniform dose distribution across the junction region at the reference depth.

One of the common clinical situations where the matching of electron and photon beams is required is the treatment of head and neck cancers. The treatment usually involves the irradiation of the primary tumor and the cervical lymph nodes. After the tolerance dose of the spinal cord is reached using opposed lateral photon beams, the lateral fields are reduced off the spinal cord. The treatment of the anterior neck along with the primary tumor is continued using the reduced photon beams, whereas the posterior neck overlying the spinal cord is treated with lateral electron fields. This requires the matching of an electron field with two opposed photon fields. Figure 4 compares the isodose distributions of the treatment plans in the transverse section of a head and neck cancer patient when the electron and photon beams were matched directly (a) and when dynamic intensity modulation was used for the photon beams (b). When the electron and unmodulated photon beams were matched directly, hot spots greater than 15% above the prescribed dose were seen in the abutting region. This was reduced to ~5% when the proposed technique was used with markedly better dose homogeneity in the abutting region.

The treatment plan for a follicular lymphoma involving the right pleura using the proposed technique is displayed in Fig. 5. The patient positioning was prone. In order to reduce radiation dose to the critical structures as much as possible, the posterior part of the chest wall was treated using a 9 MeV electron beam, which was matched with two 15 MV opposed photon beams to treat the medial part of the tumor, with gantry angles of 200° (RPO) and 20° (LAO). A third photon beam was added at a gantry angle of 150° (LPO) and was directed at the deep medial part of the tumor in order to reduce the entrance dose from the LAO beam. The LPO beam did not match with the electron beam and carried a low weight due to its passage through the spinal cord. Figure 5 shows good tumor coverage with a maximum hot spot in the abutting region of only 107%, compared with a hot spot of more than 118% when electron and unmodulated photon beam abutting was attempted. This plan also provided much better sparing of the critical structures than a regular 7-field IMRT-only plan, with only marginal increase in dose inhomogeneity to the target due to the electron field. The technique has also been applied to the breast treatment with favorable results [7].

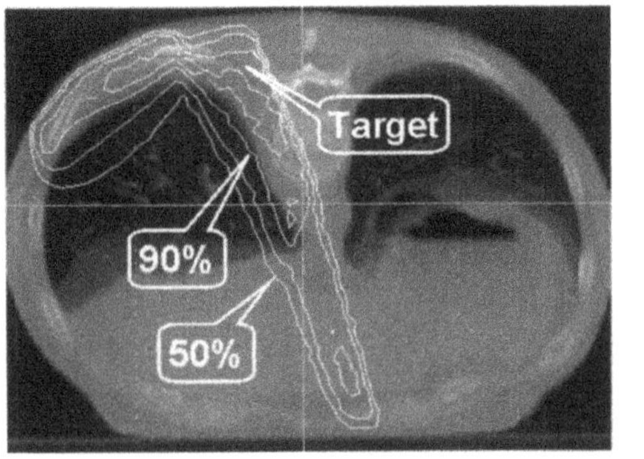


**Figure 5:** Isodose distribution in a transverse section of the treatment plan of a patient diagnosed with Stage IV follicular lymphoma involving the right pleura. The treatment plan involved a 9 MeV electron beam and 3 intensity modulated photon beams with gantry angles of 200° (right-posterior-oblique), 150° (left-posterior-oblique), and 20° (left-anterior-oblique). The maximum hot spot in the abutting region of the electron and photon beams is about 107%

## Conclusion

A technique for optimizing the combined electron and IMRT treatment plans was demonstrated. In its simplest application, the technique can be used to match photon and electron fields in order to reduce the hot and/or cold spots in the abutting region. It uses a computer controlled MLC to broaden the penumbra of the photon beam that abuts the electron beam in such a way that it compliments the electron penumbra at a specific depth or in the target volume. Because of the broadened photon penumbra, the dose homogeneity in the abutting region becomes less sensitive to setup errors. This new application of IMRT provides a unique opportunity to fully explore the two different treatment modalities and may result in better sparing of critical structures for certain classes of tumors. It allows one to design patient-specific intensity profiles in various clinical circumstances and suggests a strong potential for general clinical application.

## References

[1] Korevaar E W, Heijmen B J M, *et al.* 1999. Mixing intensity modulated electron and photon beams: combining a steep dose fall-off at depth with sharp and depth-independent penumbras and flat beam profiles. *Phys. Med. Biol.* **44** 2171-2181.

[2] Sidhu N P S and Smith C J. 1995. Dosimetric effects of matching electron fields with Cobalt 60 fields in the management of head and neck cancer. *Medical Dosimetry.* **20** 19-24.

[3] Johnson J M and Khan F M. 1994. Dosimetric effects of abutting extended source to surface distance electron fields with photon fields in the treatment of head and neck cancers. *Int. J. Radiat. Oncol., Biol., Phys.* **28** 741-747.

[4] Kalend M, Zwicker R D, *et al.* 1985. A beam-edge modifier for abutting electron fields. *Medical Physics.* **12** 793-798.

[5] Li J G, Xing L, Boyer A L, *et al.* 1999. Matching photon and electron fields with dynamic intensity modulation. *Medical Physics.* **26** 2379-2384.

[6] Xing L, Li J G, Pugachev A, *et al.* 1999. Estimation theory and model parameter selection for therapeutic treatment plan optimization. *Medical Physics.* **26** 2348-2358.

[7] Li J G, Williams S S, Boyer A L, Xing L. Breast-conserving radiation therapy using combined electron and IMRT technique. 1999. *Int. J. Radiat. Oncol., Biol., Phys.* **45** (Suppl. 1) 312.

# A comparison of IMRT planning systems in the treatment of colon-rectal cancer

**Wolfram U. Laub, Di Yan, Michael Sharpe, Joost Nuyttens, John Robertson and John Wong**

Department of Radiation Oncology, William Beaumont Hospital, Royal Oak, MI, USA

## Introduction

Adjuvant post-operative radiotherapy and chemotherapy has been shown to significantly reduce the risk of both pelvic and distant failure, with an improved survival rate. However small bowel toxicity due to treatment of rectal cancer is common. About 30% of patients receiving adjuvant post-operative radiation therapy (RT) were found to have acute diarrhea [1], leading to breaks and/or early termination of therapy. An increased incidence of long-term bowel disfunction has also been reported for RT patients, including more frequent bowel movements and/or incontinence [2]. Any reduction in the volume of small bowel irradiated may improve the tolerance to therapy. The potential use of IMRT to reduce the volume of small bowel irradiated during both post-operative and pre-operative RT for rectal cancer has recently been shown. However, IMRT treatment planning is relatively difficult for those patients. In general, the PTV is large and has a concave shape, with the small bowel in very close proximity. Therefore, the intensity profile calculated from an inverse planning could be complicated to deliver.

In this study, we report the results of a comparison of three different inverse-planning systems used to create IMRT treatment plans for rectal cancer patients. The qualtity of resulting treatment plans in this challenge clinical situation is considered with respect to the resulting dose-volume histograms (DVHs), the calculated dose distributions and the number of field segments necessary for step& shoot delivery.

## Material and methods

Treatment planning CT scans were obtained for 4 patients with rectal cancer. All patients had CT compatible small bowel contrast. They were positioned prone in a rigid foam cradle with an abdominal cut-out area, and instructed to have a full bladder. The clinical target volume (CTV) and small bowel were outlined. The planning target volume (PTV) was defined as CTV + 3mm margin. Four plans were calculated for each patient: conventional three-field plan and 3 IMRT plans with five equispaced 18MV photon beams in each case. The IMRT plans were calculated with the treatment planning systems:

i. KonRad (scientific Version 1.2 beta, MRC-Systems, Heidelberg)
ii. Hyperion (Dept. of Medical Physics, Tuebingen)
iii. Hyperion + beam-weight optimization of Pinnacle Version 5.1b.

After the optimization procedure in KonRad [4,5] and Hyperion was finished, the calculated intensity profiles were translated into MLC segments, deliverable on ELEKTA linear accelerators. A minimum beam resolution of 1x1cm was choosen for the translation. Tolerance levels of 5-7% were choosen for the maximum deviation between calculated intensity profiles and intensity profiles resulting from the translation into step&shoot fields.

The step&shoot fields were then used to create an IMRT-treatment plan in Pinnacle Version 4.2f and to recalculate the dose distribution and the according DVHs.

The isocenter was specified to receive 100% of the description dose of 45Gy, with the 95% isodose line encompassing the PTV and no more than plus 110% inhomogeneity within the target volume. Table 1 shows parameters as set in the used treatment-planning systems during the optimization procedures:

| | Pinnacle | KonRad | Hyperion [3] |
|---|---|---|---|
| PTV | Max. 48Gy (weight 2-4), Min. 43Gy (weight 2-3) | Max. 48Gy (weight 2-4), Min. 43Gy (weight 2-5) | $d_{eff} \geq 45$Gy (isoeffective dose), weight 6 |
| Small bowel | Max. 45Gy (weight 2), 90% of vol. <40Gy (weight 1), 60% of vol. <30Gy (weight 0.5) | Max. 45Gy (weight 1) + DVH constraints | $d_{eff} \leq 33$Gy (isoeffective dose), weight 8 |
| Rest of normal tissues | Max. 43Gy (weight 0.5) | Max. 45Gy (weight 1) | $d_{eff} \leq 45$Gy (isoeffective dose), weight 12 |

**Table 1:** Parameters for optimization.

It can be seen that objectives of dose-volume were defined for optimizations in KonRad, while biological objectives were applied in Hyperion. In addition, a smoothing method for intensity profiles is included in the optimization searching for Hyperion. Instead of the steepest descent method and a least square optimization as in KonRad, the conjugate gradient method and a biological target function are used in Hyperion for optimization. All inverse-planning systems use fast pencil-beam algorithms for dose calculation. The dose distribution of the final step&shoot treatment plans was recalculated with the adaptive-convolve method in Pinnacle.

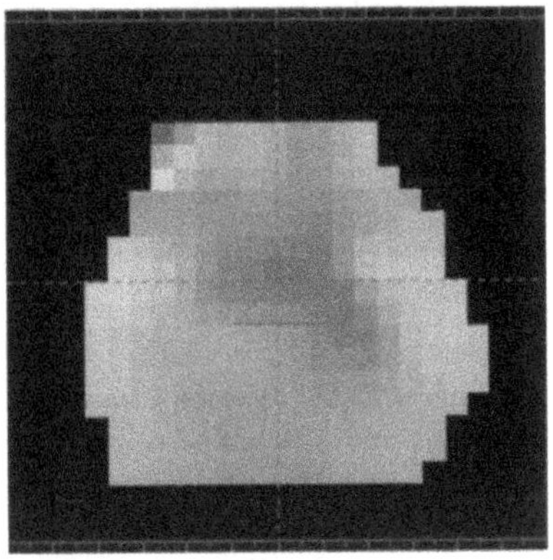

**Figure 1:** Intensity profiles as calculated in i. KonRad and ii. Hyperion (from left to right).

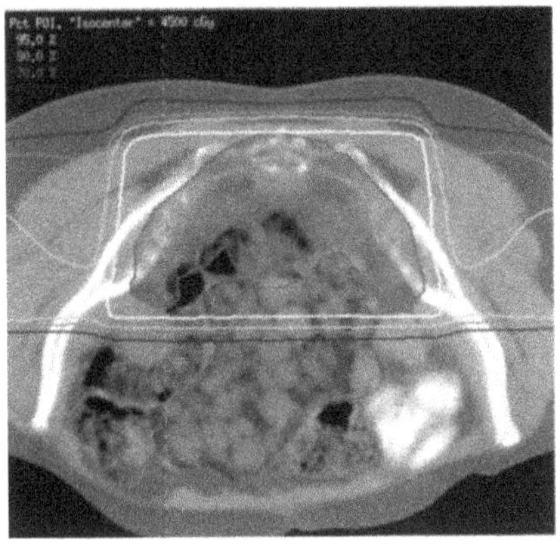

**Figure 2:** Dose distribution of a conventional three field plan. From the inner to the outer: 95%, 80%, 70% and 50% isodose lines. PTV and small bowel are outlined.

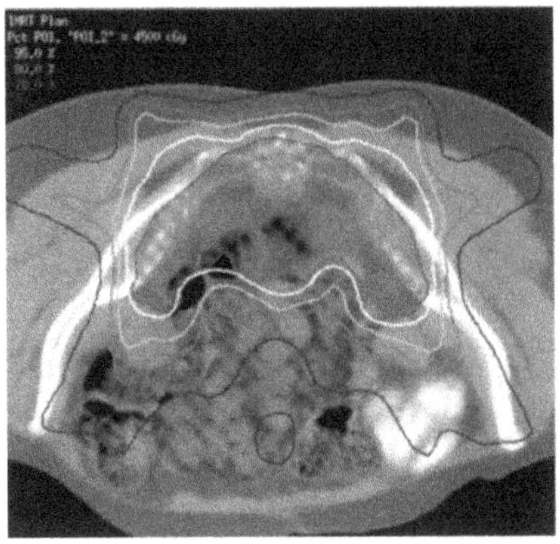

**Figure 3:** Dose distribution of IMRT plan as calculated in KonRad. From the inner to the outer: 95%, 80%, 70% and 50% isodose lines. PTV and small bowel are outlined.

## Results and discussion

Intensity profiles calculated from the inverse planning tools show a general agreement. However, as expected, intensity profiles from Hyperion are more smooth than intensity profiles from KonRad. Figure 1 shows a typical intensity profile calculated by both inverse planning systems for a beam with gantry angle 0 degree.
IMRT plans created in KonRad fullfilled the given objectives well. The small bowel volume irradiated to a dose 95% of the isocenter dose was reduced by about 70% compared to conventional treatment planning [Fig. 2 and 3]. However, parameter adjustment for the objectives and the DVH-constraints was necessary and therefore several optimizations had to be run for each patient. Nevertheless, the complete procedure of creating a treatment plan in KonRad, optimization in KonRad, translation of calculated intensity profiles into step&shoot fields and recalculation of dose distribution in Pinnacle took only about 2h. The number of resulting MLC segments was above 120. No constraints for the smoothness of intensity profiles can be specified in KonRad during the optimization process to decrease this number. Spikes at the edges of intensity profiles rather increase the number of MLC segments and lead to very small field segments with large offsets. Because the calculation of monitor units for such fields is difficult and therefore can be inaccurate and because of the MLC segmentation, unacceptable hotspots in the PTV were sometimes found after the recalculation of the dose distribution in Pinnacle. One explanation for spikes could be, that KonRad does not take into account scattering when changing fluence values and backprojecting dose to fluence. Another reason for spikes could be, that KonRad uses circular finite sized pencil beams to calculate the dose contributions of the quadratic matix elements of intensity profiles.
IMRT plans created in Hyperion also fullfilled the given objectives well. The objectives did not have to be changed for each patient and the complete procedure of making an IMRT plan with Hyperion took only about 1.5h. Because of the smoothness is part of the objective and incorporated in the optimization searching, the number of resulting step&shoot fields was reduced to be less than 60. Consequently, the time needed to recalculate the dose distribution in Pinnacle was shorter. More importantly, the IMRT plans from Hyperion were more clinically practical regarding the total delivering time.
Because of the MLC segmentation and monitor units conversion which most likely deviated the original optimization result, a beam weight optimization was also performed in Pinnacle, using the MLC segments obtained from the IMRT plan. It was found that a beam weight optimization,

which in general took a few minutes, can slightly improve the dose distribution.

## Conclusion

This study shows, that IMRT can substantially reduce small bowel irradiation for patients with rectal cancer. However, IMRT treatment by means of step&shoot delivery is only clinically practical, if the number of step&shoot fields does not lead to unacceptable long treatment times. To limit the number of step&shoot fields, intensity profiles must be as smooth as possible. Therefore, including an intensity profile smoothing function in the objective is necessary. Deliverable IMRT plans for patients with rectal cancer were calculated from Hyperion, following the procedure: optimize in Hyperion, translate calculated intensity profiles into step&shoot fields and recalculate dose distribution and DVHs in Pinnacle. A beam weight optimization of the step&shoot fields was found to also improve the treatment plan, because of the deviation of MLC segmentation, and the uncertainties in the conversion of intensity values into monitor units.
Therefore, future version of inverse planning system should include the MLC segmentation and the monitor unit conversion into the optimization procedure. For further improvement of the rectal cancer treatments, more study will also be needed to incorporate the mobility of the small bowel during treatment course into the intensity optimization.

## References

[1] Miller R C, Martenson J A, Sargert D J et al 1998 Acute treatment-related diarrhea during postoperative adjuvant therapy for high-risk rectal carcinoma *Int J Radiation Onc. Biol. Phys.* Vol. **15** No **3** 593-598
[2] Tepper E T, O'Connell M L, Petroni G R et al 1997 Adjuvant postoperative fluorouracil-modulated chemotherapy combined with pelvic radiation therapy for rectal cancer: initial results of intergroup 0114 J of Clinical Oncology, Vol. 15 No 5 2030-2039
[3] Alber M, Nusslin F 1999 An objective function for radiation treatment optimization based on local biological measures Phys Med Biol Vol 44 No2 479-493
[4] Bortfeld T, Stein, J. Preiser, K. 1997 Clinically relevant intensity modulation optimization using physical criteria Proc. of the XII$^{th}$ ICCR Salt Lake City USA 1-4
[5] Preiser K, Bortfeld T, Hartwig K, Schlegel W, Stein J 1997 A new program for inverse radiotherapy planning Proc. of the XII$^{th}$ ICCR Salt Lake City USA 425-428

# A Clinically Oriented Inverse Planning Implementation

**Alonso R. Arellano[1], Timothy D. Solberg[1,2], Jorge Llacer[3]**

[1]UCLA Department of Radiation Oncology, [2]Jonsson Comprehensive Cancer Center, 200 UCLA Medical Plaza, Suite B265, Los Angeles, CA 90095-6951, and EC Engineering Consultants, Los Gatos, CA 95032

## Introduction

Intensity Modulated Radiation Therapy (IMRT) has become a very promising cancer therapy modality. Since its clinical introduction a few years ago [1-2] it has attracted great interest from both researchers and clinicians. The four key elements to the successful clinical implementation of IMRT are a) inverse treatment planning, b) plan delivery, c) plan delivery verification, and d) patient positioning. This paper will discuss the first of these essential areas of IMRT. There are several aspects of the current clinical inverse treatment planning implementations that need improvement, in particular, the number and type of pre-optimization parameters asked of the planner and the control that the inverse treatment planning algorithm has over the treatment planning process. Current implementations of inverse treatment planning often require too many pre-optimization parameters. While some of these are clinically relevant, such as dose volume constraints, others, such as start/end grain, number of iterations, and $kT_o$/beam have no clinical meaning. These parameters are more applicable to research activities than to a clinical implementation of inverse treatment planning. Once the parameters have been supplied, the inverse treatment planning algorithm will try to find a solution. The solution found may not always be realizable because by trying to meet all given parameters it may have tried to solve an ill-conditioned problem. Ill-conditioned problems arise when the given parameters define a physically unachievable situation such as requesting a lower dose to an OAR than is possible given the current geometric setup. A large number of required pre-optimization parameters tends to increase the probability of defining an ill-conditioned problem, especially when dealing with non-clinical pre-optimization parameters. Once a solution is calculated, the planner/physician is force to accept the plan or restart the optimization process, thus relinquishing control of the optimization process to the computer.

The work presented here will discuss a more clinical oriented inverse treatment planning implementation than the current approaches. First, few and only clinically relevant pre-optimization parameters are asked of the planner. This greatly reduces the uncertainty in the definition of the optimization problem. Second, the inverse treatment planning algorithm used not only calculates the optimized solution with the given parameters but also provides several alternative optimized solutions to the same problem by both relaxing and strengthing the dose volume constraints given. By having multiple optimized solutions to the same problem, our clinical implementation of inverse treatment planning meets two objectives. The first objective is to assure the planner/physician that specifying a precise amount of OAR sparing prior to the optimization process is not critical. The second objective is to give the planner/ physician a choice of optimized plans thus regaining control of the optimization process. The third key element of our clinical implementation of inverse treatment planning is that additional plan evaluation tools are provided to the planner/physician to aid in deciding which of the plans presented, including the conformal plan, is more beneficial to the patient.

## Material and methods

The anatomy used to investigate our clinical implementation of inverse treatment planning is shown by the left image of figure 1. It consists of a planning target volume (PTV) located on the left side of a patient's brain adjacent to the brainstem, identified as the organ at risk (OAR). A conformal plan was first done with four conformal beams incident at 235, 270, 315, and 345 degrees. The result of the conformal plan is shown on

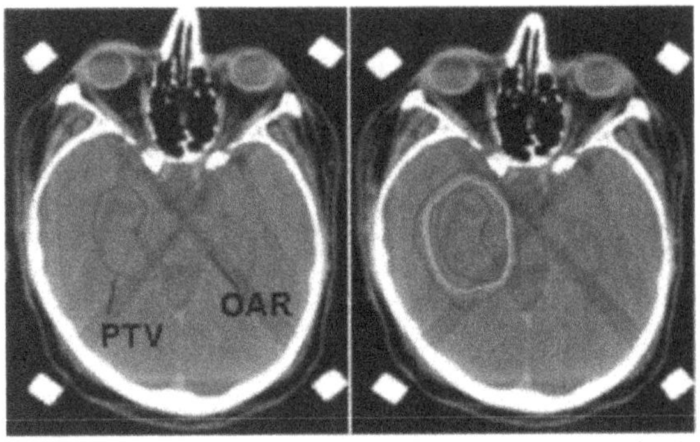


**Figure 1 Left:** Anatomical layout for problem optimized
**Right:** 4 Field Conformal Plan

the right side of figure 1. This calculation provided the seed dosimetric information necessary to conduct our inverse treatment planning. The inverse treatment planning algorithm used for this work is based on the maximum likelihood estimator (MLE) used in image reconstruction [3] and is a variant of the dynamic penalized likelihood (DPL) method [4]. The objective function used by the inverse algorithm is the log of a target function consisting of two terms. The first is an MLE term that maximizes the likelihood of obtaining the target dose, $d_i$ at each voxel

$$L(\bar{d} \mid \bar{w}) = \sum_{i \in D}\left[-\sum_j F_{ij} w_j + d_i \log\left(\sum_j F_{ij} w_j\right) - \log(d_i!)\right] - \sum_{i \in S} \beta_i \left(\sum_j F_{ij} w_j - s_j\right)^2$$

within the PTV ($i \in D$). The second is a dynamic penalization term that penalizes the intensity, $w_j$, of those pencil beams that deliver a dose, $F_{ij}w_j$, to the OAR voxels ($i \in S$) higher than the limiting dose, $s_i$. $F_{ij}$ is the dose deposition coefficient within voxel i, per pencil beam j, with unit intensity $w_j = 1.0$.

It is not uncommon for current clinical implementations of inverse treatment planning using dose volume constraints to ask the planner for hard constraints such as minimum and maximum dose, soft constraints such as a maximum allowable volume to receive a minimum dose and a maximum allowable volume to receive a maximum dose and mean doses desired. These constraints are required for each PTV and OAR in the problem in addition to non-clinical parameters. The clinical implementation presented in this paper uses only three dose volume soft constraints instead of the 10 to 12 needed in the current clinical implementations. These are the two volume percent soft constraints for the PTV and the maximum allowed volume to receive a maximum dose soft constraint for the OAR. Since our inverse treatment planning algorithm will maximize the probability of obtaining the desired dose at each voxel of the PTV while minimizing the dose to the OAR during each iteration, the two PTV constraints are not used as optimization constraints but as stopping conditions that halt the optimization process once either/both conditions are violated. By using fewer and more clinically relevant pre-optimization parameters, the risk of defining an unsolvable problem is reduced and a greater latitude is given to the planner/physician in defining the problem. The more parameters an inverse planning algorithm tries to meet during the optimization process, the greater the probability of defining an unsolvable problem and the greater search space for an optimized solution. In the event that an ill-conditioned problem is defined, the MLE, the basis for our inverse treatment planning algorithm, will converge even under such conditions [5]. By having multiple optimized solutions for the same problem, the planner/physician is able to compare the optimized solutions and the conformal solution and decide which of the plans best suits the patient under consideration. This gives the control of the treatment planning process back to the planner/physician and takes it away from the computer.

To aid the planner/physician in making a decision as to which of the optimized plans, including the conformal plan, is best suited to treat the patient, four evaluation tools were added to our clinical inverse treatment planning in addition to the commonly used tools such as isodose line contours and dose volume histograms. We have added dosimetric evaluations tools, conformity and uniformity index, and radio-biological evaluation tools, normal tissue complication probability and equivalent uniform dose. The conformity index is a ratio of two volumes that quantifies the amount of surrounding normal tissue being irradiated to the same intensity as the PTV in order

$$Conformity\ Index = \frac{ISO\ VOLUME_{PTV}}{PTV\ VOLUME}$$

to irradiate it to the desired dose. The numerator of this ratio is the volume enclosed by the maximum isodose line covering the entire PTV volume while the denominator is the PTV volume. The minimum quotient of this ratio is 1.0 for the best conformal plan. As the ratio increases above 1.0, the plan becomes less conformal. The uniformity index is a ratio of two volumes quantified as areas under the PTV's dose volume histogram. The ratio is subtracted from 1.0 for consistency and it quantifies the amount of dose uniformity within the PTV.

$$Uniformity\ Index = 1 - \frac{fall-off\ area}{total\ area}$$

The ratio is defined as the fall-off area divided by the total area under the PTV's dose volume histogram. The fall-off area is measured from the minimum dose not irradiating 100% of the PTV up to the maximum dose irradiating the PTV. The ratio ranges from 0.0 to 1.0, with 1.0 defining the best possible PTV uniformity. The normal tissue complication probability (NTCP) was calculated from Lyman's model [6] using Emami et. al. dose tolerance data [7], with Kutcher et. al. dose volume histogram reduction method [8], and Burman et. al. analytic fitting parameters [9] to the sigmoid dose curve of the tolerance data. Because the accuracy of the NTCP calculation is a direct function of the accuracy of the tolerance data, the NTCP was used as a radio-biological ranking tool identifing which plans are more likely to cause complications. The calculated NTCP for the same problem, under the same irradiation conditions serves well for this purpose although the exact probability of complication may not be known until further research is done on dose tolerance data. The equivalent uniform dose (EUD) was calculated as outlined by Niemierko [10].

## Results and discussion

Using the anatomy of figure 1, an optimization problem was constructed with a desired dose of 5400 cGy to the PTV and 3240 cGy to the OAR. This corresponds to 60% of the PTV dose. Two stopping conditions were used. First condition was that no more than 90% of the PTV volume should receive a

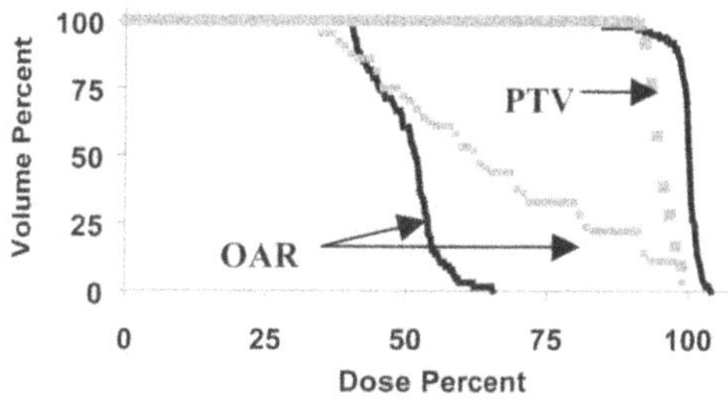


**Figure 2:** Dose volume histogram for conformal plan (broken lines) vs. inverse plan #1 (solid lines)

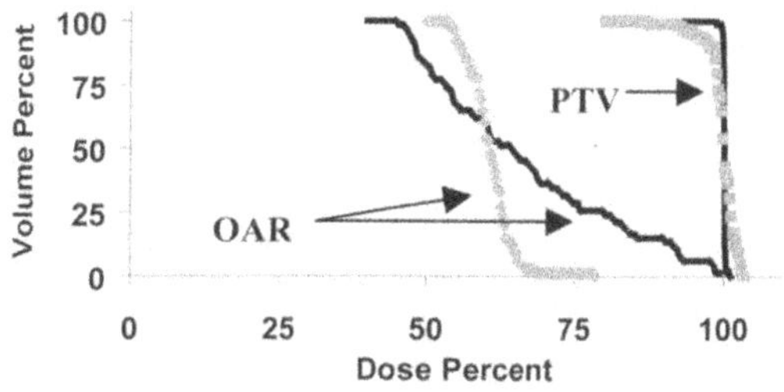


**Figure 3:** Dose volume histogram for inverse plan #2 (broken lines) vs. inverse plan #3 (solid lines)

dose less than 90% of desired dose. The second condition was that no more than 10% of the PTV volume should receive a dose more than 110% of desired dose. The inverse planning algorithm's first calculated optimized solution is plan#1 which met the desired results. Next, the inverse planning algorithm calculated plan #2 and plan #3 (Figure 3). Plan #2 improved the PTV dose uniformity by achieving a homogeneous dose distribution within the OAR. Plan #3 achieves the best possible dose conformity and uniformity, given the current geometric set up, by totally ignoring the OAR. Lastly, the inverse treatment planning algorithm calculated plan #4 (Figure 4 ) by aggressively sparing the OAR

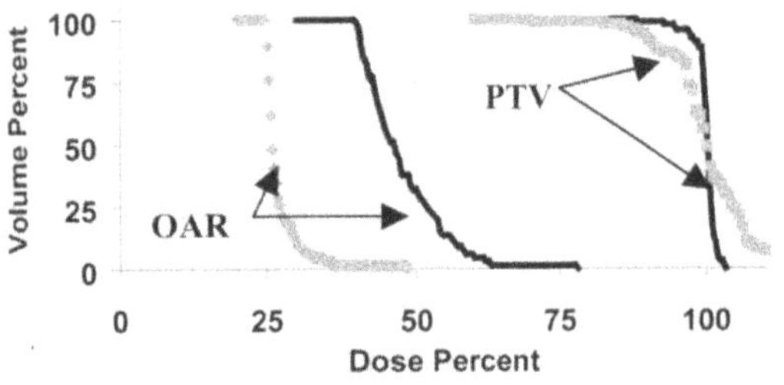


**Figure 4:** Dose volume histogram for inverse plan #4 (broken lines) vs. inverse plan #5 (solid lines)

| | Dosimetric | | Biological | |
|---|---|---|---|---|
| Plan | Conformity | Uniformity | EUD | NTCP |
| Conformal | 1.7 | 0.95 | 50.5 Gy | 99% |
| Inverse #1 | 2.1 | 0.83 | 52.4 Gy | 23% |
| Inverse #2 | 2.2 | 0.87 | 53.2 Gy | 66% |
| Inverse #3 | 1.5 | 0.98 | 53.9 Gy | 99% |
| Inverse #4 | 2.7 | 0.70 | 48.6 Gy | 0% |
| Inverse #5 | 1.9 | 0.88 | 53.6 Gy | 20% |

**Table 1:** Results of dosimetric and radio-biological evaluation tools as calculated from dose volume histogram data for conformal and multiple inverse plans for the same problem.

and allowing both stopping conditions to be violated. In plan #5 the OAR is moderately spared by stopping the optimization process when the first condition is violated (Figure 4). The results of the four evaluation tools for each of the inverse treatment plans as well as the conformal plan are shown in table 1.

Plan#1 which adheres to the pre-optimization parameters is not neccesary the best plan although it does spare the OAR. It also has a better tumor control according to EUD than the conformal plan. Plan #2 has a similar conformity as plan #1 with a better uniformity and tumor control but more likely to cause normal tissue complications. Plan#3 has the best conformity, uniformity and tumor control, however, is the most probable to cause normal tissue complications. The least likely plan to cause normal tissue complications is plan#4, but it has the worse conformity, uniformity, and tumor control. Judging from the results of these four evaluation tools, plan#5 is the best overall plan. It shows the most acceptable compromise of all issues. It is important to notice that plan#5 would not have been found with the set pre-optimization parameters. It is the ability of the inverse algorithm to modify the pre-optimization parameters to find alternative solutions that gave us access to the best solution.

## Conclusion

The research presented in this paper on inverse treatment planning investigates how it can be better implemented into a clinical setting. We have concluded that a better clinical implementation of inverse treatment planning requires three essential steps. First, the inverse planning algorithm should require few and clinical revelant pre-optimization parameters. Second, the control over the optimization process should belong to the planner/physician. Third, additional plan evaluation tools need to be incorporated for better inverse plan evaluations to aid the planner/physician to better serve the patient.

## References

[1]Ling, C.C., Burman, C., Chui, C.S., LoSasso, T., Mohan, R., Spirou, S., Stein, J., Wu, Q., Kutcher, G.J., Leibel, S., et. al., 1997 Implementation of photon IMRT with dynamic MLC for the treatment of prostate cancer, in The Theory & Practice of Intensity-Modulated Radiation Therapy (ed. Sternick, E.S.) pp.219.

[2]Carol, M.P., Peacock$^{TM}$: 1995 A system for planning and rotational delivery of intensity-modulated fields, Int Jo of Imaging Systems and Technology 6, 56-61.

[3]Shepp L.A., Vardi Y., 1982 Maximum likelihood reconstruction for emission tomography, IEEE Trans. Med. Imaging MI-1 113-121.

[4]Llacer, J., 1997 Inverse radiation treatment planning using the Dynamic Penalized Likelihood Method. Med Phys 24: 1751-64.

[5]Vardi T., Lee D., 1993 From image deblurring to optimal investments: Maximum Likelihood Solutions for positive linear inverse problems J.R. Stat. Soc. B55 pp 569-612.

[6]Emami, B., Lyman, J., Brown, A., Coia, L., Goitein, M., Munzenrider, J.E., Shank, B., Solin, L.J., Wesson, M., 1991 Tolerance of Normal Tissue to Therapeutic Radiation, Int J Radiat Oncol Biol Phys. 21, 109-122.

[7]Lyman, J.T., 1985 Complication probability as assessed from dose volume histograms. Rad Res. 104:S-13 – S-19.

[8]Kutcher, G.J., Burman, C., Brewster, L., Goitein, M., Mohan, R., 1991 Histogram reduction method for calculating complication probabilities for three-dimensional treatment planning evaluations. Int J Radiat Oncol Biol Phys 21: 137-146.

[9]Burman, C., Kutcher, G.J., Emami, B., Goittein, M., 1991 Fitting of normal tissue tolerance data to an analytic function. Int J Radiat Oncol Biol Phys 21: 123-135.

[10]Niemierko, A., 1997 Reporting and analyzing dose distributions: A concept of equivalent uniform dose. Med Phys 24(1): 103-110.

# Incorporating clinical factors in plan optimization

**Daniel McShan, Marc Kessler, and Benedick Fraass**

Department of Radiation Oncology, The University of Michigan, Ann Arbor, Michigan

## Introduction

Numerous clinical factors which are typically ignored in plan optimization can affect the choice of treatment plans or can compromise the realization of a treatment plan over the course of a treatment. For example, plan complexity and time constraints can affect the preference in choice of plans, while factors such as setup errors and organ motion can compromise the resulting delivered dose distribution. In this work, we describe methodologies which allow the investigation of many of these factors as part of a generalized plan optimization system.

## Material and methods

A generalized plan optimization research system (called "UMOpt") has been developed[1-2]. This system includes the ability to script multiple session treatments (Fig. 1) and to optimize a new plan using prior delivered dose distributions.

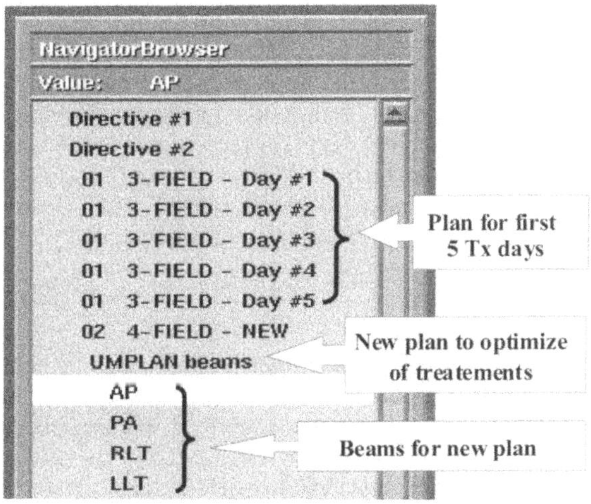


**Figure 1:** Optimization including multiple session treatments

The system allows modification of beam and anatomy geometries on a session by session basis, allowing the system to predict "dose to date" scenerios under actual or simulated conditions. Furthermore, the system utilizes a flexible scoring system based on costlets[1] which has been extended to include other factors (such as treatment delivery time and effort/complexity factors ) for use in ranking treatment plans. The optimization system uses simulated annealing to achieve an optimal solution.

The software has been developed to run on Compaq Alpha OpenVMS systems using the AVS (Advanced Visualization System) graphical framework. The system is developed in a highly modular form using a bulk shared memory allocation scheme for sharing data between modules.

## Results

A number of different clinical issues are important to the overall result which can be obtained with any optimization system. A summary of such issues in shown in Table 1 below.

| Clinical Issue | Reasons for Incorporating into Optimization |
|---|---|
| Geom. uncertainties | Affects dose predictions |
| Treatment efficiency | Would like to achieve most efficient treatments |
| Safety | Need to avoid collision, reduce peripheral rad. |
| Dosim. inaccuracies | Affects dose predictions |
| Biological,clinical model uncertainties | Affects scoring predictions |
| Clinical response feedback | Can necessitate change in target or normal tissue prescription or optimization trade-offs |

**Incorporating geometrical uncertainties.** The inclusion of geometrical uncertainties is non-trivial for plan optimization. In the simplest case, where we know the specifics of the geometrical errors, we can construct the specific geometrical situations and accurately compute the resulting dose distribution and resulting evaluation scores. Within the UMOpt system, anatomy is represented through a point sample distribution which can be geometrically transformed according the known error predictions. Even under the influence of distortions this method will work provided we assume that volume is conserved and that the anatomy moves in a stable connected fashion. In most situations, however, there are at best only estimates of the uncertainties. For this situation, we have begun investigation of various techniques ranging from convolutions which smear out the dose sampled by each region of interest to "Monte Carlo" algorithms which directly simulate dose delivery over an entire treatment course by sampling configurations for each planned fraction[4,5].

**Treatment efficiency.** The initial model used for treatment efficiency is the minimization of estimated treatment delivery time. Time estimates are included in the optimization using a costlet[1] (a component of the cost function) which is a function of treatment delivery time. The shape and importance of this costlet's response are defined by parameters, including acceptable treatment time (which can be defined by summarizing treatment times (by site) for patient treatments). The costlet thus involves a constraint on time as well as a cost which pushes the result towards shorter times and penalizes extremely complex plans which require long treatment times.

**Time/fractionation.** Incorporation of explicit treatment schedules into the optimization framework is needed to consider time-dose-fractionation issues. The initial method to be used makes use of the linear quadratic model (the most commonly accepted method for fractionation effects). Several methods for specifying time and fraction size will be explored. The most flexible of these is to define each individual fraction and specify the relative time of delivery and fraction size, however, if other factors remain constant then the computation of bio-effective doses involving a fixed fractionation schedule does not require calculation of each individual fraction. This simplification may not, however, be appropriate when motion or other issues are considered.

**Safety.** Safety concerns always play a role, often implicit, in plan optimization. Concerns range from collision to peripheral dose effects. Collision issues are handled in UMOpt with an optimization loop step which performs a configuration check of each new proposed solution to make sure the solution is viable. This includes checking for possible or near collisions between gantry, table or patient based on vendor-specific machine models[3]. Other safety issues like peripheral dose concerns will be also be studied. Since few calculational algorithms calculate leakage, electron contamination or peripheral doses accurately, if at all, at long distances from the target, then sensitive organs (lens, testes, etc.) may need special dose-volume assessments to help the optimization properly avoid those structures.

**Dosimetric inaccuracy.** Calculated dosimetric predictions are typically only accurate to between 1 and 3 percent of the maximum predicted dose, and can often be much worse in interfaces or difficult geometries. Since all calculational algorithms make speed-accuracy trade-offs, the system uses several methods to incorporate these inaccuracies, including an error map to correct the dose before scoring or to modify particular costlet weights or calculations. Error maps to be studied include 1) a map of general calculational error estimates which change with depth, intensity gradients, patient density or geometry changes, 2) a map composited from individual beam-oriented error maps, and 3) intermittently performing a higher accuracy calculation to create specific error maps.

**Biological/clinical model uncertainties.** Biological models and their parameters are probably the least exact factors included in the optimization process. The uncertainties in these estimates introduce confidence limits into the costlet function outputs which can be used to terminate optimization loops. One method for incorporate of these uncertainties is explicit mathematical error propagation, but numerical estimates of errors will be investigated as well. Ultimately, model estimates must include confidence limits and the optimization control will use those confidence limits in the control of the optimization: it will provide cut-off limits for optimization loops, and variance analysis may make it possible to more quickly achieve a solution.

**Clinical response feedback.** In some cases, prescription/plan changes are required due to clinical responses of the patient (e.g., inflation of a collapsed lung, tumor shrinkage, decreasing blood counts forcing protection of bone marrow). Optimization in such cases is challenging due to possibly dramatic changes in volumes and positions. Two general classes of issues are expected: 1) a significant change in anatomical basis for the plan, where a new imaging study would be used to define the new geometry, followed by the use of geometry warping techniques, and 2) a clinical response which forces a change in the optimization directive (basic anatomy remains constant). In both situations, the optimization system must support the anatomic and dosimetric compositing of the various situations, as well as analysis which takes into account the fractionation and anatomy distortion issues.

## Discussion

A challenge to fully automating the planning of radiotherapy is to develop plans which are not only optimized but also are realizable and practical in the clinic. Most current systems for optimization do not include a number of clinically relavent factors, thus leading to plans which are unrealistically optimized. For example, geometrical uncertainities in the form of daily patient setup errors as well as organ motion may substantially degrade the optimality of a given plan. This is particularly true in situations involving nearby normal tissue structures. Since the effects of geometrical errors on a given plan will depend on the specific beam arrangements, some beam arrangements may be less prone to geometrical uncertainties and those plans may be preferable to what would be achieved using a plan that has been optimized based on a static representation of the anatomy. A great deal of work studying these issues will be required to fully incorporate all these issues into routine clinical plan optimization.

## Summary

We have described a new research system that will be used to investigate the incorporation of important clinical factors into automated plan optimization. We hypothesize that these considerations will lead to the development of treatment plans which are more optimal within the constraints of clinical realities. Clearly not all factors will represent the same degree of importance or influence on the choice of plans and a carefull analysis of the dependencies on treatment site, treatment techniques, and levels of technology must be included.

## References


1. ML Kessler, JJH Kim, DL McShan, BA Fraass: A general framework for interactive and automated treatment plan optimization, part I: evaluators, modifiers, and costlets. Med Phys **25**: [Abstract], 1998.
2. DL McShan, BA Fraass, ML Kessler: Intensity modulation using beamlets. Med Phys 25: A149, 1998 [Abstract].
3. ML Kessler, DL McShan, BA Fraass: A computer-controlled conformal radiotherapy system. III: Graphical simulation and monitoring of treatment delivery. *International Journal of Radiation Oncology, Biology, Physics* **33**: 1173-80, 1995.
4. Lujan AE, Larsen EW, Balter JM, Ten Haken RK: A method for incorporating organ motion due to breathing into 3D dose calculations. *Med Phys* **26**:715-720, 1999.
5. Lujan AE, Ten Haken RK, Larsen E, Balter JM: Quantization of setup uncertainties in 3D dose calculations. *Med Phys*, in press, 1999.

# Microboost treatment of prostate tumors

**U.A. van der Heide, A.J. Nederveen, P. Hofman, J.J. Welleweerd and J.J.W. Lagendijk**

Department of Radiotherapy, University Medical Center, Heidelberglaan 100, 3584 CX Utrecht, the Netherlands.

## Introduction

Intensity modulated radiation therapy (IMRT) is considered a technique that will significantly enhance the quality of patient treatment in the near future. In our clinic we started the introduction of IMRT using commercially available inverse planning software (PLATO, Nucletron, Veenendaal, NL) and a linear accelerator with a multi-leaf collimator (SL25, Elekta Oncology Systems, Crawley UK.) that can be operated in dynamic and step-and-shoot mode. Our goal is to apply IMRT routinely for the dose escalation in prostate tumors, which affects a large group of patients in the clinic. This is motivated by the observation that dose escalation in the prostate leads to improved local control [1]. IMRT is crucial in achieving dose escalation in the tumor without increasing the level of normal tissue complications.

The conformal treatment of prostate tumors is complicated by uncertainties in the target position: Firstly, the position of the prostate varies relative to the bony anatomy from day to day Secondly, the location of tumor cells within and outside the prostate is very difficult when only CT images are available. We intend to address the first aspect of this problem by EPID imaging of opaque markers implanted in the prostate [2–5] using an a-Si flat panel imager. This guarantees that the position of the prostate is known at the start of each field. Localization of tumor cells can be improved when different imaging modalities are combined (CT, MRI, PET). In the absence of such information we treat the whole prostate as the target for dose escalation.

In this report we focus on the development of an IMRT plan for dose escalation. We use the fact that the current treatment practice leads to an acceptable low level of complications so that dose reduction in organs at risk is not a prime goal. The key element in our approach is the escalation of the dose inside the target while leaving the dose outside the target unchanged compared to current treatments [6]. A higher dose outside the target could result in complications in normal tissue, while a lower dose may compromise the control at the periphery of the tumor.

With this microboost approach we combine the benefits of the current treatment, where a fixed margin around the target is treated, with the enhanced probability of local control in the boost volume.

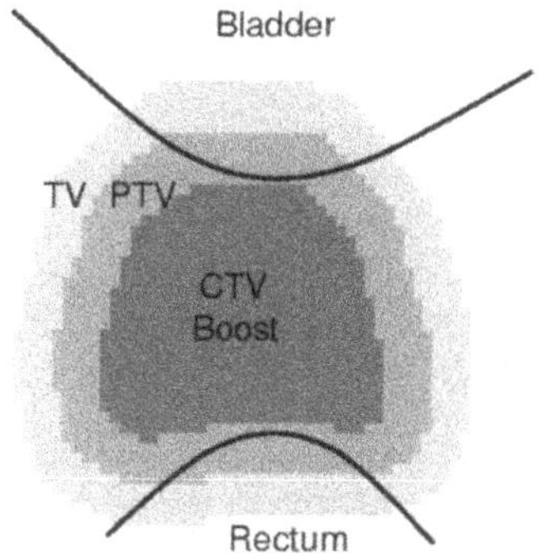


**Figure 1:** Outline of target and critical organs.

## Material and methods

On a CT the target and critical organs are outlined by the clinician (see Figure 1). The CTV includes the prostate, with seminal vesicles and microscopic intrusions. In addition, a boost volume is drawn, that coincides with the prostate without the seminal vesicles. Finally the rectum and bladder are delineated. An additional contour is generated automatically in 3D at 8 mm around the CTV. The 8 mm margin represents the planning target volume PTV. A treatment plan is generated using the PLATO planning system (Nucletron, Veenendaal, Netherlands) and its inverse treatment planning module ITP. The latter is a commercially available version of the KonRad program, developed by the Bortfeld group [7]. The ITP module optimizes the fluence for a fixed beam geometry to obtain a dose distribution that best fits a series of dose constraints. For the target volumes a maximum and minimum dose are specified, for organs at risk a maximum dose. The relative weight of these constraints is manipulated with so called 'penalties'.

The treatment currently in use in the clinic is a three-field technique with an open AP field and two lateral opposing wedge fields. Fifty Gy is delivered in 25 fractions with the field boundaries set at 15 mm around the prostate in beam's eye view. For the 20 Gy boost (in the last 10 fractions) the rectum near the seminal vesicles are blocked, leading to a reduction of the rectum dose. This technique results in a homogeneous dose of 70 Gy inside the boost volume, falling to about 35 Gy towards the field boundaries at a 15 mm distance. Between 10 and 20% of the rectum receives a dose higher than 66 Gy, while the maximum dose is 70 Gy.

To date we are investigating what beam geometry (number of beams, beam angles) and which number of intensity levels in the fluence are minimally required to get an IMRT plan that matches our requirements. Here we present first results with a three-beam geometry (gantry angles 0, 100 and 260°), with dynamic delivery of the fluence (effectively giving an infinite number of intensity levels in the fluence).

## Results and discussion

The microboost plan intends to mimic the dose distribution of the current plan, while escalating the dose to the boost volume to 80 Gy. Thus, a dose of 70 to 80 Gy is required in the boost volume and a dose of 66 to 70 Gy to the remainder of the PTV. In the current treatment plans the dose falls off to 35 Gy towards the field boundaries set at 15 mm around the CTV. In order to achieve such a gradual decline in dose, a new contour is generated in 3D at 15 mm around the CTV. This margin is referred to as the treated volume (TV) (see Figure 1). The dose is allowed to fall off from 66 at the boundary of the PTV to 35 Gy towards the outside in the rest of the TV. Bladder and rectum overlap with the PTV and TV. However, they don't overlap with the boost volume. Thus, if the constraints on PTV and TV outside the boost volume are met, the risk of overdosage in rectum and bladder is also averted. Therefore, we don't include constraints for these organs at risk in the inverse planning procedure.

In Figure 2 the dose-volume histograms for a current treatment plan (dashed curves) and the microboost plan (solid curves) are compared. The CTV in the microboost plan (Figure 2a) receives a dose of up to 80 Gy, while the conventional plan shows a homogeneous dose of 70 Gy. Note that the seminal vesicles are not included in the boost volume, leading to a dip in the DVH of the CTV for the microboost plan. In Figure 2b the dose volume histograms are shown for the shell of PTV around the CTV, and the shell of TV around the PTV. For the PTV the DVH for both plans is comparable. This demonstrates that the dose escalation is indeed limited to the CTV. The dose in the shell of treated volume TV around the PTV (between 8 and 15 mm around the CTV) lies between 30 and 68 Gy in the microboost plan, while the current plan shows a slightly broader dose distribution. Although these distributions are not the same, the gradual decline in dose is clearly reproduced in the microboost plan.

The DVH for the rectum is again virtually identical in both plans. This corroborates the claim that the dose constraint for the rectum can be met through the constraints on the PTV and TV shells. We consider this a valuable property of this treatment plan. It provides a way to circumvent the complication that the position and shape of the rectum (and bladder) exhibit large variations from day to day. Nevertheless one must assume that the anterior wall of the rectum stays in close contact with the prostate despite the internal motions. Consequently, it is important to ensure that the dose of 80 Gy in the boost volume is not in fact delivered outside this volume as a result of set-up errors and internal motions. Thus a robust system for position verification of the prostate is required.

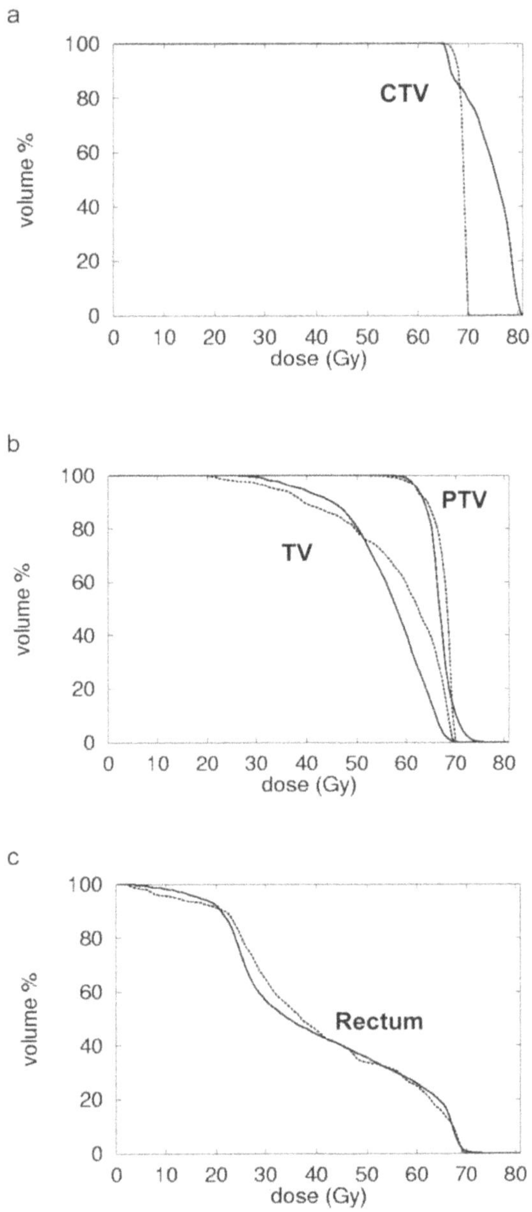


**Figure 2:** Dose-volume histograms for current treatment plan (dashed lines) and microboost plan (solid lines)

## Acknowledgements

This study is supported by Nucletron, Veenendaal NL, and Elekta Oncology Systems, Crawley, UK.

## References

[1] Zelefsky M J et al. 1998 Dose escalation with three-dimensional conformal therapy affects the outcome in prostate cancer *Int. J. Radiat. Oncol. Biol. Phys* **41** 491–500.

[2] Beard J B et al. 1996 Analysis of prostate and seminal vesicle motion implications for treatment planning *Int. J. Radiat. Oncol. Biol. Phys* **34** 451–458.

[3] van Herk M et al. 1995 Quantification of organ motion during conformal radiotherapy of the prostate by three dimensional image registration *Radiother. Oncol* **37** 35-42.

[4] Balter M B et al. 1995 Automated localization of the prostate at the time of treatment using implanted radiopaque markers: technical feasibility *Int. J. Radiat. Oncol. Biol. Phys* **33** 1281–1286.

[5] Nederveen A J et al. 1999 Detection of fiducial gold markers for automatic on-line megavoltage position verifaction using a marker extraction kernel (MEK), *submitted to Int. J. Radiat. Oncol. Biol. Phys.*

[6] Lagendijk J J W and Hofman P 1999 The microboost concept for the improvement of local control of solid tumors *Radth. Oncol.* **51** S2.

[7] Bortfeld T and Schlegel W 1993 Optimization of beam orientations in radiation therapy: some theoretical considerations. *Phys. Med. Biol.* **38** 291–304.

# Application of some regularization methods to the radiosurgery inverse problem

**Pascal Grandjean, Dimitri Lefkopoulos, Catherine Dejean, Hanna El-Balaa, Fredéric Julia and Michel Schlienger**

Tenon hospital - radiation-oncology department - 4 rue de la Chine 75020

## Introduction

The calculated dose distribution $D$, can be expressed in the abbreviated operator form : $M \; W = D$ (1)

This problem (eq. 1) may be considered as an inverse problem in which $M$ represents the dose kernel, $D$ represents the prescribed conformational dose distribution and $W$ is the unknown weighting of the elementary beams. In other words, we must find which weight of each minibeam (elementary beams ) has to be used when the desired dose distribution is to be achieved ? However, this problem is in general ill-posed for several reasons :

1. The problem has no exact solution. So, the aim is modified to that of delivering a specified high dose to the target volume and as low a dose as possible elsewhere.

2. In the discretization procedure (the number of beams $NB$ and the number of dose points $NPD$) may lead to an ill-conditioned matrix $M$. Any attempt to solve the system directly, e.g by Gaussian elimination, is likely to produce an oscillatory solution or poor approximations of eq. (1).

3. The effects of round-off error in numerical computations lead to highly oscillatory behaviour.

To obtain meaningful approximation, one has to resort to a "filtering" process or a regularization method. A regularization method replaces an ill-posed problem by an associated well-posed problem provided this analysis yields physically acceptable approximations to the given ill-posed problem. The purpose of this work is to study four regularization methods from the viewpoint of filtering in the singular system [1] : (i) the singular value decomposition truncation (SVDT), (ii) the Twomey-Tikhonov (TT), (iii) the iterative Landweber (LND) and (iv) the iterative Twomey-Tikhonov (ITT) methods. This analysis in the singular system has the advantage to provide a quantitative procedure of studying the effects of iterative techniques.

## Material and methods

### The radiosurgery irradiation system

The stereotactic radiosurgery is carried out with a linear accelerator generating minibeam X-rays of 15 MV. We add circular collimators which produce fields of 6 mm to 20 mm diameter in steps of 2 mm at the isocenter. We use a Talairach stereotactic frame and a Betti chair. This work is not limited to our stereotactic irradiation device but could be applied to all stereotactic systems (Gamma Knife, Linac with lying and sitting position).

### The radiosurgery irradiation modelization

The discretized representation of the stereotactic irradiation space is represented as a half-sphere situated in the superior half of the cranium; the half sphere center is situated to the linac isocenter which coincides with the subvolume center. It is covered by 19 irradiation plans passing through the Right-Left axis of the stereotactic system and varying from $\phi$ = -90° (Posterior) to $\phi$ = +90° (Anterior) with an angular sampling of 10°. Each arc, discretized in 19 minibeams, is defined by the rotation of 180° of the linear accelerator from $\theta$ = -90° (Right) to $\theta$ = +90° (Left).

The calculation of a mono-isocentric dose in a 3-D matrix situated inside the head of the patient can be written by the following linear equations system:

$$D_i = \sum_{j=1}^{NB} M_{i,j} W_j \quad \text{for i} = 1 \text{ to } NDP \qquad (2)$$

where $D_i$ is the dose value computed in the voxel $i$ and $W_j$ the j[th] minibeam weighting.

### Description of the regularization methods into the singular system

$M$ is a real $NDP \; x \; NB$ matrix decomposed into two orthogonal bases [1] $U = [u_1, \cdots, u_{NDP}] \in \Re^{NDPxNDP}$ and $V = [v_1, \cdots, v_{NB}] \in \Re^{NBxNB}$ such that :

$$U^T MV = diag(\sigma_1, \cdots, \sigma_r) \in \Re^{NDPxNB} \text{ with } r = \min\{NDP, NB\} \qquad (3)$$

$\sigma_1 \geq \sigma_2 \geq \cdots \geq \sigma_r \geq 0$ are the singular values of $M$. $u_1, \cdots, u_{NDP}$ and $v_1, \cdots, v_{NB}$ are the left and right singular vectors. The singular vectors $(u_n, v_n)$ associated with large values are characterized as high order singular components.

The condition number $CN$ characterizes quantitatively the ill-conditionning of the matrix and is defined as follows :

$$CN = \frac{\sigma_1}{\sigma_p} \quad \text{with } CN \geq 1 \quad \text{and } \sigma_p \neq 0 \qquad (4)$$

When the problem is ill-conditioned, well conditioned or perfectly conditioned, $CN$ is respectively large, small or 1.

In Radiosurgery, we have observed that high order singular vectors are high frequency vectors [2-4]. One way of avoiding these situations is to impose a smoothness requirement which would have the effect of filtering out the oscillatory contributions from the high frequency singular functions. The four presented regularization techniques can be represented as a filter $F$ over the singular components as follows :

$$W_N = \sum_{n=1}^{N} F(regul.param.)\frac{1}{\sigma_n}\langle D,u_n\rangle v_n\ ,\ N=1,\cdots,NB \quad (5)$$

The filters $F$ and the corresponding regularization parameters are presented in table 1. The principal advantage of this analysis, is that it provides a quantitative procedure of studying the effects of iterative methods and designs the filter which after a finite number of iterations $k$ achieves a suitable effect. $N$, $\beta$, $\gamma_{TT}$ , $\gamma_{ITT}$ and $k$ are the regularization parameters.

| Method | Filter |
|---|---|
| SVDT | $F_{SVDT}(\alpha,\sigma_n) = \begin{cases} 1, \sigma_n^2 \geq \alpha \\ 0, \sigma_n^2 < \alpha \end{cases}$ |
| TT | $F_{TT}(\gamma_{TT},\sigma_n) = \frac{\sigma_n^2}{\sigma_n^2 + \gamma_{TT}}\quad ,\sigma_n^2 + \gamma_{TT} \neq 0$ |
| LND | $F_{LND}(\beta,k,\sigma_n) = 1-(1-\beta\sigma_n^2)^k$ |
| ITT | $F_{ITT}(\gamma_{ITT},k,\sigma_n) = 1-\left(\frac{\gamma_{ITT}}{\gamma_{ITT}+\sigma_n^2}\right)^k$ |

**Table 1:** The singular component filter of four presented techniques.

## Results and discussion

**The studied experimentations**
In this work, we investigated the number of dose points $NDP$ so as to obtain a compromise between computation times and the quality of the reconstructed solutions. $NDP$ depends on the dimension of the dose matrix size $MS$ and the dose voxel size $VS$. So, we studied the following different configurations : $MS$=$64^3$ $mm^3$ with $VS$=1, 2, 4 and 8 mm (spelled respectively M1, M2, M3 and M4) as well as $VS$=2 mm with $MS$=80, 64, 32 and $24^3$ $mm^3$ (spelled respectively M5, M2, M6 and M7). The 20 mm diameter collimator was used to obtain more ill-conditioned M matrices. The number of minibeam $NB$ was 361 (19 arcs x 19 minibeams per arc).

**The SVD analysis**
In table 2, we observe that the condition number $CN$ was found minimal for the M2 configuration ($MS$=$64^3$ $mm^3$, $VS$=2mm) whereas it increases considerably for under-sampling configurations (M4) and slightly for over-sampling configurations (M1 and M5). The general behavior of the singular values specter and singular vector are presented in previous articles [2,4].

| M1 | M2 | M3 | M4 | M5 | M6 | M7 |
|---|---|---|---|---|---|---|
| 58204 | 10783 | 16352 | 5,32E6 | 65553 | 15256 | 24062 |

**Table 2 :** Condition number $CN$ for different $MS$ and $VS$ sizes.

**The dose prescription**
$D$ represents the desired dose distribution generated by the lesion 3-D matrix in a practical case. The lesion voxels are set to 100% and the outside lesion voxels to 0%. $D$ can be also the Previsional Dose Matrix (PDM) calculated from a well know Previsional Weighting Vector (PWV) as it is in this experimentation. This test procedure permits to easily compare different algorithms. The PWV used for the experimental configurations simulates the irradiation of an elliptic lesion oriented to 15° left and 25° anterior.

**Comparative study of differents regularization algorithms**
The accuracy of the solutions $W^*$ reconstructed by the regularization algorithms is measured by the quantity :

$$\delta = \left(\frac{\sum_{j=1}^{NB}\left(PWV_j - W_j^*\right)^2}{NB}\right)^{\frac{1}{2}} \quad (6)$$

In table 3, we present the minimal $\delta$ for the 4 techniques SVDT, TT, LND and ITT after varying the regularization parameters. Negative weights are truncated to zero because negative dose are not permitted. However, the number of negative weights and their amplitude were found small in amplitude. The importance of the negative weigths increases with the increasing of the number of singular components taking into account in the computation of the solution.

| | M1 | M2 | M3 | M4 | M5 | M6 | M7 |
|---|---|---|---|---|---|---|---|
| SVDT | 9.56 | 8.67 | 12.90 | 17.80 | 8.17 | 15.50 | 19.61 |
| TT | 7.16 | 7.54 | 11.98 | 15.01 | 6.77 | 14.22 | 17.03 |
| LND | 7.70 | 9.62 | 12.93 | 14.89 | 7.19 | 14.69 | 17.53 |
| ITT | 7.72 | 8.01 | 12.39 | 14.74 | 7.04 | 14.64 | 17.51 |

**Table 3 :** Optimum reconstruction errors $\delta$opt x 100 for the different dose kernels and algorithms SVDT, TT, LND and ITT.

The results obtained with the four techniques show that the minimal error $\delta$ is found for a large matrix size and a voxel size $VS$=1mm or 2 mm (configurations M1, M2 and M5). Slight better results are obtained for the modulated filters (techniques TT, LND and ITT) compared to the rectangular filter (technique SVDT). This is more true when the dose space is over-sampled or under-sampled. However, taking into account the convergence of a great number of minibeams in one point this improvement is considered small when the dose distribution is computed. So, we can consider that the four techniques gives similar results for our application. However, are similar the filters corresponding to the 4 techniques ?

In figure 1, we present the singular component filters corresponding to the four techniques only for the configurations M2, M4 and M5. We have observed that the filters generated for the different techniques are similar for any studied configurations. The intersection of the TT, LND and ITT filters is around 50% with the SVDT filter except for the M5 and M7 configurations. All these configurations show that regularization is needed as the last singular components are removed or weakly weigthed to obtain an acceptable solution. For information, the error $\delta \times 100$ increases up to about 60% for all the configurations when all the singular components are considered.

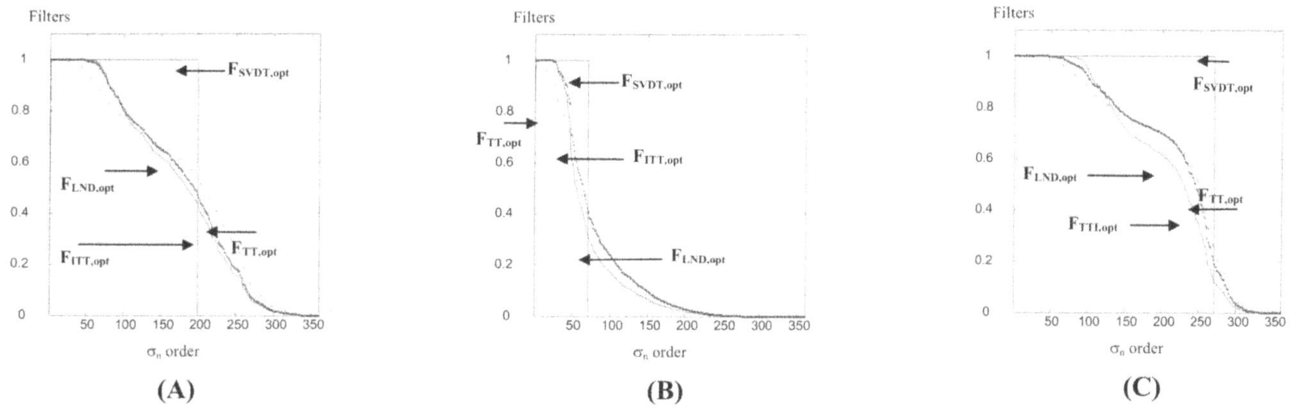


**Figure 1 :** The optimal filters corresponding to the SVDT, TT, LND, ITT techniques : **(A)** M2 kernel ; **(B)** M4 kernel and **(C)** M5 kernel.

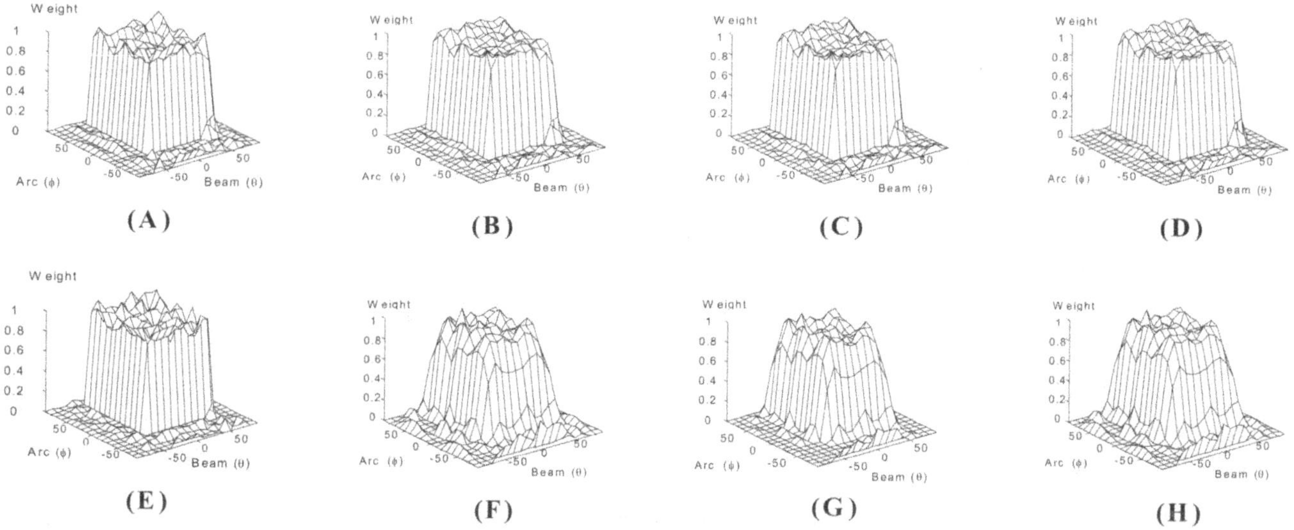


**Figure 2 :** The optimal reconstructed weighting vectors (RWV) corresponding to the 4 techniques : **(A-D)** M2 kernel using the SVDT, TT, LND and ITT techniques respectively; **(E-H)** M4 kernel using the SVDT, TT, LND and ITT techniques respectively.

In figure 2, we can observe similar reconstructed solutions close to the PWV between the four techniques for the configurations M2 and M4. However, we note that for the configurations M3, M4, M6 and M7 the solutions contain oscillations for the zero weight areas and the limits of the unit weight area is ill reconstructed.

## Conclusion

We have studied qualitatively and quantitatively the behavior of the different filters as function of their smoothing parameters *N*, *β*, $\gamma_{TT}$ , $\gamma_{ITT}$ and the quantitative effect on the solution accuracy for different dose space samplings. The M2 configuration seems to be a compromise between computations time (depending on the number of dose points *NPD*) and the reconstruction quality. However in real cases, the matrix size *MS* can be adjusted to the size of the target to be irradiated taking into account a surrounding margin to protect organs at risks and healthy tissues. The M2 configuration is used for real cases [2] and gives good results. The four techniques have shown their capacity to give acceptable approximations solution and their adaptability to our problem.

## References

[1] Strand O. N. 1974 Theory and methods related to the singular function expansion and Landweber's iteration for integral equation of the first kind. *SIAM J. Numer. Anal.* **11** 798-825

[2] Grandjean P., Platoni K., Lefkopoulos D., Merienne L. and Schlienger M. 1998 Use of a general inverse technique for the conformational stereotactic treatment of complex intra-cranial lesions. *Int. J. Radiat. Oncol. Biol. Phys.* **41**. 69-76

[3] Grandjean P. 1998 Optimisation de la distribution de dose en radiothérapie conformationnelle basée sur l'analyse en valeurs singulières (SVD) (University René Descartes - Paris V) PhD Doctoral Thesis.

[4] Lefkopoulos D., Grandjean P., Laouar A. and Schlienger M. 1995 Study of the ill-conditionning of a radiosurgical irradiation space using the singular value decomposition. *Int. J. of Imaging Science and technology* **6** 104-113

# Modelling the Effects of IMRT Delivery: Constraints and Incorporation of Beam Smoothing into Inverse Planning

**Joao Seco, Phil M. Evans and Steve Webb**

Joint Department of Physics, Institute of Cancer Research and Royal Marsden Hospital, NHS Trust, Downs Road, Sutton, UK
Email: joao@icr.ac.uk

## Introduction

The problem of obtaining the optimal treatment plan parameters (such as type and energy of radiation, number and direction of beams, intensity profiles etc) for a prescribed dose distribution in radiotherapy is designated as the inverse problem. As indicated in [1], with the emphasis on obtaining the optimum intensity modulated beams (IMB), many inverse planning systems have ignored constraints applied to the *functional form of the IMBs themselves*.

There are various reasons why smooth IMBs may be preferable to non-smoothed/unconstrained IMBs [1]: (i) they may be less sensitive to patient movement, (ii) they may be more favourable to the DMLC delivery technique, (iii) they may be preferred on the physchological basis that they are 'less unlike conventional open or wedge fields' and thus represent a smaller paradigm shift. Additionally, smoothed inverse planning can also be advantageous to static MLC, compensator, and possibly other delivery techniques, since leaf/collimator leakage, beam-on time and number of IMB sub-fields may be reduced.

The present study reports the effects of the MIMiC delivery constraints and beam smoothing on inverse planning for a prostate tumour. The technique modelled in this paper builds on previous work [1], developed for the NOMOS MIMiC, where a static-mode delivery of 9 coplanar beams was used.

The inverse problem of obtaining the optimum IMBs, for the prostate tumour site, was customized to the MIMiC static-mode delivery technique via an interpreter, which was applied to the IMBs during the optimization calculation every certain number of iteration events. The interpreter would generate a new, customized, dose matrix from which the simulation would proceed. For every other event, the beam bixels would be delivered considering them as independent single bixels.

After analysing how the NOMOS MIMiC interpreter influences the optimum IMBs solution, the effects of applying a smoothing median window filter (MWF) synchronized and non-synchronized with the delivery interpreter was studied.

## Material and methods

The study was performed for a prostate patient using an "in-house"-developed IMRT program customized, via an interpreter, to the NOMOS MIMiC delivery technique. The interpreter was based on the Dose Calculation in the Peacock Plan [2] manual that accompanies the MIMiC.

The Peacock Plan dose calculation model allows the radiation beam to be geometrically divided into a finite number of finite-size (on the order of 1 x 1 $cm^2$ at the isocentre) smaller pencil beam elements.

The dose calculation algorithm includes the scattering contributions from neighbouring beam bixels to the dose within the primary beam of a single pencil beam. The dose at any point in a single pencil beam, i.e., with all other leaves completely closed, changes when other leaves open. The scatter contribution from multiple adjacent bixels is described by a relative output factor (ROF) at central axis, which increases from 0.85, for a single open bixel, to 1.00, for a 2 x 20 $cm^2$ field. For off-axis open bixels, an additional off-axis ratio is used as defined by Khan *et al* [3] for asymmetric collimators.

The developed IMRT program generates an initial "back-projected" dose matrix and beam intensity profile from which it starts the inverse planning. The initial intensity of each beam bixel is proportional to the number of PTV voxels in its view divided by the maximum value of all the number of PTV voxels viewed by all of the bixels for the various beams (cf. eqn. (1)):

$$\mathbf{I(i_b \in BIXELS\,, b \in BEAMS) = C^* \frac{PTV\ voxels}{MAX(\forall_{i_b\, and\, b} PTV\ voxels)}}\ , \quad (1)$$

where $\mathbf{I(i_b,b)}$ is the intensity of bixel $\mathbf{i_b}$ of beam **b**, **BIXELS** is the set of all the applied bixels per beam, **BEAM** is the set of all the applied beams, **PTVvoxels** is the number of PTV voxels within the view of bixel $\mathbf{i_b}$ of beam **b** and **C** is the proportionality constant. The constant, C, is calculated such that, after delivering all the initial bixel intensities (by considering C=1 in eqn.(1)), the highest dose observed in the PTV region is scaled up to 64 Gy, the dose to be delivered to the PTV, by a factor C.

The IMRT beam intensity modulation optimization is achieved using physical criteria taking the DVH approach described by Bortfeld *et al* [4]. In this approach, DVH constraints are applied to the PTV and OARs regions yielding a global cost function (CF) described by the following equation:

$$\mathbf{CF = \Sigma_k\, w_k\, \Sigma_j\, (C_{[0,\Delta Dk]}\, \{D_{kj} - D^{DVH}{}_k\})^2}\ , \quad (2)$$

where $\mathbf{\Sigma_k}$ represents the sum over the $k^{th}$ VOI with weighting factor $\mathbf{w_k}$, $\mathbf{\Sigma_j}$ represents the sum over the $j^{th}$ voxel within the $k^{th}$-VOI, the $\mathbf{C_{[0,\Delta Dk]}}$ is defined as

$$C_{[a,b]}\{x\} = \begin{cases} x, \text{for} \ldots a \le x \le b \\ 0, \text{for} \ldots \text{otherwise} \end{cases}, \quad (3)$$

and $\mathbf{D}^{\mathbf{DVH}}{}_{\mathbf{k}}$ is a DVH constraint which is applied to the $k^{th}$-VOI, with $\mathbf{\Delta D_k}$ representing the excess dose in relation to this DVH constraint. The optimum IMBs are obtained by minimizing the global cost function described in eqn.(3) assuming that we wish to deliver a dose between 62.5 Gy and 66.0 Gy to the PTV, associated with the relative dose interval of [97.7%,103.1%] (where 100% corresponds to 64 Gy). For all PTV voxels with dose below 62.5 Gy a penalty value of 10 was applied. While for all PTV voxels with dose above 66.0 Gy the applied penalty value was 500.

The analysis of the effects of the NOMOS MIMiC delivery constraints and beam smoothing on inverse planning, with the "in-house" code, was divided into two studies.

Study 1: consisted of studying the influence of the NOMOS MIMiC delivery constraints on inverse planning.

The developed simulation generated optimum IMBs, for different frequencies, at which the MIMiC interpreter was applied. The interpreter was always applied to the initial back-projected beam profile and at frequencies of 1000, 2000, 3000, 4000, 6000 and 12000 events of a total of 12000 events. The patient grid was constituted by 128x128x8 voxels (associated with 8 slices of 128x128 pixels) of 3.89x3.89x5.00 mm$^3$, where the patient was assumed to be in a supine position. A static-mode MIMiC delivery was assumed for 27 applied beams distributed in three groups of 9 coplanar beams. The first group of coplanar beams irradiated the two central CT slices of the patient. While, the remaining groups of coplanar of beams were displaced inferiorly and superiorly of 1 cm, such that two CT slices of patient were irradiated per group. An additional two slices, without the PTV region, were considered on either side of the planning slices to incorporate the effects of scattered dose. The coplanar beams were placed every 40° clockwise starting at 0°, which corresponds to an anterior delivery.

For every iteration, a small random intensity (positive or negative in value) was added to a bixel $\mathbf{i_b}$ of a beam $\mathbf{b}$, both randomly selected. The new bixel intensity was then delivered considering it as a single independent bixel with ROF of 0.85 (scatter factor associated with all neighbouring bixels closed, as described previously).

Study 2: consisted of studying the effects of applying a smoothing MWF synchronized and non-synchronized with the delivery interpreter.

The grid was comprised of 128x128x4 voxels (4 slices of 128x128 pixels) with the same single voxel volume as the previous set-up. There were 9 beams uniformly distributed around the central 2 slices (every 40° clockwise, starting at 0° which correspond to an anterior delivery), with two additional slices placed one either side of the central ones.

In this study, the MIMiC interpreter was applied to the initial "back-projected" beam profile and at a frequency of 2000 events, which was fixed for the whole of study 2. While, the smoothing MWF was applied at frequencies of 500, 800, 1000, 1200, 1500, 2000, 2400, 3000, 4000, 5000, 6000 and 7000 events of a total of 12000 iterations.

The simulation proceeds in a similar fashion to that described in study 1, where each bixel was delivered considering single bixel delivery, except when the MIMiC interpreter is applied. For the smoothing filter the beam intensities were smoothed by a MWF and then delivered considering single bixel delivery.

## Results and discussion

**Study 1:**

The weighted mean dose (MEAN_D) and the standard deviation (SD) were calculated, for each IMRT plan, for the PTV and OARs, and are presented in the following table.

| | **MIMiC Interpreter applied at the following intervals** | | | | | |
|---|---|---|---|---|---|---|
| **MEAN_D ±1 SD** | 1000 | 2000 | 3000 | 4000 | 6000 | 12000 |
| PTV | 63.57 ± 2.11 | 63.58 ± 2.16 | 63.71 ± 2.18 | 63.63 ± 2.11 | 63.21 ± 2.09 | 64.92 ± 2.25 |
| RECTUM | 33.02 ± 14.01 | 34.39 ± 13.77 | 34.05 ± 13.94 | 33.89 ± 14.25 | 33.61 ± 14.23 | 34.95 ± 14.45 |
| BLADDER | 26.15 ± 16.03 | 27.25 ± 16.03 | 27.11 ± 15.86 | 27.20 ± 16.31 | 27.12 ± 15.95 | 28.26 ± 16.45 |
| **%CF** | **1.58** | **3.50** | **9.98** | **10.38** | **8.71** | **>100** |

**%CF = 100 x ($\mathbf{CF_{after}}$-$\mathbf{CF_{before}}$)/$\mathbf{CF_{before}}$**

**Table 1**: The MEAN_D and SD values obtained per run for the PTV and OARs (data values correspond to 12000 iterations for each run with interpreter applied at intervals shown). The **%CF** represents the variation of the CF, before and after applying the final MIMiC interpreter.

The values presented in table 1 indicate that, the mean dose obtained at the end of the simulation, to the PTV and OAR regions, is approximately independent of the interval frequency at which the interpreter is applied. However, the change in the cost function value (described by %CF) varies significantly with the interval frequency at which the interpreter is applied. If the interpreter is applied with a frequency of 12000 events, the mean dose to the PTV and OARs is respectively 2% and 4% higher than the values of all the other frequency intervals. This higher dose delivered to the PTV voxels produces a much higher $\mathbf{CF_{after}}$ value, since some of the voxels are irradiated with dose in excess of 66 Gy (the upper dose PTV-DVH constraint) and therefore, receive a penalty of 500.

The %CF obtained at frequencies of 1000 and 2000 events indicate that a customized inverse plan can be generated without having to apply a delivery interpreter after every iteration. However, the frequency at which the delivery should be applied may depend on the IMRT program used and on the dimensions of the dose space and the bixel space to optimize.

**Study 2:**

Since we are interested in studying the effects of applying a MWF, we have fixed the frequency at which the MIMiC interpreter is applied to 2000 events. In Figure 1, we present the mean dose delivered to the PTV and it's SD for runs of 12000 events and for different frequencies at which the smoothing filter was applied.

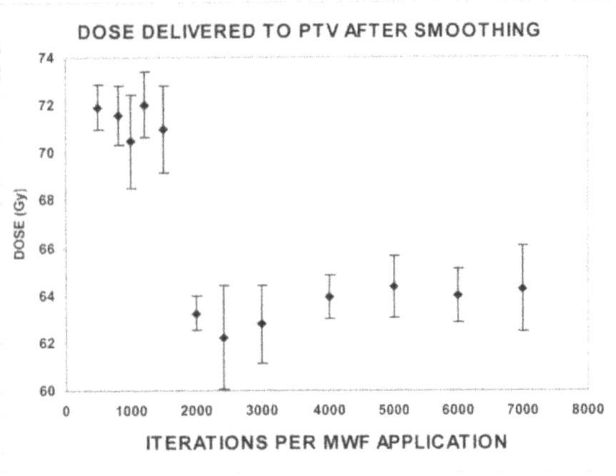


**Figure 1:** The MEAN_D and 1 SD values obtained per run for the PTV (data values correspond to 12000 iterations for each run with interpreter applied every 2000 events and the smoothing filter at frequencies shown).

Figure 1 indicates that, for smoothing filter frequencies below that of the MIMiC interpreter (which in this case is 2000 events) the dose to the PTV does not converge to within the desired dose interval of 62.5-66.0 Gy. If however, smoothing occurs at frequencies greater or equal to that of the MIMiC interpreter, various distinct end situations may occur.

If the smoothing frequency is *synchronized* with the MIMiC interpreter frequency (associated with the 2000 event frequency), the mean dose to the PTV converges to within the dose interval 62.5-66.0 Gy. Furthermore, more than 99% of the total PTV voxels receive a dose with 95% and 107% of the planned 64 Gy dose. If the smoothing filter is *weakly-synchronized* (associated with the 4000 and the 6000 event frequency) with the MIMiC interpreter, the mean dose converges to the PTV and the number PTV voxels within the ICRU limits still exceeds 99% of the total voxels. However, for *partial-synchronization* (associated with the 2400 and 3000 event frequency) or *no-synchronization* (associated with the 5000 and 7000 event frequency) the percentage of the total PTV voxels receiving a dose within the ICRU dose limits drops to the minimum of 75%. Therefore, synchronizing (or weakly-synchronizing) the smoothing frequency with the MIMiC interpreter frequency does not significantly affected the convergence of the inverse plan.

In table 2, the smoothing parameters obtained for the synchronized and weakly-synchronized frequencies are presented. The values correspond to the percentage of bixels which form neighbouring bixel clusters, of size **k**, of approximately equally intensity. For the 2000, 4000 and 6000 smoothing frequencies, the number of adjacent open bixels was increased when compared to the no-smoothed case. This is expected since, many bixels are clustered together into groups of 2, 3 or 4 of, approximately, equal intensity. As expected, the 2000 case yields smoother final IMB intensities, due to the large number of N(k) bixel clusters.

| SMOOTHING PARAMETERS | | | | | |
|---|---|---|---|---|---|
| **SM FREQ. (%)** | N(1) % | N(2) % | N(3) % | N(4) % | N(5) % |
| No smoothing | 96.69 | 3.31 | 0.00 | 0.00 | 0.00 |
| 6000 | 64.46 | 29.75 | 2.48 | 3.31 | 0.00 |
| 4000 | 60.33 | 34.71 | 4.96 | 0.00 | 0.00 |
| 2000 | 59.50 | 24.79 | 12.40 | 3.31 | 0.00 |

**Table 2**: N(k), k=1..5 represents the number of groups of **k** adjacent bixels (on the same line) with there bixel intensity within 0.5% of the mean intensity of all the concerned **k** bixels.

However, there is very little difference between the 2000 and the 4000 cases and even between the 2000 and the 6000. Therefore, further studies are needed, with larger patient set-ups (and consequently with a larger BIXEL/BEAM space), to analyse the main advantages and disadvantages of weakly-synchronizing or synchronizing beam smoothing with the MIMiC interpreter.

## Conclusion

A method of incorporating the delivery constraints into IMRT planning was developed and evaluated, where the MIMiC delivery model was used as a vehicle for the evaluation.

The dose statistics obtained (cf. table 1) for the customized IMRT plan do not change significantly with the delivery constraints, but the cost function does. Further analysis is needed to establish what are the consequences of this strong dependence of the cost function.

For the smoothing MWF study, the synchronization of the delivery technique with the filter was shown to have the advantage of allowing the convergence of the inverse problem. In addition, the smoothing frequency seemed not to affect the end result of the IMRT plan.

We propose to investigate the benefits of applying the planning method, described in the present paper, to other delivery techniques for which they are expected to be more advantageous.

## References

[1]Webb S, Convery DJ and Evans PM 1998 Inverse planning with constraints to generate smoothed intensity-modulated beams *Phys. Med. Biol.* **43** 2785-2794,

[2]Bleier AR, Carol MP, Curran ME, Kania AA, Scherch JD and Sternick ES 1996 Dose Calculation in Peacock Plan, NOMOS Corporation,

[3]Khan FM, Gerbi GJ, Deibel FC 1986 Dosimetry of asymmetric X-ray collimators *Med. Phys.* **13** 936,

[4]Bortfeld T, Stein J and Preiser K 1997 Clinically relevant intensity modulation optimization using physical criteria *Proc. Of the XII. ICCR meeting in Salt Lake City*, 27-30

# Simplification of IMRT intensity maps by means of 1-D and 2-D median-filtering during the iterative calculation

**Andreas Kessen, Karl-Heinz Grosser and Thomas Bortfeld**
DKFZ-Heidelberg, Im Neuenheimer Feld 280, D-69120 Heidelberg

## Introduction

In inverse planning the calculated intensity maps are often not applicable without further modification due to their filigree structure. One well known representative of this phenomenon are the so called "hotspots". This article describes an approach to solve this problem using median-filtering.(cf. [1])

The median filter ist a special case of the rank value filter[2]. The advantage of this non-linear filter operation is the preservation of edges while "hotspots" as well as "blackspots" are cut off and replaced by the median value of their neighbourhood.

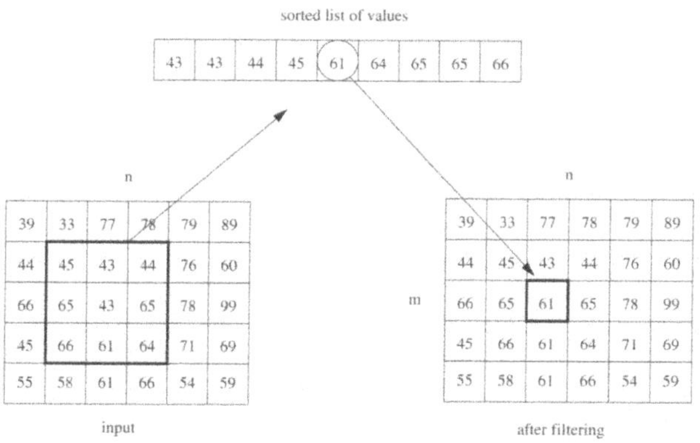


**Figure 1:** 3x3 median filter

## Methods and Materials

We modified the existing KonRad IMRT software to use a median filter which is variable in two dimensions. The filtering takes place after each optimisation step and before the break-condition (improvement of the objective function) is calculated. The algorithm is so flexible that one can even change the size of the filter during the iteration in order to study the response of the system.

Any filter bigger than the trivial filter ($1x1$) will have a problem at the boundary of the fluence map, because the filter laps over border of the intensity map into the undefined area outside. The values outside the intensity map are assumed to contribute no intensity at all and are so set to zero. The application of the "pure" median filter can cause drastic changes in the intensity maps. We had to realize that even the smallest 2-D filter ($3x3$) does cut off too much information so that the convergence was not warranted any more. Therefore, we implemented another slightly different algorithm that is used on all 2-D median filtering described below:

$$I(x,y) = \frac{1}{2}\left(I(x,y) + m(x,y,\delta x,\delta y)\right).$$

Here $m(x,y,\delta x,\delta y)$ is the filtered intensity value at position $x,y$ with the filter width of $\delta x$ and the filter height of $\delta y$. This second algorithm evaluates the median value but then does not substitute the old value with the median value, but takes the average of the median and the old value. By doing this we do not simply cut off the "hotpots", we cut off just half of what could have been cut off. This reduces the effect of the filter and preserves the convergent behaviour of the algorithm.

The data used for the calculation is taken from patients treated in Heidelberg with plans obtained from KonRad. This makes a comparison of filtered and unfiltered intensity maps possible. We tested the filter on Prostate, Mamma and Meningioma patients.

All DVHs and profiles shown in the figures are discretized with five equidistant dose values in order to be applicable with multiple-static MLC-shaped fields.

### When to use median filtering

There are several ways to implement filtering. We tested three filtering sequences described below:

**Median filtering during each iteration step.** For 1-D filters this showed even faster convergence than without a filter. When using a 2-D filter (e.g. $3x3$) the algorithm showed an unpredictable behaviour of alternating values of the objective function which could not lead to any useable result without any further modification of the filter algorithm.

**Intermitted use.** The filter is normally swiched off and just swiched on at special occasions (e.g. every second step in the iteration). The intermitted use results in an alternating value of the objective function. Comparing the objective function value with the previous value normally shows an improvement. Due to filtering the "improvement" is negative. The IMRT-Software normally uses the improvement as a break condition which is now obsolete because of this alternating behaviour.

**Use of the filter at the end of the iteration.** When the filter is used in the final step only, the quality of the result dramatically decreases. The algorithm allowed the buildup of hotspots to get the best possible result. Therefore a lot of information of the solution is "stored" in these points. The median filter then just cuts off this very relevant information.

A direct comparison of the objective function values is shown in figure .

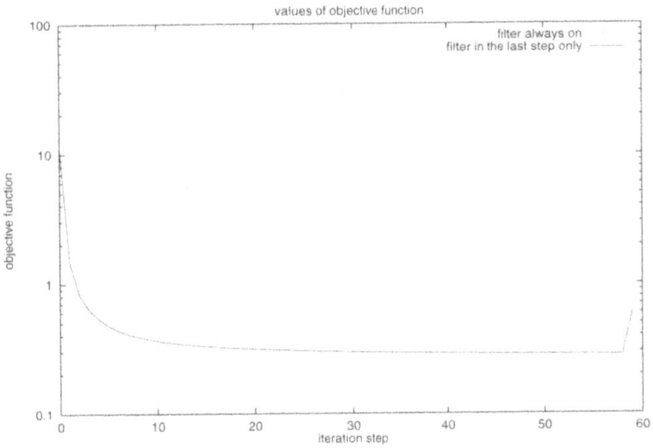


**Figure 2:** comparison of objective function values

### Filter size

When implementing the filter we allowed variable filter sizes as long as they were uneven in both length and width in order to keep the center of the rank-value list well defined. It only took very few tests to realize that a two dimensional filter with more than $3x3$ elements used on a standard resolution fluence map is not useful: We only got large areas in different intensities which led to poor looking DVHs (as shown in figure 4 and 5). In the following we compared the smallest possible 2-D filter ($3x3$) with one dimensional filters ($1x5$), "normal" resolution intensity maps and high-resolution-intensity maps.

When using this filter the resulting fluence maps showed only very few different values, which covered larger areas. The enlargement of the filter lead towards an intensity map that could have been described as a direct projection of the target volume into the map layer with the same intensity. The target function as well as the DVHs we obtained were unusable but showed the effect of the filter in an impressive way and led us to the high resolution fluence maps.

The area filter reduced the number of different intensities in the affected area to almost one. The next logical step was to use a line-filter on a high-resolution intensity map. The MLC leaf positioning allows a resolution down to millimeters in the isocenter layer which is not used in inverse treatment planning because the optimization algorithm normally uses all elements and fills them with the apropriate intensity regardless of the problems in practical application in radiotherapy. By using the line median filter it is possible to reduce the fragmentation of the maps. Using a $2mm$ resolution in leaf-movement-axis while using an $11x1$ filter with the same orientation the smallest structures are still in the order of $1cm$ x $1cm$. But now the boundary is much better adapted to the target.

## Results

The DVHs achieved with filtering using the $11x1$ technique were comparable to the ones without filter and in a few cases even slightly better due to the higher resolution. The following three figures show data of a Meningioma patient.

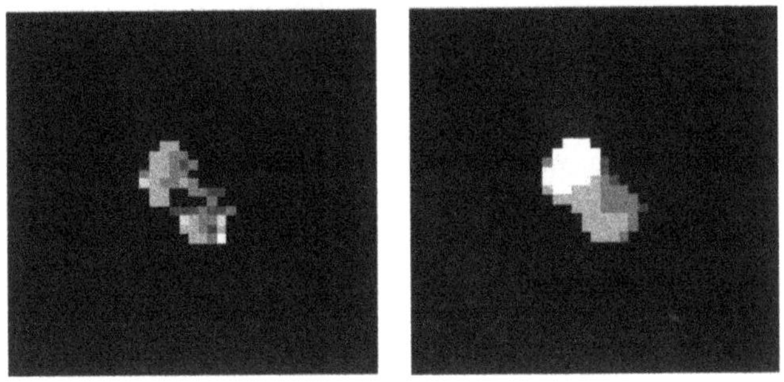

**Figure 3:** Example for the 2-D filter: one beam of a Meningioma patient calculated with and without the 2-D filter. left⇔without any filter; right⇔ with an $3x3$ filter. These fluence maps refer to the DVHs shown in figure 4 and 5

The DVH for the target looks good while the DVH for the organ at risk is not acceptable for the $3x3$ filter.

In figure 6 three fluence maps of a Prostate treatment plan are shown. Even though the grayscale may be unrecognizeable you can still see the margin of the 1-D filtered map is not as angular as the others.

## Discussion

For the application of treatment plans with multiple static flields a segmentation of the intensity maps has to take place. The decisive factor for the minimal number of static fields used for the application is the shape of the intensity distribution of one leaf in an MLC. Each intensity peak has to be irradiated separately. In general a smooth looking distribution needs less static fields and is therefore faster. (see [4] [5],[6])

Secondly the treatment planner can more easily understand and accept the calculated fluence maps because of their simple looking structure.
After filtering there are no unwanted "hotspots" anymore at best there are "hot areas".

One could think of an alternative discretisation routine: the 2-D median filter reduced the number of different intensities in one map, which almost equals a discretisation. These preset intensities could then be taken for the real discretisation. But then the values would not be equidistant anymore which would make the use of existing algorithms

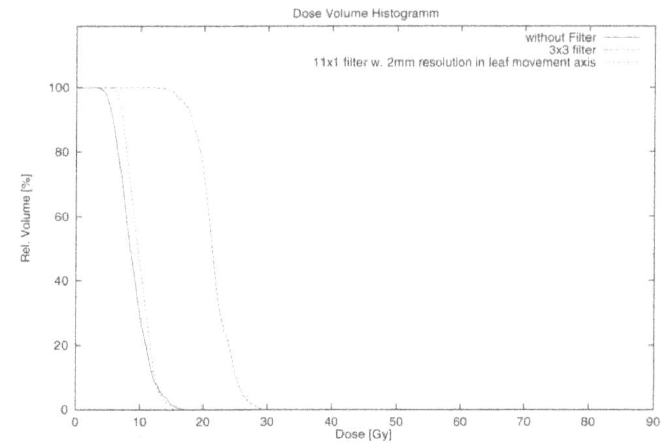


**Figure 4:** Meningioma: DVH for one organ at risk (here: left eye)

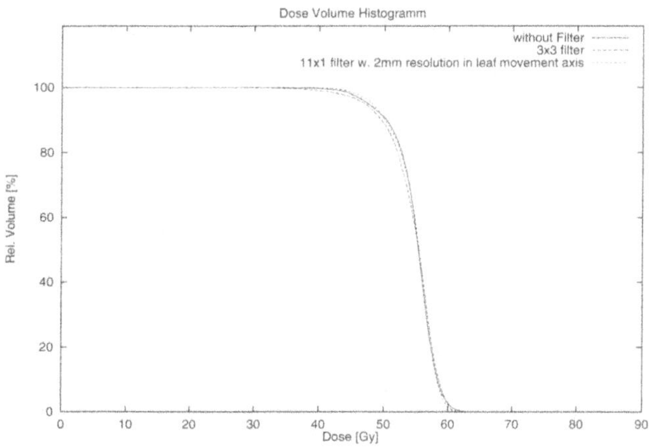


**Figure 5:** Meningioma: DVH for the target volume

for multiple static field treatment obsolete due to their dependence on the equidistance of the intensities.

## Conclusion

We implemented a flexible median filter into an existing planning software and compared different filter dimensions. The median filter should not be used at the end of the optimization, but after each single step to give the algorithm an opportunity to compensate the changes to the fluence map.

Pure 2-D median filters seem to bee unusable beacuse of convergence problems. With a simple odification convergence can be achieved but the the results are worse than without any filter.

We also found that the optimum filter dimensions depend on the specific case.

The number of segments necessary for multiple static field treatment are expected to be lower, because the maps are much smoother. To proove this additional work has to be done. The resulting degree of saved treatment delivery time will be subject of further investigation.

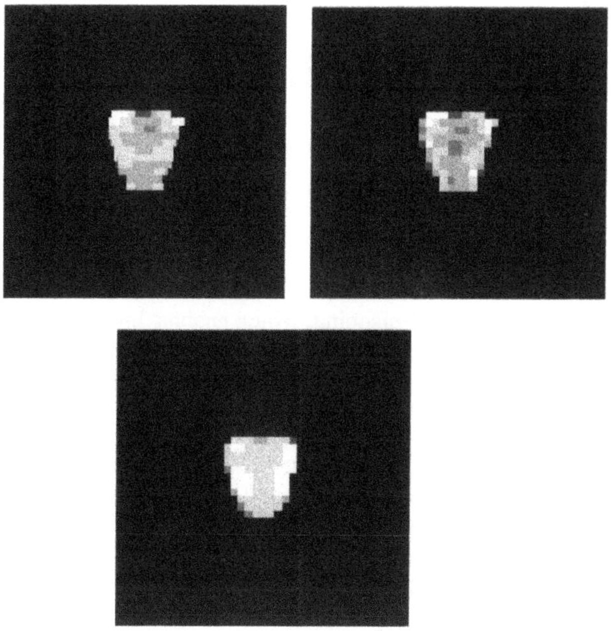

**Figure 6:** Example: One intensity map caculated with different filtering algorithms: top left⇔without any filter; top right⇔with an $11x1$ ; bottom⇔$3x3$ filter

## References


[1] Webb S. 1998, *Inverse planning with constaints to generate smoothed intensity-modulated beams*, Phys. Med. Biol. **43** (1998) 2785-2794

[2] Jähne, Bernd: *Digitale Bildverarbeitung.* Springer Verlag. Heidelberg, 1997.

[3] S. Spirou, S.A. Leibel, T. LoSasso, R. Mohan, T. Bortfeld, L. Reinstein, C.C. Ling, H.W. X., C. Burman, W. Qiuwen, C.S. Chui, M. Zelefsky,G.J. Kutcher, Z. Fuks,*Conformal radiation treatment of prostate cancer using inversely-planned intensity-modulated photon beams produced with dynamic multileaf collimation*

[4] Thomas R. Bortfeld, Darren L. Kahler, Timothy J. Waldron and Arthur L. Boyer *X-ray field compensation with multileaf collimators* Int. J. Radiation Oncology Biol. Phys. **28** No.3 pp 723-730,1994

[5] Que Q, *Comparison of algorithms for multileaf collimator field segmentation*, Med.Phys. 1999;26:2390-2396

[6] Siochi, R A C: *Minimizing static intensity modulation delivery time using an intensity solid paradigm*,Int J Rad. Oncol. Biol. Phys. 1999;43:671-680.

# Errors in inverse treatment planning based on inaccurate dose calculation

**Robert Jeraj**[1] **and Paul Keall**[2]

[1]Jožef Stefan Institute, Ljubljana, Slovenia and [2]Medical College of Virginia, Richmond, VA, USA

## Introduction

Inverse treatment planning, which enables intensity modulated radiation treatment (IMRT), is quickly entering into clinical practice. One of the key ingredients of any inverse, as well as conventional treatment planning systems, is the used dose calculation algorithm. Ideally, the dose calculation algorithm should be accurate and fast; however, there is always some trade off between accuracy and speed. Most of the current inverse treatment algorithms use fast dose calculation algorithms, usually based on pencil beam or convolution/superposition approach [1-4]. These algorithms work well for many clinical cases, but there are some examples where systematic errors of several percent may occur [5,6]. On the other hand, Monte Carlo based dose calculations are known for their accuracy, but they are also burdened with some statistical error, which introduces different type of problems [7].

The main aim of this study was to identify the errors in inverse treatment planning caused with the use of an inaccurate dose calculation algorithm and to determine the magnitude of the errors for the convolution/superposition type of dose calculation on different clinical examples and using different objectives.

## Material and methods

Errors of the non-Monte Carlo based dose calculation algorithms can be determined either comparing the calculations to an experiment or to Monte Carlo calculations. Because comparison to the experiment is not always possible, especially not for real clinical cases, the calculations have to be compared to more accurate Monte Carlo calculations. However, to do this, both, non-Monte Carlo and Monte Carlo planning systems have to be properly commissioned.

The inverse treatment planning system used in this study was the 'Monte Carlo based inverse treatment planning algorithm' (MCI) [8]. MCI is a two-dimensional inverse treatment planning algorithm based on Monte Carlo dose calculations. It uses simulated annealing for optimisation. To simulate a non-Monte Carlo inverse treatment planning system, the Monte Carlo bixels (narrow beams) were exchanged with the convolution bixels. This convolution based inverse treatment planning algorithm will be referred to as CI.

The Monte Carlo dose calculations were performed using the Monte Carlo treatment planning system at Medical College of Virginia (MCV), which has been successfully commissioned [9]. Statistical error in MCI plans was less than 0.3% of $D_{max}$.

As an example of a non-Monte Carlo dose calculation, the collapsed cone convolution [10] in the ADAC• Pinnacle[3] treatment planning system was used.

Three different typical clinical cases were used in our study: head and neck, lung and prostate. These sites were chosen to examine different geometry types with different geometry complexities and different level of expected convolution systematic errors.

In addition, two different types of physical (dose based) objective functions with different hard constraints (upper/lower dose limits) were used. One was of the square form, with quadratic penalties for all tissues

$$OF = \sum_T \frac{C_T}{N_T} \sum_{i \in T} (d_i - D_T)^2 , \qquad (1)$$

while in the second type, the quadratic penalties in the tumour were replaced with exponential penalties (on the basis of the linear-quadratic model)

$$OF = \frac{C_T}{N_T} \sum_{i \in T} (e^{|d_i - D_T|} - 1) + \sum_{T'} \frac{C_{T'}}{N_{T'}} \sum_{i \in T'} (d_i - D_{T'})^2 \qquad (2)$$

$C_T$ is the weight of a tissue type $T$ and $d_i$ is the dose in a voxel $i$ of type $T$. $D_T$ is the desired dose in a tissue type $T$ and $N_T$ the number of voxels of type $T$. In the exponential/quadratic form, $T$ represents tumour tissue and $T'$ all other tissues.

## Results and discussion

Before starting the comparison, Monte Carlo and convolution bixels were compared for all three geometries. Example for the lung example is shown in Figure 1.

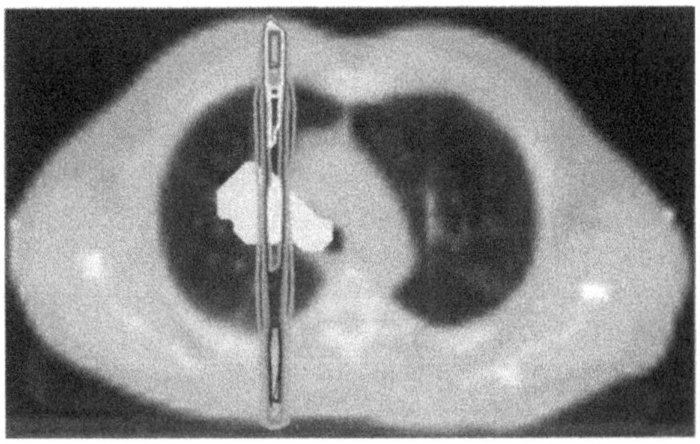

**Figure 1:** Comparison between Monte Carlo (bold) and convolution (narrow) bixels used in the study. Differences can hardly be seen and are of the order of a percent of $D_{max}$. Slightly higher/lower differences were observed in the head and neck/prostate examples.

• ADAC Laboratories, Milpitas, CA 95035.

Use of inaccurate dose calculation in inverse treatment planning introduces two errors in the plan. One is a **systematic error** because of the inaccuracy of the dose calculation itself. Second is a **convergence error** because the planning algorithm converges to the optimal solution for the inaccurate dose calculation, which is different from the optimal solution for the accurate dose calculation.

Our study is illustrated with the head and neck example. Different plans are shown in Figure 2. Figure 2a represents an MCI plan and Figure 2b a CI plan. When the CI plans is recalculated with the Monte Carlo bixels, the plan as shown in Figure 2c is obtained. Note underdose of the tumour in some parts (over 95% dose in the tumour was required). To check convergence to the global minimum the CI plan (2b) was reoptimised and the resultant plan is shown in Figure 2d. Note the similarity between Figures 2a and 2d compared to 2b.

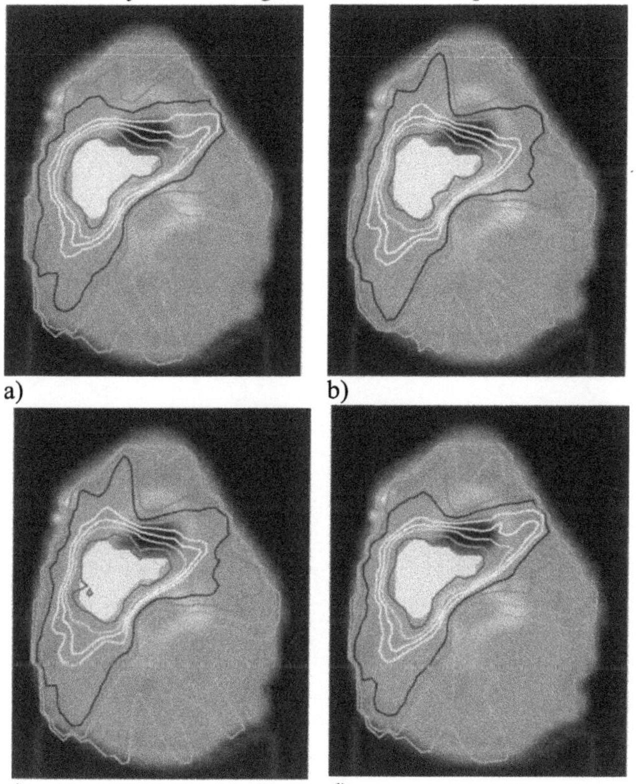

a) b) c) d)

**Figure 1:** Example of different inverse treatment plans for the head and neck tumour site. MCI plan (a), CI plan (b), recalculated CI plan (c) and reoptimised CI plan (d). Note the similarity between (a) and (d) and underdose in the tumour in (c). The tumour was reqired to receive the dose above 95%. The 95% isodose is represented with the red line.

For all three cases, different types of objective functions and different hard constraints all four types of plans were calculated. The systematic error of a plan was determined by subtracting the CI plan from the recalculated CI plan. The convergence error was determined by subtracting the recalculated CI plan from the MCI plan. Because the convergence error is meaningful only if the convergence to the global minimum (or at least vicinity) is ensured, the MCI convergence error was determined by subtracting the reoptimised CI plan from the MCI plan. This error appears because of the finite number of iterations used in the simulated annealing optimisation.

Summary of the systematic and convergence errors for different plans is given in Tables 1 and 2, respectively. The errors are standard deviations of the differences in the plans.

| | Head&neck | Lung | Prostate |
|---|---|---|---|
| **Tumour** | 2.3 | 1.5 | 1.2 |
| **Other tissue** | 1.5 | 1.4 | 1.1 |

**Table 1:** Convolution systematic error in % of $D_{max}$ for different treatment sites. Given are absolute errors.

| | Head&neck | Lung | Prostate |
|---|---|---|---|
| **Tumour** | 4-7 | 3-6 | 3-6 |
| **Other tissue** | 3-6 | 3-6 | 3-6 |

**Table 2:** Convolution convergence error in % of $D_{max}$ for different treatment sites. Given are approximate ranges of the absolute errors.

Several interesting conclusions can be drawn from the results. The systematic errors of the plans are insensitive to the used objective function. As expected, the largest, but still relatively small errors were observed in the head and neck example. However, even such relatively small systematic errors may represent severe violation of the required criteria as shown in Figure 2c.

The convergence errors, on the other hand, strongly depend on the posed objectives. Especially hard constraints (limiting the dose in the tumour/critical structures) may introduce severe convergence errors. The MCI convergence errors were determined to be approximately 0.5-1% of $D_{max}$ for the tumour and 0.5-3% outside the tumour depending on the objective function.

It should be noted that the quoted error values are absolute errors in units of percent $D_{max}$. For tumour, the values approximately correspond to the relative errors, while for other than tumour tissues, the relative errors are much higher (up to 8% systematic and 30% convergence errors were observed). Clinical significance of these errors has not been addressed; however it is to expect that for some tumour sites, shapes, nearby critical structures and posed objectives, these errors may be significant.

In our study one of the most accurate non-Monte Carlo dose calculation algorithms (collapsed cone convolution) was used. It is to expect that if other less accurate dose calculations (e.g. pencil beams) were used, much higher errors would appear.

## Conclusion

In our study, errors in inverse treatment planning algorithms, based on inaccurate dose calculations, were addressed and investigated.

Two types of errors were identified, systematic error because of the inaccuracy of the dose calculation and convergence error because of the convergence to the global minimum for the inaccurate dose calculation, which is different from the minimum of the accurate dose calculation. While the systematic error is not dependent on the chosen objectives, the convergence error shows strong dependence. The systematic errors for the collapsed cone convolution dose calculations, which were used in our study, are of the order of 1-3% in the tumour and slightly less outside, while the convergence errors are of the order of 3-8% of $D_{max}$.

## References

[1] T. Bortfeld, W. Schlegel and B. Rein 1993, Decomposition of pencil beam kernels for fast dose calculation in three-dimensional treatment planning, Med. Phys. 20, 311-318.

[2] Mackie T R, Holmes T W, Swedloff S et al 1993, Tomotherapy: A new concept for the delivery of dynamic conformal radiotherapy, Med. Phys. 20(6), 1709-1719.

[3] Preiser K, Bortfeld T, Harwig K, Schlegel W and Stein J, A new program for inverse radiotherapy planning, Proceedings of the International Conference on the Use of Computers in Radiation Therapy, Utah, USA, 425-428.

[4] Holmes T, Bleier A, Carlo M, Curran B et al 1998 The CORVUS dose model revealed, Med. Phys. 25(7), A144.

[5] Mohan R 1997, Why Monte Carlo?, Proceedings of the International Conference on the Use of Computers in Radiation Therapy, Utah, USA, 16-18.

[6] Nahum A E 1997, Conformal therapy needs Monte-Carlo dose computation, Proceeding of Challenges in Conformal Radiotherapy, Nice, 1-11.

[7] Jeraj R and Keall P J 1999, Effect of noise on Monte Carlo based inverse treatment planning, To be submitted to Phys. Med. Biol.

[8] Jeraj R and Keall P J, Monte Carlo based inverse treatment planning, Phys. Med. Biol. 44, (1999), 1885-1896.

[9] Keall P J, Siebers J V and Mohan R, Acceptance testing and commissioning tests for a Monte Carlo-based photon dose calculation algorithm, Medical College of Virginia Internal Report, 1999.

[10] Ahnesjö A 1989, Collapsed cone convolution of radiant energy for photon dose calculation in heterogeneous media, Med. Phys. 16(4), 577-592.

# Defining margins for systematic rotations and translations: A probability based geometrical approach

**Peter Remeijer, Coen Rasch, Joos V. Lebesque and Marcel van Herk**

The Netherlands Cancer Institute, Antoni van Leeuwenhoek Huis, Plesmanlaan 121, 1066 CX, Amsterdam, The Netherlands

## Introduction

In the ICRU 50 report, a formalism is provided to account for geometrical uncertainties in treatment planning. In this formalism, the geometrical uncertainties are incorporated by adding a margin to the clinical target volume (CTV), thus yielding the planning target volume (PTV).
When designing margins, it is imperative to distinguish between random (day-to-day) and systematic (mean patient position, different for each patient) geometrical uncertainties, because their impact on the dose received by the CTV is quite different. Random deviations blur the dose distribution, hence their effect is limited. Systematic deviations shift the dose distribution, which might lead to severe underdosage.
Since the geometrical uncertainties do not only consist of translations, but also include rotations, rotations should be included in the margin design as well. The effect of random translations and rotations can easily be incorporated in the dose distribution by convolving the planned dose with their distributions. For the systematic uncertainties, the way to include rotations is not clear, and only few studies have addressed this problem. We propose a method, which is an extension of the well known rolling ball algorithm, which uses the probability distribution of the systematic rotations and translations. Furthermore, we will compare this method with existing margin generation algorithms.

## Material and methods

Systematic translations along the three principal axes (x, y, z) can be characterized by their standard deviations, $\Sigma_x$, $\Sigma_y$, and $\Sigma_z$,. A statistically correct procedure to account for these translations in treatment planning [1], assuming that the CTV is a rigid body, is the use of a confidence ellipsoid with radii $\alpha\Sigma_x$, $\alpha\Sigma_y$, $\alpha\Sigma_z$, to determine the possible positions of the CTV in a population of patients. The PTV is then given by the envelope of all these positions. Note that this PTV does not incorporate the random deviations. For that purpose the dose should be convoluted with the probability distributions of the random deviations, and this convoluted dose should conform the PTV. For simplicity we will not do this here and will regard the PTV as a PTV for systematic deviations only. The parameter $\alpha$ is an expansion factor which is given by the 3-D chi-squared distribution. For a 90 % confidence interval, $\alpha$ is equal to 2.5.
We have extended this procedure, often referred to as the rolling ball algorithm, to include rotations as well (hence 6 degrees of freedom, 3 translations and 3 rotations). This was achieved by defining a confidence interval for all 6 degrees of freedom of the CTV (i.e. a 6-D ellipsoid) and determining the envelope of all possible CTV positions within this confidence interval.

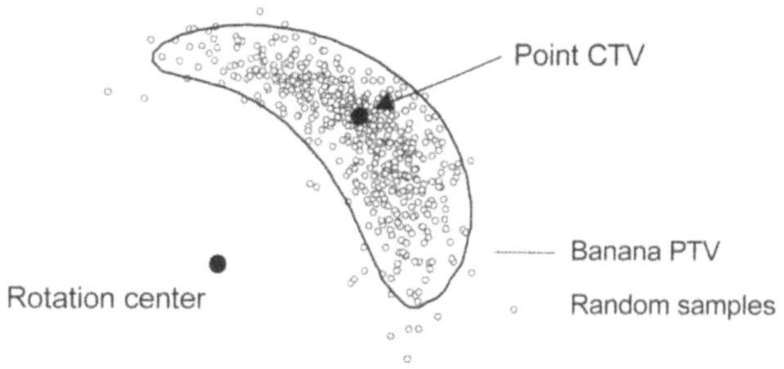


**Figure 1:** Example of a banana PTV, constructed for a point-shaped CTV in 2-D. The gray points are randomly displaced CTVs, using the known probability distributions of the systematic translations and rotations.

The method, which we call the banana method due to the characteristic shape of the confidence interval it creates (Figure 1), is exact for a point CTV with arbitrary rotations and translations and for a finite size CTV with rotations or translations only. Analogue to the rolling ball algorithm, this method also uses an expansion factor $\alpha$. For the limiting cases mentioned before, $\alpha$ should be equal to 2.5 for a 90 % confidence interval. For other cases, some adjustment of $\alpha$ is necessary to obtain a 90 % confidence interval.
The accuracy of the banana method was compared with two existing expansion methods: the rolling ball algorithm (ignoring rotations), and the convolution, or coverage probability method [2]. The latter method uses a 3-D CTV grid, with voxels valued one inside and zero outside the CTV. On this grid a convolution with the distribution of the translations and rotations is performed. Subsequently the PTV is determined by selecting all pixels with values higher than a certain iso-probability value $\beta$.
The comparison was done as follows. First, PTVs were determined using the three methods for a number of CTV shapes (a sphere, a sphere with an extension, and a real prostate case, Figure 2). Second, the probability that the CTV is inside

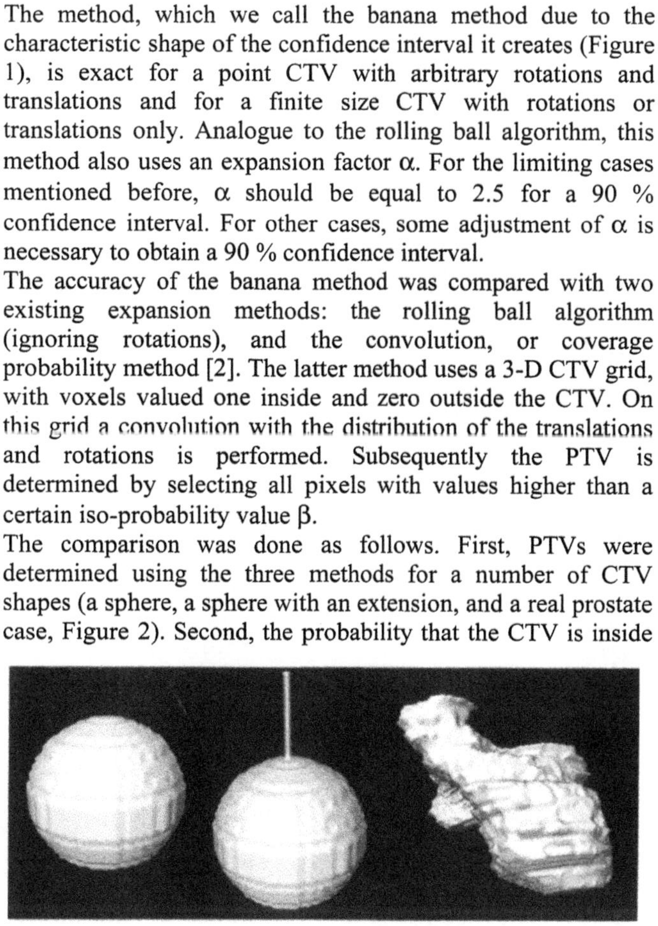

**Figure 2:** Three dimensional rendering of the shapes used to determine the accuracy of the expansion methods. From left to right, a sphere (r = 3 cm), a sphere with an extension (r = 3 cm), and a CTV of a prostate.

the PTV (in short, the success rate) was experimentally determined with a Monte Carlo sampling method (analogue to the method depicted in Figure 1). The standard deviations of the translations and rotations we used were $\Sigma_x = 1.7$ mm, $\Sigma_y = 2.4$ mm, $\Sigma_z = 2.4$ mm, $\Sigma_{rx} = 4.0°$, $\Sigma_{ry} = 1.3°$, $\Sigma_{rz} = 2.1°$ [3][4]. The rotation center was taken at (0, 0, 0) for the sphere, (0, 0, -2) for the sphere with an extension, and at the apex of the prostate.

| | Rolling ball | Coverage prob. | Banana |
|---|---|---|---|
| Sphere | 90 % | 88 % | 89 % |
| Ext. Sphere | 55 % | 59 % | 85 % |
| CTV #1 | 38 % | 56 % | 83 % |

**Table 1:** The probability that the CTV will be inside the PTV for different shapes and methods. The expansion parameters were chosen such that theoretically a sphere without rotation or a rotation around the center would yield a 90 % success rate ($\alpha = 2.5$, $\beta = 0.006$). The probabilities were experimentally determined using 1000 random samples, which leads to a standard error of about 1 %.

## Results and discussion

Table 1 gives the probability that the CTV will be inside the PTV for different shapes and methods. Using the expansion parameters that yield a 90 % success rate for a sphere ($\alpha = 2.5$, $\beta = 0.006$), the banana method gives the best results for all shapes. On average, a success rate (excluding the results for the sphere) of 84 %, 58 %, 47 % was obtained, using the banana method, coverage probability and rolling ball, respectively. When the expansion parameters were adjusted such that the PTVs had the same volume for all methods, the respective average probabilities were 84 %, 70 % and 69 %.

Thus, given an equal volume of the PTV, these results show that the banana method is favorable in terms of the success rate. Furthermore, the choice of the expansion parameter (which is the factor $\alpha$ in the case of the rolling ball and banana algorithm and the iso-probability level $\beta$ for the coverage probability method) is less sensitive to the actual shape of the CTV. While the other methods will go down as low as 38 % for other shapes than a sphere, the banana method obtains a minimum success rate of 83 % for all shapes we tested (Table 1).

## Conclusion

The banana algorithm provides a straightforward way to include the effects of systematic rotations in the PTV. Compared to other algorithms the method is less sensitive to the shape of the CTV and for an equal volume the probability that the CTV is inside the PTV is larger.

## References


[1] van Herk M, Remeijer P, Rasch C, Lebesque JV, 1999, Int. J. Radiat. Oncol. Biol. Phys. Submitted.

[2] Stroom JC, de Boer HCJ, Huizenga H, Visser AG, 1999, Int. J. Radiat. Oncol. Biol. Phys. **43**, 905-919.

[3] van Herk M, Bruce A, Kroes G, Shouman T, Touw A, Lebesque JV, 1995, Int. J. Radiat. Oncol. Biol. Phys. **33**, 1311-1320.

[4] Bel A, van Herk M, Lebesque JV, 1996, Med. Phys. **23**, 1537-1547.


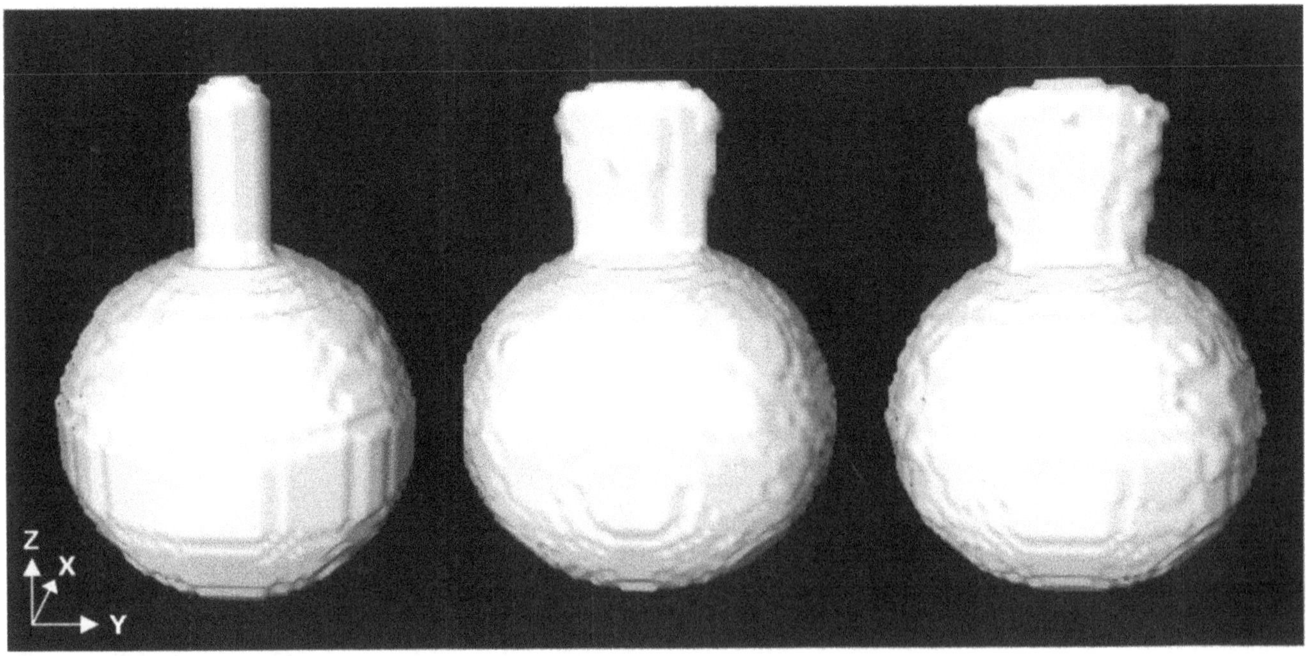


**Figure 3:** From left to right, PTVs of the sphere with extension obtained with the rolling ball method, the coverage probability method and the banana method. The differences are mainly in the way the extension is handled. The rolling ball algorithm does not account for rotations and therefore only a uniform expansion is done. The coverage probabilty method handles rotations to a large extent, but underestimates the margin due to the sharpness of the extension. The banana method yields a PTV which best ensures 90 % probability that the CTV will be inside the PTV.

# An optimal off-line set-up correction protocol based on numerical simulations with measured set-up data of 600 prostate cancer patients

**J.C.J. de Boer and B.J.M. Heijmen**

Daniel den Hoed Cancer Center/University Hospital Rotterdam, Groene Hilledijk 301, Rotterdam, The Netherlands. E-mail:boer@kfih.azr.nl

## Introduction

The application of a well-defined protocol for set-up corrections based on portal images is a prerequisite for obtaining a verifiable level of final positioning accuracy. In case of an off-line correction protocol (OP), patient position data obtained from previous fractions are applied to improve the set-up in subsequent fractions. Therefore, OPs aim at reduction of systematic and not random errors, which is a useful approach because the former errors have a larger impact on geometrical treatment planning margins than the former.[1] Bel *et al.*[2] have studied a 'shrinking action level' (SAL) protocol, in which the action level decreases as the square root of the number of measurements. They studied the trade-off between workload and accuracy for various parameter selections. This OP has become much used in the Netherlands, and it is to date the only protocol for which clinical studies with truly large amounts of patients have been reported[3]. Also in our hospital, the SAL protocol has been applied to ~2000 patients and for various tumor sites. These data were obtained, however, at only two gantries since broad application of the SAL protocol is still hampered by the rather large amount of images to be obtained and analyzed, specifically if weekly check measurements are incorporated[3] (note that for 3D applications, at least 2 but usually 3 images per fraction are required). In this paper, we therefore investigate a simplified OP based on the premise that the workload generated by the OP is determined by the number of images to be acquired and analyzed and not by the actual set-up corrections. This premise is based on experience: for off-line corrections, a table shift is performed each day once the patient has been positioned on the original tattoos with lasers. With a reliable digital table read-out, this shift requires only a few seconds of extra treatment time, whereas the careful analysis of 2 or more portal images (which vary quite strongly in quality from patient to patient) may require several minutes.

We retrospectively simulated the simplified OP to measured set-up data of 600 prostate cancer patients, which is considered an ideal group for OPs due to the small random set-up errors. We compare the results to those obtained when applying the most optimal (in the sense of limited number of measurements) SAL protocol to the same data.

## Material and methods

### Definition of quantities

For a patient $p$, who is treated without a correction protocol, and for fraction $f$, the set-up deviation measured in a portal image along axis $X$ is $x_{pf}$. Let the mean of a quantity $Q$ over a set of measurements $m$ be $\langle Q\rangle_m$ and the unbiased estimate of the standard deviation over that set be $SD_m$ ($Q$). Then, the mean set-up error for patient $p$ is $S_{p,X} = \langle x_{pf}\rangle_f$ and the random (fraction-to-fraction) error $\sigma_{p,X} = SD_f\,(x_{pf})$. The patient population can now be characterized by[2] the "systematic error" $\Sigma_X = SD_p\,(S_{p,X})$ and the "random error" $\sigma_X = (\langle\sigma_{p,X}{}^2\rangle_p)^{1/2}$ (this definition of systematic and random errors includes the measurement errors since in practice their effect on the OP cannot be distinguished from true set-up errors.) If an OP is applied, which generates corrections $\delta x_{pf}$, the measured data will become $x_{pf}' = x_{pf} + \delta x_{pf}$ (we assume that the table corrections are executed with a negligible error, which is true for the data presented below: the measured table read-out error was 0.1±0.3 mm (1 SD)). For data obtained with a correction protocol, we may then directly derive $x_{pf}$, the data that would have been obtained if no OP was applied, from $x_{pf}'$. In addition, we calculate the systematic error "after correction" using $S_{p,X} = \langle x_{pf}'\rangle_T$ where $T$ indicates that when corrections are applied, the available measurements must be weighed appropriately with the actual time between measurements. Similar quantities are obtained for the $Y$ (cran-caud) and $Z$ (ventro-dorsal) directions. The average 3D set-up error $d_p$ for patient $p$ is the length of the vector $V_p = (S_{p,X}, S_{p,Y}, S_{p,Z})$. Note that off-line protocols are only aimed at reducing systematic errors $\Sigma$, not $\sigma$.

### SAL protocol

Details on this OP may be found in Bel *et al.*[2] In short, an initial action level ($\alpha$) and a maximum number of measurements, ($N_{max}$) are selected. After $n$ analyzed fractions, the length of the mean set-up vector $V_n$ is calculated and compared with the 'shrinking' action-level $\alpha/\sqrt{n}$, which reflects the increased accuracy with which the systematic error is measured as $n$ increases. If $V_n > \alpha/\sqrt{n}$, then a set-up correction equal to $-V_n$ is applied in subsequent fractions and the protocol restarts with $n = 1$. If $N_{max}$ subsequent measurements can be obtained for which $V_n < \alpha/\sqrt{n}$, the protocol has finished. Note that multiple corrections may be detected with this protocol. We will denote a specific SAL OP by SAL($\alpha$/mm,$N_{max}$). In many applications, the SAL is followed by a second phase, which in our hospital is a weekly measurement which is added to a running average and tested against a fixed action-level.[3] The second phase strongly increases the number of images required and hence we do not consider it in the current study.

### Simplified 'no action level' protocol

For this protocol, we accept exactly 1 correction for each patient. The average set-up vector after $N_{max}$ measurements is calculated and applied as a set-up correction for each patient.

Because it is known *a priori* that each patient is corrected and that this correction is always based on $N_{max}$ measurements without a test on its magnitude, it will be referred to as the 'no action level' protocol (NAL($N_{max}$)). For patients with isotropic and identical (for each patient) normally distributed random errors ($\sigma_X = \sigma_Y = \sigma_Z \equiv \sigma_{iso}$), we derive that the cumulative distribution of $d_p$ for the NAL($N_{max}$) protocol is given by:

$$\text{fraction}(d_p > x\sigma_{iso}/\sqrt{N_{max}}) = (2/\pi)^{1/2} x \exp(-x^2/2) + 1 - \text{erf}(x/\sqrt{2}),$$

where 'erf' is the standard error function. This distribution, which is independent of the magnitude of the systematic errors, will be referred to as 'analytical'. It is also the *optimal* cumulative distribution that may be achieved with $N_{max}$ measurements and 1 correction, in the sense that the average vector which is applied as a correction is the optimal unbiased estimate of the true systematic error.

### Patient data and protocol simulation

We analyzed set-up measurements of patients treated for prostate cancer with a 3 field technique. These patients had been verified with SAL(9,4) or SAL(8,3) protocols with a second phase. The 600 patients we selected satisfied the following criterion: 3D data were available (i.e., portal images of 2 lateral beams and 1 AP beam per fraction were analyzed) for at least 8 fractions per patient (this is the minimum number of fractions for the above SAL parameters and 30 treatment fractions if no measurements are missing). In this patient group, the average number of measured fractions, $\langle N_{meas}\rangle_p$ = 10.1 and $SD_p(N_{meas})$ = 1.8, sufficient for the simulations described below.

We subtracted the effect of the OP according to the method described above, and so obtained a database of measured uncorrected set-up deviations $\{x_{pf}, y_{pf}, z_{pf}\}$ consisting of over 6000 data points. Next, we applied the SAL (with various parameters) and NAL protocols to $\{x_{pf}, y_{pf}, z_{pf}\}$ to investigate the impact on the distribution of systematic errors and the expected workload. For the time weighing necessary in calculating $\Sigma$ in case of an OP, the assumptions were that (1) the measurements used for the OP are all obtained in the first subsequent fractions and (2) there are 30 fractions in total. For instance, if for a certain patient the OP is finished after 3 measurements, the weight of the first 3 measurements is 3/30 and of the subsequent (on average ≈ 7) measurements is 27/30. Set-up corrections for which all three vector components were ≤ 1 mm were not counted nor applied. All processing was performed with routines written in the Interactive Data Language (IDL).

## Results and discussion

### Protocol comparison for an equal number of measurements

Figure 1 shows the cumulative distribution of the 3D vector lengths without and with OPs. Obviously, a significant improvement is achieved with the NAL protocol for $N_{max}$ = 3, which may also be appreciated from the distribution parameters in Table 1. The random errors $\sigma_X$, $\sigma_Y$, and $\sigma_Z$ are all close to 2 mm and so the random error distribution may be considered isotropic. Indeed, the curve of the analytical distribution for $N_{max}$ = 3 in Figure 1 closely resembles the distribution of the NAL(3). The tail of the latter distribution is slightly wider, partly because in reality a spectrum of patient random errors occurs. The similarity of the NAL(3) distribution to the analytical distribution also implies that, for the patient population under consideration, the NAL correction is applicable to the entire treatment period of about 6 weeks without additional measurements being necessary: the application of a correction based on the first 3 measurements to the, on average, 7 remaining fractions per patient (which are distributed quite homogeneously in time over the full treatment period), yields a cumulative distribution close to the analytically expected result in the absence of time trends. In fact, from the analytical distribution we expect $\Sigma$ = 1.2 mm for all 3 directions, which compares well with the results of the NAL protocol in Table 1.

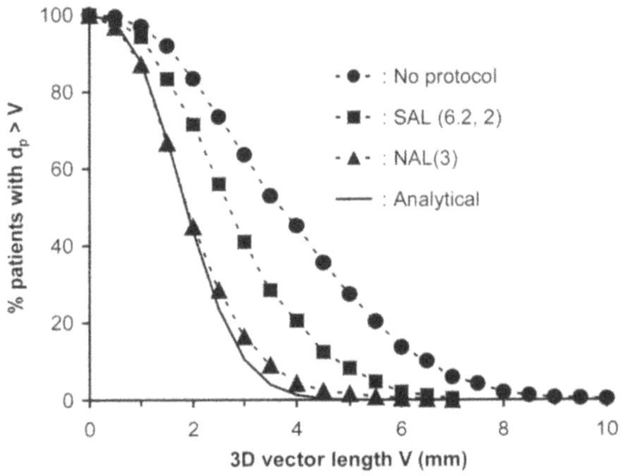


**Figure 1:** Cumulative distributions of the mean set-up vector length with and without the application of an OP with (for the case of the SAL protocol, on average) 3 measurements/patient

We have sought SAL protocols which yield (i) the same average number of measured fractions as NAL(3) (i.e., $\langle N_{meas}\rangle$ = 3) and (ii) a fraction of patients with more than 2 detected corrections ≤ 10%. The latter constraint is a matter of practicality: a large fraction of multiple corrections indicates that the initial action level is too small, yielding inaccurate corrections due to random errors. However, because of the dispersion in $\sigma_p$, multiple corrections for some patients are hard to avoid in the SAL protocol. For the specific patient distribution we studied, the one non-trivial solution meeting the above constraints was SAL(6.2, 2).

| | No OP | NAL(3) | SAL(6.2, 2) |
|---|---|---|---|
| $d_p$ > 5 mm (%) | 27 | 1.7 | 8.2 |
| $\Sigma_X$ (mm) | 2.2 | 1.3 | 1.8 |
| $\Sigma_Y$ (mm) | 2.2 | 1.2 | 1.7 |
| $\Sigma_Z$ (mm) | 2.5 | 1.4 | 1.9 |

**Table 1:** Population set-up distribution parameters for the distributions plotted in Figure 1.

As indicated by Figure 1 and Table 1, the final set-up with the SAL protocol is significantly less accurate for the same (average) required amount of image acquisition and analysis workload. The fraction of patients for which corrections are necessary is only 0.4, but the number of detected corrections per patient shows a large spread and is on average 0.6.

**Comparison for restricted multiple correction detection**

From the above, it is clear that the SAL protocol does not perform well for a small number of measurements. We next investigate how well SAL protocols perform if we only apply the constraint that the fraction of patients with > 2 correction detections ≈ 10%, i.e. we try to find those SAL parameters which yield a reasonably fast and accurate estimate of the significant systematic errors. In Figure 2 we show the results of three SAL protocols which meet this requirement. We did not study SAL protocols with $N_{max} > 4$ as we are still investigating OPs with a small number of measured fractions, whereas for $N_{max} = 4$, already $\langle N_{meas} \rangle = 6.2$. Obviously, the SAL(5.7, 2) protocol, for which $\langle N_{meas} \rangle$ is close to that of NAL(3) (Table 2), yields a significantly worse accuracy than the NAL protocol, as can also be judged from Table 2. Even the SAL $N_{max} = 4$ protocol, with a doubled acquisition and analysis workload compared to the NAL protocol, performs slightly worse in terms of final accuracy although the majority of patients will have a set-up correction with this OP.

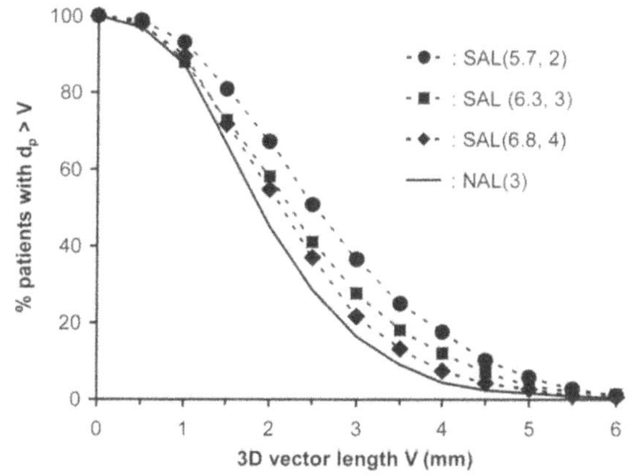


**Figure 2:** Cumulative distributions of the mean set-up vector length for several OPs.

| | NAL(3) | SAL(5.7,2) | SAL(6.3,3) | SAL(6.8,4) |
|---|---|---|---|---|
| $\Sigma_X$ (mm) | 1.3 | 1.7 | 1.5 | 1.4 |
| $\Sigma_Y$ (mm) | 1.2 | 1.6 | 1.5 | 1.4 |
| $\Sigma_Z$ (mm) | 1.4 | 1.8 | 1.6 | 1.5 |
| $\langle N_{meas} \rangle$ | 3 | 3.3 | 4.8 | 6.2 |
| % cor | 100 | 49 | 55 | 59 |

**Table 2:** Population distribution parameters for various OPs (see text), the average number of measurements involved and the fraction of patients that require a correction (% cor). For the SAL protocol: a patient with multiple detected corrections counts as 1 patient with a correction since the workload associated with correcting the set-up is not increased by multiple detections.

## Conclusion

Optimal set-up corrections based on a small number of portal images may be achieved with the simple NAL protocol described above. Although we studied the NAL protocol for a group of prostate cancer patients, the above conclusion will apply to any group with relatively small random errors $\sigma$: the NAL protocol with $N_{max}$ measurements effectively reduces the systematic errors to $\sigma/\sqrt{N_{max}}$, independent of the initial distribution of systematic errors. For the patient group we studied, we found that 3 measurements are indicative of the full treatment period of ~ 6 weeks, rendering the NAL protocol particularly efficient and yielding a minimum workload in terms of image acquisition and analysis. The much applied shrinking action level protocol yields less than optimal results, specifically for a small (~ 3) number of measurements per patient and we found no SAL protocol which generated the accuracy of the NAL protocol for both a small number of measurements and limited triple correction detections. This is due to the fact that (i) the corrections of the SAL protocol are on average based on less than $N_{max}$ measurements yielding less accurate estimates of the systematic error than the NAL protocol and (ii) the protocol is re-started after each correction (partly this is a necessity because of (i)) requiring a relatively large amount of fractions to be imaged. As a result, the SAL protocol therefore requires a 'tailoring' of parameters, e.g. using simulations based on knowledge of the systematic and random set-up errors[2] to maintain a limited workload. For the NAL protocol the workload is determined only by $N_{max}$, and the required $N_{max}$ follows directly from the desired final accuracy level and the magnitude of the random set-up errors.

## References

[1] Stroom JC, de Boer JCJ, Huizenga H and Visser AG 1999 Inclusion of geometrical uncertainties in radiotherapy treatment planning by means of coverage probability *Int. J. Rad. Onc. Biol. Phys.* **43** 905-919

[2] Bel A, van Herk M, Bartelink M and Lebesque V 1993 A verification procedure to improve patient set-up accuracy using portal images *Rad. Onc.* **29** 253-260

[3] Bel A, Vos PH, Rodrigus PTR *et al.* 1996 High-precision prostate cancer irradiation by clinical application of an offline patient setup verification procedure, using portal imaging *Int. J. Rad. Onc. Biol. Phys.* **35** 321-332

This work was financially supported by the Dutch Cancer Society (Grant DDHK 96-1258).

# Verification of dynamic MLC beam delivery using electronic portal imaging

**Mike Partridge[1], J Richard N Symonds-Tayler[1] and Philip M Evans[1]**

[1]Joint Department of Physics, Institute of Cancer Research / Royal Marsden NHS Trust, Downs Road, Sutton, SM2 5PT, UK.

## Introduction

The use of intensity-modulated beams in radiotherapy as been shown to have the potential to deliver highly conformal dose distributions, which enable high doses to be delivered to target volumes, whilst minimising the dose to surrounding critical structures. One method of delivering such intensity-modulated beams that is currently of great interest is the use of the dynamic multileaf collimator (MLC).

A typical dynamic MLC delivery may requite each individual leaf and diaphragm to follow a different, complex trajectory while the radiation beam is on. This represents a radical departure from established clinical practice. The verification of such a delivery and the quality assurance (QA) of dynamic MLC systems therefore poses a major challenge that must overcome for safe commissioning and routine operation[1].

Dosimetric and mechanical verification studies of dynamic MLC treatments have been demonstrated using film[2] and, more recently, using electronic portal imaging devices (EPIDs). There are two main methods of using EPIDs for dynamic MLC verification: (i) leaf tracking[3,4], where a rapid sequence of frames are recorded and the collimator positions measured from each frame are compared to those prescribed, and (ii) integrated intensity measurement[5], where the fluence incident on the imager is integrated over the entire beam delivery and compared to that predicted.

Leaf tracking measurements are relatively simple and provide the possibility of automatic or manual on-line intervention if the measured collimator trajectories differ from those prescribed. The major complication with this type of measurement, however, is the requirement to know the cumulative dose delivered at the moment when each frame is acquired. This is because collimator position must be specified in terms of delivered dose, rather than time, to allow for variation in output dose rate of the linac. Understanding the content of integrated intensity images is much more difficult. Here we have the combined action of the intensity modulation, absorption and scatter by the patient and the response of the imaging system to account for. Camera-based EPIDs have been shown to have a highly non-linear and field size dependent optical cross-talk signal[6,7] that must be corrected for.

In this paper both leaf tracking and dosimetric verification measurements are demonstrated from a modified Theraview imager (QADOS, Camberley, UK). We describe the modifications made to permit the recording of delivered dose in each frame and to reduce the optical cross talk and show sample results.

## Materials and method

Theraview camera-based flurorscopic EPIDs attached to Elekta SL series linacs were used for all measurements shown here. Two in-house modifications were made to the commercially available imaging system.

### Dose display board

The first modification enables the cumulative delivered dose to be determined for each frame recorded. This simplest way of achieving this, without accessing the imager's computerised data acquisition sytem, was to mount a display board inside the imaging system just above the plane of the scintillation screen and at one edge of the field of view of the camera. The display board is comprised of a linear array of 40 LEDs arranged as four decade counters, and 8 field marker LEDs to help alignment. The board counts the digital pulses generated every $1/64^{th}$ of a monitor unit by the SL linacs. The dose value in each frame can be automatically read out with a simple, unsupervised image processing routine.

### Anti-scatter grid

Multiple optical reflections between the scintillation screen and the 45° mirror in EPID generate a non-linear and field-size dependent "glare" signal. If we consider a primary fluence distribution from the scintillation screen $D(x',y')$ emitted at angle $\phi$, being reflected by the mirror back onto the scintillator and scattering through angle $\theta$, the first-order scatter signal $S(x,y)$, contributed to the image is given by[6]:

$$S(x,y)=\frac{1}{2\pi}\sum_{x'}\sum_{y'}D(x',y')\frac{\cos\phi\cos\theta}{r^2},$$

where $r$ is the optical path length between emission and scattering. (Note: the above assumes perfect Lambertian scattering and an infinite 45° mirror, but is a reasonable approximation in this case[7].) These optical reflections can be removed from the image mathematically by deconvolution[5] or physically using an anti-scatter grid. For the work presented in this paper a layer of 3M light control film (3M Corporation, St Paul, MN, USA) was placed in contact with the scintillation screen, reducing the non-linear glare signal to a roughly uniform background[7].

## Results and discussion

### Dose display board

Figure 1 shows a preliminary image from the Theraview EPID with the dose display board. The cumulative dose is indicated by the pattern of LEDs down the left hand side of the image. The eight "marker" LEDs are clearly visible, as are the values shown by the bottom two decades. In the top two decades, the

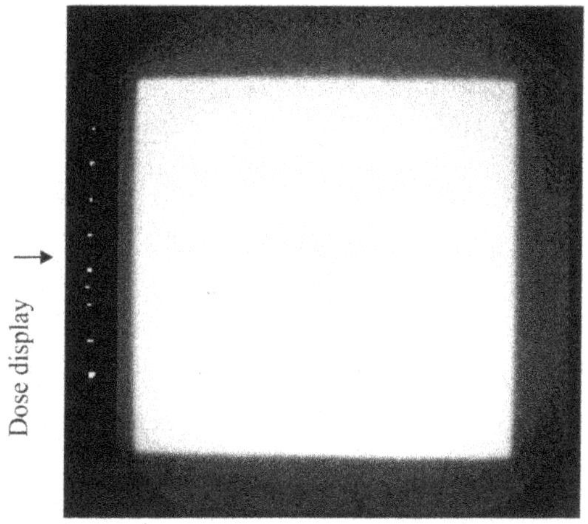


**Figure 1:** Example of dose display image.

count rate is too fast to be resolved, so single LED positions are not seen. The dose display board is designed with a programmable divider on the pulsed input, so the range can be adjusted by pre-scaling the input. The intrinsic resolution of this method is limited by the integration time of the EPID. The above image was acquired with a dose rate of 100 MU/min and a camera integration time of 0.25 s, giving a dosimetric resolution of 0.4 MU. This is perfectly sufficient for dynamic MLC delivery verification by leaf-tracking[3].

**Anti-scatter grid**

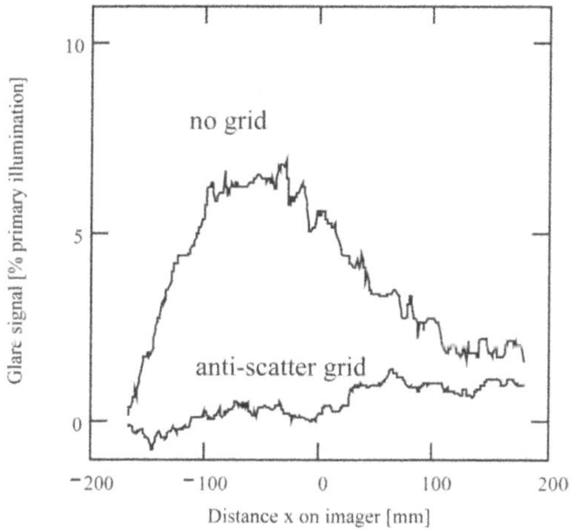


**Figure 2:** The effect of adding an anti-scatter grid.

A sheet of 3M light control film was placed directly in contact with the scintillation screen inside the EPID. The film is essentially a louvre grid with a series of opaque parallel strips set normal to the plane of the film in a transparent matrix. By orienting the strips parallel to the line of intersection of the scintillation screen and mirror, the glare signal is reduced from a strongly peaked function of field size (figure 2, upper trace) to a uniform background (figure 2, lower trace). The profiles in figure 2 are shown along the central axis of the imager in the GT direction (normal to the plane of the gantry) for a 250×300 mm field (all distances are quoted in the plane of the imager). The intersection of the mirror and scintillation screen is at $x = -200$ mm.

Glare signals of 12-13% of the primary fluence are seen for flood-field images (400×400 mm at the plane of the imager)[7] but the peak scatter signal drops off roughly linearly with field area. For the small field sizes proposed for many dynamic MLC treatments, the optical scatter contribution is typically less than 2% of the primary fluence. For accurate integrated intensity measurements therefore, the flood-field calibration images should be corrected to remove the optical scatter signal and thus prevent the introduction of systematic errors.

## Conclusions

It has been demonstrated that intensity modulated field delivery using dynamic multileaf collimation can be verified by either leaf-tracking or integrated intensity measurements. Both types of measurement have been demonstrated on a modified commercially available electronic portal imaging system.

Leaf tracking measurements are relatively simple to perform and, in the event of a delivery error, can give precise information about where and when the error occurred with the possibility of real-time on-line intervention. Integrated intensity measurements provide an off-line method of quality assurance, verifying that the dose delivered corresponds to that planned. Indentifying whether a discrepancy between prescribed and delivered dose is due to a delivery error or patient movement in a clinical case remains technically difficult.

**Acknowledgement**
This work was funded by the Cancer Research Campaign [CRC].

## References

[1] Webb S 1997 *The physics of conformal therapy: advances in technology* 1st ed. (IoP Press, Bristol, UK)
[2] Wang X, Spirou S, LoSasso T, Stein J, Chui C S and Mohan R 1996 Dosimetric verification of intensity-modulated fields *Med. Phys.* **23** 317-27
[3] Partridge M, Evans P M, Mosleh-Shirazi A and Convery D 1998 Independent verification using portal imaging of intensity-modulated beam delivery by the dynamic MLC technique *Med. Phys.* **25** 1872-79
[4] James H, Atherton S, Budgell G, Kirby M and Williams P 1999 Verification of dynamic multileaf collimation using an electronic portal imaging device *Radiother. Oncol.* **51** S25
[5] Pasma K, Dirkx M, Kroonwijk M, Visser A and Heijmen 1999 Dosimetric verification of intensity modulated fields produced with dynamic multileaf collimation using an electronic portal imaging device *Radiother. Oncol.* **51** S33
[6] Munro P, Bouius D C, Mosley J, Martin L Zhang Y and Jaffray D A 1998 Glaring errors in transit dosimetry Proc. 5th Int. Workshop on Electronic Portal Imaging, Phoenix Arizona 128-9
[7] Partridge M, Evans P M and Symonds-Tayler J R N 1999 Optical scattering in camera-based electronic portal imaging *Phys. Med. Biol.* **44** 2381-96

# Cone-beam computed tomography on a medical linear accelerator using a flat-panel imager

**David A. Jaffray[1], Jeffrey H. Siewerdsen[1], Burkhard Groh[1,2], Douglas G. Drake[1], John W. Wong[1], Alvaro A. Martinez[1]**

[1]Department of Radiation Oncology, William Beaumont Hospital, 3601 W. Thirteen Mile Rd., Royal Oak, MI 48073, USA
[2]Deutsches Krebsforschungszentrum, Medical Physics E0400, Im Neuenheimer Feld 280, 69120 Heidelberg, Germany

## Introduction

A major roadblock to the full exploitation of radiation's therapeutic effect is the lack of geometric precision that can be maintained over the fractionated course of therapy. Numerous factors are responsible for this imprecision, and significant effort has been applied to quantifying and controlling the geometric uncertainties. The motivation for increased precision is clear: by increasing the precision of field placement, the prostate can be confidently irradiated with a smaller and more conformal radiation field, thereby reducing the probability of complications in surrounding normal tissues. The reduced probability of complication allows the oncologist to pursue higher radiation doses, thereby improving efficacy while maintaining complication rates at a manageable level.

In recent years, signficant advances have been made in understanding the factors affecting geometric precision and in developing on-line and off-line strategies to reduce these uncertainties. These approaches operate, for the most part, on radiographic (portal) images acquired at the time of treatment. Investigators have also demonstrated that a significant source of uncertainty in treating some sites, such as the prostate, arise from the motion of the target and normal structures with respect to the bony anatomy. Reducing this uncertainty requires an imaging system that is capable of detecting the target and normal structures. Furthermore, such a system must also be capable of producing multiple images over the course of treatment – preferably with the patient in treatment position. In this report, an approach based upon cone-beam CT (CBCT) is employed to acquire on-line volumetric CT images in the reference frame of the treatment machine. In previous reports, the development of the cone-beam method has been described for a CCD-based kV imaging system integrated onto a medical linear accelerator.[1] Subsequent investigation were performed using a more efficient detector based-upon an amorphous silicon flat-panel imager. These investigations were performed on a test-bed and demonstrate the CT imaging performance that can be achieved with these detectors.[2] In this article, recent results of our investigations using the test-bed are reported and the transfer of the flat-panel imager to a medical linear accelerator for CBCT is described.

## Material and methods

### i. FPI-based CBCT on a test-bed

A system was constructed to measure the CT imaging performance that could be achieved with a detector based upon flat-panel imaging technology. This system is described in detail elsewhere.[2] Briefly, the system consists of a 20.5x20.5 $cm^2$ flat-panel imager (EG&G Heimann RID 512-400 A0 - 512 x 512 array of 400 μm photodiodes, 133 $mg/cm^2$ thick $Gd_2O_2S$:Tb phosphor screen) that has been rigidly set in a geometry that mimics that of the kV imaging system of our medical linear accelerator. The imager is read out synchronously with the computer-controlled firing of an x-ray tube (300,000 HU tube, MSI-800 generator) and the rotation of the object of interest. A frame time (and inter-exposure period) of 3200 ms was used for the data reported here. This system was used to measure the CT imagng performance that could be achieved with flat-panel technology. An image produced with this system is shown in Figure 1.

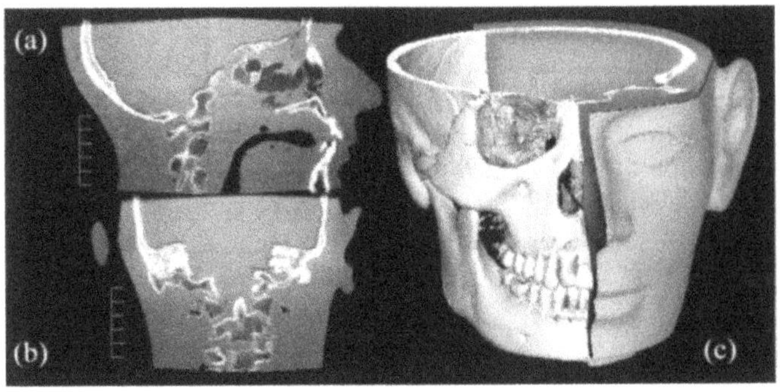


Figure 1. Flat-panel imager CBCT images of an anthropomorphic head phantom acquired on the test-bed: (a) sagittal, (b) coronal, and (c) volume-rendering, all shown at half-resolution (0.5 x 0.5 x 0.5 $mm^3$ voxels) and acquired at 120 kVp. These results illustrate preliminary tests of using the FPI in an offset-detector geometry for CBCT. Preliminary to implementation of a reconstruction algorithm for offset geometry and to demonstrate the performance of the CBCT prototype for large objects, these data were acquired with the FPI translated off-axis by +-90 mm, with the projection images from each automatically combined to give 300 projections (512 x 1090 pixels each, with FOV increased by a factor of ~1.88). Overall, the images demonstrate excellent spatial resolution in features of the bony anatomy.

Estimates of CT imaging performance were made based upon the signal and noise and transfer characteristics of the x-ray detectors.[3] The detective quantum efficiency (DQE) of conventional CT detectors was compared to that of the flat-panel detector used in the test-bed investigations. Additional calculations were performed to estimate the performance of a new generation flat-panel imager that incorporates the current state of this technology. The results of these calculations are shown in Figure 2 with details of the calculations described in the caption. These investigations demonstrate that a CBCT system that incorporates a state-of-the-art flat-panel imager (Figure 2, curve c) should be capable of producing images that are comparable to a conventional CT scanner. It is important to recognize that these calculations provide no estimate for the impact of x-ray scatter that will be present in the CBCT imaging geometry. Further investigations are necessary to address this issue.

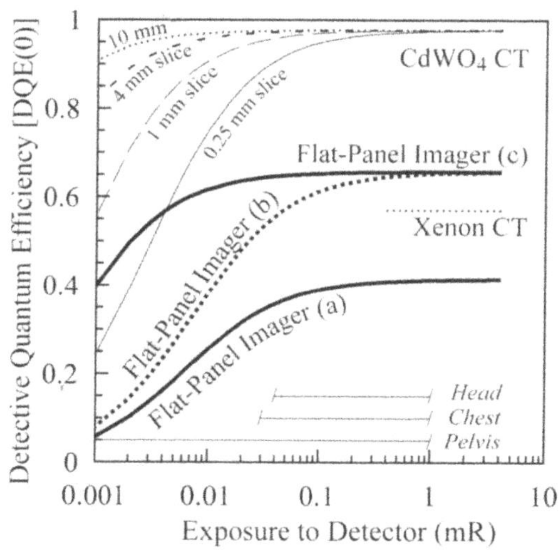


Figure 2. Detective quantum efficiency calculated as a function of exposure for various detector systems in CBCT and conventional (slice-based) CT. Horizontal brackets labeled "Head," "Chest," and "Pelvis" designate the approximate exposure range for these sites. The bold curve (a) represents the DQE(0) for the current flat-panel CBCT prototype and shows that for exposures less than ~0.1 mR, the DQE declines due to the fairly high level of additive electronic noise (~13,000 e). Incorporation of an enhanced x-ray converter (e.g., 250 mg/cm$^2$ CsI:Tl) improves the DQE as shown in the bold dotted curve (b). Improving the additive noise as well (e.g., reducing the amplifier noise to 3000 e) increases the DQE as shown in curve (c) and approaches the theoretical limit of the system. The DQE(0) for conventional CT scanners based on Xenon or $CdWO_4$ detectors is also shown. The Xenon provides ~57% quantum detection efficiency, with performance at low exposures dependent on the intrinsic gain and noise (not shown). A state-of-the-art scanner based on $CdWO_4$ detectors provides DQE~99% at high exposures and for thick (e.g., 5-10 mm) slices. However, the gain and additive noise are such that the system exhibits strong exposure dependence for thinner slices (since these properties were sacrificed in favor of fast temporal response), resulting in DQE that is less than that of the flat-panel imager [curve (c)] at the lowest exposures, for equivalent slice thickness.

**ii. FPI-based cone-beam CT on a medical linear accelerator equipped with a kV x-ray source**

The flat-panel imager employed in the investigations described above was transferred to an Elekta SL20 that is equipped with a kilovoltage x-ray source (Figure 3). Mounted orthogonal to the treatment beam are the flat-panel imager (EG&G Heimann RID 512-400 A0) and the x-ray tube (Eureka Rad-92 in a Varian Sapphire housing). Similar to the test-bed, the process of image acquisition is performed under computer control. The x-ray generator (Innerscan-Ideal, Innerscan Inc., Chicago) is controlled via an RS-232 port and the gantry angle is monitored via an analog link to the accelerator. Gantry rotation can be performed either by hand-pendant from behind a shield or through the assisted motion features of the SL20 accelerator.

A test phantom was imaged consisting of an 11 cm water-filled cylinder containing low-contrast electron density inserts (from the RMI 465 phantom): solid water (CT# 1001); breast (CT# 945); brain (CT# 1005); CB3 resin (CT# 1002); liver (CT# 1082); and polyethylene (CT# 897). A total of 500 projection images were acquired over a 360° rotation at 100 kVp (0.625 mAs per projection). Of the 500 images acquired during the scanning process, 427 were used in the volume reconstruction, since variations in the speed of the gantry rotation during the scan resulted in projections being acquired at variable projection increments. The 427 projections used were selected to minimize the variance between actual projection angle and back-projection angle. The standard deviation in projection angle after this process was 0.3°.

The mechanical flex in the imaging system is known to be substantial and was measured using a reference BB placed at a known mechanical offset from the treatment isocenter. The measured trajectory of the BB in the projection images traces a sinusoidal pattern of amplitude equal to twice the offset. The residuals of a sinusoidal fit to the measured trajectories are the flex due to non-circular motion and provide a straightforward means for flex compensation and is applied with the Feldkamp reconstruction algorithm[4].

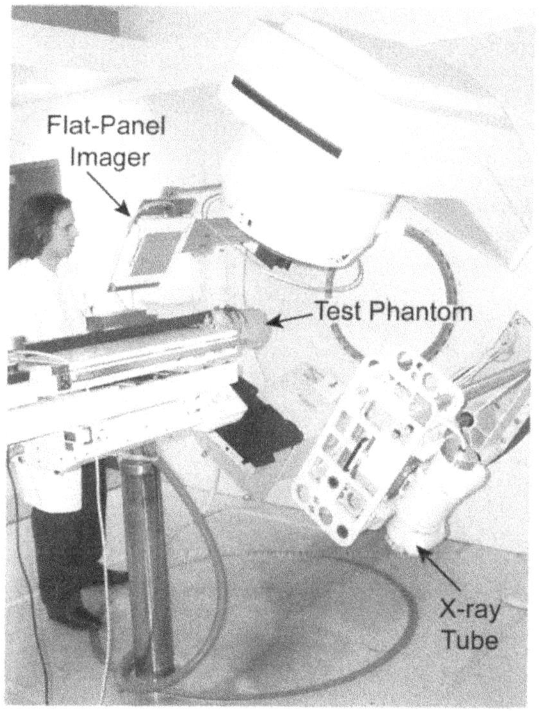


Figure 3. Photograph of the prototype FPI-based CBCT system implemented on a medical linear accelerator (Elekta SL-20). A test phantom containing low-contrast inserts was placed at isocenter. The small detector used in these tests limits the field of view to ~13 cm in diameter. This is to be addressed in the clinical implementation through the use of a large (40cmx40cm), offset detector.

## Results and discussion

Analysis of the measured trajectory of the reference BB reveals a significant range of motion in both the lateral and longitudinal directions. Furthermore, this motion possesses considerable high-frequency angular-dependence. The lateral motion ranges over ~5 pixels (2 mm), giving consistent displacement at 0° and 360°, whereas the longitudinal displacement is ~7 pixels (2.8 mm) and is discontinuous from 360° to 0° due to the corkscrew motion of the drum gantry. These data are used in the reconstruction process to adjust the back-projection trajectories. It should be noted that this algorithm does not properly accommodate the discontinuity caused by the corkscrew motion of the source; however the discontinuity is small (~1.2 mm). Adjustments to the bearing assembly of the linac can be made to reduce this effect.

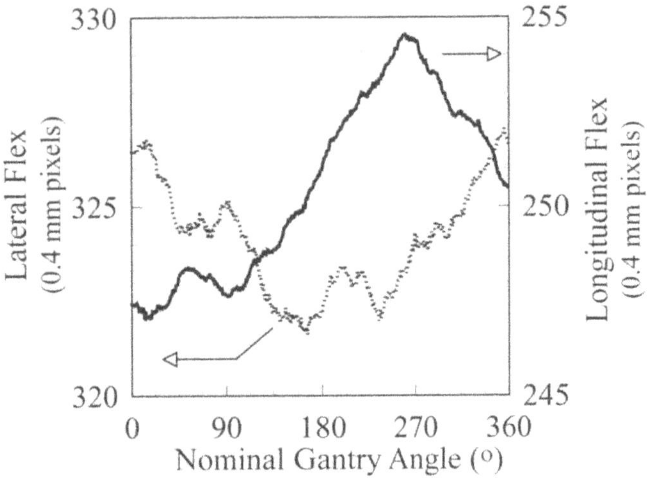


Figure 4. Measured flex corrections as a function of gantry angle for linac-based kV cone-beam CT. Flex is shown in units of pixel (0.4 mm). Lateral flex refers to motion orthogonal to the axis of rotation (AOR); longitudinal flex is orthogonal is parallel to the AOR.

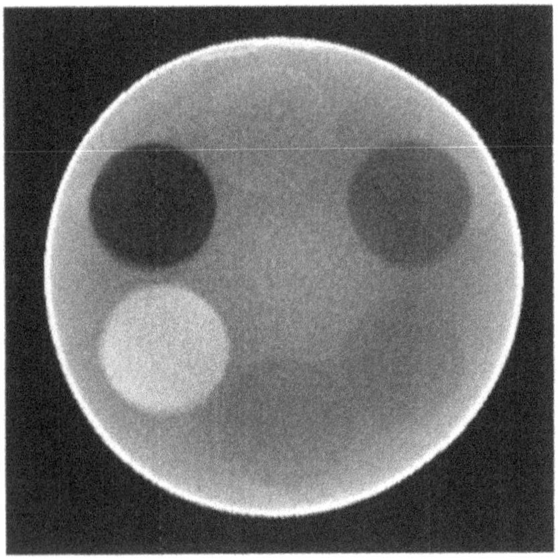

Figure 5. CBCT image of the contrast phantom as acquired on the kV imaging system implemented on the medical linear accelerator. This image was reconstructed using the estimates for mechanical flex acquired with scans of the reference BB, as described above. The voxels in this image are 0.25 x 0.25 x 3 $mm^3$ . The image was produced from 427 projections (100 kVp, 204 mAs of total charge, ~1300 mR in-air on the axis of rotation) over 360°. The inserts are: (in clock-wise order from the top) solid water (CT# 1001); breast (CT# 945); brain (CT# 1005); CB3 resin (CT# 1002); liver (CT# 1082); and polyethylene (CT# 897).

The results of the kV CBCT scans performed on the medical linear accelerator are shown in Figure 5. Overall, the image demonstrates excellent contrast sensitivity, nearly indistinguishable from that demonstrated on the prototype test-bed, which in turn demonstrated constrast sensitivity comparable to a conventional CT scanner for equivalent dose and slice thickness. Subtle artifacts due imprecision in the projection angles are evident in the reconstruction. The success of the flex compensation algorithm is demonstrated in the well defined outer rim of the phantom. More detailed studies of flex with smaller markers and higher contrast will be used to assess the performance of the flex correction.

## Conclusion

The development of a CBCT imaging system for guiding therapy shows great promise. At the onset of our investigations, there were three major confounding factors that were perceived as road-blocks to implementation of this technology. These are: sufficient x-ray efficiency of a 2-D detector, non-rigidity of the linear accelerator gantry, and the presence of increased x-ray scatter in the cone-beam geometry. Our results to date suggest that issues of detector performance and flex can be addressed. Further investigations will be necessary to address the question of the importance of x-ray scatter.

## Acknowledgement

This research was funded in part by the Prostate Cancer Research Program Grant #DAMD-17-98-1-8497, the National Cancer Institute (CA66074), and Elekta Oncology Systems. B. Groh would like to thank the German Academic Exchange Service for funding his stay at William Beaumont Hospital.

## References

[1] Jaffray D A, Drake D G, Moreau M, Martinez A A, Wong J W 1999 A radiographic and tomographic imaging system integrated into a medical linear accelerator for localization of bone and soft-tissue targets *Int J Radiat Oncol Biol Phys* 3 773-789

[2] Jaffray D A, Siewerdsen J H, Drake D G 1998 Performance of a volumetric CT scanner based upon a flat-panel imager *in Medical Imaging 1999: Physics of Medical Imaging, J.M. Boone and J.T. Dobbins III Eds., Proceedings of SPIE* Vol. 3336, 316-324

[3] Siewerdsen J H, Antonuk L E, El-Mohri Y, Yorkston J, and Huang W, "Signal, noise power spectrum, and detective quantum efficiency of indirect-detection flat-panel imagers for diagnostic radiology," Med. Phys. 25(5) 614-628 (1998).

[4] Feldkamp L A, Davis L C, Kress J W 1984 Practical cone-beam algorithm *J Opt Soc Am* 1 612-619

# MV and kV cone-beam CT on a medical linear accelerator

**Burkhard A. Groh [1,2], Jeffrey H. Siewerdsen[1], Douglas G. Drake[1], John W. Wong[1], David A. Jaffray[1]**

[1]Department of Radiation Oncology, William Beaumont Hospital, 3601 W. Thirteen Mile Rd., Royal Oak, MI 48073, USA
[2]Deutsches Krebsforschungszentrum, Medical Physics E0400, Im Neuenheimer Feld 280, 69120 Heidelberg, Germany

## Introduction

The use of intensity modulated radiotherapy (IMRT) with its power to create highly conformal dose distributions emphasizes the role of margins in radiotherapy. In sites where day-to-day organ movements are present image-guided (IG) therapy offers the possibility for reduced margins and dose escalation. Such image guidance systems must meet certain requirements: it must be operated in the treatment room, minimally invasive for the patient, fast enough not to significantly prolong treatment time, free from distortions, and capable of differentiating soft tissue. A strong candidate for such an IG system is integrated CT. Several investigators have proposed two possible methods. One uses the megavoltage (MV) source of the linear accelerator [8,9] the other an additional kilovoltage (kV) source [6].
While theory clearly indicates that kV is far better in terms of signal-to-noise ratio (SNR) per unit dose, no investigation has been undertaken to bridge the theory with realistic kV and MV detectors. This paper benchmarks the theory at kV and MV using well characterized kV and MV flat-panel imagers (FPI). These investigations allow quantitative comparison of the performance of IG systems for both energy ranges.

## Material and Methods

**Theoretical estimation of performance:**
A prediction of the SNR in the reconstructed image of a water cylinder is given by the following equation [9]

$$(1) \qquad SNR = \sqrt{\frac{\eta \varepsilon^3 \Delta z \mu_0^{\ 2} D}{K E \mu_{en} \exp(\mu_0 d / 2)}}$$

where ε is the FWHM of the pointspread function of the detector and Δz the slice thickness. $\mu_0$ and $\mu_{en}$ are the linear attenuation and the energy transfer coefficients for water [3]. D is the central dose to the phantom, E the energy of the primary photons, and d is the diameter of the cylinder. K describes the noise transfer through the used filter in the reconstruction (equal to 1.82 for the Hamming filter) [1]. η is the quantum detection efficiency, calculated analytically for the kV FPI [3], and simulated using Monte Carlo methods for the MV panel [4]. The theory was also used to calculate the SNR of a standard CT Xenon gas detector with an MV efficiency of 1% [8] and a fluoroscopic CsI system with $\eta \approx 18$ % [7].

**Measurement of SNR performance:**
To measure the SNR a phantom was built from an 11 cm plastic cylinder filled with water in the upper half and with six 3 cm diameter cylinders made from tissue equivalent materials inserted in the lower half. The inserts are visible in the reconstructed images in Fig 4, starting in the upper left with liver (electron density relative to water: 1.05) and going clockwise to polyethylene (0.945), solid water (1.0), breast (0.98), brain (1.039) and resin (1.02) in clockwise order. From a slice or averaged slices from the pure water bath the mean and standard deviation in voxel values were determined and the SNR calculated.

**MV cone-beam CT (CBCT)**
All recorded images were dark and gain-corrected by subtracting an averaged dark field and then dividing the image by an averaged open field, which was normalized to a mean value of 1. A small number of defect pixels were filtered. To correct for variations in the intensity of the photon source, the signal of 9 pixels outside the phantom shadow was used as a reference signal.

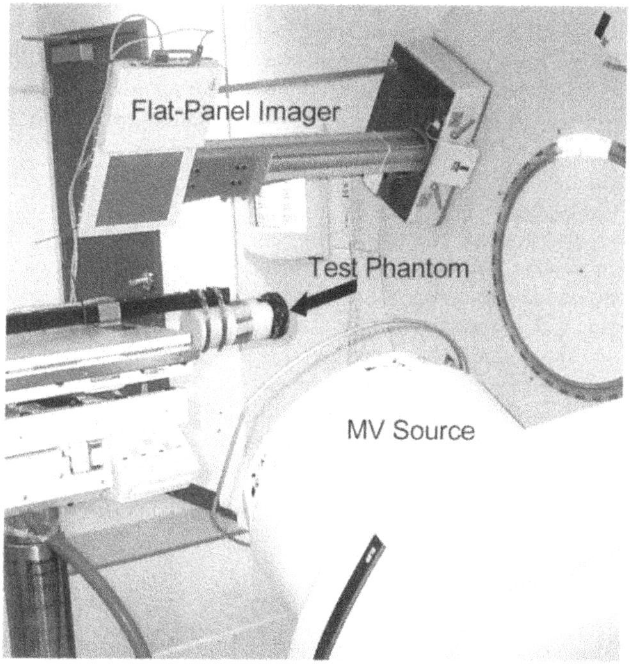


**Figure 1:** MVCT-system with the flat-panel imager, the MV source and the cylindrical phantom attached to the table.

A picture of the MV system is shown in figure 1 consisting of an Elekta SL20 medical linear accelerator and MV flat-panel imager. For all images 6 MV photons were used at a dose rate of 6 MU/min and the gantry speed was 6 or 12 min/revolution. For each image the actual gantry angle was recorded.
The detector (Heimann RID 256-L) incorporates a Kodak Lanex Fast Back $Gd_2O_2S$:Tb phosphor (133 mg/cm$^2$) and a 1 mm copper plate. The phosphor is directly coupled to a photodiode array made from amorphous silicon. The array consists of 256 x 256 square pixels with a pixel pitch of 800 µm. Possible readout times are 79 ms, 100 ms, 200 ms, 400 ms, 800 ms, 1600 ms and 3200 ms. The FPI was operated asynchronously

from the accelerator; therefore the problem of interference between radiation pulses and detector readout was solved in the following way. A fixed pulse repetition time (160 ms) was chosen for the accelerator, and the integration times of the detector were set according to that. As the integration times 800 ms and 1600 ms are multiples of 160, it was assured that exactly 4 or 9 pulses hit the detector. Using 200 ms integration time 1 pulse or 2 pulses could hit the detector, therefore frames where two pulses hit the detector were determined offline and rejected. In this case the dose to the phantom was actually 4 times higher than the dose used for imaging.
The detector was mounted to the drum of the accelerator 159 cm from the source. The phantom was placed at iso center, i.e. 100 cm from the source. The dose to the center of the phantom was computed to be 0.0156 cGy per pulse.
The mechanical flex in the imaging system was measured by placing a ball bearing (bb) 6 mm below iso center and recording 2000 images over 360°. From the images, the bb was extracted using a threshold, and its centroid was calculated. From this path of the bb a sinusoidal describing its relative motion due to the 6 mm offset was subtracted to obtain the actual flex. The phase and the offset of the sinusoidal were derived from a fit to the data.
The volumes were reconstructed using the FDK algorithm [2] after the backprojection ray was corrected for flex by using the data from the bb measurement. Images were reconstructed with voxel size of 0.5 x 0.5 x 0.5 mm$^3$, corresponding to the 800 µm pixel pitch of the MV flat-panel imager.

**kV cone-beam CT (CBCT)**

The kV system consists of a benchtop which mimics the accelerator geometry [5]. This system consists of 3 components: an x-ray tube, a rotation stage, and a flat-panel imager. All components are computer controlled. The x-ray tube (General Electric Maxi-ray 75) is a 300 kHU tube with a minimum filtration of 1.5 mm Al and an additional filtration of 0.127 mm Cu. A 100 kVp beam was used, with a mean energy of ~60 keV. The flat-panel imager (EG&G Heimann RID 512-400 A0) incorporates a 512x512 array of a-Si:H photodiodes and TFTs at a pixel pitch of 400 µm. The x-ray converter was a Kodak Lanex Fast Back screen. The imager was operated at an integration time of 3200 ms and synchronized with the x-ray tube.

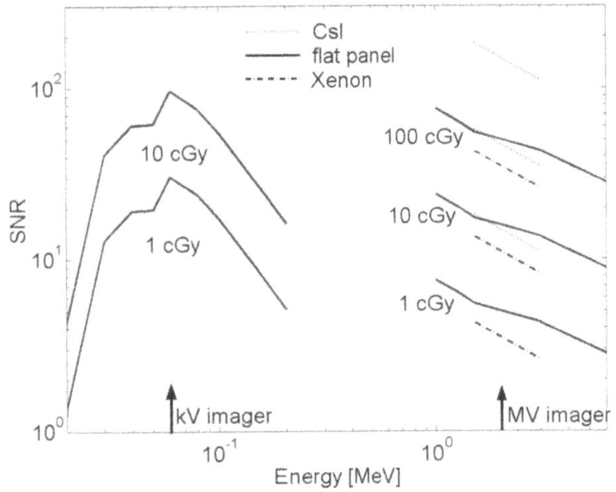


**Figure 2:** Theoretical prediction of SNR vs. energy for the kV flat-panel (at 2 dose levels: 1 and 10 cGy) and for three different MV detectors (at 3 dose levels: 1, 10 and 100 cGy). The arrows indicate the approximate energy for the SNR results in figure 3.

## Results and discussion

| Integration time | 200 ms | 800 ms | 1600 ms |
|---|---|---|---|
| Pulses per view | 1 | 4 | 9 |
| # of frames recorded/used | 2000/374 | 600/428 | 600/437 |
| Dose per revol. | 36 | 36 | 72 |
| Estimated dose | 5.8 cGy | 26.7 cGy | 61.3 cGy |
| SNR for 1 slice | 2.9 | 9.6 | 14.4 |
| For 2 averaged slices | 3.6 | 11.7 | 17.7 |
| For 10 averaged slices | 7.3 | 30.8 | 34.0 |

**Table 1:** Parameters for the MV SNR measurements.

Figure 2 shows the theoretical predictions of the SNR for the kV and MV flat-panel imagers and for two other MV detectors. Two dose levels are shown for the kV and three for the MV calculations. The calculations were done assuming a 25 cm diameter water cylinder, a slice thickness of 5 mm and 0.5 x 0.5 mm$^2$ voxel size. The curves roughly show that at least a reduction in dose by an order of magnitude is achievable when switching from MV to kV, although a very high efficient fluoroscopic CsI detector may reduce that gap.
The results for the SNR measurements as a function of dose are shown in figure 3. Circles represent the MV data and stars the kV data. The solid line is the predicted theoretical performance for assumed mean energies of 2 MeV and 60 keV respectively. The agreement for higher dose levels is excellent in both energy regimes. Although the overestimation of the SNR value for the low dose in the MV case may be due to the presence of additive noise (not accounted for in equation 1), this trend is reversed in the kV case. Therefore the small discrepancies in prediction and measurement may be the result of simplifying assumptions in the model, e.g. using a mean energy for polychromatic spectra.
The reconstructions of the contrast phantom are shown in figure 4 with a slice thickness of 5 mm. As the cylinder was clamped to a metal post in the MV system it is not perfectly round, compared to the kV image, where the cylinder was standing upright. In the two high dose images the four highest contrast objects are clearly visible. In the 5.8 cGy image liver and polyethylene are the only inserts which are detectable at all. Figure 4 d) shows a reconstruction from the kV system, where all the inserts are visible. Even the solid water insert is detectable because of a small contrast difference at its edges. The brain insert appears to be darker than the water, which suggests a slight disproportionality between reconstructed values and electron density.

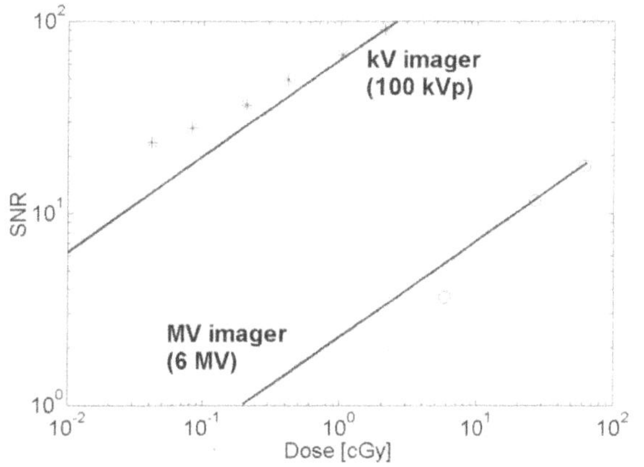


**Figure 3:** Measured SNR for 3 dose levels with the MV flat-panel (circles) and for 6 dose levels with the kV panel (stars). The solid line show the theoretical predictions. Voxel size was 0.5 x 0.5 x 1 $mm^3$.

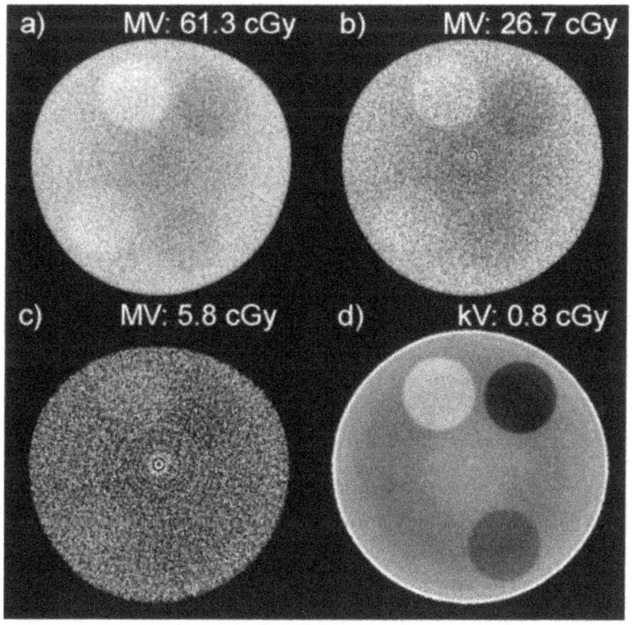


**Figure 4:** MV-images of the contrast phantom with a pixel size of 0.5 x 0.5 $mm^2$ and a slice thickness of 5 mm done with different dose levels (a), (b) and (c), kV-image (d). The ring artifacts in the MV images indicate instabilities in the flat-panel imager.

## Conclusion

The theoretical model for SNR prediction proved to be a useful tool for the evaluation of kV and MV detectors for CT. Furthermore this investigations clearly shows the advantage of kV over MV in terms of SNR per unit dose, when using state-of-the-art flat-panel imagers. The theory predicts that using fluoroscopic CsI imaging systems may help to overcome this disadvantage in MVCT.

## Acknowledgement

This research was funded in part by the Prostate Cancer Research Program Grant #DAMD-17-98-1-8497, the National Cancer Institute (CA66074), and Elekta Oncology Systems. B. Groh would like to thank the German Academic Exchange Service for funding his stay at William Beaumont Hospital.

## References

[1] Chesler D A, Riederer S J, Pelc N J 1977 Noise due to photon counting statistics in computed X-ray tomography *J. Computer Assisted Tomography* 1 64-74

[2] Feldkamp L A, Davis L C, Kress J W 1984 Practical cone-beam algorithm *J Opt Soc Am* 1 612-619

[3] Hubbell J H and Seltzer S M 1997 Tables of X-Ray Mass Attenuation Coefficients and Mass Energy-Absorption Coefficients (version 1.02), [Online]. Available: *http://physics.nist.gov/xaamdi* [1999, December 6]. National Institute of Standards and Technology, Gaithersburg, MD.

[4] Jaffray D A, Battista J J, Fenster A, Munro P 1994 Monte Carlo studies of x-ray energy absorption and quantum noise in megavoltage transmission radiography, *Med. Phys.* 21 45-60

[5] Jaffray D A, Siewerdsen J H, Drake D G 1998 Performance of a volumetric CT scanner based upon a flat-panel imager *in Medical Imaging 1999: Physics of Medical Imaging, J.M. Boone and J.T. Dobbins III Eds., Proceedings of SPIE* Vol. 3336, 316-324

[6] Jaffray D A, Drake D G, Moreau M, Martinez A A, Wong J W 1999 A radiographic and tomographic imaging system integrated into a medical linear accelerator for localization of bone and soft-tissue targets *Int J Radiat Oncol Biol Phys* 3 773-789

[7] Mosleh-Shirazi M A, Evans P M, Swindell W, Webb S. Partridge M 1998 A cone beam megavoltage CT scanner for treatment verification in conformal radiotherapy *Radiother. Onc.* 48 319-328

[8] Ruchala K J, Olivera G H, Schloesser E A, Mackie T R 1999 Megavoltage CT on a tomotherapy system *Phys Med Biol* 44 2597-2621

[9] Swindell W, Simpson R G, Oleson J R, Chen C, Grubbs E A 1983 Computed tomography with a linear accelerator with radiotherapy applications *Med. Phys.* 10 416-420

# Quantitative cone beam megavoltage CT

**L Spies, M Ebert, B A Groh, B M Hesse, and T Bortfeld**
Deutsches Krebsforschungszentrum, Heidelberg, Germany

## Introduction

In recent years there has been increasing interest in cone beam megavoltage CT (MVCT) using the photon beam of a treatment machine and an electronic portal imaging device (EPID), see e. g. [1]. So far this technique has been investigated with respect to its potential in patient set-up control, which requires high contrast and adequate spatial resolution ([2] and references therein).

However, for a quantitative verification of the dose delivered to the patient the three-dimensional (3D) electron density distribution at time of treatment has to be accurately known. We believe that this information can be obtained from cone beam MVCT. Scatter, which is always present in transmission imaging, may limit the accuracy. Furthermore, the method of Feldkamp, Davis and Kress (FDK) [3], which currently is the only established cone beam reconstruction technique, is not exact and thus may lead to reconstruction artefacts.

In this study an algorithm is presented, which calculates 3D electron density distributions based on a scatter correction of portal images. Moreover, the suitability of the FDK algorithm for application in cone beam MVCT is analysed. Inaccuracies arising from mechanical instabilities of the detector-gantry assembly during a gantry rotation is not a matter of this paper, since there are appropriate correction methods available elsewhere in the literature [4].

## Material and methods

### EPID and imaging geometry

We use a camera-based EPID, the BIS[1] with a converter comprising a 1 mm thick copper plate bonded to 134 mg $cm^{-1}$ $Gd_2O_2S$:Tb phosphor. Images are digitized into 10 bit and consist of 512 × 512 pixels with a pixel size of 0.6 × 0.6 $mm^2$. The phantom in use is a water-equivalent ball of 9 cm radius. The central slice is equipped with inserts of several materials (for details see legend to Fig. 2). The inserts are 3 cm in diameter and 1 cm thick. The centre of the ball is in the isocentre of the linac. The phantom is rotated in a stationary 6 MV cone beam. Images are taken in increments of 3° resulting in 120 2D profiles for the full revolution. The integration time is 1.6 s to make use of the full dynamic range of the detector. The field size in the isocentre plane is 20 × 20 $cm^2$. The detector is placed 30 cm from the isocentre. After an off-set correction the profiles are normalized to an open field measurement, taken without phantom, resulting in 120 transmittance maps.

[1]Beam Image System (BIS) 710, Wellhöfer-Dosimetrie, Schwarzenbruck, Germany.

### Scatter estimation

Scatter is estimated by convolving the input beam profile with analytically derived scatter kernels. The inhomogeneity of the phantom is taken into account in the kernel via the radiological thickness map [5]. Scatter kernels are separated into a single scatter and a multiple scatter component. Single scattering is treated exactly. Double and

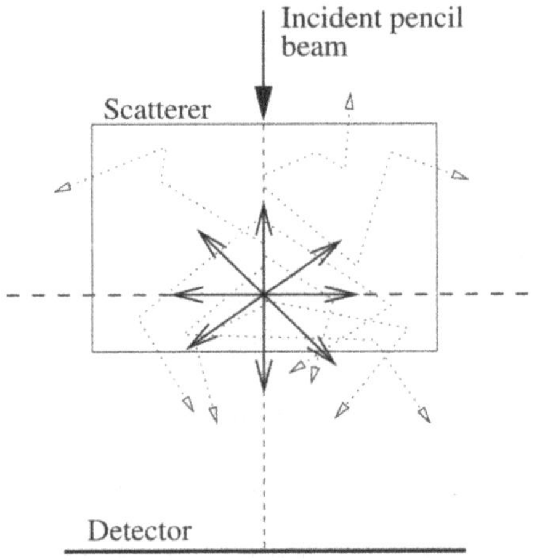


**Figure 1:** Dotted line show possible pathways of multiple scattered radiation from a pencil-like input beam. Solid arrows illustrate the approximation. The intersection point of the horizontal and the vertical dashed line is the site of the *multiple-scatter* source.

higher-order scattering, summarized as multiple scattering in what follows, is approximated by an isotropic distribution, emerging form a source located at a certain depth along the incident pencil beam. This depth is estimated theoretically to be at 73 per cent of the total radiological thickness, $L$. The multiple scatter kernel has then a simple form

$$K_{ms}(L) = \frac{P_{ms}(L)}{4\pi} \cdot \frac{\boldsymbol{r} - \boldsymbol{r}_{ms}}{|\,\boldsymbol{r} - \boldsymbol{r}_{ms}\,|^3} \cdot \hat{\boldsymbol{e}}_\perp. \tag{1}$$

Here, $\boldsymbol{r}$ is the position, where the radiation is recorded. The vector $\boldsymbol{r}_{ms}$ points to the source of the isotropic distribution and $\hat{\boldsymbol{e}}_\perp$ is the unit vector normal to the detector surface. The parameter $P_{ms}$ is the probability that an incoming photon exits the phantom as a multiply scattered photon. For radiological thicknesses up to 20 cm, $P_{ms}(L) = 0.24\ cm^{-1} \cdot L$, is a good approximation. Monte Carlo calculations using the GEANT package [6] were performed to simulate the detector response of the BIS. The calculations show that the converter overestimates strongly multiply scattered radiation of low energy. Additionally, the mean detector response to multiply scattered radiation as a function of phantom thickness is needed. This quantity has also been delivered by means of a Monte Carlo analysis. For more details on the model and its implementation we refer to [7].

### 3D tomographic reconstruction

The FDK algorithm suits ideally to our cone-beam geometry and delivers an approximative inversion to the 3D X-ray transform. It is based on the following steps:

1. Pre-weighting of all profiles (as descriped in [3]),
2. row-wise 1D filtering of all profiles either in spatial or in frequency domain (in this study we employ a convolution with a Shepp-Logan kernel in spatial domain),
3. weighted 3D backprojecting of all profiles into the reconstruction volume.

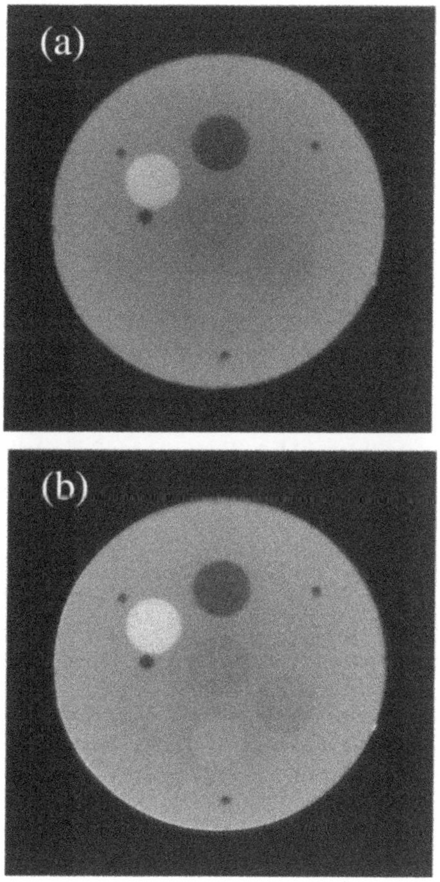


**Figure 2:** Tomographic reconstruction of the central phantom slice of the ball (the electron density relative to water is 1.01) without (a) and with a scatter correction (b). The inserts are (beginning at 12 o'clock in clockwise order): lung (0.29), water, fat (0.90), spongy bone (1.08), muscle (1.02), cortical bone (1.71), and fat in the central region.

FDK reconstruction is exact in the plane defined by the source orbit only. Outside this plane reconstruction artefacts may arise. To quantify these artefacts a large uniform ball of 25 cm radius located in the isocentre of the linac is reconstructed from synthetic transmission data provided for the detector plane of the experimental set-up. All reconstructions are performed voxel-driven on a cubic grid with $1 \times 1 \times 1\,\mathrm{mm}^3$ resolution.

## Results and discussion

An algorithm has been developed to reconstruct 3D electron density distributions. The algorithm works as follows:

1. A quadratic calibration of all collected profiles with data acquired under narrow beam condition is performed [8]. It converts the transmittance map, $t$, to radiological thicknesses, $L$. In mathematical notations:
$$L^{(1)} = \mathcal{P}^{-1}(t)\,. \qquad (2)$$
The calibration operator, $\mathcal{P}^{-1}$, compensates beam-hardening. Since scatter is not corrected for $L^{(1)}$ is only a first approximation to the radiological thickness. To include scatter an iterative process, summarized by
$$L^{(n)} = \mathcal{P}^{-1}\left(t - \mathcal{S}\left(L^{(n-1)}\right)\right), \qquad (3)$$
has to be performed. Here, $\mathcal{S}\left(L^{(n-1)}\right)$ is the scatter distribution calculated for a given radiological thickness map $L^{(n-1)}$, as described above.
2. After each iteration step a tomographic reconstruction can be performed. It turns out that for megavoltage energies the inverse X-ray transform, $\mathcal{R}^{-1}$, relates radiological thicknesses to electron densities relative to water
$$\delta_{\mathrm{e}}^{(n)} = \mathcal{R}^{-1}\left(L^{(n)}\right). \qquad (4)$$

We observe that after three iterations the scatter distribution converges, hence further iterations do not alter the radiological thickness maps significantly. In Fig. 2a the reconstruction of the set $L^{(1)}$ (not scatter-corrected) is displayed. Fig. 2b shows the scatter-corrected slice, reconstructed from the set $L^{(3)}$. By eye examination we see that a scatter correction removes a dome-like structure from the image. Although contours become sharper muscle is hardly detectable. However, we report a significant yield in accuracy for the reconstructed electron densities, Fig. 3. A scatter correction reduces the discrepancy of 30% to about 10% for soft tissue. Fat is located at different positions in the phantom to show the effect of a scatter correction. As a result we observe a smaller discrepancy in reconstructed electron densities for fat tissue at different locations.

The performance of the FDK algorithm in axial direction is illustrated in Fig. 4. We observe a reconstructed density

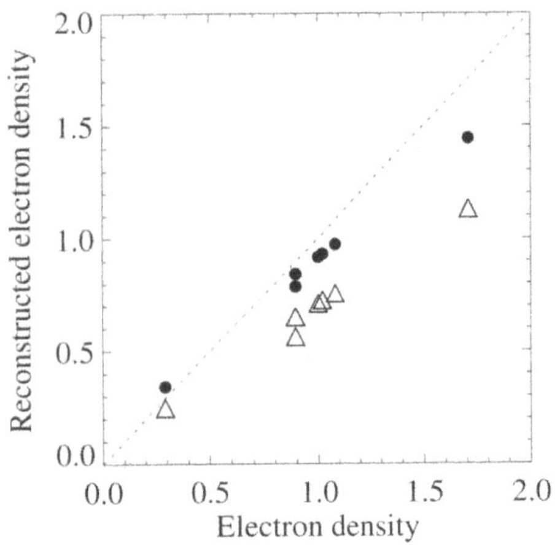


**Figure 3:** The reconstructed electron density, extracted from Fig. 2, as a function of the true electron densities is shown. The dashed line is the ideal. (△) are the electron densities without scatter correction. After correction we obtain electron densities, indicated by (•).

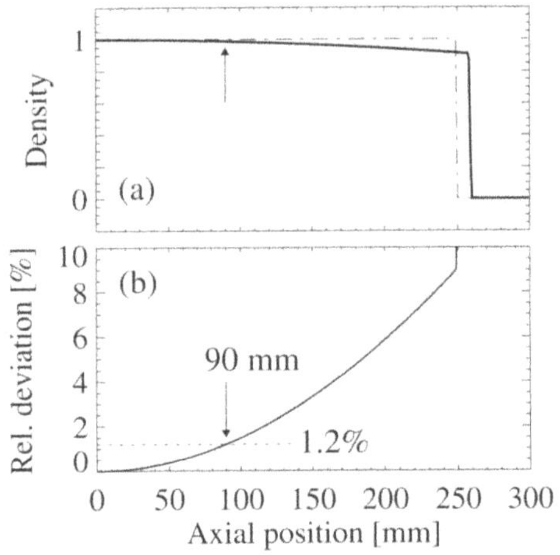


**Figure 4:** Reconstruction of an uniform ball from synthetic data. The upper plot shows the ideal shape (dash-dotted line) in comparison to the reconstruction result (solid line) in axial direction. In the lower plot the relative deviation between ideal and reconstructed profile is displayed. Arrows indicate the artefact level of the experiment.

which falls below the expected one. The level of underestimation increases with incresing axial distance. For 90 mm (corresponds to a cone beam angle of 5°), which is the radius of the ball used experimentally, the relative deviation is about 1%. Moreover, we observe distortions in the reconstructed shape, which result in a displacement of the phantom edge by 4% for a ball of 250 mm in radius.

## Conclusion

An iterative procedure, developed for scatter correction in cone beam MVCT, improves the accuracy of the reconstructed data significantly. Convergence is obtained within a small number of steps. However, rotational symmetric scatter kernels are not well-suited for phantoms, which comprise large inhomogeneities. Especially multiple-scatter kernels are strongly affected, since scattered photons travel a relatively long distance within the phantom and hence are more sensitive to the phantom composition. Moreover, the converter of the BIS strongly overestimates multiply scattered photons of low energy. As a consequence an approximation based on an isotropic distribution is insufficient if a higher degree of accuracy is sought.

Reconstruction artefacts, such as distortions and too low densities, play a role if large objects are scanned. However, for object dimensions on the scale of the experimental phantom deficiencies in scatter control dominate over reconstruction artefacts in cone beam MVCT.

## References

[1] Midgley S, Millar R M, and Dudson J 1998 A feasibility study for megavoltage cone beam CT using a commercial EPID *Phys Med Biol* **43** 155–169

[2] Ruchala K J, Olivera G H, Schloesser E A, and Mackie T R 1999 Megavoltage CT on a tomotherapy system *Phys Med Biol* **44** 2597–2621

[3] Feldkamp L A, Davis L C, and Kress J W 1984 Practical cone-beam algorithm *J Opt Soc Am* **1** 612–619

[4] Mosleh-Shirazi M A, Evans P M, Swindell W, Webb S, and Partridge M 1998 A cone-beam megavoltage CT scanner for treatment verification in conformal radiotherapy *Radiother Oncol* **48** 319–328

[5] Hansen V N, Swindell W, and Evans P M 1997 Extraction of primary signal from EPIDs using only forward convolution *Med Phys* **24** 1477–1484

[6] GEANT – Detector description and simulation tool, CERN Program Library, Long Writeup W5013, CERN Geneva, Switzerland, 1994

[7] Spies L 1999 On scatter in megavoltage X-ray transmission imaging, Doctoral thesis, University of Heidelberg

[8] Morton E J, Swindell W, Evans P M, and Lewis D G 1991 A linear array scintillation crystal-photodiode detector for megavoltage imaging *Med Phys* **18** 681–691

# Quality assurance of a videogrammetric system for computer-controlled non-invasive patient positioning for fractionated radiosurgery

**H. Treuer[1], M. Hoevels[1], N. Veeser[1], A. Gierich[1], M. Kocher[2], C. Lappe[3], S. Helfert[3], O. Pastyr [3], W. Schlegel[3], R.-P. Müller[2], and V. Sturm[1]**

[1]Dept. for Stereotaxy, U. of Cologne [2]Dept. for Radiotherapy, U of Cologne, and [3]German Cancer Research Center, Heidelberg, Germany

## Introduction

Stereotactic radiosurgery is a well established method for the treatment of small arterio-venous malformations and intra-cranial tumours. The dose distributions are characterised by steep dose gradients and have to be applied with high spatial accuracy. Therefore, radiosurgery is given to an invasively fixed patient in a single session. Compared to single dose irradiation fractionation has some radiobiological advantages and allows an extension of treatment indications. The main problem of fractionation is the loss in spatial accuracy due to the fact, that identical re-fixation of the stereotactic frame over a period of several weeks is not possible and that fixation and positioning with masks is often not precise enough for radiosurgery [1].

## Material and methods

A *frameless* high precision system for fractionated linac radiosurgery has been designed (Patient Position Sensor Unit PPSU). The method is based on the precise *initial* localisation and positioning of the target using an invasive fixation of the patient in the stereotactic frame. The system developed consists of (1) a videogrammetric position sensor, infra-red illumination and an landmark system with individual shaped dento-maxillary fixation, (2) a computer controlled table top, and (3) a patient management system (Fig.1 and 2).

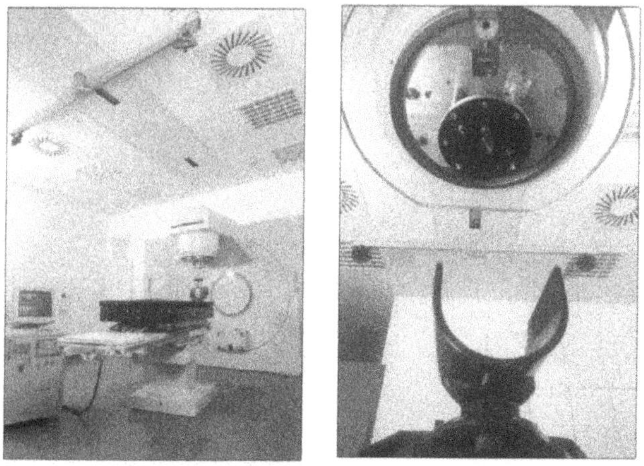

**Figure 1:** Room view with stereo cameras, PPSU computer and table top (left) and head holder and stereotactic collimator and stereo cameras (rght)

Fractionated stereotactic radiosurgery starts –like single dose irradiation– with the invasive fixation of the head in the stereotactic frame, stereotactic imaging, target localisation, dose planning and adjustment of the patient at the linac. But instead of applying the full dose the patient position at the linac is registered by measuring the landmark position of the mouth piece videogrammetrically. At the following fractions the patient is fixed non-invasively and the target points are adjusted automatically to the isocenter by the system according to the data of the initial positioning. During irradiation, the patient position is controlled and may be corrected manual or automatically.

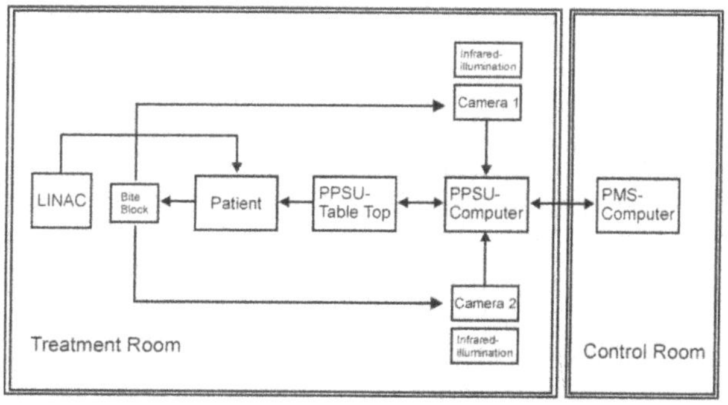


**Figure 2:** Block diagram of the PPSU with feedback control loop

A quality assurance program for fractionated radiosurgery with the PPSU has been developed. It consists of test for determination of the initial status of the system and of tests checking the constancy of the system. Therefore, a set of test phantoms has been developed: (1) Calibration phantom for determination of the camera parameters, control of camera position with respect to the room lasers and for determination of the long term stability, (2) test phantom for the stability of mouth piece and landmark system, (3) xyz-drive for determination of the linearity of the measurement system, (4) oscillator for determination of the control parameters of the feedback control loop, (5) film box with positioning device for determination and control of the accuracy of positioning with respect to the radiation isocenter, (6) head phantom for determination of the overall accuracy of the system for fractionated radiosurgery (Fig. 3 and 4).

## Results and discussion

Measurement of the *long term stability* of the position sensor shows a constancy of ±0.1 mm within a period of 72 h. Measurement of the *constancy* of positioning with respect to the radiation isocenter shows deviations less than ±0.3 mm in a period of several weeks. This is the same range as the accuracy of positioning of a film box to lasers manually.

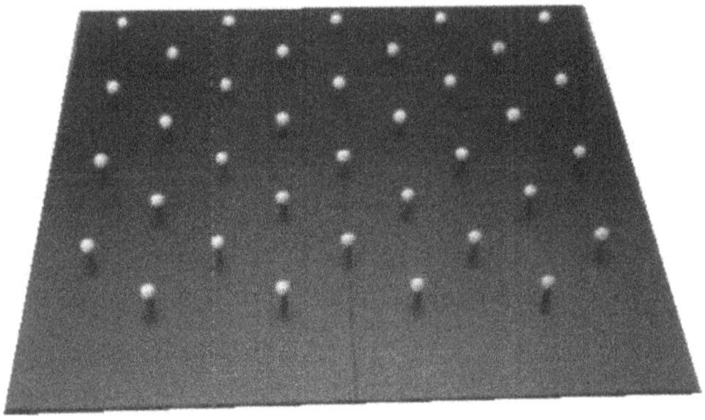

**Figure 3**: Calibration phantom for room lasers and camera system

The frequency of measurement depends on the segmentation algorithm and is 60 Hz in maximum. The *time delay* of the feedback control loop is ≈0.09 s for the correction of horizontal displacements and ≈0.15 s for vertical displacements. The maximal *speed* of the table top is 17 mm/s in horizontal directions and 3.3 mm/s in vertical direction. The *attenuation factor* defined as the ratio of the average deviation with closed and with open feedback loop (for amplitudes of 1 mm) is 0.1 at 1 Hz, 0.25 at 0.2 Hz and 0.4 at 0.5 Hz (Fig. 5a).
The *repositioning accuracy* of the mouth piece at the patient is 0.28 mm ±0.14 mm [2].
The *overall accuracy* of the system is better than 1 mm i.e. the spatial shift of the filmdosimteric (GafChromic) measured dose distribution compared to the calculated dose distribution (STP3) has been less than 1 mm in three test runs. This result includes the errors in target localisation, dose planning, initial positioning with the stereotactic positioning device, repositioning with the PPSU, linac irradiation and computer aided film dosimetry (Fig 5b).

## Conclusion

The developed system for computer-controlled non-invasive patient positioning is highly accurate and reliable. It allows the identical repositioning of a patient over a period of several weeks with an accuracy better than 0.5 mm. The overall accuracy is better than 1 mm. Thus the method is as accurate as single dose radiosurgery. Methods for verification of patient set-up using port films are currently investigated.

## References

[1] Menke M, Hirschfeld F, Mack M, Pastyr O, Sturm V, and Schlegel W 1994 Photogrammetric accuracy measurement of head holder systems for fractionated radiotherapy *Int. J. Rad. Oncol. Biol. Phys.* **29** 1147-1155

[2] Lappe C, Helfert S, Braun M, Pastyr O, Sturm V, and Schlegel W 1997 *A videogrammetric system for computer-controlled non-invasive patient positioning*, Proc. XIIth Int. Conf. on the Use of Computers in Radiation Therapy, Salt Lake City, Utah, 168-171

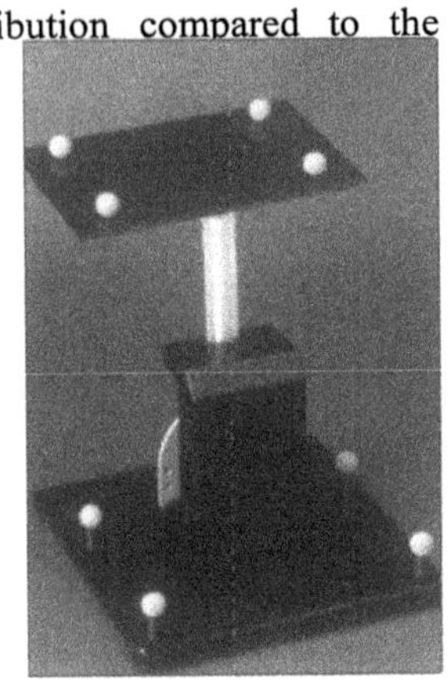

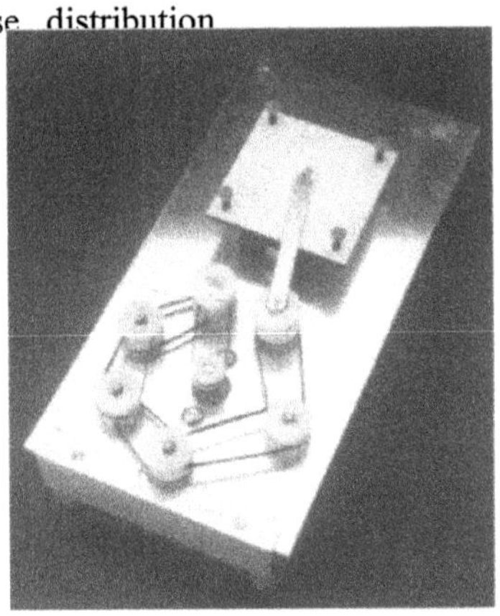

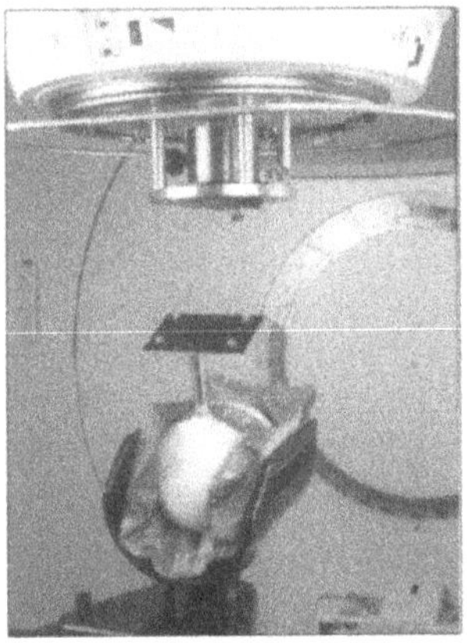

**Figure 4:** Control phantom for bite plate and landmark system (left), oscillator (center) and head phantom with landmark system (right)

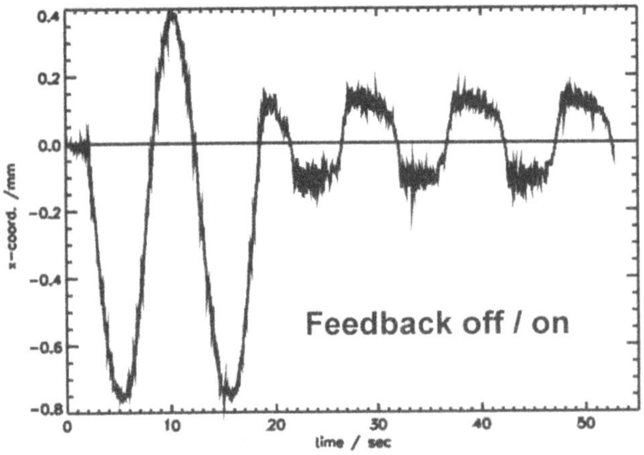


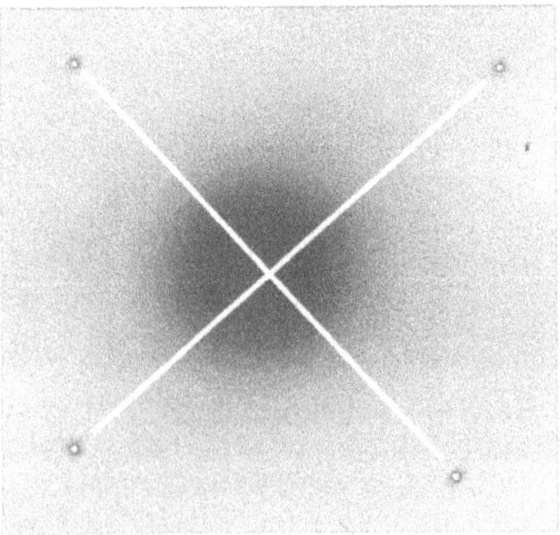

**Figure 5:** Measurement with the oscillator and open/closed feedback control loop (left) and measurement of the overall accuracy with GafChromic film and two lines emphasizing the target point (right).

# Initial experience with a system for automated patient positioning

**Rex Boone and Timothy Solberg**

Department of Radiation Oncology, University of California Los Angeles, Los Angeles, CA

## Introduction

Conformal radiation therapy promises to deliver high tumor doses while sparing nearby tissue. Full realization of this promise, however, requires accurate and convenient patient positioning. Methods for positioning cranial targets rely on the rigidity of this body region. This work investigates a novel approach for positioning extracranial targets based on the location of IR reflective markers attached to the patient's skin. Both phantom and volunteer tests assess the accuracy and reproducibility of the system. Volunteer tests suggest that in addition to positioning the patient, the system might also track his breathing cycle for gating of the linear accelerator. The system promises to strengthen the weak link in the chain of conformal radiation therapy, patient positioning. While conventional accuracy is between 5-10 mm[1], this system positions a target to within 2-3 mm of the isocenter.

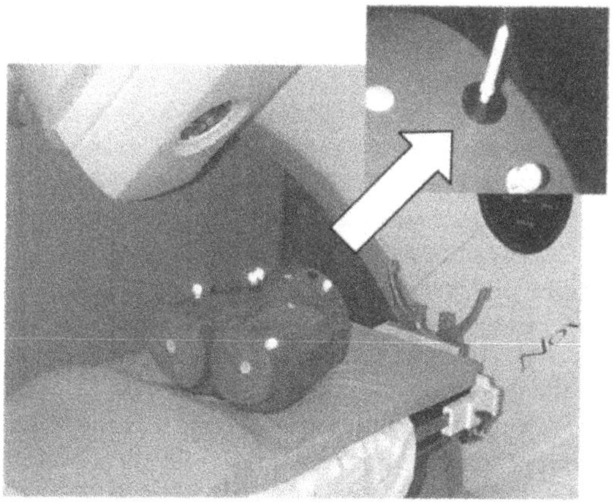

**Figure 1:** Torso phantom with markers and target attached.

## Material and methods

Two infrared tracking cameras separated by approximately 3 m mount on the ceiling of the treatment room. LEDs around the lenses of each camera emit IR towards the isocenter of the linac at a distance between 2-5 m. A coating on the spherical markers with a diameter of 13 mm reflects IR back to the cameras. The spherical markers form circular images in each camera plane. Software algorithms determine the center of each image. Based on the 2D coordinates of the centers, additional algorithms calculate the 3D coordinates of the markers through the techniques of photogrammetry.[2] At a frequency over 20 Hz, the system determines the coordinates of each marker within 0.3 mm.

An initial simulation places the target at the isocenter of the linac. The system locates and stores this position relative to the IR markers. Vector geometry allows it to reposition the target at the isocenter; averaging algorithms improve the accuracy. The system can automatically drive the couch into position or the user can manually position it based on the computer display.

The spherical markers screw onto a flat plastic base that attaches to a surface with adhesive. For the first tests, markers attached to a plastic torso phantom in Figure 1. A small plastic nipple also attached to the phantom served as a target. The displacement of the nipple from the intersection of the lasers determined the positioning accuracy of the system. The accuracy of the system was determined with both stationary and shifting markers.

In addition to positioning based on an initial simulation, the system can establish a coordinate system relative to the marker positions measured from CT. At the center of each marker, a small metal sphere appears on the CT scan without artifacts. The treatment planning software recognizes these markers and transfers their relative positions to the positioning software. Figure 2 displays an axial slice through the torso phantom at the target; the markers in other slices appear as small dots.

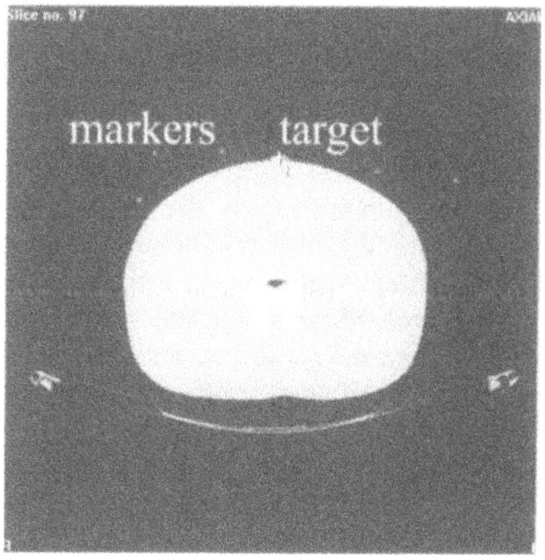


**Figure 2:** CT treatment plan to target based on marker positions.

Next, the markers and target attached to the skin of several volunteers. Because exhalation is the most reproducible position in the breathing cycle,[3] initial setup of the volunteers occurred during exhalation. In addition, a couch-mounted vacuum bag held the volunteers in a rigid position for the measurements. The cradle attached to the couch and its sloped sides and ridged back held the vacuum bag in place. Marks on the volunteer's skin aligned with marks on the bag to place the volunteer in a reproducible position. Additional marks drawn around the plastic base of each marker repositioned the markers on the volunteers' skin between measurements. Once the target was in position, displacements of the markers from their initial positions were also recorded. Recording during exhalation minimized the motion due to breathing. Thus, measurement of marker position estimated skin shifts, body shifts, and reattachment errors. One set of measurements positioned volunteers during several trials on a single day. Markers were removed and reattached between measurements. For another set of measurements, volunteers returned over several days to simulate treatment of a patient. Each day, the skin marks were redrawn to place the markers in the same spot during the next day.

Markers were also attached to the thermoplastic masks of several stereotactic and head-and-neck patients. The rigid surface of the mask should provide accuracy comparable to results on the torso phantom. During the first day of treatment, the therapists accurately set the stereotactic patient into position based on stereotactic information. The IR system then acquired a simulation of the markers and target based on this initial position. Over the course of treatment, the IR system measured the displacement of the target from the isocenter after the therapists had positioned the patient.

Measurements were made on the head-and-neck masks without the patients present. Three BBs marked the intersections of the lasers with the mask during the simulation. A target was planned at the intersections of lines joining these BBs. Separate targets were also planned to each BB. The treatment planning system determined the position of the targets relative to IR markers attached to the mask in the CT scan. Without the patient, the masks were positioned so that the lasers intersected the BBs. The IR system then measured the displacement of the target from the isocenter in a number of trials. Then, the system positioned the mask so that each target BB was at the isocenter. The displacement in each direction was measured and a total displacement calculated.

## Results and discussion

Stationary markers on the surface of a rigid torso phantom provided the best positioning accuracy. The mean displacement of the target from the isocenter after repositioning by the system was 0.5 mm with any number of markers. CT localization of the markers and target increased this mean value to 1.0 mm. The accuracy with stationary markers did not depend on number or location of markers.

Shifting the markers on the surface of the phantom increased displacement of the target from the isocenter. Small (2.5 mm) and large (5.0 mm) random shifts of all markers on the surface of the phantom result in Figure 3. The system returned the target to the isocenter based on the shifted marker positions. Accuracy improved with number of markers. Results did not differ significantly for simulation or CT positioning.

Figure 4 graphs the displacement of markers with breathing at several locations on the skin surface of one volunteer. Positioning began on exhalation. During succeeding exhalations, the markers and isocenter returned within 1 mm of their initial positions on all volunteers. Bony areas moved less than 1 mm while the stomach moved over 10 mm. The chest region showed wide variations between 2-5 mm with shallow breathing among these volunteers in agreement with other work.[4]

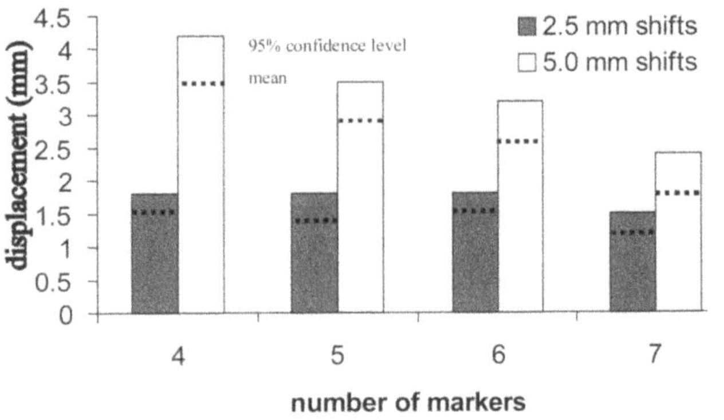


**Figure 3:** Positioning accuracy with shifting markers on phantom.

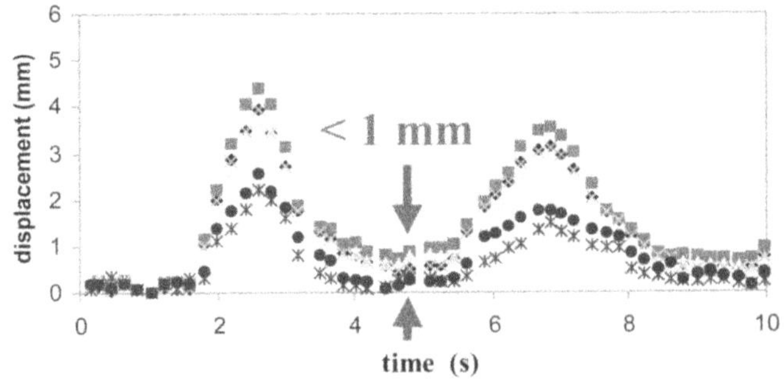


**Figure 4:** Marker shift with breathing on one volunteer.

Table 1 displays the positioning results for three volunteers with trials over several days. The accuracy for all trials was better than 3 mm. Trials over several days were not significantly worse than trials on a single day.

The system also tracked the position of each marker. With the target in position, marker positions were compared against the initial values. Because exhalation minimized shifts due to breathing, the displacement estimated skin shift and marker placement errors. The couch-mounted vacuum bag limited shifts to less than 2 mm and improved positioning accuracy. Without the apparatus, marker shifts exceeded 5 mm.

| | Volunteer | | |
|---|---|---|---|
| day | A | B | C |
| 1 | 0.9 | 1.8 | 1.9 |
| 2 | 1.0 | 1.4 | |
| 3 | 1.6 | 1.2 | 1.2 |
| 4 | | 1.9 | |
| 5 | | 2.1 | 1.8 |
| 6 | | 3.0 | |
| 7 | | | |
| 8 | | | 1.6 |

**Table 1:** System accuracy (mm) on volunteers over several days.

Because the markers do not move on the surface of the stereotactic masks, simulation measurements in Table 2 show mean accuracy of about 1 mm. Positioning of the rigid torso phantom produced similar results. At the same time, a small phantom checked the isocenter position before each treatment. Five IR markers attached to this phantom. Lines scored on each side of the block align it accurately with the lasers. Daily positioning errors of the phantom were much less than 1 mm.

| | displacement (mm) | |
|---|---|---|
| **patient** | **mean** | **95% level** |
| **A** | 0.71 | 0.92 |
| **B** | 0.67 | 1.05 |
| **iso check** | 0.24 | 0.29 |

**Table 2:** Positioning accuracy of stereotactic masks in simulation.

The system positioned the head-and-neck masks based on CT information. In Table 3, the accuracy is between 1-2 mm for the target BBs and 2-3 mm for the isocenter. Localization of the isocenter depends on accurate localization of three BBs, and so the error is slightly larger. The system positioned the same isocenter phantom above to better than 1 mm based on a CT scan of the phantom. These results also agree with tests on the rigid torso phantom.

| **patient** | | **mean** | **95% level** |
|---|---|---|---|
| **C** | | | |
| | iso | 2.16 | 2.42 |
| | BB | 1.20 | 1.52 |
| **D** | | | |
| | iso | 2.43 | 2.84 |
| | BB | 1.86 | 2.04 |
| **iso check** | | 0.93 | 1.11 |

**Table 3:** Positioning accuracy for head-and-neck masks in CT.

## Conclusion

Tests indicate that a positioning system attaching IR reflective markers to the patient's skin for localization of a target is both accurate and convenient. The system automatically positions the target to within a few millimeters of the isocenter over several trials. Accuracy on the thermoplastic masks approaches that on the torso phantom with stationary markers. Based on these results, a few patients who could not be positioned with conventional stereotactic methods have been positioned with markers attached to masks. Future work will assess the accuracy of the system in clinical situations involving extracranial targets. It will also use the system for gated radiation therapy based on movement of the marks with breathing.

## References

[1] Rudat V et al. 1994 Influence of positioning error on 3D conformal dose distributions during fractionated radiotherapy *Rad Ther Onc* **33** 56-63

[2] Atkinson K ed. 1996 Close Range Photogrammetry and Machine Vision

[3] Balter J et al. 1998 Improvement of CT-based treatment-planning models of abdominal targets using static exhale imaging *Int J Rad OncBio Phys* **41** 939-943

[4] Kubo H et al. 1996 Respiration gated radiotherapy treatment: a technical study *Phys Med Biol* **41** 83-91

[5] Rogus D et al. 1999 Accuracy of a photogrammetry-based patient positioning and monitoring system for radiation therapy *Med Phys* **26** 721-728

# Implementation of a System for Precision, Automated Daily Target Volume Positioning

**Dale W. Litzenberg[1], James Balter, Kwok Lam, Daniel McShan, and Randall Ten Haken**

[1]The University of Michigan Department of Radiation Oncology, Ann Arbor, Michigan, 48109-0010

## Introduction

It is hypothesized that with precise target volume localization, Planning Target Volume (PTV) margins may be reduced, leading to reduced complications by increased sparing of adjacent normal tissues. A system has been implemented for precise, daily localization and positioning of the target volume within a patient. This system is an integrated extension of our Computer Controlled Radiotherapy System (CCRS) which was developed in-house. In recent years the technology to build such a system has been available but lack of integration prevented it from being a practical clinical system. This system employs orthogonal digital radiographs, obtained using room mounted diagnostic X-ray tubes and a digital flat panel imager, to localize radio-opaque markers implanted at the periphery of the target volume. Three-dimensional marker positions are extracted from the images and compared to known reference positions, obtained from CT data, to find a six-degree-of-freedom correctional transformation which may be applied automatically.

## Materials and Methods

In this section we will describe the architecture of the system, it's integration into CCRS and the basic properties of the sub-systems.

### System Architecture

The system is designed around an independent modular architecture and shown schematically in Figure 1. Communication between modules is implemented through predefined text strings. Such a design allows independent modules to be modified and upgraded to new technology without affecting other systems. Modules must be designed so that if another module is not available or malfunctioning, an alternative path or technique may be implemented. Communication between modules is typically by means of Berkeley Sockets on a protected network.

### Tilt and Roll Sub-System

The Tilt and Roll Table [1, 2] allows two additional rotational degrees of freedom for correcting target volume orientation. The Tilt and Roll capabilities of the table are accessed and controlled through the Tilt and Roll Server. This server contains a geometrical model of the table, monitors the current position of the table and its state, and calculates table position correction parameters based on the measured target volume transformation.

### Imaging Sub-System

Target volume position is measured using two diagnostic X-ray tubes and a digital imager. The X-ray tubes are mounted on the ceiling and the wall with the ceiling tube 9 degrees off AP, 190 cm from isocenter, and the wall tube 5 degrees below lateral, 290 cm from isocenter. These locations are separated by 86 degrees and help visually differentiate anatomy and marker locations in the direction longitudinal to the view. A dot graticule is mounted to each X-ray tube to provide a projected reference geometry at isocenter.

An amorphous silicon flat panel imager with a 30 cm x 40 cm active area and 127 micron pixel pitch is used to acquire images. The imager is manually moved to the appropriate location for each image. A suite of image manipulation tools, including windowing and histogram equalization, is available to optimize image quality. The images are originally 2304 pixels x 3200 pixels at 2 bytes per pixel. These are reduced to 512 pixels by 711 pixels at 1 byte per pixel for use in the user interface.

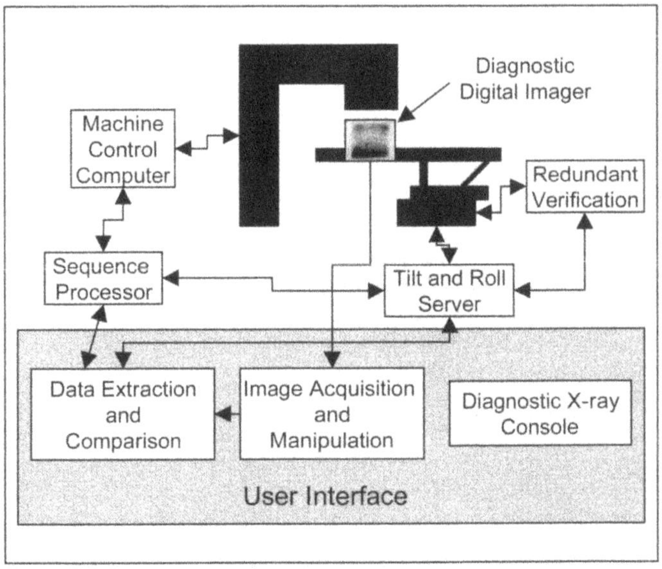


**Figure 1:** Schematic architecture of the Target-of-the-Day Positioning System.

### User Interface

The graphical user interface (GUI) [4] presents the AP and the lateral images as shown in Figure 2. Buttons provide tools for finding the dot graticules and markers in the images. After isocenter and the markers have been identified in the images, the 3-dimensional marker locations may be calculated and compared to the stored reference positions. (Reference positions are determined by localizing the implanted markers in the planning CT volume data set.) The correctional target volume transfomation is presented to the user. The user may decide to correct translations only or both translations and rotations. If only translations are corrected the changes are sent to the Sequence Processor (SP) and implemented by pendant controls. If translations and rotations are corrected, the measured target volume transformation is sent to the Tilt and Roll Server which calculates and returns the changes in table position to return the target volume to isocenter and account for the rotations about a non-isocenteric point (ie. the universal joint under the center of the table.) These changes in table position are sent to the SP which initiates the translational and table floor rotation corrections and sends a command to the Tilt and Roll Server to initiate the other rotational corrections.

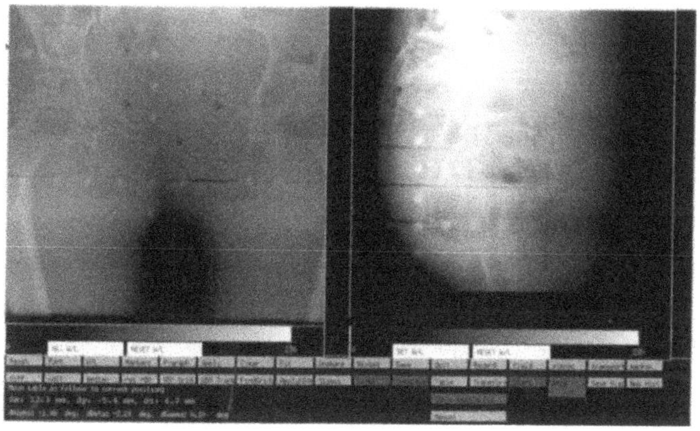

**Figure 2:** The graphical user interface with AP and lateral images.

## Results and discussion

This system is currently in use for a daily prostate positioning protocol as well as part of a focal liver protocol combined with Active Breathing Control. A trial is currently being developed to apply this system to fractionated acoustic neuroma treatments. Patient setup and target volume position correction takes approximately 5 minutes for the prostate protocol. Initial patient setup time could be reduced since the patient does not have to be precisely localized; only immobilized and placed in the field of view of the imager. After the patient is placed on the immobilized, image acquistion takes about one minute as the imager must be manually placed, and moved between images. Image manipulation, scaling and storage takes an additional two minutes. Localizing the dot graticules and markers and finding the correctional transformation in the user interface takes approximately thirty seconds. Applying computer controlled target volume corrections takes about 10 seconds. Software is being developed which will incorporate the necessary image acquistion, manipulation, and analysis capabilities into a single graphical user interface application. Once in place, the system will be easier to use, more automated and further reduce the setup correction time by approximately two minutes.

Studies, in which a phantom was offset by known translations and rotations, indicate a positioning accuracy of roughly +/- 0.2 cm in each translation and +/- 1.0 degree in each rotation. This includes an uncertainty of roughly +/- 0.1 cm and +/- 0.5 degrees in the determined correctional transformation. The remaining translational uncertainty is primarily due to limitations of the table translation control system which has one millimeter position resolution.

Issues that require further investigation include an evaluation of the positioning accuracy in patients where there is a non-rigid target volume geometry. Changes in tumor size and migration of the markers will reduce the repositioning accuracy. Based on the results of this evaluation, Planning Target Volume (PTV) margins may be reduced to spare adjacent normal tissue and reduce complications. In turn, this may allow higher doses to be delivered to improve local tumor control at some sites [5].

## Conclusion

A system has been implemented for precise, daily localization and positioning of the target volume within a patient. This system allows daily on-line target volume position correction with six degrees of freedom. Its accuracy in phantoms is approximately +/- 0.2 cm in each translation and +/- 1.0 degree in each rotation. The current implementation of this system allows the patient to be setup, the target volume position corrected and ready to treat in approximately 5 minutes. This is made possible by the integration of the sub-systems into a semi-automated system, with an interface to a computer controlled radiotherapy system.

## References

[1] Hornick D C, Litzenberg D W, Lam K L, Balter J M, Hetrick J, and Ten Haken R K, "A tilt and roll device for automated correction of rotational setup errors," *Med. Phys.*, **25(9),** 1739-40, September 1998.

[2] Litzenberg D W, Balter J M, Hornick D C, Lam K L, and Ten Haken R K, "A mathematical model for correcting patient setup errors using a tilt and roll device," *Med. Phys.*, **26(12),** December, 1999.

[3] Lam K L, Ten Haken R K, McShan D L, Thorton Jr. A F, "Automated determination of patient setup errors in radiation therapy using spherical radio-opaque markers," *Med. Phys*., **20(4),** Jul/Aug, 1145-52, 1993.

[4] Balter J, Chen G T Y, Pelizzari C A: "Correlation of projection radiographs in radiation therapy using open curve and point pairs", Med Phys **19**, 329-334, 1992.

[5] Balter J, Chen G T Y, Pelizzari C A, Krishnasamy S, Rubin S, Vijayakumar S, "Online repositioning during treatment of the prostate, A study of potential limits and gains," *Int J Rad Onc Biol Phys* **27**, 137-143, 1993.

# Using routine portal images to detect internal organ motion in prostate cancer patients; a simulation

**Joep C. Stroom,[1] Kasper L. Pasma,[1] Peter C.M. Koper,[2] and Ben J.M. Heijmen.[1]**

Daniel den Hoed Cancer Center, University Hospital Rotterdam, [2]Department of Radiotherapy, [1]Division of Clinical Physics, Groene Hilledijk 301, 3075 EA Rotterdam, The Netherlands. **E-mail:** stroom@kfih.azr.nl.

## Introduction

Geometrical uncertainties in external radiotherapy consist for a large part of set-up errors and internal organ motion. Set-up deviations can be derived from portal images acquired during the treatment. The gray shades in those images reflect the irradiated radiological thicknesses and bony structures are therefore highly visible. Determining the position of the bony anatomy relative to the reference situation yields the set-up deviation. In routine portal images of pelvic fields, the most visible objects besides bony structures are gas pockets in the rectum. These gas pockets might indicate the position of the ventral rectum wall, which is expected to have a good correlation with the prostate position because of their close proximity. In Fig. 1 the idea behind this correlation is

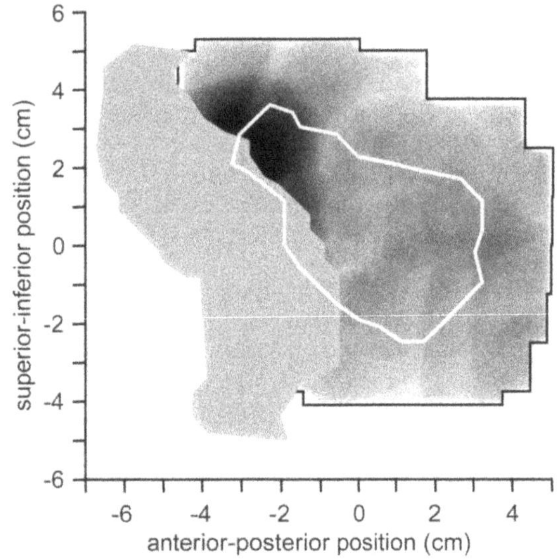


**Figure 1** The beams-eye-view (BEV) contours of the planned rectum and CTV of a prostate cancer patient superimposed on a lateral portal image used for set-up verification. The dark spot in the image indicates a gas pocket that extends outside the rectum. This implies that the local rectum wall, and probably the prostate, moved in a ventral direction.

visualized. Kroonwijk *et al* already pointed out that gas pockets in portal images can reveal internal organ motion.[1] They did however not specify how this could be used in practice. In this abstract, a method for using the imaged gas pockets for quantitative determination of the rectum wall and prostate position is proposed. Compared to other methods which make use of e.g. radio-opaque markers or multiple CT data, this method is non-invasive and little extra work is required; portal images are already routinely made for set-up verification in our institute.

## Material and methods

In order to verify whether gas pockets in clinical portal images can be used to quantitatively predict rectum wall and prostate movement, simulations have been performed using previously obtained multiple CT scans acquired during treatment of 15 prostate cancer patients.[2] In Fig. 2 a schematic outline of the study set-up is depicted. Firstly, the 4 CT data sets per patient were matched and resliced in 3D to remove the set-up

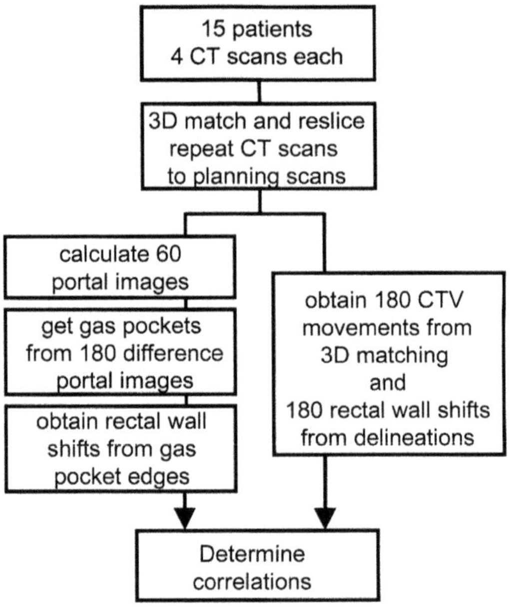


**Figure 2** Schematic outline of the study set-up.

deviations. In all scans the clinical target volume (CTV) and rectum were delineated. Secondly, portal images for the left lateral beams were simulated from the resliced data sets by calculation of so-called radiological thickness images (RTIs), in which the pixel values indicate the radiologic thickness in cm. In order to automatically detect gas pockets, difference images (dRTIs) between two scans (a repeat scan and a reference scan) were created for all combinations per patient. To avoid that a gas pocket in the repeat scan is neutralized by a gas pocket in the reference scan, the rectum in the *reference* scan was automatically filled with water-equivalent CT values before calculation of the reference RTI (i.e. gas pockets were removed). The gas pocket edges were automatically detected in the dRTIs and subsequently used to estimate the local rectum wall shifts between two scans (see Fig. 3). Thirdly, the "true" rectum wall shifts between two scans were measured by comparing rectum delineations in reference and repeat CT scan. Corresponding movements of the center-of-mass (COM) of the prostate were determined from 3D chamfer matching. Finally, the rectum wall shifts as determined in the portal images were correlated with the true rectum wall shifts and with the prostate COM movement.

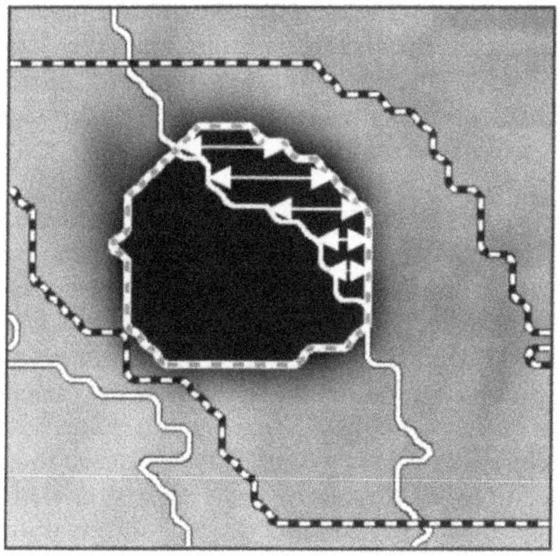

**Figure 3** Determination of the rectum wall shift in a dRTI. The search area (outer dashed contour) to find gas pockets is limited by rectum (white contour) and prostate (not indicated) projections. The gas pocket is automatically detected by searching for all pixels connected to the pixel with the minimal value that remain below a user defined threshold. The resulting gas pocket is indicated by the lightly dashed contour. The rectum wall shift is estimated as the average AP shift along the cranio-caudal length of the gas pocket, as indicated by the arrows.

## Results

Fig. 4 shows a dRTI with a significant prostate shift between two CT scans of the same patient, due to the appearance of a gas pocket. In this dRTI the BEV projection of the respective prostates and rectums are indicated. In the repeat scan the rectum is clearly larger than in the reference scan. Also, a rather large gas pocket is visible, the ventral edge of which corresponds nicely to the rectum wall in the repeat scan. Hence the edge of the gas pocket gives a good estimate of the position of the rectum wall. Moreover, the two prostate projections indicate a clear ventral shift of the prostate which in turn corresponds nicely to the rectum wall shift.

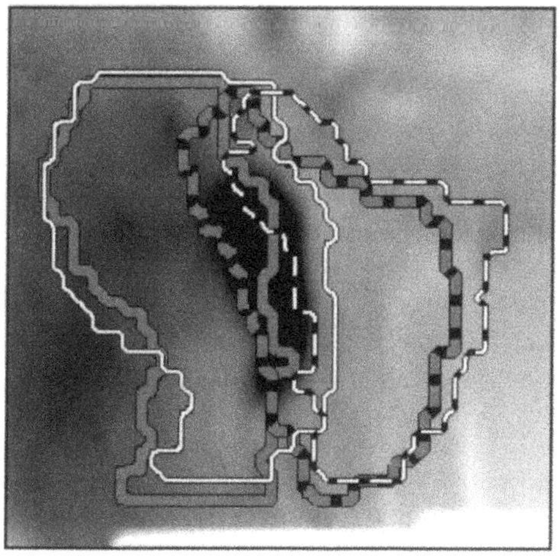

**Figure 4** Example of a prostate motion that can be detected by a gas pocket in the difference RTI. BEV projection of rectums are indicated by solid lines, prostates by dashed lines. In the dRTIs the reference organs are indicated by thick gray lines, the repeat organs by thin white lines.

In Fig. 5 the rectum wall shifts as derived from gas pockets in dRTIs, are plotted against the true rectum wall shift. The thickness threshold that was used for gas pocket detection was equal to the optimal value of 2 cm. Lower values generated too many false positive gas pockets, higher values reduced the number of detected gas pockets and the efficacy of the method. The excellent correlation, r = 0.97, implies that if a gas pocket is detected in a lateral portal image, one is able to predict the position of the local rectum wall accurately. The

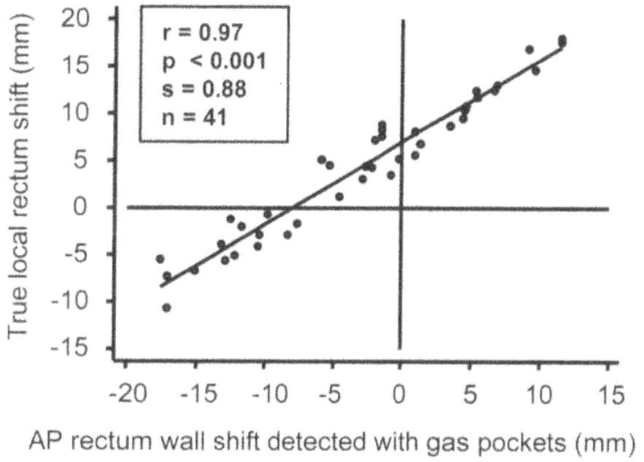


**Figure 5** The correlation between true local rectum wall shifts and rectum wall shifts detected using gas pockets in dRTIs. Ventral shifts are positive and dorsal shifts negative. Indicated are the correlation coefficient (r), the statistical significance (p), the slope of the curve (s), and the number of measurements (n).

offset of the straight fit from zero (ca. 7 mm) is due to the fact that the gas pocket edge is always more dorsal then the true rectum wall due to the thickness of the wall itself and due to the threshold that is used to detect the gas pocket.

In Fig. 6 the measured AP rectum wall shifts (with threshold equal to 2 cm) that were corrected for offsets and tilted rectum walls, are plotted versus the corresponding AP translations of the prostate COM measured by 3D matching. One possible explanation for the correlation (r=0.88) and the slope (s=0.68) not being equal to 1 is that the translation of the prostate COM has been plotted against a local rectum wall shift, and for instance prostatic rotations have not been taken into account. Furthermore, especially near the cranial part of the prostate (where most gas pockets are observed), there can be a relatively wide separation between prostate and rectum, i.e. the rectum may shift locally without moving the prostate.

Visible inspection of the 60 CT scans revealed that 17 scans had gas pockets. Therefore maximally 51 internal organ motions might have been detected instead of the 41 as shown in Figs. 5 and 6. Considering a total of 180 internal organ motions, only 23 % could be detected using gas pockets. However, when only the ventral prostate shifts are considered,

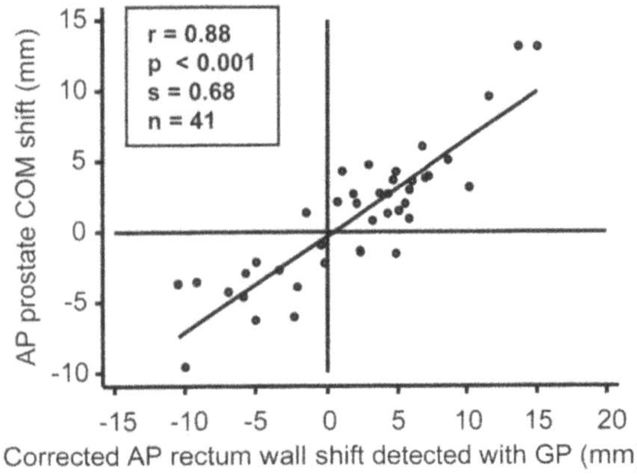


**Figure 6** The correlation between AP movements of the COM of the prostate, as measured with 3D chamfer matching, and rectum wall shifts detected from gas pockets in the dRTIs. The applied rectum wall shifts were corrected for the slope of the rectum wall near the gas pockets and the threshold dependent distance between the true rectum wall and the gas pocket edge.

40 % (4 of 10) larger than 5 mm was accompanied by a detected gas pocket, and all shifts (3) larger than 7 mm were detected. This is due to the fact that large ventral shifts imply a large increase in rectum volume which are more likely to be accompanied by gas pockets. For the same reason, dorsal prostate movements are less likely to be detected, which explains the asymmetrical shape of Fig. 6. In clinical practice one might be particularly interested in ventral shifts because those imply movement of the rectum, which is the most critical structure for prostate treatments, into the treatment field. In our institute, the ventral shifts dominate because rectum laxation is used before acquisition of the planning CT scan. The detection probability for the 45 shifts with respect to the clinical planning CTs only, confirm this: 50 % (3 of 6) of shifts larger than or equal to 5 mm is detected.

## Discussion

In order to use clinical portal images to quantify internal organ movement, the "repeat" portal image as acquired with e.g. an EPID should be comparable to the reference image as derived from the CT data. This implies that the clinical portal dose image should be converted to a reference RTI, or vice versa. Pasma *et al* have indicated that RTIs can be derived from portal images obtained with a CCD camera based fluoroscopic EPID.[3] The clinical images will generally be noisier than the simulated RTIs used in this study, which might make the smaller gas pockets invisible. Furthermore, if too many artifacts appear, the threshold for gas pocket detection might have to be increased. This would decrease the number of detected gas pockets, but the largest and most significant ones would still be caught.

If a rectum wall shift from the reference situation is found using the dRTI, two different strategies may be followed before the rest of the fraction is given. The first strategy is aimed at sparing the rectum which can at some (boost) stage of the treatment get a higher priority than adequate irradiation of the prostate. In case the ventral gas pocket wall in the dRTI indicates that the rectum wall has moved into the treatment field, a correction of the table position or the lateral treatment fields (e.g. MLCs) can be applied to shield the rectum wall. The second strategy primarily aims at an accurate irradiation of the prostate. If a rectum wall shift is observed, the fit in Fig. 6 can be used to determine the probable prostate movement. The isocenter of the lateral beams can then be moved accordingly before the rest of the fraction dose is applied. Considering the limited accuracy of the fit, action might be undertaken only in case of larger prostate shifts (e.g. > 4 mm).

In the future, methods may be investigated to increase the detection probability (i.e. the gas pocket frequency). Nevertheless, even if only a limited percentage of prostate movements is correctable, the size of the safety margins and treatment portals might be decreased. For instance, the overall standard deviation of the AP prostate COM movements for the 45 shifts from the planning CT scans in this study was 3.8 mm. If the detected gas pockets would have been used to correct the prostate position (in 11 cases), this standard deviation would reduce to 2.8 mm. If we assume the planning margin equal to about 2 times this overall standard deviation[4] (and if we neglect other sources of uncertainties), a margin reduction of 2 mm would be justified.

## Conclusion

An accurate, quick and non-invasive method was proposed for determination of internal organ motion in prostate cancer patients with an EPID. A study based on multiple CT data indicated that gas pockets in routine portal images might be used to detect the ventral rectum wall and the prostate COM position. Since not all organ motions are caused by gas pockets, not all movements can be detected, but the method is especially sensitive for the larger movements. Hence, clinical portal images which were up till now only used for set-up correction, might with little extra effort also be used to correct field shapes for internal organ motions. Further clinical study is required.

## References

[1] Kroonwijk M, Pasma K L, Quint S, Koper P C M, Visser A G and Heijmen B J M 1998 In-vivo dosimetry for prostate cancer patients using an electronic portal imaging device (EPID); demonstration of internal organ motion *Radiother. Oncol.* **49**, 125-132

[2] Stroom J C, Koper P C, Korevaar G A, van Os M, Janssen M, Levendag P C and Heijmen B J M 1999 Internal organ motion in prostate cancer patients treated in prone and supine position *Radiother. Oncol.* **51**, 237-248

[3] Pasma K L, Kroonwijk M, van Dieren E B, Visser A G, and Heijmen B J M 1999 Verification of compensator thicknesses using a fluoroscopic electronic portal imaging device *Med. Phys.* **26**, 1524-1529

[4] Stroom J C, de Boer J C J, Huizenga H, and Visser A G 1999 Inclusion of geometrical uncertainties in radiotherapy treatment planning by means of coverage probability *Int. J. Radiat. Oncol. Biol. Phys.* **43**, 905-919

# Preliminary evaluation of a non-invasive ultrasound prostate localization device

J. Markman[1], D.A. Low[1], R. LaLonde[2], R. Halperin[3], J.M. Michalski[1], and J.A. Purdy[1]

[1]Mallinckrodt Institute of Radiology. St. Louis, Missouri , [2]Western Pennsylvania Hospital. Pittsburgh, Pennsylvania, and [3]Cross Cancer Institute. Edmonton, Canada

## Introduction

Three-dimensional conformal radiotherapy (3DCRT) is increasingly being used in the treatment of prostate cancer. Published clinical studies show that 3DCRT can allow for dose escalation to the prostate, tighter conformal fields, and satisfactory normal tissue toxicity [1]. However, the traditional solution of increasing prostate tumor volumes to account for localization and organ motion uncertainties gives the possibility of increasing normal tissue toxicity. Studies suggest that mean internal motion of the prostate relative to the bony anatomy can be as large as 5 mm along a major axis[2]. Daily setup procedures also introduce errors in prostate localization. Studies have indicated a shift in the position of the beams relative to bony anatomy, with variations up to 1 cm [3,4]. Online radiographic portal imaging can reduce the variation in daily setup error but cannot account for physiologic motion of the prostate. The ideal approach would setup patients for treatment based on the prostate position at time of treatment. The BAT ultrasound localization device (produced by NOMOS) has been developed to noninvasively locate the prostate and position it as close to its position in the CT-treatment plan (relative to isocenter) as possible. If proven to be precise and accurate, the BAT device can minimize the setup error, ultimately allowing for tighter margins and more effective treatment.

This study characterizes the precision and accuracy of the BAT system using CT-scans obtained immediately after the ultrasound readings. Phantom and patient data was obtained to evaluate systematic errors in the process. The post-ultrasound CT-scans were also used to confirm the proper placement of the planning contours superimposed on the ultrasound images.

## Material and methods

The BAT system consists of an ultrasound probe attached to a three-dimensional digitizer, allowing the device to determine the probe's position and orientation. In the treatment room, the digitizer is registered to both isocenter and the treatment couch. Ultrasound images of the phantom can then be registered to the CT-dataset from the treatment plan, and a couch move is predicted which will move the target and/or dose contours to the same position as they are in the plan relative to isocenter. This process can be repeated as necessary.

Commissioning tests have been done with both an ultrasound phantom and patients undergoing 3DCRT. To measure the precision and accuracy of the system in a controlled environment, a phantom was purposefully misaligned by independently measured precise distances along the three principal axes. The QA phantom provided with the system was modified with scribe marks to allow proper alignment to isocenter. A CT scan of the phantom was taken and a 3 cm spherical target was contoured and downloaded to the BAT device. In the treatment room, the phantom is aligned to isocenter using the scribe lines and then secured to the treatment couch. Couch movements were used to misalign the phantom. The couch movements in the lateral and cephalo-caudad direction are controlled and measured using a immobilizing device consisting of orthogonal rack-and-pinion drive mechanisms with corresponding linear digital position readouts. The A-P movements were controlled with a similar device modified to measure vertical movement. Accuracy of both devices has been previously measured at 0.08-0.10 mm [5]. The digital readouts give the offset on the three axes. The BAT was then used to determine the motion needed to return the target to its position in the treatment plan. Offsets were taken along the three principal axes, and at the corners of a 1.5 cm cube centered at isocenter. Multiple measurements were taken at isocenter to determine systematic error in the system. The experiment was repeated over a series of days to investigate precision.

Patients undergoing 3DCRT were recruited to test the BAT in a clinical setting. The offset predicted by the BAT was compared against the offset obtained from a CT-scan taken immediately after the ultrasound measurement. Each patient's treatment plan CT-scan and contours were downloaded to the BAT device. To register the BAT to the CT-scanner coordinate system, an aluminum structure (built in-house) with docking device was securely attached to the head of the couch and aligned to the lasers. Patients were positioned on the couch immediately below the aluminum docking device and adjustments made for treatment in the usual manner. The ultrasound measurements and contour alignments were performed, followed immediately by a CT-scan. This procedure was repeated 5 times for each patient.

To determine the true offset of the prostate relative to the treatment plan, the target volume was contoured for each post-ultrasound CT-scan. To insure consistency, all the contouring was performed by the treatment physician. To increase alignment accuracy, each target surface was triangulated and new contour points were chosen to uniformly cover the surface (Figure 1). The offset was determined by comparing the reinterpolated treatment plan and post-ultrasound contours through center-of-mass compisons. Additionally, the post-ultrasound contours were projected onto the ultrasound to validate the precise placement of the contours on an ultrasound image during the alignment process.

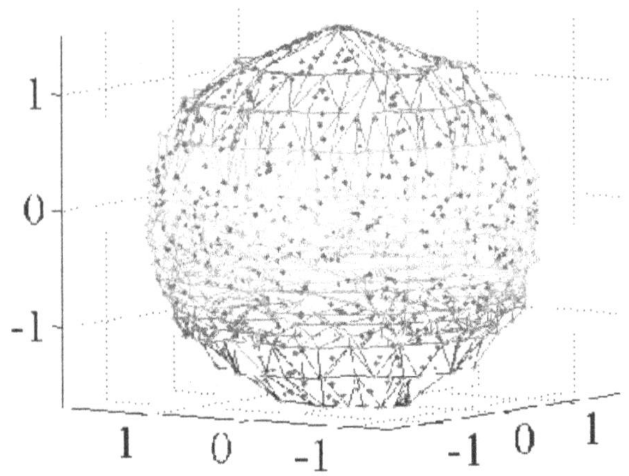


**Figure 1:** Triangulated Phantom Target Surface

## Results and discussion

Each session with the phantom began with 10 measurements at isocenter to determine the systematic offset for that session. The mean error and standard deviation of the isocenter measurements are shown in Figure 2. The systematic offset differed from session to session and was the dominant part of the error at all points. The S-I direction was clearly the most inconsistent, which is most likely due to the 3mm distance between contour slices.

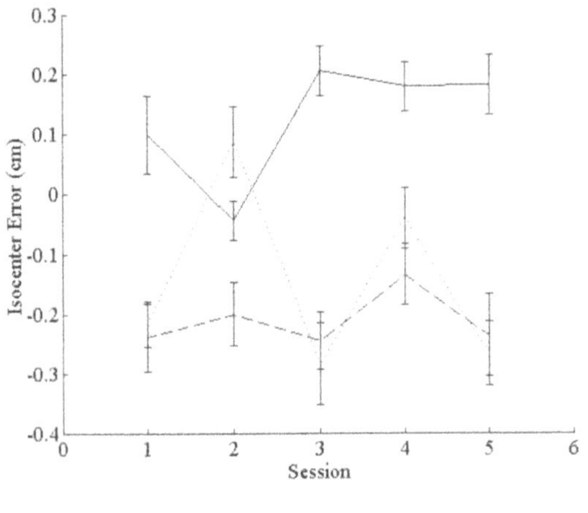


**Figure 2:** Mean isocenter error for each phantom session. solid: lateral, dashed:A-P,dotted:S-I

The systematic error of each session was removed from the analysis by subtracting the mean values in Figure 2 from the remaining measurements. The measurements were also corrected by determining the rigid-body transformation matrix that minimized the mean error in a least-squares sense. The sizes of the errors are tabulated in Figure 3. After corrections were made, a majority of the measurements showed less than 1 mm error.

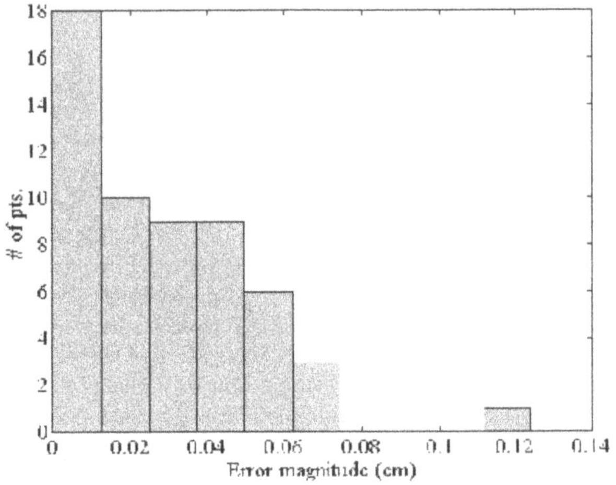


**Figure 3:** True offset versus corrected measured offset

Patient data is collection is ongoing and has been collected for only three of ten patients at this point. Table 1 shows the BAT alignment data and true offsets for one patient. The data collected so far indicates that the largest error occurs in the lateral direction, most likely due to the poor visualization of the hyperechoic tissue in that direction on the axial image.

The localization process depends strongly on the ability of the therapist to both obtain quality images and overlay the contours in the correct position. The post-ultrasound contours are being used to gather information on the optimal placement of the contours on the image. An example is shown in Figure 4. Note how the contour traces the white area near the bladder in both images. If consistent through the entire patient dataset, this information can be used to guide the therapist in aligning the patient during treatment.

## Conclusion

The intrinsic positional precision of the BAT in a controlled environment is sufficient to support future clinical investigations. The registration system should be modified to

| | BAT prediction | | | CT-measured | | |
|---|---|---|---|---|---|---|
| | Lateral | Ant-Pos | Sup-Inf | Lateral | Ant-Pos | Sup-Inf |
| Alignment 1 | -0.16 | 1.34 | -1.40 | -0.88 | 1.38 | -1.36 |
| Alignment 2 | 0.11 | 1.03 | -1.47 | -1.11 | 1.22 | -1.00 |
| Alignment 3 | -0.15 | 0.94 | -1.42 | -0.87 | 1.20 | -0.95 |
| Alignment 4 | -0.05 | 0.75 | -1.30 | -1.12 | 1.32 | -1.06 |
| Alignment 5 | 0.46 | 1.06 | -1.30 | -0.83 | 1.13 | -1.16 |

**Table 1:** Sample patient data for clinical trial(cm). Mean difference = (-1.00 0.23 0.27) cm.

Standard Deviation = (0.27 0.21 0.19) cm.

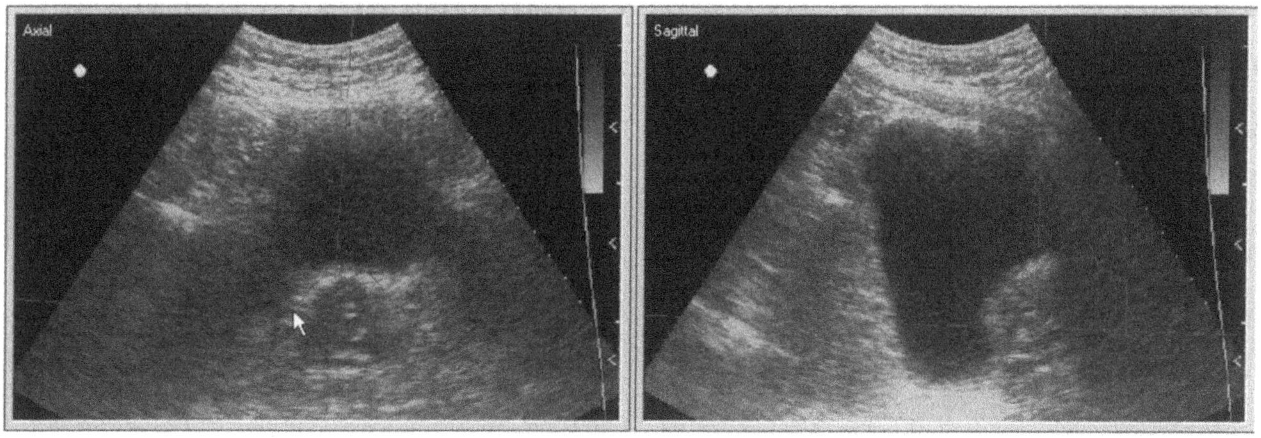


**Figure 4:** Ultrasound Image with true position of prostate spliced in

reduce intrasession systematic errors. CT-scans taken at the time and place of alignment can be used to accurately quantify the accuracy of ultrasound in identifying prostate boundaries. Ongoing clinical trials suggest that the BAT may improve localization errors in the prostate.

## Acknowledgements

This work supported in part by an industrial grant from NOMOS corp.

## References

[1] Leibel et al, Int J Radiat Oncol Biol Phys 1994 **28:1**,55-65
[2] Balter et al, Int. J. Radiat. Oncol. Biol. Phys.1995:**31:1**, 113-118
[3] Greer et al, Int J Radiat Oncol Biol Phys 1998 **41:5** 1193-9
[4] van Herk et al, Int. J. Radiat. Oncol. Biol. Phys 1995 **33:5**, 1311-1320
[5] Low et al, Int J Radiat Oncol Biol Phys 1999 Aug 1 **45:1** 193-203

# Ultrasound guided percutaneous radiotherapy of prostate cancer

**P. Kneschaurek, H. Geinitz, F.B. Zimmermann**

Klinik für Strahlentherapie, Klinikum rechts der Isar

## Introduction

The number of patients treated by radiation therapy of localized prostate cancer (PC) increases significantly because of the high incidence and detection of PC due to an increasing mean age of men as well as an increasing use of laboratory tests (PSA). Different clinical studies could demonstrate a better local tumor control with higher total doses. Because the risk of severe side effects decreases with decreasing the volume irradiated with high doses of these organs the margin between the CTV and the PTV should be as small as possible. It is well known, that the prostate shifts with different filling of both the rectum and the bladder. In most cases the definition of the target volume is based on one initial CT-scan. The expected movement of the prostate during the next 7 to 8 weeks of treatment is taken into account by determining the planning target volume (PTV) in such a manner that the clinical target volume (CTV) is enclosed by the 95% isodose in at least 95% of the treatment sessions. A safety margin of 8 to 15 millimeters around the CTV (e.g. the prostate) is usually included when defining the PTV. This margin can only be reduced if the exact shape and position of the CTV is known during or directly before the radiation treatment. In this paper we investigate the use of ultrasound (US) to increase the accuracy of patient setup for prostate cancer[1].

## Material and methods

The US positioning system is an add-on to the BrainLab ExacTrac patient positioning system. This system uses reflecting markers fixed to the patients skin for patient setup. After fixation of the markers CT-slices of the pelvis were taken with a thickness of 5 mm and a table feed of 5 mm. The prostate as the clinical target volume was contoured in every slice. The isocenter and the shape of the beams with the safety margins were defined using the beta-version of the BrainSCAN planning system. The position of the isocenter relative to the body markers was calculated and transferred to the ExacTrac system in the irradiation vault. We could demonstrate that the position of the isocenter relative to the center of gravity of the markers does not depend very sensitive to the displacement of a single marker if more than 5 markers are used [2].
The ExacTrac system uses two infrared cameras in the treatment room to detect the the position of the body markers. Before using the system it has to be calibrated in the room coordinate system. This is performed by tools supplied by BrainLab. After the calibration the ExacTrac system is able to determine the position of the reflecting markers in room coordinates. The US system has to be calibrated in room coordinates in a second step. A special applicator with three infrared reflectable markers was firmly connected to the head of the ultrasound probe. The ultrasound was calibrated with a US phantom that contains guide wires in a tissue equivalent US gel. The position of the US-Phantom in the treatment room is detected by the ExacTrac system with the help of three reflecting markers at known position on the outside of the US phantom. The US echoes of the wires inside the phantom are interactively marked on the US image. Because the exact position of the wires are known in room coordinates, the position of the US image plane can be calculated. The system is than able to calculate the position of the US plane by detecting the position of the reflecting markers attached to the US probe. After calibration the following data are available to the ExacTrac system:
The position of the patient and the localization of the CT-defined isocenter of the prostate.
The position of the isocenter of the linear accelerator.
The position of the ultrasound probe as well as the direction and orientation of the scanning beam.
The patient is set up with the help of the ExacTrac system. Then the ultrasound imaging is performed in two different directions (e.g. axial and sagital). The images are stored. The system displays the US-images and two reconstructed CT-images in the identical plane. The contour of the prostate has been marked on CT and is displayed also on the US-images. This contours can be shifted by the mouse to the exact position of the prostate seen on US. After this has been performed the ExacTrac system allows to shift the patient to the correct position, so that the target point in the center of the prostate and the isocenter of the linac coincide.

## Results and discussion

Before using the system clinically we tested its accuracy with a custom made phantom. This phantom contained different structures in a water bath which could be detected both with CT and US. After performing a CT scan with 5 reflecting markers attached to the phantom the data were transferred to the BrainScan planning system and the target an the isocenter defined. This information was then transferred to the ExacTrac system in the treatment room. Two different situations have been tested. Firstly we misaligned the phantom on the treatment table by a known amount. The above described US procedure was then performed an the Target marked on the CT was shifted to the position seen on the US images. After having done this ExacTrac calculates the needed shifts of the phantom in all directions. The shift can interactively be performed using ExacTrac and the reflecting markers. The deviation between planned and actual position after this shift was smaller than 3 mm in all directions. In a second test we aligned the phantom correctly and simulated an organ shift by using a different internal structure as target. After readjusting the phantom with the help of the ExacTrac system we determined the deviation of this target from the isocenter. The deviations measured have always found to be smaller than 3 mm.

After this initial tests we used this system for patient setup. The additional time requirement for positioning the patient using the ultrasound was in mean

5 minutes for calibration of the system (which has to be done just once a day independent of the number of treated patients),

3 minutes for the ultrasound detection of the prostate in two directions, axial and sagittal,

2 minutes for defining the prostate in the planning computer

3 minutes for the correction of the patients position according to the data of the planning computer.

In a first evaluation we tested the reproducibility of the procedure with two independent acting physicians who were familiar with ultrasound imaging. Both physicians defined the target volume twice a day with a time gap of 7 minutes using the ultrasound probe. The patient did not leave the treatment position during the whole procedure. The mean error in the axial, the sagital and the coronal direction was 2.0 mm (0-3.5 mm), 2.0 mm (0-2 mm), 2.0 mm (1-5 mm).

## Conclusion

We conclude that an ultrasound guided radiation treatment is feasible and not very time consuming. It will further be evaluated in the treatment of localized prostate cancer as well as in liver metastases. Nevertheless, there are some pitfalls in this system: In very obese patients and in cases of an emptied bladder the visualization of the prostate might be hindered. An extreme pressure with the ultrasound head and an extremely overdistended bladder will dislocate the prostate deep into the small pelvis.

On the other hand recent improvements in ultrasound imaging like digital processing of the signals, 3-dimensional ultrasound, or contrast harmonic imaging might further increase the precision of ultrasound and enhance the use in radiation treatment.

## References

[1] Lattanzi J, McNeeley S, Pinover W. Horwitz E, Das I, Schultheiss TE, Hanks GE 1999 A comparison of daily CT localisation to a daily ultrasound-basedsystem in prosate cancer. *Int.J. Rad. Onc. Biol. Phys.* **43**:719-725

[2] Geinitz H, Zimmermann F, Kuzmany A, Kneschaurek P 2000 Daily CT planning during boost irradiation of prostate cabcer: feasibility, time requirements and technical prerequisites. *Strahlentherapie und Onkologie*, to be published

# Whole Body Frame for the Target Localization with CCTV Camera System and Fluoroscopy

W.K. Chung[1], B. Yi[1], E.K. Choi[1], J.H. Kim[1], S.D. Ahn[1], C.K. Min[1], D.I.Shin[2], H. Chang[1]

[1]Dept. of Radiation Oncology, [2]Dept. of Medical Engineering,
Asan Medical Center, University of Ulsan, College of Medicine, Seoul, 138-736, Korea

## Introduction

State of art radiation treatment such as the radiosurgery, conformal therapy and the IMRT strongly require the reliable target localization method which considers the organ motions as well.

In order to obtain the accurate localization, a realiable and reproducible setup method is necessary. The coordinate based target localization is well known technique for the intra-cranial radiosurgery with the stereotactic frame system. But, due to the organ motions, a precise extra-cranial localization has been regarded as a very difficult goal to achieve[1, 2]. There are a few reports about the internal target localization with radio-opaque material [3] and about the localization with skin image detection [4]. But the non-invasive real time target localization method has not been well established yet. The target localization technique considering organ movement has been developed for the purpose of utilization in 3D conformal radiotherapy, IMRT and whole body radiosurgery. Whole body frame is designed for body immobilization with the stereotactic coordinate system. Two CCD cameras and a fluoroscopic unit are used for the detection of the movement of surface markers and internal markers.

## Material and methods

A whole body stereotactic frame is designed for the immobilization of interested body region. Figure 1 shows the body frame. With this frame one can easily find the coordinates of the target either from an axial CT image or from the orthogonal X-ray image set. Two CCD cameras are mounted on the camera-mounting unit over the body frame. LED's are attached on body surface and provides the cameras with the visualization position changes of the surface markers on body surface.

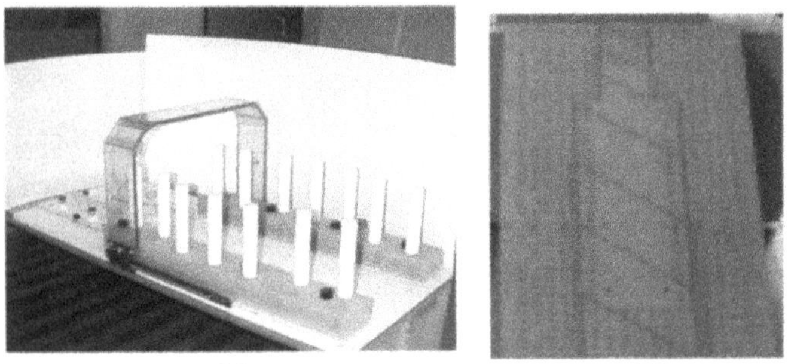

(a) (b)

**Figure 1:** Side views of the whole body frame (a) and coordinate system engraved (b).

These position changes are analyzed into the variation of 3-dimensional coordination and are monitored all the time during the treatment for the prediction of the internal target motions from the external patient positioning markers. For tracing internal target motion, a fluoroscopic unit is used for detecting the motions of surface LED markers and the internal target simultaneously. Correlation of motions between surface markers and internal markers is established and then we can predict the location of the target from the skin marker coordinates with this correlation. Two CCD cameras and a fluoroscopic unit are interfaced to control PC, which analyzes two related images of markers into 3-dimentional coordination and tests motion tolerances. Figure 2 shows a schematic diagram of this target localization system. A fluoroscopy and camera system are used when the simulation procedure. The correlation function between the skin marker and the target (or internal marker) is obtained at this procedure. Only camera system is used during treatment, since we can predict the organ location from the skin marker coordinate.

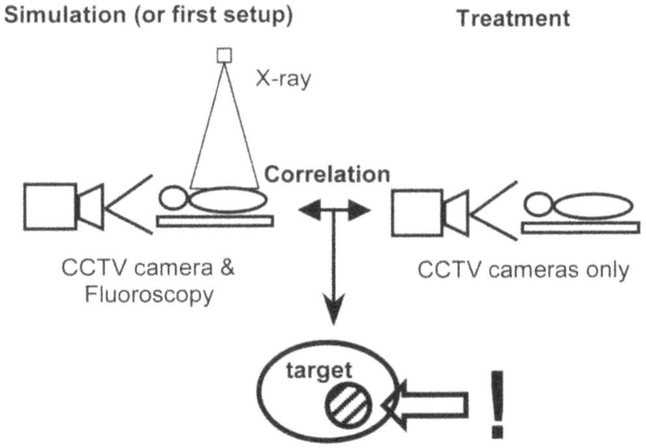


**Figure 2:** Schematic diagrams of the system

## Results and discussion

Setup verification system is customized with two CCD cameras, their supporting frame, a fluoroscopic unit and an algorithm for detecting dynamic position of internal target. Correlation of motions is determined through the surface marker position and internal target localization. An algorithm is built for handling images from CCD cameras and for determining target motion tolerance by the correlation. Figure 3 shows how to determine the target coordinate from an axial CT image. It is essential to obtain the customized correlation function for each patients. Figure 4 shows the images from the

fluoroscoic X-ray units. The correlation could be calculacted from the rectangular coordinates of the skin markers and the anatomical land markers.
Further correlation study should be continued between the skin markers and the various internal anatomic sites. Present semi-automatic procedure may be evolved into full-automatic control system for the determination of internal target motion and its tolerance in next step

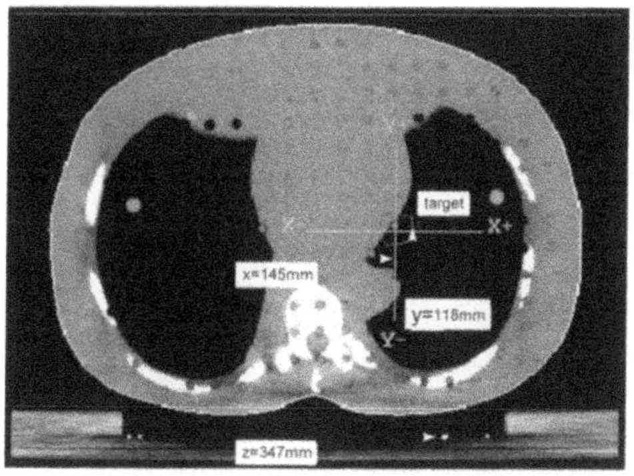


**Figure 3:** Humanoid phantom on the whole body frame

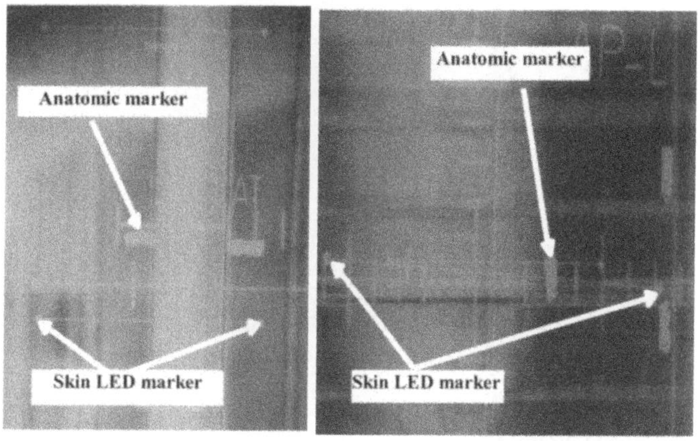


**Figure 4:** The fluoroscopic images of land markers for the correlation determination.

## Conclusion

To improve clinical results of the conformal radiotherapy, the IMRT and the whole body radiosurgery, a new system of tracing dynamic movement of internal target is designed and constructed. Localization of target as well as patient positioning may be performed through the detection of the surface markers using CCD cameras and fluoroscopic unit. For this purpose, correlation of motions is established between LED surface markers and internal markers.

This lead to minimization of patient setup error and detection of the motion of interested internal organ, resulting in determination of more accurate PTV.

## References

[1] Blomgren H, Lax I, Naslund I, Svanstrom R. Stereotactic high dose fraction radiation therapy of extracranial tumors using an accelerator. *Acta Oncol* 1995 : 34. 861
[2] Lax I, Blomgren H, Naslund I, Svanstrom R. Stereotactic Radiotherapy of Malignancies in the Abdomen. *Acta Oncol* 1994 : 33(6). 677
[3] Balter M, Lam K, Sandler H, Littles J, Bree L, Ten Haken R. Automated localization of the prostate at the time of treatment using implanted radiopaque markers : Technical Feasibility. *Int J Radiat Oncol Biol, Phys* 1995 ; 33 : 1281
[4] Menke M., Hirschfeld F. et al. Photogrammaetric accuracy measurements of head holder systems used for fractionated radiotherapy. *Int J Radiat Oncol Biol, Phys* 1994 ; 29(5) : 1147- 1155

# Studies for On-line Registration of Different Quality Images in Radiation Therapy

**S. Eulenstein[1], A. Friedrich[1], J. Vlad[1], W. Wlodarczyk[1], P. Wust[1]**
[1]Strahlenklinik, Charite Campus Virchow Klinikum
Augustenburger Platz 1, D-13353 Berlin, Germany

## Abstract

Radiation therapy of prostate cancer requires high geometric accuracy of dose delivery. Numerical tools have been developed and investigated in order to detect and correct on-line positioning errors. This control is based on registration of low-quality portal images (PI) and high-quality digitally reconstructed radiographs (DRR). Various image processing tools to better delineate the bony structures in phantom and patients were investigated. Furthermore, different similarity measures and optimization procedures were investigated to achieve the best registration as fast as possible. The best results have been achieved using mutual information as similarity measure and Powell's method as optimizer.

## 1 Introduction and Purpose

With the introduction of conformal and 3-D irradiation techniques in radiation therapy higher requirements on geometric accuracy in treatment delivery are posed. An example for such a critical treatment is the irradiation of the prostate cancer, where positionning errors considerably degrade the therapeutic ratio and put at risk sensitive organs such as rectum and bladder. Therefore on-line verification and correction of dose delivery is increasingly demanded by radiation oncologists.

The intended approach is to compare the low-dose PI recorded just before the high-dose treatment irradiation with DRRs derived from the treatment plan and to correct appropriately the setup parameters of accelerator. Unfortunately, such an automatic alignment fails in most cases because of poor quality of PIs. Therefore, some operator handlings such as eg. manual pre-contouring of PIs is often required, so disqualifying the method from the desired on-line application.

The purpose of this contribution is to develop numerical tools for on-line registration of positionning errors in radiotherapy of prostate cancer based on PIs and to verify them in phantom and patients. Special attention was drawn to different similarity measures in combination with some image quality improving procedures applied to PIs and DRRs.

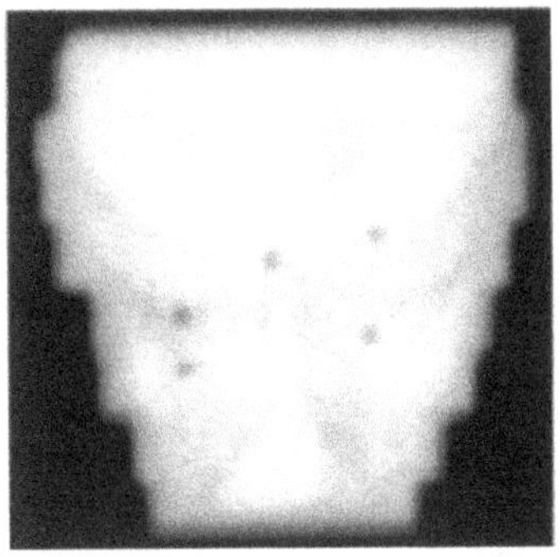

Figure 1. Typical PI of a patient with ILM implanted in the prostate.

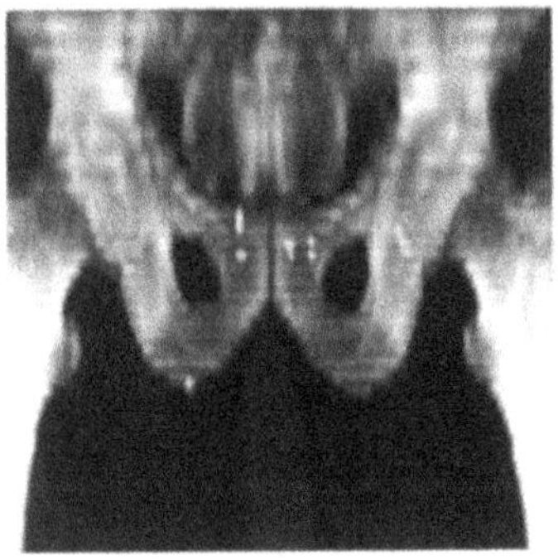

Figure 2. DRR corresponding to Fig. 1.

## 2 Methods

Any registration study at patients under radiation treatment suffers from lack of an absolute reference for assessment of displacements and their correction. Therefore, development and investigation of registration procedures was first performed using the pelvic part of the Alderson phantom. That allows for simulation of behaviour of bony structures throughout all steps of computer tomography (CT) planning, simulation and treatment (PI). This bony structures occur on PI as hardly visible (Fig. 1) or on DRR as clearly visible (Fig. 2) delineated bony landmarks (BLM). In addition, three radio-opaque gold seeds occurring as point-like internal landmarks (ILM) were used.

The automatic recognition of ILM in phantom and patients is relatively simple in both, DRR and PI. Therefore, using two orthogonal PI projections and applying the rigid body transformation, the 3-D registration based on ILM can be easily performed. As a criterion for the quality of the registration the mean square error (MSE) was used.

In the phantom experiment, this result of the ILM based registration forms a reference for the BLM based registration studies. In this contribution we investigated only the 2-D registration of frontal images (DRR and PI). As criteria for the quality of this BLM based registration different similarity measures typical for grey- scale images were used [1].

**Mean Square Error (MSE)**

$$M = \frac{1}{N}\sum_{i,j}(I_{PI}(i,j) - I_{DRR}(i,j))^2$$

$N$ is the number of pixels in each of the images. This measure is effective if the intensities of both images, $\bar{I}_{PI}$ and $\bar{I}_{DRR}$, are similar.

**Normalised Cross Correlation (NCC)**

$$R = \frac{\sum_{i,j}(I_{PI}(i,j) - \bar{I}_{PI})(I_{DRR}(i,j) - \bar{I}_{DRR})}{\sqrt{\sum_{i,j}(I_{PI}(i,j) - \bar{I}_{PI})^2}\sqrt{\sum_{i,j}(I_{DRR}(i,j) - \bar{I}_{DRR})^2}}$$

$\bar{I}_{PI}$ and $\bar{I}_{DRR}$ are the mean values of the image intensities.

**Mutual Information (MI)**

$$S = \sum_{x,y} p(x,y)\log\frac{p(x,y)}{p(x)p(y)}$$

$p(x)$ and $p(y)$ denote the probability distributions in DRR and PI grey-scale images and $p(x,y)$ is the joint probability distribution.

In order to reduce the large discrepancy in image quality of DRR and PI the following procedures (IQP) for similarizing image quality of PI and DRR were used:

**IQP1:** contrast limited adaptive histogram equalization of PI

**IQP2:** Sobel filter on DRR and PI and treshold

**IQP3:** noise reducing using blur filter before Sobel filter and threshold

The following procedures for multi-dimensional optimization (OP) were used:

**OP1:** conjugate gradient method (CGM) [2]

**OP2:** Powell's method (PM) [2]

**OP3:** QuickProp method based on neuronal networks (QPM)[3]

The similarity measures for 2-D registration of the frontal images were investigated in form of a cost function spanned over the square of 21 x 21 pixels. Criteria for comparison of similarity measures were: distance D of achieved BLM based optimum of the cost function from the ILM based optimum and area A closed by the 95 % isoline decay from the optimum. Registration procedure using the best similarity measure was applied to align the patient data and remaining positioning errors, such as translation shifts and quaternions representing the rotational errors, were evaluated.

## 3 Results

The cost functions of the registration are relatively flat and even the best achieved optimum differs slightly from the absolute optimum. Some examples for the worst (a), moderate (b) and the best registration results (c) in form of cost functions are shown in Fig. 3. All these results are summarized in Table 1.

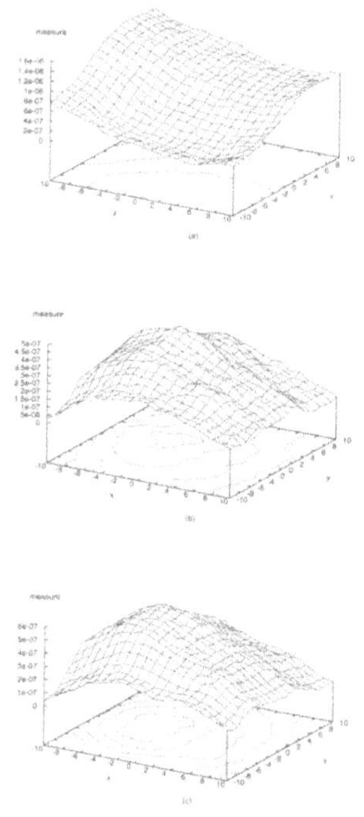

Figure 3. Cost function of MI (a), MI+IQP2 (b) and MI+ IQP3 (c).

Applying the best registration procedure (MI + IQP3 + OP2) to the patient data results showed in Fig. 4 and 5 as well as in Table 2 were achieved.

## 4 Conclusions

In this paper we investigated procedures for on-line registration of PI and DRR. The achieved accuracy in patient data is quite well. Some improvements are expected when lateral projections will be included and the 2-D registration will be extended to the entire 3-D registration.

**Table 1:** Comparison of similarity measures in form of D (norm) and A (pixel number)

| | MSE | MSE+IQP2 | MSE+IQP3 | NCC | NCC+IQP2 | NCC+IQP3 | MI | MI+IQP2 | MI+IQP3 |
|---|---|---|---|---|---|---|---|---|---|
| D | 10.77 | 5 | 9.22 | 10.19 | 5 | 5.38 | 10.77 | 4.24 | 4.12 |
| A | - | 40 | 34 | - | 42 | 54 | - | 14 | 34 |

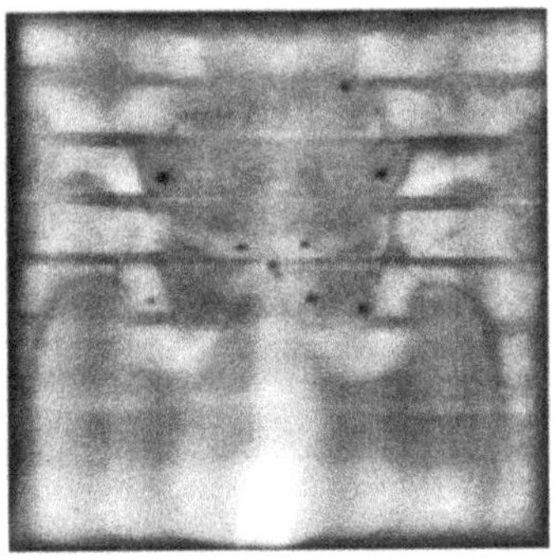

Figure 4. PI of the Alderson phantom with ILM visible as black points.

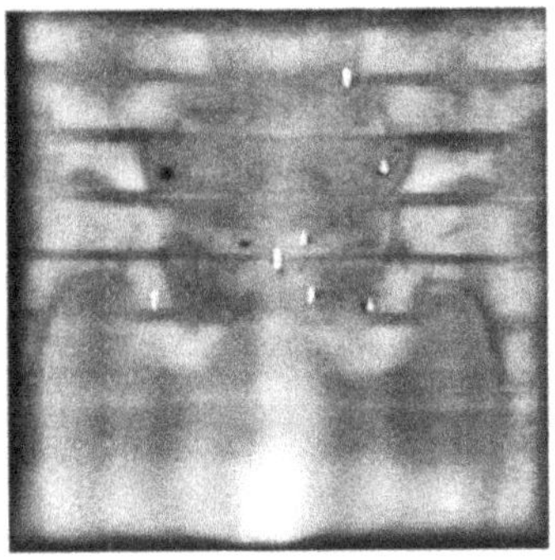

Figure 5. PI of Fig. 4 with additional ILM of DRR (white) showing complete alignement of ILM and BLM after registration.

**Table 2:** Setup errors between BLM and ILM found after registration using the procedure of MI + IQP3 + OP2

| | Translation | | | Rotation | | |
|---|---|---|---|---|---|---|
| | x | y | z | Gantry | Kollim | Table |
| result of ILM | 0.68 | -11.01 | -0.80 | 0.56 | 119.97 | -122.35 |
| result of BLM | 0.67 | -9.05 | -0.60 | 1.36 | 170.24 | -171.17 |
| error | | 1.95 mm | | | 0.91 | |

## Acknowledgement

This work has been supported by Deutsche Forschungsgemeinschaft (Sfb 273)

## References

[1] G. P. Penney, J. Weese, J.A. Little, P. Desmedt, D. LG Hill, D. J. Hawkes, "A comparision of similarity measures for use in 2D-3D medical image registration", *IEEE Trans. Med. Imaging* **17(8)**:586-599, 1998

[2] W. H. Press, , S. A. Teukolsky, W. T. Vetterling, W. P. Flannery, "Numerical Recipes in C: The Art of Scientific Computing", 2nd Edition, Cambridge University Press, 1992

[3] T. Rohlfing, J. Beier, O.Schulte, N. Hosten, R. Felix, "Multimodale Registierung mit effizienten Lernverfahren fr neuronale Netze", in: T. Lehmann (Editor), *"Bildverarbeitung fr die Medizin: Algorithmen - Systeme - Anwendungen"*, pp. 323-327, Springer Berlin, 1998

# Experimental study of six parameter patient registration from helical MV fan-beam data

**Edward Fitchard[1], Gustavo Olivera,2[1], Kenneth Ruchala[1],Jeff Kapatoes[2], Ralf Hinderer[2], Paul Reckwerdt[1], and Rock Mackie,2[1]**
[1]Tomotherapy Inc. 2228 Evergreen Road, Middleton WI, (53562-4241), USA, and [2]Department of Medical Physics University of Wisconsin-Madison 1300 University Ad. Madison WI 53705, USA

## Introduction

Tomotherapy, a cancer treatment method capable of delivering dose to difficult tumor geometries, require precise patient positioning or registration. The initial objective for the tomotherapy registration problem was to obtain distance errors less than ±2 mm and angular errors less than ±2°.

It has previously been established[1-4] that registration with $x, y$, and roll can be obtained with errors much less than ±1 mm and $i \pm 1°$ respectively. Recent experiments demonstrate that the method also works for full six parameter offsets. Some of the results are shown in Table 1.

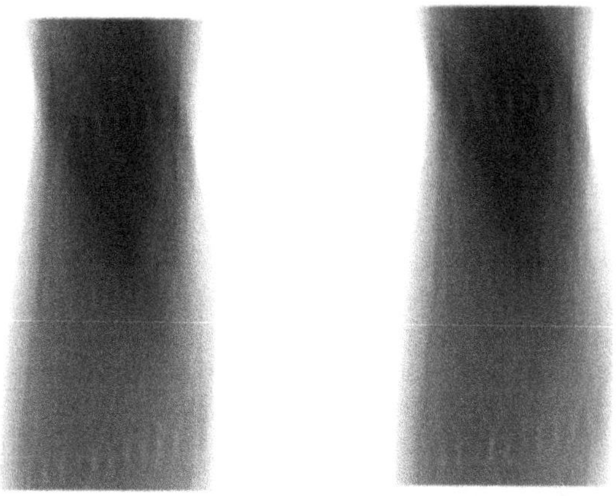

**Figure 1:** Two helical fan-beam sinograms with a relative offset.

## Results and discussion

The algorithm inputs fraction and reference helical fan-beam sinograms (see Fig. 1) and performs the following steps:

1. covert each helical fan-beam sinograms to a closely spaced stacks of axial sinograms,
2. integrate over detector and gantry angle to produce two functions of $z$,
3. cross correlate these function to determine the $z$ offset,
4. $z$ correct the stacks of axial sinograms,
5. correlate corresponding $z$-corrected axial slices to determine the roll offset,
6. roll correct the stacks of axial sinograms,
7. $x$ and $y$ correlate corresponding axial sinograms from the top and bottom of the stacks,
8. use the $xy$ offsets and the separation between the top and bottom axial sinograms to compute the pitch and yaw offsets,
9. iterate if necessary,
10. return the six offsets.

Table 1 summarizes the comparison of experiment and algorithm for over a hundred different Rando phantom offsets. The numbers tabulated under the columns marked $\sigma_x, \sigma_y, \sigma_z, \sigma_{pitch}, \sigma_{yaw}$, and $\sigma_{roll}$ are the standard deviations of the difference between the experimentally measured offsets and the offsets returned by the registration algorithm. These numbers contain both experimental and algorithm errors so they represent an upper limit on the algorithm error. The last two columns in the table are obtained by statistically summing respectively the three linear and three angular errors and multiplying by two to obtain the 95% confidence level. The rows label the types of data collected. The first two rows are offsets in respectively the $x$ only and $y$ only directions. For this data the experimental error was small (±0.01 mm). This is reflected in the smaller experimental plus algorithm error for these measurements. The third row, $z$ only, contains the largest individual error. The experimental error for these measurements is comparable, or only slightly larger than, the $x$ and $y$ experimental errors indicating that this is mostly algorithm error which i is understandable, because the functions involved do not have compact support and the distance traversed in the $z$ direction is small, less than 10 cm which limits the density variation in the correlation. Recent enhancements to the $z$, (e.g., changing from a full scan to a half scan helical to axial interpolation scheme), offset part of the algorithm have reduced this error. However, that data is still being analysised so it is not shown in Table 1. The pitch offset calculation involves two $y$ offsets and a $z$ offset, so the error in this measurement should be about three to four times greater than the $y$ only error, which is approximately consistent with the results. The roll only errors are small, except for the $z$ direction as expected. The last row shows measurements

**Registration Algorithm STD of 6 Parameter Data**

| | Offset (mm) | | | Offset (deg) | | | 95 % Conf. Lev. | |
|---|---|---|---|---|---|---|---|---|
| Offset Type | $\sigma_x$ | $\sigma_y$ | $\sigma_z$ | $\sigma_{pitch}$ | $\sigma_{yaw}$ | $\sigma_{roll}$ | $2\sigma$ (mm) | $2\sigma$ (deg) |
| x only | 0.06 | 0.07 | 0.40 | 0.07 | 0.07 | 0.37 | 0.82 | 0.77 |
| y only | 0.04 | 0.03 | 0.44 | 0.04 | 0.04 | 0.15 | 0.89 | 0.32 |
| z only | 0.19 | 0.66 | 0.43 | 0.94 | 0.66 | 0.16 | 1.6 | 2.32 |
| pitch only | 0.36 | 0.31 | 0.63 | 0.48 | 0.29 | 0.20 | 1.58 | 1.19 |
| roll only | 0.07 | 0.19 | 0.31 | 0.26 | 0.19 | 0.10 | 0.74 | 0.67 |
| 6 parameter | 0.3 | 0.3 | 0.5 | 0.4 | 0.4 | 0.4 | 1.4 | 1.4 |

**Table 1:** Tabulation of the experimental plus algorithm error computed from fan-beam helical sinograms of a Rando phantom.

in which all six experimental parameters are changed. This is the most difficult data to collect experimentally. The error contains component from each of the six offsets. If the component errors were systematic and additive the '6 parameter' row would read (1.1,1.6,2.8,2.3,1.5,1.2). Since the values obtained are significantly less than this we conclude that the component error tend to cancel.

## Conclusion

In conclusion, the experiments conducted to date indicate the registration algorithm will produce errors that are less than the specification of ±2 mm and ±2° to the 95% confidence level. There are several minor improvement to the algorithm that are under investigation which should further improve these results.

## References

[1] Smith J A, Jones R and Miller B S 1999 The imaginary title *Journal title* **15** 1–10

[2] Registration of Synthetic Tomotherapy Projection Data Sets Using Cross-Correlation, E. E. Fitchard, J. S. Aldridge, P. J. Reckwerdt, T. R. Mackie 1998 *Phys Med. Bio.* **43** 1645-1657.

[3] Six parameter patient registration directly from projection data, E. E. Fitchard, J. S. Aldridge, P. J. Reckwerdt, G. H. Olivera T. R. Mackie, and a. Iosevich 1999a *Nuc. Instr. and Meth. in Phys. Res. A* **421** 342-351.

[4] Lu, W., *et al., Image/patient registration from (partial) projection data by Fourier phase matching method.* Phys. in Med. and Biol., 1999. **44**: p.2029-2048.

[5] Registration using tomographic projection files, E. E. Fitchard, J. S. Aldridge, K. Ruchala, G. Fang, J. Balog, D. W. Pearson, G. H. Olivera, E. A. Schloesser, D. Wenman, P. J. Reckwerdt, and T. R. Mackie 1999b *Phys Med. Bio.* **44** 495-507.

# Computer assisted decision making after portal imaging

**Tomas Kron[1,2], Chris Hamilton[1], Claire Hood[2], Chris Wratten[1] and Jim Denham[1,3]**

[1] Newcastle Mater Misericordiae Hospital, Waratah, NSW 2298, Australia, [2] University of Newcastle, Department of Physics, Callaghan, NSW 2306, Australia, [3] University of Newcastle, Faculty of Medicine, Callaghan, NSW 2306, Australia

## Introduction

The verification of patient positioning during radiotherapy relies on the comparison of portal iamges to a reference image which may be a simulator film or a digitally reconstructed radiograph (DRR) from the computerised treatment planning system. While the comparison has been traditionally done by physicians and/or radiation therapists, much research has been undertaken in recent years to determine the differences between simulator and portal images utilising automatic and quantitative systems (1-4). The outcome is a numerical value for the shift and/or rotation of the treatment field as determined in each portal image in relation to the simulator image.

Less effort has directed towards the question of what to do in a particular case when a discrepancy of a certain magnitude has been detected. However, this is the task which has to be performed within a very short time if on-line verification of conformal treatment approaches is desired. At present, the decision to move the patient is often intuitive and leads to much variability in practice. The variability may depend in part on differences in equipment in different institutions, however, it also reflects a different attitude and approach by different clinicians to correct for perceived errors in treatment delivery (5).

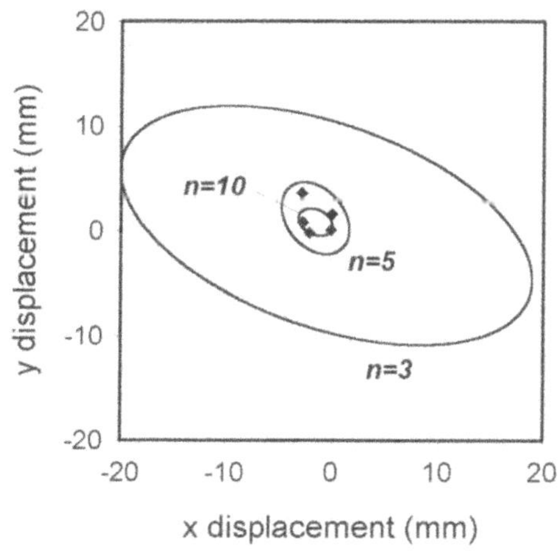


**Figure 1:** Graphical representation of model III. Shown is the x and y displacement of five portal images (symbols) as compared to the reference image. The 95% confidence ellipses depicted here get smaller as the number of images for their determination increases.

### Decision making models

Several algorithms utilising mathematical and statistical assumptions have been developed to objectively diagnose systematic treatment errors (6-9). They are based on one or more portal images of an individual patient and may take machine performance and historical data from the treatment centre into account. Most of these models also assume that the data are normally distributed and consider x and y displacement to be independent of each other.

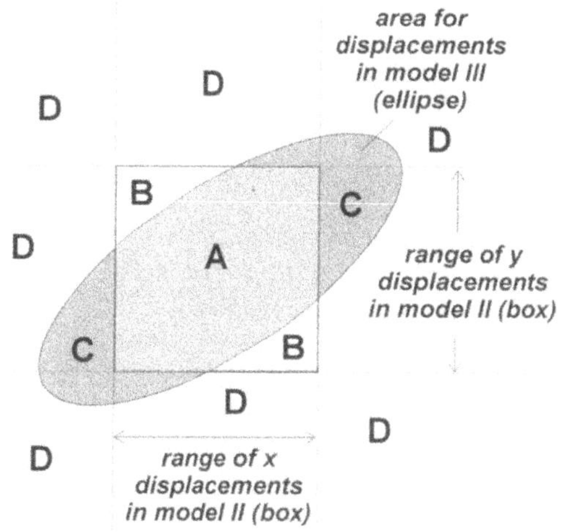


**Figure 2:** Comparison of a model II (2 x one-dimensional) and model III (two-dimensional) for decision making. If the centre of the reference image is in area A both models agree that no patient movement is required. In area D both models diagnose a field misplacement while in B and C only one of the two models diagnoses a problem.

Table 1 summarises three types of decision making models. The 'standard' model (I) - exemplified in a paper by Bel et al (6) - assumes shifts in different dimensions to be independent of each other and uses historical data to define action criteria for patient movement. It requires the user to determine action levels for different treatment scenarios from past clinical experience. These action levels are then equally applied to all new patients who are treated according to the particular scenario.

The 'individual/box' model (II) determines the random variation of set-up for each individual patient and derives the action level from this. This proceedure requires at least two portal images and utilises the t-statistics to account for the insufficient knowledge of the actual distribution.

Model III (ellipse) allows in addition to a variation of random displacement from patient to patient, a correlation between the movements in the two dimensions of the image. This would occur eg. when the patient is rotated: x and y displacements are always linked. Model III is illustrated in figure 1. The decision making space is determined by Hotelling's statistic (10). If in two dimensions a value is outside a given ellipse it can be

| | I: Standard | II: Individual/Box | III: Individual/Ellipse |
|---|---|---|---|
| Assumptions of the model | - Normal distribution,<br>- Independent dimensions,<br>- Historical data appropriate | - Normal distribution,<br>- Independent dimensions,<br>- Every patient different | - Normal distribution,<br>- Correlation possible,<br>- Every patient different |
| Determination of random uncertainty and action levels | - From historical data<br>- Calculated for **2** independent **one**-dimensional 95% confidence envelopes | - For each individual patient<br>- Calculated for **2** independent **one**-dimensional 95% confidence envelopes | - For each individual patient<br>- Calculated for **1 two-**dimensional 95% confidence envelopes |
| Example from literature | (6) | | (7, 9) |
| Number of images required | At least 1, preferably 2 | At least 2, preferably more | At least 3, preferably more |
| Statistics used | Gaussian | t distribution | Hotelling's statistic |

**Table 1:** Comparison of decision making models

assumed to be statistically different from the rest of the distribution. The size of the ellipse is determined by the number of measurements (ie. the number of portal images taken) and the required confidence level. The x and y co-ordinates of the confidence ellipse are calculated from the deviations between each portal image and reference image, $\Delta x_i$ and $\Delta y_i$ (11). For n portal films the variances, $v_x=\Sigma(\Delta x_i^2)/(n-1)$ and $v_y=\Sigma(\Delta y_i^2)/(n-1)$ and the covariance $v_{xy}=\Sigma(\Delta x_i * \Delta y_i)/(n-1)$ are calculated. For an angle $\alpha$, the x and y co-ordinates are:

$$x = <\Delta x> + K\,(v_x - (v_{xy}^2 / v_y))^{1/2} \cos\alpha + K\,(v_{xy}^2 / v_y)^{1/2} \sin\alpha$$

$$y = <\Delta y> + K\ v_y^{1/2} \sin\alpha$$

with $<\Delta x>$ and $<\Delta y>$ being the mean deviation between portal and reference image. For 5 portal images and a 90% confidence level the statistical parameter K is 1.706.

It was the aim of the present study to compare models II and III using a normal distribution of systematic and random displacements in two dimensions. Model I was not included.

## Material and methods

A spreadsheet program (MS-Excel) was developed to model portal image displacement from a reference image. No rotation or scaling errors were considered. The model samples two systematic variations, Sx and Sy, from a normal distribution with a given standard deviation, SS. Then it samples five additional points using a second normal distribution with a different standard deviation, SR. This random variation is added to the systematic displacement determined before and the five resulting points used as input for the decision making model. This situation represents the acquisition of five portal images of a patient. The aim is to determine the systematic variation (which should be corrected for) on the background of the random variations.

Models II and III were employed to determine the decision making space as illustrated in figure 2 based on five 'portal images'. The confidence level for each of the two dimensions in model II was 95% (two sided). A t-distribution for 4 degrees of freedom was chosen with the resulting width of the range determined from the standard deviation $\sigma$ of the n measurements as $\sigma * t * n^{-0.5}$. This results in an overall confidence level of 0.95 * 0.95 = 0.9025 for model II. Consequently, the confidence level for the ellipse in model III was chosen to be 90%. The confidence ellipse was calcualted using the equations given above. A variety of different combinations of random and 'systematic' variations were sampled and the location of the box (model II) and ellipse (model III) in relation to the centre of the reference image recorded. Four different situations were distinguished as illustrated in figure 2. Each run contained at least 5000 events (ie. 5000 'patients').

## Results and discussion

The results of the modelling are shown in figure 3. The horizontal axis shows the ratio between the systematic and random distribution of the sampling range, SS/SR. The absolute values of SS and SR do not affect the results. On the left hand of the graph the systematic variation is small and one would expect both models to encompass the centre of the reference image (area A in figure 2). On the right site the random variation is small compared to the systematic variation and all models should diagnose a move (area D).

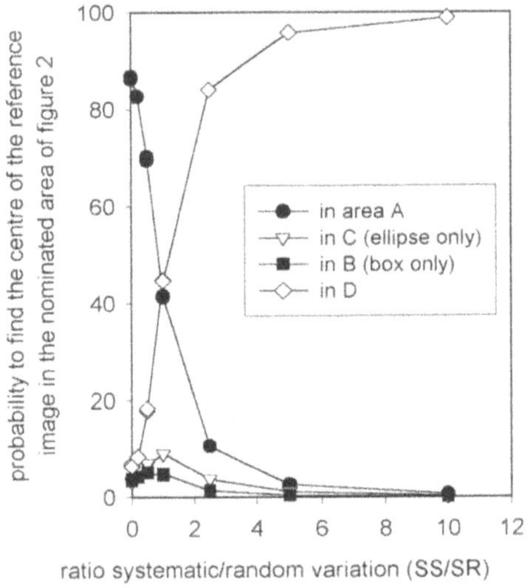


**Figure 3:** Probability to find the centre of the reference image in a certain area of the decision making space illustrated in figure 2.

The difference between the two models becomes evident in the range where systematic and random variations are of the same order of magnitude. In a review of systematic and random displacement S. Shalev found that most studies reported that both were approximately the same with a tendency for the systematic variation to be larger (12). The difference between the models found in the present simulation can be seen in figure 4. It displays the ratio of problems diagnosed by model III (ellipse) versus model II (box).

As can be seen the difference between the models is not large. The drop in the ratio below 1 (ie. model II diagnoses more displacements) is in part due to the reduced number of degrees of freedom in the two-dimensional model III. If more than five portal images are evaluated this difference diminishes. When the systematic variation from the reference centre is significantly larger than the random variation, both models are equivalent in their pick-up rate.

Two things can also be noted:
a) The modelling did not include any correlation between different dimensions. Both systematic and random variations were normally distributed with a chosen standard deviation, SS and SR. Any correlation between the two dimensions in the random variations would favour model III because an elongated ellipse will encompass the data better than a box.
b) The modelling does not allow any conclusions in regards to true or false findings. It merely detects the ability of a particular model to diagnose a systematic displacement of a certain order of magnitude on the background of random variations of another order of magnitude.

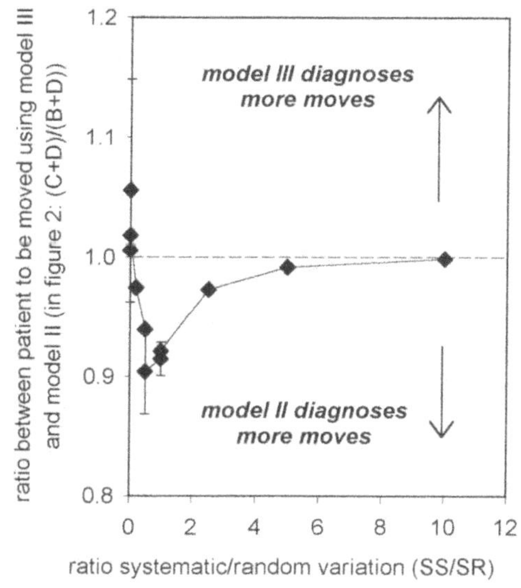


**Figure 4:** Ratio of systematic dislocations diagnosed by model III as compared to model II.

# Conclusion

In the modelling of systematic and random variations a two times one-dimensional model (model II) was found to be slightly more sensitive than a truly two dimensional decision making model III. Both models can easily be incorporated into a software package which could assist an operator to reach a quick decision about a particular patient directly after the acquision of an image. As the difference between the two approaches is small in the present modelling, it seems to be appropriate to use the two dimensional model which would be advantageous if the patient movement in the two dimensions of the image is correlated.

# References

[1] Meertens H, Bijhold J, and Strackee J 1990 A method for the measurement of field placement errors in digital portal images *Phys. Med. Biol.* **35** 299-323

[2] Jones S, and Boyer A 1991 Investigation of an FFT-based correlation technique for verification of treatment set-up. *Med. Phys.* **18** 1116-1125

[3] van Herk M, Bel A, Gilhuijs K, and Vijlbrief R 1993 A comprehensive system for the analysis of portal images. *Radiother. Oncol.* **29** 221-229

[4] Gilhuijs K, and van Herk M 1993 Automatic on-line inspection of patient set-up in radiation therapy using digital portal images. *Med. Phys.* **20** 667-677

[5] Morgan T, Banks D, and Kagan R 1998 Radiation therapy port films: a quality assurance study. *Int. J. Radiat. Oncol. Biol. Phys.* **42** 223-227

[6] Bel A, van Herk M, Bartelink H, and Lebesque J 1993 A verification procedure to improve patient set-up accuracy using portal images. *Radiother. Oncol.* **29** 253-260

[7] Denham J, Dally M, Hunter K, et al. 1993 Objective decision making following a portal film: the results of a pilot study. *Int. J. Radiat. Oncol. Biol. Phys.* **26** 869-876

[8] Shalev S, and Gluhchev G 1994 Decision rules for the correction of field set-up parameters. *Med. Phys.* **21** 952

[9] Kron T, Hamilton C, Wratten C, and Denham J 1999 A two-dimensional decision making model after comparing portal and reference images. *Med. Phys.* **26** 1131

[10] Morrison D 1976 *Multivariate statistical methods.* 2nd edition. New York: McGraw Hill, p 128-134

[11] See A, Kron T, Johansen J, Hamilton C, Bydder S, Hawkins J, Roff M and Denham J 1999 Decision making models in the analysis of portal films: a clinical pilot study. *Australas. Radiol.* (in print)

[12] Shalev S 1996 On-line portal imaging: contributions and limitations in clinical practice. *Front. Radiat. Ther. Oncol.* **29** 156-167.

# Digital Enhancement of Portal Images by Anisotropic Diffusion

**Konrad W. Leszczynski and Susan G. Boyko**

Department of Medical Physics, Northeastern Ontario Regional Cancer Centre, 41 Ramsey Lake Road, Sudbury, P3E 5J1, Canada

## Introduction

Despite the wide availability of electronic portal imaging devices (EPIDs) in radiation therapy centres, their clinical use remains limited. This is mainly due to the difficulties in visual or computerized analysis of electronic portal images, which stem from their inherent poor quality in terms of low contrast and high noise levels. Analysis of portal images for the purpose of geometric verification of radiotherapy treatments involves extraction of anatomical reference features. This process can be facilitated by selectively removing noise from homogeneous areas in an image and preserving edges between different anatomical areas. The present study examines the application of advanced digital image processing methods, based on the concept of anisotropic diffusion, to enhancement of electronic portal images.

## Material and methods

The inherent drawback of conventional, linear digital filters is that the resulting image blurring and de-emphasis of image features always accompany noise removal. Non-linear filters are generally more suitable for feature preserving image enhancement. In recent years a new class of non-linear filters has been proposed [1, 2], which is based on the numerical solution of partial differential equations describing the process of non-linear anisotropic diffusion:

$$\frac{\partial I(x,y,t)}{\partial t} = div(g(\nabla I)\nabla I)$$

In the above, $I(x,y,t)$ represents the image function subjected to the diffusion process, and the diffusion coefficient, $g(\nabla I)$, is a decreasing function of the image gradient, $\nabla I$. In this way, the diffusion process is inhibited around the edges, where the image gradient is high. The results presented here were obtained with $g(\nabla I)$ having the functional form as proposed by Perona and Malik [1].

Enhancement by anisotropic diffusion (AD) was applied to the electronic portal images of ten patients treated with 23 MV X-rays for cancer of the prostate. Small field portal images pose a particularly difficult challenge to portal verification. The efficacy of the AD filtering was quantitatively evaluated in two ways. Firstly, a signal to noise measure for pelvic bony features was calculated in original and enhanced images. This measure was derived from averages and standard deviations of pixel values within small regions defined over bony features and the adjacent homogenous soft tissue areas. Secondly, the reproducibility of visual feature extraction in original and filtered images was quantified. For this purpose, an experienced observer was asked to draw reference anatomical features in each of the original and enhanced images twice. The difference between the repeated feature extraction was quantified in terms of relative shifts and rotations using an image registration technique [3].

## Results and discussion

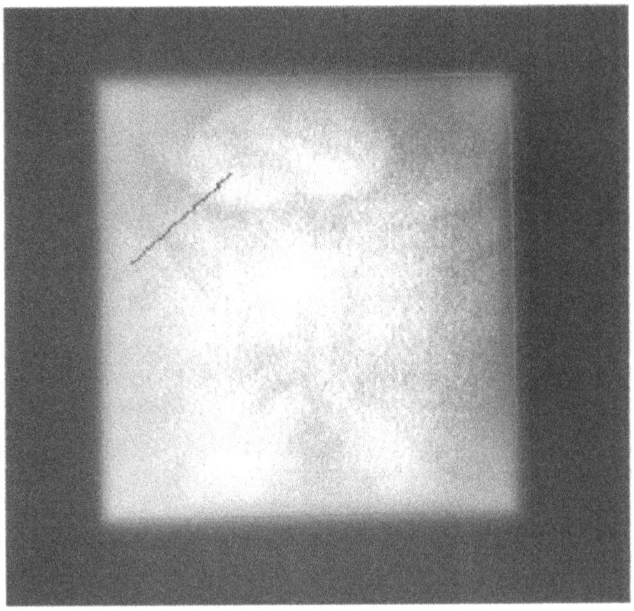

**Figure 1a:** A portal image of a prostate field before applying the AD filter. The diagonal line in the upper-left quadrant of the image indicates the position of the pixel intensity profiles shown in Figure 2.

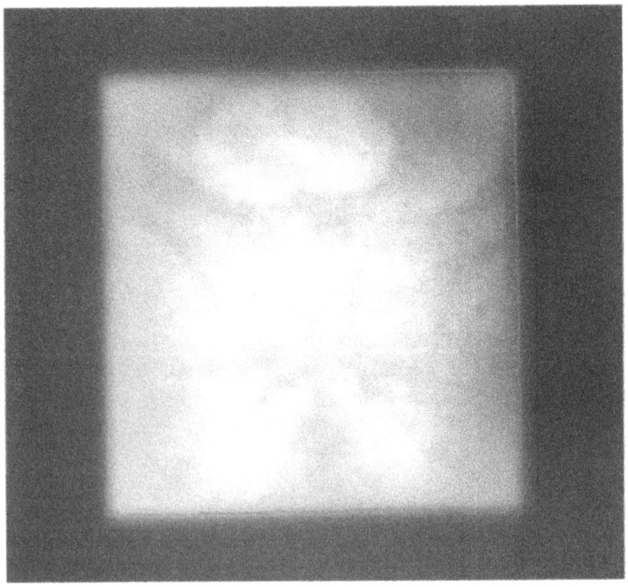

**Figure 1b:** The same portal image after AD filtration.

An example of a portal image of a prostate field before and after filtering with anisotropic diffusion is shown in Figure 1. For better visual presentation the contrast in both images was enhanced using the selective Contrast Limited Adaptive Histogram Equalization [4].

To better illustrate the edge preserving noise removal by the AD filter, pixel intensity profiles were taken across a bony anatomy feature, as indicated in Figure 1a. The profiles from the original and the AD-filtered image are plotted in Figure 2.

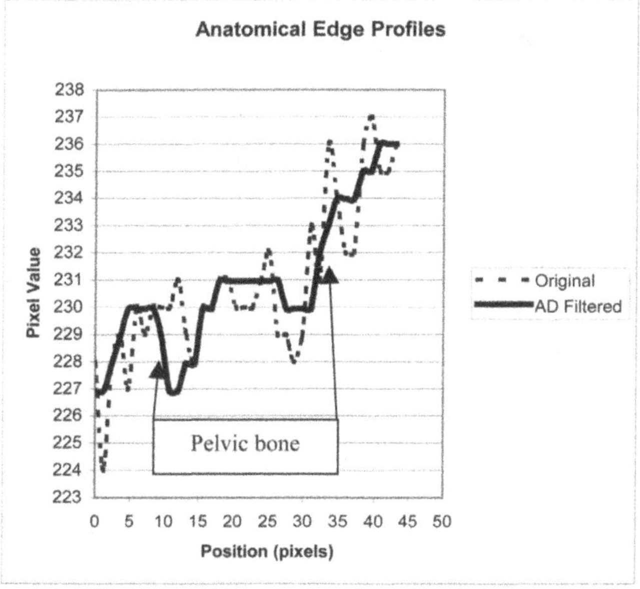


**Figure 2:** Pixel intensity profiles across an anatomical reference feature before and after filtering with AD.

Measurements of the signal to noise index associated with the anatomical features indicated a significant improvement after AD filtering. The index increased by a factor of 2.75, on average.

The reproducibility of visual feature extraction was quantified by translational and rotational displacements of features extracted from the same images in two separate trials. These displacements were reduced from the maximum of 1.2 mm (~ 2 pixels) before the enhancement to a maximum of 0.6 mm (~ 1 pixel) after AD filtering.

## Conclusion

Anisotropic Diffusion has been shown to be a useful method of digital enhancement of electronic portal images. It improves the detectability of anatomical features by suppressing noise without reducing contrast. It also leads to better reproducibility of visual feature extraction.

## References

[1] Perona P and Malik J 1990 Scale-space and edge detection using anisotropic diffusion *IEEE Trans. on PAMI* **12** 629-39

[2] Black M J, Sapiro G, Marimont D H and Heeger D 1998 Robust anisotropic diffusion *IEEE Trans. On Image Proc.* **7** 421-32

[3] Leszczynski K W, Loose S and Boyko S 1998 An image registration scheme applied to verification of radiation therapy *British Journal of Radiology* **71** 413-26

[4] Leszczynski K, Shalev S and Cosby S 1992 The enhancement of radiotherapy verification images by an automated edge detection technique *Medical Physics* **19** 611-21

# Evaluation of a New Relocatable Head Fixation System

**Arthur J. Olch, Robert S. Lavey**

Radiation Oncology Program, Childrens Hospital Los Angeles, 4650 Sunset Blvd., Los Angeles, CA, USA

## Introduction

Precision fractionated 3D conformal and intensity modulated radiotherapy is dependent on reproducability of the position of the radiation fields with respect to the target to the maximum extent feasible. Prior experience with the daily set-up variation with the thermoplastic mask systems in current clinical use has been reported to be 2-5 mm[1]. Thermoplastic masks also often become ill-fitting and require adjustment over the course of radiation therapy in patients receiving concurrent steroid therapy for brain tumors. To improve patient postioning reproducibility and comfort, a new relocatable head immobilization system (HeadFix, Medical Intelligence, Schwabmunchen, Germany) has been used for fractionated radiation therapy of children and adolescents with tumors of the brain or head and neck at Childrens Hospital Los Angeles since April 1999. This abstract describes the new head immobilization system and reports on a comparison of positioning reproducibility between the new system and a standard thermoplastic mask system in 29 patients with primary brain tumors under 18 years of age.

## Materials and Methods

The head fixation system in this report is a highly modified version of a previously reported device (1). Head fixation is based on a custom impression of the patient's maxillary teeth and hard palate fixed to a plastic dental tray (bite block). A vacuum applied through the bite block secures it to the maxillary structures. Any malplacement of the bite block is indicated by a decrease in pressure on a gauge attached to the vacuum pump placed on the treatment couch. A set of hollow carbon fiber vertical support posts attached to a baseplate at the bottom and connected by a horizontal plate at the top has been substituted for the bulky aluminum hydraulic arms of the previously reported version to permit beams to be directed through them with minimal attenuation. The two extension arms of the bite block are secured in the vertical position to the 3-dimensionally adjustable connecting plate. The bite block remains assembled with the horizontal connecting plate as a single unit throughout the patient's radiation therapy course. The baseplate in the new system has been greatly reduced in size and weight to an open hollow frame by removing all carbon fiber material unnecessary for structural integrity. This baseplate is mounted to pins on the S-frame (MedTec, Orange City, Iowa) extension attachment to the Varian Exact couch. Thus, radiation fields can be directed through almost any portion of the system with only a few percent attenuation. A leveling screw has been added to the superior-most aspect of the baseplate. 1 mm in diameter metal balls were embedded into the center spine of the baseplate as lateral reference markers. A laser localizer box with fiducials is attached to the baseplate for targeting and daily setup. Etched horizontal and vertical white lines on the side and top plates of the box aid in visualizing the laser lines projected on the plates for patient setup. 1 mm metal balls are embedded at 4 cm intervals in the white lines of the side plates as reference markers on CT scans and simulation and port films.

The Uni-frame system, consisting of a thermoplastic mesh sheet bonded to a rigid frame and clamped to a lucite baseplate (MedTec, Orange City, Iowa) was used for comparison. Laser locating marks were made on tape applied to the mask for daily field setup.

The study group consists of twenty-nine children aged 2-16 years given fractionated external beam radiation therapy for a primary brain tumor at Childrens Hospital Los Angeles between 1997-99. The course of therapy was either opposed laterals or 3 to 6 conformal fields in 18-38 fractions given once daily, five days per week. Patients under age 6 were generally sedated for treatment. The Uni-frame system was anlayzed for 17 patients treated prior to November 1999 and the HeadFix system was analyzed for 12 patients treated between April-November 1999. The age, sex, and sedation distribution was similar for patients treated with the two systems. Measurements of field position relative to bony anatomical

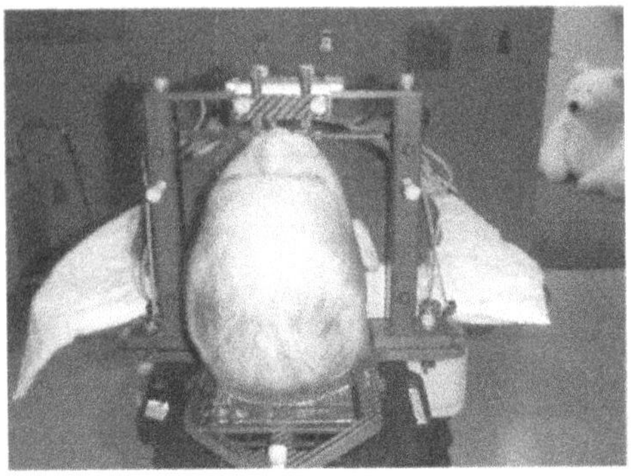

**Figure 1:** HeadFix bite block attached to rigid carbon fiber framed mounted on couch extension.

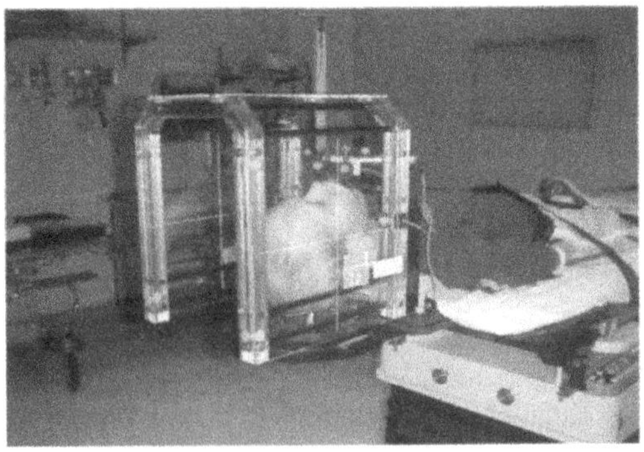

**Figure 2:** Laser localizer box attached to frame.

landmarks in the head were made on between 1-8 (mean=3.8) anterior-posterior and 3-9 (mean=5.4) lateral port films for each mask patient and between 2-8 (mean=5.8) anterior-posterior and 2-8 (mean=6.2) lateral port films for each HeadFix patient. Films were taken weekly during the course of treatment on each patient and compared to the orthogonal pair of simulation films. The field size on all films was 10 cm x 10 cm. The most frequent bony landmarks used were the sella, base of skull, orbits, sinuses, and cranial surface. The distance from the edge of the field to the anatomical reference point was measured to within 0.5 mm and recorded. Deviations were recorded in the lateral direction for the anterior-posterior films and in the anterior-posterior and superior-inferior directions for the lateral films. The deviations reported include device repositioning error, anatomical reference point misidentification error (<1 mm) and laser alignment error. The latter may be due to either a small misalignment of the lasers themselves (<.7mm) or human error in matching the laser line with the marks on the HeadFix or Uniframe systems (<.5 mm).

## Results and Discussion

The results of the comparison are shown in Table 1. The mean deviation in any one direction per patient was 0.8-1.2 mm for HeadFix system and 1.6-2.2 mm for the Uni-frame system. The mean 3D deviation per patient for the Headfix system was 1.8±0.6 mm compared to 3.5±0.9 mm for the Uni-frame system (p=0.01). The patient's head was relocatable to within 1 mm in any direction in 62-82% of HeadFix films and 41-48% of Uni-frame patient films (Table 2). Changes in position of greater than 3 mm in any direction were seen on 0-5% of HeadFix compared to 13-22% of the Uni-frame films.

The HeadFix system was found to have several advantages over the Uni-frame system in pediatric clinical use in addition to the measured improvement in field position reproducibility. The simple attachment procedure and lack of adjustment or measurement prior to treatment make set-up time with the HeadFix system short. The lack of contact with the soft tissues of the head by the HeadFix system permitted better visualization of all facial structures, eliminated the thermoplastic bolus effect on skin and scalp, and better accomodated patients with nasogastric or endotracheal tubes and sedated patients with oral or nasal airways. Facial swelling due to steroid use and hair loss during radiation therapy did not affect the HeadFix system, while it often required spacers to be removed, cutting slits in the thermoplastic mesh, or resimulation with the Uni-frame system

Other relocatable fixation systems, either commercial or institutionally developed, are reported in the literature (1-6). Some of these use masks as well as mouthpieces. They report mean 3D repositioning deviations of about 1 mm. They all have in common a metal framework, using either a ring or metal hydraulic arms. On the contrary, the HeadFix system is all carbon fiber, permitting any deliverable beam angle to be used with minimal attenuation. For example, inferior beam angles are useful in 3D conformal therapy but are frequently disallowed by the other relocatable systems because they would pass through the metal structure. We have had little problem using these beam angles with the HeadFix system. In addition, other systems may not be suitable for use on children due to size constraints. We have used the HeadFix system on children as young as 2 years old with good results.

One should note that the results reported here are based on the use of a new system on our first 12 cases. We have noted that our methodology has improved as we learned how to best apply the mouthpiece and position the patient within the system. In addition, our results include all sources of error which are always present when evaluating reproducability from inspection of the film record. We expect our results of positional reproducibility to improve as we gain more experience, converging on the 1 mm 3D error value.

| | Lateral | Ant-Post | Sup-Inf | 3D |
|---|---|---|---|---|
| HeadFix | 0.9±0.6 | 0.8±0.6 | 1.2±0.5 | 1.8±0.6 |
| Mask | 1.6±0.9 | 2.2±1.2 | 1.7±1.0 | 3.5±0.9 |

**Table 1:** Positional deviations (mm) ± SD for Headfix vs. Uni-frame mask patients.

| Deviation | Lateral | | Ant-Post | | Sup-Inf | |
|---|---|---|---|---|---|---|
| (mm) | HeadFix | Mask | HeadFix | Mask | HeadFix | Mask |
| <=1 | 74% | 48% | 82% | 41% | 62% | 41% |
| >1, <=2 | 16% | 32% | 18% | 29% | 30% | 31% |
| >2, <=3 | 9% | 8% | 0% | 10% | 3% | 12% |
| >3, <=4 | 1% | 6% | 0% | 7% | 5% | 12% |
| >4, <=5 | 0% | 5% | 0% | 7% | 0% | 2% |
| >5 | 0% | 2% | 0% | 8% | 0% | 2% |

**Table 2:** Distribution of positional deviations for Headfix vs. Uni-frame mask films.

## Conclusion

In 12 patients, the HeadFix system has been demonstrated to be superior to the thermoplastic mask system for immobilizing and relocating the head for fractionated treatments, with a total 3D positional accuracy of 1.8±0.6 mm. Besides its improved relocatability, it provides practical advantages that improve both patient comfort and quality of the treatment compared to mask systems or other relocatable head frames. We have used it exclusively on children, awake or sedated, and find that it is a valuable patient positioning tool when delivering fractionated radiation therapy with standard or conformal treatment plans. As we use HeadFix to treat more patients, we will continue to analyze orthogonal film data to further assess its positional accuracy.

## References

[1] Sweeney R, Bale R, Vogele M, Nevinny-Stickel M, Bluhm A, Auer T, Hessenberger G, Lukas P 1998 Repositioning accuracy: Comparison of a noninvasive head holder with thermoplastic mask for fractionated radiotherapy and a case report Int J. Radiation Oncology Biol. Phys. **41** 475-483

[2] Rosenberg I, Alheit H, Beardmore C, Lee K S, Warrington A P, Brada M 1999 Patient position reproducibility in fractionated stereotactic radiotherapy: an update after changing dental impression material Radiotherapy & Oncology 239-240

[3] Kooy H M, Dunbar S F, Tarbell N J, Mannarino E, Ferarro N, Shusterman S, Bellerive M, Finn L, Mcdonough C V, Loeffler J S 1994 Adaptation and verification of the relocatable Gill-Thomas-Cosman frame in stereotactic radiotherapy Int J. Radiation Oncology Biol. Phys. 685-691
[4] Scott T W, Beach J L, Mendiondo OA 1997 A precision repeat localization head freame for fractionated stereotactic radiotherapy Medical Dosimetry **22** 5-8
[5] Theodorou K, Kappas C, Tsokas C 1998 A new non-invasive and relocatable immobilization frame for fractionated stereotactic radiotherapy Radiotherapy & Oncology **47** 313-317
[6] Bale R J, Vogele M, Freysinger W, Gunkel A R, Martin A, Bumm K, Thumfart W F 1997 A minimally invasive head holder to improve the performance of frameless stereotactic surgery Laryngoscope **107** 1-5

# Author Index

# Index

www.ingramcontent.com/pod-product-compliance
Ingram Content Group UK Ltd.
Pitfield, Milton Keynes, MK11 3LW, UK
UKHW051047131026
476584UK00003B/68
* 9 7 8 3 5 4 0 6 7 1 7 6 3 *